the calorie carb and fat bible 2011

Juliette Kellow BSc RD, Lyndel Costain BSc RD & Laurence Beeken

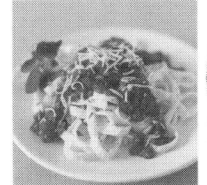 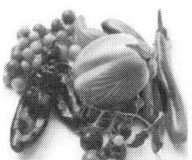 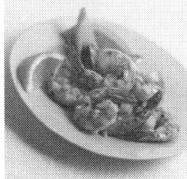 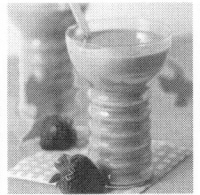 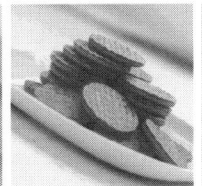 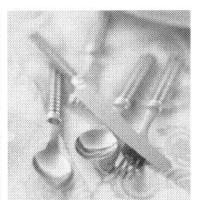

The UK's Most Comprehensive Calorie Counter

The Calorie, Carb & Fat Bible 2011

Published by:
Weight Loss Resources Ltd
29 Metro Centre
Woodston,
Peterborough
PE2 7UH.

Tel: 01733 345592
www.weightlossresources.co.uk

Companies and other organisations wishing to make bulk purchases of the Calorie, Carb and Fat Bible should contact their local bookstore or Weight Loss Resources direct.

Whilst every effort has been made to ensure accuracy, the publishers cannot be held responsible for any errors or omissions.

ISBN 978-1-904512-09-7   613.23
                          434847

Authors: Lyndel Costain BSc RD
          Juliette Kellow BSc RD
          Laurence Beeken, Weight Loss Resources

Database Editor: Laurence Beeken

Design & Layout: Jonathan Lansdown

Printed and bound in Finland by:
Bookwell Oy

Contents

Losing weight – the easy way

Juliette Kellow BSc RD

CHINESE TAKEAWAYS, curries, chocolate, chips and a glass of wine! Imagine being told the best diet to help you lose weight includes all these foods and more. It sounds too good to be true, doesn't it? But the truth is, these are exactly the types of foods you can still enjoy if you opt to lose weight by counting calories.

But you'd be forgiven for not knowing you can still eat all your favourite foods *and* lose weight. In recent years, endless trendy diets that cut carbs, boost protein intake or skip entire groups of foods, have helped to make dieting a complicated business. Added to this, an increasing number of celebrities and so-called nutrition experts have helped mislead us into thinking that dieting is all about restriction and denial. Is it any wonder then that most of us have been left feeling downright confused and miserable about what we should and shouldn't be eating to shift those pounds?

Dieting doesn't have to be complicated or an unhappy experience. In fact, there's really only one word you need to remember if you want to shift those pounds healthily and still eat all your favourite foods. And that's CALORIE!

It's calories that count

When it comes to losing weight, there's no getting away from the fact that it's calories that count. Ask any qualified nutrition expert or dietitian for advice on how to fight the flab and you'll receive the same reply: quite simply you need to create a calorie deficit or shortfall. In other words, you need to take in fewer calories than you use up so that your body has to draw on its fat stores to provide it with the energy it needs to function properly. The result: you start losing fat and the pounds start to drop off!

Fortunately, it couldn't be easier to create this calorie deficit. Regardless of your age, weight, sex, genetic make up, lifestyle or eating habits, losing weight is as simple as reducing your daily calorie intake slightly by modifying your diet and using up a few more calories by being slightly more active each day.

Better still, it's a complete myth that you need to change your eating and exercise habits dramatically. You'll notice I've said you need to reduce your calorie intake 'slightly' and be 'slightly' more active. It really is just LITTLE differences between the amount of calories we take in and the amount we use up that make BIG differences to our waistline over time. For example, you only need to consume one can of cola more than you need each day to gain a stone in a year. It's no wonder then that people say excess weight tends to 'creep up on them'.

10 simple food swaps you can make every day (and won't even notice!)

Make these simple swaps every day and in just 4 weeks you'll lose 7lb!

SWAP THIS...	FOR THIS...	SAVE...
300ml full-fat milk (195 calories)	300ml skimmed milk (100 calories)	95 calories
1tsp butter (35 calories)	1tsp low-fat spread (20 calories)	15 calories
1tbsp vegetable oil (100 calories)	10 sprays of a spray oil (10 calories)	90 calories
1tsp sugar (16 calories)	Artificial sweetener (2 calories)	14 calories
1tbsp mayonnaise (105 calories)	1tbsp fat-free dressing (10 calories)	95 calories
Regular sandwich (600 calories)	Low-fat sandwich (350 calories)	250 calories
Can of cola (135 calories)	Can of diet cola (1 calorie)	134 calories
Large (50g) packet of crisps (250 calories)	Small (25g) packet of crisps (125 calories)	125 calories
1 chocolate digestive (85 calories)	1 small chocolate chip cookie (55 calories)	30 calories
1 slice thick-cut wholemeal bread (95 calories)	1 slice medium-cut wholemeal bread (75 calories)	20 calories
	TOTAL CALORIE SAVING:	868 calories

The good news is the reverse is also true. You only need to swap that daily can of cola for the diet version or a glass of sparking water and you'll lose a stone in a year – it really is as easy as that!

Of course, most people don't want to wait a year to shift a stone. But there's more good news. To lose 1lb of fat each week you need to create a calorie deficit of just 500 calories a day. That might sound like a lot, but you can achieve this by simply swapping a croissant for a wholemeal fruit scone, a regular sandwich for a low-fat variety, a glass of dry white wine for a gin and slimline tonic and using low-fat spread on two slices of toast instead of butter. It is also important to become more active and increase your level of exercise. Losing 1lb a week, amounts to a stone in 14 weeks, or just under 4 stone in a year!

Taking control of calories

By now you've seen it really is calories that count when it comes to shifting those pounds. So it should be no surprise that a calorie-controlled diet is the only guaranteed way to help you shift those pounds – and that's a scientific fact! But better still, a calorie-controlled diet is one of the few that allows you to include anything, whether it's pizza, wine or chocolate. A healthy diet means including a wide range of foods (see 'Healthy Eating Made Easy' page 32).

And that's where this book can really help. Gone are the days when it was virtually impossible to obtain information about the calorie contents of foods. This book provides calorie information for more than 22,000 different branded and unbranded foods so that counting calories has never been easier.

The benefits of counting calories
☐ *It's guaranteed to help you lose weight providing you stick to your daily calorie allowance*
☐ *You can include favourite foods*
☐ *No foods are banned*
☐ *It's a great way to lose weight slowly and steadily*
☐ *Nutrition experts agree that it's a proven way to lose weight*

Calorie counting made easy

Forget weird and wacky science, complicated diet rules and endless lists of foods to fill up on or avoid every day! Counting calories to lose weight couldn't be easier. Quite simply, you set yourself a daily calorie allowance to help you lose between ½-2lb (¼-1kg) a week and then add up the calories of everything you eat and drink each day, making sure you don't go over your limit.

To prevent hunger from kicking in, it's best to spread your daily calorie allowance evenly throughout the day, allowing a certain amount of calories for breakfast, lunch, dinner and one or two snacks. For example, if you are allowed 1,500 calories a day, you could have 300 calories for breakfast, 400 calories for lunch, 500 calories for dinner and two snacks or treats of 150 calories each. You'll find more detailed information on p26-31 (Your step-by-step guide to using this book and shifting those pounds).

QUESTION
What affects the calorie content of a food?

ANSWER:
Fat, protein, carbohydrate and alcohol all provide the body with calories, but in varying amounts:

- *1g fat provides 9 calories*

- *1g alcohol provides 7 calories*

- *1g protein provides 4 calories*

- *1g carbohydrate provides 3.75 calories*

The calorie content of a food depends on the amount of fat, protein and carbohydrate it contains. Because fat provides more than twice as many calories as an equal quantity of protein or carbohydrate, in general, foods that are high in fat tend to contain more calories. This explains why 100g of chips (189 calories) contains more than twice as many calories as 100g of boiled potato (72 calories).

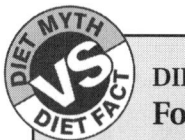

DIET MYTH:
Food eaten late at night stops you losing weight

DIET FACT:

It's not eating in the evening that stops you losing weight. It's consuming too many calories throughout the day that will be your dieting downfall! Providing you stick to your daily calorie allowance you'll lose weight, regardless of when you consume those calories. Nevertheless, it's a good idea to spread your calorie allowance throughout the day to prevent hunger from kicking in, which leaves you reaching for high-calorie snack foods.

Eat for good health

While calories might be the buzz word when it comes to shifting those pounds, it's nevertheless important to make sure your diet is healthy, balanced and contains all the nutrients you need for good health. Yes, you can still lose weight by eating nothing but, for example, chocolate, crisps and biscuits providing you stick to your calorie allowance. But you'll never find a nutrition expert or dietitian recommending this. And there are plenty of good reasons why.

To start with, an unbalanced diet is likely to be lacking in essential nutrients such as protein, vitamins, minerals and fibre, in the long term putting you at risk of nutritional deficiencies. Secondly, research proves that filling up on foods that are high in fat and/or salt and sugar can lead to many different health problems. But most importantly, when it comes to losing weight, it's almost impossible to stick to a daily calorie allowance if you're only eating high-calorie foods.

Filling up on lower-calorie foods also means you'll be able to eat far more with the result that you're not constantly left feeling unsatisfied. For example, six chocolates from a selection box contain around 300 calories, a lot of fat and sugar, few nutrients – and are eaten in just six mouthfuls! For 300 calories, you could have a grilled skinless chicken breast (packed with protein and zinc), a large salad with fat-free dressing (a great source of fibre, vitamins and minerals), a slice of wholemeal bread with low-fat spread (rich in fibre and B vitamins) and a satsuma (an excellent source of vitamin C). That's a lot more food that will take you a lot more time to eat! Not convinced? Then put six chocolates on one plate, and the chicken, salad, bread and fruit on another!

Bottom line: while slightly reducing your calorie intake is the key to losing weight, you'll be healthier and far more likely to keep those pounds off if you do it by eating a healthy diet *(see 'Healthy Eating Made Easy' page 32).*

Eight steps to a healthy diet

1 *Base your meals on starchy foods.*

2 *Eat lots of fruit and vegetables.*

3 *Eat more fish.*

4 *Cut down on saturated fat and sugar.*

5 *Try to eat less salt - no more than 6g a day.*

6 *Get active and try to be a healthy weight.*

7 *Drink plenty of water.*

8 *Don't skip breakfast.*   SOURCE: FSA www.eatwell.gov.uk

Fat facts

Generally speaking, opting for foods that are low in fat can help slash your calorie intake considerably, for example, swapping full-fat milk for skimmed, switching from butter to a low-fat spread, not frying food in oil and chopping the fat off meat and poultry. But don't be fooled into believing that all foods described as 'low-fat' or 'fat-free' are automatically low in calories or calorie-free. In fact, some low-fat products may actually be higher in calories than standard products, thanks to them containing extra sugars and thickeners to boost the flavour and texture. The solution: always check the calorie content of low-fat foods, especially for things like cakes, biscuits, crisps, ice creams and ready meals. You might be surprised to find there's little difference in the calorie content when compared to the standard product.

Uncovering fat claims on food labels

Many products may lure you into believing they're a great choice if you're trying to cut fat, but you need to read between the lines on the labels if you want to be sure you're making the best choice. Here's the lowdown on what to look for:

LOW FAT	by law the food must contain less than 3g of fat per 100g for solids. These foods are generally a good choice if you're trying to lose weight.
REDUCED FAT	by law the food must contain 25 percent less fat than a similar standard product. This doesn't mean the product is low-fat (or low-calorie) though! For example, reduced-fat cheese may still contain 14g fat per 100g.
FAT FREE	the food must contain no more than 0.5g of fat per 100g or 100ml. Foods labelled as Virtually Fat Free must contain less than 0.3g fat per 100g. These foods are generally a good choice if you're trying to lose weight.
LESS THAN 8% FAT	this means the product contains less than 8g fat per 100g. It's only foods labelled 'less than 3% fat' that are a true low-fat choice.
X% FAT FREE	claims expressed as X% Fat Free shall be prohibited.
LIGHT OR LITE	claims stating a product is 'light' or 'lite' follows the same conditions as those set for the term 'reduced'.

10 easy ways to slash fat (and calories)

1   Eat fewer fried foods – grill, boil, bake, poach, steam, roast without added fat or microwave instead.

2   Don't add butter, lard, margarine or oil to food during preparation or cooking.

3   Use spreads sparingly. Butter and margarine contain the same amount of calories and fat – only low fat spreads contain less.

4   Choose boiled or jacket potatoes instead of chips or roast potatoes.

5   Cut off all visible fat from meat and remove the skin from chicken before cooking.

6   Don't eat too many fatty meat products such as sausages, burgers, pies and pastry products.

7   Use semi-skimmed or skimmed milk instead of full-fat milk.

8   Try low-fat or reduced-fat varieties of cheese such as reduced-fat Cheddar, low-fat soft cheese or cottage cheese.

9   Eat fewer high-fat foods such as crisps, chocolates, cakes, pastries and biscuits.

10   Don't add cream to puddings, sauces or coffee.

Getting Ready for Weight Loss Success

Lyndel Costain BSc RD

THIS BOOK not only provides tools to help you understand more about what you eat and how active you are, but guidance on how to use this information to develop a weight loss plan to suit your needs. Getting in the right frame of mind will also be a key part of your weight control journey, especially if you've lost weight before, only to watch the pounds pile back on.

The fact is that most people who want to lose weight know what to do. But often there is something that keeps stopping them from keeping up healthier habits. The same may be true for you. So what's going on? For many it's a lack of readiness. When the next diet comes along with its tempting promises it's so easy to just jump on board. But if you have struggled with your weight for a while, will that diet actually help you to recognise and change the thoughts and actions that have stopped you shifting the pounds for good?

Check out your attitude to weight loss programmes

Before starting any new weight loss programme, including the Weight Loss Resources approach, ask yourself:

Am I starting out thinking that I like myself as a person right now?	(YES or NO)
OR I feel I can only like myself once I lose weight?	(YES or NO)
Do I want to stop overeating, but at the same time find myself justifying it – in other words I want to be able to eat what I want, but with no consequences?	(YES or NO)
Do I believe that I need to take long-term responsibility for my weight?	(YES or NO)
OR Am I relying on 'it' (the diet) to do it for me?	(YES or NO)

Keep these questions, and your replies, in mind as you read through this chapter.

Next Steps

You may have already assessed the healthiness of your weight using the BMI guide on page 37. If not, why not do it now, remembering that the tools are a guide only. The important thing is to consider a weight at which you are healthy and comfortable – and which is realistic for the life you lead *(see opposite - What is a healthy weight?).*

The next step is to have a long hard think about why you want to lose weight. Consider all the possible benefits, not just those related to how you look. Psychologists have found that if we focus only on appearance we are less likely to succeed in the long-term. This is because it so often reflects low self-esteem or self-worth – which can sabotage success – as it saps confidence and keeps us stuck in destructive thought patterns. Identifying key motivations other than simply how you look - such as health and other aspects of physical and emotional well being - is like saying that you're an OK person right now, and worth making changes for. Making healthy lifestyle choices also has the knock on effect of boosting self-esteem further.

Write down your reasons for wanting to lose weight in your Personal Plan *(see page 42)* – so you can refer back to them. This can be especially helpful when the going gets tough. It may help to think of it in terms of what your weight is stopping you from doing now. Here's some examples: to feel more confident; so I can play more comfortably with my kids; my healthier diet will give me more energy; to improve my fertility.

What is a Healthy Weight?

With all the 'thin is beautiful' messages in the media it can be easy to get a distorted view about whether your weight is healthy or not. However, as the BMI charts suggest, there is no single 'ideal' weight for anybody. Research also shows that modest amounts of weight loss can be very beneficial to health and are easier to keep off. Therefore, health professionals now encourage us to aim for a weight loss of 5-10%. The ideal rate of weight loss is no more than 1-2 pounds (0.5-1kg) per week – so averaging a pound a week is great, and realistic progress.

The health benefits of modest weight loss include:

☐ *Reduced risk of developing heart disease, stroke and certain cancers*

☐ *Reduced risk of developing diabetes and helping to manage diabetes*

☐ *Improvements in blood pressure*

☐ *Improvements in mobility, back pain and joint pain*

☐ *Improvements with fertility problems and polycystic ovarian syndrome*

☐ *Less breathlessness and sleep/snoring problems*

☐ *Increased self esteem and control over eating*

☐ *Feeling fitter and have more energy*

Are You Really Ready to Lose Weight?

When you think of losing weight, it's easy just to think of what weight you'd like to get to. But weight loss only happens as a result of making changes to your usual eating and activity patterns – which allow you to consume fewer calories than you burn *(see 'It's calories that count' page 5)*.

So here comes the next big question. Are you really ready to do it? Have you thought about the implications of your decision? If you have lost weight in the past, and put it all back on - have you thought about why that was? And how confident do you feel about being successful this time?

To help you answer these questions, try these short exercises.

Where would you place yourself on the following scales?

Importance

How important is it to you, to make the changes that will allow you to lose weight?

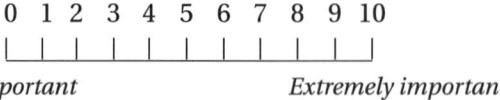

Not at all important   Extremely important

If you ranked yourself over half way along the scale then move on to the next question. If you were half way or less along the scale, you may not be mentally ready to make the required changes to lose weight. To further explore this, go to 'The Pros and Cons of Weight Loss' (page 17).

Confidence

How confident are you in your ability to make the changes that will allow you to lose weight?

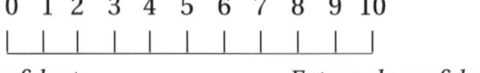

Not at all confident   Extremely confident

Now ask yourself (regarding your confidence ratings):

1. Why did I place myself here?

2. What is stopping me moving further up the scale (if anything)?

3. What things, information, support would help me move further up the scale? (if not near 10)

If you aren't sure about answers to question 3, then keep reading for some pointers.

The Pros and Cons of Weight Loss

Making lifestyle changes to lose weight is simpler if there are lots of clear benefits or pros, for example, clothes fit again, more energy, helps back pain - but there will also be associated downsides or cons. For example, some may feel it interferes with their social life, or don't have the time to plan meals or check food labels. Or overeating can help, if only temporarily, as a way of coping with unwanted feelings. Being overweight allows some people to feel strong and assertive, or to control their partner's jealousy. So in these cases there are downsides to losing weight, even if the person says they are desperate to do it.

If you are aware of the possible downsides, as well as the pros, you will be better prepared to deal with potential conflicts. Understanding what could be (or were with past weight loss efforts) barriers to success gives you the chance to address them. This boosts confidence in your ability to succeed this time, which in turn maintains your motivation.

Have a go at weighing up the pros and cons using the charts below and on page 18. Some examples are included. If you decide that the pros outweigh the cons, then great. You can also use the cons as potential barriers to plan strategies for *(see page 42)*. If you find it's the other way around, this may not be the best time to actively lose weight. Try the exercise again in a month or so.

Making Lifestyle Changes to Lose Weight Now

CONS *e.g. Must limit eating out, take aways*	PROS *e.g. Feel more energetic, slimmer*

Not Making Changes Now – how would I feel in 6 months time?

PROS *e.g. Haven't had to worry about failing; Still able to eat take aways a lot*	CONS *e.g. Probably gained more weight; Back pain may be worse*

To change your weight, first change your mind

To lose weight you may already have a list of things to change, such as eating more fruit and veg, calculating your daily calorie intake, going for a walk each morning or buying low fat options. Others could also give you tips to try. But knowing what to do isn't the same as feeling motivated or able to do it. To be effective, you have to believe the changes are relevant, do-able and worth it.

What you think, affects how you feel, and in turn the actions you take.

Self-efficacy

In fact, research is telling us that one of the most important factors that influences weight loss success are your feelings of 'self-efficacy'. Self-efficacy is a term used in psychology to describe a person's belief that any action they take will have an effect on the outcome. It reflects our inner expectation that what we do will lead to the results we want. Not surprisingly, high levels of self-efficacy can enhance motivation, and allow us to deal better with uncertainty and conflict, and recovery from setbacks. But low levels, can reduce our motivation. We fear that whatever we do will not bring about our desired goal. This can lead self-defeating thoughts or 'self-talk', which make it hard to deal with set-backs, meaning we are more likely to give up. Here's some examples.

Examples: Low self-efficacy

'*No matter how carefully I diet, I don't lose weight . . .*'

'*I have eaten that chocolate and as usual blown my diet, so I may as well give up now.*'

'*I had a rich dessert – I have no willpower to say no. I can't stand not being able to eat what I want.*'

If you have a strong sense of self-efficacy, your mindset and 'self-talk' will be more like:

Examples: High self-efficacy

'*I know from previous weight loss programmes, that if I stay focussed on what I am doing I do lose weight. I have always expected to lose too much too quickly which frustrates me. I know that I will lose weight if I keep making the right changes, and this time it is important to me.*'

'*The chocolate bar won't ruin my diet, but if I think it has and keep on eating, then my negative self-talk will. So I will get back on track.*'

'*I don't like having to eat differently from others, but losing weight is very important to me, so I **can** stand it. After all, the world won't stop if I say no to dessert, and I will feel great afterwards. If I think about it, I am not hungry so would just feel bloated and guilty if I ate it.*'

Willpower is a Skill

Many people feel that they just need plenty of willpower or a good telling off to lose weight. But willpower isn't something you have or you don't have. Willpower is a skill. Like the dessert example on page 19, it's a sign that you've made a conscious choice to do something, because you believe the benefits outweigh any downsides. In reality everything we do is preceded by a thought. This includes everything we eat. It just may not seem like it because our actions often feel automatic *(see 'Look out for trigger eating' page 21).*

When it comes to weight loss, developing a range of skills – including choosing a lower calorie diet, coping with negative self-talk and managing things that don't go to plan - will boost your sense of self-efficacy to make the changes you want. This is especially important because we live in such a weight-promoting environment.

Our weight-promoting environment

We are constantly surrounded by tempting food, stresses that can trigger comfort eating and labour-saving devices that make it easy not to be physically active. In other words, the environment we live in makes it easy to gain weight, unless we stop and think about the food choices we make and how much exercise we do. In fact, to stay a healthy weight/maintain our weight, just about all of us need to make conscious lifestyle choices everyday. This isn't 'dieting' but just part of taking care of ourselves in the environment we live in.

It is also true that some people find it more of a challenge than others to manage their weight, thanks to genetic differences in factors such as appetite control, spontaneous activity level and emotional responses to food – rather than metabolic rate, as is often believed. The good news is that with a healthy diet and active lifestyle a healthier weight can still be achieved. But do talk to your doctor if you feel you need additional support.

Coping with Common Slimming Saboteurs

Lyndel Costain BSc RD

Look out for 'trigger' eating

Much of the overeating we do or cravings we have are actually down to unconscious, habitual, responses to a variety of triggers. These triggers can be external, such as the sight or smell of food, or internal and emotion-led, such as a response to stress, anger, boredom or emptiness. Your food diary (see page 43) helps you to recognise 'trigger' or 'non-hungry' eating which gives you the chance to think twice before you eat (see below).

Get some support

A big part of your success will be having someone to support you. It could be a friend, partner, health professional, health club or website. Let them know how they can help you most.

Make lapses your ally

Don't let a lapse throw you off course. You can't be, nor need to be perfect all the time. Doing well 80-90% of the time is great progress. Lapses are a normal part of change. Rather than feel you have failed and give up, look at what you can learn from a difficult day or week and use it to find helpful solutions for the future.

Understand why you eat

When I ask people what prompts them to eat, hunger usually comes down near the bottom of their list of reasons. Some people struggle to remember or appreciate what true hunger feels like. We are lucky that we have plenty of food to eat in our society. But its constant presence makes it harder to control what we eat, especially if it brings us comfort or joy.

If you ever find yourself in the fridge even though you've recently eaten, then you know hunger isn't the reason but some other trigger. The urge to eat can be so automatic that you feel you lack willpower or are out of control. But it is in fact a learned or conditioned response. A bit like Pavlov's dogs. He rang a bell every time he fed them, and from then on, whenever they heard the bell ring they were 'conditioned' to salivate in anticipation of food.

Because this 'non-hungry' eating is learned, you can reprogramme your response to the situations or feelings that trigger it. The first step is to identify when these urges strike. When you find yourself eating when you aren't hungry ask yourself 'why do I want to eat, what am I feeling?' If you aren't sure think back to what was happening before you ate. Then ask yourself if there is another way you can feel better without food. Or you could chat to your urge to eat in a friendly way, telling it that you don't want to give into it, you have a planned meal coming soon, and it's merely a learned response. Whatever strategy you choose, the more often you break into your urges to eat, the weaker their hold becomes.

Practise positive self-talk

Self-talk may be positive and constructive (like your guardian angel) or negative and irrational (like having a destructive devil on your shoulder).

If you've had on-off battles with your weight over the years, it's highly likely that the 'devil' is there more often. 'All or nothing' self-talk for example, 'I ate a "bad food" so have broken my diet', can make you feel like a failure which, can then trigger you into the action of overeating and/or totally giving up *(see 'Diet-binge cycle' page 23)*. One of the most powerful things about it is that the last thoughts we have are what stays in our mind. So if we think 'I still look fat' or 'I will never be slim', these feelings stay with us.

To change your self-talk for the better, the trick is to first recognise it's happening (keeping a diary really helps, *see Keep a Food Diary, page 29*). Then turn it around into a positive version of the same events *(see Self-efficacy, page 18)* where the resulting action was to feel good and stay on track. Reshaping negative self-talk helps you to boost your self-esteem and feelings of self-efficacy, and with it change your self-definition - from someone who can't 'lose weight' or 'do this or that', to someone 'who can'. And when you believe you can…

The Diet – Binge Cycle

If this cycle looks familiar, use positive self-talk, and a more flexible dietary approach, to help you break free.

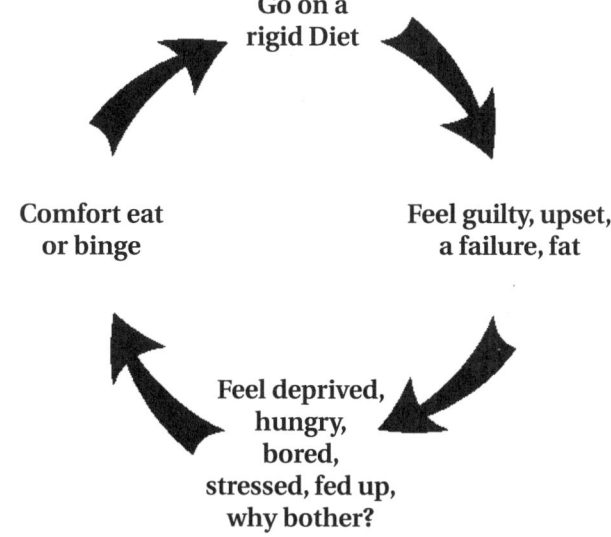

Go on a
rigid Diet

Feel guilty, upset,
a failure, fat

Feel deprived,
hungry,
bored,
stressed, fed up,
why bother?

Comfort eat
or binge

Really choose what you want to eat

This skill is like your personal brake. It also helps you to manage 'trigger/ non-hungry' eating and weaken its hold. It legalises food and stops you feeling deprived. It helps you to regularly remind yourself why you are making changes to your eating habits, which keeps motivation high. But it doesn't just happen. Like all skills it requires practise. Sometimes it will work well for you, other times it won't – but overall it will help. Basically, ask yourself if you really want to eat that food in front of you. This becomes the prompt for you to make a conscious choice, weighing up the pros and cons or consequences of making that choice, and feeling free to have it, reject it or just eat some. Remembering all the while that you can eat this food another time if you want to.

Action Planning

Successful people don't just wait for things to happen. They believe in themselves, plan ahead, take action and then refine their plan until it gets, and keeps on getting the results they want. Successful slimmers use a very similar approach. They don't rely on quick-fixes or magic formulas, but glean information from reliable sources to develop a plan or approach that suits their needs, tastes and lifestyle. Thinking of weight management as a lifelong project, which has a weight loss phase and a weight maintenance phase, is also a route to success.

When the Going Gets Tough - Staying on Track

If things start to go off track, don't panic. Learning new habits takes time. And life is never straightforward so there will be times when it all seems too much, or negative 'self- talk' creeps in to try and drag you back into old ways. So if the going gets tough:

- Value what you've achieved so far, rather than only focus on what you plan to do.

- Look back at your reasons to lose weight and refer to the list often .

- Don't expect to change too much, too quickly. Take things a step at a time.

- Accept difficulties as part of the learning and skill building process.

- Enjoy a non-food reward for achieving your goals (including maintaining your weight).

- Use recipes and meal ideas to keep things interesting.

- Talk to your supporters and get plenty of encouragement. This is really vital!

Strategies of Successful Slimmers

Thanks to research conducted by large studies such as the US National Weight Control Registry and the German Lean Habits Study, we now know more about what works best for people who have lost weight and successfully kept it off. So be inspired!

The key elements of success are to:

- Believe that you can control your weight and the changes involved are really worth it.

- Stay realistic and value what you have achieved rather than dwell on a weight you 'dream' of being.

- Be more active – plan ways to fit activity into your daily life – aim for 1 hour of walking daily.

- Plan ahead for regular meals and snacks, starting with breakfast.

- Choose a balanced, low-fat diet with plenty of fruit and vegetables *(see Healthy Eating Made Easy, page 32).*

- Watch portion size and limit fast food.

- Sit down to eat and take time over meals, paying attention to what you are eating.

- Have a flexible approach – plan in and enjoy some favourite foods without guilt.

- Recognise and address 'all or nothing' thinking and other negative 'self-talk'.

- Keep making conscious choices.

- Learn to confront problems rather than eat, drink, sleep or wish they would go away.

- Enlist ongoing help and support from family, friends, professionals or websites.

- Regularly (at least once a week but not more than once daily) check your weight.

- Take action before your weight increases by more than 4-5lb (2kg).

- Accept that your weight management skills need to be kept up long-term.

- Take heart from successful slimmers, who say that it gets easier over time.

Your step-by-step guide to using this book and shifting those pounds

Juliette Kellow BSc RD and Rebecca Walton

1. Find your healthy weight

Use the weight charts, body mass index table and information on pages 36-43 to determine the right weight for you. Then set yourself a weight to aim for. Research shows it really helps if you make losing 10% of your weight your first overall target. It also brings important health benefits too *(see 'What is a Healthy Weight?' page 15)*. You can break this down into smaller manageable steps, for example, 3kg/6.5lbs at a time. If 10% is too much, then go for a 5% loss – this has important health benefits too. In fact, just keeping your weight stable is a great achievement these days, because of our weight-promoting environment *(see page 20)*.

Waist Management

In addition to BMI, another important way to assess your weight is by measuring your waist just above belly button level. It is especially useful for men as they tend to carry more excess weight around their bellies, but women should test it out too. Having excess weight around your middle (known as being 'apple-shaped') increases your risk of heart disease and type 2 diabetes. A simple way to stay aware of your waist is according to how well, or otherwise, skirts and trousers fit. Talk to your doctor about any weight and health concerns.

WAIST MEASUREMENT

	Increased Health Risk	High Risk to Health
Women	32-35in (81-88cm)	more than 35in (88cm)
Men	37-40in (94-102cm)	more than 40in (102cm)

2. Set a realistic time scale

With today's hectic lifestyles, everything tends to happen at breakneck speed, so it's no wonder that when it comes to losing weight, most of us want to shift those pounds in an instant. But it's probably taken years to accumulate that extra weight, with the result that it's unrealistic to expect to lose the excess in just a few weeks! Instead, prepare yourself to lose weight slowly and steadily. It's far healthier to lose weight like this. But better still, research shows you'll be far more likely to maintain your new, lower weight.

If you only have a small amount of weight to lose, aim for a weight loss of around 1lb (½kg) a week. But if you have more than 2 stone (28kg) to lose, you may prefer to aim for 2lb (1kg) each week. Remember though, it's better to keep going at 1lb (½kg) a week than to give up because trying to lose 2lb (1kg) a week is making you miserable! The following words may help you to keep your goal in perspective:

'Never give up on a goal because of the time it will take to achieve it – the time will pass anyway.'

Weight Fluctuations

Weight typically fluctuates on a day to day basis. You know that shock/ horror feeling when you weigh yourself in the morning then later in the day, or after a meal out, and it looks like youve gained pounds in hours! But this is due to fluid not fat changes. Real changes in body fat can only happen more gradually (remember, to gain 1lb you need to eat 3500 calories more than you usually do). Don't be confused either by seemingly very rapid weight loss in the first week or so.

When calorie intake is initially cut back, the body's carbohydrate stores in the liver and muscles (known as glycogen) are used up. Glycogen is stored with three times its weight in water, meaning that rapid losses of 4.5- 6.6lb (2 -3 kg) are possible. These stores can be just as rapidly refilled if normal eating is resumed. True weight loss happens more gradually and this book helps you to lose weight at the steady and healthy rate of no more than 1-2 lbs per week.

3. Calculate your calorie allowance

Use the calorie tables on pages 39-40 to find out how many calories you need each day to maintain your current weight. Then use the table below to discover the amount of calories you need to subtract from this amount every day to lose weight at your chosen rate. For example, a 35 year-old woman who is moderately active and weighs 12 stone (76kg) needs 2,188 calories a day to keep her weight steady. If she wants to lose ½lb (¼kg) a week, she needs 250 calories less each day, giving her a daily calorie allowance of 1,938 calories. If she wants to lose 1lb (½kg) a week, she needs 500 calories less each day, giving her a daily calorie allowance of 1,688 calories, and so on.

TO LOSE...	Cut your daily calorie intake by	In three months you could lose...	In six months you could lose...	In one year you could lose...
½lb a week	250	6.5lb	13lb	1st 12lb
1lb a week	500	13lb	1st 12lb	3st 10lb
1½lb a week	750	1st 5.5lb	2st 11lb	5st 8lb
2lb a week	1,000	1st 12lb	3st 10lb	7st 6lb

TO LOSE...	Cut your daily calorie intake by	In three months you could lose...	In six months you could lose...	In one year you could lose...
¼kg a week	250	3.25kg	6.5kg	13kg
½kg a week	500	6.5kg	13kg	26kg
¾kg a week	750	9.75kg	19.5kg	39kg
1kg a week	1,000	13kg	26kg	52kg

4. Keep a food diary

Writing down what you eat and drink and any thoughts linked to that eating helps you become more aware of your eating habits. Recognising what is going on helps you feel in control and is a powerful way to start planning change. Keeping a food diary before you start to change your eating habits will also help you identify opportunities for cutting calories by substituting one food for another, cutting portion sizes of high-calorie foods or eating certain foods less often. Simply write down every single item you eat or drink during the day and use this book to calculate the calories of each item. Then after a few days of eating normally, introduce some changes to your diet to achieve your daily calorie allowance. Remember to spread your daily calorie allowance fairly evenly throughout the day to prevent hunger. You'll find a template for a daily food and exercise diary on page 43. Try to use it as carefully as you can as research shows that people who do, do best.

Top Tip

If you only fill in your main food diary once a day, keep a pen and notepad with you to write down all those little extras you eat or drink during the day – that chocolate you ate in the office, the sliver of cheese you had while cooking dinner and the few chips you pinched from your husband's plate, for example! It's easy to forget the little things if they're not written down, but they can make the difference between success and failure.

QUESTION: Why are heavier people allowed more calories than those who have smaller amounts of weight to lose?

ANSWER: This confuses a lot of people but is easily explained. Someone who is 3 stone overweight, for example, is carrying the equivalent of 42 small packets of butter with them everywhere they go – up and down the stairs, to the local shops, into the kitchen. Obviously, it takes a lot more energy simply to move around when you're carrying that extra weight. As a consequence, the heavier you are, the more calories you need just to keep your weight steady. In turn, this means you'll lose weight on a higher calorie allowance. However, as you lose weight, you'll need to lower your calorie allowance slightly as you have less weight to carry around.

5. Control your portions

As well as making some smart food swaps to cut calories, it's likely you'll also need to reduce your serving sizes for some foods to help shift those pounds. Even 'healthy' foods such as brown rice, wholemeal bread, chicken, fish and low-fat dairy products contain calories so you may need to limit the amount you eat. When you first start out, weigh portions of foods like rice, pasta, cereal, cheese, butter, oil, meat, fish, and chicken rather than completing your food diary with a 'guesstimated' weight! That way you can calculate the calorie content accurately. Don't forget that drinks contain calories too, alcohol, milk, juices and sugary drinks all count.

6. Measure your success

Research has found that regular weight checks do help. Weighing yourself helps you assess how your eating and exercise habits affect your body weight. The important thing is to use the information in a positive way – to assess your progress - rather than as a stick to beat yourself up with. Remember that weight can fluctuate by a kilogram in a day, for example, due to fluid changes, premenstrually, after a big meal out, so weigh yourself at the same time of day and look at the trend over a week or two.

People who successfully lose weight and keep it off, also tend to continue weighing themselves at least once a week, and often daily (but not in an obsessive way), because they say it helps them stay 'on track'. Probably because they use it as an early warning system. People who weigh themselves regularly (or regularly try on a tight fitting item of clothing) will notice quickly if they have gained a couple of kilograms and can take action to stop gaining more. Checking your weight less often can mean that you might discover one day that you gained 6kg. That can be pretty discouraging, and it might trigger you to just give up.

Top Tip

Don't just focus on what the bathroom scales say either – keep a record of your vital statistics, too. Many people find it doubly encouraging to see the inches dropping off, as well as the pounds!

7. Stay motivated

Each time you lose half a stone, or reach your own small goal – celebrate! Treat yourself to a little luxury – something new to wear, a little pampering or some other (non-food) treat. It also helps replace the comfort you once got from food and allows you to take care of yourself in other ways. Trying on an item of clothing that used to be tight can also help to keep you feeling motivated. Make sure you keep in touch with your supporters, and if the going gets tough take another look at the 'Coping with Slimming Saboteurs' section. Once you've reviewed how well you've done, use this book to set yourself a new daily calorie allowance based on your new weight to help you lose the next half stone *(see point 3 - page 28 - Calculate your calorie allowance)*.

8. Keep it off

What you do to stay slim is just as important as what you did to get slim. Quite simply, if you return to your old ways, you are likely to return to your old weight. The great thing about calorie counting is that you will learn so much about what you eat, and make so many important changes to your eating and drinking habits, that you'll probably find it difficult to go back to your old ways – and won't want to anyway. It's still a good idea to weigh yourself at least once a week to keep a check on your weight. The key is to deal with any extra pounds immediately, rather than waiting until you have a stone to lose *(see page 30)*. Simply go back to counting calories for as long as it takes to shift those pounds and enjoy the new slim you. Page 25 has more information about how successful slimmers keep it off.

QUESTION: Do I need to stick to exactly the same number of calories each day or is it OK to have a lower calorie intake during the week and slightly more at the weekend?

ANSWER: The key to losing weight is to take in fewer calories than you need for as long as it takes to reach your target, aiming for a loss of no more than 2lb (1kg) a week. In general, most nutrition experts recommend a daily calorie allowance. However, it's just as valid to use other periods of time such as weeks. If you prefer, simply multiply your daily allowance by seven to work out a weekly calorie allowance and then allocate more calories to some days than others. For example, a daily allowance of 1,500 calories is equivalent to 10,500 calories a week. This means you could have 1,300 calories a day during the week and 2,000 calories a day on Saturday and Sunday.

Healthy Eating Made Easy

Juliette Kellow BSc RD

GONE ARE THE DAYS when a healthy diet meant surviving on bird seed, rabbit food and carrot juice! The new approach to eating healthily means we're positively encouraged to eat a wide range of foods, including some of our favourites – it's just a question of making sure we don't eat high fat, high sugar or highly processed foods too often.

Eating a healthy diet, together with taking regular exercise and not smoking, has huge benefits to our health, both in the short and long term. As well as helping us to lose or maintain our weight, a healthy diet can boost energy levels, keep our immune system strong and give us healthy skin, nails and hair. Meanwhile, eating well throughout life also means we're far less likely to suffer from health problems such as constipation, anaemia and tooth decay or set ourselves up for serious conditions in later life such as obesity, heart disease, stroke, diabetes, cancer or osteoporosis.

Fortunately, it couldn't be easier to eat a balanced diet. To start with, no single food provides all the calories and nutrients we need to stay healthy, so it's important to eat a variety of foods. Meanwhile, most nutrition experts also agree that mealtimes should be a pleasure rather than a penance. This means it's fine to eat small amounts of our favourite treats from time to time.

To help people eat healthily, the Food Standards Agency recommends eating plenty of different foods from four main groups of foods and limiting the amount we eat from a smaller fifth group. Ultimately, we should eat more fruit, vegetables, starchy, fibre-rich foods and fresh products, and fewer fatty, sugary, salty and processed foods.

The following guidelines are all based on the healthy eating guidelines recommended by the Food Standards Agency.

Bread, other cereals and potatoes

Eat these foods at each meal. They also make good snacks.

Foods in this group include bread, breakfast cereals, potatoes, rice, pasta, noodles, yams, oats and grains. Go for high-fibre varieties where available, such as wholegrain cereals, wholemeal bread and brown rice. These foods should fill roughly a third of your plate at mealtimes.

TYPICAL SERVING SIZES

- *2 slices bread in a sandwich or with a meal*
- *a tennis ball sized serving of pasta, potato, rice, noodles or couscous*
- *a bowl of porridge*
- *around 40g of breakfast cereal*

Fruit and vegetables

Eat at least five portions every day.

Foods in this group include all fruits and vegetables, including fresh, frozen, canned and dried products, and unsweetened fruit juice. Choose canned fruit in juice rather than syrup and go for veg canned in water without added salt or sugar.

TYPICAL PORTION SIZES

- *a piece of fruit eg apple, banana, pear*
- *2 small fruits eg satsumas, plums, apricots*
- *a bowl of fruit salad, canned or stewed fruit*
- *a small glass of unsweetened fruit juice*
- *a cereal bowl of salad*
- *3tbsp vegetables*

Milk and dairy foods

Eat two or three servings a day.

Foods in this group include milk, cheese, yoghurt and fromage frais. Choose low-fat varieties where available such as skimmed milk, reduced-fat cheese and fat-free yoghurt.

TYPICAL SERVING SIZES

* *200ml milk*

* *a small pot of yoghurt or fromage frais*

* *a small matchbox-sized piece of cheese*

Meat, fish and alternatives

Eat two servings a day

Foods in this group include meat, poultry, fish, eggs, beans, nuts and seeds. Choose low-fat varieties where available such as extra-lean minced beef and skinless chicken and don't add extra fat or salt.

TYPICAL SERVING SIZES

* *a piece of meat, chicken or fish the size of a deck of cards*

* *1-2 eggs*

* *3 heaped tablespoons of beans*

* *a small handful of nuts or seeds*

Healthy Eating on a plate

A simple way to serve up both balance and healthy proportions is to fill one half of your plate with salad or vegetables and divide the other half between protein-rich meat, chicken, fish, eggs or beans, and healthy carbs (potatoes, rice, pasta, pulses, bread or noodles).

Fatty and sugary foods

Eat only small amounts of these foods

Foods in this group include oils, spreading fats, cream, mayonnaise, oily salad dressings, cakes, biscuits, puddings, crisps, savoury snacks, sugar, preserves, confectionery and sugary soft drinks.

TYPICAL SERVING SIZES:

- *a small packet of sweets or a small bar of chocolate*
- *a small slice of cake*
- *a couple of small biscuits*
- *1 level tbsp mayo, salad dressing or olive oil*
- *a small packet of crisps*

Useful Tools

Body Mass Index

The Body Mass Index (BMI) is the internationally accepted way of assessing how healthy our weight is. It is calculated using an individual's height and weight. Use the Body Mass Index Chart to look up your BMI, and use the table below to see what range you fall into.

BMI Under 18.5	Underweight
BMI 18.5-25	Healthy
BMI 25-30	Overweight
BMI 30-40	Obese
BMI Over 40	Severely Obese

This is what different BMI ranges mean.

- **Underweight:** you probably need to gain weight for your health's sake. Talk to your doctor if you have any concerns, or if you feel frightened about gaining weight.

- **Healthy weight:** you are a healthy weight, so aim to stay in this range (note that most people in this range tend to have a BMI between 20-25).

- **Overweight:** aim to lose some weight for your health's sake, or at least prevent further weight gain.

- **Obese:** your health is at risk and losing weight will benefit your health.

- **Severely obese:** your health is definitely at risk. You should visit your doctor for a health check. Losing weight will improve your health.

Please note that BMI is not as accurate for athletes or very muscular people (muscle weighs more than fat), as it can push them into a higher BMI category despite having a healthy level of body fat. It is also not accurate for women who are pregnant or breastfeeding, or people who are frail.

Body Mass Index Table

HEIGHT IN FEET / INCHES

WEIGHT IN STONES / LBS	4'6	4'8	4'10	5'0	5'2	5'4	5'6	5'8	5'10	6'0	6'2	6'4	6'6	6'8	6'10
6st 7	22.0	20.5	19.1	17.8	16.7	15.7	14.7	13.9	13.1	12.4	11.7	11.1	10.6	10.0	9.5
7st 0	23.7	22.1	20.6	19.2	18.0	16.9	15.9	15.0	14.1	13.3	12.6	12.0	11.4	10.8	10.3
7st 7	25.4	23.6	22.0	20.6	19.3	18.1	17.0	16.0	15.1	14.3	13.5	12.8	12.2	11.6	11.0
8st 0	27.1	25.2	23.5	22.0	20.6	19.3	18.1	17.1	16.1	15.2	14.4	13.7	13.0	12.3	11.8
8st 7	28.8	26.8	25.0	23.3	21.8	20.5	19.3	18.2	17.1	16.2	15.3	14.5	13.8	13.1	12.5
9st 0	30.5	28.4	26.4	24.7	23.1	21.7	20.4	19.2	18.1	17.2	16.2	15.4	14.6	13.9	13.2
9st 7	32.2	29.9	27.9	26.1	24.4	22.9	21.5	20.3	19.2	18.1	17.1	16.2	15.4	14.7	14.0
10st 0	33.9	31.5	29.4	27.4	25.7	24.1	22.7	21.4	20.2	19.1	18.0	17.1	16.2	15.4	14.7
10st 7	35.6	33.1	30.8	28.8	27.0	25.3	23.8	22.4	21.2	20.0	18.9	18.0	17.0	16.2	15.4
11st 0	37.3	34.7	32.3	30.2	28.3	26.5	24.9	23.5	22.2	21.0	19.8	18.8	17.9	17.0	16.2
11st 7	39.0	36.2	33.8	31.6	29.6	27.7	26.1	24.6	23.2	21.9	20.7	19.7	18.7	17.8	16.9
12st 0	40.7	37.8	35.2	32.9	30.8	28.9	27.2	25.6	24.2	22.9	21.6	20.5	19.5	18.5	17.6
12st 7	42.3	39.4	36.7	34.3	32.1	30.1	28.3	26.7	25.2	23.8	22.5	21.4	20.3	19.3	18.4
13st 0	44.0	41.0	38.2	35.7	33.4	31.4	29.5	27.8	26.2	24.8	23.5	22.2	21.1	20.1	19.1
13st 7	45.7	42.5	39.6	37.0	34.7	32.6	30.6	28.8	27.2	25.7	24.4	23.1	21.9	20.8	19.8
14st 0	47.4	44.1	41.1	38.4	36.0	33.8	31.7	29.9	28.2	26.7	25.3	23.9	22.7	21.6	20.6
14st 7	49.1	45.7	42.6	39.8	37.3	35.0	32.9	31.0	29.2	27.6	26.2	24.8	23.5	22.4	21.3
15st 0	50.8	47.3	44.0	41.2	38.5	36.2	34.0	32.0	30.2	28.6	27.1	25.7	24.4	23.2	22.0
15st 7	52.5	48.8	45.5	42.5	39.8	37.4	35.2	33.1	31.2	29.5	28.0	26.5	25.2	23.9	22.8
16st 0	54.2	50.4	47.0	43.9	41.1	38.6	36.3	34.2	32.3	30.5	28.9	27.4	26.0	24.7	23.5
16st 7	55.9	52.0	48.5	45.3	42.4	39.8	37.4	35.2	33.3	31.4	29.8	28.2	26.8	25.5	24.2
17st 0	57.6	53.6	49.9	46.6	43.7	41.0	38.6	36.3	34.3	32.4	30.7	29.1	27.6	26.2	25.0
17st 7	59.3	55.1	51.4	48.0	45.0	42.2	39.7	37.4	35.3	33.3	31.6	29.9	28.4	27.0	25.7
18st 0	61.0	56.7	52.9	49.4	46.3	43.4	40.8	38.5	36.3	34.3	32.5	30.8	29.2	27.8	26.4
18st 7	62.7	58.3	54.3	50.8	47.5	44.6	42.0	39.5	37.3	35.3	33.4	31.6	30.0	28.6	27.2
19st 0	64.4	59.9	55.8	52.1	48.8	45.8	43.1	40.6	38.3	36.2	34.3	32.5	30.8	29.3	27.9
19st 7	66.1	61.4	57.3	53.5	50.1	47.0	44.2	41.7	39.3	37.2	35.2	33.3	31.7	30.1	28.6
20st 0	67.8	63.0	58.7	54.9	51.4	48.2	45.4	42.7	40.3	38.1	36.1	34.2	32.5	30.9	29.4
20st 7	69.4	64.6	60.2	56.3	52.7	49.4	46.5	43.8	41.3	39.1	37.0	35.1	33.3	31.6	30.1
21st 0	71.1	66.2	61.7	57.6	54.0	50.6	47.6	44.9	42.3	40.0	37.9	35.9	34.1	32.4	30.9
21st 7	72.8	67.7	63.1	59.0	55.3	51.9	48.8	45.9	43.3	41.0	38.8	36.8	34.9	33.2	31.6
22st 0	74.5	69.3	64.6	60.4	56.5	53.1	49.9	47.0	44.4	41.9	39.7	37.6	35.7	34.0	32.3
22st 7	76.2	70.9	66.1	61.7	57.8	54.3	51.0	48.1	45.4	42.9	40.6	38.5	36.5	34.7	33.1
23st 0	77.9	72.5	67.5	63.1	59.1	55.5	52.2	49.1	46.4	43.8	41.5	39.3	37.3	35.5	33.8
23st 7	79.6	74.0	69.0	64.5	60.4	56.7	53.3	50.2	47.4	44.8	42.4	40.2	38.2	36.3	34.5
24st 0	81.3	75.6	70.5	65.9	61.7	57.9	54.4	51.3	48.4	45.7	43.3	41.0	39.0	37.0	35.3
24st 7	83.0	77.2	71.9	67.2	63.0	59.1	55.6	52.3	49.4	46.7	44.2	41.9	39.8	37.8	36.0
25st 0	84.7	78.8	73.4	68.6	64.2	60.3	56.7	53.4	50.4	47.6	45.1	42.8	40.6	38.6	36.7
25st 7	86.4	80.3	74.9	70.0	65.5	61.5	57.8	54.5	51.4	48.6	46.0	43.6	41.4	39.4	37.5
26st 0	88.1	81.9	76.3	71.3	66.8	62.7	59.0	55.5	52.4	49.5	46.9	44.5	42.2	40.1	38.2
26st 7	89.8	83.5	77.8	72.7	68.1	63.9	60.1	56.6	53.4	50.5	47.8	45.3	43.0	40.9	38.9
27st 0	91.5	85.1	79.3	74.1	69.4	65.1	61.2	57.7	54.4	51.5	48.7	46.2	43.8	41.7	39.7
27st 7	93.2	86.6	80.8	75.5	70.7	66.3	62.4	58.7	55.4	52.4	49.6	47.0	44.7	42.4	40.4
28st 0	94.9	88.2	82.2	76.8	72.0	67.5	63.5	59.8	56.4	53.4	50.5	47.9	45.5	43.2	41.1
28st 7	96.5	89.8	83.7	78.2	73.2	68.7	64.6	60.9	57.5	54.3	51.4	48.7	46.3	44.0	41.9
29st 0	98.2	91.4	85.2	79.6	74.5	69.9	65.8	62.0	58.5	55.3	52.3	49.6	47.1	44.8	42.6
29st 7	99.9	92.9	86.6	80.9	75.8	71.1	66.9	63.0	59.5	56.2	53.2	50.5	47.9	45.5	43.3

Weight Chart

Underweight
BMI less than 18.5

HEALTHY
WEIGHT
BMI 18.5-25

Overweight
BMI 25-30

Obese
BMI 30-40

Severely
Obese
BMI 40 or more

BMI: 10 11 12 13 14 15 16 17 18 19 20 21 22 23 24 25 26 27 28 29 30 31 32 33 34 35 36 37 38

Height:
6ft 6" / 197.5cm
6ft 5" / 195cm
6ft 4" / 192.5cm
6ft 3" / 190cm
6ft 2" / 187.5cm
6ft 1" / 185cm
6ft 0" / 182.5cm
5ft 11" / 180cm
5ft 10" / 177.5cm
5ft 9" / 175cm
5ft 8" / 172.5cm
5ft 7" / 170cm
5ft 6" / 167.5cm
5ft 5" / 165cm
5ft 4" / 162.5cm
5ft 3" / 160cm
5ft 2" / 157.5cm
5ft 1" / 155cm
5ft 0" / 152.5cm
4ft 11" / 150cm
4ft 10" / 147.5cm
4ft 9" / 145cm
4ft 8" / 142.5cm
4ft 7" / 140cm
4ft 6" / 137.5cm

Weight:
4st 7lb / 29kg
5st 0lb / 32kg
5st 7lb / 35kg
6st 0lb / 38kg
6st 7lb / 41kg
7st 0lb / 45kg
7st 7lb / 48kg
8st 0lb / 51kg
8st 7lb / 54kg
9st 0lb / 57kg
9st 7lb / 60kg
10st 0lb / 64kg
10st 7lb / 67kg
11st 0lb / 70kg
11st 7lb / 73kg
12st 0lb / 76kg
12st 7lb / 79kg
13st 0lb / 83kg
13st 7lb / 86kg
14st 0lb / 89kg
14st 7lb / 92kg
15st 0lb / 95kg
15st 7lb / 98kg
16st 0lb / 102kg
16st 7lb / 105kg
17st 0lb / 108kg
17st 7lb / 111kg
18st 0lb / 114kg
18st 7lb / 118kg
19st 0lb / 121kg
19st 7lb / 124kg
20st 0lb / 127kg
20st 7lb / 130kg
21st 0lb / 133kg
21st 7lb / 137kg
22st 0lb / 140kg
22st 7lb / 143kg
23st 0lb / 146kg
23st 7lb / 149kg

Calories Required to Maintain Weight
Adult Females

ACTIVITY LEVEL / AGE

WEIGHT IN STONES / LBS	VERY SEDENTARY			MODERATELY SEDENTARY			MODERATELY ACTIVE			VERY ACTIVE		
	<30	30-60	60+	<30	30-60	60+	<30	30-60	60+	<30	30-60	60+
7st 7	1425	1473	1304	1544	1596	1412	1781	1841	1630	2138	2210	1956
8st 0	1481	1504	1338	1605	1629	1450	1852	1880	1673	2222	2256	2008
8st 7	1537	1535	1373	1666	1663	1487	1922	1919	1716	2306	2302	2059
9st 0	1594	1566	1407	1726	1696	1524	1992	1957	1759	2391	2349	2111
9st 7	1650	1596	1442	1787	1729	1562	2062	1996	1802	2475	2395	2163
10st 0	1706	1627	1476	1848	1763	1599	2133	2034	1845	2559	2441	2214
10st 7	1762	1658	1511	1909	1796	1637	2203	2073	1888	2644	2487	2266
11st 0	1819	1689	1545	1970	1830	1674	2273	2111	1931	2728	2534	2318
11st 7	1875	1720	1580	2031	1863	1711	2344	2150	1975	2813	2580	2370
12st 0	1931	1751	1614	2092	1897	1749	2414	2188	2018	2897	2626	2421
12st 7	1987	1781	1648	2153	1930	1786	2484	2227	2061	2981	2672	2473
13st 0	2044	1812	1683	2214	1963	1823	2555	2266	2104	3066	2719	2525
13st 7	2100	1843	1717	2275	1997	1861	2625	2304	2147	3150	2765	2576
14st 0	2156	1874	1752	2336	2030	1898	2695	2343	2190	3234	2811	2628
14st 7	2212	1905	1786	2397	2064	1935	2766	2381	2233	3319	2858	2680
15st 0	2269	1936	1821	2458	2097	1973	2836	2420	2276	3403	2904	2732
15st 7	2325	1967	1855	2519	2130	2010	2906	2458	2319	3488	2950	2783
16st 0	2381	1997	1890	2580	2164	2047	2976	2497	2362	3572	2996	2835
16st 7	2437	2028	1924	2640	2197	2085	3047	2535	2405	3656	3043	2887
17st 0	2494	2059	1959	2701	2231	2122	3117	2574	2449	3741	3089	2938
17st 7	2550	2090	1993	2762	2264	2159	3187	2613	2492	3825	3135	2990
18st 0	2606	2121	2028	2823	2298	2197	3258	2651	2535	3909	3181	3042
18st 7	2662	2152	2062	2884	2331	2234	3328	2690	2578	3994	3228	3093
19st 0	2719	2182	2097	2945	2364	2271	3398	2728	2621	4078	3274	3145
19st 7	2775	2213	2131	3006	2398	2309	3469	2767	2664	4162	3320	3197
20st 0	2831	2244	2166	3067	2431	2346	3539	2805	2707	4247	3366	3249
20st 7	2887	2275	2200	3128	2465	2383	3609	2844	2750	4331	3413	3300
21st 0	2944	2306	2235	3189	2498	2421	3680	2882	2793	4416	3459	3352
21st 7	3000	2337	2269	3250	2531	2458	3750	2921	2836	4500	3505	3404
22st 0	3056	2368	2303	3311	2565	2495	3820	2960	2879	4584	3552	3455
22st 7	3112	2398	2338	3372	2598	2533	3890	2998	2923	4669	3598	3507
23st 0	3169	2429	2372	3433	2632	2570	3961	3037	2966	4753	3644	3559
23st 7	3225	2460	2407	3494	2665	2608	4031	3075	3009	4837	3690	3611
24st 0	3281	2491	2441	3554	2699	2645	4101	3114	3052	4922	3737	3662
24st 7	3337	2522	2476	3615	2732	2682	4172	3152	3095	5006	3783	3714
25st 0	3394	2553	2510	3676	2765	2720	4242	3191	3138	5091	3829	3766
25st 7	3450	2583	2545	3737	2799	2757	4312	3229	3181	5175	3875	3817
26st 0	3506	2614	2579	3798	2832	2794	4383	3268	3224	5259	3922	3869
26st 7	3562	2645	2614	3859	2866	2832	4453	3307	3267	5344	3968	3921
27st 0	3618	2676	2648	3920	2899	2869	4523	3345	3310	5428	4014	3973
27st 7	3675	2707	2683	3981	2932	2906	4594	3384	3353	5512	4060	4024
28st 0	3731	2738	2717	4042	2966	2944	4664	3422	3397	5597	4107	4076
28st 7	3787	2768	2752	4103	2999	2981	4734	3461	3440	5681	4153	4128

Calories Required to Maintain Weight
Adult Males

ACTIVITY LEVEL / AGE

WEIGHT IN STONES / LBS	VERY SEDENTARY			MODERATELY SEDENTARY			MODERATELY ACTIVE			VERY ACTIVE		
	<30	30-60	60+	<30	30-60	60+	<30	30-60	60+	<30	30-60	60+
9st 0	1856	1827	1502	2010	1979	1627	2320	2284	1878	2784	2741	2254
9st 7	1913	1871	1547	2072	2026	1676	2391	2338	1933	2870	2806	2320
10st 0	1970	1914	1591	2134	2074	1724	2463	2393	1989	2955	2871	2387
10st 7	2027	1958	1636	2196	2121	1772	2534	2447	2045	3041	2937	2454
11st 0	2084	2001	1680	2258	2168	1820	2605	2502	2100	3127	3002	2520
11st 7	2141	2045	1724	2320	2215	1868	2677	2556	2156	3212	3067	2587
12st 0	2199	2088	1769	2382	2262	1916	2748	2611	2211	3298	3133	2654
12st 7	2256	2132	1813	2444	2310	1965	2820	2665	2267	3384	3198	2720
13st 0	2313	2175	1858	2506	2357	2013	2891	2719	2322	3470	3263	2787
13st 7	2370	2219	1902	2568	2404	2061	2963	2774	2378	3555	3329	2854
14st 0	2427	2262	1947	2630	2451	2109	3034	2828	2434	3641	3394	2920
14st 7	2484	2306	1991	2691	2498	2157	3106	2883	2489	3727	3459	2987
15st 0	2542	2350	2036	2753	2545	2205	3177	2937	2545	3813	3525	3054
15st 7	2599	2393	2080	2815	2593	2253	3248	2992	2600	3898	3590	3120
16st 0	2656	2437	2125	2877	2640	2302	3320	3046	2656	3984	3655	3187
16st 7	2713	2480	2169	2939	2687	2350	3391	3100	2711	4070	3721	3254
17st 0	2770	2524	2213	3001	2734	2398	3463	3155	2767	4155	3786	3320
17st 7	2827	2567	2258	3063	2781	2446	3534	3209	2823	4241	3851	3387
18st 0	2884	2611	2302	3125	2828	2494	3606	3264	2878	4327	3917	3454
18st 7	2942	2654	2347	3187	2876	2542	3677	3318	2934	4413	3982	3520
19st 0	2999	2698	2391	3249	2923	2591	3749	3373	2989	4498	4047	3587
19st 7	3056	2741	2436	3311	2970	2639	3820	3427	3045	4584	4112	3654
20st 0	3113	2785	2480	3373	3017	2687	3891	3481	3100	4670	4178	3721
20st 7	3170	2829	2525	3434	3064	2735	3963	3536	3156	4756	4243	3787
21st 0	3227	2872	2569	3496	3112	2783	4034	3590	3211	4841	4308	3854
21st 7	3285	2916	2614	3558	3159	2831	4106	3645	3267	4927	4374	3921
22st 0	3342	2959	2658	3620	3206	2880	4177	3699	3323	5013	4439	3987
22st 7	3399	3003	2702	3682	3253	2928	4249	3754	3378	5098	4504	4054
23st 0	3456	3046	2747	3744	3300	2976	4320	3808	3434	5184	4570	4121
23st 7	3513	3090	2791	3806	3347	3024	4392	3862	3489	5270	4635	4187
24st 0	3570	3133	2836	3868	3395	3072	4463	3917	3545	5356	4700	4254
24st 7	3627	3177	2880	3930	3442	3120	4534	3971	3600	5441	4766	4321
25st 0	3685	3220	2925	3992	3489	3168	4606	4026	3656	5527	4831	4387
25st 7	3742	3264	2969	4054	3536	3217	4677	4080	3712	5613	4896	4454
26st 0	3799	3308	3014	4116	3583	3265	4749	4135	3767	5699	4962	4521
26st 7	3856	3351	3058	4177	3630	3313	4820	4189	3823	5784	5027	4587
27st 0	3913	3395	3103	4239	3678	3361	4892	4243	3878	5870	5092	4654
27st 7	3970	3438	3147	4301	3725	3409	4963	4298	3934	5956	5158	4721
28st 0	4028	3482	3191	4363	3772	3457	5035	4352	3989	6042	5223	4787
28st 7	4085	3525	3236	4425	3819	3506	5106	4407	4045	6127	5288	4854
29st 0	4142	3569	3280	4487	3866	3554	5177	4461	4101	6213	5354	4921
29st 7	4199	3612	3325	4549	3913	3602	5249	4516	4156	6299	5419	4987
30st 0	4256	3656	3369	4611	3961	3650	5320	4570	4212	6384	5484	5054

Calories Burned in Exercise

This table shows the approximate number of extra* calories that would be burned in a five minute period of exercise activity.

ACTIVITY	CALORIES BURNED IN 5 MINUTES	ACTIVITY	CALORIES BURNED IN 5 MINUTES
Aerobics, Low Impact	25	Situps, Continuous	17
Badminton, Recreational	17	Skiing, Moderate	30
Cross Trainer	30	Skipping, Moderate	30
Cycling, Recreational, 5mph	17	Squash Playing	39
Dancing, Modern, Moderate	13	Tennis Playing, Recreational	26
Fencing	24	Toning Exercises	17
Gardening, Weeding	19	Trampolining	17
Hill Walking, Up and Down, Recreational	22	Volleyball, Recreational	10
Jogging	30	Walking, Uphill, 15% Gradient, Moderate	43
Kick Boxing	30	Walking Up and Down Stairs, Moderate	34
Netball Playing	23	Walking, 4mph	24
Rebounding	18	Weight Training, Moderate	12
Roller Skating	30	Yoga	13
Rowing Machine, Moderate	30		
Running, 7.5mph	48		

*Extra calories are those in addition to your normal daily calorie needs.

My Personal Plan

Date:

Body Mass Index:

Weight:

Waist Measurement:

Height:

Body Fat % (if known)

10% Weight Loss Goal:

Current weight	16stone (224lb)	100kg
- 10% weight	1stone 8½lb (22½lb)	10kg
= 10% loss goal	14stone 5½lb (201½lb)	90kg

My smaller weight targets on the way to achieving my 10% goal will be:

Reasons why I want to lose weight:

Changes I will make to help me lose weight:
Diet:

Activity:

Potential saboteurs or barriers will be:

Ways I will overcome these:

My supporters will be:

I will monitor my progress by:

I will reward my progress with:
In the short term:

In the long term:

Food and Exercise Diary

Date:
/ /

Daily Calorie Allowance: Ⓐ

Food/Drink Consumed	Serving Size	Calories

Total calories consumed Ⓑ

Exercise/Activity	No. mins	Calories

Calories used in exercise Ⓒ

Calorie balance Ⓓ

You are aiming for your Calorie Balance (Box D) to be as close to zero as possible - ie. you consume the number of calories you need.

Your Daily Calorie Allowance (Box A) should be set to lose ½-2lb (¼-1kg) a week, or maintain weight, depending on your goals.

Daily Calorie Allowance (A) *plus* Extra Calories used in Exercise (C) *minus* Total Calories Consumed (B) *equals* Calorie Balance (D)

$A + C - B = D$

You can also write down any comments or thoughts related to your eating if you want to.

Food Information

Nutritional Information

CALORIE AND FAT values are given per serving, plus calorie and nutrition values per 100g of product. This makes it easy to compare the proportions of fat, protein, carbohydrate and fibre in each food.

The values given are for uncooked, unprepared foods unless otherwise stated. Values are also for only the edible portion of the food unless otherwise stated. ie - weighed with bone.

Finding Foods

The Calorie, Carb & Fat Bible has an Eating Out section which is arranged alphabetically by brand. In the General Foods and Drinks A-Z most foods are grouped together by type, and then put in to alphabetical order. This makes it easy to compare different brands, and will help you to find lower calorie and/or fat alternatives where they are available.

This format also makes it easier to locate foods. Foods are categorised by their main characteristics so, for example, if it is bread, ciabatta or white sliced, you'll find it under "Bread".

Basic ingredients are highlighted to make them easier to find at a glance. You'll find all unbranded foods in bold - making the index easier to use, whether it's just an apple or all the components of a home cooked stew.

There are, however, some foods which are not so easy to categorise, especially combination foods like ready meals. The following pointers will help you to find your way around the book until you get to know it a little better.

FILLED ROLLS AND SANDWICHES - Bagels, baguettes, etc which are filled are listed as "Bagels (filled)" etc. Sandwiches are under "Sandwiches".

CURRIES - Popular types of curry, like Balti or Jalfrezi, are listed under their individual types. Unspecified or lesser known types are listed under their main ingredient.

BURGERS - All burgers, including chicken-type sandwiches from fast-food outlets, are listed under "Burgers". CHIPS & FRIES - Are listed separately, depending on the name of the particular brand. All other types of potato are listed under "Potatoes".

SWEETS & CHOCOLATES - Well-known brands, eg. Aero, Mars Bar, are listed under their brand names. Others are listed under "Chocolate" (for bars) and "Chocolates" (for individual sweets).

READY MEALS - Popular types of dishes are listed under their type, eg. "Chow Mein", "Casserole", "Hot Pot", etc. Others are listed by their main ingredient, eg. "Chicken With", "Chicken In", etc.

EATING OUT & FAST FOODS - By popular demand this edition has the major eating out and fast food brands listed separately, at the back of the book. They are alphabetised first by brand, then follow using the same format as the rest of the book.

Serving Sizes

Many ready-meal type foods are given with calories for the full pack size, so that an individual serving can be worked out by estimating the proportion of the pack that has been consumed. For example, if you have eaten a quarter of a packaged pasta dish, divide the calorie value given for the whole pack by 4 to determine the number of calories you have consumed. Where serving sizes are not appropriate, or unknown, values are given per 1oz/28g. Serving sizes vary greatly from person to person and, if you are trying to lose weight, it's very important to be accurate – especially with foods that are very high in calories such as those that contain a fair amount of fat, sugar, cream, cheese, alcohol etc.

Food Data

Nutrition information for basic average foods has been compiled by the Weight Loss Resources food data team using many sources of information to calculate the most accurate values possible. Some nutrition information for non-branded food records is from The Composition of Foods 6th Edition (2002). Reproduced under licence from The Controller of Her Majesty's Stationary Office. Where basic data is present for ordinary foodstuffs such as 'raw carrots'; branded records are not included.

Nutrition information for branded goods is from details supplied by retailers and manufacturers, and researched by Weight Loss Resources staff. The Calorie Carb & Fat Bible contains data for over 1400 UK brands, including major supermarkets and fast food outlets.

The publishers gratefully acknowledge all the manufacturers and retailers who have provided information on their products. All product names, trademarks or registered trademarks belong to their respective owners and are used only for the purpose of identifying products.

Calorie & nutrition data for all food and drink items are typical values.

Caution

The information in The Calorie, Carb and Fat Bible is intended as an aid to weight loss and weight maintenance, and is not medical advice. If you suffer from, or think you may suffer from a medical condition you should consult your doctor before starting a weight loss and/or exercise regime. If you start exercising after a period of relative inactivity, you should start slowly and consult your doctor if you experience pain, distress or other symptoms.

Weights, Measures & Abbreviations

ABBREVIATIONS

kcal	*kilocalories / calories*
prot	*protein*
carb	*carbohydrate*
sm	*small*
med	*medium*
av	*average*
reg	*regular*
lge	*large*
tsp	*teaspoon*
tbsp	*tablespoon*
dtsp	*dessertspoon*

BRAND ABBREVIATIONS USED

ASDA
Good for You	*GFY*

MARKS & SPENCER — *M & S*
Count on Us	*COU*

MORRISONS
Better For You	*BFY*

SAINSBURY'S
Be Good to Yourself	*BGTY*
Way to Five	*WTF*
Taste the Difference	*TTD*

TESCO
Healthy Eating	*HE*
Healthy Living	*HL*

WAITROSE
Perfectly Balanced	*PB*

	Measure INFO/WEIGHT	per Measure KCAL	FAT	Nutrition Values per 100g / 100ml KCAL	PROT	CARB	FAT	FIBRE
ABSINTHE								
Average	*1 Shot/35ml*	*127.0*	*0.0*	*363*	*0.0*	*38.8*	*0.0*	*0.0*
ACKEE								
Canned, Drained, Average	*1oz/28g*	*42.0*	*4.0*	*151*	*2.9*	*0.8*	*15.2*	*0.0*
ADVOCAAT								
Average	*1 Shot/35ml*	*91.0*	*2.0*	*260*	*4.7*	*28.4*	*6.3*	*0.0*
AERO								
Bar, Milk, Giant, Nestle*	1 Giant/125g	674.0	39.0	539	6.6	57.7	30.9	2.2
Bar, Milk, Medium, Nestle*	1 Med Bar/43g	232.0	13.0	539	6.6	57.7	30.9	2.2
Bar, Milk, Snacksize, Nestle*	1 Bar/20.5g	110.0	7.0	537	6.6	55.9	31.9	2.2
Bar, Milk, Standard, Nestle*	1 Std Bar/31g	165.0	10.0	531	6.3	56.9	30.9	0.8
Minis, Nestle*	1 Bar/11g	57.0	3.0	518	6.8	58.1	28.7	0.8
Mint, Nestle*	1 Bar/46g	245.0	14.0	533	4.9	61.2	29.8	0.4
Mint, Snack Size, Nestle*	1 Bar /20.5g	112.0	7.0	548	7.7	55.3	32.8	0.9
ALFALFA SPROUTS								
Raw, Average	*1 Serving/80g*	*19.0*	*1.0*	*24*	*4.0*	*0.4*	*0.7*	*1.7*
ALMONDS								
Blanched, Average	*1oz/28g*	*171.0*	*15.0*	*610*	*24.9*	*7.1*	*53.5*	*8.5*
Cocoa Dusted, Organic, Green & Black's*	1 Pack/110g	585.0	40.0	532	7.8	42.8	36.7	7.6
Flaked, Average	*1oz/28g*	*172.0*	*15.0*	*613*	*24.9*	*6.5*	*54.3*	*7.6*
Flaked, Toasted, Average	*1oz/28g*	*176.0*	*16.0*	*629*	*24.6*	*5.8*	*56.4*	*7.5*
Ground, Average	*1 Serving/10g*	*62.0*	*6.0*	*625*	*24.0*	*6.6*	*55.8*	*7.4*
Marcona, Average	*1 Serving/100g*	*608.0*	*54.0*	*608*	*22.1*	*13.0*	*53.7*	*9.7*
Sugared, Co-Op*	1 Almond/6g	25.0	1.0	455	7.0	74.0	14.0	2.0
Toasted, Average	*1oz/28g*	*178.0*	*16.0*	*634*	*24.9*	*6.6*	*56.4*	*6.6*
Whole, Average	*1 Serving/20g*	*122.0*	*11.0*	*612*	*23.4*	*21.2*	*54.8*	*8.4*
ALOO TIKKI								
Indian Selection, Tesco*	1 Serving/23g	49.0	3.0	211	2.3	20.1	13.5	3.5
Mini, from Indian Snack Selection, Sainsbury's*	1 Piece/25g	44.0	2.0	175	4.8	22.1	7.5	3.9
Mini, Indian Selection, Somerfield*	1 Serving/25g	49.0	2.0	199	4.5	30.3	6.6	0.2
ANCHOVIES								
Drained, Finest, Tesco*	1 Fillets/3g	7.0	0.0	220	21.3	0.8	14.6	0.5
Fillets in Olive Oil, Sainsbury's*	1 Anchovy/10g	18.0	1.0	185	23.7	0.1	10.0	0.1
Fillets, Tesco*	1 Serving/15g	34.0	2.0	226	25.0	0.0	14.0	0.0
in Oil, Canned, Drained, Average	*1 Serving/30g*	*58.0*	*3.0*	*194*	*22.9*	*0.0*	*11.3*	*0.0*
Marinated, Sainsbury's*	¼ Pot/44g	78.0	4.0	177	22.0	2.0	9.0	0.1
Provencale, Finest, Tesco*	1 Anchovy/10g	20.0	1.0	201	22.0	0.0	12.6	0.0
Salted, Finest, Tesco*	1 Serving/10g	9.0	0.0	93	18.2	0.0	2.2	0.0
ANGEL DELIGHT								
Banana Flavour, Kraft*	1 Sachet/59g	289.0	12.0	490	2.5	72.0	21.0	0.0
Banana Toffee Flavour, No Added Sugar, Kraft*	1 Sachet/59g	292.0	16.0	495	4.8	58.5	26.5	0.0
Butterscotch Flavour, Kraft*	1 Sachet/59g	280.0	11.0	475	2.4	73.5	19.0	0.0
Butterscotch Flavour, No Added Sugar, Kraft*	1 Sachet/47g	226.0	11.0	480	4.5	61.0	24.0	0.0
Chocolate Flavour, Kraft*	1 Sachet/67g	305.0	12.0	455	3.7	69.5	18.0	0.4
Forest Fruit Flavour, Kraft*	1 Sachet/59g	289.0	13.0	490	2.5	71.5	21.5	0.0
Raspberry Flavour, Kraft*	1 Sachet/59g	289.0	12.0	490	2.5	72.0	21.0	0.0
Raspberry Flavour, No Added Sugar, Kraft*	1 Sachet/59g	292.0	15.0	495	4.8	59.5	26.0	0.0
Strawberry Flavour, Kraft*	1 Sachet/59g	286.0	12.0	485	2.5	71.0	21.0	0.0
Strawberry Flavour, No Added Sugar, Kraft*	1 Sachet/47g	230.0	12.0	490	4.8	59.0	26.5	0.0
Tangerine Flavour, No Added Sugar, Kraft*	1 Sachet/59g	292.0	16.0	495	4.8	58.0	27.0	0.9
Toffee Flavour, Kraft*	1 Sachet/59g	283.0	12.0	480	2.6	70.0	21.0	0.0
Vanilla Ice Cream Flavour, Kraft*	1 Sachet/59g	289.0	13.0	490	2.5	71.5	21.5	0.0
Vanilla Ice Cream Flavour, No Added Sugar, Kraft*	1 Sachet/59g	295.0	16.0	500	4.8	59.5	27.0	0.0

A

	Measure INFO/WEIGHT	per Measure KCAL	per Measure FAT	Nutrition Values per 100g / 100ml KCAL	PROT	CARB	FAT	FIBRE
ANGEL HAIR								
Pasta, Spaghetti, Sainsbury's*	1 Serving/100g	357.0	2.0	357	12.3	73.1	1.7	2.5
ANTIPASTO								
Artichoke, Sainsbury's*	1 Serving/50g	67.0	6.0	135	2.0	3.6	12.5	2.3
Mixed Mushroom, Sainsbury's*	¼ Jar/72g	70.0	6.0	97	2.7	1.4	9.0	3.7
Mixed Pepper, Sainsbury's*	½ Jar/140g	48.0	2.0	34	1.3	4.2	1.3	3.5
Parma Ham, from Selection Platter, TTD, Sainsbury's*	1 Serving/100g	236.0	13.0	236	29.9	0.1	12.9	0.0
Parma, Salami Milano, Bresaola, Finest, Tesco*	¼ Pack/30g	118.0	8.0	395	36.0	0.5	27.3	0.0
Roasted Pepper, Drained, Tesco*	1 Jar /170g	127.0	9.0	75	0.9	5.5	5.5	4.1
Seafood, Drained, Sainsbury's*	½ Jar/84g	150.0	10.0	178	14.3	4.1	11.6	1.4
Sun Dried Tomato, Sainsbury's*	¼ Jar/70g	275.0	25.0	393	4.5	13.4	35.7	6.2
APPLES								
Bites, Average	1 Pack/118g	58.0	0.0	49	0.3	11.6	0.1	2.2
Braeburn, Average	*1 Apple/165g*	*79.0*	*0.0*	*48*	*0.4*	*11.3*	*0.1*	*1.8*
Cape, Tesco*	1 Apple/100g	50.0	0.0	50	0.4	11.8	0.1	1.8
Cooking, Baked with Sugar, Flesh Only, Average	*1 Serving/140g*	*109.0*	*0.0*	*78*	*0.5*	*20.1*	*0.1*	*1.7*
Cooking, Raw, Peeled, Average	*1oz/28g*	*10.0*	*0.0*	*35*	*0.3*	*8.9*	*0.1*	*1.6*
Cooking, Stewed with Sugar, Average	*1 Serving/140g*	*104.0*	*0.0*	*74*	*0.3*	*19.1*	*0.1*	*1.2*
Cooking, Stewed without Sugar, Average	*1 Serving/140g*	*46.0*	*0.0*	*33*	*0.3*	*8.1*	*0.1*	*1.5*
Cox, English, Average	*1 Apple/108g*	*53.0*	*0.0*	*49*	*0.4*	*11.6*	*0.1*	*2.2*
Discovery, Average	*1 Apple/182g*	*95.0*	*0.0*	*52*	*0.3*	*13.8*	*0.2*	*2.4*
Dried, Average	*1 Pack/250g*	*554.0*	*1.0*	*221*	*1.0*	*57.3*	*0.3*	*6.6*
Empire, Average	*1 Serving/100g*	*48.0*	*0.0*	*48*	*0.4*	*11.8*	*0.1*	*2.0*
Fuji, Organic, Sainsbury's*	1 Apple/130g	61.0	0.0	47	0.4	11.8	0.1	1.8
Gala, Average	*1 Apple/152g*	*74.0*	*0.0*	*49*	*0.4*	*11.5*	*0.1*	*1.4*
Golden Delicious, Average	*1 Med/102g*	*49.0*	*0.0*	*48*	*0.4*	*11.5*	*0.1*	*1.7*
Granny Smith, Average	*1 Sm/125g*	*62.0*	*0.0*	*50*	*0.4*	*11.9*	*0.1*	*2.0*
Green, Average, Raw	*1oz/28g*	*13.0*	*0.0*	*47*	*0.3*	*11.3*	*0.1*	*1.7*
Mackintosh, Red, Average	*1 Apple/165g*	*81.0*	*0.0*	*49*	*0.2*	*12.8*	*0.3*	*1.8*
Pink Lady, Average	*1 Apple/125g*	*62.0*	*0.0*	*49*	*0.4*	*11.7*	*0.1*	*1.8*
Sliced, Average	*1oz/28g*	*14.0*	*0.0*	*49*	*0.4*	*11.6*	*0.1*	*1.8*
APPLETISE								
Schweppes*	1 Glass/200ml	98.0	0.0	49	0.0	11.8	0.0	0.0
APRICOTS								
& Prunes, in Fruit Juice, Breakfast, Sainsbury's*	1 Pot/150g	133.0	0.0	89	1.1	21.2	0.1	0.7
Canned, in Syrup, Average	*1oz/28g*	*18.0*	*0.0*	*63*	*0.4*	*16.1*	*0.1*	*0.9*
Dried, Average	*1 Apricot/10g*	*17.0*	*0.0*	*171*	*3.6*	*37.4*	*0.5*	*6.3*
Dried, Soft, Average	*1 Serving/100g*	*208.0*	*0.0*	*208*	*3.2*	*47.7*	*0.5*	*6.6*
Halves, in Fruit Juice, Average	*1 Can/221g*	*87.0*	*0.0*	*40*	*0.5*	*9.2*	*0.1*	*1.0*
Organic, Whole, Graze*	1 Pack/50g	94.0	0.0	188	4.8	43.4	0.7	7.7
Raw, Flesh Only, Average	*1 Apricot/37g*	*19.0*	*0.0*	*52*	*1.5*	*12.0*	*0.4*	*2.1*
Raw, Weighed with Stone, Average	*1 Apricot/40g*	*19.0*	*0.0*	*48*	*1.4*	*11.1*	*0.4*	*2.0*
ARCHERS*								
Aqua, Peach, Archers*	1 Bottle/275ml	206.0	0.0	75	0.3	5.1	0.0	0.0
Peach (Calculated Estimate), Archers*	1 Shot/35ml	91.0	0.0	260	0.0	0.0	0.0	0.0
ARROWROOT								
Fresh, Average	*1 Root/33g*	*21.0*	*0.0*	*64*	*4.2*	*13.3*	*0.0*	*1.2*
ARTICHOKE								
Chargrilled, in Olive Oil, Cooks Ingredients, Waitrose*	1 Serving/40g	52.0	5.0	129	1.7	2.7	12.3	2.7
Hearts, Canned, Drained, Average	*½ Can/117g*	*35.0*	*0.0*	*30*	*1.9*	*5.4*	*0.0*	*2.1*
Hearts, Marinated & Grilled, Waitrose*	1 Serving/50g	57.0	5.0	114	3.0	3.0	10.0	3.0
Hearts, Sliced, with Extra Virgin Olive Oil, Waitrose*	1 Serving/40g	24.0	2.0	59	1.3	4.4	4.0	7.0
In Oil, Tesco*	1 Piece/15g	18.0	2.0	120	2.0	2.2	11.0	7.5
Raw, Fresh, Average	*1oz/28g*	*13.0*	*0.0*	*47*	*3.3*	*10.5*	*0.1*	*5.4*

ARTICHOKES

	Measure INFO/WEIGHT	per Measure KCAL	per Measure FAT	Nutrition Values per 100g / 100ml KCAL	PROT	CARB	FAT	FIBRE
Chargrilled, In Olive Oil, TTD, Sainsbury's*	¼ Pack/70g	242.0	25.0	346	1.2	5.1	36.1	0.0

ASAFOETIDA

Schwartz*	1 Serving/100g	271.0	2.0	271	6.5	56.2	2.2	0.0

ASPARAGUS

Boiled, in Salted Water, Average	*5 Spears/125g*	*32.0*	*1.0*	*26*	*3.4*	*1.4*	*0.8*	*1.4*
British, with Butter, Tesco*	1 Serving/50g	26.0	2.0	52	2.6	1.6	4.0	2.0
Canned, Average	*1 Can/250g*	*47.0*	*0.0*	*19*	*2.3*	*2.0*	*0.2*	*1.6*
Raw, Trimmed, Average	*1 Serving/80g*	*20.0*	*0.0*	*25*	*2.9*	*2.0*	*0.6*	*1.7*

AUBERGINE

Baby, Tesco*	1 Aubergine/50g	7.0	0.0	15	0.9	2.2	0.4	2.3
Baked Topped, M & S*	1 Serving/150g	165.0	12.0	110	2.4	7.4	7.7	0.9
Fried, Average	*1oz/28g*	*85.0*	*9.0*	*302*	*1.2*	*2.8*	*31.9*	*2.3*
in Hot Sauce, Yarden*	1 Serving/35g	96.0	9.0	273	1.5	8.8	25.8	0.0
Marinated & Grilled, Waitrose*	½ Pack/100g	106.0	10.0	106	1.0	3.0	10.0	2.0
Parmigiana, M & S*	1 Pack/350g	332.0	19.0	95	4.6	7.6	5.3	1.1
Raw, Fresh, Average	*1 Sm/250g*	*37.0*	*1.0*	*15*	*0.9*	*2.2*	*0.4*	*2.0*

AVOCADO

Flesh Only, Average	*1 Med/145g*	*275.0*	*28.0*	*190*	*1.9*	*1.9*	*19.5*	*3.4*

	Measure INFO/WEIGHT	per Measure KCAL	FAT	Nutrition Values per 100g / 100ml KCAL	PROT	CARB	FAT	FIBRE
BACARDI*								
*37.5% Volume, Bacardi**	*1 Shot/35ml*	**72.0**	**0.0**	**207**	**0.0**	**0.0**	**0.0**	**0.0**
*40% Volume, Bacardi**	*1 Shot/35ml*	**78.0**	**0.0**	**222**	**0.0**	**0.0**	**0.0**	**0.0**
Breezer, Apple, Half Sugar, Crisp, Bacardi*	1 Bottle/275ml	121.0	0.0	44	0.0	3.7	0.0	0.0
Breezer, Cranberry, Bacardi*	1 Bottle/275ml	154.0	0.0	56	0.0	7.1	0.0	0.0
Breezer, Lemon, Diet, Bacardi*	1 Bottle/275ml	96.0	0.0	35	0.0	1.2	0.0	0.0
Breezer, Lime, Bacardi*	1 Bottle/275ml	181.0	0.0	66	0.0	9.1	0.0	0.0
Breezer, Orange & Vanilla, Diet, Bacardi*	1 Bottle/275ml	96.0	0.0	35	0.0	1.2	0.0	0.0
Breezer, Orange, Bacardi*	1 Bottle/275ml	179.0	0.0	65	0.0	8.2	0.0	0.0
Breezer, Orange, Diet, Bacardi*	1 Bottle/275ml	80.0	0.0	29	0.0	0.0	0.0	0.0
Breezer, Pineapple, Bacardi*	1 Bottle/275ml	170.0	0.0	62	0.0	8.6	0.0	0.0
BACON								
Back, Dry Cured, Average	*1 Rasher/31g*	**77.0**	**5.0**	**250**	**28.1**	**0.3**	**15.1**	**0.3**
Back, Dry Fried Or Grilled, Average	*1 Rasher/25g*	**76.0**	**5.0**	**304**	**26.5**	**0.1**	**21.9**	**0.0**
Back, Lean, Average	*1 Rasher/33g*	**57.0**	**4.0**	**173**	**16.3**	**0.1**	**12.0**	**0.5**
Back, Smoked, Average	*1 Rasher/25g*	**66.0**	**5.0**	**265**	**20.9**	**0.0**	**19.9**	**0.0**
Back, Smoked, Lean, Average	*1 Rasher/25g*	**41.0**	**1.0**	**163**	**28.2**	**1.1**	**5.0**	**0.2**
Back, Smoked, Rindless, Average	*1 Rasher/25g*	**60.0**	**4.0**	**241**	**21.0**	**0.1**	**17.4**	**0.0**
Back, Tendersweet, Average	*1 Rasher/25g*	**63.0**	**4.0**	**250**	**29.8**	**0.4**	**14.3**	**0.0**
Back, Unsmoked, Average	*1 Rasher/32g*	**78.0**	**6.0**	**243**	**21.3**	**0.4**	**17.3**	**0.0**
Back, Unsmoked, Rindless, Average	*1 Rasher/23g*	**56.0**	**4.0**	**241**	**22.5**	**0.0**	**16.9**	**0.0**
Chops, Average	*1oz/28g*	**62.0**	**4.0**	**222**	**22.3**	**0.0**	**14.8**	**0.0**
Collar Joint, Lean & Fat, Boiled	*1oz/28g*	**91.0**	**8.0**	**325**	**20.4**	**0.0**	**27.0**	**0.0**
Collar Joint, Lean & Fat, Raw	*1oz/28g*	**89.0**	**8.0**	**319**	**14.6**	**0.0**	**28.9**	**0.0**
Collar Joint, Lean Only, Boiled	*1oz/28g*	**53.0**	**3.0**	**191**	**26.0**	**0.0**	**9.7**	**0.0**
Fat Only, Cooked, Average	*1oz/28g*	**194.0**	**20.0**	**692**	**9.3**	**0.0**	**72.8**	**0.0**
Fat Only, Raw, Average	*1oz/28g*	**209.0**	**23.0**	**747**	**4.8**	**0.0**	**80.9**	**0.0**
Gammon Rasher, Lean Only, Grilled	*1oz/28g*	**48.0**	**1.0**	**172**	**31.4**	**0.0**	**5.2**	**0.0**
Lardons, Smoked, Sainsbury's*	1 Serving/200g	476.0	31.0	238	21.4	0.1	15.4	0.1
Lean Only, Fried, Average	*1 Rasher/25g*	**83.0**	**6.0**	**332**	**32.8**	**0.0**	**22.3**	**0.0**
Lean Only, Grilled, Average	*1 Rasher/25g*	**73.0**	**5.0**	**292**	**30.5**	**0.0**	**18.9**	**0.0**
Lean, Average	*1oz/28g*	**40.0**	**2.0**	**142**	**19.6**	**0.9**	**6.7**	**0.2**
Loin Steaks, Grilled, Average	*1 Serving/120g*	**229.0**	**12.0**	**191**	**25.9**	**0.0**	**9.7**	**0.0**
Medallions, Average	*1 Rasher/18g*	**27.0**	**1.0**	**151**	**29.3**	**0.9**	**3.3**	**0.1**
Middle, Fried	*1 Rasher/40g*	**140.0**	**11.0**	**350**	**23.4**	**0.0**	**28.5**	**0.0**
Middle, Grilled	*1 Rasher/40g*	**123.0**	**9.0**	**307**	**24.8**	**0.0**	**23.1**	**0.0**
Middle, Raw	*1 Rasher/43g*	**104.0**	**9.0**	**241**	**15.2**	**0.0**	**20.0**	**0.0**
Rindless, Average	*1 Rasher/20g*	**30.0**	**2.0**	**150**	**18.5**	**0.0**	**8.5**	**0.0**
Smoked, Average	*1 Rasher/28g*	**46.0**	**2.0**	**166**	**24.7**	**0.2**	**7.3**	**0.0**
Smoked, Crispy, Cooked, Average	*1 Serving/10g*	**46.0**	**3.0**	**460**	**53.0**	**2.1**	**26.9**	**0.0**
Smoked, Rindless, Average	*1 Rasher/20g*	**21.0**	**1.0**	**106**	**19.8**	**0.0**	**3.0**	**0.0**
Streaky, Average	*1oz/28g*	**76.0**	**6.0**	**270**	**20.0**	**0.0**	**21.0**	**0.0**
Streaky, Cooked, Average	*1 Rasher/20g*	**68.0**	**6.0**	**342**	**22.4**	**0.3**	**27.8**	**0.0**
BACON VEGETARIAN								
Rashers, Cheatin', The Redwood Co*	1 Rasher/16g	32.0	1.0	196	25.9	7.3	7.3	0.5
Rashers, Tesco*	1 Rasher/20g	41.0	2.0	203	22.5	3.3	11.1	3.9
Realeat*	1 Rasher/19g	49.0	1.0	260	27.0	25.0	5.8	1.6
Streaky Style Rashers, Tesco*	1 Rasher/8g	17.0	1.0	215	23.7	5.0	10.6	2.2
Strips, Morningstar Farms*	1 Strip/8g	30.0	2.0	375	12.5	12.5	28.1	6.2
BAGEL								
Bacon, & Soft Cheese, Boots*	1 Serving/148g	481.0	25.0	325	12.0	31.0	17.0	2.2
Cream Cheese, & Salmon, Smoked, M & S*	1 Bagel/23g	64.0	3.0	280	10.9	31.7	12.2	2.9
Cream Cheese, M & S*	1 Bagel/23g	79.0	5.0	352	7.8	31.0	21.8	1.8
Ham, & Pesto, COU, M & S*	1 Pack/173g	259.0	2.0	150	11.1	23.5	1.4	1.7

	Measure INFO/WEIGHT	per Measure KCAL	per Measure FAT	Nutrition Values per 100g / 100ml KCAL	PROT	CARB	FAT	FIBRE
BAGEL								
Smoked Salmon, & Cream Cheese, Handmade, Tesco*	1 Bagel/162g	380.0	13.0	235	13.1	27.7	7.8	1.5
Smoked Salmon, & Cream Cheese, M & S*	1 Bagel/19g	43.0	1.0	230	14.0	26.7	7.1	1.8
Soft Cheese, & Salmon, Smoked, American, Sainsbury's*	1 Bagel/131g	356.0	16.0	272	8.3	31.8	12.4	1.7
Soft Cheese, & Salmon, Smoked, Finest, Tesco*	1 Pack/173g	396.0	10.0	229	13.1	31.2	5.8	1.7
Tuna, & Salad, BGTY, Sainsbury's*	1 Bagel/170g	325.0	7.0	191	10.4	26.0	4.2	1.0
Turkey, & Cranberry, Bagelmania*	1 Pack/198g	325.0	7.0	164	9.0	24.5	3.7	1.1
Turkey, Pastrami & American Mustard, Shapers, Boots*	1 Bagel/146g	296.0	5.0	203	11.0	32.0	3.4	1.4
BAGUETTE								
All Day Breakfast, Darwins Deli*	1 Serving/184g	498.0	22.0	271	13.4	31.9	11.7	0.0
Cheese, & Ham, Snack 'n' Go, Sainsbury's*	1 Baguette/178g	383.0	9.0	215	12.6	29.6	5.1	1.9
Cheese, & Tomato, Tesco*	1 Baguette/108g	243.0	8.0	225	9.7	29.3	7.7	1.8
Cheese, Mixed, & Spring Onion, Asda*	1 Pack/190g	629.0	35.0	331	9.5	32.1	18.3	1.3
Cheese, Tomato, & Basil, Asda*	¼ Baguette/42g	138.0	6.0	329	10.0	40.8	14.0	1.3
Chicken, & Mayonnaise, Asda*	1 Pack/190g	407.0	17.0	214	9.7	30.5	8.7	1.3
Chicken, & Salad, Asda*	1 Serving/158g	326.0	9.0	206	9.0	29.0	6.0	2.1
Chicken, & Salad, Shapers, Boots*	1 Baguette/132g	222.0	3.0	168	11.0	27.0	2.0	1.5
Chicken, & Spicy Tomato, Snack, Sainsbury's*	1 Baguette/160g	344.0	6.0	215	14.1	31.2	3.7	2.2
Chicken, & Stuffing, Hot, Sainsbury's*	1 Baguette/227g	543.0	16.0	239	13.7	29.6	7.2	0.0
Chicken, Honey & Mustard, BGTY, Sainsbury's*	1 Pack/187g	340.0	4.0	182	11.0	30.0	2.0	0.0
Chicken, Tikka, Asda*	1 Pack/190g	439.0	18.0	231	10.4	32.8	9.4	1.3
Chicken, Tikka, Hot, Sainsbury's*	1 Pack/190g	386.0	12.0	203	8.5	28.4	6.1	0.0
Egg Mayonnaise, & Cress, Cafe, Sainsbury's*	1 Pack/100g	480.0	20.0	480	13.8	60.2	20.4	0.0
Ham, & Salad, with Mustard Mayonnaise, Sainsbury's*	1 Baguette/100g	412.0	16.0	412	17.6	49.6	15.9	0.1
Ham, & Turkey, Asda*	1 Baguette/360g	774.0	18.0	215	11.6	30.7	5.1	1.3
Prawn Mayonnaise, Asda*	1 Pack/190g	399.0	9.0	210	9.1	32.5	4.9	1.3
Prawn, French, Shell*	1 Baguette/63g	171.0	7.0	272	9.7	32.4	11.5	0.0
Steak, & Onion, Snack 'n' Go, Sainsbury's*	1 Baguette/177g	398.0	9.0	225	14.3	30.6	5.0	2.2
Tuna, Crunch, Shapers, Boots*	1 Pack/138g	315.0	5.0	228	14.0	35.0	3.5	3.1
Tuna, Melt, Sainsbury's*	1 Serving/204g	373.0	8.0	183	11.3	25.8	3.9	0.0
BAILEYS*								
Glide, Baileys*	1 Serving/200ml	212.0	2.0	106	0.0	18.0	1.2	0.0
*Irish Cream, Original, Baileys**	*1 Glass/37ml*	*121.0*	*5.0*	*327*	*3.0*	*25.0*	*13.0*	*0.0*
BAKE								
Aubergine & Mozzarella Cheese, BGTY, Sainsbury's*	1 Pack/360g	194.0	7.0	54	3.0	6.0	2.0	1.3
Aubergine & Mozzarella, Finest, Tesco*	1 Pack/400g	288.0	14.0	72	3.6	6.7	3.4	2.6
Aubergine & Spinach, BGTY, Sainsbury's*	1 Pack/360g	148.0	6.0	41	2.2	4.0	1.8	1.3
Bean & Pasta, Asda*	1 Pack/450g	598.0	22.0	133	5.0	17.0	5.0	1.7
Broccoli & Cheese, M & S*	1 Pack/400g	380.0	23.0	95	4.8	5.6	5.7	1.1
Cauliflower & Broccoli Bake, Tesco*	½ Pack/250g	177.0	10.0	71	2.8	5.8	4.1	1.0
Cheese & Spinach, Tesco*	1 Bake/140g	269.0	11.0	192	4.5	26.0	7.8	1.4
Cheesy Broccoli, Asda*	1 Pack/400g	400.0	18.0	100	4.5	10.6	4.4	1.4
Chicken & Mushroom, COU, M & S*	1 Serving/360g	324.0	8.0	90	7.3	10.3	2.3	1.1
Chicken & Pasta, BGTY, Sainsbury's*	1 Pack/400g	394.0	10.0	98	9.0	10.0	2.5	2.5
Chicken Spiralli, M & S*	1 Serving/400g	400.0	15.0	100	7.9	9.1	3.8	1.1
Chicken, Bacon & Potato, British Classics, Tesco*	½ Pack/375g	435.0	17.0	116	7.0	12.2	4.4	1.4
Chicken, Tomato & Mozzarella, Birds Eye*	1 Pack/285g	370.0	5.0	130	7.1	14.3	1.9	0.3
Chicken, Tomato, & Mascarpone, HL, Tesco*	1 Serving/400g	468.0	11.0	117	7.6	15.5	2.7	0.8
Cod & Prawn, COU, M & S*	1 Pack/400g	320.0	8.0	80	6.5	8.8	2.0	1.0
Creamy Peppercorn, Vegetarian, Tesco*	1 Serving/140g	322.0	17.0	230	3.6	27.0	12.0	1.2
Fish & Vegetable, Youngs*	1 Serving/375g	446.0	24.0	119	5.6	10.0	6.3	1.3
Fish Dinner, Light & Easy, Youngs*	1 Pack/385g	370.0	13.0	96	6.4	9.7	3.5	1.6
Fish, Broccoli & Sweetcorn, Light & Easy, Youngs*	1 Pack/240g	187.0	6.0	78	8.6	5.7	2.3	0.6
Fish, Haddock, Smoked, Light & Easy, Youngs*	1 Pack/310g	242.0	7.0	78	6.4	8.0	2.3	0.9

	Measure INFO/WEIGHT	per Measure KCAL	per Measure FAT	Nutrition Values per 100g / 100ml KCAL	PROT	CARB	FAT	FIBRE
BAKE								
Fish, with Carrots & Peas, Light & Easy, Youngs*	1 Pack/240g	168.0	4.0	70	8.3	5.4	1.7	1.4
Haddock, Smoked, Light & Easy, Youngs*	1 Pack/300g	234.0	7.0	78	6.4	8.0	2.3	0.9
Haddock, Smoked, Luxury, Light & Easy, Youngs*	1 Pack/355g	390.0	17.0	110	7.5	9.2	4.8	0.6
Minced Beef & Root Vegetable, COU, M & S*	1 Pack/400g	320.0	12.0	80	6.6	6.0	2.9	3.0
Mushroom, Leek & Cheddar, Asda*	1 Pack/400g	348.0	18.0	87	3.7	8.1	4.4	1.9
Mushroom, Leek & Spinach, Cumberland, Sainsbury's*	1 Pack/450g	518.0	24.0	115	3.6	12.9	5.4	1.2
Penne Bolognese, BGTY, Sainsbury's*	1 Pack/400g	492.0	11.0	123	7.0	17.7	2.7	1.3
Penne Bolognese, Sainsbury's*	1 Pack/397g	603.0	28.0	152	7.6	14.8	7.0	2.0
Potato, Cheese, & Onion, Tesco*	1 Pack/400g	376.0	20.0	94	2.4	10.0	4.9	1.0
Potato, Mushroom & Leek, M & S*	1 Serving/225g	225.0	13.0	100	3.5	10.0	5.9	2.0
Potato, Tomato & Mozzarella, M & S*	1 Bake/450g	585.0	34.0	130	5.2	9.8	7.6	1.8
Potato, with Cheese & Leek, Aunt Bessie's*	½ Pack/275g	300.0	14.0	109	3.4	12.7	5.0	2.7
Roast Onion & Potato, COU, M & S*	1 Pack/450g	337.0	6.0	75	1.9	13.6	1.3	1.5
Roast Potato, Cheese & Onion, Asda*	½ Pack/200g	288.0	16.0	144	4.2	14.0	8.0	1.1
Salmon & Broccoli, Youngs*	1 Bake/375g	409.0	19.0	109	6.3	9.6	5.1	1.3
Salmon & Prawn, M & S*	1 Bake/329g	460.0	31.0	140	7.4	6.6	9.5	0.7
Smoked Haddock & Prawn, BGTY, Sainsbury's*	1 Pack/350g	318.0	2.0	91	7.5	13.6	0.7	1.1
Spicy Bean & Potato, Safeway*	1 Pack/386g	405.0	12.0	105	3.9	14.2	3.2	2.1
Spicy Chickpea & Apricot, Safeway*	1 Pack/400g	340.0	11.0	85	2.2	12.5	2.9	3.1
Vegetable & Lentil, Somerfield*	1 Pack/350g	318.0	6.0	91	4.9	13.8	1.8	2.5
Vegetable, M & S*	1 Pack/300g	210.0	8.0	70	1.9	8.9	2.7	1.6
Vegetable, Multigrain, Grassington's Food Co*	1 Bake/106g	148.0	4.0	140	4.9	22.4	3.4	5.0
BAKING POWDER								
Average	*1 Tsp/2g*	*3.0*	*0.0*	*163*	*5.2*	*37.8*	*0.0*	*0.0*
BAKLAVA								
Average	1 Serving/100g	393.0	21.0	393	5.0	46.0	21.0	0.0
BALTI								
Chicken & Mushroom, Tesco*	1 Serving/350g	325.0	10.0	93	12.3	4.2	3.0	0.7
Chicken Ceylon, Finest, Tesco*	1 Pack/400g	588.0	38.0	147	14.4	0.9	9.5	5.0
Chicken Tikka, & Wedges, HL, Tesco*	1 Pack/450g	391.0	10.0	87	6.0	10.7	2.2	1.3
Chicken Tikka, Finest, Tesco*	½ Pack/200g	280.0	17.0	140	15.8	1.1	8.6	3.2
Chicken, & Rice, M & S*	1 Pack/400g	380.0	6.0	95	6.9	14.1	1.5	1.2
Chicken, Asda*	1 Pack/450g	324.0	10.0	72	8.0	5.0	2.2	0.0
Chicken, Indian Takeaway, Iceland*	1 Pack/402g	362.0	19.0	90	7.8	4.0	4.8	0.7
Chicken, M & S*	½ Pack/175g	245.0	15.0	140	13.0	2.0	8.7	1.7
Chicken, Ready Meals, M & S*	1oz/28g	34.0	2.0	120	10.2	4.7	6.5	1.6
Chicken, Sainsbury's*	½ Pack/200g	222.0	11.0	111	11.6	3.6	5.6	1.3
Chicken, Takeaway, Sainsbury's*	1 Pack/400g	404.0	18.0	101	10.4	4.8	4.5	1.4
Chicken, Tesco*	1 Pack/460g	662.0	26.0	144	6.1	17.4	5.6	1.6
Chicken, with Garlic & Coriander Naan, Frozen, Patak's*	1 Pack/375g	431.0	19.0	115	6.3	11.1	5.0	1.1
Chicken, with Naan Bread, Perfectly Balanced, Waitrose*	1 Pack/375g	450.0	13.0	120	12.1	9.7	3.6	2.8
Chicken, with Naan Bread, Sharwood's*	1 Pack/375g	529.0	23.0	141	7.3	14.1	6.2	2.2
Chicken, with Pilau Rice, Asda*	1 Pack/504g	625.0	25.0	124	5.0	15.0	4.9	1.2
Chicken, with Pilau Rice, Light Choices, Tesco*	1 Pack/400g	440.0	5.0	110	6.3	17.4	1.3	1.8
Chicken, with Pilau Rice, Weight Watchers*	1 Pack/329g	306.0	4.0	93	6.9	13.4	1.3	1.2
Chicken, with Potato Wedges, HL, Tesco*	1 Pack/450g	387.0	9.0	86	6.0	10.8	2.1	1.1
Chicken, with Rice, Curry Break, Patak's*	1 Pack/220g	198.0	6.0	90	4.7	11.6	2.8	0.0
Chicken, with Rice, Patak's*	1 Pack/370g	440.0	13.0	119	6.1	16.7	3.5	1.7
Prawn, Budgens*	1 Pack/350g	374.0	25.0	107	5.6	5.2	7.1	1.3
Vegetable & Rice, Tesco*	1 Pack/450g	378.0	7.0	84	2.0	15.6	1.6	1.3
Vegetable, Asda*	½ Can/200g	206.0	12.0	103	2.2	10.0	6.0	2.5
Vegetable, GFY, Asda*	1 Pack/450g	324.0	4.0	72	1.9	14.0	0.9	1.5
Vegetable, Indian Meal for 2, Finest, Tesco*	½ Pack/150g	144.0	11.0	96	1.6	6.1	7.2	2.9

	Measure INFO/WEIGHT	per Measure KCAL	FAT	Nutrition Values per 100g / 100ml KCAL	PROT	CARB	FAT	FIBRE
BAMBOO SHOOTS								
Canned, Average	*1 Sm Can/120g*	*11.0*	*0.0*	*9*	*1.1*	*0.9*	*0.1*	*0.9*
BANANA								
Raw, Flesh Only, Average	*1 Sm/95g*	*90.0*	*0.0*	*95*	*1.2*	*20.9*	*0.3*	*4.2*
Raw, Weighed with Skin, Average	*1 Lge/185g*	*176.0*	*1.0*	*95*	*1.2*	*20.9*	*0.3*	*4.2*
BANANA CHIPS								
Average	*1oz/28g*	*143.0*	*9.0*	*511*	*1.0*	*59.9*	*31.4*	*1.7*
BANGERS & MASH								
& Beans, Blue Parrot Cafe, Sainsbury's*	1 Pack/300g	354.0	13.0	118	5.3	14.8	4.2	2.1
Asda*	1 Pack/400g	636.0	28.0	159	9.0	15.0	7.0	1.6
Bitesize, Birds Eye*	1 Pack/316.7g	285.0	9.0	90	2.7	13.3	2.9	1.5
Loved By Kids, M & S*	1 Pack/225g	191.0	7.0	85	5.4	8.1	3.3	1.2
Meal for One, M & S*	1 Pack/431g	560.0	34.0	130	4.7	9.5	7.9	1.1
Morrisons*	1 Pack/300g	306.0	15.0	102	3.0	12.3	4.9	0.8
Sausage, & Cabbage Mash, Eat Smart, Safeway*	1 Pack/400g	340.0	10.0	85	6.4	9.0	2.5	1.3
BARS								
All Bran, Apple, Kellogg's*	1 Bar/40g	158.0	8.0	395	8.0	48.0	19.0	5.0
All Bran, Honey & Oat, Kellogg's*	1 Bar/27g	99.0	2.0	366	6.0	67.0	8.0	12.0
All Fruit, Frusli, Passion Fruit, Jordans*	1 Bar/30g	92.0	0.0	307	1.3	74.0	0.7	5.0
All Fruit, Frusli, Strawberry, Jordans*	1 Bar/30g	94.0	0.0	313	2.3	81.3	0.3	5.0
Almond & Apricot, Weight Watchers*	1 Bar/34g	151.0	7.0	443	8.6	55.9	19.4	5.2
Almond, Apricot, & Mango, M & S*	1 Bar/50g	205.0	7.0	410	9.0	60.2	14.8	5.0
Am, Breakfast Muffin, Apple & Sultana, McVitie's*	1 Bar/45g	168.0	8.0	373	4.4	54.9	16.7	1.6
Am, Cereal, Apple, McVitie's*	1 Bar/40g	160.0	5.0	400	4.3	65.4	13.5	3.1
Am, Cereal, Apricot, McVitie's*	1 Bar/30g	146.0	6.0	486	6.5	68.8	20.5	0.5
Am, Cereal, Berry, McVitie's*	1 Bar/30g	146.0	6.0	486	6.5	68.8	20.5	0.5
Am, Cereal, Fruit & Nut, McVitie's*	1 Bar/35g	167.0	8.0	477	6.6	64.9	21.4	3.4
Am, Cereal, Grapefruit, McVitie's*	1 Bar/35g	136.0	3.0	389	5.1	70.9	9.4	3.1
Am, Cereal, Orange Marmalade, McVitie's*	1 Bar/40g	151.0	7.0	377	4.5	53.2	18.0	1.7
Am, Cereal, Raisin & Nut, McVitie's*	1 Bar/35g	148.0	6.0	422	6.4	62.1	16.4	2.4
Am, Cereal, Strawberry, McVitie's*	1 Bar/35g	138.0	4.0	395	5.7	70.5	10.1	2.7
Am, Granola, Almond, Raisin & Cranberry, McVitie's*	1 Bar/35g	133.0	4.0	380	7.1	62.9	11.4	4.0
Am, Muesli Fingers, McVitie's*	1 Bar/35g	154.0	7.0	440	6.0	59.8	19.6	3.1
Apple & Blackberry, Fruit Bake, McVitie's*	1 Bar/35g	124.0	3.0	354	2.7	73.8	7.2	1.2
Apple Pie, Nak'd*	1 Bar/68g	221.0	6.0	325	6.8	57.2	8.7	7.3
Apple, Fruit Bake, Go Ahead, McVitie's*	1 Bar/35g	124.0	3.0	354	2.7	73.8	7.2	1.2
Apple, Granola, McVitie's*	1 Bar/35g	128.0	3.0	366	6.6	63.1	9.7	4.3
Apricot & Almond, Yoghurt Coated, Eat Natural*	1 Bar/50g	228.0	12.0	456	5.7	52.8	24.7	5.7
Banana Break, Breakfast in a Bar, Jordans*	1 Bar/40g	152.0	4.0	381	5.7	69.1	9.1	5.0
Banana, Apricot, & Milk Chocolate, Lunchies, Eat Natural*	1 Bar/30g	108.0	2.0	362	3.7	71.8	6.7	4.0
Banoffee, Weight Watchers*	1 Bar/18g	68.0	1.0	379	6.3	77.0	5.1	3.0
Biscuit, Chocolate Mint, Penguin, McVitie's*	1 Bar/25g	133.0	7.0	531	5.4	65.0	27.7	1.5
Biscuit, Chocolate Orange, Penguin, McVitie's*	1 Bar/25g	133.0	7.0	531	5.4	65.0	27.7	1.5
Biscuit, Chocolate, Penguin, McVitie's*	1 Bar/25g	130.0	7.0	520	5.2	62.4	27.7	2.4
Blue Riband, 99 Calories, Nestle*	1 Bar/19g	99.0	5.0	513	4.8	66.4	25.3	0.0
Blue Riband, Double Choc, Nestle*	1 Bar/22g	113.0	6.0	513	4.8	66.4	25.3	1.1
Blue Riband, Nestle*	1 Bar/21g	104.0	5.0	495	4.5	64.5	24.5	1.0
Blueberry, Weight Watchers*	1 Bar/25g	91.0	2.0	365	4.5	74.9	7.4	2.2
Breakfast, Cherry, Oats & More, Nestle*	1 Bar/30g	109.0	2.0	363	6.0	70.2	6.5	3.6
Brunch, Cranberry & Orange, Cadbury*	1 Bar/35g	154.0	6.0	440	5.9	67.7	15.9	0.0
Brunch, Hazelnut, Cadbury*	1 Bar/35g	160.0	7.0	460	7.0	60.5	21.4	2.2
Brunch, Snack, Raisin, Cadbury*	1 Bar/35g	150.0	5.0	430	5.6	66.4	15.5	1.8
Caramel Crisp, Go Ahead, McVitie's*	1 Bar/33g	141.0	4.0	428	4.8	75.1	12.0	0.8
Caramel Crunch, Go Ahead, McVitie's*	1 Bar/24g	106.0	3.0	440	4.7	76.6	13.8	0.8

B

BARS

Measure INFO/WEIGHT	per Measure KCAL	FAT	Nutrition Values per 100g / 100ml KCAL	PROT	CARB	FAT	FIBRE

	Measure INFO/WEIGHT	per Measure KCAL	FAT	KCAL	PROT	CARB	FAT	FIBRE
Caramel Wafer, Weight Watchers*	1 Bar/18g	79.0	4.0	427	5.7	64.7	20.2	1.9
Cashew Cookie, Gluten Free, Nak'd*	1 Bar/35g	143.0	8.0	410	10.0	46.0	23.0	0.0
Cereal & Milk, Nesquik, Nestle*	1 Bar/25g	108.0	4.0	433	6.2	68.5	14.9	1.0
Cereal, 3 Berries & Cherries, Dorset Cereals*	1 Bar/35g	127.0	2.0	363	5.7	73.9	4.9	5.2
Cereal, 3 Fruit, Nuts & Seeds, Dorset Cereals*	1 Bar/35g	136.0	4.0	389	7.4	66.6	10.3	6.2
Cereal, Apple & Blackberry, with Yoghurt, Alpen*	1 Bar/29g	117.0	3.0	404	5.4	71.8	10.6	5.0
Cereal, Apple & Raisin, Harvest, Quaker Oats*	1 Bar/22g	87.0	3.0	396	5.0	70.0	11.5	4.0
Cereal, Blueberry Flavour, Breakfast, Sweet Mornings*	1 Bar/38g	152.0	5.0	399	4.5	66.0	13.0	2.5
Cereal, Cheerios & Milk Bar, Nestle*	1 Bar/22g	92.0	3.0	416	7.6	66.1	13.5	2.0
Cereal, Chewy Apple, Fruitus, Lyme Regis Foods*	1 Bar/35g	132.0	4.0	378	5.4	64.8	10.8	5.4
Cereal, Choc Chip & Nut, Chewy & Crisp, Sainsbury's*	1 Bar/27g	129.0	7.0	476	8.8	51.8	26.0	4.4
Cereal, Chocolate & Orange, Fitnesse, Nestle*	1 Bar/24g	87.0	1.0	370	4.7	76.2	5.1	3.8
Cereal, Chocolate & Pear, Fitnesse, Nestle*	1 Bar/24g	88.0	1.0	374	4.7	76.3	5.5	3.2
Cereal, Chocolate & Raisin, Geobar, Traidcraft*	1 Bar/35g	138.0	2.0	394	4.6	81.7	5.5	1.9
Cereal, Chocolate Chip, Special K, Kellogg's*	1 Bar/21g	84.0	1.0	401	9.0	76.0	7.0	1.5
Cereal, Chocolate, Geobar, Traidcraft*	1 Bar/35g	146.0	3.0	417	3.9	79.5	9.3	0.0
Cereal, Cinnamon Grahams, Nestle*	1 Bar/25g	106.0	4.0	426	7.2	66.2	14.7	1.9
Cereal, Coconut, Original Crunchy, Jordans*	1 Bar/30g	141.0	7.0	470	6.5	60.0	22.7	6.2
Cereal, Cranberry & Orange, Weight Watchers*	1 Bar/28g	102.0	1.0	365	4.5	77.6	4.1	2.3
Cereal, Crunchy Granola, Apple Crunch, Nature Valley*	1 Bar/21g	92.0	3.0	440	7.3	69.0	15.0	5.7
Cereal, Fruit & Nut Break, Jordans*	1 Bar/37g	138.0	4.0	374	7.0	63.2	10.4	8.1
Cereal, Fruit & Nut with Milk Chocolate, Alpen*	1 Bar/29g	124.0	4.0	427	7.1	67.8	14.1	4.0
Cereal, Fruit & Nut, Alpen*	1 Bar/28g	110.0	3.0	394	6.6	69.6	9.9	5.0
Cereal, Fruit & Nut, Chewy Trail Mix, Nature Valley*	1 Bar/30g	114.0	3.0	379	7.7	63.2	10.6	7.3
Cereal, Frusli, Absolutely Apricot, Jordans*	1 Bar/33g	120.0	3.0	365	5.0	63.8	10.0	6.3
Cereal, Frusli, Blueberry Burst, Jordans*	1 Bar/30g	118.0	3.0	392	5.8	70.1	9.8	5.1
Cereal, Frusli, Cranberry & Apple, Jordans*	1 Bar/30g	118.0	3.0	393	5.7	70.0	10.0	5.3
Cereal, Frusli, Raisin & Hazelnut, Jordans*	1 Bar/30g	117.0	4.0	390	5.8	64.3	12.2	4.5
Cereal, Frusli, Red Berries, Jordans*	1 Bar/30g	113.0	2.0	378	5.1	71.7	7.9	4.5
Cereal, Frusli, Tangy Citrus, Jordans*	1 Bar/33g	124.0	3.0	376	4.4	67.7	9.8	4.8
Cereal, Frusli, Wild Berries, Jordans*	1 Bar/30g	118.0	3.0	392	5.7	70.0	9.8	5.0
Cereal, Golden Grahams, Nestle*	1 Bar/25g	106.0	3.0	425	6.5	68.8	13.7	0.0
Cereal, Hazelnut & Pistachio, Go Ahead, McVitie's*	1 Bar/30g	117.0	3.0	389	4.8	66.5	11.5	2.5
Cereal, Hazelnut & Sultana, Organic, Seeds of Change*	1 Bar/29g	116.0	4.0	399	5.9	65.5	12.6	5.1
Cereal, Marmite*	1 Bar/25g	93.0	2.0	372	18.5	56.2	8.1	6.0
Cereal, Milk Chocolate, Weetos, Weetabix*	1 Bar/20g	88.0	3.0	440	5.9	70.9	14.7	1.6
Cereal, Mint Chocolate, Kellogg's*	1 Bar/22g	88.0	2.0	401	4.5	74.0	10.0	3.5
Cereal, Mixed Berry, Go Ahead, McVitie's*	1 Bar/35g	134.0	2.0	383	4.6	77.1	6.3	3.1
Cereal, Muesli Break, Breakfast in a Bar, Jordans*	1 Bar/46g	178.0	5.0	387	5.9	66.6	10.8	4.3
Cereal, Muncho Chocolate & Coconut, Orco*	1 Bar/21g	93.0	3.0	441	5.0	71.4	15.0	0.0
Cereal, Oat & Raisin, Soft Oaties, Nutri-Grain, Kellogg's*	1 Bar/40g	173.0	6.0	432	6.0	66.0	16.0	3.5
Cereal, Oats & More, Chocolate, Nestle*	1 Bar/30g	118.0	3.0	395	6.8	68.3	10.5	3.4
Cereal, Protein Flapjack, Cherry Crunch, Trek*	1 Bar 56g	241.0	11.0	430	18.2	47.0	19.8	3.0
Cereal, Raisin & Apricot, Weight Watchers*	1 Bar/28g	100.0	1.0	358	6.8	72.2	4.6	3.2
Cereal, Raisin & Nut Snack Bar, Benecol*	1 Bar/25g	97.0	3.0	390	3.9	68.5	11.1	2.0
Cereal, Redberry & Chocolate, Sveltesse, Nestle*	1 Bar/25g	97.0	2.0	389	5.4	69.2	9.9	6.8
Cereal, Roast Hazelnut, Organic, Jordans*	1 Bar/33g	150.0	7.0	455	8.0	56.7	21.8	7.8
Cereal, Strawberry with Yoghurt, Alpen*	1 Bar/29g	119.0	3.0	409	5.7	72.6	10.6	0.0
Cereal, Strawberry, Fitness, Nestle*	1 Bar/24g	89.0	2.0	378	4.9	73.8	7.0	4.1
Cereal, Sultana & Honey, Jordans*	1 Bar/36g	130.0	3.0	361	6.0	65.9	8.2	9.2
Cereal, Super High Fibre, Dorset Cereals*	1 Bar/35g	149.0	6.0	425	9.6	60.8	16.0	7.1
Cereal, Tropical Fruit & Nut, Organic, Dove's Farm*	1 Bar/40g	196.0	5.0	490	6.5	63.3	11.5	5.3
Cherries, & Almonds, & a Yoghurt Coating, Eat Natural*	1 Bar/45g	200.0	10.0	444	6.6	58.8	21.1	3.6

BARS

INFO/WEIGHT	per Measure KCAL	per Measure FAT	KCAL	PROT	CARB	FAT	FIBRE

| | Measure INFO/WEIGHT | per Measure KCAL FAT | Nutrition Values per 100g / 100ml KCAL PROT CARB FAT FIBRE |

Item	INFO/WEIGHT	KCAL	FAT	KCAL	PROT	CARB	FAT	FIBRE
Cherry & Coconut Low Fat Fingers, Ok*	1 Bar/35g	119.0	1.0	339	4.1	75.0	2.5	2.0
Chocolate & Caramel, Lo Carb, Boots*	1 Bar/28g	101.0	3.0	359	2.8	82.0	11.0	1.8
Chocolate & Orange, Crispy, Free From, Sainsbury's*	1 Bar/30g	132.0	5.0	440	4.8	68.2	16.2	1.2
Chocolate & Orange, Crispy, Shapers, Boots*	1 Bar/22g	93.0	3.0	425	3.6	77.0	12.0	0.8
Chocolate & Orange, Shapers, Boots*	1 Bar/26g	98.0	3.0	378	4.2	73.0	13.0	1.5
Chocolate & Raspberry, COU, M & S*	1 Bar/25g	90.0	1.0	360	5.4	78.2	2.7	3.2
Chocolate & Toffee, Free From, Sainsbury's*	1 Bar/30g	139.0	5.0	465	4.8	71.0	18.0	0.8
Chocolate Banana, Recovery, Mule Refuel*	1 Bar/65g	253.0	6.0	390	21.0	56.0	9.0	2.0
Chocolate Brownie, Big Softies, to Go, Fox's*	1 Bar/25g	87.0	1.0	348	5.5	74.9	2.9	0.0
Chocolate Caramel Whip, Weight Watchers*	1 Bar/25g	88.0	3.0	353	2.7	72.4	10.8	1.0
Chocolate Caramel, Weight Watchers*	1 Bar/20g	80.0	2.0	400	5.0	70.0	12.5	0.0
Chocolate Creme, Endulge, Atkins*	1 Bar/14g	70.0	5.0	504	12.5	38.6	34.3	2.5
Chocolate Crisp, Weight Watchers*	1 Bar/25g	94.0	3.0	378	4.8	66.8	10.2	1.6
Chocolate Date, Recovery, Mule Refuel*	1 Bar/65g	261.0	6.0	401	20.0	58.0	10.0	2.0
Chocolate Decadence, Atkins*	1 Bar/60g	227.0	12.0	378	27.1	30.7	20.4	11.6
Chocolate Flavour Almond, Carbolite*	1 Bar/28g	124.0	10.0	438	8.7	52.0	36.0	3.8
Chocolate Truffle, M & S*	1 Bar/35g	168.0	11.0	480	5.9	41.7	32.5	8.3
Chocolate, Crisp, Weight Watchers*	1 Bar/25g	92.0	3.0	369	5.4	75.1	10.2	0.8
Chocolate, Double Cream, Nestle*	1 Bar/47g	250.0	15.0	531	8.5	54.8	30.9	0.0
Chocolate, Double, Dark, Zone Perfect*	1 Bar/45g	190.0	6.0	422	24.5	44.9	12.2	2.0
Chocolate, Fruit & Nut, M & S*	1 Bar/50g	235.0	12.0	470	6.5	57.1	24.1	2.5
Chocolate, Polar, Sainsbury's*	1 Bar/25g	133.0	7.0	533	5.5	63.0	28.6	1.2
Chocolate, Soya, Dairy Free, Free From, Sainsbury's*	1 Bar/50g	274.0	17.0	548	10.8	47.5	35.0	4.3
Chocolate, Toffee Pecan, M & S*	1 Bar/36g	179.0	10.0	498	4.9	58.3	27.3	0.7
Chocolate, Wild & Whippy, Tesco*	1 Bar/18g	78.0	3.0	447	3.7	72.0	16.0	0.8
Coco Pops, & Milk, Kellogg's*	1 Bar/20g	85.0	3.0	423	7.0	70.0	13.0	1.0
Cocoa Loco, Nak'd*	1 Bar/30g	100.0	3.0	332	8.0	55.0	10.0	7.0
Cocoa Mole, Larabar*	1 Bar/51g	190.0	9.0	373	7.8	56.9	17.6	9.8
Cocoa Orange, Gluten Free, Nak'd*	1 Bar/35g	131.0	7.0	373	9.0	48.0	20.0	0.0
Coconut Chocolate Crisp, Weight Watchers*	1 Bar/25g	89.0	3.0	356	3.6	71.2	10.4	3.2
Coconut Cream Pie, Larabar*	1 Bar/48g	200.0	10.0	417	6.2	56.2	20.8	10.4
Coconut Whip, Weight Watchers*	1 Bar/20g	81.0	3.0	404	2.4	70.6	14.1	1.5
Cookie, Apple Crumble, COU, M & S*	1 Bar/27g	90.0	1.0	335	5.8	72.6	2.6	2.3
Corn Flakes, & Chocolate Milk, Kellogg's*	1 Bar/40g	176.0	6.0	440	9.0	66.0	16.0	2.0
Cranberry & Honey, Soft & Chewy, Sunny Crunch*	1 Bar/30g	115.0	2.0	382	6.0	73.1	8.3	3.1
Cranberry & Raisin, Geobar, Traidcraft*	1 Bar/35g	131.0	3.0	374	3.7	72.6	8.0	2.3
Cranberry, Crunch, Cambridge Diet*	1 Bar/50g	152.0	5.0	305	23.7	28.7	10.6	17.9
Crazy Caramel, Tesco*	1 Bar/40g	192.0	9.0	480	3.9	64.0	23.0	1.0
Creme Brulee Chocolate, M & S*	1 Bar/36g	178.0	11.0	495	4.4	54.0	29.2	0.4
Crispy Lemon Yoghurt, Carb Minders*	1 Bar/60g	240.0	9.0	400	33.3	38.3	15.0	3.3
Crispy Raspberry, Carb Minders*	1 Bar/60g	240.0	9.0	400	35.0	40.0	15.0	1.7
Crunchy Caramel, Tesco*	1 Bar/21g	98.0	5.0	467	4.6	56.0	25.0	1.4
Crunchy Crispy Treat, Kids, Tesco*	1 Bar/24g	109.0	5.0	453	3.6	62.5	20.9	1.5
Crunchy Granola, Oats 'n Honey, Nature Valley*	1 Bar/21g	97.0	3.0	460	8.3	70.4	16.1	6.2
Crunchy Nut, Chocolate Peanut Crisp, Kellogg's*	1 Bar/35g	169.0	9.0	483	12.0	53.0	25.0	3.5
Dark Chocolate, Cranberries, & Macadamias, Eat Natural*	1 Bar/45g	221.0	14.0	492	5.6	47.3	31.2	5.5
Dark Chocolate, Cranberry, Organic, Biona*	1 Bar/40g	162.0	6.0	405	6.2	53.5	14.7	0.0
Date & Fig, Lyme Regis Foods*	1 Bar/42g	143.0	5.0	341	7.0	52.0	11.7	9.3
Date & Fruit, Lyme Regis Foods*	1 Bar/42g	169.0	7.0	402	7.3	58.2	15.5	8.9
Date & Walnut, Eat Natural*	1 Bar/50g	220.0	10.0	441	8.0	57.1	20.1	3.3
Energy, Cocoa Brownie, Trek*	1 Bar/68g	216.0	4.0	318	17.0	51.0	6.0	0.0
Fair Break, Traidcraft*	1 Bar/22g	116.0	6.0	528	6.0	63.0	28.0	0.0
Fig & Mango, The Food Doctor*	1 Bar/35g	113.0	3.0	323	9.7	53.6	7.7	13.4

BARS

INFO/WEIGHT	Measure per Measure		Nutrition Values per 100g / 100ml				
	KCAL	FAT	KCAL	PROT	CARB	FAT	FIBRE
Food Bar, Apple & Walnut, The Food Doctor*	1 Bar/35g	117.0	4.0	333	10.8	46.8	11.4	15.3
Four Fruits, Organic, Trophy, The Village Bakery*	1 Bar/43g	150.0	3.0	353	3.8	71.2	5.9	4.2
Four Seeds, Organic, Trophy, The Village Bakery*	1 Bar/43g	164.0	4.0	385	8.1	68.7	8.7	2.5
Frosties, & Milk, Kellogg's*	1 Bar/25g	102.0	3.0	408	7.0	71.0	11.0	1.0
Frosties, Chocolate, Kellogg's*	1 Bar/25g	103.0	3.0	412	6.0	72.0	12.0	1.6
Fruit & Fibre, Whole Grain, Sainsbury's*	1 Bar/27g	109.0	3.0	405	6.2	70.1	11.1	3.8
Fruit & Nut, Eat Natural*	1 Bar/50g	223.0	11.0	446	11.6	49.8	22.3	5.3
Fruit & Nut, Ginger Snap, Larabar*	1 Bar/51g	220.0	14.0	431	9.8	47.1	27.4	9.8
Fruit & Nut, Multigrain, Jordans*	1 Bar/40g	164.0	6.0	410	7.0	59.1	16.2	5.7
Fruit & Nut, Organic, Eat Natural*	1 Bar/50g	244.0	15.0	488	10.2	42.9	30.6	0.0
Fruit 'n' Fibre Bakes, with Sultanas, Kellogg's*	1 Bar/40g	146.0	5.0	365	4.5	58.0	13.0	9.0
Fruit 'n' Fibre, Kellogg's*	1 Bar/25g	95.0	2.0	380	5.0	71.0	9.0	5.0
Fruit to Go, Apple Wildberry, Evernat*	1 Bar/14g	49.0	0.0	350	1.4	85.7	0.0	5.7
Fruit, Apple, Hellema*	1 Bar/33g	127.0	2.0	384	4.5	74.0	7.5	2.0
Fruit, Apple, Trimlyne*	1 Bar/27g	88.0	1.0	326	4.5	69.6	2.7	3.8
Fruit, Date, Oskri Organics*	1 Bar/43g	120.0	1.0	279	2.3	74.4	2.3	7.0
Fruit, Nut & Seed Bars, The Village Bakery*	1 Bar/25g	93.0	2.0	373	5.7	73.7	6.2	0.1
Fruit, Strawberry, Fruitina*	1 Bar/15g	43.0	0.0	289	1.9	61.9	1.1	12.2
Fruit, with Apricot, Castus*	1 Bar/25g	75.0	1.0	300	2.0	63.0	4.5	9.0
Fruits of the Forest, Advantage, Atkins*	1 Bar/60g	224.0	10.0	374	31.0	32.9	17.4	7.7
Fruitsome, Citrus, Rowntree's*	1 Bar/35g	140.0	5.0	400	4.1	65.1	13.7	2.3
Fruity Cereal Bar, Free From, Sainsbury's*	1 Bar/25g	100.0	3.0	399	4.4	72.3	10.2	2.6
Fruity Cereal, Go, Soreen*	1 Bar/40g	141.0	2.0	352	5.7	73.9	4.8	0.0
Fruity, Oat, Low Fat, Organic, Dove's Farm*	1 Bar/40g	142.0	1.0	354	5.0	71.5	2.7	2.4
Fudge Mallow Delight, Whipple Scrumptious, Wonka*	1 Bar/38g	205.0	12.0	537	4.6	59.2	31.3	0.6
Ginger & Oat, Chocolate Covered, Snack, Waitrose*	1 Bar/27g	120.0	5.0	444	4.2	65.0	18.6	2.1
Ginger Truffle, Waitrose*	1 Bar/38g	187.0	12.0	493	4.4	46.7	32.1	1.1
Ginger, Perfectly Balanced, Waitrose*	1 Bar/25g	92.0	1.0	367	4.9	79.3	3.3	3.3
Goodies, Cereal & Fruit, Apricot, Organic, Organix*	1 Bar/30g	122.0	6.0	408	7.2	55.3	20.4	6.2
Granola, Crunchy, Roasted Almond, Nature Valley*	1 Bar/42g	193.0	8.0	459	8.1	65.6	18.2	3.7
Granola, Peanut Butter, Quaker Oats*	1 Bar/28g	110.0	3.0	393	7.1	64.3	12.5	3.6
Granola, with Peanut Butter, Natco*	1 Bar/29g	129.0	4.0	445	10.0	69.0	14.1	5.5
Groove, Lemon, Alpen*	1 Bar/32g	124.0	2.0	389	5.6	78.4	5.9	1.9
Groove, Sassy Strawberry, Alpen*	1 Bar/32g	124.0	2.0	386	5.6	78.8	5.4	1.9
Harvest Cheweee, Apple & Raisin, Quaker Oats*	1 Bar/22g	89.0	3.0	405	5.5	68.0	12.0	3.0
Harvest Cheweee, Choc Chip, Quaker Oats*	1 Bar/22g	95.0	4.0	430	5.5	68.0	16.0	3.5
Harvest Cheweee, Toffee, Quaker Oats*	1 Bar/22g	94.0	3.0	427	5.0	68.0	15.0	3.0
Harvest Cheweee, White Chocolate Chip, Quaker Oats*	1 Bar/22g	93.0	3.0	425	6.0	67.0	15.5	3.5
Hazelnut Sandwich, Finn Crisp*	1 Bar/25g	134.0	8.0	535	7.0	50.0	34.0	0.0
Honey Rice Crisp, Lower Fat, Go Ahead, McVitie's*	1 Bar/22g	90.0	2.0	411	3.9	75.8	10.2	1.1
Honey, Natural, Trail Mix, Kallo*	1 Bar/40g	196.0	13.0	490	15.7	40.9	33.2	5.7
K-Time, Honey Nut Crunch, Kellogg's*	1 Bar/33g	128.0	1.0	382	5.0	82.7	2.5	1.8
K-Time, Mixed Berry, Kellogg's*	1 Bar/28g	104.0	1.0	372	4.9	80.1	2.2	3.8
Lemon, Larabar*	1 Bar/51g	210.0	11.0	412	11.8	51.0	21.6	5.9
Luna, Chocolate Pecan Pie, Luna*	1 Bar/48g	180.0	5.0	375	20.8	50.0	9.4	2.1
Luna, Nutz Over Chocolate, Luna*	1 Bar/48g	180.0	5.0	375	20.8	50.0	9.4	2.1
Luxury, Absolute Nut, Jordans*	1 Bar/45g	251.0	19.0	557	12.7	33.3	41.4	7.0
Luxury, Cranberry & Almond, Jordans*	1 Bar/50g	217.0	10.0	434	8.6	56.6	19.2	5.8
Luxury, Exotic Fruit & Nut, Jordans*	1 Bar/50g	196.0	3.0	393	5.0	69.1	5.4	4.8
Macadamia & Fruit, Eat Natural*	1 Bar/50g	242.0	15.0	485	7.3	44.6	30.8	0.0
Mango & Brazil, Tropical Wholefoods*	1 Bar/40g	172.0	8.0	429	4.7	61.4	19.1	4.2
Maple & Pecan, Crunchy, Jordans*	1 Bar/33g	153.0	8.0	464	7.7	56.8	22.9	6.5
Maple & Pecan, Organic, Jordans*	1 Bar/25g	101.0	3.0	405	5.5	66.2	13.1	3.2

BARS

INFO/WEIGHT	Measure KCAL	FAT	KCAL	PROT	CARB	FAT	FIBRE
Meal Replacement, Bar, Peanut Crunch, Cambridge Diet*	1 Bar/50g	173.0	7.0	346	26.7	27.0	14.6	14.8
Milk Chocolate Chip & Hazelnut, Snack, Benecol*	1 Bar/25g	99.0	3.0	395	4.7	64.5	13.1	2.5
Milk Chocolate Coated Orange Flavour, Energy, Boots*	1 Bar/70g	274.0	7.0	391	5.2	70.0	10.0	2.8
Mint Chocolate Whip, Weight Watchers*	1 Bar/20g	80.0	2.0	402	3.6	74.0	9.9	0.7
Mint, Double Take, Sainsbury's*	1 Bar/20g	107.0	6.0	534	7.2	56.9	30.8	1.3
Mixed Berry, Trek, Natural Balance Foods*	1 Bar/68g	204.0	1.0	300	15.6	56.5	2.2	6.0
Mixed Nut Feast, Eat Natural*	1 Bar/50g	278.0	20.0	556	18.8	28.0	41.0	0.0
Muesli, Apricot & Almond, Carmen's*	1 Bar/45g	190.0	8.0	423	10.4	50.6	18.2	7.4
Muesli, Cherry & Milk, Sirius*	1 Bar/25g	104.0	3.0	417	7.2	71.3	11.4	3.9
Muesli, Cookie Coach*	1 Bar/75g	289.0	8.0	385	6.8	65.1	11.1	0.0
Multigrain, Apple & Sultana, Jordans*	1 Bar/40g	141.0	2.0	353	4.4	70.0	6.2	4.8
Multigrain, Cranberry & Raspberry, Jordans*	1 Bar/37g	135.0	2.0	364	4.8	71.3	6.6	4.8
Multigrain, Fruit & Nut, Jordans*	1 Bar/40g	164.0	6.0	410	7.0	59.1	16.2	5.7
Nine Bar, Mixed Hemp Seed, Original, Wholebake*	1 Bar/50g	281.0	19.0	562	18.6	38.5	38.5	4.7
Nine Bar, Nutty, Wholebake*	1 Bar/50g	277.0	20.0	555	18.3	29.9	40.6	5.2
Nutri-Grain, Apple, Kellogg's*	1 Bar/37g	131.0	3.0	355	4.0	67.0	9.0	4.0
Nutri-Grain, Blackberry & Apple, Kellogg's*	1 Bar/37g	131.0	3.0	355	4.0	67.0	9.0	4.0
Nutri-Grain, Blueberry, Kellogg's*	1 Bar/37g	130.0	3.0	351	4.0	66.0	9.0	4.0
Nutri-Grain, Cherry, Kellogg's*	1 Bar/37g	129.0	3.0	348	4.0	67.0	8.0	4.0
Nutri-Grain, Chocolate Chip, Chewy, Kellogg's*	1 Bar/25g	103.0	3.0	413	4.5	73.0	12.0	2.5
Nutri-Grain, Chocolate, Kellogg's*	1 Bar/37g	136.0	4.0	367	4.5	66.0	10.0	4.0
Nutri-Grain, Elevenses, Choc Chip, Kellogg's*	1 Bar/45g	179.0	6.0	397	4.0	66.0	13.0	2.0
Nutri-Grain, Elevenses, Ginger, Kellogg's*	1 Bar/45g	168.0	4.0	373	5.0	68.0	9.0	3.0
Nutri-Grain, Elevenses, Raisin, Kellogg's*	1 Bar/45g	164.0	4.0	364	5.0	66.0	9.0	3.5
Nutri-Grain, Honey Oat & Raisin, Chewy, Kellogg's*	1 Bar/25g	98.0	2.0	393	3.5	78.0	8.0	2.5
Nutri-Grain, Oat Bakes, Cherry, Kellogg's*	1 Bar/50g	204.0	7.0	408	4.5	66.0	14.0	2.5
Nutri-Grain, Oat Bakes, Totally Oaty, Kellogg's*	1 Bar/50g	205.0	7.0	411	5.0	64.0	15.0	3.0
Nutri-Grain, Raspberry, Kellogg's*	1 Bar/37g	131.0	3.0	355	4.0	67.0	9.0	4.0
Nutri-Grain, Strawberry, Kellogg's*	1 Bar/37g	131.0	3.0	355	4.0	67.0	9.0	3.5
Nuts & Choc Chip, Asda*	1 Bar/27g	127.0	6.0	471	8.0	58.0	23.0	2.8
Nutty Crunch Surprise, Wonka*	1 Bar/37g	202.0	12.0	543	4.9	58.7	32.1	0.9
Nutty Nougat Caramel, Tesco*	1 Bar/20g	99.0	5.0	493	8.5	54.0	27.0	2.4
Oat, Mixed Berry, Quaker Oats*	1 Bar/38g	137.0	3.0	360	6.8	64.5	8.8	8.0
Oat, Original with Golden Syrup, Quaker Oats*	1 Bar/38g	139.0	4.0	366	7.1	64.5	9.5	7.9
Oat, Quaker Oats*	1 Bar/38g	137.0	3.0	360	6.8	64.5	8.8	8.0
Oats, Raisins, Honey & Apricots, Geobar, Traidcraft*	1 Bar/35g	132.0	3.0	376	5.3	69.0	8.8	3.5
Oaty with Cranberry & Blueberry, Tesco*	1 Bar/38g	141.0	3.0	370	5.5	69.0	7.5	6.2
Optivita, Berry Oat, Kellogg's*	1 Bar/28g	101.0	2.0	360	7.0	68.0	7.0	9.0
Orange Crunch, Go Ahead, McVitie's*	1 Bar/23g	99.0	3.0	430	4.1	78.0	12.8	0.8
Orange Truffle, M & S*	1 Bar/33g	177.0	11.0	535	6.6	55.6	31.9	1.4
Orchard Fruits & Yoghurt, Fruit & Fibre, Sainsbury's*	1 Bar/27g	102.0	2.0	379	5.9	75.3	6.0	4.1
Original, Crunchy, Honey & Almond, Jordans*	1 Bar/30g	139.0	7.0	463	8.3	56.7	22.7	6.7
Peach & Raspberry, Low GI, Solo Slim, Rosemary Conley*	1 Bar/35g	115.0	1.0	329	26.9	46.7	4.0	9.4
Peach, Apricot & Almond, Altu*	1 Bar/40g	158.0	5.0	395	7.9	65.2	11.4	4.3
Peanut & Caramel Whip, Weight Watchers*	1 Bar/20g	76.0	3.0	381	4.4	73.7	13.7	1.2
Peanut, Cashew & Thai Sweet Chilli, Altu*	1 Bar/40g	172.0	8.0	430	14.7	47.0	20.3	3.1
Peanut, Raisin & Chocolate, Weight Watchers*	1 Bar/25g	97.0	3.0	388	7.6	60.0	11.2	12.8
Pear & Ginger, Fruit Break, Lyme Regis Foods*	1 Bar/42g	160.0	9.0	381	2.7	45.4	20.9	9.9
Pecan Apricot & Peach, M & S*	1 Bar/50g	255.0	18.0	510	9.3	38.2	35.5	4.9
Pecan Pie, Larabar*	1 Bar/45g	200.0	14.0	444	6.7	48.9	31.1	8.9
Penguin, Chukka, McVitie's*	1 Bar/28g	135.0	6.0	481	6.1	65.1	21.8	0.0
Protein Pack, X-Treme, with White Chocolate, Inkospor*	1 Bar/35g	136.0	3.0	388	32.0	43.0	10.0	0.3
Protein, Chocolate Chewy Crisp, Pro-Bar Xs*	1 Bar/70g	239.0	5.0	341	44.0	6.0	6.5	12.0

B

	Measure INFO/WEIGHT	per Measure KCAL	FAT	Nutrition Values per 100g / 100ml KCAL	PROT	CARB	FAT	FIBRE
BARS								
Protein, Peanut Chewy Crisp, Chemical Protein Pro-Xs*	1 Bar/70g	243.0	5.0	347	42.9	5.5	7.5	12.5
Raisin & Apricot, Geobar, Traidcraft*	1 Bar/35g	132.0	3.0	376	5.3	69.0	8.8	3.5
Raisin & Hazelnut, Weight Watchers*	1 Bar/24g	95.0	2.0	396	5.0	71.2	10.0	2.9
Raisin & Oatmeal, Breakfast Snack, Tesco*	1 Bar/38g	133.0	4.0	355	5.6	56.8	11.7	2.8
Raisin, Munch, Tesco*	1 Bar/30g	126.0	4.0	420	5.4	66.3	14.8	3.8
Raspberry, Fruit Bake, Go Ahead, McVitie's*	1 Bar/35g	124.0	3.0	354	2.7	73.8	7.2	1.2
Rice Crisp, Cranberry & Orange, Go Ahead, McVitie's*	1 Bar/22g	92.0	2.0	417	3.9	77.0	10.4	1.0
Rice Krispies & Milk, Kellogg's*	1 Bar/20g	83.0	2.0	416	7.0	71.0	12.0	0.3
Rice, Crispy Orange, Milk Chocolate, Reduced Fat, Tesco*	1 Bar/22g	95.0	3.0	432	3.6	75.4	12.7	0.4
Rich Toffee, Weight Watchers*	1 Bar/26g	83.0	3.0	319	3.6	52.3	10.6	0.8
Roasted Nut, Chewy & Crisp, Sainsbury's*	1 Bar/27g	120.0	7.0	446	10.1	46.6	24.3	3.9
Roasted Peanut, Weight Watchers*	1 Bar/25g	104.0	3.0	415	9.6	65.3	12.8	3.7
Sandwich, Chocolate, Rik & Rok*	1 Bar/22g	105.0	4.0	477	6.5	70.0	19.0	0.0
Sandwich, Milk Chocolate, Smart Price, Asda*	1 Bar/25g	132.0	7.0	528	6.0	63.0	28.0	0.0
Sandwich, Milk Chocolate, Value, Tesco*	1 Bar/26g	130.0	6.0	504	5.4	64.5	24.9	2.4
School, Apple, Fruit Bowl*	1 Bar/20g	67.0	1.0	337	0.7	75.0	3.0	6.0
School, Apricot, Fruit Bowl*	1 Bar/20g	67.0	1.0	337	0.7	75.0	3.0	6.0
School, Blackcurrant, Fruit Bowl*	1 Bar/20g	67.0	1.0	337	0.7	75.0	3.0	6.0
School, Cherry, Fruit Bowl*	1 Bar/20g	67.0	1.0	337	0.7	75.0	3.0	6.0
Slow Fig & Macadamia, Southern Alps, Slow Puck*	1 Bar/45g	200.0	7.0	444	4.0	70.2	16.4	4.4
Slow Mango, Apple & Almond, Southern Alps*	1 Bar/45g	214.0	12.0	476	10.4	50.7	26.0	0.0
Smarties, Nestle*	1 Bar/45g	238.0	13.0	528	6.2	58.2	30.0	0.9
Special Fruit Muesli, Jordans*	1 Bar/40g	140.0	2.0	349	5.0	68.8	6.0	5.0
Special K, Apple & Pear, Kellogg's*	1 Bar/23g	92.0	2.0	400	8.0	73.0	8.0	2.0
Special K, Bliss Bar, Raspberry & Chocolate, Kellogg's*	1 Bar/22g	88.0	2.0	399	4.0	74.0	10.0	4.0
Special K, Chocolate Chip, Kellogg's*	1 Bar/22g	90.0	2.0	401	9.0	76.0	7.0	1.5
Special K, Fruits of the Forest, Kellogg's*	1 Bar/22g	87.0	2.0	397	8.0	74.0	8.0	2.5
Special K, Peach & Apricot, Kellogg's*	1 Bar/21g	84.0	2.0	400	8.0	73.0	9.0	2.5
Special K, Red Fruits, Kellogg's*	1 Bar/22g	84.0	1.0	390	8.0	78.0	5.0	1.5
Special Muesli, Jordans*	1 Bar/40g	152.0	5.0	379	6.0	61.6	12.1	5.8
Strawberry, Breakfast, Carb Control, Tesco*	1 Bar/37g	144.0	9.0	389	7.0	40.5	23.2	4.0
Strawberry, Morning Shine, Atkins*	1 Bar/37g	145.0	8.0	392	28.9	24.9	21.6	14.1
Strawberry, Organic, Seeds of Change*	1 Bar/26g	102.0	2.0	390	5.4	75.7	7.3	0.0
Strawberry, Shapers, Boots*	1 Bar/22g	75.0	2.0	343	2.5	77.0	11.0	0.9
Sultana, Apple & Yoghurt, Balance, Sainsbury's*	1 Bar/27g	104.0	2.0	387	6.1	77.4	5.9	2.3
Superfoods, Jordans*	1 Bar/45g	171.0	5.0	379	7.0	63.3	10.9	6.7
Three Musketeer, Candy, Mars*	1 Bar/60g	260.0	8.0	430	3.3	76.2	13.2	1.7
Toffee & Banana, Weight Watchers*	1 Bar/18g	67.0	1.0	372	6.1	77.2	3.9	1.7
Toffee Crunch, Simply Lite, Perfect Days*	1 Bar/51g	200.0	9.0	392	23.5	49.0	17.6	9.8
Tracker, Breakfast, Banana, Mars*	1 Bar/37g	176.0	8.0	476	4.7	63.3	22.6	9.4
Tracker, Breakfast, Lemon, Mars*	1 Bar/26g	124.0	6.0	477	4.6	64.3	22.4	0.0
Tracker, Chocolate Chip, Mars*	1 Bar/37g	178.0	9.0	480	6.8	58.0	23.6	3.8
Tracker, Forest Fruits, Mars*	1 Bar/26g	123.0	6.0	474	4.6	64.1	22.2	0.0
Tracker, Yoghurt, Mars*	1 Bar/27g	133.0	6.0	491	6.3	64.2	23.2	0.0
Triple Dazzle, Wonka*	1 Bar/39g	195.0	10.0	504	5.9	61.9	25.9	0.0
Very Berry, Cookie, Big Softies, Fox's*	1 Bar/26g	85.0	1.0	325	5.7	69.7	2.5	2.5
BASIL								
Dried, Ground	*1 Tsp/1.4g*	*4.0*	*0.0*	*251*	*14.4*	*43.2*	*4.0*	*0.0*
Fresh, Average	*1 Tbsp/5g*	*2.0*	*0.0*	*40*	*3.1*	*5.1*	*0.8*	*0.0*
BATTER MIX								
for Pancakes & Yorkshire Puddings, McDougalls*	1 Pancake/38g	83.0	4.0	218	6.3	24.8	10.4	1.9
for Yorkshire Puddings & Pancakes, Tesco*	1 Serving/17g	34.0	0.0	200	2.3	43.3	1.5	2.5
Green's*	1 Bag/125g	296.0	9.0	237	8.7	34.3	7.2	0.0

	Measure INFO/WEIGHT	per Measure KCAL	FAT	Nutrition Values per 100g / 100ml KCAL	PROT	CARB	FAT	FIBRE
BATTER MIX								
Pancake, Buttermilk, Krusteaz*	3 Pancakes/16g	57.0	1.0	352	11.3	66.0	4.7	3.4
Pancake, Sainsbury's*	1 Pancake/63g	96.0	1.0	152	6.5	27.4	1.8	3.1
Smart Price, Asda*	1 Pack/128g	268.0	6.0	209	8.0	34.0	4.5	2.7
Tesco*	1 Pack/130g	467.0	2.0	359	12.3	74.4	1.4	7.7
BAY LEAVES								
Dried, Average	*1 Tsp / 0.6g*	*2.0*	*0.0*	*313*	*7.6*	*48.6*	*8.4*	*0.0*
BEAN SPROUTS								
Mung, Canned, Drained, Average	*1 Serving/90g*	*9.0*	*0.0*	*10*	*1.6*	*0.8*	*0.1*	*0.7*
Mung, Raw, Average	*1oz/28g*	*9.0*	*0.0*	*31*	*2.9*	*4.0*	*0.5*	*1.5*
Mung, Stir-Fried in Blended Oil, Average	*1 Serving/90g*	*65.0*	*5.0*	*72*	*1.9*	*2.5*	*6.1*	*0.9*
Raw, Average	*1 Serving/150g*	*45.0*	*0.0*	*30*	*3.0*	*5.9*	*0.2*	*1.8*
BEANS								
Aduki, Cooked in Unsalted Water, Average	*1 Tbsp/30g*	*37.0*	*0.0*	*123*	*9.3*	*22.5*	*0.2*	*5.5*
Aduki, Dried, Raw	*1 Tbsp/30g*	*82.0*	*0.0*	*272*	*19.9*	*50.1*	*0.5*	*11.1*
Baked & Vegetarian Sausages, In Tomato Sauce, Asda*	½ Can/210g	204.0	4.0	97	7.4	12.5	1.9	8.4
Baked, & Jumbo Sausages, Asda*	1 Serving/210g	317.0	15.0	151	7.0	15.0	7.0	2.6
Baked, & Pork Sausages, Sainsbury's*	1 Serving/210g	248.0	9.0	118	5.7	13.9	4.4	3.4
Baked, & Sausage, Asda*	½ Can/205g	252.0	8.0	123	6.0	16.0	3.9	3.0
Baked, & Sausage, GFY, Asda*	1 Serving/217g	178.0	6.0	82	4.7	10.0	2.6	1.8
Baked, & Sausages, Meatfree, Sainsbury's*	1 Can/420g	500.0	17.0	119	8.0	12.6	4.0	2.7
Baked, Barbecue, Smokey, Beanz, Heinz*	1 Can/420g	332.0	1.0	79	4.9	14.3	0.2	3.8
Baked, Curried, Average	*½ Can/210g*	*203.0*	*2.0*	*96*	*4.8*	*17.2*	*0.9*	*3.6*
Baked, Curry, Beanz, Heinz*	1 Can/200g	204.0	3.0	102	4.8	18.0	1.3	4.0
Baked, HL, Tesco*	1 Can/420g	315.0	2.0	75	4.3	12.1	0.5	3.8
Baked, in a Tomato Sauce, Reduced Sugar & Salt, Asda*	½ Tin/210.7g	158.0	1.0	75	4.6	13.0	0.5	4.5
Baked, in Tomato Sauce, Average	*1 Can/400g*	*346.0*	*2.0*	*86*	*4.8*	*15.9*	*0.5*	*3.3*
Baked, in Tomato Sauce, Beanz, Heinz*	½ Can/208g	164.0	0.0	79	4.7	12.9	0.2	3.7
Baked, in Tomato Sauce, Healthy Range, Average	*½ Can/210g*	*143.0*	*0.0*	*68*	*3.9*	*12.8*	*0.2*	*2.8*
Baked, in Tomato Sauce, Organic, Beanz, Heinz*	1 Can/415g	299.0	1.0	72	4.7	12.8	0.2	3.8
Baked, in Tomato Sauce, Reduced Sugar & Salt	*½ Can/210g*	*159.0*	*1.0*	*75*	*4.5*	*13.6*	*0.3*	*3.8*
Baked, Jalfrezi, Mean, Beanz, Heinz*	1 Serving/195g	135.0	3.0	69	4.5	9.8	1.3	3.6
Baked, Mexican, Mean, Beanz, Heinz*	½ Can/208g	158.0	1.0	76	5.0	12.9	0.5	4.0
Baked, Sweet Chilli, Mean, Beanz, Heinz*	½ Can/195g	142.0	1.0	73	4.5	13.0	0.3	3.6
Baked, Tikka, Mean, Beanz, Heinz*	1 Serving/195g	172.0	6.0	88	4.8	10.6	3.0	3.5
Baked, with Chicken Nuggets, Beanz, Heinz*	1 Can/200g	210.0	6.0	105	6.7	12.4	3.1	3.2
Baked, with Hidden Veg, Beanz, Heinz*	½ Can/208g	156.0	1.0	75	4.7	13.5	0.3	4.1
Baked, with Lea & Perrins Sauce, Beanz, Heinz*	1 Can/415g	303.0	1.0	73	4.8	13.1	0.2	3.8
Baked, with Spicy Meatballs, Beanz, Heinz*	1 Can/400g	372.0	10.0	93	5.8	12.0	2.4	2.9
Baked, with Steak Chunks, Beanz, Heinz*	1 Can/415g	340.0	3.0	82	6.9	12.1	0.7	3.5
Baked, with Vegetable Sausages, Beanz, Heinz*	1 Sm Can/200g	210.0	7.0	105	6.0	12.2	3.6	2.9
Black, Cooked, Average	*1 Cup/172g*	*227.0*	*1.0*	*132*	*8.8*	*23.7*	*0.5*	*8.7*
Black, Dried, Average	*1 Serving/100g*	*341.0*	*1.0*	*341*	*21.6*	*62.4*	*1.4*	*15.2*
Blackeye, Canned, Average	*1 Can/172g*	*206.0*	*1.0*	*119*	*8.4*	*19.7*	*0.7*	*3.3*
Blackeye, Dried, Raw	*1oz/28g*	*87.0*	*0.0*	*311*	*23.5*	*54.1*	*1.6*	*8.2*
Borlotti, Canned, Average	*1oz/28g*	*29.0*	*0.0*	*103*	*7.6*	*16.9*	*0.5*	*4.7*
Borlotti, Dried, Raw, Average	*1 Serving/100g*	*335.0*	*1.0*	*335*	*23.0*	*60.0*	*1.2*	*24.7*
Broad, Canned, Drained, Average	*1 Can/195g*	*136.0*	*1.0*	*70*	*6.9*	*9.2*	*0.6*	*6.8*
Broad, Dried, Raw, Average	*1oz/28g*	*69.0*	*1.0*	*245*	*26.1*	*32.5*	*2.1*	*27.6*
Broad, Frozen, Sainsbury's*	1 Serving/80g	64.0	0.0	80	7.9	10.7	0.6	6.5
Broad, in Water, Drained, Asda*	1 Serving/98g	73.0	0.0	75	7.4	10.1	0.5	7.1
Broad, Weighed with Pod, Raw, Average	*1oz/28g*	*17.0*	*0.0*	*59*	*5.7*	*7.2*	*1.0*	*6.1*
Butter, Canned, Average	*1oz/28g*	*22.0*	*0.0*	*79*	*5.9*	*12.9*	*0.5*	*4.0*
Butter, Dried, Boiled, Average	*1oz/28g*	*30.0*	*0.0*	*106*	*7.2*	*18.6*	*0.6*	*5.2*

	Measure INFO/WEIGHT	per Measure KCAL	per Measure FAT	Nutrition Values per 100g / 100ml KCAL	PROT	CARB	FAT	FIBRE
BEANS								
Butter, Dried, Raw, Average	1oz/28g	81.0	0.0	290	19.1	52.9	1.7	16.0
Cannellini, Canned, Average	1oz/28g	26.0	0.0	94	7.2	15.0	0.5	5.7
Chilli, Canned, Average	1 Can/420g	381.0	3.0	91	5.2	15.8	0.7	4.3
Edamame, Sainsbury's*	1 Serving/150g	211.0	10.0	141	12.3	6.8	6.4	4.2
Edamame, Shelled, Frozen, Raw, Average	1 Serving/80g	88.0	4.0	110	10.2	8.6	4.7	4.8
Flageolet, Canned, Average	1 Can/265g	235.0	2.0	89	6.7	14.0	0.6	3.5
French, Boiled, Average	1 Serving/150g	37.0	0.0	25	2.3	3.8	0.0	3.7
French, Canned, Average	1oz/28g	6.0	0.0	22	1.6	3.5	0.3	2.5
French, Raw	1oz/28g	7.0	0.0	24	1.9	3.2	0.5	2.2
Green, Cut, Average	1oz/28g	6.0	0.0	22	1.7	3.7	0.2	2.1
Green, Fine, Average	1 Serving/75g	18.0	0.0	24	1.8	3.4	0.4	2.6
Green, Sliced, Average	1oz/28g	6.0	0.0	23	1.9	3.5	0.2	2.1
Green, Sliced, Frozen, Average	1 Serving/50g	13.0	0.0	26	1.8	4.4	0.1	4.1
Green, Whole, Average	1oz/28g	6.0	0.0	22	1.6	3.0	0.4	1.7
Haricot, Dried, Boiled in Unsalted Water	1oz/28g	27.0	0.0	95	6.6	17.2	0.5	6.1
Haricot, Dried, Raw	1oz/28g	80.0	0.0	286	21.4	49.7	1.6	17.0
Haricot, in Water, Canned, Tesco*	½ Can/117.5g	76.0	1.0	65	5.7	9.0	0.5	7.8
Kidney, Red, Canned, Average	½ Can/90g	92.0	1.0	102	7.8	16.7	0.6	5.6
Kidney, Red, Dried, Boiled in Unsalted Water	1oz/28g	29.0	0.0	103	8.4	17.4	0.5	6.7
Kidney, Red, Dried, Raw	1oz/28g	74.0	0.0	266	22.1	44.1	1.4	15.7
Kidney, White, Dry, Raw, Unico*	½ Cup/80g	270.0	1.0	337	22.5	61.2	1.1	21.2
Mixed, Canned, Average	1 Can/300g	300.0	3.0	100	6.7	15.6	1.2	4.1
Mixed, Spicy, Average	1 Serving/140g	108.0	1.0	77	4.8	13.4	0.5	3.9
Mung, Whole, Dried, Boiled in Unsalted Water	1oz/28g	25.0	0.0	91	7.6	15.3	0.4	3.0
Mung, Whole, Dried, Raw	1oz/28g	78.0	0.0	279	23.9	46.3	1.1	10.0
Pinto, Dried, Boiled in Unsalted Water	1oz/28g	38.0	0.0	137	8.9	23.9	0.7	0.0
Pinto, Dried, Raw	1oz/28g	92.0	0.0	327	21.1	57.1	1.6	14.0
Refried, Average	1 Serving/215g	162.0	2.0	75	4.6	12.7	0.7	1.7
Runner, Average	1 Serving/80g	16.0	0.0	20	1.4	2.8	0.4	2.2
Soya, Dried, Average	1oz/28g	104.0	5.0	370	34.2	15.4	18.3	19.6
Soya, Dried, Boiled in Unsalted Water	1oz/28g	39.0	2.0	141	14.0	5.1	7.3	6.1
Soya, Frozen, Birds Eye*	1 Serving/80g	120.0	5.0	150	12.3	11.0	6.3	4.0
Soya, in Water, Salt Added, Sainsbury's*	1 Serving/100g	102.0	7.0	102	4.0	5.1	7.3	6.1
BEEF								
Brisket, Raw, Lean	1oz/28g	39.0	2.0	139	21.1	0.0	6.1	0.0
Brisket, Raw, Lean & Fat	1oz/28g	61.0	4.0	218	18.4	0.0	16.0	0.0
Cooked, Sliced, From Supermarket, Average	1 Slice/35g	35.0	1.0	101	17.4	2.6	2.4	0.4
Flank, Pot-Roasted, Lean	1oz/28g	71.0	4.0	253	31.8	0.0	14.0	0.0
Flank, Pot-Roasted, Lean & Fat	1oz/28g	87.0	6.0	309	27.1	0.0	22.3	0.0
Flank, Raw, Lean	1oz/28g	49.0	3.0	175	22.7	0.0	9.3	0.0
Flank, Raw, Lean & Fat	1oz/28g	74.0	6.0	266	19.7	0.0	20.8	0.0
for Casserole, Lean, Diced, Average	1oz/28g	35.0	1.0	126	23.0	0.0	3.8	0.0
Fore Rib, Lean & Fat, Average	1oz/28g	40.0	2.0	143	21.7	0.0	6.2	0.2
Fore Rib, Raw, Lean	1oz/28g	41.0	2.0	145	21.5	0.0	6.5	0.0
Fore Rib, Roasted, Lean	1oz/28g	66.0	3.0	236	33.3	0.0	11.4	0.0
Fore Rib, Roasted, Lean & Fat	1oz/28g	84.0	6.0	300	29.1	0.0	20.4	0.0
Grill Steak, Average	1 Steak/170g	501.0	39.0	295	19.3	2.1	23.2	0.1
Grill Steak, Peppered, Average	1 Serving/172g	419.0	24.0	243	23.6	5.2	14.2	0.3
Joint, for Roasting, Average	1oz/28g	38.0	1.0	134	24.5	1.4	3.4	0.2
Joint, Sirloin, Roasted, Lean	1oz/28g	53.0	2.0	188	32.4	0.0	6.5	0.0
Joint, Sirloin, Roasted, Lean & Fat	1oz/28g	65.0	4.0	233	29.8	0.0	12.6	0.0
Mince, Cooked, Average	1 Serving/75g	214.0	15.0	286	23.9	0.0	20.3	0.0
Mince, Extra Lean, Raw, Average	1 Serving/100g	131.0	5.0	131	21.0	0.0	5.3	0.0

BEEF	Measure INFO/WEIGHT	per Measure KCAL	FAT	KCAL	PROT	CARB	FAT	FIBRE
Mince, Extra Lean, Stewed	1oz/28g	50.0	2.0	177	24.7	0.0	8.7	0.0
Mince, Lean, Raw, Average	1oz/28g	49.0	3.0	175	22.0	0.0	9.7	0.0
Mince, Raw, Average	1oz/28g	67.0	5.0	239	18.7	0.2	18.0	0.1
Mince, Steak, Extra Lean, Average	1oz/28g	37.0	2.0	131	20.5	0.4	5.6	0.0
Mince, Steak, Raw, Average	1 Serving/125g	317.0	25.0	254	17.2	0.0	20.0	0.0
Mince, Stewed	1oz/28g	59.0	4.0	209	21.8	0.0	13.5	0.0
Peppered, Sliced, Average	1 Slice/20g	26.0	1.0	129	18.2	1.3	5.6	1.0
Roast, Sliced, Average	1 Slice/35g	48.0	1.0	136	26.1	0.4	3.6	0.2
Salt, Average	1 Serving/70g	80.0	2.0	114	21.7	1.0	2.5	0.1
Salted, Dried, Raw	1oz/28g	70.0	0.0	250	55.4	0.0	1.5	0.0
Silverside, Pot-Roasted, Lean	1oz/28g	54.0	2.0	193	34.0	0.0	6.3	0.0
Silverside, Pot-Roasted, Lean & Fat	1oz/28g	69.0	4.0	247	31.0	0.0	13.7	0.0
Silverside, Raw, Lean	1oz/28g	38.0	1.0	134	23.8	0.0	4.3	0.0
Silverside, Raw, Lean & Fat	1oz/28g	60.0	4.0	215	20.4	0.0	14.8	0.0
Silverside, Salted, Boiled, Lean	1oz/28g	52.0	2.0	184	30.4	0.0	6.9	0.0
Silverside, Salted, Boiled, Lean & Fat	1oz/28g	63.0	3.0	224	27.9	0.0	12.5	0.0
Silverside, Salted, Raw, Lean	1oz/28g	39.0	2.0	140	19.2	0.0	7.0	0.0
Silverside, Salted, Raw, Lean & Fat	1oz/28g	64.0	5.0	227	16.3	0.0	18.0	0.0
Steak, Braising, Braised, Lean	1oz/28g	63.0	3.0	225	34.4	0.0	9.7	0.0
Steak, Braising, Braised, Lean & Fat	1oz/28g	69.0	4.0	246	32.9	0.0	12.7	0.0
Steak, Braising, Lean, Raw, Average	1oz/28g	40.0	1.0	144	24.8	0.0	5.0	0.0
Steak, Braising, Raw, Lean & Fat	1oz/28g	45.0	2.0	160	20.7	0.0	8.6	0.0
Steak, Economy, Average	1oz/28g	53.0	2.0	190	26.9	1.2	8.7	0.4
Steak, Fillet, Cooked, Average	1oz/28g	54.0	2.0	191	28.6	0.0	8.5	0.0
Steak, Fillet, Lean, Average	1oz/28g	42.0	2.0	150	21.0	0.0	7.3	0.0
Steak, Fillet, Lean, Cooked, Average	1oz/28g	52.0	2.0	186	28.6	0.0	7.9	0.0
Steak, Frying, Average	1 Steak/110g	128.0	3.0	116	23.7	0.0	2.5	0.0
Steak, Rump, Cooked, Average	1oz/28g	69.0	4.0	245	29.1	0.5	14.1	0.0
Steak, Rump, Grilled, Rare, Lean	1 Steak/227g	381.0	16.0	168	26.5	0.0	6.9	0.0
Steak, Rump, Lean, Cooked, Average	1oz/28g	50.0	2.0	179	31.0	0.0	6.1	0.0
Steak, Rump, Raw, Lean	1oz/28g	35.0	1.0	125	22.0	0.0	4.1	0.0
Steak, Rump, Raw, Lean & Fat	1oz/28g	49.0	3.0	174	20.7	0.0	10.1	0.0
Steak, Sirloin, Fried, Rare, Lean	1oz/28g	53.0	2.0	189	28.8	0.0	8.2	0.0
Steak, Sirloin, Fried, Rare, Lean & Fat	1oz/28g	65.0	4.0	233	26.8	0.0	14.0	0.0
Steak, Sirloin, Grilled, Medium-Rare, Lean	1oz/28g	49.0	2.0	176	26.6	0.0	7.7	0.0
Steak, Sirloin, Grilled, Medium-Rare, Lean & Fat	1oz/28g	60.0	4.0	213	24.8	0.0	12.6	0.0
Steak, Sirloin, Grilled, Rare, Lean	1oz/28g	46.0	2.0	166	26.4	0.0	6.7	0.0
Steak, Sirloin, Grilled, Rare, Lean & Fat	1oz/28g	60.0	4.0	216	25.1	0.0	12.8	0.0
Steak, Sirloin, Grilled, Well-Done, Lean	1oz/28g	63.0	3.0	225	33.9	0.0	9.9	0.0
Steak, Sirloin, Grilled, Well-Done, Lean & Fat	1oz/28g	72.0	4.0	257	31.8	0.0	14.4	0.0
Steak, Sirloin, Raw, Lean	1oz/28g	38.0	1.0	135	23.5	0.0	4.5	0.0
Steak, Sirloin, Raw, Lean & Fat	1oz/28g	56.0	4.0	201	21.6	0.0	12.7	0.0
Stewed Steak, Average	1 Serving/220g	258.0	10.0	117	15.8	3.3	4.6	0.0
Stewing Steak, Lean & Fat, Raw, Average	1oz/28g	41.0	2.0	146	22.1	0.0	6.4	0.0
Stewing Steak, Raw, Lean	1oz/28g	34.0	1.0	122	22.6	0.0	3.5	0.0
Stewing Steak, Stewed, Lean	1oz/28g	52.0	2.0	185	32.0	0.0	6.3	0.1
Stewing Steak, Stewed, Lean & Fat	1oz/28g	57.0	3.0	203	29.2	0.0	9.6	0.0
Stir Fry Strips, Raw, Average	1 Serving/125g	146.0	3.0	116	23.5	0.0	2.5	0.3
Topside, Lean & Fat, Average	1oz/28g	61.0	3.0	219	27.5	0.0	12.2	0.0
Topside, Raw, Lean	1oz/28g	32.0	1.0	116	23.0	0.0	2.7	0.0
Wafer Thin Sliced, Cooked, Average	1 Slice/10g	13.0	0.0	129	24.5	0.5	3.2	0.1
BEEF &								
Beer, Princes*	½ Can/205g	215.0	6.0	105	14.0	5.5	3.0	0.0

B

	Measure INFO/WEIGHT	per Measure KCAL	FAT	Nutrition Values per 100g / 100ml KCAL	PROT	CARB	FAT	FIBRE
BEEF &								
Black Bean, Sizzling, Oriental Express*	1 Pack/400g	420.0	8.0	105	7.2	14.0	2.1	2.1
Black Bean, with Rice, Weight Watchers*	1 Pack/320g	288.0	4.0	90	5.0	14.6	1.3	0.1
Macaroni, Lean Cuisine*	1 Serving/269g	310.0	9.0	115	7.4	14.1	3.3	1.1
Mashed Potato, Braised, Sainsbury's*	1 Pack/434g	425.0	14.0	98	7.6	9.4	3.3	0.8
Onions, Minced, Asda*	½ Can/196g	314.0	20.0	160	13.0	4.6	10.0	0.1
Onions, with Gravy, Minced, Lean, Sainsbury's*	1 Sm Can/198g	285.0	14.0	144	17.0	3.1	7.0	0.2
Potatoes, Minced, Light Choices, Tesco*	1 Pack/350g	210.0	3.0	60	4.6	7.7	0.9	2.1
Yorkshire Pudding, Minced, Sainsbury's*	1 Pack/350g	374.0	12.0	107	8.4	10.7	3.4	1.1
BEEF BOURGUIGNON								
Extra Special, Asda*	1 Serving/300g	279.0	11.0	93	9.3	5.7	3.7	0.7
Finest, Tesco*	½ Pack/300g	247.0	8.0	82	9.9	4.8	2.6	0.5
BEEF BRAISED								
& New Potatoes, GFY, Asda*	1 Pack/448g	242.0	6.0	54	8.1	2.2	1.4	3.1
Steak, & Cabbage, COU, M & S*	1 Pack/380g	323.0	10.0	85	8.3	6.7	2.6	1.9
Steak, & Carrots, Mini Favourites, M & S*	1 Serving/200g	140.0	5.0	70	8.0	4.2	2.5	1.3
Steak, & Mash, GFY, Asda*	1 Pack/400g	260.0	3.0	65	3.4	11.0	0.8	0.7
Steak, & Mash, HL, Tesco*	1 Pack/450g	418.0	12.0	93	7.0	10.2	2.7	0.7
Steak, & Red Wine, Veg Mash, HL, Tesco*	1 Pack/500g	360.0	13.0	72	5.1	6.9	2.7	1.2
Steak, with Colcannon Mash, Tesco*	1 Pack/450g	477.0	16.0	106	9.5	9.0	3.5	0.9
Tender, Pub Specials, Birds Eye*	1 Pack/450g	243.0	4.0	54	5.5	6.1	0.8	1.8
BEEF CANTONESE								
Sainsbury's*	½ Pack/175g	199.0	2.0	114	5.5	20.1	1.3	0.5
BEEF CHASSEUR								
& Potato Mash, BGTY, Sainsbury's*	1 Pack/450g	387.0	11.0	86	7.8	8.4	2.4	1.3
Somerfield*	1 Serving/275g	287.0	7.0	104	14.8	5.2	2.7	2.1
BEEF CHILLI								
Crispy, Cantonese, Chilled, Sainsbury's*	1 Pack/250g	682.0	39.0	273	11.4	22.1	15.5	1.9
Crispy, Tesco*	1 Pack/250g	472.0	17.0	189	10.8	21.0	6.9	0.5
Sweet, Asda*	1 Pack/400g	356.0	4.0	89	7.8	12.3	0.9	1.9
BEEF DINNER								
British Cuisine, Tesco*	1 Pack/433g	390.0	10.0	90	6.3	10.0	2.3	2.3
Roast, Iceland*	1 Serving/340g	354.0	13.0	104	8.5	9.1	3.7	1.6
Roast, Sainsbury's*	1 Pack/400g	356.0	7.0	89	6.5	12.0	1.7	1.9
Tesco*	1 Pack/400g	380.0	11.0	95	6.1	10.1	2.8	1.7
BEEF ESCALOPE								
BGTY, Sainsbury's*	1 Serving/300g	321.0	6.0	107	22.1	0.1	2.1	0.1
BEEF HOT & SOUR								
Chef's Selection, M & S*	1 Pack/329g	395.0	17.0	120	9.2	8.4	5.3	1.3
with Garlic Rice, BGTY, Sainsbury's*	1 Pack/400g	428.0	7.0	107	5.9	17.0	1.7	0.6
with Vegetable Rice, COU, M & S*	1 Pack/400g	360.0	6.0	90	5.5	14.4	1.4	0.6
BEEF IN								
Ale Gravy, Chunky, Birds Eye*	1 Pack/340g	272.0	7.0	80	7.4	8.3	2.0	1.5
Ale with Mushrooms, BGTY, Sainsbury's*	1 Pack/251g	193.0	4.0	77	10.2	5.6	1.5	0.4
Black Bean Sauce, Chinese, Tesco*	1 Pack/400g	396.0	12.0	99	9.1	8.7	3.1	0.5
Black Bean Sauce, M & S*	1 Pack/350g	402.0	22.0	115	8.9	5.7	6.4	1.1
Black Bean, with Egg Noodles, M & S*	1 Pack/400g	460.0	6.0	115	8.6	16.7	1.5	1.8
Black Pepper Sauce & Egg Fried Rice, Tesco*	1 Pack/451g	622.0	25.0	138	7.0	15.2	5.5	1.2
Black Velvet Porter, Diet Chef Ltd*	1 Meal/300g	201.0	4.0	67	8.2	6.0	1.2	2.1
Burgundy Red Wine, GFY, Asda*	1 Pack/405g	348.0	8.0	86	8.0	9.0	2.0	1.1
Creamy Peppercorn Sauce, Steak, Tesco*	1 Steak/150g	189.0	8.0	126	16.5	2.6	5.5	0.1
Gravy, Roast, Birds Eye*	1 Pack/227g	177.0	4.0	78	13.4	2.2	1.7	0.0
Gravy, Sliced, Iceland*	1 Pack/200g	172.0	3.0	86	12.1	5.9	1.6	0.3
Gravy, Sliced, Sainsbury's*	1 Serving/125g	100.0	2.0	80	13.5	2.6	1.8	0.2

	Measure INFO/WEIGHT	per Measure KCAL	FAT	Nutrition Values per 100g / 100ml KCAL	PROT	CARB	FAT	FIBRE
BEEF IN								
Gravy, Sliced, Tesco*	1 Serving/200g	152.0	4.0	76	11.3	3.1	2.1	0.2
Madeira & Mushroom Gravy, Sliced, Finest, Tesco*	1 Pack/400g	536.0	25.0	134	15.2	4.3	6.2	1.0
Oriental Sauce, Lean Cuisine, Findus*	1 Pack/350g	420.0	9.0	120	4.5	20.0	2.5	1.5
Oyster Sauce, Asda*	1 Serving/100g	82.0	4.0	82	7.0	4.4	4.0	1.7
Peppercorn Sauce, & Mashed Potato, Weight Watchers*	1 Pack/400g	312.0	8.0	78	5.0	10.0	2.0	1.0
Red Wine Sauce, Milson's Kitchen, Aldi*	1 Pack/400g	256.0	6.0	64	5.6	9.6	1.5	2.1
Red Wine, & Spinach Mash, Low Saturated Fat, Waitrose*	1 Pack/380g	338.0	7.0	89	9.3	8.8	1.9	1.4
Strips, Chilli Sauce, Tesco*	1 Pack/166g	290.0	8.0	175	23.2	9.6	4.7	0.0
Tuscan Chianti, Bighams*	½ Pack/300g	132.0	11.0	44	5.1	4.3	3.6	1.4
Velvet Porter, with Potatoes, Look What We Found*	1 Pack/300g	201.0	4.0	67	8.2	6.0	1.2	2.1
BEEF WELLINGTON								
Extra Special, Asda*	1 Serving/218g	605.0	37.0	277	11.0	20.0	17.0	0.9
Finest, Tesco*	1/3 Pack/216g	525.0	34.0	243	13.0	12.3	15.7	1.5
Sainsbury's*	1 Serving/175g	472.0	27.0	270	14.7	18.0	15.5	0.4
BEEF WITH								
Black Bean Sauce, Chilli, Sainsbury's*	1 Pack/300g	336.0	14.0	112	8.7	8.6	4.8	1.0
Diane Sauce, Rump Steak, Tesco*	1 Steak/165g	181.0	8.0	110	15.1	1.1	4.9	0.3
Honey & Black Pepper, Waitrose*	1 Pack/350g	325.0	7.0	93	9.1	9.4	2.1	1.8
Horseradish & Mustard Crust, Joint, Easy, Waitrose*	1/5 Pack/110g	153.0	6.0	139	20.9	2.5	5.1	0.7
Horseradish Dressing, Slow Cooked, HL, Tesco*	1 Pack/356g	285.0	10.0	80	5.4	7.5	2.9	1.4
Onion & Gravy, Minced, Princes*	1 Serving/200g	342.0	24.0	171	9.9	5.5	12.2	0.0
Onions & Gravy, Minced, Tesco*	1 Can/198g	224.0	10.0	113	14.0	2.8	5.1	0.8
Oyster Sauce, Ooodles of Noodles, Oriental Express*	1 Pack/425g	378.0	6.0	89	4.9	14.2	1.3	1.5
Peppercorn Sauce, Rib Eye Joint, Sainsbury's*	•1 Serving/181g	299.0	13.0	165	22.2	3.4	7.0	0.1
Peppercorn Sauce, Steak, Just Cook, Sainsbury's*	½ Pack/128g	174.0	7.0	136	17.7	3.4	5.7	1.2
Peppercorn Sauce, Steak, Simply Cook, Tesco*	½ Pack /167g	242.0	13.0	145	15.3	2.1	7.9	0.2
Red Wine Sauce, Rump Steak, Tesco*	1 Serving/150g	180.0	9.0	120	17.2	0.1	5.7	3.3
Red Wine Sauce, Steaks, Just Cook, Sainsbury's*	½ Pack/70g	83.0	2.0	118	20.0	2.0	3.3	0.2
Rigatoni Pasta, Chianti Ragu, Simply Fuller Longer, M & S*	1 Pack/400g	440.0	14.0	110	8.5	11.0	3.6	1.8
Shiraz Wine Sauce, Pot Roast, Finest, Tesco*	1 Pack/350g	350.0	9.0	100	14.1	5.1	2.6	0.9
Vegetables & Gravy, Minced, Birds Eye*	1 Pack/178g	155.0	6.0	87	9.1	5.1	3.4	0.6
Vegetables & Mashed Potato, Braised, BGTY, Sainsbury's*	1 Pack/450g	330.0	6.0	73	6.5	8.9	1.3	1.2
Vegetables, Tesco*	1 Pot/300g	102.0	3.0	34	2.9	3.3	1.0	1.1
BEER								
Ale, Bottled, Old Speckled Hen*	1 Bottle/330ml	148.0	0.0	45	0.0	0.0	0.0	0.0
Bitburger*	1 Bottle/500ml	205.0	0.0	41	0.4	2.5	0.0	0.0
Bitter, Canned, Average	*1 Can/440ml*	*141.0*	*0.0*	*32*	*0.3*	*2.3*	*0.0*	*0.0*
Bitter, Draught, Average	*1 Pint/568ml*	*182.0*	*0.0*	*32*	*0.3*	*2.3*	*0.0*	*0.0*
Bitter, Keg, Average	*1 Pint/568ml*	*176.0*	*0.0*	*31*	*0.3*	*2.3*	*0.0*	*0.0*
Bitter, Low Alcohol, Average	*1 Pint/568ml*	*74.0*	*0.0*	*13*	*0.2*	*2.1*	*0.0*	*0.0*
Brown Ale, Bottled, Average	*1 Bottle/330ml*	*99.0*	*0.0*	*30*	*0.3*	*3.0*	*0.0*	*0.0*
Guinness Extra Stout, Bottled*	*1 Bottle/500ml*	*215.0*	*0.0*	*43*	*4.0*	*0.0*	*0.0*	*0.0*
Guinness, Draught*	*1 Pint/568ml*	*210.0*	*0.0*	*37*	*0.3*	*3.2*	*0.0*	*0.0*
Guinness, Stout*	*1 Pint/568ml*	*170.0*	*0.0*	*30*	*0.4*	*3.0*	*0.0*	*0.0*
Kilkenny, Diageo*	1 Pint/568ml	210.0	0.0	37	0.3	3.0	0.0	0.0
Low Calorie, Low Carb, Cobra*	1 Bottle/330ml	96.0	0.0	29	0.1	1.3	0.0	0.0
Mackeson, Stout	*1 Pint/568ml*	*205.0*	*0.0*	*36*	*0.4*	*4.6*	*0.0*	*0.0*
Mild, Draught, Average	*1 Pint/568ml*	*136.0*	*0.0*	*24*	*0.2*	*1.6*	*0.0*	*0.0*
Non Alcoholic, Cobra*	1 Bottle/330ml	79.0	0.0	24	0.8	2.0	0.0	0.0
Non Alcoholic, Wrigleys*	1 Serving/355ml	58.0	0.0	16	0.3	3.7	0.0	0.0
Premium, Lager, San Miguel*	1 Bottle/330ml	148.0	0.0	45	0.3	3.7	0.0	0.0
Raspberry, Framboise, Lindemans*	1 Serving/355ml	185.0	0.0	52	0.0	8.8	0.0	0.0
Resolution, Low Carb, Marstons*	1 Glass/250ml	77.0	0.0	31	0.3	0.6	0.1	0.0

B

	Measure INFO/WEIGHT	per Measure KCAL	FAT	Nutrition Values per 100g / 100ml KCAL	PROT	CARB	FAT	FIBRE
BEER								
Ultra, Michelob*	1 Bottle/275ml	88.0	0.0	32	0.0	0.9	0.0	0.0
Weissbier, Alcohol Free, Erdinger*	1 Bottle/500ml	125.0	0.0	25	0.4	5.3	0.0	0.0
BEETROOT								
& Roasted Red Onion, M & S*	1 Serving/125g	94.0	3.0	75	1.5	12.6	2.1	2.5
Baby, Pickled, Average	*1oz/28g*	*10.0*	*0.0*	*37*	*1.7*	*7.2*	*0.1*	*1.2*
Cooked, Boiled, Drained, Average	*1 Serving/100g*	*44.0*	*0.0*	*44*	*1.7*	*10.0*	*0.2*	*2.0*
Pickled, in Sweet Vinegar, Average	*1oz/28g*	*16.0*	*0.0*	*57*	*1.2*	*12.8*	*0.1*	*1.5*
Pickled, in Vinegar, Average	*1 Serving/50g*	*19.0*	*0.0*	*37*	*1.6*	*7.5*	*0.1*	*1.2*
Raw, Average	*1oz/28g*	*9.0*	*0.0*	*32*	*1.5*	*6.0*	*0.1*	*1.8*
BHAJI								
Aubergine & Potato, Fried in Vegetable Oil, Average	1oz/28g	36.0	2.0	130	2.0	12.0	8.8	1.7
Cabbage & Pea, Fried in Vegetable Oil, Average	1oz/28g	50.0	4.0	178	3.3	9.2	14.7	3.4
Cauliflower, Fried in Vegetable Oil, Average	1oz/28g	60.0	6.0	214	4.0	4.0	20.5	2.0
Mushroom, Fried in Vegetable Oil, Average	1oz/28g	46.0	5.0	166	1.7	4.4	16.1	1.3
Okra, Bangladeshi, Fried in Butter Ghee, Average	1oz/28g	27.0	2.0	95	2.5	7.6	6.4	3.2
Onion, Asda*	1 Bhaji/49g	96.0	5.0	196	6.0	20.0	10.0	2.0
Onion, Indian Meal for One, Tesco*	1 Bhaji/100g	204.0	7.0	204	5.5	29.2	7.3	1.3
Onion, Indian Starter Selection, M & S*	1 Bhaji/22g	65.0	5.0	295	5.7	15.8	23.3	2.8
Onion, Indian, Mini, Asda*	1 Bhaji/18g	33.0	2.0	186	4.9	19.0	10.0	6.0
Onion, Mini Indian Selection, Tesco*	1 Bhaji/23g	40.0	2.0	172	6.1	15.4	9.5	4.6
Onion, Mini, Snack Selection, Sainsbury's*	1 Bhaji/22g	49.0	3.0	226	4.1	17.4	15.5	3.5
Onion, Mini, Tesco*	1 Bhaji/23g	48.0	2.0	210	7.3	26.7	8.2	1.3
Onion, Sainsbury's*	1 Bhaji/38g	93.0	5.0	245	6.5	24.7	13.4	6.4
Onion, Waitrose*	1 Bhaji/45g	124.0	9.0	276	4.7	17.5	20.8	2.5
Onion, with Tomato & Chilli Dip, M & S*	1 Bhaji/54g	111.0	6.0	205	4.1	21.1	11.7	3.6
Potato & Onion, Fried in Vegetable Oil, Average	1oz/28g	45.0	3.0	160	2.1	16.6	10.1	1.6
Potato, Onion & Mushroom, Fried, Average	1oz/28g	58.0	5.0	208	2.0	12.0	17.5	1.5
Potato, Spinach & Cauliflower, Fried, Average	1oz/28g	47.0	4.0	169	2.2	7.1	15.1	1.4
Spinach & Potato, Fried in Vegetable Oil, Average	1oz/28g	53.0	4.0	191	3.7	13.4	14.1	2.3
Spinach, Fried in Vegetable Oil, Average	1oz/28g	23.0	2.0	83	3.3	2.6	6.8	2.4
Turnip & Onion, Fried in Vegetable Oil, Average	1oz/28g	36.0	3.0	128	1.3	7.1	10.9	2.2
Vegetable, Fried in Vegetable Oil, Average	1oz/28g	59.0	5.0	212	2.1	10.1	18.5	2.4
BHUNA								
Chicken Tikka, Tesco*	1 Pack/350g	437.0	23.0	125	11.3	5.0	6.7	0.9
Chicken, & Rice, Sainsbury's*	1 Pack/501g	696.0	32.0	139	7.3	13.3	6.3	1.5
Chicken, Curry, Tesco*	1 Serving/300g	396.0	23.0	132	11.4	4.5	7.6	0.5
Chicken, Indian Takeaway, Tesco*	1 Pack/350g	437.0	28.0	125	8.3	4.6	7.9	2.2
Chicken, with Naan Bread, Sharwood's*	1 Pack/375g	465.0	19.0	124	6.8	12.8	5.1	2.8
Lamb, & Rice, Sainsbury's*	1 Pack/500g	619.0	26.0	124	7.4	11.6	5.3	2.0
Prawn, Co-Op*	1 Pack/400g	300.0	16.0	75	3.0	6.0	4.0	1.0
Prawn, Tandoori, Indian, Sainsbury's*	½ Pack/200g	152.0	8.0	76	5.5	4.5	4.0	1.7
BIERWURST								
Average	*1 Slice/10g*	*25.0*	*2.0*	*252*	*14.4*	*0.9*	*21.2*	*0.0*
BILBERRIES								
Fresh, Raw	*1oz/28g*	*8.0*	*0.0*	*30*	*0.6*	*6.9*	*0.2*	*1.8*
BILTONG								
Average	*1 Serving/25g*	*64.0*	*1.0*	*256*	*50.0*	*0.0*	*4.0*	*0.0*
BIRYANI								
Chicken Tikka, & Lentil Pilau, Simply Fuller Longer, M & S*	1 Pack/400g	440.0	12.0	110	9.5	12.0	2.9	2.3
Chicken Tikka, BGTY, Sainsbury's*	1 Pack/400g	384.0	4.0	96	7.1	14.6	1.0	1.5
Chicken Tikka, Northern Indian, Sainsbury's*	1 Pack/450g	697.0	26.0	155	9.4	16.5	5.7	1.2
Chicken Tikka, with Basmati Rice, Sharwood's*	1 Pack/373g	481.0	16.0	129	6.3	16.2	4.3	0.9
Chicken, COU, M & S*	1 Pack/400g	360.0	8.0	90	6.9	10.8	2.1	1.9

	Measure INFO/WEIGHT	per Measure KCAL	FAT	Nutrition Values per 100g / 100ml KCAL	PROT	CARB	FAT	FIBRE
BIRYANI								
Chicken, Easy Steam, HL, Tesco*	1 Pack/400g	424.0	7.0	106	7.0	15.5	1.8	0.6
Chicken, Indian, Asda*	1 Pack/450g	778.0	22.0	173	9.0	23.0	5.0	0.7
Chicken, Light Choices, Tesco*	1 Serving/450g	495.0	10.0	110	7.0	15.0	2.3	3.4
Chicken, Weight Watchers*	1 Pack/330g	308.0	4.0	93	6.2	14.6	1.1	0.6
Lamb, HL, Tesco*	1 Pack/400g	560.0	18.0	140	5.1	19.0	4.4	3.1
Seafood, M & S*	1 Pack/450g	619.0	26.0	138	7.1	14.4	5.7	1.7
Vegetable, & Rice, Sainsbury's*	½ Pack/125.0g	229.0	5.0	183	4.4	32.4	4.0	0.7
Vegetable, HL, Tesco*	1 Pack/450g	454.0	9.0	101	2.7	17.9	2.1	1.6
Vegetable, Perfectly Balanced, Waitrose*	1 Serving/350g	238.0	1.0	68	2.6	14.0	0.2	2.7
Vegetable, Sainsbury's*	1 Serving/225g	328.0	18.0	146	2.4	16.3	7.9	1.1
Vegetable, Waitrose*	1 Pack/450g	486.0	18.0	108	2.8	15.2	4.0	2.2
Vegetable, with Rice, Patak's*	½ Pack/125g	194.0	2.0	155	3.6	32.9	1.5	1.2
BISCUITS								
Abbey Crunch, McVitie's*	1 Biscuit/9g	43.0	2.0	477	6.0	72.8	17.9	2.5
Abernethy, Simmers*	1 Biscuit/12g	61.0	3.0	490	5.7	69.2	21.9	0.0
Ace Milk Chocolate, McVitie's*	1 Biscuit/24g	122.0	6.0	510	6.1	66.2	24.5	1.6
After Eight, Nestle*	1 Biscuit/5g	26.0	1.0	525	6.5	62.6	27.7	1.5
All Butter, Tesco*	1 Biscuit/9g	44.0	2.0	486	6.3	63.5	23.0	1.9
Almond Butter Thins, Extra Special, Asda*	1 Biscuit/4g	15.0	0.0	375	5.0	60.0	12.5	2.5
Almond Fingers, Tesco*	1 Finger/46g	180.0	7.0	391	6.2	58.4	14.7	1.0
Almond Thins, Continental, Tesco*	1 Biscuit/3g	15.0	0.0	450	6.7	72.8	14.7	3.1
Almond Thins, Sainsbury's*	1 Biscuit/3g	13.0	0.0	430	7.0	80.3	9.0	1.0
Almond, Thins, Morrisons*	1 Biscuit/3.6g	16.0	1.0	450	6.7	72.8	14.7	3.1
Almond, Thins, TTD, Sainsbury's*	1 Biscuit/4g	16.0	1.0	450	6.7	72.8	14.7	3.1
Amaretti, Doria*	1 Biscuit/4g	17.0	0.0	433	6.0	84.8	7.8	0.0
Amaretti, M & S*	1 Biscuit/6g	30.0	1.0	480	9.6	71.3	17.2	3.8
Amaretti, Sainsbury's*	1 Biscuit/6g	27.0	1.0	450	6.5	80.5	11.3	1.1
Animals, Milk Chocolate, Cadbury*	1 Biscuit/19g	94.0	4.0	493	6.6	69.8	20.9	0.0
Animals, Mini Packs, Cadbury*	1 Pack/25g	123.0	5.0	491	6.7	70.7	20.2	0.0
Animals, Minis, Cadbury*	1 Biscuit/2g	10.0	0.0	480	6.5	68.5	20.1	0.0
Apple & Blackberry, Oat Squares, Go Ahead, McVitie's*	1 Bar/40g	137.0	4.0	343	4.5	63.7	9.5	4.2
Apple & Cinnamon Thins, Finest, Tesco*	1 Biscuit/5g	22.0	1.0	470	5.9	71.7	17.5	1.5
Apple & Raspberry, Minis, Officially Low Fat, Fox's*	1 Bag/40g	140.0	1.0	350	3.9	76.9	2.7	3.8
Apple & Sultana, Go Ahead, McVitie's*	1 Biscuit/15g	56.0	1.0	386	6.0	72.7	7.9	3.3
Apple Crumble, Officially Low Fat, Fox's*	1 Biscuit/23g	85.0	1.0	365	5.4	80.4	2.4	2.5
Apple Strudel, Big Softies, Fox's*	1 Biscuit/23g	80.0	0.0	348	5.3	77.0	1.6	2.8
Apricot, Low Fat, M & S*	1 Biscuit/23g	79.0	1.0	343	6.1	69.6	4.4	7.8
Arrowroot, Thin, Crawfords*	1 Biscuit/7g	35.0	1.0	473	7.4	76.7	15.2	2.2
Banana Milk Shake, Creams, Safeway*	1 Biscuit/13.0g	60.0	2.0	460	5.6	70.9	16.8	1.8
Belgian Chocolate, Selection, Finest, Tesco*	1 Biscuit/10g	51.0	3.0	515	6.0	62.0	27.0	3.0
Belgian Chocolate, Thins, Extra Special, Asda*	1 Biscuit/9g	44.0	2.0	503	7.0	67.0	23.0	0.2
Belgian Milk Chocolate, M & S*	1 Biscuit/12.2g	60.0	2.0	490	6.2	70.1	20.3	2.5
Bisc & Bounty, Master Foods*	1 Bar/25g	131.0	8.0	526	4.8	52.3	33.0	0.0
Bisc & M&m's, Master Foods*	1 Biscuit/17g	90.0	5.0	527	5.8	59.2	29.6	0.0
Bisc & Mars, Master Foods*	1 Bar/27g	141.0	8.0	523	5.3	61.4	28.5	0.0
Bisc & Twix, Master Foods*	1 Bar/27g	140.0	8.0	520	5.2	61.1	28.3	0.0
Blackcurrant with Wheat Bran, Bisca*	1 Biscuit/7.5g	31.0	1.0	420	6.0	72.0	12.0	5.5
Blueberry & Vanilla, Oaty, Weight Watchers*	1 Biscuit/22g	101.0	4.0	460	7.1	65.6	18.8	4.2
BN, Chocolate Flavour, McVitie's*	1 Biscuit/18g	83.0	3.0	460	6.6	71.0	16.7	2.6
BN, Strawberry Flavour, McVitie's*	1 Biscuit/18g	71.0	1.0	395	5.6	78.0	6.8	0.0
BN, Vanilla Flavour, McVitie's*	1 Biscuit/18g	85.0	3.0	470	5.9	74.0	16.6	1.2
Boasters, Hazelnut & Choc Chip, McVitie's*	1 Biscuit/16g	88.0	5.0	549	7.0	55.5	33.3	2.4
Bourbon Creams, Asda*	1 Biscuit/14g	67.0	3.0	482	5.0	66.0	22.0	3.4

B

BISCUITS

	Measure INFO/WEIGHT	per Measure KCAL	per Measure FAT	Nutrition Values per 100g / 100ml KCAL	PROT	CARB	FAT	FIBRE
Bourbon Creams, Sainsbury's*	1 Biscuit/13g	60.0	2.0	476	5.7	70.4	19.1	1.7
Bourbon Creams, Tesco*	1 Biscuit/14g	68.0	3.0	485	5.4	66.2	21.6	3.4
Bourbon Creams, Value, Multipack, Tesco*	1 Biscuit/13g	62.0	3.0	494	5.9	68.0	22.8	1.7
Bourbon, Trufree*	1 Biscuit/12g	61.0	3.0	512	4.0	70.0	24.0	2.0
Brandy Snaps	1oz/28g	122.0	6.0	437	2.5	64.0	20.3	0.8
Butter, Covered in Dark 70% Chocolate, Green & Black's*	1 Biscuit/12g	62.0	4.0	520	7.1	5.6	29.4	0.1
Butter, Crinkle Crunch, Fox's*	1 Biscuit/11g	50.0	2.0	460	5.8	69.8	17.5	2.4
Butter, Thins, Belgian Chocolate, The Best, Safeway*	1 Biscuit/10g	49.0	2.0	487	6.4	64.0	22.8	0.8
Cafe Noir, McVitie's*	1 Biscuit/9.3g	39.0	1.0	420	4.5	87.0	5.5	1.1
Cantucci, with Honey, Loyd Grossman*	1 Biscuit/7g	31.0	1.0	450	9.5	66.3	16.3	0.9
Cantuccini, Sainsbury's*	1 Biscotti/8g	35.0	1.0	440	10.4	63.1	16.2	4.4
Cantuccini, with Almonds, Average	1 Biscotti/30g	130.0	5.0	433	10.0	60.0	16.7	3.3
Caramel Crunch, Go Ahead, McVitie's*	1 Bar/24g	106.0	3.0	440	4.7	76.6	13.8	0.8
Caramelised, Lotus*	1 Biscuit/9g	44.0	2.0	488	5.0	72.0	20.0	0.8
Caramels, Milk Chocolate, McVitie's*	1 Serving/17g	81.0	4.0	478	5.6	65.8	21.4	1.8
Cheddars, Real Cheddar Cheese, Jacob's*	1 Biscuit/4g	19.0	1.0	509	11.6	53.2	27.7	2.7
Cheese Melts, Carr's*	1 Biscuit/5g	22.0	1.0	479	11.9	58.2	22.0	2.2
Cheese Sandwich, Ritz*	1 Biscuit/9g	50.0	3.0	530	9.5	55.0	30.2	2.0
Cheese Savouries, Sainsbury's*	1 Serving/50g	268.0	15.0	536	11.6	53.3	30.6	2.5
Cherry Bakewell, Handfinished, M & S*	1 Biscuit/40g	200.0	10.0	495	5.9	62.1	24.0	0.5
Choc Chip, Paterson's*	1 Biscuit/17g	79.0	4.0	474	5.6	64.0	21.6	3.1
Chocahoops, Cadbury*	1 Biscuit/13g	65.0	3.0	510	5.8	62.7	26.4	0.0
Choco Leibniz, Dark Chocolate, Bahlsen*	1 Biscuit/14g	69.0	4.0	493	6.8	59.0	26.0	5.1
Choco Leibniz, Milk, Bahlsen*	1 Biscuit/10g	51.0	3.0	515	7.9	63.4	25.5	0.0
Choco Leibniz, Orange Flavour, Bahlsen*	1 Biscuit/14g	70.0	4.0	504	7.9	58.5	26.4	0.0
Chocolate & Coconut, Duchy Originals*	1 Biscuit/13g	68.0	4.0	543	6.3	52.1	34.4	2.6
Chocolate Break, Plain Chocolate, Tesco*	1 Biscuit/21g	112.0	6.0	535	6.7	61.2	29.2	3.8
Chocolate Chip & Peanut, Trufree*	1 Biscuit/11g	55.0	3.0	496	4.0	66.0	24.0	2.0
Chocolate Fingers, Caramel, Cadbury*	1 Finger/8g	39.0	2.0	490	5.8	63.2	23.8	0.0
Chocolate Fingers, Milk, Cadbury*	1 Biscuit/6g	31.0	2.0	515	6.8	60.8	27.1	1.7
Chocolate Fingers, Milk, Extra Crunchy, Cadbury*	1 Biscuit/5g	25.0	1.0	505	6.6	66.2	23.6	0.0
Chocolate Fingers, Plain, Cadbury*	1 Biscuit/6g	30.0	2.0	508	6.2	60.6	26.8	0.0
Chocolate Flavour, Taillefine, Lu*	1 Biscuit/8g	33.0	1.0	408	5.8	70.8	10.8	5.8
Chocolate Florentine, M & S*	1 Serving/39g	195.0	10.0	500	7.4	64.5	24.9	1.7
Chocolate Ginger, Organic, Duchy Originals*	1 Biscuit/12g	64.0	4.0	518	4.6	59.7	29.0	2.1
Chocolate Ginger, Thorntons*	1 Biscuit/19g	96.0	5.0	512	5.9	58.2	28.4	0.0
Chocolate Kimberley, Jacob's*	1 Biscuit/20g	86.0	3.0	428	3.9	64.4	17.2	1.1
Chocolate Mousse Meringue, Occasions, Sainsbury's*	1 Biscuit/47g	245.0	14.0	522	5.6	55.7	30.7	3.2
Chocolate Seville, Thorntons*	1 Biscuit/19g	97.0	5.0	512	5.7	59.0	28.1	0.0
Chocolate Teddy, Arnotts*	1 Biscuit/17g	80.0	3.0	478	6.6	69.3	19.2	2.0
Chocolate Toffee, Crunch, Moments, McVitie's*	1 Biscuit/17g	89.0	5.0	520	5.6	62.3	27.6	1.7
Chocolate Viennese, Fox's*	1 Biscuit/16g	85.0	5.0	530	6.7	56.6	30.7	1.7
Chocolate, Belgian Chocolate, Weight Watchers*	1 Biscuit/18g	87.0	4.0	481	7.1	61.8	22.8	4.5
Chocolinis, Milk Chocolate, Go Ahead, McVitie's*	1 Biscuit/12g	56.0	2.0	466	7.7	77.2	14.0	2.0
Chocolinis, Plain Chocolate, McVitie's*	1 Biscuit/12g	56.0	2.0	468	6.9	77.0	14.7	2.6
Christmas Shapes, Assorted, Sainsbury's*	1 Biscuit/15g	77.0	4.0	525	5.2	59.0	29.8	1.7
Classic, Creams, Fox's*	1 Biscuit/14g	72.0	4.0	516	4.4	65.2	25.8	1.7
Classic, Milk Chocolate, Fox's*	1 Biscuit/13g	67.0	3.0	517	6.1	64.9	24.0	1.6
Coconut Crinkle, Sainsbury's*	1 Biscuit/11g	54.0	3.0	500	6.4	59.6	26.2	3.7
Coconut Ring, Asda*	1 Biscuit/8g	37.0	2.0	486	6.0	66.0	22.0	2.6
Coconut Rings, Tesco*	1 Biscuit/9g	44.0	2.0	485	6.2	66.1	21.7	2.6
Cracked Black Pepper, Savoury, Weight Watchers*	1 Serving/16g	71.0	3.0	446	8.3	59.2	19.5	9.4
Cranberry & Pumpkin Seed, BGTY, Sainsbury's*	1 Biscuit/17g	68.0	3.0	410	7.2	56.6	17.1	13.9

BISCUITS

	Measure INFO/WEIGHT	per Measure KCAL	per Measure FAT	Nutrition Values per 100g / 100ml KCAL	PROT	CARB	FAT	FIBRE
Cranberry & Sunflower Seed, Oaty, Weight Watchers*	1 Biscuit/22g	103.0	5.0	469	7.5	62.4	21.0	5.3
Cranberry with Hip & Honey, Bisca*	1 Biscuit/7.5g	31.0	1.0	410	6.5	69.0	12.0	6.5
Cranberry, Crispy Slices, Light Choices, Tesco*	1 Biscuit/14.5g	54.0	1.0	370	6.0	76.0	3.9	5.5
Crunchy Caramel, Tesco*	1 Bar/21g	98.0	5.0	467	4.6	56.0	25.0	1.4
Custard Creams, 25% Less Fat, Asda*	1 Biscuit/10g	47.0	2.0	474	6.0	72.0	18.0	1.2
Custard Creams, 25% Less Fat, Sainsbury's*	1 Biscuit/13g	59.0	2.0	469	5.8	72.7	17.3	1.3
Custard Creams, 25% Less Fat, Tesco*	1 Biscuit/13g	59.0	2.0	473	5.8	72.2	17.9	1.2
Custard Creams, Asda*	1 Biscuit/11.9g	59.0	3.0	495	5.0	67.0	23.0	2.0
Custard Creams, BGTY, Sainsbury's*	1 Biscuit/12g	56.0	2.0	473	5.8	72.2	17.9	1.2
Custard Creams, Crawfords*	1 Biscuit/11g	57.0	3.0	517	5.9	69.2	24.1	1.5
Custard Creams, Jacob's*	1 Biscuit/16g	77.0	3.0	481	5.3	68.0	20.9	1.6
Custard Creams, Sainsbury's*	1 Biscuit/13g	67.0	3.0	514	5.5	70.4	23.4	1.6
Custard Creams, Smart Price, Asda*	1 Biscuit/13g	61.0	3.0	486	6.0	69.0	21.0	1.6
Custard Creams, Tesco*	1 Biscuit/13g	65.0	3.0	510	5.7	65.7	24.7	1.5
Custard Creams, Trufree*	1 Biscuit/12g	60.0	3.0	501	3.5	70.0	23.0	1.0
Custard Creams, Value, Tesco*	1 Biscuit/11g	51.0	2.0	450	7.2	72.5	14.3	3.0
Dark Chocolate All Butter, M & S*	1 Biscuit/15g	72.0	4.0	480	6.9	52.4	27.2	11.4
Dark Chocolate Ginger, M & S*	1 Biscuit/21g	105.0	6.0	505	5.0	58.8	27.6	4.2
Dark Chocolate Gingers, Border*	1 Biscuit/17g	74.0	3.0	445	4.4	61.4	20.1	2.9
Digestive, 25% Less Fat, Asda*	1 Biscuit/16g	73.0	3.0	455	7.3	69.8	16.3	2.6
Digestive, 25% Less Fat, Tesco*	1 Biscuit/14g	65.0	2.0	462	7.3	71.0	16.5	3.8
Digestive, BGTY, Sainsbury's*	1 Biscuit/15g	70.0	3.0	468	7.4	71.0	17.2	3.8
Digestive, Caramels, Milk Chocolate, McVitie's*	1 Biscuit/17g	81.0	4.0	478	5.6	65.1	21.7	2.3
Digestive, Caramels, Plain Chocolate, McVitie's*	1 Biscuit/17g	82.0	4.0	481	5.7	65.5	22.1	2.1
Digestive, Chocolate	1 Biscuit/ 17g	84.0	4.0	493	6.8	66.5	24.1	2.2
Digestive, Chocolate Chip, Asda*	1 Biscuit/14g	68.0	3.0	491	6.0	65.0	23.0	2.9
Digestive, Chocolate, Cadbury*	1 Biscuit/17g	85.0	4.0	495	6.8	62.3	24.4	0.0
Digestive, Cracker Selection, Tesco*	1 Biscuit/12g	56.0	2.0	464	7.1	65.2	19.4	4.3
Digestive, Crawfords*	1 Biscuit/12g	58.0	2.0	484	7.1	68.8	20.0	3.4
Digestive, Creams, McVitie's*	1 Biscuit/12g	60.0	3.0	502	5.6	68.2	23.0	2.1
Digestive, Dark Chocolate, McVitie's*	1 Biscuit/17g	82.0	4.0	487	6.0	61.6	24.0	4.0
Digestive, Economy, Sainsbury's*	1 Biscuit/13g	65.0	3.0	498	6.8	66.3	22.8	3.3
Digestive, Finger, Reduced Fat, Sainsbury's*	1 Finger/8g	39.0	2.0	482	6.8	63.6	22.2	3.2
Digestive, Fingers, Morrisons*	1 Finger/8g	39.0	2.0	482	6.8	63.6	22.2	3.2
Digestive, GFY, Asda*	1 Biscuit/14g	65.0	2.0	461	6.0	71.0	17.0	3.6
Digestive, Happy Shopper*	1 Biscuit/13g	64.0	3.0	498	6.8	66.3	22.8	3.3
Digestive, High Fibre, Reduced Sugar, M & S*	1 Biscuit/13g	60.0	3.0	460	6.5	59.3	21.7	9.4
Digestive, Hovis*	1 Biscuit/6g	27.0	1.0	447	10.2	60.0	18.5	4.4
Digestive, Jacob's*	1 Biscuit/14g	67.0	3.0	479	6.6	65.7	21.1	3.4
Digestive, Lemon & Ginger, McVitie's*	1 Biscuit/15g	72.0	3.0	480	6.7	66.7	20.7	2.7
Digestive, Light, McVitie's*	1 Biscuit/15g	65.0	2.0	437	7.3	69.5	14.4	3.6
Digestive, McVitie's*	1 Biscuit/15g	70.0	3.0	470	7.2	62.7	21.5	3.6
Digestive, Milk Chocolate Mint, McVitie's*	1 Biscuit/17g	81.0	4.0	487	6.7	62.6	23.4	2.9
Digestive, Milk Chocolate, 25% Less Fat, Tesco*	1 Biscuit/17g	79.0	3.0	466	7.4	69.0	17.8	2.6
Digestive, Milk Chocolate, 25% Reduced Fat, McVitie's*	1 Biscuit/17g	78.0	3.0	459	7.2	68.6	17.3	3.2
Digestive, Milk Chocolate, GFY, Asda*	1 Biscuit/17g	78.0	3.0	457	7.0	69.0	17.0	3.2
Digestive, Milk Chocolate, Homewheat, McVitie's*	1 Biscuit/17g	83.0	4.0	486	6.0	61.5	24.0	4.0
Digestive, Milk Chocolate, M & S*	1 Biscuit/17g	85.0	4.0	505	6.1	62.2	26.0	2.6
Digestive, Milk Chocolate, Mini, McVitie's*	1 Bag/25g	124.0	6.0	496	6.6	61.9	24.7	2.9
Digestive, Milk Chocolate, Mini, Tesco*	1 Pack/30g	153.0	8.0	510	6.6	59.8	27.1	1.8
Digestive, Milk Chocolate, Sainsbury's*	1 Biscuit/17g	87.0	6.0	511	6.9	65.9	36.8	2.5
Digestive, Milk Chocolate, Tesco*	1 Biscuit/17g	84.0	4.0	497	6.8	62.4	24.5	2.7
Digestive, Milk Chocolate, Trufree*	1 Biscuit/12g	63.0	3.0	521	4.0	70.0	25.0	2.0

BISCUITS

INFO/WEIGHT	Measure per Measure KCAL	FAT	Nutrition Values per 100g / 100ml KCAL	PROT	CARB	FAT	FIBRE
Digestive, Oat, Weight Watchers*	1 Biscuit/11g 50.0	2.0	457	6.0	66.3	18.6	6.9
Digestive, Organic, Sainsbury's*	1 Biscuit/12g 60.0	3.0	483	6.6	60.9	23.7	5.8
Digestive, Organic, Tesco*	1 Biscuit/13g 60.0	3.0	464	7.7	66.3	20.8	4.6
Digestive, Plain	1 Biscuit/14g 66.0	3.0	471	6.3	68.6	20.9	2.2
Digestive, Plain Chocolate, Asda*	1 Biscuit/17g 84.0	4.0	500	7.0	64.0	24.0	3.2
Digestive, Plain Chocolate, Tesco*	1 Biscuit/17g 85.0	4.0	499	6.2	63.5	24.4	2.8
Digestive, Plain Chocolate, Value, Tesco*	1 Biscuit/14g 71.0	4.0	497	6.5	62.2	24.7	3.1
Digestive, Plain, M & S*	1 Biscuit/16g 80.0	4.0	490	6.5	62.7	23.8	3.3
Digestive, Reduced Fat, M & S*	1 Biscuit/16g 75.0	3.0	480	7.2	73.3	17.5	3.4
Digestive, Reduced Fat, McVitie's*	1 Biscuit/15g 70.0	2.0	467	7.1	72.8	16.3	3.4
Digestive, Reduced Fat, Tesco*	1 Biscuit/16g 70.0	3.0	453	7.0	69.1	16.6	3.4
Digestive, Smart Price, Asda*	1 Biscuit/14g 67.0	3.0	465	6.0	65.3	20.0	3.1
Digestive, Sweetmeal, Asda*	1 Biscuit/14g 68.0	3.0	499	7.0	66.0	23.0	3.5
Digestive, Sweetmeal, Sainsbury's*	1 Biscuit/14g 72.0	3.0	498	6.0	66.4	23.1	3.3
Digestive, Sweetmeal, Tesco*	1 Biscuit/18g 80.0	3.0	444	8.4	70.0	14.5	3.1
Digestive, Trufree*	1 Biscuit/10g 45.0	2.0	454	2.1	71.0	21.0	2.4
Digestive, Value, Tesco*	1 Biscuit/15g 73.0	3.0	490	6.9	64.0	22.4	3.3
Digestive, with Wheatgerm, Hovis*	1 Biscuit/12g 37.0	2.0	306	6.2	66.8	18.5	5.8
Digestives, Milk Chocolate, McVitie's*	1 Biscuit/17g 84.0	4.0	488	6.7	62.7	23.4	2.9
Dips, Toffee, KP Snacks*	1 Pot/32g 171.0	10.0	534	4.4	62.2	29.7	1.2
Double Choc Chip, Trufree*	1 Biscuit/11g 58.0	3.0	523	3.0	67.0	27.0	1.8
Extremely Chocolatey Orange, M & S*	1 Biscuit/24g 120.0	6.0	510	7.5	59.9	26.5	2.7
Figfuls, Go Ahead, McVitie's*	1 Biscuit/15g 54.0	1.0	355	4.2	76.8	4.6	2.9
First Class, Bahlsen*	1 Serving/125g 711.0	45.0	569	7.5	53.4	36.2	0.0
Florentines, Sainsbury's*	1 Florentine/8g 40.0	2.0	506	10.0	47.2	30.8	7.0
for Cheese, Bran Cracker, Christmas, Tesco*	1 Biscuit/28g 127.0	5.0	454	9.7	62.8	18.2	3.2
for Cheese, Chive Cracker, Christmas, Tesco*	1 Biscuit/28g 125.0	4.0	448	9.3	66.6	16.0	2.4
for Cheese, Cornish Wafer, Christmas, Tesco*	1 Biscuit/28g 148.0	9.0	530	8.0	56.8	31.2	2.4
for Cheese, Cream Cracker, Christmas, Tesco*	1 Biscuit/28g 118.0	4.0	421	9.9	71.9	12.7	5.1
for Cheese, Digestive, Hovis, Christmas, Tesco*	1 Biscuit/28g 127.0	5.0	453	4.2	74.6	18.2	7.0
for Cheese, Poppy Snack, Christmas, Tesco*	1 Biscuit/28g 129.0	5.0	461	10.0	64.4	18.2	3.1
for Cheese, Sesame Carlton, Christmas, Tesco*	1 Biscuit/28g 133.0	6.0	476	9.1	61.5	21.5	2.7
for Cheese, Whole Grain, Christmas, Tesco*	1 Biscuit/28g 128.0	5.0	458	9.0	63.9	18.5	4.1
Fruit & Fibre, Breakfast, Belvita, Nabisco*	1 Biscuit/13g 56.0	2.0	430	7.5	64.0	16.0	7.8
Fruit Shortcake, McVitie's*	1 Biscuit/8g 37.0	2.0	464	5.7	65.1	20.1	2.7
Fruit Shortcake, Sainsbury's*	1 Biscuit/8g 39.0	2.0	483	5.9	69.6	20.1	2.1
Fruit Shortcake, Tesco*	1 Biscuit/9g 43.0	2.0	473	5.8	70.1	18.8	1.9
Fruit Shrewsbury, Mini Pack, Paterson's*	1 Biscuit/17g 81.0	4.0	483	4.9	64.9	22.7	1.9
Fruit, All Butter, Sainsbury's*	1 Biscuit/9g 45.0	2.0	477	5.6	66.0	21.2	1.9
Fruity Iced, Blue Parrot Cafe, Sainsbury's*	1 Pack/20g 83.0	1.0	415	6.0	82.0	7.0	1.1
Fruity Oat, Dove's Farm*	1 Biscuit/17g 79.0	4.0	471	7.6	62.7	21.1	4.0
Fudge Flavour Choc Chip, Go Eat*	1 Biscuit/15g 76.0	4.0	510	6.5	59.2	27.4	1.7
Galettes, Bonne Maman*	1 Serving/90g 460.0	22.0	511	6.0	65.7	25.0	0.0
Garibaldi, Asda*	1 Biscuit/10g 39.0	1.0	375	4.7	68.5	9.1	2.2
Garibaldi, Sainsbury's*	1 Biscuit/9g 35.0	1.0	389	5.7	67.1	10.9	3.3
Garibaldi, Tesco*	1 Biscuit/10g 40.0	1.0	400	4.7	74.0	9.1	2.2
Garibaldi, Waitrose*	1oz/28g 109.0	3.0	389	5.7	67.1	10.9	1.3
Ginger Crinkle Crunch, Fox's*	1 Biscuit/12g 50.0	1.0	435	4.7	75.3	12.5	1.6
Ginger Crinkle, Sainsbury's*	1 Biscuit/11g 53.0	3.0	486	6.2	63.8	22.9	2.9
Ginger Crunch Creams, Fox's*	1 Biscuit/14g 73.0	4.0	518	4.6	64.8	26.7	0.0
Ginger Crunch, Hand Baked, Border*	1 Biscuit/12g 54.0	2.0	470	4.7	71.4	20.4	0.0
Ginger Crunches, Organic, Against the Grain*	1 Biscuit/15g 71.0	3.0	474	2.8	65.6	23.0	1.2
Ginger Nuts, Asda*	1 Biscuit/10g 45.0	1.0	447	5.0	73.0	15.0	0.0

BISCUITS

	Measure INFO/WEIGHT	per Measure KCAL	FAT	Nutrition Values per 100g / 100ml KCAL	PROT	CARB	FAT	FIBRE
Ginger Nuts, Milk Chocolate, McVitie's*	1 Biscuit/14g	68.0	3.0	489	5.8	71.8	19.9	1.5
Ginger Nuts, Tesco*	1 Biscuit/8g	36.0	1.0	450	5.8	73.1	14.7	2.0
Ginger Snap, BGTY, Sainsbury's*	1 Biscuit/12g	51.0	1.0	427	6.5	78.2	9.8	1.8
Ginger Snap, Fox's*	1 Biscuit/8g	35.0	1.0	443	4.6	77.1	12.8	1.5
Ginger Snap, Less Than 10% Fat, Sainsbury's*	1 Biscuit/12g	51.0	1.0	424	6.5	78.9	9.1	1.9
Ginger Snap, Sainsbury's*	1 Biscuit/11g	47.0	2.0	445	5.3	73.0	14.7	2.2
Ginger Snaps, Trufree*	1 Biscuit/11g	51.0	2.0	467	2.5	76.0	17.0	1.5
Ginger Thins, Anna's*	1 Biscuit/2g	10.0	0.0	480	6.0	67.0	20.0	0.4
Ginger Thins, Asda*	1 Biscuit/5g	23.0	1.0	462	6.0	73.0	16.0	1.9
Ginger, Safeway*	1 Biscuit/12g	55.0	2.0	456	5.9	73.9	15.3	1.7
Ginger, Traditional, Fox's*	1 Biscuit/8g	33.0	1.0	404	4.4	70.1	11.7	1.4
Gingered, Duchy Originals*	1 Biscuit/16g	74.0	3.0	472	6.0	64.8	21.0	2.5
Gingernut	1 Biscuit/11g	50.0	2.0	456	5.6	79.1	15.2	1.4
Golden Crunch Creams, Fox's*	1 Biscuit/15g	75.0	4.0	515	4.7	64.8	26.3	1.2
Golden Crunch, Bronte*	1 Biscuit/14.6g	69.0	3.0	474	5.1	62.5	22.6	0.0
Golden Crunch, Go Ahead, McVitie's*	1 Biscuit/9g	38.0	1.0	419	7.7	75.2	9.7	2.1
Golden Crunch, Paterson's*	1 Biscuit/15g	69.0	3.0	474	5.1	62.5	22.6	4.8
Golden Shortie, Jacob's*	1 Biscuit/11g	54.0	3.0	492	6.0	64.9	23.2	0.0
Golden Syrup, McVitie's*	1 Biscuit/12g	63.0	3.0	508	5.1	67.3	24.2	2.2
Happy Faces, Jacob's*	1 Biscuit/16g	78.0	4.0	485	4.8	66.1	22.3	1.6
Hazelnut Crispies, Occasions, Sainsbury's*	1 Biscuit/7g	36.0	2.0	518	6.0	64.3	26.3	0.0
Hazelnut Meringue, Sainsbury's*	1 Biscuit/6g	24.0	1.0	404	5.0	43.0	23.5	1.1
Hob Nobs, Chocolate Creams, McVitie's*	1 Biscuit/12g	60.0	3.0	503	6.7	60.3	26.1	4.0
Hob Nobs, Light, 25% Reduced Fat, McVitie's*	1 Biscuit/14g	62.0	2.0	435	8.1	64.6	16.1	6.2
Hob Nobs, McVitie's*	1 Biscuit/14.4g	67.0	3.0	466	7.1	60.8	21.7	5.5
Hob Nobs, Milk Chocolate, McVitie's*	1 Biscuit/19g	92.0	4.0	479	6.8	60.7	23.3	4.5
Hob Nobs, Milk Chocolate, Mini, McVitie's*	1 Pack/25g	121.0	6.0	483	6.6	61.3	23.5	4.4
Hob Nobs, Munch Bites, McVitie's*	1 Pack/40g	203.0	10.0	508	6.8	63.4	25.2	2.8
Hob Nobs, Plain Chocolate, McVitie's*	1 Biscuit/16g	81.0	4.0	498	6.7	63.3	24.3	4.2
Hob Nobs, Vanilla Creams, McVitie's*	1 Biscuit/12g	60.0	3.0	501	6.1	62.3	25.2	3.6
Honeycomb Nibbles, High Lights, Cadbury*	1 Bag/16g	75.0	3.0	465	6.2	73.4	16.2	1.8
Iced Gems, Jacob's*	1 Portion/30g	116.0	1.0	388	5.0	85.5	2.9	1.5
Jaffa Cakes, Asda*	1 Cake/12g	43.0	1.0	368	4.7	67.5	8.8	1.9
Jaffa Cakes, Blackcurrant, McVitie's*	1 Cake/12g	45.0	1.0	371	4.8	69.7	8.1	2.3
Jaffa Cakes, Dark Chocolate, M & S*	1 Cake/11g	45.0	2.0	395	3.7	64.9	13.2	2.8
Jaffa Cakes, Dark Chocolate, Mini, M & S*	1 Cake/5g	20.0	1.0	410	3.9	62.8	15.8	1.9
Jaffa Cakes, Free From, Asda*	1 Cake/12g	42.0	1.0	340	5.8	62.6	7.4	8.0
Jaffa Cakes, Lemon & Lime, McVitie's*	1 Cake/12.2g	45.0	1.0	370	4.7	69.5	8.1	2.1
Jaffa Cakes, Lunch Box, McVitie's*	1 Cake/7g	26.0	1.0	395	4.2	74.3	9.0	1.4
Jaffa Cakes, McVitie's*	1 Cake/12g	45.0	1.0	374	4.8	70.6	8.0	2.1
Jaffa Cakes, Mini Roll XI, McVitie's*	1 Cake/44g	169.0	5.0	384	3.5	66.9	11.4	0.0
Jaffa Cakes, Mini Roll, McVitie's*	1 Cake/30g	115.0	3.0	382	3.5	67.2	11.0	1.3
Jaffa Cakes, Mini, Asda*	1 Cake/5g	21.0	1.0	412	3.9	63.0	16.0	1.9
Jaffa Cakes, Mini, Bags, McVitie's*	1 Cake/5g	20.0	1.0	396	4.2	65.0	13.1	3.5
Jaffa Cakes, Mini, Orange Pods, McVitie's*	1 Cake/40g	150.0	3.0	380	4.3	71.2	8.7	3.5
Jaffa Cakes, Mini, Tesco*	1 Cake/5g	19.0	1.0	380	4.0	64.0	12.0	2.0
Jaffa Cakes, Plain Chocolate, Sainsbury's*	1 Cake/13g	50.0	1.0	384	4.4	73.3	8.1	1.3
Jaffa Cakes, Sainsbury's*	1 Cake/11g	41.0	1.0	373	4.3	69.3	8.8	2.0
Jaffa Cakes, Smart Price, Asda*	1 Cake/11.5g	43.0	1.0	374	4.3	69.0	9.0	2.0
Jaffa Cakes, Value, Tesco*	1 Cake/11g	42.0	1.0	370	4.8	67.6	8.8	1.9
Jam Creams, Jacob's*	1 Biscuit/15g	75.0	3.0	486	5.0	67.4	21.8	1.6
Jam Rings, Crawfords*	1 Biscuit/12g	56.0	2.0	470	5.5	73.0	17.2	1.9
Jam Sandwich Creams, M & S*	1 Biscuit/17g	80.0	4.0	485	5.7	64.5	22.6	1.8

B

BISCUITS

	Measure INFO/WEIGHT	per Measure KCAL	FAT	Nutrition Values per 100g / 100ml KCAL	PROT	CARB	FAT	FIBRE
Jam Sandwich Creams, Sainsbury's*	1 Biscuit/16g	77.0	3.0	486	5.0	67.0	21.8	1.6
Jammie Dodgers, Minis. Lunchbox, Burton's*	1 Pack/20g	90.0	3.0	452	5.5	72.7	14.7	2.5
Jammie Dodgers, Original, Burton's*	1 Biscuit/19g	83.0	3.0	437	5.1	69.5	15.9	1.9
Jestives, Milk Chocolate, Cadbury*	1 Biscuit/17g	86.0	4.0	506	6.4	64.4	24.8	0.0
Kimberley, Bolands*	1 Biscuit/16g	72.0	2.0	449	5.1	82.6	10.9	1.4
Lebkuchen, Sainsbury's*	1 Biscuit/10g	39.0	1.0	400	5.7	76.1	8.0	1.3
Lemon Butter, Thins, Sainsbury's*	1 Biscuit/13g	65.0	4.0	515	5.3	60.7	27.9	2.2
Lemon Curd Sandwich, Fox's*	1 Biscuit/14g	69.0	3.0	494	4.7	66.2	23.4	1.3
Lemon Puff, Jacob's*	1 Biscuit/13g	69.0	4.0	533	4.3	58.8	31.2	2.8
Lemon Thins, Sainsbury's*	1 Biscuit/10g	47.0	2.0	468	5.6	72.3	17.3	1.7
Lemon, All Butter, Half Coated, Finest, Tesco*	1 Biscuit/17g	84.0	4.0	505	5.6	60.4	26.9	3.6
Lincoln, McVitie's*	1 Biscuit/8g	41.0	2.0	514	6.3	69.0	23.6	2.0
Lincoln, Sainsbury's*	1 Biscuit/8g	40.0	2.0	479	7.2	66.1	20.6	2.1
Malt, Basics*	1 Biscuit/8g	36.0	1.0	470	7.1	73.6	15.7	0.0
Malted Milk, Asda*	1 Biscuit/8g	39.0	2.0	490	7.0	66.0	22.0	2.0
Malted Milk, Chocolate, Tesco*	1 Biscuit/10g	52.0	2.0	500	6.7	64.4	24.0	1.9
Malted Milk, Milk Chocolate, Asda*	1 Biscuit/11g	56.0	3.0	509	7.0	64.0	25.0	1.7
Malted Milk, Sainsbury's*	1 Biscuit/8g	40.0	2.0	488	7.1	65.5	21.9	2.0
Malted Milk, Tesco*	1 Biscuit/9g	43.0	2.0	490	6.6	66.7	21.8	2.0
Marie, Crawfords*	1 Biscuit/7g	33.0	1.0	475	7.5	76.3	15.5	2.3
Melts, Carr's*	1 Biscuit/4g	20.0	1.0	468	11.0	58.3	21.2	4.9
Milk & Cereals, Breakfast, Belvita, Nabisco*	1 Biscuit/13g	58.0	2.0	445	8.7	69.0	15.0	3.6
Milk Chocolate, All Butter, M & S*	1 Biscuit/14g	70.0	4.0	490	7.9	57.4	25.5	1.4
Milk Chocolate, Assortment, Cadbury*	1 Serving/10g	51.0	3.0	510	6.8	61.0	26.4	0.0
Milk Chocolate, Tesco*	1 Biscuit/25g	135.0	7.0	535	6.4	62.1	29.0	1.8
Mini Assortment, M & S*	1 Biscuit/2.5g	12.0	1.0	480	6.1	63.9	22.5	2.8
Mint, Plain Chocolate, Tesco*	1 Biscuit/25g	136.0	7.0	538	5.1	63.0	29.5	1.7
Mint, Viscount*	1 Biscuit/13g	73.0	4.0	552	5.1	60.6	28.8	1.3
Mixed Seed & Honey, Oaty, Weight Watchers*	1 Biscuit/22g	106.0	5.0	482	9.2	59.0	23.2	4.9
Morning Coffee, Asda*	1 Biscuit/5g	22.0	1.0	455	8.0	72.0	15.0	2.4
Morning Coffee, Tesco*	1 Biscuit/5g	22.0	1.0	450	7.6	72.3	14.5	2.4
Nice, Asda*	1 Biscuit/8g	38.0	2.0	480	6.0	68.0	21.0	2.4
Nice, Cream, Tesco*	1 Serving/10g	50.0	2.0	503	5.3	66.2	24.1	1.9
Nice, Fox's*	1 Biscuit/9g	39.0	2.0	450	6.3	62.4	19.4	5.0
Nice, Jacob's*	1 Biscuit/7g	33.0	1.0	471	6.1	68.5	19.2	1.8
Nice, Sainsbury's*	1 Biscuit/8g	40.0	2.0	486	5.9	68.3	20.9	2.7
Nice, Value, Multipack, Tesco*	1 Biscuit/8g	39.0	2.0	485	6.5	68.0	20.8	2.4
Nice, Value, Tesco*	1 Biscuit/5g	24.0	1.0	489	6.9	64.6	22.6	2.4
Nobbles, Milk Chocolate, Trufree*	1 Biscuit/13g	67.0	4.0	513	7.4	55.7	29.0	4.0
Oat & Chocolate Chip, Cadbury*	1 Biscuit/16.5g	80.0	4.0	485	6.9	60.2	23.9	4.2
Oat & Wholemeal, Crawfords*	1 Biscuit/14g	67.0	3.0	482	7.7	64.2	21.6	4.8
Oat & Wholemeal, Dbc Foodservice*	1 Biscuit/14g	67.0	3.0	466	7.1	60.8	21.7	5.5
Oat Crunch, Weight Watchers*	1 Biscuit/11.5g	52.0	2.0	448	7.4	65.2	17.8	6.1
Oat Digestives, Nairn's*	1 Biscuit/11.4g	50.0	2.0	437	12.0	57.8	17.5	7.8
Oat, Fruit & Spice, Nairn's*	1 Biscuit/10g	43.0	1.0	425	7.8	65.3	14.7	7.6
Oat, Mixed Berries, Nairn's*	1 Biscuit/10g	43.0	1.0	430	7.7	67.0	14.6	5.9
Oat, Santiveri*	1 Biscuit/5g	23.0	1.0	428	10.0	58.8	17.0	7.0
Oat, Stem Ginger, Nairn's*	1 Biscuit/10g	43.0	2.0	434	8.8	65.6	15.2	6.1
Oaten, Organic, Duchy Originals*	1 Biscuit/16g	71.0	3.0	441	9.8	62.3	16.9	5.3
Oatmeal Crunch, Jacob's*	1 Biscuit/8g	37.0	1.0	458	6.8	65.9	18.6	3.6
Oatmeal, Asda*	1 Biscuit/12g	54.0	3.0	470	6.0	62.0	22.0	6.0
Orange Chocolate, Organic, Duchy Originals*	1 Biscuit/13g	64.0	4.0	509	5.5	60.0	28.0	3.0
Orange Sultana, Go Ahead, McVitie's*	1 Biscuit/15g	58.0	1.0	400	5.1	75.7	8.1	3.0

BISCUITS

	Measure INFO/WEIGHT	per Measure		Nutrition Values per 100g / 100ml				
		KCAL	FAT	KCAL	PROT	CARB	FAT	FIBRE
Parmesan Cheese, Sainsbury's*	1 Biscuit/3g	18.0	1.0	553	14.7	56.4	29.9	1.8
Party Rings, Iced, Fox's*	1 Biscuit/6g	29.0	1.0	459	5.1	75.8	15.0	0.0
Peanut Butter, American Style, Sainsbury's*	1 Biscuit/13g	63.0	3.0	504	5.2	68.7	23.1	2.2
Petit Beurre, Stella Artois*	1 Biscuit/6g	26.0	1.0	440	9.0	73.0	15.0	0.0
Pink Wafers, Crawfords*	1 Biscuit/7g	36.0	2.0	521	2.5	68.6	26.5	1.1
Pink Wafers, Sainsbury's*	1 Biscuit/8g	36.0	2.0	486	4.6	64.2	23.4	1.7
Puffin, Chocolate, Asda*	1 Biscuit/25g	133.0	7.0	533	5.0	63.0	29.0	1.2
Puffin, Orange, Asda*	1 Biscuit/25g	133.0	7.0	529	5.0	62.0	29.0	2.2
Redcurrant Puffs, Eat Well, M & S*	1 Biscuit/7g	32.0	1.0	470	5.6	67.7	19.8	2.0
Rich Shorties, Asda*	1 Biscuit/10g	50.0	2.0	486	6.0	66.0	22.0	2.0
Rich Tea Creams, Fox's*	1 Biscuit/11g	52.0	2.0	456	5.3	62.7	20.4	1.4
Rich Tea Finger, Tesco*	1 Finger/5g	23.0	1.0	451	7.4	72.9	14.4	2.3
Rich Tea Fingers, Morrisons*	1 Finger/4g	18.0	1.0	448	7.2	72.5	14.3	3.0
Rich Tea, 25% Less Fat, Tesco*	1 Biscuit/10g	43.0	1.0	435	7.1	77.0	11.0	1.3
Rich Tea, Asda*	1 Biscuit/10g	45.0	1.0	447	7.0	71.0	15.0	2.3
Rich Tea, Basics, Sainsbury's*	1 Biscuit/8g	35.0	1.0	450	7.1	71.3	15.2	2.9
Rich Tea, BGTY, Sainsbury's*	1 Biscuit/10g	43.0	1.0	430	7.8	75.9	10.6	2.4
Rich Tea, Classic, McVitie's*	1 Biscuit/8g	38.0	1.0	453	7.1	71.2	15.5	2.9
Rich Tea, Light, McVitie's*	1 Biscuit/8g	36.0	1.0	431	7.5	75.0	11.3	3.1
Rich Tea, Low Fat, M & S*	1 Biscuit/9g	40.0	1.0	435	8.3	76.7	10.5	2.4
Rich Tea, Milk Chocolate Covered, Cadbury*	1 Biscuit/12g	60.0	3.0	490	6.6	67.6	21.4	0.0
Rich Tea, Milk Chocolate, Sainsbury's*	1 Biscuit/13g	66.0	3.0	504	6.3	68.5	22.7	2.1
Rich Tea, Plain Chocolate, Sainsbury's*	1 Biscuit/13g	65.0	3.0	497	6.6	66.0	23.0	2.6
Rich Tea, Sainsbury's*	1 Biscuit/8g	34.0	1.0	440	7.2	72.7	13.4	3.0
Rich Tea, Tesco*	1 Biscuit/10g	45.0	2.0	454	7.4	71.5	15.4	2.3
Rich Tea, Value, Tesco*	1 Biscuit/8g	35.0	1.0	453	7.2	72.4	15.0	2.3
Riva Milk, McVitie's*	1 Biscuit/25g	136.0	8.0	540	6.4	57.7	31.5	1.6
Rocky Rounds, Caramel, Fox's*	1 Biscuit/15g	72.0	3.0	480	6.2	62.3	22.9	1.1
Rocky, Chocolate & Caramel, Fox's*	1 Biscuit/21.1g	107.0	4.0	507	6.9	60.3	19.3	15.5
Rocky, Chocolate, Fox's*	1 Biscuit/24.5g	125.0	7.0	510	7.3	58.7	27.0	1.7
Rolo, Nestle*	1 Biscuit/22g	110.0	6.0	498	5.4	62.0	25.4	0.6
Rosemary & Raisin, M & S*	1 Biscuit/7g	35.0	2.0	490	5.1	62.5	24.1	1.8
Rosemary & Thyme, Savoury, Weight Watchers*	1 Biscuit/8g	33.0	1.0	419	8.1	55.0	18.7	13.1
Savoury, Gluten, Wheat & Dairy Free, Sainsbury's*	1 Biscuit/17g	77.0	3.0	467	11.7	65.1	17.7	2.4
Savoury, Organic, M & S*	1 Biscuit/7g	28.0	1.0	395	7.0	58.4	14.6	8.7
Shortcake Ring, Creations, Fox's*	1 Biscuit/20g	105.0	6.0	515	7.8	59.1	27.4	1.0
Shortcake, Asda*	1 Biscuit/14g	73.0	4.0	518	5.0	66.0	26.0	2.0
Shortcake, Caramel, Mini, Finest, Tesco*	1 Biscuit/15g	74.0	4.0	493	4.3	56.3	27.8	1.0
Shortcake, Caramel, Mr Kipling*	1 Biscuit/36g	182.0	10.0	506	4.2	57.6	28.8	1.3
Shortcake, Caramel, Squares, M & S*	1 Square/40g	190.0	10.0	475	5.5	59.7	23.9	1.0
Shortcake, Caramel, Tesco*	1 Biscuit/45g	217.0	12.0	482	4.6	57.8	25.8	0.5
Shortcake, Caramel, The Handmade Flapjack Company*	1 Biscuit/75g	383.0	23.0	511	4.6	54.3	30.6	0.0
Shortcake, Crawfords*	1 Biscuit/10g	53.0	3.0	518	6.4	68.1	24.4	2.0
Shortcake, Dutch, M & S*	1 Biscuit/17g	90.0	5.0	530	5.7	58.2	30.6	0.9
Shortcake, Fruit Biscuits, Crawfords*	1 Biscuit/8g	34.0	2.0	419	5.4	55.9	19.3	2.4
Shortcake, Jacob's*	1 Biscuit/10g	48.0	2.0	485	6.7	65.6	21.8	2.0
Shortcake, Organic, Waitrose*	1 Biscuit/13g	64.0	3.0	495	5.8	63.0	24.4	1.8
Shortcake, Sainsbury's*	1 Biscuit/11g	53.0	5.0	479	6.1	65.3	47.2	2.5
Shortcake, Snack, Cadbury*	1 Biscuit/10g	52.0	3.0	520	7.0	62.6	26.8	0.0
Shortcake, with Real Milk Chocolate, Cadbury*	1 Biscuit/15g	75.0	4.0	500	6.3	65.8	23.5	0.0
Shorties, Cadbury*	1 Biscuit/15g	77.0	4.0	511	6.5	67.3	24.0	0.0
Shorties, Fruit, Value, Tesco*	1 Serving/10g	46.0	2.0	457	5.7	69.3	17.4	3.0
Shorties, Rich Highland, Tesco*	1 Biscuit/10g	48.0	2.0	485	6.1	65.3	21.7	2.6

	Measure INFO/WEIGHT	per Measure KCAL	per Measure FAT	Nutrition Values per 100g / 100ml KCAL	PROT	CARB	FAT	FIBRE
BISCUITS								
Shorties, Rich, Tesco*	1 Biscuit/10g	48.0	2.0	484	6.4	65.6	21.8	2.0
Shorties, Sainsbury's*	1 Biscuit/10g	50.0	2.0	500	6.4	69.8	21.8	2.0
Signature Collection, Cadbury*	1 Biscuit/15g	79.0	4.0	530	6.2	60.1	29.5	0.0
Sports, Fox's*	1 Biscuit/8.5g	41.0	2.0	483	6.7	67.0	20.0	2.0
Stem Ginger, Brakes*	1 Biscuit/12.5g	62.0	3.0	495	5.6	62.6	24.7	0.0
Sticks, Chocolate, COU, M & S*	1 Biscuit/4g	15.0	0.0	370	10.4	77.0	2.6	4.4
Strawberry, Cream Tease, McVitie's*	1 Biscuit/19g	97.0	5.0	510	4.8	65.9	25.2	1.2
Sugar Wafers, Vanilla, Flavoured, Triunfo*	1 Biscuit/10.4g	53.0	3.0	511	4.1	70.1	24.3	0.6
Sultana & Cinnamon, Weight Watchers*	1 Biscuit/11.5g	51.0	2.0	441	4.3	72.3	15.0	3.0
Tangy Jaffa Viennese, Creations, Fox's*	1 Biscuit/17g	76.0	3.0	447	5.0	63.5	19.2	0.9
Taxi, McVitie's*	1 Biscuit/27g	134.0	7.0	504	4.2	63.3	26.0	0.7
Teddy Bear, Mini, M & S*	1 Biscuit/16.8g	80.0	4.0	475	5.4	62.6	22.7	3.2
Toffee Chip Crinkle Crunch, Fox's*	1 Biscuit/11g	51.0	2.0	460	4.6	69.6	18.2	0.0
Treacle Crunch Creams, Fox's*	1 Biscuit/13g	65.0	3.0	502	4.5	65.3	24.8	1.4
Triple Chocolate, Fox's*	1 Biscuit/21g	100.0	5.0	478	5.7	57.3	25.1	2.5
Viennese Creams, Raspberry, M & S*	1 Biscuit/17g	90.0	5.0	520	4.6	60.4	28.6	1.3
Viennese Creams, Strawberry, M & S*	1 Biscuit/17g	80.0	4.0	485	6.4	63.0	22.2	1.7
Viennese Finger, Mr Kipling*	1 Finger/32g	167.0	10.0	523	4.3	54.9	31.8	0.0
Viennese Whirl, Chocolate, Border*	1 Biscuit/19g	96.0	4.0	512	6.5	61.9	23.2	0.0
Viennese Whirl, Fox's*	1 Biscuit/25g	129.0	7.0	518	6.7	60.1	27.8	0.0
Viennese, Jaffa, M & S*	1 Biscuit/17g	80.0	4.0	465	5.9	61.1	21.7	0.9
Viennese, Sandwich, Chocolate, M & S*	1 Biscuit/15g	80.0	5.0	535	7.2	58.0	30.6	1.7
Wafer, Vanilla, Loacker*	1 Pack/45g	231.0	13.0	514	7.5	58.0	28.0	0.0
Water, Average	1oz/28g	123.0	3.0	440	10.8	75.8	12.5	3.1
Water, High Bake, Jacob's*	1 Biscuit/5g	22.0	0.0	414	10.5	76.4	7.4	3.0
Water, Table, Carr's*	1 Biscuit/7.5g	30.0	1.0	400	9.9	73.1	7.5	4.1
White Chocolate, M & S*	1oz/28g	150.0	8.0	535	6.8	60.8	29.3	0.7
Wholemeal Brans, Fox's*	1 Biscuit/20g	90.0	4.0	451	8.5	58.8	20.2	7.5
Yorkie, Nestle*	1 Biscuit/25g	127.0	7.0	510	6.7	60.4	26.8	1.3
Yumbles, Oat Nibbles, Organic, McVitie's*	1 Biscuit/11g	50.0	3.0	449	7.9	53.2	22.7	6.6
BISON								
Raw	*1oz/28g*	*31.0*	*1.0*	*109*	*21.6*	*0.0*	*1.8*	*0.0*
Roasted	*1oz/28g*	*41.0*	*1.0*	*143*	*28.4*	*0.0*	*2.4*	*0.0*
BITTER LEMON								
Low Calorie, Tesco*	1 Glass/200ml	6.0	0.0	3	0.1	0.3	0.1	0.1
Sainsbury's*	1 Glass/250ml	45.0	0.0	18	0.1	4.4	0.1	0.1
Schweppes*	1 Glass/250ml	85.0	0.0	34	0.0	8.2	0.0	0.0
BLACK PUDDING								
Average	*1 Serving/40g*	*101.0*	*6.0*	*252*	*10.2*	*19.0*	*14.9*	*0.6*
BLACKBERRIES								
Fresh, Raw, Average	*1oz/28g*	*8.0*	*0.0*	*29*	*0.8*	*6.0*	*0.3*	*1.5*
in Fruit Juice, Average	*½ Can/145g*	*52.0*	*0.0*	*36*	*0.6*	*7.9*	*0.2*	*1.3*
BLACKCURRANTS								
Fresh, Raw	*1oz/28g*	*8.0*	*0.0*	*28*	*0.9*	*6.6*	*0.0*	*3.6*
in Fruit Juice, Average	*1 Serving/30g*	*11.0*	*0.0*	*37*	*0.6*	*8.6*	*0.1*	*2.4*
Stewed with Sugar	*1oz/28g*	*16.0*	*0.0*	*58*	*0.7*	*15.0*	*0.0*	*2.8*
Stewed without Sugar	*1oz/28g*	*7.0*	*0.0*	*24*	*0.8*	*5.6*	*0.0*	*3.1*
BLINIS								
Cocktail, M & S*	½ Pack/81g	154.0	2.0	190	6.3	35.9	2.3	2.0
Sausage, Cocktail, Waitrose*	1 Blini/16g	30.0	0.0	190	6.3	35.9	2.3	2.0
Smoked Salmon, M & S*	1oz/28g	67.0	4.0	240	11.9	18.9	13.0	1.8
BLUEBERRIES								
Chocolate Covered, Waitrose*	1 Serving/25g	120.0	6.0	481	4.0	65.6	22.4	3.0

B

	Measure INFO/WEIGHT		per Measure		Nutrition Values per 100g / 100ml				
			KCAL	FAT	KCAL	PROT	CARB	FAT	FIBRE
BLUEBERRIES									
Dried, Whitworths*	1 Pack/75g		226.0	0.0	301	0.9	74.2	0.1	11.4
Fresh, Raw, Average	*1 Serving/80g*		*43.0*	*0.0*	*53*	*0.8*	*12.6*	*0.3*	*2.1*
Frozen, Sainsbury's*	1 Serving/80g		26.0	0.0	32	0.6	6.9	0.2	1.8
BOAR									
Wild, Raw, Average	*1 Serving/200g*		*244.0*	*7.0*	*122*	*21.5*	*0.0*	*3.3*	*0.0*
BOILED SWEETS									
Average	1oz/28g		92.0	0.0	327	0.0	87.1	0.0	0.0
Blackcurrant & Liquorice, Co-Op*	1 Sweet/8g		32.0	0.0	405	0.9	91.0	5.0	0.0
Cherry Drops, Bassett's*	1 Sweet/5g		18.0	0.0	390	0.0	98.1	0.0	0.0
Clear Fruits, Sainsbury's*	1 Sweet/7g		26.0	0.0	372	0.1	92.9	0.0	0.0
Cough Sweets, Fundays, Bassett's*	1oz/28g		107.0	0.0	383	0.0	94.9	0.0	0.0
Fruit Drops, Co-Op*	1 Sweet/6g		24.0	0.0	395	0.2	98.0	0.0	0.0
Fruit Rocks, Assorted, M & S*	1oz/28g		107.0	0.0	381	0.0	95.2	0.0	0.0
Fruit Sherbets, Assorted, M & S*	1 Sweet/8g		34.0	1.0	425	0.0	89.7	7.3	0.0
Lockets, Mars*	1 Pack/43g		165.0	0.0	383	0.0	95.8	0.0	0.0
Mentho-Lyptus, Cherry, Sugar Free, Hall's*	1 Lozenge/3.6g		8.0	0.0	234	0.0	62.4	0.0	0.0
Mentho-Lyptus, Extra Strong, Hall's*	1 Lozenge/4g		14.0	0.0	389	0.0	96.9	0.0	0.0
Pear Drops, Bassett's*	1 Sweet/4g		16.0	0.0	390	0.0	96.4	0.0	0.0
Soothers, Blackcurrant, Hall's*	1 Lozenge/4.5g		16.0	0.0	365	0.0	91.4	0.0	0.0
Soothers, Cherry, Hall's*	1 Pack/45.2g		165.0	0.0	365	0.0	91.3	0.0	0.0
BOK CHOY									
Tesco*	1 Serving/100g		11.0	0.0	11	1.0	1.4	0.2	1.2
BOLOGNESE									
Beef, 2 Minute Meals, Sainsbury's*	1 Pack/200g		144.0	7.0	72	4.2	5.6	3.6	1.8
Beef, Asda*	1 Pack/392g		412.0	20.0	105	8.0	7.0	5.0	0.0
Beef, Diet Chef Ltd*	1 Serving/300g		246.0	7.0	82	7.7	7.6	2.3	3.4
Extra Meaty, M & S*	1oz/28g		25.0	1.0	90	10.4	5.5	2.7	0.0
Fusilli, Ready Meals, M & S*	1oz/28g		38.0	2.0	135	7.0	13.1	6.2	1.0
Meatless, Granose*	1 Pack/400g		400.0	16.0	100	8.0	8.0	4.0	0.0
Pasta Shells, Canned, 98% Fat Free, BGTY, Sainsbury's*	½ Can/200g		174.0	4.0	87	5.5	11.5	2.1	0.7
Penne, Heinz*	1 Pack/300g		213.0	3.0	71	3.8	11.8	0.9	0.6
Shells, Italiana, Weight Watchers*	1 Can/395g		280.0	5.0	71	5.2	9.6	1.3	0.7
Tagliatelle, Weight Watchers*	1 Serving/300g		300.0	5.0	100	5.5	15.4	1.8	0.1
Vegetarian, M & S*	1 Pack/360g		360.0	13.0	100	4.5	12.5	3.5	2.1
BOMBAY MIX									
Average	1oz/28g		141.0	9.0	503	18.8	35.1	32.9	6.2
BON BONS									
Apple, Lemon & Strawberry, Co-Op*	¼ Bag/50g		202.0	2.0	405	1.0	88.0	5.0	0.0
Bassett's*	1 Sweet/7g		28.0	0.0	417	1.1	85.4	7.5	0.0
Fruit, Bassett's*	1 Serving/7g		25.0	0.0	380	0.1	94.2	0.0	0.0
Lemon, Bassett's*	1 Sweet/7g		30.0	1.0	425	0.0	83.7	9.8	0.0
BOOST									
Standard Bar, Cadbury*	1 Bar/60.5g		305.0	17.0	510	5.8	57.0	28.5	0.9
Treat Size, Cadbury*	1 Bar/24g		130.0	7.0	535	5.3	59.6	30.5	0.0
with Glucose & Guarana, Cadbury*	1 Bar/61g		314.0	18.0	515	5.5	56.7	29.5	0.0
with Glucose, Cadbury*	1 Bar/60.5g		315.0	18.0	521	5.6	58.0	29.4	4.0
BOUILLON									
Beef, Benedicta*	1 fl oz/30ml		22.0	0.0	73	7.5	9.5	0.5	0.0
Chicken, Benedicta*	1 fl oz/30ml		22.0	1.0	75	4.0	8.0	3.0	5.6
Fish, Benedicta*	1 fl oz/30ml		21.0	0.0	69	7.5	9.0	0.3	0.0
Powder, Miso, Marigold*	1 Tsp/5g		12.0	0.0	248	7.0	34.0	9.3	1.4
Powder, Swiss Vegetable, Green Tub, Marigold*	1 Tsp/5g		12.0	0.0	243	10.5	29.4	8.1	0.7
Vegetable, Benedicta*	1 fl oz/30ml		30.0	0.0	101	7.5	17.0	0.3	0.0

B

	Measure INFO/WEIGHT	per Measure KCAL	FAT	Nutrition Values per 100g / 100ml KCAL	PROT	CARB	FAT	FIBRE
BOUILLON								
Vegetable, Herbamare Concentre*	1 Serving/5g	15.0	1.0	298	4.6	13.5	25.4	0.3
BOUNTY								
Calapuno, Mars*	1 Pack/175g	919.0	55.0	525	6.3	54.3	31.4	0.0
Dark, Mars*	1 Funsize/29g	137.0	8.0	471	3.2	54.1	26.8	0.0
Milk, Mars*	1 Funsize/29g	137.0	7.0	471	3.7	56.4	25.6	0.0
BOURNVITA								
Powder, Made Up with Semi-Skimmed Milk	1 Mug/227ml	132.0	4.0	58	3.5	7.8	1.6	0.0
Powder, Made Up with Whole Milk	1 Mug/227ml	173.0	9.0	76	3.4	7.6	3.8	0.0
BOVRIL								
Beef Extract, Bovril*	1 Tsp/5g	10.0	0.0	197	10.8	29.3	4.1	0.0
Chicken Savoury Drink, Bovril*	1 Serving/13g	16.0	0.0	129	9.7	19.4	1.4	2.1
BOYSENBERRIES								
Canned, in Syrup	*1oz/28g*	*25.0*	*0.0*	*88*	*1.0*	*20.4*	*0.1*	*1.6*
BRANDY								
37.5% Volume, Average	*1 Shot/35ml*	*72.0*	*0.0*	*207*	*0.0*	*0.0*	*0.0*	*0.0*
40% Volume, Average	*1 Shot/35ml*	*78.0*	*0.0*	*222*	*0.0*	*0.0*	*0.0*	*0.0*
Cherry, Average	*1 Shot/35ml*	*89.0*	*0.0*	*255*	*0.0*	*32.6*	*0.0*	*0.0*
BRAZIL NUTS								
Average	*6 Whole/20g*	*137.0*	*14.0*	*687*	*15.5*	*2.9*	*68.3*	*4.9*
Milk Chocolate, Tesco*	1 Nut/8g	47.0	3.0	585	9.9	38.0	43.7	1.9
BREAD								
50/50, Wholemeal & White, Medium Sliced, Kingsmill*	1 Slice/40g	90.0	1.0	225	9.9	41.2	2.3	4.9
Apple Sourdough, Gail's*	1 Slice/50g	118.0	0.0	236	7.5	43.9	0.7	4.3
Apricot & Sesame Seed, Lifefibre*	1 Slice/43g	148.0	4.0	344	8.1	55.0	10.3	6.2
Arabic, El Amar Bakery*	1 Serving/110g	318.0	1.0	289	11.6	57.9	1.2	0.0
Bagel, Caramelised Onion & Poppyseed, Waitrose*	1 Bagel/86g	222.0	2.0	258	9.7	49.2	2.5	2.4
Bagel, Chocolate Chip, Mini, Ixxy's*	1 Bagel/35.5g	89.0	1.0	251	9.3	49.4	1.8	3.7
Bagel, Cinnamon & Raisin, New York Bagel Co*	1 Bagel/85g	215.0	2.0	253	7.7	51.1	2.0	4.5
Bagel, Cinnamon & Raisin, Tesco*	1 Bagel/85g	223.0	2.0	262	10.3	51.0	1.9	2.1
Bagel, Granary, Bagel Factory*	1 Bagel/99.9g	288.0	2.0	288	11.9	57.4	2.1	4.5
Bagel, High Bran & Seed, with Cranberry, The Food Doctor*	1 Bagel/85g	212.0	2.0	250	10.8	47.4	1.9	6.7
Bagel, Mini, Sainsbury's*	1 Bagel/25g	67.0	0.0	268	11.2	52.4	1.6	2.8
Bagel, Multigrain, Mini, Ixxy's*	1 Bagel/39g	105.0	1.0	270	9.2	50.3	3.5	6.3
Bagel, Multigrain, Sainsbury's*	1 Bagel/113g	293.0	4.0	259	10.0	49.6	3.1	2.0
Bagel, Onion, New York Bagel Co*	1 Bagel/85g	222.0	2.0	261	10.6	50.3	1.9	3.1
Bagel, Onion, Tesco*	1 Bagel/85g	233.0	2.0	274	10.5	52.4	2.4	1.9
Bagel, Original, Organic, New York Bagel Co*	1 Bagel/85g	220.0	1.0	259	9.3	52.2	1.4	4.1
Bagel, Plain, Average	*1 Bagel/78g*	*215.0*	*1.0*	*276*	*10.7*	*53.6*	*1.5*	*0.0*
Bagel, Poppy Seed, New York Bagel Co*	1 Bagel/85g	233.0	2.0	274	11.4	50.8	2.8	3.2
Bagel, Rye, Bagel Factory*	1 Bagel/85g	279.0	1.0	329	14.5	64.3	1.5	6.2
Bagel, Sesame Seed, GFY, Asda*	1 Bagel/84g	227.0	2.0	271	11.0	51.0	2.5	2.6
Bagel, Sesame, M & S*	1 Bagel/87g	240.0	3.0	275	10.2	51.2	3.2	2.1
Bagel, Sesame, New York Bagel Co*	1 Bagel/85g	226.0	3.0	266	10.3	49.2	3.1	4.0
Bagel, White, Asda*	1 Bagel/86g	227.0	3.0	264	10.0	49.0	3.1	0.0
Bagel, White, Original, Weight Watchers*	1 Bagel/66g	142.0	1.0	215	9.5	42.4	0.8	10.7
Bagel, Wholemeal, Multiseed, M & S*	1 Bagel/84g	215.0	6.0	255	13.1	35.4	6.6	8.3
Baguette, Cheese, & Onion, Asda*	¼ Loaf/42g	154.0	7.0	366	12.0	39.8	17.6	1.3
Baguette, Crusty Brown, M & S*	½ Loaf/71.1g	160.0	1.0	225	9.8	42.7	1.6	6.3
Baguette, French, Tesco*	1 Serving/60g	144.0	1.0	240	7.8	49.5	1.2	3.4
Baguette, Garlic, Reduced Fat, Asda*	¼ Loaf/43g	107.0	3.0	249	8.1	39.9	6.3	2.7
Baguette, Granary, Co-Op*	1 Serving/60g	150.0	1.0	250	20.0	46.0	2.5	6.0
Baguette, Harvester, French Style, Somerfield*	1 Serving/110g	276.0	2.0	251	10.6	47.9	1.9	3.7
Baguette, Mediterranean Herb, Sainsbury's*	1 Serving/60g	203.0	9.0	339	8.5	40.8	15.7	2.3

BREAD

INFO/WEIGHT	Measure	per Measure KCAL	FAT	Nutrition Values per 100g / 100ml KCAL	PROT	CARB	FAT	FIBRE
Baguette, Part Baked, Classique, Deli France, Delifrance*	1 Pack/250g	745.0	3.0	298	9.8	54.8	1.2	2.7
Baguette, Paysanne, Stonebaked, Asda*	1/6 Loaf/46g	119.0	1.0	259	10.0	48.0	3.0	3.3
Baguette, Ready to Bake, Sainsbury's*	½ Baguette/62g	150.0	1.0	242	7.8	49.7	1.3	2.8
Baguette, Soft Bake, Somerfield*	1 Serving/60g	170.0	1.0	284	10.3	57.3	1.5	1.9
Baguette, Sourdough, la Brea Bakery*	1 Serving/60g	160.0	0.0	266	8.8	56.1	0.7	1.8
Baguette, White, Homebake, Tesco*	1 Baguette/135g	331.0	2.0	245	7.8	49.7	1.3	2.5
Baguette, White, Ready to Bake, Asda*	1 Serving/60g	168.0	1.0	280	10.0	56.0	1.8	2.6
Baguette, White, Sainsbury's*	1 Serving/50g	131.0	1.0	263	9.3	53.1	1.5	2.7
Baguette, White, Sandwich, Somerfield*	1 Serving/60g	155.0	1.0	259	9.4	52.1	1.4	1.7
Baguette, Wholemeal, Part Baked, Asda*	½ Baguette/75g	176.0	1.0	235	8.2	47.7	1.3	3.0
Baguette, Wholemeal, Part Baked, Mini, Landgut*	½ Baguette/25g	56.0	0.0	223	7.5	46.0	1.0	0.0
Baps, Brown, Large, Asda*	1 Bap/58g	140.0	1.0	242	10.0	47.0	1.6	0.0
Baps, Brown, Malted Grain, Large, Tesco*	1 Bap/93g	228.0	3.0	245	9.9	42.7	3.3	5.3
Baps, Cheese Top, Sainsbury's*	1 Bap/75g	218.0	6.0	291	12.1	41.6	8.5	2.0
Baps, Floured, M & S*	1 Bap/60g	168.0	4.0	280	11.5	46.8	6.2	2.0
Baps, Giant Malted, Sainsbury's*	1 Bap/109g	282.0	5.0	260	8.6	45.7	4.8	5.7
Baps, Multigrain, Tesco*	1 Serving/98g	238.0	3.0	244	8.7	45.1	3.2	1.9
Baps, White Sandwich, Kingsmill*	1 Bap/80g	209.0	3.0	261	10.1	46.2	4.0	2.2
Baps, White, Floured, Waitrose*	1 Bap/60g	147.0	1.0	244	8.0	48.6	2.0	1.1
Baps, White, Giant, Sainsbury's*	1 Bap/86g	235.0	3.0	273	8.3	51.7	3.7	3.4
Baps, White, Giant, Waitrose*	1 Bap/104g	260.0	4.0	250	9.5	45.0	3.6	4.8
Baps, White, Large, Tesco*	1 Bap/95g	252.0	4.0	265	8.7	46.2	4.5	2.4
Baps, White, Sliced, Large, Asda*	1 Bap/58g	148.0	1.0	255	10.0	50.0	1.7	0.0
Baps, White, Soft, Floured, M & S*	1 Bap/63g	176.0	4.0	280	11.5	46.8	6.2	2.0
Baps, White, Warburton's*	1 Bap/57g	144.0	2.0	252	9.8	43.4	4.3	2.7
Baps, Wholemeal, Giant, Rathbones*	1 Bap/110g	230.0	2.0	209	9.4	39.0	1.9	8.0
Baps, Wholemeal, Large, Tesco*	1 Bap/95g	223.0	4.0	235	10.5	39.1	4.1	7.6
Baps, Wholemeal, Tesco*	1 Bap/46g	104.0	2.0	227	9.6	41.4	5.3	5.6
Baps, Wholemeal, Waitrose*	1 Bap/67g	156.0	3.0	234	10.6	37.2	4.8	6.7
Best of Both, Farmhouse, Hovis*	1 Slice/44g	99.0	1.0	226	9.5	40.0	3.1	4.9
Best of Both, White, Wheatgerm, Sliced, Hovis*	1 Med Slice/40g	86.0	1.0	214	9.0	40.4	1.8	5.0
Black Olive, Finest, Tesco*	1 Serving/72g	184.0	5.0	255	9.7	39.7	6.4	2.9
Bloomer, COU, M & S*	1 Slice/33g	78.0	0.0	235	9.5	45.5	1.5	3.6
Bloomer, Multi Seed, Organic, Sainsbury's*	1 Serving/60g	160.0	4.0	266	10.9	40.3	6.8	8.8
Bloomer, Multi Seed, Sliced, M & S*	1 Slice/54g	150.0	4.0	280	10.5	43.6	7.2	3.1
Bloomer, Multiseed, Finest, Tesco*	1 Slice/50g	100.0	2.0	200	12.8	28.4	3.8	11.1
Bloomer, Multiseed, TTD, Sainsbury's*	1 Slice/50g	119.0	2.0	239	12.0	39.7	3.6	8.8
Bloomer, Soft Grain, M & S*	1 Slice/34g	80.0	1.0	235	9.5	45.5	1.5	3.6
Bloomer, Vienna, M & S*	1oz/28g	79.0	1.0	281	9.6	55.8	2.1	2.7
Bloomer, White, Sliced, Waitrose*	1 Slice/50g	129.0	1.0	259	8.5	52.1	1.8	2.6
Bloomer, Wholemeal, Organic, M & S*	1 Slice/50g	110.0	2.0	220	10.2	35.5	4.2	6.4
Brioche, Continental Classics*	1 Roll/35g	122.0	3.0	349	8.2	58.3	9.3	0.0
Brioche, Finest, Tesco*	1 Roll/52g	207.0	12.0	398	10.8	38.3	22.4	2.0
Brioche, Loaf, Butter, Sainsbury's*	1/8 Loaf/50g	173.0	5.0	347	8.0	55.0	10.5	2.2
Brioche, Rolls, Butter, Tesco*	1 Serving/35g	127.0	4.0	363	8.6	56.0	11.4	3.7
Brioche, Rolls, Tesco*	1 Roll/26g	92.0	3.0	349	8.5	54.0	11.0	0.0
Brown, Danish, Sliced, Weight Watchers*	1 Slice/20.4g	44.0	0.0	216	11.3	38.7	2.0	7.3
Brown, Danish, Warburton's*	1 Slice/21g	44.0	0.0	213	11.1	38.9	1.9	7.2
Brown, Farmhouse, Linwoods*	1 Slice/25g	56.0	0.0	225	7.3	44.4	1.7	5.8
Brown, Gluten & Wheat Free, Sliced	1 Slice/25g	56.0	1.0	224	3.4	41.0	5.2	9.4
Brown, Gluten Free, Genius*	1 Slice/35g	97.0	5.0	277	6.7	42.2	13.3	9.5
Brown, Good Health, Warburton's*	1 Slice/35g	79.0	1.0	226	10.3	39.6	2.9	7.2
Brown, Granary Malted, thick Sliced, Waitrose*	1 Slice/40g	95.0	1.0	238	9.4	44.8	2.3	5.1

B

B

BREAD

	Measure INFO/WEIGHT	per Measure KCAL	FAT	Nutrition Values per 100g / 100ml KCAL	PROT	CARB	FAT	FIBRE
Brown, Harvest, M & S*	1oz/28g	67.0	1.0	240	8.8	44.5	2.7	3.7
Brown, High Fibre, Ormo*	1 Slice/24g	57.0	1.0	239	9.2	42.9	2.6	7.5
Brown, Honey & Oat Bran, Vogel*	1 Serving/100g	220.0	4.0	220	7.9	39.2	4.5	5.7
Brown, Irwin's Bakery*	1 Slice/64g	137.0	0.0	214	10.4	41.8	0.6	6.1
Brown, Kingsmill Gold, Seeds & Oats, Kingsmill*	1 Slice/45g	126.0	4.0	280	12.2	35.6	9.8	4.9
Brown, Malted, Farmhouse Gold, Morrisons*	1 Slice/38g	94.0	1.0	248	8.2	49.6	1.4	3.0
Brown, Medium Sliced	*1 Slice/34g*	*74.0*	*1.0*	*218*	*8.5*	*44.3*	*2.0*	*3.5*
Brown, Mixed Grain, Original, Vogel*	1 Slice/45g	102.0	1.0	227	9.8	47.1	1.2	6.4
Brown, Multi Grain, Wheat Free, Gluten Free	1 Slice/33.2g	76.0	2.0	229	5.1	40.8	5.1	5.6
Brown, Sainsbury's*	1 Slice/34g	81.0	1.0	239	8.4	46.8	2.1	4.2
Brown, Seeded Batch, Large Loaf, 800g, Warburton's*	1 Slice/45.8g	132.0	4.0	288	12.3	39.7	8.9	6.0
Brown, Sliced, By Brennans, Weight Watchers*	1 Slice/20g	42.0	0.0	209	9.5	38.1	2.1	5.8
Brown, Sliced, Free From, Tesco*	1 Slice/45g	121.0	4.0	268	5.4	43.2	8.2	3.6
Brown, Soda, M & S*	1 Slice/40g	92.0	1.0	229	9.2	43.6	3.6	4.9
Brown, Soy & Linseed, Vogel*	1 Slice/50g	116.0	2.0	232	11.2	33.3	4.9	7.0
Brown, Sunflower & Barley, Vogel*	1 Slice/50g	120.0	3.0	240	8.8	39.9	6.1	5.4
Brown, Thick Slice, Tesco*	1 Serving/50g	109.0	1.0	219	10.3	38.9	2.5	5.3
Brown, Thick, Warburton's*	1 Slice/38g	80.0	1.0	211	9.4	39.2	1.8	6.2
Brown, Thin Sliced, Sainsbury's*	1 Slice/29g	65.0	1.0	225	8.2	43.8	1.9	3.9
Brown, Toasted, Average	*1 Med Slice/24g*	*65.0*	*1.0*	*272*	*10.4*	*56.5*	*2.1*	*4.5*
Brown, Toastie, Thick Sliced, Kingsmill*	1 Slice/44g	101.0	1.0	230	9.5	40.5	3.3	4.7
Brown, Wholemeal, Healthy Choice, Warburton's*	1 Slice/23.8g	55.0	1.0	231	10.4	40.7	2.5	6.5
Buns, Burger, American Style, Sainsbury's*	1 Bun/50g	131.0	2.0	261	10.5	45.6	4.1	3.6
Buns, Burger, Sainsbury's*	1 Bun/56g	154.0	3.0	275	9.2	47.8	5.2	4.1
Buns, Burger, Sesame, Sliced, Tesco*	1 Bun/60g	168.0	4.0	280	7.9	47.3	6.6	2.1
Buns, Burger, with Sesame Seeds, Co-Op*	1 Bun/55g	143.0	3.0	260	9.0	44.0	5.0	2.0
Buns, White, Burger, Waitrose*	1 Serving/64g	169.0	2.0	264	10.0	47.2	3.9	2.7
Buns, White, Stay Fresh, Tesco*	1 Bun/56g	152.0	4.0	271	7.5	45.5	6.6	0.0
Challah, Average	*1 Slice/50g*	*143.0*	*4.0*	*286*	*8.9*	*53.6*	*7.1*	*3.6*
Cholla, Average	*1/10 Loaf/154g*	*421.0*	*14.0*	*274*	*6.9*	*40.8*	*9.3*	*1.0*
Ciabatta Stick, Organic, M & S*	1 Stick/140g	315.0	2.0	225	8.9	48.5	1.4	4.2
Ciabatta, Black Olive, Part Baked, Sainsbury's*	¼ Ciabatta/67g	172.0	3.0	257	8.8	46.8	3.8	2.4
Ciabatta, Finest, Tesco*	1/6 Ciabatta/45g	124.0	3.0	275	10.4	44.8	5.9	2.7
Ciabatta, Garlic & Herb, GFY, Asda*	¼ Ciabatta/60g	137.0	1.0	230	8.8	43.2	2.4	1.0
Ciabatta, Garlic, Mini, Italiano, Tesco*	½ Ciabatta/47g	150.0	7.0	320	8.2	38.5	14.6	2.8
Ciabatta, Garlic, TTD, Sainsbury's*	1 Serving/67g	199.0	8.0	298	8.3	38.7	12.2	3.1
Ciabatta, Green Olive, Tesco*	¼ Ciabatta/70g	155.0	3.0	222	7.4	38.2	4.4	1.9
Ciabatta, Italian Style, Safeway*	¼ Ciabatta/75g	193.0	3.0	258	8.9	47.7	3.5	2.2
Ciabatta, Italian Style, Waitrose*	1 Ciabatta/89g	231.0	1.0	260	10.7	51.2	1.3	2.2
Ciabatta, Olive & Rosemary, Mini, Tesco*	1 Pack/75g	319.0	8.0	425	17.8	63.0	10.9	3.6
Ciabatta, Olive, Safeway*	1 Serving/25g	59.0	1.0	238	8.2	43.7	3.4	2.3
Ciabatta, Part Baked, Half, Sainsbury's*	½ Ciabbatta/67g	174.0	2.0	260	8.9	47.7	3.7	2.2
Ciabatta, Plain, Tesco*	¼ Ciabatta/73g	174.0	3.0	240	9.8	41.5	3.9	2.4
Ciabatta, Ready to Bake, M & S*	1 Serving/150g	393.0	6.0	262	10.3	48.1	4.1	2.1
Ciabatta, Ready to Bake, Sainsbury's*	½ Ciabatta/66g	172.0	2.0	260	8.9	47.7	3.7	2.2
Ciabatta, Spicy Topped, Finest, Tesco*	1 Serving/73g	163.0	4.0	223	9.2	34.0	5.5	1.7
Ciabatta, Square, Bake At Home, Part Baked, Asda*	1 Roll/59.9g	157.0	2.0	262	8.4	49.1	3.5	2.1
Ciabatta, Sun Dried Tomato & Basil, Tesco*	¼ Ciabatta/75g	193.0	4.0	257	8.9	42.4	5.7	2.4
Ciabatta, Tomato & Basil, GFY, Asda*	1 Serving/55g	143.0	1.0	260	9.0	51.0	2.2	0.0
Ciabatta, Tomato & Mozzarella, Iceland*	1 Ciabatta/150g	373.0	15.0	249	10.0	29.6	10.1	3.3
Ciabatta, TTD, Sainsbury's*	¼ Pack/68g	185.0	4.0	274	10.4	44.8	5.9	2.7
Cinnamon Swirl, Asda*	1 Serving/25g	87.0	3.0	349	6.0	52.0	13.0	1.6
Cottage Loaf, Stonebaked, Asda*	1 Serving/67g	155.0	1.0	232	10.0	45.0	1.3	3.2

BREAD

	Measure INFO/WEIGHT	per Measure KCAL	FAT	Nutrition Values per 100g / 100ml KCAL	PROT	CARB	FAT	FIBRE
Crostini, Olive Oil, TTD, Sainsbury's*	1 Roll/4g	16.0	0.0	409	11.4	72.2	8.3	3.3
Danish, White, Medium Sliced, Tesco*	1 Slice/20g	47.0	0.0	234	9.4	45.4	1.7	3.3
Danish, White, Thick Sliced, Tesco*	1 Slice/24g	60.0	1.0	250	9.7	47.4	2.3	2.9
Farl, Irish Soda, Irwin's Bakery*	1 Farl/150g	334.0	5.0	223	4.0	44.0	3.4	2.3
Farmhouse, Poppy Seed, Crusty, Loaf, M & S*	1 Slice/40g	104.0	1.0	260	9.4	47.6	3.3	2.3
Farmhouse, with Oatmeal, Batch, Finest, Tesco*	1 Slice/50g	122.0	2.0	245	10.5	40.8	4.3	4.9
Fiery Green Pepper & Cheese, The Best, Safeway*	¼ Loaf/75g	180.0	3.0	240	12.3	38.4	4.1	3.4
Fig & Almond, Bröderna Cartwright*	4 Slices/100g	267.0	7.0	267	9.2	39.7	7.5	0.0
Flatbread, Garlic & Herb, Tear & Share, Sainsbury's*	¼ Bread/68g	201.0	6.0	297	10.9	42.5	9.3	3.7
Flatbread, Garlic, BGTY, Sainsbury's*	¼ Bread/56g	177.0	6.0	316	9.6	46.6	10.1	2.7
Flatbread, Garlic, Tesco*	1 Serving/83g	249.0	9.0	302	6.7	45.3	10.4	3.0
Flatbread, Tomato & Garlic, Italian Style, Iceland*	1 Serving/75g	195.0	9.0	260	6.3	32.3	11.8	2.4
Flatbread, Tomato & Garlic, Sainsbury's*	1/3 Bread/73g	191.0	5.0	261	8.4	41.7	6.7	3.4
Focaccia, Mini, Sun Dried Tomato & Basil, Sainsbury's*	1oz/28g	90.0	4.0	321	8.0	41.8	13.6	0.0
Focaccia, Onion & Herb, Tesco*	½ Pack/190g	547.0	24.0	288	8.7	35.2	12.5	3.7
Focaccia, Oregano, The Best, Safeway*	1 Serving/56g	150.0	3.0	270	9.1	45.0	5.7	1.8
Focaccia, Roast Cherry Tomato & Olive, GFY, Asda*	½ Pack/148g	350.0	6.0	237	9.0	41.0	4.1	2.8
Focaccia, Roasted Onion & Cheese, M & S*	1 Serving/89g	240.0	4.0	270	10.4	45.7	4.6	2.8
Focaccia, Safeway*	1/6 Bread/47g	131.0	3.0	279	9.5	46.9	5.9	3.4
Fougasse, Caramelised Onion & Cheese, Tesco*	1oz/28g	80.0	2.0	284	11.1	43.1	6.3	3.5
Fougasse, Garlic & Gruyere, TTD, Sainsbury's*	¼ Bread/76g	219.0	7.0	288	9.5	42.6	8.9	2.9
French	1.5" Slice/45g	110.0	0.0	244	8.9	53.3	0.0	2.2
French Stick, Average	*1 Serving/60g*	*162.0*	*2.0*	*270*	*9.6*	*55.4*	*2.7*	*1.5*
Fruit & Cinnamon Loaf, Finest, Tesco*	1 Slice/37g	134.0	5.0	363	6.4	54.6	13.2	1.5
Fruit Loaf, Apple & Cinnamon, Soreen*	1 Serving/10g	31.0	0.0	307	6.9	60.5	4.2	0.0
Fruit Loaf, Apple, M & S*	1 Slice/39g	100.0	1.0	255	8.5	51.9	1.5	3.3
Fruit Loaf, Banana, Soreen*	1 Slice/25g	78.0	1.0	313	6.8	60.9	4.7	0.0
Fruit Loaf, Luxury, Christmas, Soreen*	1 Serving/28g	85.0	1.0	303	4.5	66.6	2.1	0.0
Fruit Loaf, Mixed Berry, Weight Watchers*	1 Slice/34g	79.0	1.0	231	7.6	44.3	2.6	7.7
Fruit Loaf, Mother's Pride*	1 Slice/36g	92.0	1.0	256	8.2	49.3	2.9	2.6
Fruit Loaf, Sliced, Asda*	1 Serving/33g	89.0	1.0	269	8.0	51.0	3.7	2.9
Fruit Loaf, Sliced, Sainsbury's*	1 Slice/40g	104.0	1.0	260	8.9	47.9	3.6	2.4
Fruit Loaf, Sliced, Tesco*	1 Slice/36g	100.0	2.0	278	6.9	51.2	5.1	3.7
Fruit Loaf, Sultana & Cherry, Sainsbury's*	1 Slice/50g	178.0	6.0	357	2.7	59.0	12.2	1.7
Fruit Loaf, with Strawberry, Summer, Warburton's*	1 Slice/35g	92.0	1.0	262	7.7	50.3	3.3	3.0
Fruit, Raisin Swirl, Sun-Maid*	1 Slice/33g	95.0	2.0	287	8.3	50.4	5.8	2.6
Fruited, Malt Loaf, Weight Watchers*	1 Serving/23g	68.0	0.0	294	8.9	60.2	1.9	3.6
Fruited, Richly, Waitrose*	1 Serving/34g	95.0	2.0	279	10.4	49.3	4.5	3.1
Garlic & Cheese Slices, Italiano, Tesco*	1 Slice/31.3g	95.0	4.0	304	9.0	39.7	11.8	2.6
Garlic Slices, Asda*	1 Slice/26.8g	88.0	3.0	328	8.0	46.2	12.4	2.8
Garlic, & Cheese, Tesco*	1 Serving/143g	490.0	24.0	343	9.4	38.5	16.8	2.0
Garlic, & Herb, Giant Feast, Sainsbury's*	1 Serving/50g	158.0	6.0	317	8.0	42.1	12.9	2.6
Garlic, & Herb, Tear & Share, Tesco*	1 Serving/73g	217.0	9.0	300	6.3	40.0	12.7	1.7
Garlic, & Parsley, Tesco*	1 Loaf/230g	699.0	27.0	304	9.0	41.0	11.6	2.7
Garlic, & Tomato, Pizza, Italiano, Tesco*	½ Bread/140g	405.0	15.0	289	7.5	40.5	10.8	2.5
Garlic, 25% Less Fat, Sainsbury's*	½ Baguette/85g	268.0	12.0	315	7.8	39.4	14.0	3.1
Garlic, 30% Less Fat, Morrisons*	1 Serving/80g	231.0	7.0	289	7.9	43.8	9.2	2.7
Garlic, Baguette, 25% Less Fat, Tesco*	1 Serving/100g	292.0	11.0	292	7.0	40.7	11.3	1.8
Garlic, Baguette, 50% Less Fat, Asda*	¼ Baguette/43g	123.0	3.0	287	10.0	46.0	7.0	2.5
Garlic, Baguette, Extra Strong, Sainsbury's*	½ Baguette/85g	278.0	13.0	327	8.4	40.0	14.8	3.4
Garlic, Baguette, Frozen, GFY, Asda*	¼ Baguette/48g	132.0	4.0	277	7.0	42.0	9.0	2.7
Garlic, Baguette, Italian, Asda*	¼ Baguette/48g	173.0	9.0	364	7.0	39.0	20.0	3.4
Garlic, Baguette, Light Choices, Tesco*	¼ Baguette/52g	130.0	3.0	250	7.0	42.2	5.5	2.4

B

BREAD

	Measure INFO/WEIGHT	per Measure KCAL	per Measure FAT	Nutrition Values per 100g / 100ml KCAL	PROT	CARB	FAT	FIBRE
Garlic, Baguette, Mediterranean Herb, Tesco*	¼ Baguette/54g	181.0	9.0	335	6.9	40.3	16.3	2.3
Garlic, Baguette, Morrisons*	½ Baguette/95g	295.0	14.0	311	6.3	37.8	15.0	1.5
Garlic, Baguette, Organic, Tesco*	1 Serving/60g	192.0	8.0	320	8.5	41.1	13.5	2.5
Garlic, Baguette, Reduced Fat, Waitrose*	½ Baguette/85g	229.0	7.0	270	8.1	41.5	8.0	2.7
Garlic, Baguette, Sainsbury's*	½ Baguette/85g	342.0	16.0	403	8.9	48.6	19.2	2.3
Garlic, Baguette, Waitrose*	½ Baguette/85g	290.0	15.0	341	7.1	37.8	17.9	0.0
Garlic, Baguette, with Cheese, HL, Tesco*	1 Serving/50g	114.0	1.0	229	9.4	43.0	2.2	2.1
Garlic, Ciabatta, & Herb Butter, Sainsbury's*	½ Ciabatta/105g	345.0	16.0	329	8.5	38.8	15.5	0.0
Garlic, Ciabatta, BGTY, Sainsbury's*	½ Ciabatta/105g	306.0	13.0	291	8.7	36.2	12.4	2.7
Garlic, Ciabatta, Finest, Tesco*	1 Serving/65g	205.0	9.0	316	8.1	40.1	13.7	2.4
Garlic, Ciabatta, Hand Stretched, Sainsbury's*	¼ Pack/75g	244.0	11.0	325	8.4	41.0	14.1	2.9
Garlic, Ciabatta, HL, Tesco*	¼ Ciabatta/60g	151.0	3.0	251	8.6	44.6	4.2	2.6
Garlic, Ciabatta, Italian, Sainsbury's*	1 Serving/145g	454.0	17.0	313	10.0	41.6	11.8	2.9
Garlic, Ciabatta, Italiano, Tesco*	1 Ciabatta/65g	211.0	9.0	324	7.7	40.9	14.4	2.2
Garlic, Ciabatta, with Herbs, Weight Watchers*	1 Pack/88g	216.0	4.0	245	9.2	43.0	4.0	2.9
Garlic, Finest, Tesco*	¼ Loaf/60g	187.0	8.0	311	7.7	40.3	13.2	1.8
Garlic, Focaccia, & Onion, GFY, Asda*	¼ Focaccia/55g	150.0	2.0	272	12.0	47.0	4.0	0.0
Garlic, Focaccia, & Rosemary, Sainsbury's*	¼ Focaccia/75g	219.0	7.0	292	8.0	43.0	9.8	2.8
Garlic, Foccacia, & Rosemary, Tesco*	¼ Loaf/73g	193.0	5.0	266	9.0	42.1	6.8	3.7
Garlic, Homebake, Tesco*	1 Serving/60g	209.0	12.0	348	7.1	33.7	20.5	1.5
Garlic, Italian Style Stone Baked, Morrisons*	½ Pack/115g	420.0	22.0	365	7.9	40.4	19.1	1.9
Garlic, Micro, McCain*	½ Bread/54g	202.0	10.0	374	7.8	45.1	18.0	0.0
Garlic, Organic, Waitrose*	1 Baguette/170g	535.0	23.0	315	8.7	39.1	13.7	1.8
Garlic, Pizza Bread, Co-Op*	1 Pizza/240g	756.0	31.0	315	8.0	41.0	13.0	2.0
Garlic, Reduced Fat, Waitrose*	1 Pack/170g	551.0	19.0	324	6.9	49.4	11.0	0.9
Garlic, Slices, BGTY, Sainsbury's*	1 Slice/27g	82.0	2.0	305	9.4	48.9	8.0	2.9
Garlic, Slices, Chilled, Sainsbury's*	1 Pack/368g	1369.0	60.0	372	9.1	47.3	16.3	3.2
Garlic, Slices, GFY, Asda*	1 Slice/31g	80.0	1.0	259	8.9	48.1	3.3	3.0
Garlic, Slices, HL, Tesco*	1 Slice/52g	131.0	2.0	251	8.6	44.6	4.2	2.6
Garlic, Slices, Italian, Chilled, Tesco*	1 Slice/27g	110.0	6.0	415	6.2	46.8	22.4	2.7
Garlic, Slices, Light Choices, Tesco*	1 Slice/30g	75.0	2.0	250	7.3	42.3	5.7	2.9
Garlic, Stonebaked, M & S*	1 Loaf/85g	263.0	10.0	310	9.3	41.4	11.9	3.1
Garlic, to Share, M & S*	¼ Loaf/82g	230.0	11.0	280	6.5	33.2	13.0	1.3
Garlic, with Cheese, Asda*	1 Slice/34g	130.0	6.0	382	11.0	44.0	18.0	0.0
Granary White, Hovis*	1 Slice/44g	102.0	2.0	233	9.7	40.8	3.5	5.6
Granary, Average	*1 Slice/35g*	*82.0*	*1.0*	*235*	*9.3*	*46.3*	*2.7*	*4.3*
Granary, Baps, Large, Asda*	1 Bap/64g	143.0	1.0	224	10.0	41.0	2.2	4.3
Granary, Country, Multiseeded, Hovis*	1 Slice/44g	96.0	1.0	218	11.1	37.0	2.9	6.5
Granary, Malted, Medium Brown, Asda*	1 Slice/35g	81.0	1.0	231	9.0	43.0	2.6	3.3
Granary, Oatmeal, Hovis*	1 Slice/44.1g	104.0	1.0	236	9.2	45.3	2.1	3.1
Granary, Original, All Sizes, Hovis*	1 Sm Slice/33g	82.0	1.0	248	10.3	46.4	2.4	3.7
Granary, Seeded, Sunflower, Hovis*	1 Slice/44g	119.0	3.0	271	10.1	44.9	5.7	2.9
Granary, Thick Slice, COU, M & S*	1 Slice/25g	60.0	1.0	240	10.5	44.1	2.2	6.0
Granary, Waitrose*	1 Slice/40g	88.0	1.0	220	9.4	39.9	2.5	4.3
Granary, White, Seeded, Medium Sliced, Hovis*	1 Slice/44g	109.0	2.0	248	10.9	41.7	4.2	3.8
Granary, Wholemeal, Hovis*	1 Slice/44g	98.0	1.0	223	10.6	39.8	2.4	6.8
Granary, Wholemeal, Seeded, Medium Sliced, Hovis*	1 Slice/33g	72.0	1.0	218	11.1	37.0	2.9	6.5
Hi Bran, M & S*	1 Slice/26g	55.0	1.0	210	12.6	32.5	3.0	6.3
Hi Fibre, Seed, Lifefibre*	1 Slice/35g	109.0	4.0	313	12.5	43.6	10.1	2.7
Hot Cross Bun, Loaf, Warburton's*	1 Slice/35g	94.0	1.0	269	8.3	50.4	3.7	2.9
Khobez, Flatbread, White, Dina Foods Ltd*	1 Bread/56g	158.0	1.0	282	10.5	57.5	1.1	3.0
Lavash, Flax, Oat bran, Whole Flour, Wrap, Joseph's*	1 Serving/32g	50.0	2.0	156	15.6	21.9	6.2	9.4
Light Grain, Eat Smart, Safeway*	1 Slice/27g	65.0	1.0	245	9.7	45.5	2.5	3.5

BREAD

INFO/WEIGHT	Measure	KCAL	FAT	KCAL	PROT	CARB	FAT	FIBRE
		per Measure		Nutrition Values per 100g / 100ml				
Malt Loaf, Family, Asda*	1 Serving/20g	54.0	0.0	270	8.0	56.0	1.5	5.0
Malt Loaf, Fruity, Sliced, Soreen*	1 Slice/33g	103.0	1.0	312	7.7	65.9	2.0	0.0
Malt Loaf, Fruity, Unsliced, Soreen*	1 Serving/42g	130.0	1.0	310	7.4	65.6	2.0	2.7
Malt Loaf, Organic, Tesco*	1 Slice/28g	82.0	1.0	292	7.2	61.2	2.0	2.3
Malt Loaf, Sticky, M & S*	1 Slice/16g	47.0	0.0	295	6.9	64.9	2.3	3.1
Malt Loaf, Tesco*	1 Slice/50g	145.0	1.0	291	8.6	58.0	2.7	4.8
Malt Loaf, Value, Tesco*	1 Slice/25g	72.0	0.0	289	8.9	60.2	1.4	3.3
Malt Loaf, Weight Watchers*	1 Slice/23g	68.0	0.0	294	8.9	60.2	1.9	3.6
Malted Brown, Slice, BGTY, Sainsbury's*	1 Slice/22g	53.0	1.0	239	12.1	41.4	2.8	5.8
Malted Brown, Thick Sliced, Organic, Tesco*	1 Slice/44.4g	111.0	1.0	249	8.9	48.8	2.0	3.5
Malted Danish, Weight Watchers*	1 Slice/20.4g	49.0	0.0	241	12.3	44.5	1.7	4.3
Malted Grain, Co-Op*	1 Slice/43g	99.0	1.0	230	8.0	46.0	2.0	3.0
Malted Grain, Good As Gold, Kingsmill*	1 Slice/46.9g	114.0	1.0	243	9.5	45.4	2.6	4.2
Malted Oat, Duchy Originals*	1 Serving/80g	195.0	3.0	244	8.8	43.6	3.8	3.7
Malted Wheat, The Best, Safeway*	1 Slice/44g	103.0	1.0	235	9.1	45.6	1.8	4.7
Malted Wheatgrain, Roberts Bakery*	1 Slice/30g	79.0	1.0	265	11.0	48.0	3.3	3.6
Malted Wholegrain, Nimble*	1 Slice/22g	49.0	0.0	222	10.4	41.9	1.4	6.7
Malted, & Seeded, Batch, Organic, Waitrose*	1 Slice/50g	118.0	2.0	236	10.9	39.5	3.9	6.2
Malted, Crusty, Sainsbury's*	1 Slice/42g	109.0	1.0	259	8.6	48.6	3.3	4.4
Malted, Danish, Sliced, Warburton's*	1 Slice/19g	41.0	0.0	218	10.2	41.3	1.4	6.9
Malted, Farmhouse, Morrisons*	1 Serving/40g	94.0	1.0	235	9.1	45.6	1.8	4.7
Malted, Floury Batch, Sainsbury's*	1 Roll/68g	190.0	3.0	280	8.7	51.6	4.3	4.2
Malted, Sunblest*	1 Serving/45g	115.0	1.0	256	9.9	49.1	2.2	3.8
Malted, Wheat Loaf, Crusty, Finest, Tesco*	1 Slice/50g	115.0	1.0	230	9.8	44.2	1.5	4.4
Mediterranean Olive, Waitrose*	1 Slice/30g	82.0	3.0	273	7.4	40.1	9.2	4.9
Mediterranean Style Seed, Safeway*	1 Slice/25g	65.0	2.0	259	11.4	37.2	7.2	9.1
Mediterranean Style, M & S*	1/6 Loaf/48g	150.0	5.0	315	10.9	42.5	11.1	1.2
Milk Roll, Warburton's*	1 Slice/18g	46.0	1.0	253	11.0	45.1	2.7	2.7
Mixed Seed, Organic, Duchy Originals*	1 Slice/42.5g	114.0	3.0	269	10.9	39.1	8.1	5.3
Multigrain, Batch, Finest, Tesco*	1 Slice/49.8g	117.0	1.0	235	10.8	40.4	2.9	5.5
Multigrain, Brown, Farmhouse Baker's, M & S*	1 Slice/51g	115.0	3.0	225	13.0	31.2	5.4	5.1
Multigrain, Crusty, Finest, Tesco*	1 Slice/40g	98.0	1.0	245	9.0	44.7	3.4	5.0
Multigrain, Gluten Free, Sainsbury's*	1 Slice/17g	39.0	1.0	229	5.1	40.8	5.0	5.6
Multigrain, Sliced, Fresh And Easy*	1 Slice/40g	110.0	1.0	275	10.0	52.5	2.5	5.0
Multigrain, Soft Batch, Sainsbury's*	1 Slice/44g	106.0	3.0	242	11.3	34.5	6.5	5.6
Multigrain, Sunblest*	1 Slice/30g	76.0	1.0	254	9.0	47.0	2.5	4.5
Multigrain, Tesco*	1 Slice/31g	66.0	1.0	214	11.1	36.8	3.2	8.9
Multigrain, Thick Sliced, Tesco*	1 Slice/50g	112.0	1.0	225	8.4	42.2	2.5	3.9
Multiseed, Farmhouse, Finest, Tesco*	1 Slice /50g	135.0	4.0	270	12.5	37.0	7.7	5.8
Naan, Average	*1 Naan/130g*	*337.0*	*8.0*	*259*	*9.0*	*40.3*	*5.8*	*1.8*
Naan, Bombay Brassiere, Sainsbury's*	1 Naan/140g	372.0	4.0	266	9.8	49.6	3.1	2.9
Naan, Chilli & Mango, Finest, Tesco*	½ Naan/90g	229.0	5.0	255	8.4	41.9	5.7	3.2
Naan, Garlic & Coriander, Free From, Tesco*	1 Naan/89.6g	215.0	6.0	240	5.1	38.7	6.7	4.9
Naan, Garlic & Coriander, Fresh, Sharwood's*	1oz/28g	71.0	1.0	252	7.7	47.8	3.3	2.2
Naan, Garlic & Coriander, Large, TTD, Sainsbury's*	¼ Pack/70g	194.0	4.0	277	9.4	47.7	5.4	2.2
Naan, Garlic & Coriander, M & S*	1 Naan/150g	375.0	2.0	250	9.8	50.1	1.4	2.0
Naan, Garlic & Coriander, Mild, Patak's*	1 Naan/140g	452.0	15.0	323	9.0	47.5	10.8	0.0
Naan, Garlic & Coriander, Mini, Asda*	1 Naan/110g	320.0	13.0	291	6.9	40.2	11.4	2.5
Naan, Garlic & Coriander, Mini, Finest, Tesco*	1 Naan/50g	160.0	7.0	320	6.7	42.4	13.5	0.8
Naan, Garlic & Coriander, Mini, Long Life, Sharwood's*	1oz/28g	76.0	2.0	272	6.5	42.9	7.4	2.4
Naan, Garlic & Coriander, Mini, Sainsbury's*	1 Naan/50g	140.0	2.0	280	8.2	51.2	4.1	2.6
Naan, Garlic & Coriander, Mini, Sharwood's*	1 Naan/59g	144.0	2.0	244	7.1	46.2	3.4	2.0
Naan, Garlic & Coriander, Mini, Tesco*	1 Naan/65g	185.0	5.0	285	7.6	45.6	7.7	2.6

BREAD

Measure INFO/WEIGHT	per Measure KCAL	per Measure FAT	Nutrition Values per 100g / 100ml KCAL	PROT	CARB	FAT	FIBRE

	Measure INFO/WEIGHT	per Measure KCAL	FAT	KCAL	PROT	CARB	FAT	FIBRE
Naan, Garlic & Coriander, Mini, Weight Watchers*	1 Naan/40g	100.0	1.0	250	9.3	47.6	2.5	4.2
Naan, Garlic & Coriander, Sainsbury's*	1 Serving/130g	373.0	10.0	287	8.7	45.8	7.7	2.4
Naan, Garlic & Coriander, Tesco*	½ Naan/82.5g	235.0	6.0	285	7.6	45.6	7.7	2.6
Naan, Garlic & Coriander, TTD, Sainsbury's*	1 Serving/70g	215.0	8.0	307	7.0	43.9	11.5	2.9
Naan, Garlic & Coriander, Weight Watchers*	1 Naan/60g	155.0	3.0	259	8.9	46.0	4.3	3.4
Naan, Indian Meal for One, BGTY, Sainsbury's*	1 Serving/45g	115.0	2.0	257	10.3	44.2	4.3	2.1
Naan, Indian Meal for One, Sainsbury's*	1 Serving/50g	144.0	3.0	289	9.7	47.6	6.6	2.1
Naan, Indian Meal for Two, Sainsbury's*	1 Naan//125g	357.0	9.0	285	8.7	45.9	7.4	1.9
Naan, Keema Filled, Mini, Indian Takeaway, Safeway*	1 Naan/23g	58.0	2.0	253	10.1	38.3	6.6	2.1
Naan, Light Choices, Tesco*	1 Naan/71g	181.0	2.0	255	7.5	50.7	2.2	2.3
Naan, Long Life, Sharwood's*	1oz/28g	72.0	1.0	258	7.3	45.8	5.1	2.0
Naan, Mini, Light Choices, Tesco*	1 Naan/65g	149.0	2.0	230	8.1	42.5	2.8	2.9
Naan, Onion & Mint, M & S*	½ Naan/135g	351.0	12.0	260	8.9	35.8	8.7	2.5
Naan, Onion Bhaji, M & S*	1 Naan/140g	400.0	17.0	285	9.5	34.2	12.1	2.0
Naan, Onion Bhaji, Sharwood's*	1 Pack/130g	378.0	10.0	291	7.3	48.4	7.6	2.2
Naan, Peshwari, Finest, Tesco*	1 Naan/130g	338.0	7.0	260	8.6	43.7	5.6	4.9
Naan, Peshwari, Fresh, Sharwood's*	1oz/28g	67.0	1.0	240	6.8	41.9	5.0	2.5
Naan, Peshwari, Long Life, Sharwood's*	1oz/28g	71.0	2.0	252	6.2	42.0	6.6	2.6
Naan, Peshwari, M & S*	1 Serving/127g	394.0	13.0	310	9.2	45.8	10.1	1.9
Naan, Peshwari, Mega, Asda*	1 Naan/220g	680.0	26.0	309	7.1	43.1	12.0	2.7
Naan, Peshwari, Sainsbury's*	1 Naan/166g	511.0	18.0	308	7.1	45.1	11.0	4.7
Naan, Peshwari, Sharwood's*	1 Naan/130g	334.0	7.0	257	7.2	45.1	5.3	2.5
Naan, Peshwari, Tesco*	1 Naan/215.0g	684.0	27.0	318	7.5	48.9	12.4	4.8
Naan, Peshwari, TTD, Sainsbury's*	1 Serving/80g	247.0	10.0	309	6.3	42.5	12.6	4.4
Naan, Plain, Average	1 Naan/160g	538.0	20.0	336	8.9	50.1	12.5	1.9
Naan, Plain, GFY, Asda*	1 Naan/130g	307.0	3.0	236	8.4	45.9	2.1	2.4
Naan, Tandoori Baked, Waitrose*	1 Naan/140g	372.0	4.0	266	9.8	49.6	3.1	2.9
Naan, Tandoori, Sharwood's*	1 Naan/130g	330.0	6.0	254	7.3	45.0	5.0	2.0
Oatmeal, Batch, Finest, Tesco*	1 Slice/50g	127.0	2.0	255	10.3	43.7	4.3	4.8
Oatmeal, Farmhouse, Extra Special, Asda*	1 Slice/44g	102.0	1.0	231	11.0	41.0	2.6	6.0
Oatmeal, Farmhouse, Soft, M & S*	1 Slice/45g	110.0	2.0	245	11.1	39.5	4.4	5.2
Oatmeal, Farmhouse, Waitrose*	1 Slice/40g	110.0	2.0	276	9.4	47.9	5.2	4.6
Oatmeal, Sliced Loaf, Tesco*	1 Slice/50g	111.0	2.0	222	7.4	40.5	3.4	2.8
Olive Oval, la Brea Bakery*	1 Serving/100g	249.0	4.0	249	7.0	46.4	3.8	2.7
Olive, Waitrose*	1 Slice/28g	86.0	3.0	306	9.0	43.6	10.6	2.0
Pave, Mixed Olive, Waitrose*	1oz/28g	59.0	1.0	209	6.3	41.6	1.9	2.6
Pave, Sundried Tomato, Waitrose*	1oz/28g	76.0	0.0	271	10.8	53.4	1.6	3.3
Pave, Walnut, Sainsbury's*	1 Serving/50g	140.0	5.0	280	9.0	40.0	9.5	3.5
Petit Pain, Homebake, Mini, Tesco*	1 Roll/50g	120.0	1.0	240	7.8	48.5	1.2	3.4
Petit Pain, Organic, Tesco*	1 Roll/100g	235.0	1.0	235	7.8	49.1	0.8	1.2
Petit Pain, Part Bake, Weight Watchers*	1 Roll/50g	102.0	1.0	204	8.2	39.9	1.2	9.8
Petits Pains, Mini, Homebake, Tesco*	1 Roll/45g	110.0	1.0	245	7.8	49.7	1.3	2.5
Petits Pains, White, Ready to Bake, Sainsbury's*	1 Roll/50.4g	122.0	1.0	242	7.8	49.7	1.3	2.8
Pitta, Brown, Organic, Waitrose*	1 Pitta/60g	137.0	1.0	228	6.4	47.5	1.4	6.6
Pitta, Free From, Sainsbury's*	1 Pitta/55.1g	134.0	1.0	243	5.9	50.8	1.8	1.7
Pitta, Garlic & Coriander, Asda*	1 Pitta/55g	116.0	0.0	212	7.0	44.0	0.9	1.8
Pitta, Garlic & Herb, Tesco*	1 Pitta/60g	134.0	1.0	223	9.6	44.6	2.0	3.0
Pitta, Garlic, Morrisons*	1 Pitta/60g	149.0	1.0	249	9.7	51.1	1.8	0.0
Pitta, Garlic, Pride Valley*	1 Pitta/63g	157.0	1.0	249	9.7	51.1	1.8	2.7
Pitta, Garlic, Sainsbury's*	1 Pitta/60g	153.0	1.0	255	9.5	52.0	1.0	2.5
Pitta, Mexican, Santa Maria*	1 Pitta/66g	165.0	1.0	250	7.5	52.0	1.0	0.0
Pitta, Multi Seed & Cereal, The Food Doctor*	1 Pitta/70g	157.0	2.0	224	10.1	39.9	2.7	10.2
Pitta, Organic, Tesco*	1 Pitta/60g	124.0	1.0	206	8.3	40.2	1.4	5.7

B

BREAD

	Measure INFO/WEIGHT	per Measure KCAL	per Measure FAT	Nutrition Values per 100g / 100ml KCAL	PROT	CARB	FAT	FIBRE
Pitta, Pockets, Pride Valley*	1 Pitta/63g	151.0	1.0	239	9.3	48.4	0.9	3.2
Pitta, Pockets, Sainsbury's*	1 Serving/75g	187.0	1.0	250	8.5	52.0	1.0	3.5
Pitta, Sd Tomato, Olive & Oregano, Extra Special, Asda*	1 Pitta/74.9g	194.0	1.0	259	7.1	55.2	1.1	1.6
Pitta, Seeded, HL, Tesco*	1 Pitta/60g	153.0	4.0	255	10.8	39.4	6.0	12.8
Pitta, Sesame, Sainsbury's*	1 Pitta/59g	156.0	1.0	264	9.8	50.8	2.4	3.1
Pitta, Tex Mex Style, Mini, Morrisons*	1 Pitta/18g	43.0	0.0	240	9.2	48.7	0.9	3.3
Pitta, White Picnic, Waitrose*	1 Pitta/30g	75.0	0.0	249	10.3	49.3	1.2	3.5
Pitta, White, Average	*1 Pitta/75g*	*199.0*	*1.0*	*265*	*9.2*	*57.9*	*1.2*	*2.2*
Pitta, White, Free From, Tesco*	1 Pitta/55g	140.0	1.0	255	6.5	52.6	2.1	5.5
Pitta, White, Greek Style, Asda*	1 Pitta/50g	126.0	1.0	253	8.0	51.0	1.9	0.0
Pitta, White, Large, Tesco*	1 Pitta/90g	252.0	2.0	280	9.8	55.1	2.1	3.4
Pitta, White, M & S*	1 Pitta/61g	146.0	1.0	240	9.3	46.9	2.0	3.6
Pitta, White, Mini, Sainsbury's*	1 Pitta/30g	75.0	0.0	249	10.3	49.3	1.2	3.5
Pitta, White, Mini, Tesco*	1 Pitta/30g	84.0	1.0	280	9.8	55.1	2.1	3.4
Pitta, White, Organic, Sainsbury's*	1 Pitta/59g	150.0	1.0	254	10.3	50.7	1.1	2.5
Pitta, Wholemeal, Average	*1 Pitta/64g*	*170.0*	*2.0*	*266*	*9.8*	*55.0*	*2.6*	*7.4*
Pitta, Wholemeal, Lemon & Black Pepper, Finest, Tesco*	1 Pitta/79.6g	215.0	5.0	270	10.8	42.4	6.0	6.0
Pitta, Wholemeal, Mini, M & S*	1 Pitta/17.4g	40.0	1.0	230	11.1	39.2	3.1	7.0
Pitta, Wholemeal, Mini, Sainsbury's*	1 Pitta/30g	69.0	1.0	231	10.0	43.8	1.7	6.2
Pitta, Wholemeal, Mini, Tesco*	1 Pitta/30g	76.0	1.0	255	11.8	48.2	1.7	4.2
Pitta, Wholemeal, So Organic, Sainsbury's*	1 Pitta/60g	140.0	1.0	233	9.8	44.8	1.6	8.1
Pitta, Wholemeal, Tesco*	1 Pitta/60g	147.0	1.0	245	11.2	43.6	2.5	8.7
Pitta, Wholemeal, Waitrose*	1 Pitta/60g	145.0	1.0	242	12.4	46.0	0.9	3.1
Pitta, Wholemeal, Weight Watchers*	1 Pitta /44g	98.0	1.0	223	8.7	44.5	1.2	7.6
Pitta, Wholemeal, with Extra Virgin Olive Oil, Tesco*	1 Pitta/60g	135.0	2.0	225	8.3	41.5	2.6	5.5
Plum Fruit Loaf, Lincolnshire, Soreen*	1 Slice/25g	65.0	1.0	261	8.4	49.3	3.4	2.1
Potato & Rosemary, M & S*	1 Serving/40g	108.0	3.0	270	9.4	42.2	6.8	2.3
Potato Farls, Irish, Irwin's Bakery*	1 Farl/142g	239.0	2.0	168	3.2	35.8	1.3	2.5
Potato Farls, M & S*	1 Farl/55g	79.0	0.0	144	4.2	33.8	0.4	4.7
Potato Farls, Sunblest*	1 Farl/100g	156.0	1.0	156	3.8	33.2	0.9	1.9
Pumpernickel Rye, Kelderman*	1 Slice/50g	92.0	0.0	185	6.0	38.0	1.0	0.0
Pumpernickel, Organic, Bavarian Pumpernickel*	1 Slice/50g	90.0	0.0	180	6.0	38.0	1.0	10.0
Pumpkin Seed, Raisin & Sunflower Seed, Sainsbury's*	1 Slice/30g	76.0	1.0	255	11.6	45.9	2.8	3.4
Raisin & Pumpkin Seed, Organic, Tesco*	1 Slice/30g	76.0	2.0	253	9.7	40.6	5.8	3.8
Raisin Loaf with Cinnamon, Warburton's*	1 Slice/36g	96.0	1.0	267	7.2	51.1	3.7	3.2
Roasted Onion, M & S*	1 Slice/50g	125.0	2.0	250	9.0	46.7	3.3	2.1
Roasted Shallot & Gruyere, Safeway*	¼ Loaf/53g	150.0	4.0	285	11.2	43.1	7.3	9.1
Roll, Hot Dog, Wheat, Brownberry*	1 Roll/43g	120.0	2.0	279	9.3	48.8	4.6	2.3
Roll, Oatmeal, Co-Op*	1 Roll/70g	175.0	3.0	250	10.1	42.6	4.6	5.6
Rolls, 3 Seeded, Sandwich, Warburton's*	1 Roll/77g	242.0	7.0	314	13.3	41.2	8.7	6.0
Rolls, American Style Deli, Tesco*	1 Roll/65g	162.0	2.0	249	7.8	46.8	3.4	1.6
Rolls, Batched Sandwich, Warburton's*	1 Roll/60g	148.0	2.0	246	9.6	42.7	4.1	0.0
Rolls, Best of Both, Hovis*	1 Roll/62g	148.0	3.0	239	9.8	39.7	4.6	5.0
Rolls, Blackpool Milk, Warburton's*	1 Slice/18g	45.0	1.0	251	10.8	45.3	3.0	2.8
Rolls, Brioche, Plain Chocolate Chip, Sainsbury's*	1 Roll/35g	131.0	6.0	374	8.5	49.0	16.0	5.9
Rolls, Brioche, Sainsbury's*	1 Roll/32g	116.0	4.0	362	8.5	56.0	11.5	3.6
Rolls, Brown, Carb Control, Tesco*	1 Roll/45g	98.0	3.0	218	20.5	20.7	5.9	10.7
Rolls, Brown, Crusty	*1 Roll/50g*	*127.0*	*1.0*	*255*	*10.3*	*50.4*	*2.8*	*3.5*
Rolls, Brown, Free From, Tesco*	1 Roll/65g	174.0	5.0	268	5.4	43.2	8.2	3.6
Rolls, Brown, Malted Grain, Tesco*	1 Roll/58g	144.0	2.0	248	8.7	46.2	3.2	1.9
Rolls, Brown, Mini, M & S*	1 Serving/33g	80.0	2.0	245	9.8	35.5	7.6	3.8
Rolls, Brown, Morning, Farmfoods*	1 Roll/50g	134.0	2.0	269	12.0	47.0	3.7	4.2
Rolls, Brown, Old Fashioned, Waitrose*	1 Roll/63g	152.0	3.0	241	9.6	41.3	4.1	4.7

B

BREAD

INFO/WEIGHT	Measure	per Measure KCAL	FAT	Nutrition Values per 100g / 100ml KCAL	PROT	CARB	FAT	FIBRE
Rolls, Brown, Seeded, Organic, Sainsbury's*	1 Roll/70g	166.0	3.0	237	9.9	39.1	4.6	6.5
Rolls, Brown, Snack, Allinson*	1 Roll/44g	119.0	3.0	270	10.8	41.6	6.7	5.6
Rolls, Brown, Soft, Average	*1 Roll/50g*	*134.0*	*2.0*	*268*	*10.0*	*51.8*	*3.8*	*3.5*
Rolls, Brown, Soft, Organic, Sainsbury's*	1 Serving/70g	166.0	3.0	237	9.9	39.1	4.6	6.6
Rolls, Brown, Square, M & S*	1 Roll/105g	241.0	6.0	230	9.2	37.3	6.1	4.4
Rolls, Cheese & Tomato, Seeded, White, M & S*	1 Pack/160g	480.0	25.0	300	13.7	26.1	15.6	2.1
Rolls, Cheese Topped, Sandwich Rolls, Warburton's*	1 Roll/62g	168.0	4.0	270	12.1	40.7	6.5	2.6
Rolls, Cheese Topped, Village Green*	1 Roll/56g	159.0	4.0	284	13.1	41.2	7.4	4.8
Rolls, Ciabatta, Cheese Topped, Mini, Finest, Tesco*	1 Roll/30g	85.0	2.0	282	11.5	40.9	8.1	3.8
Rolls, Ciabatta, Garlic, Asda*	1 Roll/93g	333.0	17.0	358	9.0	40.0	18.0	2.3
Rolls, Ciabatta, M & S*	1 Roll/80g	210.0	3.0	262	10.3	48.1	4.1	2.1
Rolls, Ciabatta, Mini, Finest, Tesco*	1 Roll/30g	89.0	2.0	297	9.9	49.1	6.8	4.1
Rolls, Ciabatta, Sun Dried Tomato, Mini, Finest, Tesco*	1 Roll/30g	79.0	2.0	262	8.7	42.3	6.4	2.6
Rolls, Ciabatta, Tesco*	1 Serving/80g	208.0	2.0	260	8.6	48.2	3.1	3.3
Rolls, COU, M & S*	1 Serving/51g	120.0	1.0	235	9.8	44.0	2.3	3.4
Rolls, Country Grain, Mini, M & S*	1 Serving/31g	85.0	3.0	275	10.2	38.9	9.7	3.8
Rolls, Crisp, Original, Organic, Kallo*	1 Roll/9g	34.0	0.0	390	11.0	74.0	5.6	3.0
Rolls, Crusty, French, M & S*	1 Roll/65g	159.0	1.0	245	8.1	50.5	1.2	3.3
Rolls, Crusty, Part-Baked, Budgens*	1 Roll/50g	148.0	1.0	296	9.4	61.4	1.4	2.5
Rolls, Finger, Morrisons*	1 Roll/46g	119.0	1.0	259	10.7	50.0	1.8	2.3
Rolls, Finger, White, Sainsbury's*	1 Roll/40g	96.0	1.0	240	9.0	45.2	2.6	3.2
Rolls, Focaccia, Tesco*	1 Serving/75g	226.0	7.0	302	8.7	45.6	9.4	3.8
Rolls, Gluten Free, Antoinette Savill*	1 Serving/70g	157.0	2.0	224	1.9	48.8	2.2	1.5
Rolls, Granary Malted Wheatgrain, Soft, M & S*	1 Roll/80g	208.0	3.0	260	9.3	47.2	3.9	2.3
Rolls, Granary, Bakers Premium, Tesco*	1 Roll/65g	158.0	1.0	243	9.9	47.8	1.3	2.3
Rolls, Granary, Mini, Tesco*	1 Roll/34g	92.0	2.0	271	10.0	43.5	6.5	3.8
Rolls, Granary, Original, Hovis*	1 Roll/70g	180.0	3.0	257	10.7	44.3	4.1	5.3
Rolls, Granary, Waitrose*	1 Roll/59g	160.0	4.0	271	10.0	47.2	6.4	3.8
Rolls, Green Olive, M & S*	1 Roll/75g	210.0	4.0	280	11.2	44.0	6.0	1.8
Rolls, Hot Dog, Sliced, Asda*	1 Roll/84g	197.0	3.0	234	7.0	44.0	3.3	0.0
Rolls, Hot Dog, Tesco*	1 Roll/85g	200.0	3.0	235	7.3	44.0	3.3	1.9
Rolls, Hot Dog, Value, Tesco*	1 Serving/40g	93.0	1.0	232	8.7	45.0	1.9	2.2
Rolls, Malted Grain, Sainsbury's*	1 Roll/68g	190.0	3.0	280	8.7	51.6	4.3	4.2
Rolls, Malted Grain, Soft, Weight Watchers*	1 Roll/56.5g	142.0	1.0	251	11.7	47.1	1.8	4.2
Rolls, Malted Grain, Submarine, M & S*	1 Serving/109g	300.0	5.0	275	8.9	53.6	4.3	3.0
Rolls, Malted Wheat, Sub, Organic, Tesco*	1 Serving/108g	279.0	4.0	258	10.1	45.2	4.1	4.8
Rolls, Malted, Whole Grain Rolls, Batched, Soft, M & S*	1 Roll/80g	180.0	4.0	225	7.8	38.5	4.5	3.1
Rolls, Mini Submarine, M & S*	1 Roll/23g	63.0	1.0	275	11.4	47.7	4.9	1.1
Rolls, Mixed Seed, Deli, Tesco*	1 Roll/64.7g	165.0	2.0	255	9.4	46.8	3.3	5.2
Rolls, Morning, Tesco*	1 Roll/48g	117.0	1.0	243	10.4	44.8	2.5	4.7
Rolls, Multigrain, Torpedo, Sainsbury's*	1 Roll/112g	328.0	7.0	293	10.5	47.7	6.7	6.3
Rolls, Oatmeal, Ploughmans, GFY, Asda*	1 Roll/71.8g	181.0	3.0	252	10.0	43.0	4.4	3.9
Rolls, Oatmeal, Soft, M & S*	1 Roll/80g	224.0	5.0	280	12.3	43.4	6.4	2.7
Rolls, Pane Rustica, Waitrose*	1 Roll/114g	283.0	1.0	248	9.4	50.0	1.2	1.8
Rolls, Panini, Sainsbury's*	1 Roll/90g	249.0	6.0	276	11.0	44.1	6.2	3.0
Rolls, Panini, White, Tesco*	1 Roll/75g	210.0	5.0	280	10.1	45.2	6.1	2.7
Rolls, Part Baked, Mini, Tesco*	1 Serving/50g	120.0	1.0	240	7.8	49.5	1.2	3.4
Rolls, Poppy Seeded Knot, Waitrose*	1 Roll/60g	169.0	3.0	282	10.3	48.3	5.3	2.2
Rolls, Rye, Toasting, Good & Hot*	1 Pack/65g	143.0	1.0	220	7.3	44.6	1.1	7.1
Rolls, Scottish Morning, Morrisons*	1 Roll/60g	157.0	1.0	261	11.3	51.4	2.2	2.4
Rolls, Seed Sensations, Deli, Hovis*	1 Roll/70g	184.0	6.0	263	10.3	36.5	8.5	10.6
Rolls, Seeded, Mixed Mini Loaf Pack, M & S*	1 Roll/76g	220.0	7.0	290	10.6	39.7	9.6	4.0
Rolls, Seeded, Sandwich, Warburton's*	1 Roll/77g	242.0	7.0	314	13.3	41.2	8.7	6.0

BREAD

INFO/WEIGHT	Measure	per Measure		Nutrition Values per 100g / 100ml				
		KCAL	FAT	KCAL	PROT	CARB	FAT	FIBRE
Rolls, Snack, Mini, Tesco*	1 Roll/35g	95.0	2.0	271	19.0	43.0	6.0	4.0
Rolls, Soft, Wholemeal, Finger, M & S*	1 Roll/66g	145.0	1.0	220	12.6	38.0	2.0	5.8
Rolls, Submarine, Sainsbury's*	1 Roll/117g	305.0	5.0	261	9.1	47.4	3.9	2.4
Rolls, Sun Dried Tomato, Homebake, Tesco*	1 Roll/50g	123.0	1.0	246	11.3	44.0	3.0	0.0
Rolls, Sunflower Seed, Toasting, Good & Hot*	1 Roll/65g	162.0	3.0	250	8.5	41.0	5.0	8.0
Rolls, Tomato & Basil, Sub, COU, M & S*	1 Roll/33g	86.0	1.0	265	11.0	48.7	2.7	2.4
Rolls, White, Cheese Topped, Asda*	1 Roll/46g	121.0	2.0	264	10.0	46.0	4.4	2.0
Rolls, White, Cheese Topped, Sainsbury's*	1 Roll/75g	218.0	6.0	291	12.1	41.6	8.5	2.0
Rolls, White, Chunky, Hovis*	1 Roll/73g	173.0	2.0	237	9.4	41.7	3.3	2.5
Rolls, White, Crusty, Average	*1 Roll/50g*	*140.0*	*1.0*	*280*	*10.9*	*57.6*	*2.3*	*1.5*
Rolls, White, Crusty, Home Bake, Tesco*	1 Roll/68.5g	185.0	1.0	270	9.3	54.2	1.4	2.9
Rolls, White, Crusty, Morning, M & S*	1 Roll/65g	175.0	1.0	270	8.8	53.8	1.3	2.7
Rolls, White, Finger, Smart Price, Asda*	1 Roll/50g	121.0	1.0	242	9.0	48.0	1.6	2.1
Rolls, White, Finger, Tesco*	1 Roll/68g	170.0	2.0	250	8.5	45.8	3.5	2.1
Rolls, White, Finger, Value, Tesco*	1 Roll/50g	116.0	1.0	232	8.7	45.0	1.9	2.2
Rolls, White, Floured, Batch, Tesco*	1 Roll/76g	193.0	3.0	254	8.8	47.3	3.3	2.2
Rolls, White, Floured, Warburton's*	1 Roll/50g	123.0	2.0	247	9.8	43.3	3.8	2.7
Rolls, White, Floury Batch, Sainsbury's*	1 Roll/68g	168.0	2.0	247	8.3	47.2	2.8	2.2
Rolls, White, Floury, Roberts Bakery*	1 Roll/63.0g	160.0	2.0	254	8.4	49.5	2.5	2.0
Rolls, White, Good Health, Warburton's*	1 Roll/54g	122.0	1.0	226	9.6	42.0	2.0	4.1
Rolls, White, Hot Dog, Jumbo, Sainsbury's*	1 Roll/85g	239.0	5.0	281	7.5	49.1	6.1	2.9
Rolls, White, Hot Dog, Tesco*	1 Roll/65g	169.0	2.0	260	9.6	46.1	3.7	3.2
Rolls, White, Kingsmill*	1 Roll/60g	151.0	2.0	252	9.3	44.5	4.1	2.4
Rolls, White, Large, Sliced, Warburton's*	1 Serving/89g	230.0	4.0	258	10.1	44.4	4.5	2.7
Rolls, White, Low Price, Sainsbury's*	1 Roll/44g	107.0	1.0	243	8.9	48.2	1.6	2.1
Rolls, White, Milk, Warburton's*	1 Serving/18g	46.0	1.0	251	10.8	45.3	3.0	2.8
Rolls, White, Morning, Co-Op*	1 Roll/47g	134.0	1.0	285	12.0	53.0	3.0	2.0
Rolls, White, Old Fashioned, Waitrose*	1 Roll/64g	176.0	3.0	275	8.8	49.8	4.5	2.8
Rolls, White, Organic, Sainsbury's*	1 Roll/65g	170.0	2.0	262	8.7	49.9	3.0	1.0
Rolls, White, Part Baked, Morrisons*	1 Roll/75g	227.0	1.0	303	9.6	63.0	1.4	2.6
Rolls, White, Ploughman's, Sainsbury's*	1 Roll/65g	185.0	2.0	285	8.6	54.1	3.8	2.3
Rolls, White, Premium Soft, Rathbones*	1 Roll/65g	190.0	4.0	293	9.3	50.3	6.0	2.7
Rolls, White, Premium, Brown Hill Bakery*	1 Roll/74g	206.0	2.0	279	11.0	51.5	3.0	2.3
Rolls, White, Premium, Hovis*	1 Roll/70g	180.0	3.0	257	9.5	44.8	4.4	3.0
Rolls, White, Sandwich, Large, Warburton's*	1 Roll/88.3g	224.0	4.0	254	10.2	44.3	4.0	2.5
Rolls, White, Sandwich, Regular, Warburton's*	1 Roll/57.5g	143.0	3.0	249	9.7	42.6	4.3	2.4
Rolls, White, Scottish, Morning, Safeway*	1 Roll/40g	113.0	1.0	283	10.4	56.4	1.8	1.6
Rolls, White, Scottish, Tesco*	1 Roll/48g	117.0	1.0	243	10.4	44.8	2.5	4.7
Rolls, White, Seeded, Sainsbury's*	1 Roll/80g	217.0	5.0	271	10.9	43.4	5.9	4.8
Rolls, White, Snack, Sainsbury's*	1 Roll/67g	159.0	1.0	237	7.9	49.2	1.0	2.3
Rolls, White, Soft, Average	*1 Roll/45g*	*121.0*	*2.0*	*268*	*9.2*	*51.6*	*4.2*	*1.5*
Rolls, White, Soft, COU, M & S*	1 Roll/37g	94.0	1.0	255	10.7	47.1	2.7	1.5
Rolls, White, Soft, Farmhouse, TTD, Sainsbury's*	1 Slice/47g	111.0	1.0	235	8.1	45.4	1.7	2.9
Rolls, White, Soft, Farmhouse, Warburton's*	1 Roll/59g	147.0	3.0	250	9.7	43.0	4.4	2.5
Rolls, White, Softgrain, GFY, Asda*	1 Roll/54.0g	128.0	1.0	237	9.0	46.0	1.9	2.9
Rolls, Wholemeal	*1 Roll 45g*	*108.0*	*1.0*	*241*	*9.0*	*48.3*	*2.9*	*5.9*
Rolls, Wholemeal & White, Kingsmill*	1 Roll/60g	151.0	3.0	251	9.5	43.7	4.2	3.5
Rolls, Wholemeal with Cracked Wheat, Allinson*	1 Roll/58g	134.0	2.0	231	11.0	38.0	3.9	7.0
Rolls, Wholemeal, COU, M & S*	1 Roll/110g	225.0	3.0	205	11.3	33.4	2.8	7.1
Rolls, Wholemeal, Deli, Tesco*	1 Serving/65g	156.0	3.0	240	9.0	40.2	4.8	5.7
Rolls, Wholemeal, Floury Batch, Sainsbury's*	1 Roll/68g	152.0	2.0	223	9.9	37.8	3.4	6.5
Rolls, Wholemeal, Food Explorers, Waitrose*	1 Roll/32.0g	74.0	1.0	231	10.6	40.2	3.1	5.7
Rolls, Wholemeal, Golden, Hovis*	1 Roll/50g	111.0	2.0	223	10.5	36.5	3.9	6.8

B

BREAD

	Measure INFO/WEIGHT	per Measure KCAL	per Measure FAT	Nutrition Values per 100g / 100ml KCAL	PROT	CARB	FAT	FIBRE
Rolls, Wholemeal, HL, Tesco*	1 Roll/67.5	155.0	1.0	230	10.4	41.3	2.1	6.6
Rolls, Wholemeal, Milk, Warburton's*	1 Roll/22g	51.0	1.0	231	12.5	38.1	3.2	7.0
Rolls, Wholemeal, Mini, Assorted, Waitrose*	1 Roll/36g	84.0	2.0	236	9.0	38.1	5.3	5.2
Rolls, Wholemeal, Mini, Tesco*	1 Roll/34g	82.0	2.0	240	10.9	36.4	5.6	5.8
Rolls, Wholemeal, Oat Topped, Tesco*	1 Roll/65g	166.0	3.0	255	11.3	42.2	4.5	5.1
Rolls, Wholemeal, Oatbran, HL, Tesco*	1 Roll/56g	115.0	1.0	205	11.4	33.6	2.5	7.4
Rolls, Wholemeal, Old Fashioned, Waitrose*	1 Roll/57g	135.0	3.0	236	11.1	37.2	4.8	6.6
Rolls, Wholemeal, Organic, Sainsbury's*	1 Roll/66g	152.0	2.0	230	10.7	41.0	2.7	6.6
Rolls, Wholemeal, Organic, Tesco*	1 Roll/65g	177.0	4.0	273	10.3	44.1	6.2	5.5
Rolls, Wholemeal, Ploughman's, Sainsbury's*	1 Roll/67g	153.0	2.0	229	10.7	39.3	3.2	8.6
Rolls, Wholemeal, Sliced, Hovis*	1 Roll/60g	150.0	4.0	250	10.6	38.7	5.9	6.8
Rolls, Wholemeal, Soft, Sainsbury's*	1 Roll/60g	133.0	2.0	221	9.9	37.8	3.4	6.5
Rolls, Wholemeal, Soft, Seeded, Sainsbury's*	1 Roll/75g	193.0	6.0	257	11.8	35.6	7.4	6.2
Rolls, Wholemeal, Submarine, Tesco*	1 Roll/100g	221.0	3.0	221	9.3	39.0	3.1	5.2
Rolls, Wholemeal, Submarine, Warburton's*	1 Serving/94g	231.0	4.0	246	10.9	40.6	4.4	6.3
Rolls, Wholemeal, Sunflower & Honey, Sainsbury's*	1 Roll/85g	225.0	4.0	265	9.2	45.4	5.1	4.5
Rolls, Wholemeal, Tasty, Great Everyday, Kingsmill*	1 Roll/68.1g	158.0	3.0	232	10.6	38.8	3.8	6.5
Rolls, Wholewhite, Kingsmill*	1 Roll/63g	158.0	3.0	251	9.5	43.7	4.2	3.5
Roti, Tesco*	1 Bread/95g	256.0	5.0	269	8.4	46.4	5.5	3.2
Rye with Sunflower Seeds, Organic, Sunnyvale*	1 Slice/25g	49.0	2.0	198	5.1	30.3	6.3	7.9
Rye, Average	*1 Slice/25g*	*55.0*	*0.0*	*219*	*8.3*	*45.8*	*1.7*	*4.4*
Rye, Baltic, Organic, The Village Bakery*	1oz/28g	68.0	0.0	243	8.0	50.3	1.4	2.9
Rye, Dark, Sliced, Trianon*	1 Slice/41g	74.0	1.0	180	6.5	35.0	1.5	0.0
Rye, German Style, Bolletje*	1 Slice/60g	114.0	1.0	190	6.0	35.0	2.0	9.5
Rye, German Style, Kelderman*	1 Slice/57g	88.0	1.0	155	5.6	30.2	1.4	7.7
Rye, Light, Finest, Tesco*	1 Slice/20g	47.0	0.0	237	10.4	44.3	2.0	3.7
Rye, Organic, Waitrose*	1 Serving/100g	207.0	1.0	207	6.4	42.7	1.2	5.1
Rye, Swedish Style, Kelderman*	1 Slice/50g	92.0	2.0	185	7.2	31.5	3.2	4.3
Rye, Wheat Free, New York Deli, The Stamp Collection*	1 Slice/33g	61.0	0.0	184	6.6	43.6	1.4	7.3
Rye, Wholemeal, Organic, House Of Westphalia*	1 Slice/75g	121.0	1.0	162	5.1	32.8	1.2	7.8
Rye, Wholemeal, with Sunflower Seeds, Organic, Biona*	1 Slice/72g	144.0	3.0	202	7.1	35.0	3.7	0.0
Rye, with Sunflower Seeds, Mestemacher*	1 Slice/80g	146.0	2.0	182	6.1	32.3	3.1	0.0
Rye, with Sunflower Seeds, Organic, Schneider Brot*	1 Slice/72g	138.0	3.0	191	6.2	33.4	3.6	7.9
Soda	*1oz/28g*	*72.0*	*1.0*	*258*	*7.7*	*54.6*	*2.5*	*2.1*
Soda Farls, M & S*	1 Farl/110g	267.0	3.0	243	9.6	50.1	2.7	2.3
Soda Farls, Tesco*	1 Farl/142g	325.0	5.0	229	7.1	42.2	3.2	2.6
Soda, Fruit, M & S*	1 Slice/40g	105.0	2.0	260	5.9	51.3	4.6	2.5
Soda, M & S*	1 Slice/40g	82.0	1.0	205	8.7	39.2	1.6	4.2
Softgrain, Farmhouse, M & S*	1 Slice/25g	59.0	1.0	238	8.4	42.8	3.7	3.2
Softgrain, Medium Sliced, GFY, Asda*	1 Slice/35g	79.0	1.0	226	7.0	46.0	1.5	3.7
Softgrain, Mighty White*	1 Slice/36g	81.0	1.0	224	7.2	45.5	1.5	3.7
Sourdough	1 Med Slice/50g	144.0	1.0	289	11.7	56.4	1.8	2.4
Soya & Linseed, Burgen*	1 Slice/36g	99.0	4.0	274	15.9	29.8	10.1	6.8
Soya & Linseed, Vogel*	1 Slice/45g	107.0	3.0	238	12.2	34.0	5.9	5.4
Stoneground, Small Loaf, Organic, Sainsbury's*	1 Slice/24g	50.0	0.0	208	10.0	37.9	2.1	7.9
Sunflower & Honey, M & S*	1 Serving/67g	206.0	9.0	308	12.9	34.0	13.4	5.6
Sunflower & Honey, Organic, Cranks*	1 Slice/30g	64.0	1.0	215	11.6	37.2	3.0	8.3
Sunflower & Pumpkin Seed, Batched, Organic, Tesco*	1 Slice/30g	73.0	2.0	243	11.0	33.1	7.4	5.2
Sunflower & Pumpkin Seed, So Organic, Sainsbury's*	1 Slice/30g	76.0	2.0	254	11.4	40.0	5.4	12.9
Sunflower Seed, Bolletje, Delhaize*	1 Slice/44g	106.0	3.0	240	7.5	35.0	7.0	6.0
Sunflower, Multi-Grain, Allinson*	1 Slice/47.1g	113.0	2.0	240	9.8	39.6	4.7	3.9
Tiger Loaf, Tesco*	1 Slice/40g	96.0	1.0	239	8.7	46.6	2.0	2.6
Toaster, White, Rathbones*	1 Slice/38g	92.0	0.0	243	9.1	48.6	1.3	2.3

BREAD

	Measure INFO/WEIGHT	per Measure KCAL	FAT	Nutrition Values per 100g / 100ml KCAL	PROT	CARB	FAT	FIBRE
Tomato & Chilli, BGTY, Sainsbury's*	¼ Bread/65g	155.0	3.0	238	11.9	36.9	4.7	2.8
Tomato & Garlic, Italian Style, Morrisons*	½ Pack/155g	355.0	12.0	229	5.8	33.4	8.0	2.5
Tomato, & Herb, Tear & Share, Tesco*	¼ Pack/73g	164.0	3.0	226	6.3	40.2	4.4	2.1
Veda Malt, St Michael*	1 Serving/45g	99.0	0.0	219	7.1	45.3	1.1	2.2
Walnut, Waitrose*	1/8 Loaf/50g	169.0	8.0	339	10.0	40.6	15.2	5.9
Wheat	*1 Slice/25g*	*65.0*	*1.0*	*260*	*9.1*	*47.2*	*4.1*	*4.3*
Wheat, Tasty, Kingsmill*	1 Serving/38g	84.0	1.0	221	10.1	37.6	3.4	6.8
Wheaten, M & S*	1 Slice/33g	74.0	1.0	225	9.3	42.9	3.5	3.9
Wheaten, Sliced, Healthy, Irwin's Bakery*	1 Slice/40g	76.0	1.0	190	9.0	40.5	1.9	6.2
Wheatgerm, Hovis, Soft, Sliced, M & S*	1 Slice/23g	50.0	1.0	220	10.1	38.5	3.0	4.6
Wheatgrain, Robertson*	1 Slice/30g	90.0	1.0	300	9.3	57.3	4.0	4.0
White Seeded Batch Loaf, Truly Irresistible, Co-Op*	1 Slice/47g	129.0	3.0	275	11.6	41.1	7.2	4.3
White, Average	*1 Slice/25g*	*59.0*	*0.0*	*235*	*8.4*	*49.3*	*1.9*	*1.5*
White, Batch Loaf, Extra Special, Asda*	1 Slice/47g	109.0	1.0	233	9.0	45.0	1.9	2.2
White, Batch, Warburton's*	1 Slice/42g	98.0	1.0	233	9.8	43.6	2.1	2.7
White, Chopped Roasted Garlic, Loaf, la Brea Bakery*	1 Loaf/400g	1196.0	16.0	299	9.9	53.0	4.1	2.5
White, Classic, Medium Sliced, Hovis*	1 Slice/37.9g	91.0	1.0	240	11.4	40.3	2.3	6.5
White, Classic, Thick Sliced, Hovis*	1 Slice/50g	120.0	2.0	240	9.2	40.5	4.5	3.1
White, COU, M & S*	1 Slice/26g	60.0	1.0	231	10.6	41.9	2.3	4.6
White, Country Maid*	1 Slice/33g	76.0	1.0	229	8.5	44.1	2.1	3.0
White, Crusty, Fresh, Finest, Tesco*	1 Slice/52g	130.0	1.0	250	8.6	48.5	1.9	2.4
White, Crusty, Gold, Kingsmill*	1 Slice/27g	70.0	1.0	258	9.4	48.5	2.9	2.7
White, Crusty, Hovis*	1 Slice/44g	103.0	1.0	233	8.8	44.3	2.2	2.1
White, Crusty, Sliced Loaf, Tesco*	1 Slice/50g	116.0	1.0	233	7.4	46.0	2.1	2.0
White, Crusty, Sliced, Premium, Budgens*	1 Slice/50g	121.0	1.0	242	8.8	46.9	2.2	2.2
White, Danish Style, Thick Sliced, Light, Tesco*	2 Slices/24g	59.0	0.0	245	9.6	46.9	1.9	2.8
White, Danish, Medium Sliced, BFY, Morrisons*	1 Slice/17g	42.0	0.0	245	10.2	49.1	1.8	2.2
White, Danish, Sliced, Weight Watchers*	1 Slice/20.6g	49.0	0.0	238	10.5	45.8	1.4	2.3
White, Danish, Soft & Light, Thick Cut, Asda*	1 Slice/26g	60.0	0.0	230	9.0	45.0	1.6	2.1
White, Eat Smart, Safeway*	1 Slice/26g	60.0	0.0	230	8.8	45.0	1.8	2.3
White, Extra Thick Sliced, Kingsmill*	1 Slice/58g	135.0	1.0	232	8.8	43.8	2.4	2.8
White, Farmhouse Crusty, M & S*	1 Slice/34g	82.0	1.0	240	8.9	46.6	2.2	3.0
White, Farmhouse Gold Premium, Morrisons*	1 Slice/38g	90.0	1.0	236	8.9	47.4	1.2	2.2
White, Farmhouse, Hovis*	1 Big Slice/44g	103.0	1.0	234	8.7	44.6	2.3	2.4
White, Farmhouse, Seeded, Waitrose*	1 Serving/75g	192.0	4.0	256	10.8	40.9	5.5	5.6
White, Farmhouse, Soft, Warburton's*	1 Slice/42.7g	101.0	1.0	236	9.9	43.4	2.5	2.7
White, Fibre, Morrisons*	1 Slice/40g	96.0	1.0	240	8.0	48.4	1.7	0.3
White, Fried in Blended Oil	*1 Slice/28g*	*141.0*	*9.0*	*503*	*7.9*	*48.5*	*32.2*	*1.6*
White, Gluten & Wheat Free, Free From, Sainsbury's*	1 Slice/33g	75.0	3.0	227	1.9	35.5	8.6	1.0
White, Gluten Free, Bakers Delight*	1 Serving/28g	64.0	2.0	227	1.9	35.5	8.6	1.0
White, Gluten Free, Genius*	1oz/28g	77.0	4.0	274	5.9	40.7	14.6	11.1
White, Gold Seeded, Kingsmill*	1 Slice/44g	108.0	3.0	245	9.7	38.8	5.7	3.5
White, Golden, Square Cut, M & S*	1 Slice/40g	85.0	1.0	215	8.9	40.7	2.1	6.1
White, Good Health, Warburton's*	1 Slice/38g	84.0	1.0	220	9.4	41.6	1.8	4.1
White, Harvest Crust Premium, Ormo*	1 Slice/40g	92.0	1.0	229	9.4	47.4	1.5	2.7
White, High Fibre, Nimble*	1 Slice/22g	48.0	0.0	219	10.1	40.6	1.8	7.5
White, Invisible Crust, Hovis*	1 Slice/40g	90.0	1.0	226	8.8	44.1	1.6	2.4
White, Loaf, Crusty, Premium, Warburton's*	1 Slice/30.5g	76.0	1.0	249	10.6	46.5	2.3	2.6
White, Loaf, Danish, Asda*	1 Serving/23g	53.0	0.0	236	9.0	45.0	2.2	2.0
White, Low Carb, Sliced, Tesco*	1 Slice/16g	35.0	0.0	211	11.3	36.4	2.2	6.9
White, Medium Sliced	1 Slice/39g	93.0	1.0	238	7.5	48.5	1.6	1.8
White, Medium Sliced, Keep Fresh, Safeway*	1 Slice/34g	76.0	1.0	224	7.3	44.3	1.9	2.7
White, Medium Sliced, Long Life, Asda*	1 Slice/36g	82.0	1.0	228	8.0	45.0	1.8	2.7

BREAD

	Measure INFO/WEIGHT	per Measure KCAL	FAT	Nutrition Values per 100g / 100ml KCAL	PROT	CARB	FAT	FIBRE
White, Medium Sliced, Stay Fresh, Tesco*	1 Slice/35g	85.0	1.0	246	8.9	48.1	2.0	0.8
White, Medium Sliced, Superlife, Morrisons*	1 Slice/30g	79.0	1.0	263	9.6	47.4	3.9	2.5
White, Medium Sliced, Weight Watchers*	1 Slice/12g	30.0	0.0	247	12.5	45.2	1.9	3.2
White, Medium, Round Top, Kingsmill*	1 Slice/41.8g	97.0	1.0	232	8.8	43.8	2.4	2.8
White, Medium, Stayfresh, Tesco*	1 Slice/45g	108.0	1.0	240	8.2	47.8	1.5	3.0
White, Medium, VLH Kitchens	1 Serving/30g	72.0	1.0	241	8.4	49.3	1.9	1.5
White, Oatmeal, Allinson*	1 Slice/47g	111.0	1.0	237	9.0	43.5	3.0	2.7
White, Organic, Hovis*	1 Slice/43.9g	108.0	1.0	246	8.6	45.8	3.2	2.3
White, Organic, Sainsbury's*	1 Slice/36g	84.0	1.0	234	8.9	45.5	1.8	2.3
White, Organic, Waitrose*	1oz/28g	69.0	0.0	246	8.8	48.8	0.5	1.8
White, Plain, Scottish, Sunblest*	1 Slice/57g	133.0	1.0	233	10.1	42.3	2.6	2.8
White, Premium, M & S*	1 Slice/40g	95.0	1.0	235	8.5	45.8	1.9	2.7
White, Sandwich, Bakery, Sainsbury's*	1 Slice/50g	121.0	0.0	242	10.3	49.0	0.6	2.9
White, Sandwich, Kingsmill*	1 Slice/42g	97.0	1.0	232	8.8	43.8	2.4	2.8
White, Scottish Plain, Mother's Pride*	1 Slice/50g	113.0	1.0	227	8.7	44.6	1.5	3.0
White, Sliced, Roberts Bakery*	1 Slice/35g	87.0	1.0	249	10.0	48.0	2.1	2.5
White, Small Loaf, Classic, Hovis*	1 Slice/32.9g	75.0	1.0	228	11.4	40.3	2.3	6.5
White, Soft Batch, Sliced, Sainsbury's*	1 Slice/44.0g	102.0	1.0	232	8.2	45.4	1.9	2.3
White, Soft Crusty, M & S*	1 Slice/25g	64.0	1.0	256	9.3	49.0	2.5	2.4
White, Soft, Batch Loaf, Sliced, Tesco*	1 Slice/50g	116.0	1.0	233	7.5	46.1	2.1	2.1
White, Soft, Farmhouse, M & S*	1 Slice/25g	60.0	1.0	239	9.8	42.6	3.3	2.5
White, Soft, Gold, Kingsmill*	1 Slice/46.9g	112.0	1.0	239	8.2	44.5	3.1	2.7
White, Soft, Great Everyday, Thick Sliced, Kingsmill*	1 Slice/44g	102.0	1.0	232	9.0	44.6	2.0	2.7
White, Soft, Hovis*	1 Slice/40.2g	94.0	1.0	234	8.7	44.6	2.3	2.4
White, Soft, M & S*	1 Slice/46.7g	105.0	1.0	225	7.3	46.1	1.7	2.4
White, Soft, Organic, Warburton's*	1 Slice/27g	61.0	1.0	228	9.7	44.6	3.0	2.6
White, Soft, Sliced, Hovis*	1 Thin Slice/25g	58.0	1.0	234	8.7	44.6	2.3	2.4
White, Softgrain, Sliced, Tesco*	1 Med Slice/36g	81.0	1.0	224	7.2	45.5	1.5	3.7
White, Sour Dough, Usda Average	1 Med Slice/64g	185.0	1.0	289	11.7	56.4	1.8	2.4
White, Sourdough, Country, Oval, la Brea Bakery*	1 Slice/60g	143.0	0.0	239	8.8	49.4	0.6	1.6
White, Square, Extra Thick Sliced, Hovis*	1 Slice/67.1g	155.0	1.0	231	8.5	44.7	2.0	2.6
White, Square, Medium Sliced, Hovis*	1 Slice/40g	92.0	1.0	231	8.5	44.7	2.0	2.6
White, Square, Thick Sliced, Hovis*	1 Slice/50.2g	116.0	1.0	231	8.5	44.7	2.0	2.6
White, Stay Fresh, Tesco*	1 Slice/40g	100.0	1.0	249	8.6	48.3	2.4	1.5
White, Super Toastie, Warburton's*	1 Serving/57g	134.0	1.0	235	10.1	44.6	1.8	2.7
White, Superior English Quality, Thin Cut, Hovis*	1 Serving/73g	169.0	1.0	232	9.2	42.8	1.5	3.8
White, Thick Sliced, Fine Lady*	1 Slice/44g	113.0	1.0	254	7.8	53.1	1.2	2.3
White, Thick Sliced, Healthy, Warburton's*	1 Slice/38g	84.0	1.0	222	10.3	41.2	1.8	4.1
White, Thick Sliced, M & S*	1 Slice/42g	96.0	1.0	228	7.3	46.7	1.3	2.8
White, Thick Sliced, Organic, Tesco*	1 Slice/44g	108.0	1.0	245	8.5	46.8	2.1	3.1
White, Thick Sliced, Premium, Tesco*	1 Slice/44g	99.0	0.0	222	8.7	45.2	0.7	1.5
White, Thick Sliced, Sainsbury's*	1 Slice/44g	95.0	1.0	216	8.7	41.1	1.9	7.1
White, Thick Sliced, Square Cut, Asda*	1 Slice/44g	101.0	1.0	230	8.0	46.0	1.5	2.1
White, Thick Sliced, Staysoft, Rathbones*	1 Slice/38g	87.0	0.0	228	8.5	45.5	1.3	2.7
White, Thick Sliced, Sunblest*	1 Slice/40g	91.0	1.0	228	8.0	45.7	1.5	2.8
White, Thick Sliced, Super Toastie, Morrisons*	1 Slice/50g	128.0	1.0	257	8.7	48.9	3.0	2.1
White, Thick Sliced, Tesco*	1 Slice/44g	106.0	1.0	240	8.2	47.8	1.5	3.0
White, Thick Sliced, Warburton's*	1 Slice/28g	65.0	1.0	233	9.8	43.6	2.1	2.7
White, Thick Sliced, Warburton's, Weight Watchers*	1 Slice/29g	69.0	0.0	237	10.4	48.6	0.8	2.0
White, Thick, So Organic, Sainsbury's*	1 Slice/44.2g	102.0	1.0	231	8.2	44.6	2.2	3.1
White, Thick, Super Soft, M & S*	1 Slice/48g	115.0	1.0	240	8.7	45.3	2.6	2.5
White, Thick, Toastie, 800g Loaf, Warburton's*	1 Slice/47g	111.0	1.0	234	9.9	43.9	1.9	2.5
White, Thin Sliced, Sainsbury's*	1 Slice/29g	66.0	0.0	228	7.1	46.4	1.5	2.8

B

BREAD

	Measure INFO/WEIGHT	per Measure KCAL	FAT	Nutrition Values per 100g / 100ml KCAL	PROT	CARB	FAT	FIBRE
White, Thin Sliced, Tesco*	1 Slice/30g	68.0	0.0	228	9.5	44.5	1.3	3.4
White, Toasted, Average	*1 Slice/33g*	*87.0*	*1.0*	*265*	*9.3*	*57.1*	*1.6*	*1.8*
White, Toastie, Thick Cut, Hovis*	1 Slice/50g	115.0	1.0	230	8.5	44.7	2.0	2.5
White, Toastie, Thick, Love to Toast, Kingsmill*	1 Slice/50g	116.0	1.0	232	9.0	44.6	2.0	2.7
White, Weight Watchers*	1 Serving/5g	12.0	0.0	246	12.3	45.1	1.6	3.3
White, Whole, Extra Thick, Kingsmill*	1 Slice/57g	130.0	1.0	228	9.0	42.3	2.5	4.0
White, Whole, Kingsmill*	1 Slice/38g	87.0	1.0	230	9.0	42.9	2.5	3.4
White, Wholesome, Loaf, Sainsbury's*	1 Serving/36g	81.0	1.0	224	9.4	42.5	1.8	4.4
White, Wholesome, Medium Sliced, Asda*	1 Slice/35.0g	78.0	1.0	223	7.0	43.0	2.6	5.0
White, Wholesome, Medium Sliced, Premium, Tesco*	1 Slice/37g	85.0	1.0	232	8.9	43.9	2.3	4.2
White, Wholesome, Thick Sliced, Tesco*	1 Serving/80g	177.0	2.0	221	10.5	40.5	1.9	4.8
Whole Grain, Batch, Finest, Tesco*	1 Slice/44g	112.0	1.0	254	9.8	47.7	2.7	4.2
Whole Wheat, Harvest	1 Serving/42g	90.0	1.0	214	7.1	45.2	2.4	7.1
Whole Wheat, Nature's Own*	1 Slice/28g	66.0	1.0	236	14.3	39.3	3.6	10.7
Whole Wheat, Soft, Trader Joe's*	1 Slice/37g	70.0	1.0	189	10.8	37.8	2.7	5.4
Wholegrain, & White, Kingsmill*	1 Slice/46.9g	107.0	1.0	228	9.0	42.3	2.5	4.0
Wholegrain, Medium Sliced, Irish Pride*	1 Slice/38g	90.0	1.0	237	9.2	46.6	2.1	7.6
Wholegrain, Soft, M & S*	1 Slice/51g	115.0	3.0	225	13.0	31.2	5.4	8.2
Wholemeal Oatbran, Sliced, Tesco*	1 Slice/45g	90.0	1.0	200	10.1	35.3	1.6	7.4
Wholemeal Seeded Batch Loaf, Truly Irresistible, Co-Op*	1 Slice/47g	108.0	2.0	230	13.7	35.0	4.0	8.1
Wholemeal, & Oat Flakes, Gold, Kingsmill*	1 Slice/46.8g	103.0	2.0	220	10.0	37.3	3.4	7.0
Wholemeal, Average	*1 Slice/25g*	*54.0*	*1.0*	*215*	*9.2*	*41.6*	*2.5*	*5.8*
Wholemeal, Batch, Organic, Waitrose*	1 Slice/40g	88.0	1.0	219	10.0	38.8	2.6	7.2
Wholemeal, BGTY, Sainsbury's*	1 Slice/20g	41.0	0.0	207	12.6	36.8	1.0	7.3
Wholemeal, COU, M & S*	1 Slice/21g	45.0	1.0	213	13.6	33.7	2.6	7.0
Wholemeal, Crusty, Finest, Tesco*	1 Slice/50g	103.0	1.0	206	10.8	37.0	1.7	6.9
Wholemeal, Crusty, Kingsmill*	1 Slice/42g	104.0	2.0	247	11.2	41.1	4.2	7.0
Wholemeal, Danish, BFY, Morrisons*	1 Slice/17g	39.0	0.0	228	11.2	47.9	1.8	6.2
Wholemeal, Danish, Warburton's*	1 Slice/25g	57.0	1.0	229	13.3	38.5	2.4	7.2
Wholemeal, Economy, Sainsbury's*	1 Slice/28g	61.0	1.0	217	10.3	38.4	2.5	6.5
Wholemeal, Farmhouse Soft Golden, M & S*	1 Slice/30g	64.0	1.0	215	11.0	35.1	3.1	7.4
Wholemeal, Farmhouse, Hovis*	1 Slice/44g	91.0	1.0	207	11.0	36.0	2.2	7.1
Wholemeal, Fresher for Longer, Sainsbury's*	1 Slice/44g	98.0	2.0	222	10.9	36.2	3.7	6.5
Wholemeal, Gold, Kingsmill*	1 Slice/44g	95.0	1.0	217	10.9	36.8	2.9	7.0
Wholemeal, Golden Wheat, Kingsmill*	1 Slice/44g	97.0	1.0	221	10.9	37.8	2.9	6.0
Wholemeal, Golden, M & S*	1 Slice/30.2g	69.0	1.0	230	10.8	36.6	4.5	7.7
Wholemeal, Greggs*	1 Slice/36g	77.0	1.0	215	9.2	41.6	2.5	5.8
Wholemeal, Keep Fresh, Medium Sliced, Safeway*	1 Slice/37g	75.0	1.0	204	9.1	36.6	2.4	6.2
Wholemeal, Light, Irish Pride*	1 Slice/28.2g	68.0	0.0	241	13.3	44.1	1.3	4.5
Wholemeal, Little Brown Loaf, Unsliced, Hovis*	1 Slice/40g	86.0	1.0	216	10.0	37.8	2.7	6.8
Wholemeal, Loaf, Crusty, Farmhouse, M & S*	1 Serving/33g	75.0	1.0	230	10.1	40.7	2.7	6.3
Wholemeal, Longer Life, Medium Sliced, Sainsbury's*	1 Slice/35g	78.0	1.0	222	10.9	36.2	3.7	6.5
Wholemeal, Longer Life, Sainsbury's*	1 Slice/36g	85.0	1.0	237	10.7	41.0	3.4	6.2
Wholemeal, Medium Sliced, Fresh for a Week, Asda*	1 Slice/35g	71.0	1.0	202	9.0	36.0	2.4	7.0
Wholemeal, Medium Sliced, Great Everyday, Kingsmill*	1 Slice/40g	91.0	2.0	227	10.5	37.7	3.8	6.2
Wholemeal, Medium Sliced, M & S*	1 Slice/40g	80.0	1.0	200	10.5	32.7	3.1	6.7
Wholemeal, Medium Sliced, Organic, Asda*	1 Slice/43g	94.0	1.0	217	9.0	40.0	2.3	6.0
Wholemeal, Medium Sliced, Organic, Tesco*	1 Slice/27g	55.0	1.0	209	9.2	37.2	2.8	6.0
Wholemeal, Medium Sliced, Premium, Tesco*	1 Slice/36g	71.0	0.0	196	9.8	37.8	0.6	7.2
Wholemeal, Medium Sliced, Sainsbury's*	1 Slice/36g	77.0	1.0	214	10.3	37.8	2.4	7.4
Wholemeal, Medium Sliced, Waitrose*	1 Slice/36g	76.0	1.0	213	10.1	37.6	2.4	7.0
Wholemeal, Medium, 400g Loaf, Warburton's*	1 Slice/24g	55.0	1.0	231	10.4	40.7	2.5	6.5
Wholemeal, Medium, 800g Loaf, Warburton's*	1 Slice/40.3g	93.0	1.0	231	10.2	39.6	2.5	6.5

BREAD

	Measure INFO/WEIGHT	per Measure KCAL	FAT	Nutrition Values per 100g / 100ml KCAL	PROT	CARB	FAT	FIBRE
Wholemeal, Multi Seeded, TTD, Sainsbury's*	1 Slice/47g	110.0	3.0	234	11.7	30.7	7.2	8.1
Wholemeal, Multigrain, Sliced, Finest, Tesco*	1 Serving/50g	123.0	2.0	246	10.1	42.1	4.1	6.5
Wholemeal, Multigrain, Soft Batch, Sainsbury's*	1 Slice/44g	106.0	3.0	242	11.3	34.5	6.5	5.6
Wholemeal, Multiseed, Organic, Sainsbury's*	1 Slice/26g	75.0	3.0	289	13.8	36.6	9.7	6.0
Wholemeal, Nimble*	1 Slice/21.9g	48.0	1.0	219	12.2	37.0	2.5	6.8
Wholemeal, Oat Topped, TTD, Sainsbury's*	1 Slice/47g	109.0	1.0	232	10.0	38.5	2.8	0.3
Wholemeal, Organic, 400g Loaf, Warburton's*	1 Slice/28.2g	63.0	1.0	223	10.3	37.9	3.2	6.7
Wholemeal, Organic, Hovis*	1 Slice/44g	92.0	1.0	209	10.2	35.6	2.9	7.6
Wholemeal, Premium, Medium Slice, M & S*	1 Slice/33g	65.0	1.0	200	10.5	32.9	3.1	6.7
Wholemeal, Premium, Thick Slice, M & S*	1 Slice/50g	95.0	1.0	190	9.8	30.8	3.0	6.4
Wholemeal, Rathbones*	1 Slice/27g	57.0	0.0	211	9.4	39.2	1.8	7.1
Wholemeal, Rustic, Tin, Tesco*	1 Slice/37g	92.0	1.0	249	12.2	44.0	3.5	3.1
Wholemeal, Sliced, Gluten Free, Glutano*	1 Slice/56g	107.0	2.0	191	7.0	34.0	3.0	0.0
Wholemeal, Sliced, McCambridge*	1 Slice/38g	90.0	1.0	237	7.9	44.7	1.8	0.0
Wholemeal, Sliced, Medium, Tesco*	1 Slice/36g	79.0	1.0	220	11.0	39.1	2.2	6.6
Wholemeal, Sliced, Organic, Harvestime*	1 Slice/44g	95.0	1.0	216	9.0	38.7	2.7	5.6
Wholemeal, Soft Crusty, M & S*	1 Slice/25g	57.0	1.0	230	11.4	39.1	3.1	6.5
Wholemeal, Square Cut, Thick Sliced, Asda*	1 Slice/44g	91.0	1.0	208	10.0	37.0	2.2	6.0
Wholemeal, Stayfresh, Tesco*	1 Slice/36g	81.0	1.0	225	11.0	39.1	2.2	6.0
Wholemeal, Stoneground, 800g Loaf, Warburton's*	1 Slice/45.3g	95.0	1.0	210	10.4	35.8	2.6	6.8
Wholemeal, Stoneground, Organic, Sainsbury's*	1 Slice/29g	61.0	1.0	210	10.2	37.9	1.9	7.8
Wholemeal, Stoneground, Organic, Waitrose*	1 Sm Slice/25g	57.0	1.0	228	10.8	38.2	3.6	7.1
Wholemeal, Stoneground, Thick Sliced, Sainsbury's*	1 Slice/43.8g	92.0	1.0	210	10.2	37.9	1.9	7.8
Wholemeal, Tasty, Medium, Kingsmill*	1 Slice/40g	91.0	2.0	227	10.5	37.7	3.8	6.2
Wholemeal, Thick Sliced, Great Everyday, Kingsmill*	1 Slice/44.1g	100.0	2.0	227	10.5	37.7	3.8	6.2
Wholemeal, Thick Sliced, Keep Fresh, Safeway*	1 Slice/45g	92.0	1.0	204	9.1	36.6	2.4	6.2
Wholemeal, Thick Sliced, Organic, Tesco*	1 Slice/44g	98.0	1.0	220	8.8	38.8	2.8	5.9
Wholemeal, Thick Sliced, Premium, Tesco*	1 Serving/44g	95.0	1.0	214	10.0	40.1	1.5	5.7
Wholemeal, Thick Sliced, Sainsbury's*	1 Slice/48g	102.0	1.0	213	10.1	37.4	2.6	8.5
Wholemeal, Thick Sliced, Waitrose*	1 Slice/44g	94.0	1.0	213	10.1	37.6	2.4	7.0
Wholemeal, Thick Sliced, Weight Watchers*	1 Slice/29g	67.0	1.0	231	10.9	40.3	2.5	6.5
Wholemeal, Toasted, Average	*1 Med Slice/26g*	*58.0*	*1.0*	*224*	*8.6*	*42.3*	*2.2*	*5.8*

BREAD & BUTTER PUDDING

5% Fat, M & S*	1 Pudding/237g	367.0	10.0	155	4.4	24.8	4.2	0.4
Average	1 Serving/190g	304.0	15.0	160	6.2	17.5	7.8	0.3
BGTY, Sainsbury's*	1 Serving/125g	126.0	3.0	101	6.3	13.4	2.3	5.4
COU, M & S*	1 Pot/140g	161.0	3.0	115	6.1	18.4	2.0	0.8
GFY, Asda*	1 Serving/125g	152.0	2.0	122	7.0	20.0	1.6	1.3
Individual, M & S*	1 Pudding/130g	279.0	16.0	215	4.4	21.4	12.6	0.5
Low Fat, Individual, BGTY, Sainsbury's*	1 Pack/125g	125.0	3.0	100	6.3	13.4	2.3	5.4
Reduced Fat, Waitrose*	1 Serving/205g	299.0	5.0	146	7.4	23.3	2.6	2.0
Sticky Toffee, M & S*	1oz/28g	83.0	3.0	295	4.1	46.3	10.6	2.2

BREAD MIX

Brown, Sunflower, Sainsbury's*	1 Serving/60g	151.0	4.0	251	10.0	38.9	6.1	4.0
Cheese & Onion, Dry Mix, Sainsbury's*	1 Serving/100g	311.0	3.0	311	11.9	59.5	2.8	2.6
Ciabatta, Made Up with Water & Olive Oil, Wrights*	1 Slice/45g	113.0	2.0	251	10.0	43.6	4.0	1.8
Crusty White, Made Up, Tesco*	1 Slice/126g	316.0	2.0	251	9.4	49.3	1.8	2.5
Focaccia, Garlic & Herb, Asda*	1 Serving/125g	385.0	10.0	308	11.0	48.0	8.0	3.3
Italian Ciabatta, Sainsbury's*	1 Slice/45g	96.0	1.0	213	8.7	40.0	2.0	2.4
Italian Sun Dried Tomato & Parmesan, Sainsbury's*	1 Serving/100g	247.0	2.0	247	8.1	50.1	1.7	2.5
Mixed Grain, Sainsbury's*	1 Serving/45g	103.0	1.0	228	7.7	46.0	1.5	4.4
Parmesan & Sun Dried Tomato, Made Up, Wrights*	1 Slice/45g	103.0	1.0	229	9.3	46.0	1.3	2.4
White Loaf, Asda*	1 Slice/60g	150.0	1.0	250	10.0	49.0	1.5	3.1

B

	Measure INFO/WEIGHT	per Measure KCAL	FAT	Nutrition Values per 100g / 100ml KCAL	PROT	CARB	FAT	FIBRE
BREAD MIX								
Wholemeal, Hovis*	1 Serving/65g	148.0	3.0	227	10.0	35.8	4.8	6.8
Wholemeal, Made Up, M & S*	1 Loaf/600g	1410.0	14.0	235	11.0	42.0	2.4	5.3
BREADCRUMBS								
Average	*1oz/28g*	*98.0*	*1.0*	*350*	*10.7*	*74.8*	*1.9*	*2.5*
Golden, Paxo*	1 Serving/70g	248.0	1.0	354	11.5	73.5	1.6	3.4
BREADFRUIT								
Canned, Drained	*1oz/28g*	*18.0*	*0.0*	*66*	*0.6*	*16.4*	*0.2*	*1.7*
Raw	*1oz/28g*	*27.0*	*0.0*	*95*	*1.3*	*23.1*	*0.3*	*0.0*
BREADSTICKS								
Asda*	1 Serving/5g	21.0	0.0	412	12.0	73.0	8.0	2.9
Chive & Onion Twists, Tesco*	3 Twists/24g	115.0	5.0	480	11.6	57.6	22.1	2.2
Farleys*	1 Serving/12g	50.0	1.0	414	14.0	76.5	5.8	1.1
Grissini, Italian, Sainsbury's*	1 Breadstick/5g	20.0	0.0	408	11.6	72.9	7.8	2.9
Grissini, Thin, with Olive Oil, Forno Bianco*	1 Stick/5g	21.0	0.0	420	11.0	77.0	7.5	0.0
Grissini, Waitrose*	1 Breadstick/6g	25.0	0.0	397	12.0	72.5	6.2	3.1
Italian Original, Tesco*	1 Stick/5.5g	23.0	0.0	410	11.6	72.9	7.8	2.9
Mini, Sainsbury's*	4 Sticks/5g	20.0	0.0	404	15.6	68.7	7.4	4.8
Mini, Wheat & Gluten Free, Free From, Tesco*	1 Stick/2.7g	11.0	0.0	414	4.0	72.1	12.2	2.2
Olive, Italian, Finest, Tesco*	1 Stick/40g	170.0	5.0	424	10.5	65.0	13.6	4.8
Onion, M & S*	1 Serving/40g	166.0	6.0	415	12.6	59.6	14.1	4.8
Original, Italian, Tesco*	1 Stick/5.5g	23.0	0.0	410	11.6	72.9	7.8	2.9
Original, Organic, Kallo*	1 Breadstick/6g	24.0	0.0	393	11.8	69.5	7.6	4.7
Oven Baked, Mini, Quaker Oats*	1 Pack/35g	145.0	3.0	415	12.9	71.0	8.8	3.7
Perfectly Balanced, Waitrose*	1 Breadstick/5g	20.0	0.0	378	13.7	77.3	1.6	3.8
Pesto Flavour, Safeway*	1 Stick/6g	24.0	0.0	394	13.4	67.5	7.8	5.2
Plain, Asda*	1 Stick/5g	21.0	0.0	412	12.0	73.0	8.0	2.9
Rosemary, Asda*	1 Breadstick/7g	29.0	1.0	439	12.0	64.0	15.0	3.5
Salted, Asda*	1 Stick/8g	36.0	1.0	445	13.0	60.0	17.0	4.3
Sesame Seed Grissini, Sainsbury's*	1 Breadstick/5g	21.0	1.0	419	12.7	65.5	11.8	3.2
Torrinesi, TTD, Sainsbury's*	1 Stick/3g	13.0	0.0	411	11.0	77.0	6.5	1.1
BREAKFAST CEREAL								
3 in One, Raisin & Apple, Jordans*	1 Serving/50g	170.0	2.0	340	7.6	67.4	4.4	9.8
3 in One, Strawberry, Jordans*	1 Serving/50g	181.0	3.0	362	9.4	68.0	5.8	11.9
Advantage, Weetabix*	1 Serving/30g	105.0	1.0	350	10.2	72.0	2.4	9.0
All Bran, Apricot Bites, Kellogg's*	1 Serving/45g	126.0	1.0	279	11.0	55.0	2.5	19.0
All Bran, Asda*	1 Serving/40g	110.0	1.0	276	15.0	46.0	3.5	27.0
All Bran, Bran Flakes, & Fruit, Kellogg's*	1 Serving/40g	143.0	2.0	358	8.0	68.0	6.0	9.0
All Bran, Bran Flakes, Chocolate, Kellogg's*	1 Serving/30g	106.0	2.0	354	10.0	65.0	6.0	13.0
All Bran, Bran Flakes, Kellogg's*	1 Serving/30g	98.0	1.0	326	10.7	67.0	2.0	15.0
All Bran, Bran Flakes, Yoghurty, Kellogg's*	1 Serving/40g	141.0	2.0	353	10.0	67.0	5.0	12.0
All Bran, Fibre Plus, Kellogg's*	1 Serving/40g	112.0	1.0	280	14.0	48.0	3.5	27.0
All Bran, Fruitful, Kellogg's*	1 Serving/40g	136.0	3.0	340	12.5	57.5	7.5	0.0
All Bran, High Fibre, Morrisons*	1 Serving/40g	109.0	1.0	272	14.7	45.5	3.5	27.0
All Bran, Original, High Fibre, Kellogg's*	1 Serving/40g	112.0	1.0	280	14.0	48.0	3.5	27.0
All Bran, Splitz, Kellogg's*	1 Serving/40g	130.0	1.0	325	9.0	69.0	2.0	9.0
All Bran, Strawberry Medley, Kellogg's*	1 Serving/55g	170.0	2.0	309	9.1	80.0	2.7	1.8
Almond, Low Carb, Atkins*	1 Serving/30g	100.0	1.0	333	50.0	26.7	5.0	0.0
Almond, Oats & More, Nestle*	1 Serving/30g	119.0	3.0	398	10.7	68.7	8.9	5.5
Almond, Pecan & Cashew Muesli, Kellogg's*	1 Bowl/45g	188.0	6.0	418	11.0	62.0	14.0	8.0
Almond, Raisin & Pecan, Nature's Pleasure, Kellogg's*	1 Serving/45g	184.0	5.0	408	10.0	65.0	12.0	8.0
Alpen*, Crunchy Bran*	1 Serving/40g	120.0	2.0	299	11.8	52.3	4.7	24.8
Amaranth, Flakes, Organic, Gillian McKeith*	1 Serving/50g	198.0	2.0	396	10.0	80.0	4.0	3.0
Apple & Cinnamon Flakes, M & S*	1 Serving/30g	111.0	1.0	370	6.0	82.7	1.9	3.4

BREAKFAST CEREAL

	INFO/WEIGHT	KCAL	FAT	KCAL	PROT	CARB	FAT	FIBRE
Apple & Cinnamon, Crisp, Sainsbury's*	1 Serving/50g	216.0	7.0	433	6.2	69.1	14.7	3.4
Apple & Cinnamon, Quaker Oats*	1 Sachet/38g	136.0	2.0	358	8.0	68.0	5.5	2.5
Apple, Blackberry, & Raspberry Flakes, GFY, Asda*	1 Serving/30g	103.0	1.0	344	9.0	73.0	1.8	11.0
Apricot Wheats, Whole Grain, Tesco*	1 Serving/40g	130.0	1.0	326	7.6	70.6	1.4	8.0
Balance with Red Fruits, Sainsbury's*	1 Serving/40g	147.0	1.0	367	11.2	77.5	1.3	2.6
Balance, Sainsbury's*	1 Serving/30g	111.0	0.0	370	11.4	77.7	1.5	3.2
Banana & Toffee Crisp, Mornflake*	1 Serving/30g	133.0	5.0	443	5.7	68.8	16.1	5.4
Banana, Papaya & Honey Oat, Crunchy, Waitrose*	1 Serving/40g	170.0	5.0	426	9.6	69.8	12.0	5.5
Barley Crisp, Cocoa, Pertwood Farm*	1 Serving/30g	105.0	1.0	350	8.1	84.0	2.1	9.3
Barley Crisp, Plain, Pertwood Farm*	1 Serving/40g	142.0	1.0	356	9.4	82.7	2.3	8.2
Barley Crisp, with Maple Syrup, Pertwood Farm*	1 Serving/50g	167.0	1.0	335	7.1	86.0	1.7	6.2
Benefit Flakes, Aldi*	1 Serving/40g	148.0	1.0	370	11.4	77.7	1.5	3.2
Berry Burst, So Simple, Quaker Oats*	1 Serving/39g	144.0	2.0	370	8.0	70.0	6.0	6.5
Berry Crunchy, Sainsbury's*	1 Serving/30g	122.0	4.0	408	7.7	67.3	12.0	4.8
Bitesize, Weetabix*	1 Serving/40g	135.0	1.0	338	11.5	68.4	2.0	10.0
Blackberry & Apple, Alpen*	1 Serving/40g	140.0	2.0	349	9.2	69.4	3.8	8.3
Blueberry Wheats, Tesco*	1 Serving/50g	165.0	1.0	330	7.5	71.6	1.5	8.5
Bran Crunch, Raisin, Kellogg's*	1 Pack/80g	280.0	2.0	350	6.2	83.7	1.9	7.5
Bran Flakes, Asda*	1 Serving/47g	157.0	2.0	333	11.0	65.0	3.2	14.0
Bran Flakes, Crunchy Nut, Sainsbury's*	1 Serving/40g	203.0	4.0	507	19.7	85.7	9.5	11.0
Bran Flakes, Harvest Home, Nestle*	1 Serving/30g	99.0	1.0	331	10.2	67.1	2.4	14.1
Bran Flakes, HL, Tesco*	1 Serving/30g	100.0	1.0	335	10.2	67.0	2.4	14.1
Bran Flakes, Honey Nut, Asda*	1 Serving/50g	180.0	2.0	360	10.0	70.0	4.4	11.0
Bran Flakes, Honey Nut, Sainsbury's*	1 Serving/40g	143.0	2.0	358	9.6	70.0	4.4	11.0
Bran Flakes, Honey Nut, Tesco*	1 Serving/40g	143.0	2.0	358	9.6	70.0	4.4	11.0
Bran Flakes, Kellogg's*	1 Serving/50g	163.0	1.0	326	10.0	67.0	2.0	15.0
Bran Flakes, Morrisons*	1 Serving/25g	83.0	1.0	331	11.1	64.6	3.2	14.5
Bran Flakes, Organic, Asda*	1 Serving/30g	99.0	1.0	330	10.0	67.0	2.4	14.0
Bran Flakes, Organic, Sainsbury's*	1 Serving/30g	100.0	1.0	332	10.2	67.4	2.4	14.1
Bran Flakes, Sainsbury's*	1 Serving/30g	100.0	1.0	333	10.3	67.5	2.5	14.3
Bran Flakes, Sultana Bran, Kellogg's*	1 Serving/30g	95.0	1.0	318	8.0	67.0	2.0	13.0
Bran Flakes, Sultana, Dry, Sainsbury's*	1 Serving/30g	97.0	1.0	325	8.3	68.6	1.9	12.1
Bran Flakes, Sultana, with Milk, Sainsbury's*	1 Serving/30g	157.0	3.0	523	22.0	89.7	8.7	11.7
Bran Flakes, Tesco*	1 Serving/30g	99.0	1.0	331	10.2	67.1	2.4	14.1
Bran Flakes, Value, Tesco*	1 Serving/50g	167.0	1.0	335	10.3	67.2	2.4	14.2
Bran Flakes, Whole Grain, Sainsbury's*	1 Serving/30g	99.0	1.0	331	10.2	67.1	2.4	14.1
Bran, Natural, Sainsbury's*	1 Serving/30g	64.0	1.0	212	14.7	27.0	5.0	36.0
Breakfast Biscuits, Aldi*	4 Biscuits/60g	213.0	1.0	355	13.7	69.5	2.5	7.5
Caribbean Crunch, Alpen*	1 Serving/40g	155.0	4.0	388	8.8	67.9	9.0	4.6
Cheerios, Honey Nut, Nestle*	1 Serving/30g	112.0	1.0	374	7.0	78.3	3.7	5.2
Cheerios, Honey, Nestle*	1 Bowl/50g	184.0	1.0	369	6.6	79.2	2.8	5.8
Cheerios, Nestle*	1 Serving/30g	111.0	1.0	369	8.1	75.2	3.9	6.6
Choc & Nut Crisp, Tesco*	1 Serving/40g	185.0	8.0	462	8.3	62.5	19.9	4.8
Choco Crackles, Morrisons*	1 Serving/30g	115.0	1.0	383	5.5	84.8	2.4	1.9
Choco Flakes, Asda*	1 Serving/50g	187.0	0.0	374	6.0	86.0	0.7	2.6
Choco Flakes, Kellogg's*	1 Serving/30g	114.0	1.0	380	5.0	84.0	3.0	2.5
Choco Flakes, Sainsbury's*	1 Serving/30g	111.0	0.0	370	5.5	85.4	0.7	3.0
Choco Flakes, Tesco*	1 Serving/30g	112.0	0.0	374	5.6	86.3	0.7	2.6
Choco Hoops, Asda*	1 Serving/40g	154.0	2.0	385	7.0	79.0	4.5	4.0
Choco Hoops, Kids, Tesco*	1 Serving/30g	116.0	1.0	387	7.6	79.1	4.5	4.5
Choco Snaps, Asda*	1 Serving/30g	115.0	1.0	382	5.0	85.0	2.4	1.9
Choco Snaps, Sainsbury's*	1 Serving/30g	115.0	1.0	383	5.5	84.8	2.4	1.9
Choco Squares, Asda*	1 Serving/30g	130.0	4.0	434	10.0	67.0	14.0	4.0

BREAKFAST CEREAL

	Measure INFO/WEIGHT	per Measure		Nutrition Values per 100g / 100ml				
		KCAL	FAT	KCAL	PROT	CARB	FAT	FIBRE
Chocolate Cereal, Tesco*	1 Serving/40g	169.0	6.0	423	8.0	66.3	14.0	6.0
Chocolate Crisp, Minis, Weetabix*	1 Serving/36g	134.0	2.0	371	9.0	71.7	5.3	8.5
Chocolate Wheats, Kellogg's*	1 Serving/40g	148.0	4.0	369	10.0	62.0	9.0	12.0
Cinnamon & Apple, Sensations, Asda*	1 Serving/30g	112.0	1.0	373	10.0	72.0	5.0	7.0
Cinnamon Grahams, Nestle*	1 Serving/40g	164.0	4.0	411	4.7	76.1	9.8	4.2
Clusters, Nestle*	1 Serving/30g	111.0	1.0	371	9.3	72.6	4.8	7.4
Coco Pops, Crunchers, Kellogg's*	1 Serving/30g	114.0	1.0	380	7.0	81.0	3.5	3.0
Coco Pops, Kellogg's*	1 Serving/30g	116.0	1.0	387	5.0	85.0	3.0	2.0
Coco Pops, Mega Munchers, Kellogg's*	1 Serving/30g	112.0	1.0	375	8.0	80.0	2.5	4.5
Coco Pops, Straws, Kellogg's*	1 Straw/13g	60.0	2.0	459	9.0	72.0	15.0	2.0
Cookie Crunch, Nestle*	1 Serving/40g	154.0	1.0	385	4.6	85.3	2.8	1.8
Corn Flakes, Asda*	1 Serving/30g	111.0	0.0	370	7.0	84.0	0.7	3.0
Corn Flakes, Banana Crunch, Kellogg's*	1 Serving/40g	163.0	3.0	408	6.0	78.0	8.0	3.0
Corn Flakes, Crispy Nut, Asda*	1 Serving/30g	117.0	1.0	390	7.0	81.0	4.2	2.5
Corn Flakes, Harvest Home, Nestle*	1 Serving/25g	92.0	0.0	367	7.3	82.7	0.8	3.6
Corn Flakes, Hint of Honey, Kellogg's*	1 Serving/30g	113.0	0.0	377	6.0	87.0	0.6	2.5
Corn Flakes, Honey Nut & Cranberries, Sainsbury's*	1 Serving/40g	166.0	4.0	416	7.4	74.4	9.9	3.1
Corn Flakes, Honey Nut with Cranberries, Tesco*	1 Serving/50g	208.0	5.0	416	7.4	74.4	9.9	3.1
Corn Flakes, Honey Nut, Co-Op*	1 Serving/40g	154.0	2.0	385	7.0	81.0	4.0	1.0
Corn Flakes, Honey Nut, Harvest Home, Nestle*	1 Serving/30g	118.0	1.0	392	7.4	81.1	4.2	2.5
Corn Flakes, Kellogg's*	1 Serving/30g	112.0	0.0	372	7.0	84.0	0.9	3.0
Corn Flakes, Organic, Lima*	1 Serving/50g	177.0	0.0	355	8.3	77.7	1.0	6.4
Corn Flakes, Organic, Whole Earth*	1 Serving/40g	154.0	0.0	386	8.6	84.2	1.0	3.0
Corn Flakes, Sainsbury's*	1 Serving/25g	93.0	0.0	371	7.3	83.8	0.7	3.0
Corn Flakes, Tesco*	1 Serving/25g	93.0	0.0	371	7.3	83.8	0.7	3.0
Cornflakes, Honey Nut, Asda*	1 Serving/30g	119.0	1.0	397	7.4	81.7	4.5	2.5
Country Crisp, & Flakes, Red Berry, Jordans*	1 Serving/50g	203.0	6.0	407	7.1	68.5	11.6	7.3
Country Crisp, Four Nut Combo, Jordans*	1 Serving/50g	240.0	12.0	480	8.9	55.4	24.7	6.9
Country Crisp, Wild About Berries, Jordans*	1 Serving/50g	221.0	8.0	443	7.5	68.0	15.7	5.7
Country Crisp, with Real Raspberries, Jordans*	1 Serving/50g	214.0	8.0	429	7.5	64.1	15.8	7.1
Country Crisp, with Real Strawberries, Jordans*	1 Serving/50g	214.0	8.0	428	7.5	64.1	15.7	7.1
Country Honey, So Simple, Quaker Oats*	1 Serving/36g	134.0	2.0	373	8.5	69.0	6.5	6.0
Cranberry Wheats, Tesco*	1 Serving/40g	130.0	1.0	325	7.3	70.9	1.4	7.7
Cranberry Wheats, Whole Grain, Sainsbury's*	1 Serving/50g	162.0	1.0	325	7.3	70.9	1.4	7.7
Crispy Rice & Wheat Flakes, Asda*	1 Serving/50g	185.0	1.0	370	11.0	78.0	1.5	3.2
Crunchy Bran, Weetabix*	1 Serving/40g	122.0	1.0	306	11.9	56.6	3.6	20.0
Crunchy Choco, Crisp & Square, Tesco*	1 Serving/50g	211.0	7.0	423	8.0	66.3	14.0	6.0
Crunchy Chocolate, Carrefour*	1 Serving/40g	176.0	7.0	440	9.0	62.0	17.0	8.0
Crunchy Nut, Clusters, Honey & Nut, Kellogg's*	1 Serving/40g	174.0	6.0	435	8.0	67.0	15.7	5.0
Crunchy Nut, Clusters, Milk Chocolate Curls, Kellogg's*	1 Serving/40g	183.0	7.0	458	8.0	66.0	18.0	4.0
Crunchy Nut, Clusters, Summer Berries, Kellogg's*	1 Serving/40g	176.0	6.0	439	8.0	68.0	15.0	5.0
Crunchy Nut, Corn Flakes, Kellogg's*	1 Serving/30g	118.0	1.0	392	6.0	83.0	4.0	2.5
Crunchy Nut, Red, Kellogg's*	1 Serving/40g	138.0	1.0	346	10.0	72.0	2.0	9.0
Crunchy Oat, Golden Sun*	1 Serving/50g	205.0	6.0	411	8.6	65.0	12.9	6.2
Crunchy Oat, with Raisins, Almonds & Fruit, Tesco*	1 Serving/50g	201.0	6.0	403	8.5	63.8	12.6	6.6
Crunchy Oat, with Tropical Fruits, Tesco*	1 Serving/35g	146.0	5.0	417	7.8	65.3	13.8	6.1
Crunchy Oats, with Tropical Fruits, Jordans*	1 Serving/75g	319.0	11.0	425	8.1	65.4	14.6	6.7
Crunchy Rice & Wheat Flakes, Co-Op*	1 Serving/30g	111.0	1.0	370	11.0	78.0	2.0	3.0
Crunchy, Carb Control, Tesco*	1 Serving/35g	174.0	12.0	497	21.5	23.3	35.0	13.4
Curiously Cinnamon, Nestle*	1 Serving/30g	124.0	3.0	412	4.9	75.9	9.9	4.1
Eat Natural*	1 Serving/40g	180.0	10.0	450	12.0	45.0	25.0	6.0
Fibre 1, Nestle*	1 Serving/40g	107.0	1.0	267	10.8	50.2	2.6	30.5
Fibre Bran, Safeway*	1 Serving/48g	124.0	2.0	259	13.3	43.4	3.6	31.0

BREAKFAST CEREAL

	Measure INFO/WEIGHT	per Measure KCAL	FAT	Nutrition Values per 100g / 100ml KCAL	PROT	CARB	FAT	FIBRE
Fitnesse & Fruits, Nestle*	1 Serving/40g	148.0	0.0	370	6.6	83.4	1.1	3.4
Flakes & Grains, Exotic Fruit, BGTY, Sainsbury's*	1 Serving/30g	113.0	1.0	377	6.8	76.4	4.9	5.9
Flakes & Orchard Fruits, BGTY, Sainsbury's*	1 Serving/40g	154.0	0.0	385	13.0	80.6	1.2	4.5
Flakes, 7 Cereal, De Halm*	1 Serving/40g	139.0	1.0	347	11.3	66.7	3.4	9.0
Flakes, Multigrain, with Cranberry & Apple, Tesco*	1 Serving/30g	107.0	1.0	357	8.1	75.7	2.4	5.4
Force, Nestle*	1 Serving/40g	138.0	1.0	344	10.6	70.3	2.3	9.2
Four Berry Crisp, Organic, Jordans*	1 Serving/50g	221.0	8.0	442	7.7	67.1	15.8	5.4
Frosted Flakes, Sainsbury's*	1 Serving/30g	112.0	0.0	374	4.9	87.8	0.4	2.4
Frosted Flakes, Tesco*	1 Serving/30g	112.0	0.0	374	4.9	87.8	0.4	2.4
Frosted Wheats, Kellogg's*	1 Serving/30g	104.0	1.0	346	10.0	72.0	2.0	9.0
Frosties, Caramel, Kellogg's*	1 Serving/30g	113.0	0.0	377	5.0	88.0	0.6	2.0
Frosties, Chocolate, Kellogg's*	1 Serving/40g	158.0	2.0	394	5.0	80.0	6.0	3.5
Frosties, Kellogg's*	1 Serving/30g	111.0	0.0	371	4.5	87.0	0.6	2.0
Frosties, Reduced Sugar, Kellogg's*	1 Serving/30g	111.0	0.0	369	6.0	85.0	0.6	2.5
Fruit & Fibre, Asda*	1 Serving/40g	146.0	3.0	366	8.2	68.4	6.6	8.5
Fruit & Fibre, Flakes, Waitrose*	1 Serving/40g	143.0	2.0	357	8.2	67.2	6.2	9.9
Fruit & Fibre, Morrisons*	1 Serving/30g	110.0	2.0	366	8.8	66.5	7.2	8.5
Fruit & Fibre, Organic, Sainsbury's*	1 Serving/40g	147.0	2.0	367	10.0	72.4	4.1	7.8
Fruit & Fibre, Tesco*	1 Serving/30g	111.0	2.0	370	8.0	69.1	6.6	7.7
Fruit & Fibre, Value, Tesco*	1 Serving/40g	144.0	2.0	359	11.4	65.7	5.6	9.0
Fruit & Fibre, Whole Grain, Sainsbury's*	1 Serving/30g	108.0	2.0	361	8.1	68.7	6.0	8.9
Fruit & Nut Crisp, Minis, Weetabix*	1 Serving/40g	144.0	2.0	359	9.3	70.0	4.6	8.9
Fruit 'n' Fibre, Kellogg's*	1 Serving/40g	143.0	2.0	358	8.0	68.0	6.0	9.0
Fruit Nuts & Flakes, M & S*	1 Serving/30g	117.0	3.0	391	9.1	69.6	8.5	3.5
Golden Grahams, Nestle*	1 Serving/30g	112.0	1.0	375	6.0	81.0	3.0	3.4
Golden Honey Puffs, Tesco*	1 Serving/30g	115.0	0.0	382	6.6	86.3	1.2	3.0
Golden Nuggets, Nestle*	1 Serving/40g	152.0	0.0	381	6.2	87.4	0.7	1.5
Golden Puffs, Sainsbury's*	1 Serving/28g	107.0	0.0	383	6.6	86.3	1.2	3.0
Granola & Strawberries, with Bio Yoghurt, Rumblers*	1 Pot/168g	267.0	10.0	159	4.3	22.4	5.8	1.1
Granola, Low Fat, Home Farm*	1 Serving/55g	180.0	3.0	328	7.3	69.0	5.4	9.0
Granola, Organic, Lizi's, The GoodCarb Food Company*	1 Serving/50g	246.0	14.0	493	11.3	48.6	28.1	7.4
Granola, Original, Lizi's, The GoodCarb Food Company*	1 Serving/50g	248.0	15.0	496	10.9	46.2	29.3	10.6
Granola, Quaker Oats*	1 Serving/48g	210.0	7.0	437	10.4	72.9	14.6	6.2
Granola, Superfoods, Jordans*	1 Serving/50g	207.0	7.0	415	9.0	64.7	13.4	8.6
Granola, Treacle & Pecan, The GoodCarb Food Company*	1 Pack/50g	245.0	14.0	491	9.7	47.6	28.3	11.3
Grape Nuts, Kraft*	1 Serving/45g	155.0	1.0	345	11.5	70.0	2.0	11.0
Harvest Crunch, Nut, Quaker Oats*	1 Serving/40g	184.0	8.0	459	8.0	62.5	19.5	6.0
Harvest Crunch, Real Red Berries, Quaker Oats*	1 Serving/50g	223.0	8.0	447	7.0	66.0	17.0	4.5
Harvest Crunch, Soft Juicy Raisins, Quaker Oats*	1 Serving/50g	221.0	8.0	442	6.0	67.0	16.0	4.0
Hawaiian Crunch, Asda*	1 Serving/50g	220.0	8.0	441	8.0	64.0	17.0	6.0
Healthy Flakes, Safeway*	1 Serving/30g	111.0	0.0	371	11.0	78.4	1.5	4.3
Hi-Fibre Bran, Tesco*	1 Serving/40g	110.0	1.0	275	14.7	45.5	3.5	27.0
High Fibre Bran, Sainsbury's*	1 Serving/40g	109.0	1.0	272	14.7	45.5	3.5	27.0
High Fibre Bran, Tesco*	1 Serving/40g	110.0	1.0	275	14.7	45.5	3.5	27.0
High Fibre Bran, Waitrose*	1 Serving/40g	112.0	2.0	281	14.4	47.2	3.8	26.0
High Fibre, Alpen*	1 Serving/45g	154.0	3.0	343	7.7	62.1	7.1	14.1
High Fruit Muesli, BGTY, Sainsbury's*	1 Serving/50g	164.0	1.0	328	6.7	71.0	1.9	6.6
Honey & Nut Crisp, Mini, Weetabix*	1 Serving/40g	147.0	2.0	368	9.9	70.6	5.1	9.0
Honey Loops, Kellogg's*	1 Serving/30g	110.0	1.0	367	8.0	77.0	3.0	6.0
Honey Nut & Flakes, M & S*	1 Serving/40g	164.0	3.0	411	9.8	73.4	8.7	2.6
Honey Raisin & Almond, Crunchy, Waitrose*	1 Serving/40g	170.0	5.0	425	10.5	68.8	12.0	5.7
Honey, Oats & More, Nestle*	1 Serving/30g	114.0	2.0	379	9.7	73.1	5.3	5.9
Hooplas, Sainsbury's*	1 Serving/30g	112.0	1.0	375	6.5	78.6	3.8	4.6

BREAKFAST CEREAL

	Measure INFO/WEIGHT	per Measure KCAL	FAT	Nutrition Values per 100g / 100ml KCAL	PROT	CARB	FAT	FIBRE
Hoops, Multigrain, Asda*	1 Serving/30g	113.0	1.0	376	6.5	78.4	4.0	4.6
Hoops, Multigrain, Tesco*	1 Serving/30g	112.0	1.0	375	6.5	78.6	3.8	4.6
Hot Cereal, Flax O Meal*	1 Serving/40g	130.0	6.0	325	52.5	2.5	15.0	30.0
Hot Oat, Aldi*	1 Serving/40g	142.0	3.0	356	11.6	58.8	8.3	8.9
Hot Oats, Instant, Tesco*	1 Serving/30g	108.0	3.0	360	11.8	58.4	8.7	7.9
Hot Oats, Safeway*	1 Serving/20g	71.0	2.0	356	11.6	58.8	8.3	8.9
Hunny B's, Kellogg's*	1 Serving/28g	106.0	1.0	379	7.0	78.0	2.5	4.5
Just Right, Kellogg's*	1 Serving/40g	145.0	1.0	362	7.0	79.0	2.0	4.0
Kashi, Crunch, Seven Whole Grains, Original, Kellogg's*	1 Serving/40g	162.0	4.0	405	8.0	73.0	9.0	5.0
Kashi, Honey, Seven Whole Grains, Kellogg's*	1 Serving/30g	110.0	1.0	367	9.0	77.0	2.5	7.0
Kids, Original, Projects No1, Dorset Cereals*	1 Serving/30g	112.0	1.0	373	7.2	82.4	1.7	3.8
Krave, Chocolate & Hazelnut, Kellogg's*	1 Serving/30g	132.0	5.0	440	8.0	66.0	16.0	4.0
Malt Crunchies, Co-Op*	1 Serving/50g	167.0	1.0	335	10.0	69.0	2.0	10.0
Malted Wheaties, Asda*	1 Serving/50g	171.0	1.0	342	10.0	69.0	2.9	10.0
Malted Wheaties, New Day*	1 Serving/30g	101.0	1.0	336	10.0	69.2	2.1	0.0
Malted Wheats, Waitrose*	1 Serving/32g	110.0	1.0	343	9.7	71.7	1.9	9.9
Malties, Sainsbury's*	1 Serving/40g	137.0	1.0	343	10.0	69.2	2.9	10.0
Malty Flakes with Peach & Raspberry, BGTY, Sainsbury's*	1 Serving/40g	146.0	1.0	364	10.8	76.4	1.7	3.3
Malty Flakes with Raspberries, M & S*	1 Serving/40g	148.0	1.0	370	7.4	77.5	3.5	3.2
Malty Flakes, Peach Melba, Tesco*	1 Serving/30g	115.0	1.0	385	8.0	79.6	3.8	1.7
Malty Flakes, Tesco*	1 Serving/40g	148.0	1.0	371	11.0	78.4	1.5	4.3
Malty Flakes, with Red Berries, Tesco*	1 Serving/30g	111.0	1.0	369	9.9	78.1	1.9	3.1
Maple & Pecan Crisp, Sainsbury's*	1 Serving/50g	226.0	10.0	452	7.9	61.3	19.5	5.4
Maple & Pecan Crisp, Tesco*	1 Serving/50g	215.0	8.0	430	10.5	62.5	15.2	10.2
Maple & Pecan, Sainsbury's*	1 Serving/60g	318.0	13.0	530	13.3	69.7	22.0	5.3
Maple Flavoured, Fruit 'n' Nut, So Simple, Quaker Oats*	1 Sachet/47g	169.0	5.0	360	9.0	58.5	10.5	7.5
Maple Frosted Flakes, Whole Earth*	1 Serving/30g	112.0	0.0	375	6.2	85.6	1.0	1.6
Millet Rice Oatbran Flakes, Nature's Path*	1 Serving/56g	204.0	3.0	365	11.3	67.0	5.8	10.0
Mini Wheats, Original, Frosted, Kellogg's*	21 Biscuits/54g	190.0	1.0	352	9.3	83.3	1.8	11.1
Mini Wheats, Sainsbury's*	1 Serving/45g	157.0	1.0	348	11.8	69.9	2.3	11.8
Minibix, Weetabix*	1 Serving/40g	134.0	2.0	335	8.8	71.2	3.8	8.1
Muddles, Kellogg's*	1 Serving/30g	110.0	1.0	368	8.0	76.0	3.5	8.0
Muesli Mix, Perfect Start, Organic, The Food Doctor*	1 Serving/50g	196.0	7.0	392	12.1	55.5	14.2	7.1
Muesli, Apricot, Traidcraft*	1 Serving/30g	103.0	2.0	344	8.0	68.0	6.0	5.0
Muesli, Base, Nature's Harvest*	1 Serving/50g	179.0	3.0	358	11.0	71.2	5.1	7.4
Muesli, Berries & Cherries, Dorset Cereals*	1 Serving/70g	225.0	2.0	321	6.5	68.8	2.2	6.3
Muesli, Carb Control, Tesco*	1 Serving/35g	154.0	9.0	439	25.0	25.0	26.6	13.8
Muesli, COU, M & S*	1 Serving/60g	201.0	1.0	335	7.6	70.2	2.5	8.1
Muesli, Crunchy, Organic, Sainsbury's*	1 Serving/40g	168.0	6.0	420	10.6	62.0	14.4	9.2
Muesli, Fruit & Nut, COU, M & S*	1 Serving/40g	128.0	1.0	320	7.4	74.5	2.8	7.4
Muesli, Fruit & Nut, Jordans*	1 Serving/50g	180.0	5.0	361	8.0	61.2	9.4	7.5
Muesli, Fruit & Nut, Luxury, Sainsbury's*	1 Serving/50g	177.0	5.0	355	10.3	57.9	9.1	11.3
Muesli, Fruit & Nut, Luxury, Waitrose*	1 Serving/40g	145.0	4.0	363	9.0	60.3	9.5	6.5
Muesli, Fruit & Nut, M & S*	1 Serving/40g	128.0	1.0	320	7.4	74.5	2.8	7.4
Muesli, Fruit & Nut, Sainsbury's*	1 Serving/30g	121.0	5.0	402	10.4	51.3	17.2	9.2
Muesli, Fruit & Nut, Tesco*	1 Serving/50g	190.0	6.0	380	8.4	60.3	11.3	5.3
Muesli, Fruit & Spice, Sainsbury's*	1 Serving/50g	184.0	3.0	368	7.4	69.4	6.8	7.7
Muesli, Fruit Nut & Seed, Organic, Dorset Cereals*	1 Serving/70g	251.0	7.0	358	10.8	56.6	9.8	8.4
Muesli, Fruit Sensation, M & S*	1 Serving/50g	157.0	1.0	315	6.0	66.0	3.0	7.4
Muesli, Fruit, GFY, Asda*	1 Serving/50g	152.0	1.0	304	8.0	64.0	1.8	10.0
Muesli, Fruit, Luxury, Weight Watchers*	1 Serving/40g	127.0	1.0	318	7.2	67.7	2.0	8.1
Muesli, Fruit, Nuts & Seeds, Dorset Cereals*	1 Serving/70g	265.0	8.0	379	10.6	58.4	11.4	6.1
Muesli, Fruit, Sainsbury's*	1 Serving/40g	132.0	2.0	330	8.1	64.3	4.5	9.6

BREAKFAST CEREAL

	Measure INFO/WEIGHT	per Measure KCAL	FAT	Nutrition Values per 100g / 100ml KCAL	PROT	CARB	FAT	FIBRE
Muesli, Fruit, Waitrose*	1 Serving/30g	101.0	1.0	338	7.2	66.8	4.7	6.8
Muesli, Fruity Fibre, Jordans*	1 Serving/50g	172.0	3.0	344	7.7	64.2	6.3	8.5
Muesli, Gluten Free, Nature's Harvest, Holland & Barrett*	1 Serving/60g	234.0	8.0	390	14.1	54.1	13.0	3.3
Muesli, HL, Tesco*	1 Serving/40g	126.0	1.0	315	7.6	64.3	2.3	7.5
Muesli, Light & Crispy, Jordans*	1 Serving/50g	171.0	2.0	343	7.7	66.7	5.0	9.5
Muesli, Luxury Fruit, Perfectly Balanced, Waitrose*	1 Serving/50g	162.0	2.0	324	7.1	66.4	3.3	7.0
Muesli, Luxury Fruit, Sainsbury's*	1 Serving/50g	162.0	2.0	324	7.1	66.4	3.3	7.0
Muesli, Luxury, Finest, Tesco*	1 Serving/50g	197.0	7.0	394	8.3	60.8	13.1	5.4
Muesli, Luxury, Jordans*	1 Serving/40g	154.0	5.0	384	9.6	58.4	12.5	8.2
Muesli, Natural, No Added Sugar Or Salt, Jordans*	1 Serving/50g	160.0	2.0	321	8.9	60.7	4.7	5.2
Muesli, No Added Sugar Or Salt, Organic, Jordans*	1 Serving/50g	175.0	4.0	350	9.2	58.4	8.8	9.3
Muesli, No Added Sugar, Morrisons*	1 Serving/50g	165.0	3.0	331	11.2	64.7	5.1	6.3
Muesli, No Added Sugar, Waitrose*	1 Serving/40g	146.0	3.0	364	12.0	64.9	6.3	6.7
Muesli, No Sugar Added, Olivio*	1 Serving/55g	200.0	3.0	364	12.7	72.7	5.4	7.3
Muesli, Organic, Waitrose*	1 Serving/50g	187.0	1.0	375	10.3	59.6	1.6	8.3
Muesli, Original, Holland & Barrett*	1 Serving/30g	105.0	3.0	351	11.1	61.2	8.4	7.1
Muesli, Original, Sainsbury's*	1 Serving/60g	226.0	5.0	376	9.3	65.7	8.4	7.1
Muesli, Peach & Vanilla, Sainsbury's*	1 Serving/50g	162.0	3.0	324	7.6	61.4	5.3	7.6
Muesli, Really Nutty, Dorset Cereals*	1 Serving/70g	253.0	6.0	362	9.8	61.1	8.7	6.3
Muesli, Rich, Nature's Harvest*	1 Serving/40g	143.0	4.0	358	10.0	60.5	9.2	7.6
Muesli, Simply Delicious, Dorset Cereals*	1 Serving/70g	256.0	7.0	366	10.8	59.2	9.5	7.4
Muesli, Simply Fruity, Dorset Cereals*	1 Serving/75g	226.0	2.0	301	6.8	63.9	2.5	7.7
Muesli, Special, Fruit, Jordans*	1 Serving/50g	161.0	1.0	323	6.6	68.0	2.7	8.4
Muesli, Special, Jordans*	1 Serving/50g	183.0	5.0	366	7.9	59.5	10.7	8.5
Muesli, Super Berry, Jordans*	1 Serving/50g	174.0	4.0	348	9.0	60.8	7.6	8.1
Muesli, Super High Fibre, Dorset Cereals*	1 Serving/70g	250.0	7.0	357	8.0	60.1	9.4	8.4
Muesli, Superfoods, Jordans*	1 Serving/50g	173.0	4.0	346	9.2	60.9	7.3	10.2
Muesli, Swiss Style, No Added Salt Or Sugar, Tesco*	1 Serving/50g	177.0	3.0	355	10.9	65.1	5.4	8.2
Muesli, Swiss Style, Organic, Whole Earth*	1 Serving/50g	172.0	4.0	344	9.2	60.8	7.1	11.3
Muesli, Swiss Style, Sainsbury's*	1 Serving/50g	180.0	3.0	361	9.2	68.1	5.8	7.1
Muesli, Swiss Style, Smart Price, Asda*	1 Serving/60g	222.0	4.0	370	9.0	70.0	6.0	10.0
Muesli, Swiss Style, with Fruit, Tesco*	1 Serving/40g	144.0	2.0	360	10.4	67.4	5.3	7.4
Muesli, Tropical Fruit, Holland & Barrett*	1 Serving/60g	197.0	2.0	328	7.5	69.8	3.2	5.1
Muesli, Tropical Fruits, Jordans*	1 Serving/50g	164.0	1.0	329	6.9	68.7	2.9	7.1
Muesli, Tropical, Sainsbury's*	1 Serving/50g	182.0	3.0	365	6.5	69.4	6.8	6.4
Muesli, Tropical, Tesco*	1 Serving/50g	173.0	2.0	346	7.8	68.2	4.7	9.1
Muesli, Twelve Fruit & Nut, Sainsbury's*	1 Serving/50g	166.0	2.0	332	8.1	64.2	4.7	7.8
Muesli, Unsweetened, M & S*	1 Serving/40g	129.0	1.0	322	8.1	68.0	2.7	9.4
Muesli, Value, Tesco*	1 Serving/50g	162.0	3.0	325	10.7	58.3	5.1	14.9
Muesli, Whole Wheat, No Added Sugar & Salt, Tesco*	1 Serving/40g	154.0	5.0	386	9.5	59.1	12.4	7.4
Muesli, Whole Wheat, Organic, Asda*	1 Serving/50g	197.0	3.0	394	10.0	75.0	6.0	9.0
Muesli, Whole Wheat, Sainsbury's*	1 Serving/40g	144.0	3.0	359	11.5	60.5	7.9	8.5
Multi Fruit & Flake, COU, M & S*	1 Serving/39g	142.0	0.0	365	6.5	81.8	1.1	4.0
Multi Fruit & Flake, Perfectly Balanced, Waitrose*	1 Serving/40g	134.0	1.0	335	8.2	68.8	3.0	14.0
Multigrain Boulders, Tesco*	1 Serving/30g	112.0	0.0	375	8.2	82.3	1.3	3.6
Multigrain, Fitnesse, Nestle*	1 Serving/30g	109.0	0.0	363	8.0	79.8	1.3	5.1
Natures Whole Grains, Jordans*	1 Serving/25g	97.0	3.0	390	9.4	61.7	11.7	7.7
Nesquik, Chocolatey Corn & Rice, Nestle*	1 Serving/30g	114.0	1.0	380	7.2	79.1	3.9	5.1
No Added Sugar, Alpen*	1 Serving/40g	142.0	2.0	354	10.5	64.6	6.0	7.7
Nutty Crunch, Alpen*	1 Serving/40g	159.0	4.0	398	10.7	63.6	11.2	6.5
Nutty Crunch, Deliciously, M & S*	1 Serving/50g	238.0	11.0	476	8.8	59.6	22.5	4.4
Oat & Bran Flakes, Sainsbury's*	1 Serving/30g	97.0	2.0	324	12.2	56.0	5.7	17.7
Oat Bran, Crispies, Quaker Oats*	1 Serving/40g	153.0	3.0	383	11.0	69.0	6.5	9.0

BREAKFAST CEREAL

	Measure INFO/WEIGHT	per Measure KCAL	FAT	Nutrition Values per 100g / 100ml KCAL	PROT	CARB	FAT	FIBRE
Oat Crisp, Chocolate, Quaker Oats*	1 Serving/35g	135.0	4.0	385	10.2	57.5	11.1	12.4
Oat Crisp, Quaker Oats*	1 Serving/30g	109.0	2.0	364	10.6	60.8	6.8	12.7
Oat Crunchy, Blueberry & Cranberry, Waitrose*	1 Serving/60g	259.0	9.0	432	8.0	65.9	15.2	8.5
Oat Krunchies, Quaker Oats*	1 Serving/30g	118.0	2.0	393	9.5	72.0	7.0	5.5
Oat Meal, Medium, Heart's Content, Mornflake*	1 Serving/30g	108.0	2.0	359	11.0	60.4	8.1	8.5
Oat, Crunchy, Sainsbury's*	1 Serving/50g	226.0	10.0	453	8.2	59.3	20.3	6.6
Oat, Raisin, Nut & Honey, Crunchy, Dry, Sainsbury's*	1 Serving/50g	201.0	7.0	402	8.5	60.2	14.1	7.6
Oatbran Flakes, Nature's Path*	1 Serving/30g	124.0	1.0	414	8.7	83.0	4.7	6.7
Oatbran, Original Pure, Mornflake*	1 Serving/30g	103.0	3.0	345	14.8	49.7	9.7	15.2
Oatibix, Bitesize, Original, Weetabix*	1 Serving/36g	133.0	2.0	370	10.6	66.5	6.8	10.1
Oatibix, Flakes, Weetabix*	1 Serving/50g	190.0	3.0	381	9.5	73.2	5.6	3.5
Oatibix, Weetabix*	2 Biscuits/48g	181.0	4.0	377	12.5	63.7	8.0	7.3
Oatiflakes, with Raisin, Cranberry & Apple, Weetabix*	1 Serving/40g	135.0	0.0	338	6.7	75.0	1.2	8.6
Oatmeal, Instant, Heart to Heart, Kashi*	1 Serving/43g	150.0	2.0	349	7.0	76.7	4.6	9.3
Oatmeal, Quick Oats, Dry, Quaker Oats*	1 Serving/30g	114.0	2.0	380	14.0	66.7	6.7	10.0
Oatmeal, Scottish, Hamlyns of Scotland*	1 Portion/40g	157.0	4.0	392	11.2	66.0	9.2	7.1
Oats, Apple Flavour, Instant, Hot, Waitrose*	1 Serving/36g	141.0	2.0	392	8.1	76.4	6.0	6.7
Oats, Apple Flavour, Micro, Tesco*	1 Sachet/36g	128.0	2.0	356	6.8	70.1	5.4	5.4
Oats, Golden Syrup Flavour, Instant, Hot, Waitrose*	1 Serving/39g	153.0	2.0	393	7.8	77.4	5.8	6.0
Oats, Golden Syrup, Dry, Micro, Tesco*	1 Sachet/39g	144.0	2.0	370	7.8	71.6	5.7	6.4
Oats, Jumbo, Organic, Waitrose*	1 Serving/50g	180.0	4.0	361	11.0	61.1	8.1	7.8
Oats, Orange & Lemon Flavour, Instant, Hot, Waitrose*	1 Sachet/38g	137.0	2.0	361	8.9	68.4	5.8	8.7
Oats, Original, Instant, Hot, Waitrose*	1 Sachet/27g	97.0	2.0	359	11.0	60.4	8.1	8.5
Oats, Superfast, Mornflake*	1 Serving/40g	144.0	3.0	359	11.0	60.4	8.1	8.5
Oats, Tesco*	1 Serving/40g	142.0	3.0	356	11.0	60.0	8.0	8.0
Oats, Wholegrain, Organic, Quaker Oats*	1 Serving/25g	89.0	2.0	356	11.0	60.0	8.0	9.0
Optimum Power, Nature's Path*	1 Serving/30g	109.0	2.0	363	15.3	60.0	6.7	12.6
Optivita, Berry Oat Crisp, Kellogg's*	1 Serving/30g	107.0	1.0	357	10.0	68.0	5.0	9.0
Organic, Weetabix*	2 Biscuits/35g	116.0	1.0	331	10.9	66.8	2.2	11.0
Original, Crunchy, Raisins & Almonds, Jordans*	1 Serving/50g	203.0	6.0	407	8.7	64.0	12.9	6.6
Original, Crunchy, Tropical Fruits, Jordans*	1 Serving/50g	211.0	7.0	423	8.1	65.1	14.5	6.7
Original, Dry, Micro Oats, Tesco*	1 Sachet/27g	97.0	2.0	360	11.0	60.4	8.1	8.5
Original, Ready Brek*	1 Serving/40g	144.0	3.0	359	11.8	58.5	8.7	7.9
Original, So Simple, Quaker Oats*	1 Serving/27g	98.0	2.0	364	11.0	60.0	8.5	9.0
Original, with Raisins, Hazelnuts & Almonds, Alpen*	1 Serving/40g	144.0	2.0	359	10.5	66.6	5.8	7.3
Perfect Balance, Weight Watchers*	1 Serving/30g	90.0	1.0	300	7.8	63.3	1.7	15.6
Pomegranate & Raspberry Wheats, Tesco*	1 Serving/50g	165.0	1.0	330	7.5	71.8	1.4	8.2
Porage Oats, Old Fashioned, Thick, Scotts*	1 Serving/45g	160.0	4.0	356	11.0	60.0	8.0	9.0
Porage Oats, So Easy, Scotts*	1 Serving/30g	109.0	3.0	364	11.0	60.0	8.5	9.0
Porridge Flakes, Organic, Barkat*	1 Serving/30g	109.0	1.0	362	8.5	74.1	3.0	0.0
Porridge Oats & Bran, Co-Op*	1 Serving/40g	141.0	3.0	353	12.5	60.0	7.0	12.0
Porridge Oats, Dry Weight, Value, Tesco*	1 Serving/50g	179.0	4.0	359	11.0	60.4	8.1	8.5
Porridge Oats, Mornflake*	1 Serving/50g	179.0	4.0	359	11.0	60.4	8.1	8.5
Porridge Oats, Organic, Evernat*	1 Serving/40g	167.0	4.0	418	13.0	69.0	9.6	7.4
Porridge Oats, Organic, Jordans*	1 Serving/40g	146.0	4.0	364	11.7	58.4	9.3	9.0
Porridge Oats, Organic, Tesco*	1 Serving/28g	100.0	2.0	358	11.0	60.4	8.1	8.5
Porridge Oats, Quaker Oats*	1 Serving/45g	160.0	4.0	356	11.0	60.0	8.0	4.0
Porridge Oats, Rolled, Tesco*	1 Serving/50g	179.0	4.0	359	11.0	60.4	8.1	8.5
Porridge Oats, Scottish, Organic, Sainsbury's*	1 Serving/45g	172.0	2.0	383	10.0	74.4	5.0	7.9
Porridge Oats, Scottish, Tesco*	1 Serving/50g	179.0	4.0	359	11.0	60.4	8.1	8.5
Porridge Oats, Smart Price, Asda*	1 Serving/50g	178.0	4.0	356	11.0	60.0	8.0	8.0
Porridge Oats, Whole Oats, Jordans*	1 Serving/40g	146.0	4.0	364	11.7	58.4	9.3	9.0
Porridge Oats, with Bran, Scottish, Sainsbury's*	1 Serving/50g	190.0	2.0	380	9.6	74.1	5.0	10.3

	Measure INFO/WEIGHT	per Measure KCAL	per Measure FAT	Nutrition Values per 100g / 100ml KCAL	PROT	CARB	FAT	FIBRE
BREAKFAST CEREAL								
Porridge Oats, with Oat & Wheat Bran, HL, Tesco*	1 Sachet/30g	105.0	2.0	350	10.8	62.3	6.1	9.2
Porridge Oats, with Wheat Bran, Tesco*	1 Serving/50g	167.0	4.0	334	12.3	55.0	7.2	13.0
Porridge Oats, with Wheat Bran, Waitrose*	1 Serving/50g	168.0	4.0	336	11.2	55.8	7.6	13.0
Porridge, Apple & Raspberry, Seriously Oaty, Weetabix*	1 Serving/40g	142.0	2.0	354	8.3	63.7	6.0	7.8
Porridge, Apple, Sultana & Cinnamon, M & S*	1 Sachet/40g	144.0	3.0	360	10.3	62.3	7.5	8.6
Porridge, Chocolate, Oatibix, Weetabix*	1 Pack/40.1g	149.0	4.0	372	9.9	61.3	9.7	6.2
Porridge, Free From, Sainsbury's*	1 Serving/50g	174.0	1.0	348	8.6	72.0	3.0	3.4
Porridge, Fruity, Apple & Raisin, Dorset Cereals*	1 Serving/70g	233.0	3.0	333	9.7	62.7	4.8	8.9
Porridge, Fruity, Cranberry & Raspberry, Dorset Cereals*	1 Sachet/30g	99.0	2.0	330	10.2	58.7	6.0	12.3
Porridge, Fruity, Fruit & Nut, Dorset Cereals*	1 Serving/70g	242.0	6.0	346	9.4	59.0	8.0	8.2
Porridge, Fruity, Mixed Berries, Dorset Cereals*	1 Serving/70g	243.0	4.0	347	10.8	62.6	6.0	7.9
Porridge, Golden Honey, Oatibix, Weetabix*	1 Serving/40g	145.0	3.0	363	9.2	66.7	6.6	7.0
Porridge, Instant, Quaker Oats*	1 Serving/34g	124.0	3.0	364	11.0	60.0	8.5	9.0
Porridge, Made with Semi Skimmed Milk, Waitrose*	1 Serving/50g	277.0	7.0	554	24.6	80.4	15.0	8.6
Porridge, Manuka Honey & Apricot, Vogel*	1 Packet/35g	122.0	1.0	349	10.1	66.3	2.9	7.1
Porridge, Multigrain, Jordans*	1 Serving/40g	134.0	2.0	335	10.4	60.9	5.5	10.0
Porridge, Original, Oatibix, Weetabix*	1 Sachet/30g	104.0	2.0	347	12.5	55.6	8.3	10.1
Porridge, Original, Simply Porridge, Asda*	1 Sachet/27g	96.0	2.0	356	11.0	60.0	8.0	8.0
Porridge, Perfectly, Dorset Cereals*	1 Sachet/30g	107.0	3.0	356	11.8	58.2	8.4	11.0
Porridge, Ready Made, COU, M & S*	1 Pot/200g	180.0	4.0	90	3.9	13.3	2.2	0.9
Porridge, Real Fruit, Raisin & Apple, Jordans*	1 Serving/40g	133.0	3.0	332	9.1	58.8	6.7	7.4
Porridge, Real Fruit, Sultana & Apricot, Jordans*	1 Sachet/40g	127.0	2.0	317	8.5	57.7	5.8	7.2
Porridge, Spiced Apple, Sultana, Oatibix, Weetabix*	1 Sachet/40g	138.0	2.0	345	9.7	65.4	5.7	8.5
Porridge, Superfoods, Jordans*	1 Serving/40g	145.0	4.0	362	10.4	59.8	9.0	8.3
Porridge, Take Heart, Quaker Oats*	1 Serving/32g	194.0	6.0	606	30.9	80.3	17.8	7.8
Precise, Sainsbury's*	1 Serving/40g	148.0	1.0	371	6.4	79.9	2.9	3.5
Puffed Rice, Wholegrain, Brown, Original, Organic, Kallo*	1 Serving/25g	95.0	1.0	380	8.0	80.0	3.0	9.0
Puffed Wheat, Quaker Oats*	1 Serving/15g	49.0	0.0	328	15.3	62.4	1.3	5.6
Puffed Wheat, Tesco*	1 Serving/28g	104.0	1.0	373	13.9	72.2	3.2	5.7
Quaker Oats Crunch, Quaker Oats*	1 Serving/40g	146.0	2.0	366	9.1	71.1	5.0	7.4
Raisin & Almond, Crunchy, Jordans*	1 Serving/56g	230.0	7.0	411	8.4	66.0	12.5	5.0
Raisin & Coconut, Crunchy, Organic, Jordans*	1 Serving/50g	206.0	7.0	412	8.4	64.2	13.5	7.1
Raisin Wheats, Kellogg's*	1 Serving/30g	99.0	1.0	330	9.0	70.0	2.0	8.0
Raisin Wheats, Sainsbury's*	1 Serving/50g	166.0	1.0	332	8.2	71.5	1.5	8.0
Raisin, Bran Flakes, Asda*	1 Serving/50g	165.0	1.0	331	7.0	69.0	3.0	10.0
Raisin, Honey & Almond Crunch, Asda*	1 Serving/60g	238.0	7.0	397	8.8	64.8	11.4	7.4
Raisin, Oats and More, Nestle*	1 Serving/30g	112.0	1.0	373	8.9	73.7	4.7	5.8
Raspberry Crisp, Mornflake*	1 Serving/50g	214.0	7.0	428	6.5	68.2	14.3	6.8
Raspberry Flavour, So Simple, Quaker Oats*	1 Sachet/35g	127.0	2.0	364	8.8	67.1	6.5	7.2
Ready Brek, Banana, Weetabix*	1 Serving/40g	146.0	3.0	365	8.9	68.0	6.4	6.7
Ready Brek, Original, Weetabix*	1 Serving/40g	158.0	3.0	395	11.8	58.4	8.7	7.9
Red Berry & Almond Luxury Crunch, Jordans*	1 Serving/40g	176.0	7.0	441	8.2	60.5	18.5	6.6
Rice & Wheat Flake, Special Choice, Waitrose*	1 Serving/30g	111.0	0.0	370	11.4	77.7	1.5	3.2
Rice Krispies, Honey, Kellogg's*	1 Serving/30g	114.0	0.0	380	4.0	89.0	0.7	1.0
Rice Krispies, Kellogg's*	1 Serving/30g	114.0	0.0	381	6.0	87.0	1.0	1.0
Rice Krispies, Multi-Grain Shapes, Kellogg's*	1 Serving/30g	111.0	1.0	370	8.0	77.0	2.5	8.0
Rice Pops, Blue Parrot Cafe, Sainsbury's*	1 Serving/30g	111.0	0.0	370	7.2	82.3	1.3	2.2
Rice Pops, Organic, Dove's Farm*	1 Serving/30g	107.0	0.0	357	6.8	86.1	0.8	2.0
Rice Pops, Sainsbury's*	1 Serving/30g	114.0	0.0	381	7.4	84.8	1.3	1.5
Rice Snaps, Asda*	1 Serving/28g	105.0	0.0	376	7.0	84.0	1.3	1.5
Rice Snaps, Harvest Home, Nestle*	1 Serving/25g	94.0	0.0	378	7.4	84.2	1.3	1.5
Rice Snaps, Tesco*	1 Serving/35g	135.0	0.0	385	7.4	84.8	1.3	1.5
Ricicles, Kellogg's*	1 Serving/30g	114.0	0.0	381	4.5	89.0	0.8	0.8

BREAKFAST CEREAL

	Measure INFO/WEIGHT	per Measure KCAL	FAT	Nutrition Values per 100g / 100ml KCAL	PROT	CARB	FAT	FIBRE
Shredded Wheat, 100% Whole Grain, Nestle*	2 Biscuits/45g	153.0	1.0	340	11.6	67.8	2.5	11.8
Shredded Wheat, Bitesize, Nestle*	1 Serving/45g	157.0	1.0	350	11.8	69.9	2.6	11.9
Shredded Wheat, Fruitful, No Added Salt, Nestle*	1 Serving/40g	142.0	2.0	354	8.3	68.7	5.1	8.9
Shredded Wheat, Honey Nut, Nestle*	1 Serving/40g	151.0	3.0	378	11.2	68.8	6.5	9.4
Shredded Wheat, Triple Berry, Nestle*	1 Serving/40g	138.0	1.0	344	10.6	70.6	2.1	11.1
Shreddies, Coco, Nestle*	1 Serving/45g	161.0	1.0	358	8.4	76.5	2.0	8.6
Shreddies, Frosted, Kellogg's*	1 Serving/50g	161.0	1.0	323	0.7	78.5	1.8	4.7
Shreddies, Frosted, Nestle*	1 Serving/45g	164.0	1.0	365	7.4	80.7	1.5	6.4
Shreddies, Frosted, Variety Pack, Nestle*	1 Pack/45g	163.0	1.0	363	6.7	81.1	1.3	6.8
Shreddies, Malt Wheats, Tesco*	1 Serving/45g	151.0	1.0	335	8.3	70.7	2.1	9.7
Shreddies, Nestle*	1 Serving/45g	185.0	1.0	371	10.0	73.7	1.9	9.9
Smoothies, Strawberry, Quaker Oats*	1 Sachet/29g	117.0	3.0	402	6.5	67.0	12.0	5.5
Smoothies, Toffee, Quaker Oats*	1 Serving/30g	122.0	4.0	407	6.5	66.0	13.0	5.0
Special Crunchy Luxury, Jordans*	1 Serving/50g	205.0	7.0	411	7.6	63.8	13.9	6.5
Special Crunchy Luxury, Maple & Pecan, Jordans*	1 Serving/50g	220.0	9.0	440	9.5	61.6	17.3	7.2
Special Flakes with Peach Melba, Tesco*	1 Serving/30g	115.0	1.0	385	8.0	79.6	3.8	1.7
Special Flakes, Tesco*	1 Serving/20g	74.0	0.0	371	11.0	78.4	1.5	4.3
Special K, Bliss, Creamy Berry Crunch, Kellogg's*	1 Serving/30g	114.0	1.0	379	13.0	76.0	2.5	2.5
Special K, Bliss, Strawberry & Chocolate, Kellogg's*	1 Serving/30g	115.0	1.0	383	13.0	76.0	3.0	2.5
Special K, Choco, Kellogg's*	1 Serving/40g	160.0	3.0	400	14.0	70.0	7.0	3.5
Special K, Kellogg's*	1 Serving/30g	112.0	0.0	373	16.0	75.0	1.0	2.5
Special K, Oats & Honey, Kellogg's*	1 Serving/50g	191.0	1.0	383	13.0	77.0	2.5	3.0
Special K, Peach & Apricot, Kellogg's*	1 Serving/30g	112.0	0.0	373	14.0	77.0	1.0	2.5
Special K, Protein Plus, Kellogg's*	1 Serving/29g	100.0	3.0	345	34.5	31.0	10.3	17.2
Special K, Purple Berries, Kellogg's*	1 Serving/30g	112.0	0.0	374	13.0	77.0	1.0	3.5
Special K, Red Berries, Kellogg's*	1 Serving/30g	112.0	0.0	374	14.0	76.0	1.5	3.0
Special K, Yoghurty, Kellogg's*	1 Serving/30g	115.0	1.0	383	14.0	75.0	3.0	2.5
Start Right, Asda*	1 Serving/40g	150.0	2.0	376	8.0	74.0	6.0	5.0
Start, Kellogg's*	1 Serving/30g	112.0	1.0	375	8.0	80.0	2.5	5.0
Strawberry & Almond Crunch, M & S*	1 Serving/40g	186.0	7.0	465	8.0	66.0	18.6	4.9
Strawberry & Maltiflakes, COU, M & S*	1 Serving/40g	146.0	1.0	365	12.7	73.8	2.3	3.5
Strawberry Crisp, Asda*	1 Serving/45g	194.0	7.0	431	8.1	64.7	15.5	5.9
Strawberry, Alpen*	1 Serving/40g	144.0	2.0	359	9.4	69.5	4.8	7.9
Sugar Puffs, Quaker Oats*	1 Serving/30g	114.0	0.0	379	5.3	85.8	1.6	3.7
Sultana Bran, Asda*	1 Serving/30g	98.0	1.0	327	9.0	66.0	3.0	11.0
Sultana Bran, HL, Tesco*	1 Serving/30g	97.0	1.0	325	8.2	68.0	1.9	12.0
Sultana Bran, Morrisons*	1 Serving/30g	97.0	1.0	325	8.8	65.8	3.0	11.4
Sultana Bran, Safeway*	1 Serving/50g	162.0	1.0	324	8.2	68.6	1.9	11.6
Sultana Bran, Sainsbury's*	1 Serving/30g	97.0	1.0	324	8.2	68.6	1.9	11.6
Sultana Bran, Waitrose*	1 Serving/30g	97.0	1.0	324	8.2	68.6	1.9	11.6
Superfoods, Breakfast Flakes, Jordans*	1 Serving/40g	136.0	2.0	341	8.7	67.2	4.1	11.3
Sweet Cinnamon Flavour, So Simple, Quaker Oats*	1 Serving/33g	120.0	2.0	365	9.0	67.2	6.6	7.4
Toffee Flavour, So Simple, Quaker Oats*	1 Serving/30g	122.0	4.0	407	6.5	66.0	13.0	5.0
Triple Chocolate Crisp, Sainsbury's*	1 Serving/40g	180.0	7.0	451	7.7	63.8	18.3	6.0
Tropicana, Weight Watchers*	1 Serving/50g	120.0	0.0	240	5.1	52.0	1.0	7.0
Ultra Bran, Soya & Linseed, Vogel*	1 Serving/45g	117.0	1.0	260	15.3	45.3	1.8	33.3
Vanilla, Carb Check, Heinz*	1 Serving/35g	127.0	1.0	362	56.7	27.6	2.7	0.4
Vitality, Asda*	1 Serving/30g	111.0	0.0	370	11.0	78.0	1.5	3.2
Vitality, with Red Fruit, Asda*	1 Serving/30g	110.0	0.0	366	11.0	77.0	1.6	3.8
Vitality, with Tropical Fruit, Asda*	1 Serving/30g	112.0	1.0	373	9.0	73.0	5.0	4.9
Wall's*	1 Biscuit/19g	65.0	1.0	340	11.2	67.6	2.7	10.5
Weetaflakes, Weetabix*	1 Serving/30g	102.0	0.0	340	8.9	72.9	1.4	11.0
Weetaflakes, with Raisin, Cranberry & Apple, Weetabix*	1 Serving/40g	135.0	0.0	338	6.7	75.0	1.2	8.6

B

	Measure INFO/WEIGHT	per Measure KCAL	FAT	Nutrition Values per 100g / 100ml KCAL	PROT	CARB	FAT	FIBRE
BREAKFAST CEREAL								
Weetos, Chocolate, Weetabix*	1 Serving/30g	113.0	1.0	378	8.4	75.1	4.9	5.8
Wheat Biscuits, Morrisons*	2 Biscuits/38g	129.0	1.0	340	11.2	67.6	2.7	10.5
Wheat Biscuits, Sainsbury's*	2 Biscuits/36g	123.0	1.0	342	11.5	68.4	2.0	10.0
Wheat Bisks, Asda*	2 Biscuits/38g	128.0	1.0	338	11.5	68.4	2.0	10.0
Wheat Bisks, Banana, Mini, Asda*	1 Serving/50g	190.0	3.0	380	9.7	73.1	5.4	7.4
Wheat Flakes, Alpen*	1 Serving/40g	140.0	1.0	350	10.2	72.0	2.4	9.0
Wheats, Mini, Maple & Brown Sugar, Sainsbury's*	1 Serving/52g	99.0	1.0	190	4.0	44.0	1.0	5.0
Whole Wheat Biscuits, Dove's Farm*	1 Serving/30g	99.0	1.0	329	11.0	65.0	2.8	11.0
Whole Wheat Biscuits, Waitrose*	2 Biscuits/37g	124.0	1.0	336	11.8	68.0	1.9	10.1
Wholegrain, Apricot, Wheats, Sainsbury's*	1 Serving/50g	160.0	1.0	320	7.9	71.6	1.5	8.2
Wholegrain, Fruit & Fibre, Sainsbury's*	1 Serving/30g	109.0	2.0	363	8.1	69.1	6.0	8.9
Wholegrain, Mini Wheats, Sainsbury's*	1 Serving/40g	139.0	1.0	348	11.8	69.9	2.3	11.9
Wholegrain, Sultana Bran, Sainsbury's*	1 Serving/30g	97.0	1.0	325	8.3	68.6	1.9	12.1
Yoghurt & Raspberry, Crisp, Sainsbury's*	1 Serving/45g	191.0	7.0	424	7.5	65.2	14.8	6.4
BRESAOLA								
Della Valtellina, Sainsbury's*	1 Slice/14g	23.0	0.0	163	34.7	0.1	2.6	0.1
Finest, Tesco*	1 Serving/35g	64.0	1.0	182	36.0	0.5	4.0	0.0
M & S*	1oz/28g	56.0	2.0	200	34.6	0.0	6.8	0.0
BROCCOLI								
& Cauliflower, Crowns, TTD, Sainsbury's*	1 Serving/100g	33.0	1.0	33	4.4	1.8	0.9	2.6
& Cauliflower, Floret Mix, Fresh, Tesco*	1 Serving/80g	27.0	1.0	34	3.9	2.5	0.9	2.7
& Cauliflower, Floret Mix, Iceland*	1 Serving/100g	26.0	1.0	26	2.6	2.2	0.7	2.4
& Cheese, Morrisons*	1 Pack/350g	406.0	25.0	116	6.2	6.6	7.1	0.8
Baby Courgette & Baby Leeks, Safeway*	1oz/28g	7.0	0.0	24	2.4	2.1	0.8	2.0
Bellaverde, TTD, Sainsbury's*	1 Serving/100g	33.0	1.0	33	4.4	1.8	0.9	2.6
Cauliflower & Baby Carrots, Safeway*	1 Serving/150g	37.0	1.0	25	2.0	3.0	0.6	2.3
Cauliflower & Carrots, Frozen, Great Value, Asda*	1 Serving/100g	25.0	1.0	25	2.2	2.6	0.6	5.0
Cauliflower & Carrots, Tesco*	1 Pack/320g	112.0	2.0	35	2.5	4.9	0.6	2.3
Chinese, Kai Lan, Cooked	1 Serving/80g	18.0	1.0	22	1.4	3.8	0.7	2.5
Courgette & Peppers, COU, M & S*	1 Pack/283g	156.0	12.0	55	1.7	2.7	4.1	1.7
Green, Boiled, Average	*1 Serving/80g*	*19.0*	*1.0*	*24*	*3.1*	*1.1*	*0.8*	*2.3*
Green, Raw, Average	*1 Serving/80g*	*25.0*	*1.0*	*31*	*3.7*	*2.1*	*0.8*	*2.4*
Purple Sprouting, Boiled, Average	*1 Serving/80g*	*15.0*	*0.0*	*19*	*2.1*	*1.3*	*0.6*	*2.3*
Purple Sprouting, Raw	*1oz/28g*	*10.0*	*0.0*	*35*	*3.9*	*2.6*	*1.1*	*3.5*
Tenderstem, Finest, Tesco*	½ Pack/100g	31.0	0.0	31	4.2	3.2	0.2	3.1
Tenderstem, Ready Prepared, Raw, M & S*	1 Pack/200g	80.0	0.0	40	4.1	4.9	0.2	1.7
with a Cheese Sauce, Mash Direct*	½ Pack/150g	115.0	7.0	77	4.9	4.4	4.4	3.0
BROWNIES								
Average	1 Brownie/60g	243.0	10.0	405	4.6	0.0	16.8	0.0
Chocolate Orange, Organic, The Village Bakery*	1 Brownie/30g	126.0	7.0	421	5.0	50.5	22.2	0.9
Chocolate, Bites, Mini, Weight Watchers*	1 Brownie/9g	29.0	0.0	325	5.3	63.7	5.5	2.2
Chocolate, Cadbury*	1 Brownie/36g	145.0	6.0	403	6.1	59.7	15.8	0.0
Chocolate, Chewy, M & S*	1 Brownie/29g	130.0	6.0	455	6.5	59.8	21.1	2.0
Chocolate, Chunky, Belgian, M & S*	1 Brownie/55g	242.0	11.0	440	6.2	57.7	20.3	2.5
Chocolate, Fudgy, M & S*	1 Brownie/87g	400.0	22.0	460	4.8	56.9	25.2	3.0
Chocolate, Gu*	1 Brownie/45g	200.0	12.0	444	6.7	44.4	26.6	5.0
Chocolate, Mini Bites, Asda*	1 Brownie/15g	62.0	3.0	420	5.0	55.0	20.0	1.4
Chocolate, Sainsbury's*	1 Brownie/60g	265.0	14.0	442	4.6	55.0	22.6	1.6
Chocolate, Slices, M & S*	1 Brownie/36g	158.0	9.0	440	5.3	51.1	24.1	1.3
Chocolate, Tray Bake, Tesco*	1 Brownie/37g	155.0	7.0	420	5.5	57.1	18.4	5.7
Chocolate, Waitrose*	1 Brownie/45g	192.0	9.0	426	6.3	55.6	19.8	2.7
Chocolate, Weight Watchers*	1 Brownie/47g	143.0	2.0	304	4.8	62.5	3.8	3.2
Chocolate, Wheat & Gluten Free, Mrs Crimble's*	1 Slice/47.5g	180.0	10.0	379	4.2	47.9	20.3	1.5

	Measure INFO/WEIGHT	per Measure KCAL	per Measure FAT	Nutrition Values per 100g / 100ml KCAL	PROT	CARB	FAT	FIBRE
BROWNIES								
Double Chocolate, Mini Bites, Sainsbury's*	1 Brownie/15g	49.0	2.0	326	5.8	38.9	16.4	1.6
Pecan & Walnut, Sugar Free, Joseph's*	1 Brownie/26g	150.0	7.0	577	7.7	57.7	26.9	3.8
Praline, Mini, Finest, Tesco*	1 Brownie/12g	59.0	3.0	492	4.2	60.0	25.8	0.8
BRUSCHETTA								
Pane Italia*	1 Serving/75g	367.0	19.0	489	12.4	53.6	25.1	1.4
Ploughman's Relish, Brunchetta, Golden Vale*	1 Pack/90g	261.0	15.0	290	14.2	20.2	17.2	1.6
Red Pepper & Onion, Brunchetta, Golden Vale*	1 Pack/90g	266.0	17.0	296	14.6	17.0	19.0	1.3
Safeway*	¼ Pack/115g	420.0	7.0	365	11.8	65.5	5.8	2.8
Soft Cheese & Cranberry, Brunchetta, Golden Vale*	1 Pack/95g	200.0	9.0	211	8.2	24.8	9.0	1.3
Toasted, Olive Oil & Sea Salt, Tesco*	1 Serving/30g	126.0	5.0	420	11.5	58.7	15.5	4.5
BRUSSELS SPROUTS								
& Sweet Chestnuts, Asda*	1 Serving/100g	73.0	2.0	73	3.1	11.0	1.7	4.2
Boiled, Average	**1 Serving/90g**	**31.0**	**1.0**	**35**	**3.1**	**3.2**	**1.3**	**3.5**
Button, & Chestnuts, Tesco*	1 Serving/100g	80.0	2.0	80	3.1	12.8	1.8	4.1
Button, Raw, Average	**1 Serving/80g**	**30.0**	**1.0**	**37**	**3.5**	**2.9**	**1.3**	**3.2**
Canned, Drained	**1oz/28g**	**8.0**	**0.0**	**28**	**2.6**	**2.4**	**1.0**	**2.6**
Frozen, Morrisons*	1 Serving/200g	70.0	3.0	35	3.5	2.5	1.3	4.3
Raw, Average	**1 Serving/80g**	**29.0**	**1.0**	**37**	**3.5**	**3.3**	**1.1**	**3.0**
BUBBLE & SQUEAK								
Aunt Bessie's*	1 Serving/100g	145.0	7.0	145	2.7	17.5	7.1	1.3
Fried in Vegetable Oil	1oz/28g	35.0	3.0	124	1.4	9.8	9.1	1.5
Morrisons*	1 Serving/110g	168.0	10.0	153	2.2	16.3	8.7	0.7
Safeway*	1 Serving/200g	160.0	7.0	80	1.8	10.7	3.3	1.4
Tesco*	½ Pack/325g	292.0	13.0	90	1.6	11.3	3.9	0.9
Waitrose*	½ Pack/225g	166.0	5.0	74	1.4	11.9	2.3	2.2
BUCKWHEAT								
Average	**1oz/28g**	**102.0**	**0.0**	**364**	**8.1**	**84.9**	**1.5**	**2.1**
BULGAR WHEAT								
Dry Weight, Average	**1oz/28g**	**99.0**	**0.0**	**353**	**9.7**	**76.3**	**1.7**	**8.0**
BUNS								
American, Safeway*	1 Bun/60g	152.0	3.0	253	8.9	44.5	4.4	3.7
Bath, M & S*	1 Bun/71g	217.0	6.0	305	8.3	49.8	8.0	1.9
Bath, Tesco*	1 Bun/80g	262.0	9.0	327	8.0	48.9	11.1	5.7
Belgian, Asda*	1 Bun/133g	464.0	20.0	350	4.8	49.0	15.0	2.2
Belgian, Co-Op*	1 Bun/118g	413.0	15.0	350	5.0	54.0	13.0	2.0
Belgian, Sainsbury's*	1 Bun/110g	398.0	11.0	362	6.1	61.3	10.3	1.9
Belgian, Tesco*	1 Bun/123g	438.0	16.0	356	5.2	54.9	12.8	2.2
Chelsea	1 Bun/78g	285.0	11.0	366	7.8	56.1	13.8	1.7
Chelsea, Sainsbury's*	1 Bun/85g	239.0	4.0	281	6.9	51.6	5.2	2.9
Chelsea, Tesco*	1 Bun/85g	269.0	6.0	316	7.9	53.9	7.6	2.3
Choux, M & S*	1 Bun/78g	247.0	17.0	317	5.4	25.6	22.2	0.3
Currant	1 Bun/60g	178.0	4.0	296	7.6	52.7	7.5	0.0
Currant, HL, Tesco*	1 Bun/63g	159.0	2.0	252	7.1	50.2	2.5	2.4
Currant, Sainsbury's*	1 Bun/72g	197.0	4.0	274	7.0	50.0	5.1	2.8
Fruit, Waitrose*	1 Bun/54g	155.0	2.0	287	8.1	54.0	4.3	1.6
Hot Cross	1 Bun/50g	155.0	3.0	310	7.4	58.5	6.8	1.7
Hot Cross, Apple & Cinnamon, M & S*	1 Bun/71g	170.0	1.0	240	7.6	48.7	1.7	3.1
Hot Cross, Best of Both, Hovis*	1 Bun/65g	185.0	4.0	285	9.1	47.3	6.6	4.4
Hot Cross, Golden Wholemeal, Sainsbury's*	1 Bun/65g	180.0	4.0	277	9.9	45.4	6.2	4.3
Hot Cross, Lightly Fruited, M & S*	1 Bun/63.5g	165.0	3.0	260	8.1	45.1	5.4	4.7
Hot Cross, Reduced Fat, GFY, Asda*	1 Bun/61g	136.0	1.0	223	8.0	43.0	2.1	2.4
Hot Cross, Wholemeal, Waitrose*	1 Bun/64g	177.0	4.0	276	8.8	45.2	6.7	4.9
Iced Lemon, Tesco*	1 Bun/48g	156.0	4.0	325	5.2	56.5	8.7	1.9

B

	Measure INFO/WEIGHT	per Measure KCAL	FAT	Nutrition Values per 100g / 100ml KCAL	PROT	CARB	FAT	FIBRE
BUNS								
Iced, Filled with Raspberry Jam, M & S*	1 Bun/48g	155.0	3.0	320	6.4	58.9	6.6	1.9
Iced, Spiced Fruit, M & S*	1 Bun/90g	270.0	3.0	300	7.0	60.3	3.7	1.5
Iced, Tesco*	1 Bun/35g	117.0	3.0	334	7.0	54.8	9.6	2.5
Spiced, Carb Control, Tesco*	1 Bun/45g	96.0	2.0	214	17.6	31.4	4.2	9.2
Spiced, Perfectly Balanced, Waitrose*	1 Bun/65g	177.0	2.0	272	8.0	52.3	3.4	2.9
Swiss, Sainsbury's*	1 Bun/90g	314.0	13.0	349	5.1	49.3	14.6	1.3
Swiss, Tesco*	1 Bun/100g	334.0	12.0	334	4.0	52.8	11.9	1.4
Vanilla Iced, Soft, M & S*	1 Bun/39g	125.0	3.0	320	7.6	54.9	8.0	2.9
BURGER								
Chicken, & Fries, M & S*	1 Pack/205g	287.0	8.0	140	5.3	21.2	3.8	2.4
BURGERS								
American Style, Tesco*	1 Burger/125g	250.0	9.0	200	13.0	20.4	7.3	3.9
Beef & Mature Cheddar, Asda*	1 Burger/80g	178.0	10.0	223	21.5	6.2	12.5	0.5
Beef & Onion, Grilled, Asda*	1 Burger/81g	201.0	12.0	248	23.1	6.9	14.2	0.5
Beef Steak, British, Cooked, TTD, Sainsbury's*	1 Burger/93g	191.0	12.0	205	21.0	1.5	12.8	0.5
Beef with Onion, Sainsbury's*	1 Burger/42g	102.0	6.0	243	20.7	6.9	14.8	1.0
Beef, 100% Pure, Ross*	1 Burger/56g	128.0	10.0	229	17.1	1.4	17.1	0.0
Beef, 100%, Birds Eye*	1 Burger/41g	120.0	10.0	292	17.3	0.0	24.8	0.0
Beef, 100%, Mega, Birds Eye*	1 Burger/96g	280.0	24.0	293	17.3	0.0	24.9	0.0
Beef, 100%, Quarter Pounders, Ross*	1 Burger/74g	222.0	19.0	301	16.8	1.1	25.5	0.0
Beef, 100%, Sainsbury's*	1 Burger/44g	133.0	10.0	302	21.4	0.9	23.6	0.9
Beef, Aberdeen Angus, ¼ Pounders, TTD, Sainsbury's*	1 Serving/91g	258.0	16.0	284	29.9	2.4	17.2	0.5
Beef, Aberdeen Angus, Fresh, Waitrose*	1 Burger/113g	269.0	21.0	238	16.4	1.2	18.6	0.0
Beef, Aberdeen Angus, M & S*	1 Burger/142g	298.0	19.0	210	18.3	4.1	13.3	0.1
Beef, Aberdeen Angus, Mega, Birds Eye*	1 Burger/101g	279.0	23.0	276	16.3	2.4	22.4	0.1
Beef, Aberdeen Angus, Virgin Trains*	1 Burger/240g	695.0	38.0	290	13.5	23.8	15.7	0.0
Beef, Barbecue, Tesco*	1 Burger/114g	295.0	23.0	260	15.6	3.5	20.0	0.5
Beef, BGTY, Sainsbury's*	1 Burger/110g	177.0	6.0	161	20.8	7.1	5.5	1.1
Beef, British, Waitrose*	1 Burger/113g	279.0	21.0	247	18.6	1.2	18.6	0.0
Beef, Chargrill, Tesco*	1 Burger/114g	246.0	18.0	217	17.0	0.8	16.2	2.5
Beef, Chargrilled, Quarter Pounder, Morrisons*	1 Burger/227g	590.0	45.0	260	15.0	5.3	19.9	0.2
Beef, Filled With Gorgonzola, M & S*	1 Burger/167g	384.0	27.0	230	16.5	4.9	16.1	0.5
Beef, Flame Grilled, Dalepak*	1 Burger/44g	134.0	11.0	304	15.3	2.1	26.0	0.4
Beef, Frozen, Safeway*	1 Burger/44g	123.0	9.0	279	21.3	1.3	20.2	0.0
Beef, Giant Chargrilled, Farmfoods*	1 Burger/170g	352.0	22.0	207	17.3	5.6	12.8	1.2
Beef, Mega, Birds Eye*	1 Burger/109g	300.0	25.0	275	14.3	2.7	23.0	0.3
Beef, Organic, M & S*	1 Burger/110g	239.0	18.0	217	18.2	0.0	16.0	0.2
Beef, Original & Best, Birds Eye*	1 Burger/45.6g	115.0	9.0	252	14.1	5.1	19.5	0.4
Beef, Quarter Pounder, Chilled, Morrisons*	1 Burger/115g	228.0	14.0	198	17.2	4.4	12.1	0.2
Beef, Quarter Pounders, Flame Grilled, Tesco*	1 Burger/88g	246.0	20.0	280	13.1	4.8	23.2	0.8
Beef, Quarter Pounders, Reduced Fat, Tesco*	1 Burger/95g	171.0	12.0	180	14.0	1.8	13.0	0.8
Beef, Quarter Pounders, Steak Country*	1 Burger/68g	188.0	15.0	276	16.3	2.4	22.2	0.1
Beef, Quarter Pounders, with Onion, BGTY, Sainsbury's*	1 Burger/83g	171.0	8.0	205	26.6	3.8	9.3	0.9
Beef, Quarter Pounders, with Onion, Birds Eye*	1 Burger/114g	286.0	22.0	252	14.1	5.1	19.5	0.4
Beef, Quarter Pounders, with Onion, Sainsbury's*	1 Burger/113g	306.0	22.0	271	18.0	5.1	19.8	1.5
Beef, Sainsbury's*	1 Burger/57g	152.0	9.0	267	29.6	1.3	15.9	1.5
Beef, Scotch, Ultimate, TTD, Sainsbury's*	1 Burger/142g	284.0	12.0	200	26.0	4.7	8.6	1.0
Beef, Sundried Tomato, Grilled, Finest, Tesco*	1 Burger/99g	170.0	7.0	172	20.5	5.8	7.4	0.5
Beef, with Cheese Melt, COOK!, M & S*	1 Burger/182g	400.0	29.0	220	17.9	1.3	15.9	1.2
Beef, with Fresh Garden Herbs, Raw, TTD, Sainsbury's*	1 Burger/142g	280.0	15.0	197	21.5	4.4	10.4	1.3
Beef, with Jalapeno Chilli, Finest, Tesco*	1 Burger /205g	379.0	22.0	185	17.0	3.4	10.9	0.4
Beef, with Mediterranean Tomato & Basil, M & S*	1 Burger/169g	304.0	19.0	180	15.7	5.1	11.0	1.4
Beef, with Onion, Cooked, Ross*	1 Burger/41g	117.0	10.0	284	14.7	2.8	23.8	0.4

BURGERS

	Measure INFO/WEIGHT	per Measure KCAL	FAT	Nutrition Values per 100g / 100ml KCAL	PROT	CARB	FAT	FIBRE
Beef, with Peppermix, Danish Crown*	1 Burger/100g	250.0	19.0	250	19.0	0.0	19.0	0.0
Beef, with Potato Gratin, Weight Watchers*	1 Pack/400g	320.0	10.0	80	3.0	10.0	2.5	0.0
Beef, with Red Onion & Mustard, Finest, Tesco*	1 Burger/130g	308.0	24.0	237	17.2	0.2	18.6	2.6
Beef, with Shallots, Finest, Tesco*	1 Burger/84g	175.0	10.0	208	20.2	6.4	11.3	0.5
Beef, with West Country Cheddar, TTD, Sainsbury's*	1 Burger/112g	252.0	14.0	225	26.4	2.3	12.2	0.0
Cheeseburger, American, Tesco*	1 Burger/275g	660.0	26.0	240	13.6	24.9	9.6	1.6
Chicken Cajun, Fillet, Birds Eye*	1 Pack/180g	275.0	9.0	153	21.5	5.8	4.9	0.3
Chicken Crunch & Fries, M & S*	1 Pack/425g	915.0	48.0	215	8.8	20.8	11.2	2.1
Chicken, Breaded, Value, Tesco*	1 Burger/145g	362.0	21.0	250	12.4	16.6	14.5	1.0
Chicken, Crispy Crumb, Farmfoods*	1 Burger/242g	707.0	45.0	292	10.5	20.2	18.8	1.1
Chicken, Crunch Crumb, Tesco*	1 Burger/57g	161.0	11.0	282	12.3	15.6	18.9	0.0
Chicken, Fillet, Cajun, Weighed After Cooking, Birds Eye*	1 Burger/92g	128.0	4.0	140	20.1	4.8	4.7	0.2
Chicken, Fresh, Non Coated, Waitrose*	1 Burger/100g	141.0	4.0	141	16.0	10.4	4.0	0.9
Chicken, Golden Breadcrumbs, Frozen, Birds Eye*	1 Burger/56g	130.0	7.0	232	13.8	16.4	12.4	0.3
Chicken, Quarter Pounders, Birds Eye*	1 Burger/117g	280.0	16.0	239	13.5	15.2	13.8	0.6
Chicken, Sainsbury's*	1 Burger/46g	115.0	7.0	247	15.6	12.2	15.1	1.3
Chicken, Southern Fried, Sainsbury's*	1 Burger/52g	154.0	10.0	297	12.6	17.2	19.8	1.3
Chicken, with Sesame Seed Bun, Breaded, Tesco*	1 Burger/205g	588.0	32.0	287	10.2	26.2	15.7	2.9
Chilli, Quarter Pounders, Asda*	1 Burger/88g	221.0	14.0	252	25.0	2.0	16.0	0.5
Chilli, Quarter Pounders, Iceland*	1 Burger/84g	265.0	20.0	316	18.6	6.5	23.9	0.4
Lamb, Minted, Asda*	1 Burger/100g	234.0	14.0	234	22.0	4.9	14.0	0.3
Lamb, Minted, Quarter Pounders, Asda*	1 Burger/113.5g	241.0	14.0	212	19.2	6.1	12.3	0.0
Lamb, Quarter Pounder, Asda*	1 Burger/85g	213.0	14.0	251	20.9	5.2	16.3	0.9
Lamb, Quarter Pounders, Birds Eye*	1 Burger/112g	232.0	17.0	207	13.9	3.8	15.1	0.3
Lamb, Waitrose*	1 Burger/66.9g	99.0	5.0	148	15.7	5.4	7.0	0.9
Less Than 7% Fat, Sainsbury's*	1 Burger/102g	164.0	6.0	161	20.8	7.1	5.5	1.1
Low Fat, Iceland*	1 Burger/85g	148.0	4.0	174	27.8	5.0	4.8	1.1
Pork, Quarter Pounders, Birds Eye*	1 Burger/122g	292.0	23.0	239	13.9	3.2	19.0	0.2
Quarter Pounder, with Onion, Tesco*	1 Burger/87g	213.0	16.0	245	16.0	3.0	18.6	0.5
Quarter Pounders, 95% Fat Free, Good Choice, Iceland*	1 Burger/86g	150.0	4.0	174	27.8	5.0	4.8	1.1
Quarter Pounders, Beef, BGTY, Sainsbury's*	1 Burger/113.5g	188.0	9.0	166	16.9	6.1	8.2	1.0
Quarter Pounders, Big Country*	1 Burger/90g	271.0	21.0	301	22.1	1.8	23.1	0.0
Quarter Pounders, Chargrilled, BGTY, Sainsbury's*	1 Burger/114g	184.0	6.0	161	20.8	7.1	5.5	1.1
Quarter Pounders, Scotch Beef, Sainsbury's*	1 Burger/114g	255.0	15.0	225	22.2	3.5	13.6	0.5
Salmon, Quarter Pounders, Tesco*	1 Burger/114g	145.0	3.0	128	15.9	10.6	2.4	1.2
Salmon, Tesco*	1 Burger/100g	101.0	3.0	101	18.2	0.3	3.0	0.0
Spicy Bean, Sainsbury's*	1 Burger/110g	262.0	14.0	240	5.0	27.1	12.4	2.0
Steak, Rump, The Grill, M & S*	1 Burger/169g	330.0	21.0	195	18.7	2.6	12.2	1.1
Steak, with Cheese Melt, COOK!, M & S*	1 Burger/196g	480.0	36.0	245	18.4	2.3	18.2	0.2
Super Sized Beef, Big Bite, Birds Eye*	1 Burger/122.1g	320.0	25.0	262	13.1	6.0	20.6	1.0
Tuna, Quarter Pounders, Tesco*	1 Burger/114g	132.0	2.0	116	18.8	6.7	1.6	0.9
Tuna, Sainsbury's*	1 Serving/105g	194.0	10.0	185	20.8	3.4	9.8	1.2
Turkey, Cheeseburgers, Tesco*	1 Burger/105g	252.0	15.0	240	15.4	12.8	14.1	1.3
Turkey, Crispy Crumb, Bernard Matthews*	1 Burger/71g	222.0	14.0	313	11.3	19.3	19.8	0.9
Venison, Grilled, Tesco*	1 Burger/105g	210.0	10.0	200	22.7	5.8	9.4	0.6

BURGERS VEGETARIAN

Bean, Tesco*	1 Burger/90g	192.0	11.0	213	4.4	21.6	12.1	5.0
Black Bean, Organic, Cauldron Foods*	1 Burger/87.5g	169.0	10.0	193	9.2	13.1	11.5	8.5
Cheeseburger, Chicken Style, Safeway*	1 Burger/100g	234.0	13.0	234	16.6	11.4	13.5	3.0
Chilli, Cauldron Foods*	1 Burger/87.5g	148.0	8.0	169	11.5	8.5	9.3	3.3
Flame Grilled, Linda McCartney*	1 Burger/60g	104.0	3.0	174	17.9	13.8	5.2	3.3
Meat Free, Asda*	1 Burger/60g	138.0	6.0	230	24.0	11.0	10.0	0.3
Meat Free, Sainsbury's*	1 Burger/57g	92.0	4.0	161	19.6	3.9	7.4	4.8

	Measure INFO/WEIGHT	per Measure KCAL	FAT	Nutrition Values per 100g / 100ml KCAL	PROT	CARB	FAT	FIBRE
BURGERS VEGETARIAN								
Mexican Style, Bean, Meat Free, Tesco*	1 Burger/93.6g	206.0	9.0	220	4.9	28.2	9.3	3.9
Mushroom, Cauldron Foods*	1 Burger/88g	125.0	6.0	143	5.5	16.1	6.3	2.6
Mushroom, Meat Free, Tesco*	1 Burger/87g	151.0	9.0	173	3.6	15.3	10.8	3.7
Mushroom, Organic, Cauldron Foods*	1 Burger/88g	136.0	7.0	156	7.1	18.2	8.3	2.3
Quarter Pounders, Beef Style, Sainsbury's*	1 Burger/114g	216.0	11.0	190	20.0	6.0	9.5	2.5
Quarter Pounders, HL, Tesco*	1 Burger/102g	117.0	2.0	114	4.0	20.7	1.7	2.0
Spicy Bean, BGTY, Sainsbury's*	1 Burger/85g	123.0	2.0	145	6.9	23.3	2.7	3.1
Spicy Bean, Cauldron Foods*	1 Burger/87.5g	203.0	10.0	232	5.4	27.4	11.2	6.2
Spicy Bean, Linda McCartney*	1 Burger/85g	190.0	10.0	223	4.3	26.2	11.2	2.9
Spicy Bean, Quarter Pounder, Dalepak*	1 Burger/115g	237.0	13.0	206	4.6	22.3	10.9	2.6
Vegeburger, Linda McCartney*	1 Burger/59g	79.0	2.0	134	22.6	2.9	3.6	1.6
Vegeburger, Retail, Grilled	1oz/28g	55.0	3.0	196	16.6	8.0	11.1	4.2
BUTTER								
Brandy, Tesco*	1oz/28g	152.0	11.0	543	0.3	48.3	38.7	0.5
Brandy, with Cognac, Sainsbury's*	1/8 Pot/25g	137.0	9.0	549	0.2	44.1	37.6	0.0
Coconut, Artisana*	1 Serving/15g	53.0	6.0	353	4.0	5.0	37.0	0.0
Creamery, Average	*1 Serving/10g*	*74.0*	*8.0*	*735*	*0.5*	*0.3*	*81.3*	*0.0*
Fresh, Average	*1 Thin Spread/7g*	*51.0*	*6.0*	*735*	*0.5*	*0.4*	*81.3*	*0.0*
Garlic, Somerfield*	1oz/28g	192.0	21.0	686	1.0	2.0	75.0	0.0
Jersey, TTD, Sainsbury's*	1 Thin Spread/7g	52.0	6.0	744	0.5	0.6	82.2	0.0
Reduced Fat, Fresh, Average	*1 Thin Spread/7g*	*26.0*	*3.0*	*368*	*2.3*	*1.2*	*39.4*	*0.2*
Salted, Average	*1 Thin Spread/7g*	*51.0*	*6.0*	*729*	*0.4*	*0.3*	*81.1*	*0.0*
Spreadable, Fresh, Average	*1 Thin Spread/7g*	*51.0*	*6.0*	*730*	*0.4*	*0.3*	*80.8*	*0.0*
Spreadable, Reduced Fat, Average	*1 Thin Spread/7g*	*38.0*	*4.0*	*540*	*0.5*	*0.5*	*60.0*	*0.0*
with Crushed Garlic, Lurpak*	1 Serving/10g	70.0	7.0	700	1.0	4.0	75.0	0.0
BUTTERMILK								
Average	*1 Mug/400ml*	*177.0*	*1.0*	*44*	*4.2*	*5.9*	*0.3*	*0.0*
BUTTONS								
Chocolate, Giant, Dairy Milk, Cadbury*	1 Button/3g	15.0	1.0	525	7.7	56.7	29.9	0.7
Dairy Milk, Milk Chocolate, Cadbury*	1 Pack/32.4	170.0	10.0	525	7.7	56.7	29.9	0.7
Milk Chocolate, Asda*	1 Bag/70g	368.0	21.0	526	7.0	57.0	30.0	1.5
Milk Chocolate, M & S*	1 Pack/75g	375.0	19.0	500	8.6	59.8	25.3	1.9
Milk Chocolate, Somerfield*	1 Pack/75g	390.0	21.0	520	8.0	58.0	28.0	0.0
Milk Chocolate, Tesco*	1 Bag/70g	359.0	19.0	513	7.1	59.1	27.6	2.1
White Chocolate, Cadbury*	1 Pack/32.4g	180.0	11.0	555	4.5	58.4	33.8	0.0
White Chocolate, Co-Op*	½ Pack/35g	185.0	10.0	530	7.0	64.0	28.0	0.0
White Chocolate, Tesco*	1 Bag/70g	388.0	23.0	554	5.1	58.0	33.5	0.0

	Measure INFO/WEIGHT	per Measure KCAL	FAT	Nutrition Values per 100g / 100ml KCAL	PROT	CARB	FAT	FIBRE
CABBAGE								
& Leek, Crunchy Mix, Ready to Cook, Sainsbury's*	1 Serving/125g	34.0	1.0	27	1.9	3.7	0.5	2.6
& Leek, Tesco*	1/3 Pack/100g	28.0	1.0	28	2.2	3.2	0.7	2.4
Boiled, Average	*1 Serving/90g*	*14.0*	*0.0*	*15*	*1.0*	*2.2*	*0.3*	*1.7*
Creamed, Sainsbury's*	½ Pack/150g	88.0	6.0	59	1.5	3.9	4.2	2.3
Greens, Trimmed, Average	*1oz/28g*	*8.0*	*0.0*	*28*	*2.9*	*2.9*	*0.5*	*3.4*
Medley, Washed, Ready to Cook, Tesco*	1 Pack/200g	60.0	1.0	30	2.3	3.7	0.6	2.8
Raw, Average	*1 Serving/100g*	*21.0*	*0.0*	*21*	*1.3*	*3.1*	*0.4*	*1.8*
Red, Average	*1 Serving/90g*	*19.0*	*0.0*	*21*	*1.0*	*3.7*	*0.3*	*2.2*
Red, Braised with Red Wine, M & S*	½ Pack/150g	180.0	7.0	120	1.4	17.1	4.8	1.0
Red, Pickled, Average	*1 Serving/100g*	*26.0*	*0.0*	*26*	*0.9*	*4.6*	*0.1*	*1.5*
Red, with Apple, Braised, Sainsbury's*	½ Pack/117g	91.0	4.0	78	0.8	10.8	3.5	1.7
Savoy, Boiled in Salted Water, Average	*1 Serving/90g*	*15.0*	*0.0*	*17*	*1.1*	*2.2*	*0.5*	*2.0*
Savoy, Raw, Average	*1 Serving/90g*	*24.0*	*0.0*	*27*	*2.1*	*3.9*	*0.5*	*3.1*
Sweetheart, Tesco*	1 Serving/100g	20.0	1.0	20	1.9	1.6	0.7	2.6
White, Raw, Average	*1oz/28g*	*8.0*	*0.0*	*27*	*1.4*	*5.0*	*0.2*	*2.1*
CAKE								
Alabama Chocolate Fudge, Morrisons*	1/6 Cake/58g	195.0	6.0	337	4.5	55.1	11.0	2.3
Almond Flavoured Rounds, Country Garden Cakes*	1 Cake/45g	183.0	7.0	403	4.3	62.4	14.7	2.3
Almond Slices, GFY, Asda*	1 Slice/25g	67.0	1.0	268	4.0	56.0	3.1	0.7
Almond Slices, Lyons*	1 Slice/27g	114.0	7.0	426	7.1	41.3	25.8	1.6
Almond Slices, Mr Kipling*	1 Slice/32.5g	131.0	5.0	403	6.3	63.4	14.0	2.0
Almond Slices, Sainsbury's*	1 Serving/27g	120.0	7.0	444	5.9	45.9	26.3	1.5
Almond Slices, Weight Watchers*	1 Slice/26g	95.0	3.0	365	5.2	63.8	9.9	2.4
Almond, Slices, Weight Watchers*	1 Slice/26g	95.0	3.0	365	5.2	63.8	9.9	2.4
Angel Layer, Tesco*	1 Serving/25g	101.0	4.0	403	4.5	57.4	17.3	0.9
Angel Slices, Mr Kipling*	1 Slice/38g	153.0	7.0	403	2.9	58.8	18.3	0.6
Angel, Sainsbury's*	1/8 Cake/41g	171.0	8.0	417	4.1	55.7	19.8	0.8
Apple & Cinnamon, Oat Break, Go Ahead, McVitie's*	1 Serving/35g	122.0	2.0	349	5.2	67.2	6.6	2.6
Apple Bakes, Go Ahead, McVitie's*	1 Cake/35g	126.0	3.0	361	2.6	70.0	7.8	2.0
Apple Crumble, Slices, Weight Watchers*	1 Slice/26g	90.0	2.0	346	4.5	64.8	7.7	2.3
Apple Slice, Delightful, Mr Kipling*	1 Slice/29g	92.0	1.0	317	4.4	66.2	3.9	1.3
Apple, Bramley, & Blackberry Crumble, M & S*	1/8 Cake/56g	221.0	10.0	395	4.4	54.1	17.9	1.5
Apple, Home Style, M & S*	1 Cake/54g	189.0	8.0	350	5.3	49.4	14.7	1.5
Apricot & Almond, Bakers Delight*	1oz/28g	106.0	4.0	379	5.5	53.2	16.0	1.8
Apricot & Apple, Trimlyne*	1 Cake/50g	133.0	1.0	267	4.3	58.4	2.7	1.9
Bakewell Slices, Mr Kipling*	1 Slice/36g	163.0	7.0	454	4.2	63.4	20.4	1.2
Banana Loaf, Waitrose*	1 Slice/70g	236.0	7.0	337	5.0	55.2	10.7	1.7
Banana, The Handmade Flapjack Company*	1 Cake/75g	290.0	11.0	387	5.3	59.2	14.4	0.0
Battenberg, Mini, Mr Kipling*	1 Cake/35g	143.0	4.0	410	4.6	76.2	11.0	1.3
Battenberg, Mr Kipling*	1 Serving/38g	161.0	5.0	421	5.0	73.3	12.0	1.6
Belgian Chocolate, Slices, Weight Watchers*	1 Slice/25g	86.0	2.0	344	6.5	57.6	9.8	2.9
Birthday Present, Tesco*	1 Serving/79g	347.0	14.0	439	3.5	66.6	17.6	0.4
Birthday, M & S*	1 Serving/60g	240.0	7.0	400	2.3	70.9	11.9	0.8
Butterfly, Mr Kipling*	1 Cake/29g	114.0	6.0	392	4.4	43.4	22.2	0.6
Buttons, Happy Birthday, Cadbury*	1 Slice/50g	235.0	14.0	470	4.1	52.8	27.1	0.0
Cappuccino, Finest, Tesco*	1oz/28g	105.0	6.0	374	2.8	40.4	22.3	0.2
Caramel Slice, M & S*	1 Slice/64g	304.0	16.0	475	4.9	60.4	25.2	2.6
Caramel, Milk Chocolate, Holly Lane*	1 Cake/25g	110.0	5.0	441	6.9	57.6	20.3	1.1
Carrot & Apple, Safeway*	1 Serving/50g	157.0	6.0	315	3.2	50.4	11.2	0.8
Carrot & Orange Slices, GFY, Asda*	1 Serving/23g	77.0	1.0	334	3.4	74.0	2.7	1.0
Carrot & Orange, Finest, Tesco*	1/8 Cake/50g	205.0	10.0	410	4.6	51.2	20.5	2.1
Carrot & Orange, Light Choices, Tesco*	1/6 Cake/63g	227.0	6.0	360	3.9	64.2	9.8	1.3
Carrot & Orange, Waitrose*	1/6 Cake/47g	164.0	7.0	350	5.3	46.8	15.7	1.8

CAKE

	Measure INFO/WEIGHT	per Measure KCAL	per Measure FAT	Nutrition Values per 100g / 100ml KCAL	PROT	CARB	FAT	FIBRE
Carrot & Pecan, M & S*	1 Slice/90g	330.0	15.0	365	6.4	48.7	16.2	2.3
Carrot & Walnut, Layered, Asda*	1 Serving/42g	172.0	8.0	409	4.6	55.0	19.0	1.0
Carrot & Walnut, Mini Classics, Mr Kipling*	1 Cake/39g	172.0	10.0	440	4.5	48.6	25.2	1.0
Carrot Slices, GFY, Asda*	1 Slice/27.9g	83.0	1.0	298	2.8	66.4	2.3	2.1
Carrot Slices, Less Than 3% Fat, BGTY, Sainsbury's*	1 Slice/30g	94.0	1.0	313	3.4	68.7	2.7	2.4
Carrot Slices, Weight Watchers*	1 Slice/27g	84.0	0.0	311	2.8	73.0	0.8	0.9
Carrot Wedge, Tesco*	1 Pack/175g	532.0	28.0	304	3.9	36.6	15.8	1.5
Carrot, Entenmann's*	1 Serving/40g	156.0	8.0	391	4.1	47.4	20.5	1.5
Carrot, Farmfoods*	1/8 Cake/59g	187.0	11.0	317	3.7	35.4	17.8	1.6
Carrot, Iced, Tesco*	1 Serving/61g	246.0	12.0	404	3.1	53.7	19.6	1.6
Carrot, Mini, Weight Watchers*	1 Cake/31g	120.0	3.0	388	3.7	68.9	10.8	2.7
Carrot, Slices, Asda*	1 Slice/80g	302.0	13.0	377	3.4	53.8	16.5	1.7
Carrot, Slices, Inspirations, Mr Kipling*	Per Slice/34g	139.0	6.0	411	3.5	57.7	18.5	1.3
Carrot, Square, Margaret's Country Kitchen*	1 Cake/80g	307.0	14.0	384	3.6	54.4	16.9	2.4
Celebration, Sainsbury's*	1/12 Cake/100g	265.0	9.0	265	2.1	43.6	9.2	0.3
Cherry Bakewell, Gluten Free, Bakers Delight*	1 Cake/50g	211.0	8.0	422	2.9	66.1	16.3	0.4
Cherry Bakewell, M & S*	1 Cake/44g	185.0	8.0	420	4.5	61.7	17.7	1.0
Cherry Bakewell, Sara Lee*	1/5 Slice/70g	228.0	8.0	326	4.1	51.9	11.3	1.4
Cherry Bakewell, Slices, GFY, Asda*	1 Slice/29g	98.0	1.0	337	3.4	75.4	2.4	0.7
Cherry Bakewell, Waitrose*	1 Cake/44g	184.0	8.0	419	3.8	57.4	19.3	2.1
Cherry Bakewell, Weight Watchers*	1oz/28g	102.0	3.0	365	3.6	65.4	9.9	3.6
Cherry Bakewells, Mr Kipling*	1 Cake/45g	193.0	8.0	428	3.9	61.3	18.5	1.4
Cherry Genoa, M & S*	1oz/28g	99.0	3.0	355	4.5	59.3	10.9	1.6
Cherry, M & S*	1 Serving/75g	285.0	10.0	380	5.0	60.6	12.7	0.8
Chewy Fruity Corn Flake, Dove's Farm*	1 Bar/40g	155.0	6.0	387	5.7	64.5	14.0	4.5
Chewy Rice Pop & Chocolate, Dove's Farm*	1 Bar/35g	156.0	7.0	447	3.9	69.9	20.2	2.3
Chocolate	1oz/28g	128.0	7.0	456	7.4	50.4	26.4	0.0
Chocolate & Brandy Butter, Entenmann's*	1 Serving/39g	144.0	7.0	374	3.4	53.5	17.5	2.8
Chocolate & Orange Rolls, M & S*	1 Cake/60g	228.0	17.0	380	3.6	27.0	28.4	1.3
Chocolate & Orange Slices, GFY, Asda*	1 Serving/30g	95.0	1.0	315	3.2	70.0	2.5	1.3
Chocolate Chip, Co-Op*	1/6 Cake/63g	275.0	17.0	440	5.0	44.0	27.0	0.5
Chocolate Chip, The Cake Shop*	1 Cake/35g	178.0	11.0	508	4.7	50.2	31.5	1.1
Chocolate Egg, Small, Tesco*	1 Cake/31g	132.0	6.0	425	5.4	57.2	20.2	1.7
Chocolate Flavour Slices, GFY, Asda*	1 Slice/27.5g	71.0	1.0	257	4.3	54.0	2.6	1.4
Chocolate Flower Pot, M & S*	1 Serving/69g	295.0	13.0	430	3.8	60.8	19.3	1.5
Chocolate Fudge Slice, Waitrose*	1 Slice/60g	230.0	10.0	383	4.7	54.6	16.2	1.5
Chocolate Fudge, & Vanilla Cream, M & S*	1/6 Cake/69g	310.0	18.0	450	5.2	49.8	26.0	1.3
Chocolate Fudge, Classics, M & S*	1 Serving/71g	195.0	8.0	275	2.8	42.8	10.6	1.1
Chocolate Fudge, Entenmann's*	1 Serving/48g	173.0	7.0	361	4.4	51.8	15.1	0.9
Chocolate Fudge, M & S*	1oz/28g	109.0	5.0	390	5.3	50.2	18.4	1.1
Chocolate Log, Fresh Cream, Finest, Tesco*	1 Slice/85g	301.0	15.0	354	4.5	43.2	18.1	1.4
Chocolate Orange, Slices, Weight Watchers*	1 Slice/82g	249.0	2.0	304	4.9	64.9	2.7	2.6
Chocolate Orange, Sponge, Asda*	1 Serving/70g	297.0	18.0	425	4.9	42.9	26.0	3.0
Chocolate Roll, Sainsbury's*	1 Slice/50g	210.0	10.0	420	5.0	54.0	20.4	3.3
Chocolate Slice, Go Ahead, McVitie's*	1 Slice/32g	94.0	3.0	293	4.5	49.4	8.2	1.9
Chocolate Slices, Mr Kipling*	1 Slice/32.5g	132.0	7.0	406	5.6	50.4	20.6	2.7
Chocolate Sponge, Less Than 5% Fat, Asda*	1 Sponge/110g	198.0	4.0	180	4.4	32.0	3.8	1.1
Chocolate Sponge, Tesco*	1 Serving/35g	129.0	5.0	373	5.3	54.4	14.9	1.5
Chocolate Truffle, Extra Special, Asda*	1 Serving/103g	402.0	27.0	390	5.0	34.0	26.0	1.8
Chocolate Truffle, Mini, Finest, Tesco*	1 Cake/28g	125.0	7.0	448	5.9	52.9	23.7	0.3
Chocolate with Butter Icing, Average	1oz/28g	135.0	8.0	481	5.7	50.9	29.7	0.0
Chocolate, Champagne, Sainsbury's*	1 Serving/75g	304.0	12.0	405	2.5	62.4	16.2	0.5
Chocolate, Cup, Mini, Weight Watchers*	1 Cake/17g	72.0	4.0	422	6.1	52.0	21.1	1.8

CAKE

	Measure INFO/WEIGHT	per Measure KCAL	FAT	Nutrition Values per 100g / 100ml KCAL	PROT	CARB	FAT	FIBRE
Chocolate, Double Dream, Nestle*	1 Serving/150g	637.0	38.0	425	5.0	44.7	25.1	0.9
Chocolate, Fondants, Weight Watchers*	1 Cake/19g	70.0	2.0	368	6.1	59.0	12.0	3.2
Chocolate, Fudge, The Cake Shop*	1 Cake/37g	178.0	11.0	480	3.7	50.5	29.2	1.3
Chocolate, Individual, with Mini Eggs, Cadbury*	1 Cake/26g	119.0	6.0	455	4.6	57.5	23.1	1.3
Chocolate, Large, Happy Birthday, Tesco*	1/18 Cake/63g	249.0	12.0	396	6.2	49.3	19.3	1.8
Chocolate, Loaf, Moist, McVitie's*	1 Slice/30g	119.0	6.0	398	4.8	49.0	20.3	1.9
Chocolate, Low Fat, Safeway*	1 Slice/73g	177.0	4.0	241	5.8	45.0	4.8	1.3
Chocolate, Thorntons*	1 Serving/87g	408.0	25.0	469	5.2	47.1	28.8	0.6
Chocolate, Triple, Frozen, Majestic*	¼ Cake/58g	87.0	5.0	150	2.2	14.1	9.4	0.1
Chocolate, Viennese, M & S*	1oz/28g	105.0	4.0	375	4.4	54.1	13.6	1.6
Chocolate, White Button, Asda*	1 Cake/30g	117.0	6.0	390	5.0	44.0	21.0	2.0
Christmas Pudding Slices, Mr Kipling*	1 Slice/51g	173.0	4.0	339	3.6	62.1	7.1	1.3
Christmas Slices, Mr Kipling*	1 Slice/52g	190.0	5.0	366	3.0	68.0	8.9	0.9
Christmas Slices, Weight Watchers*	1 Slice/40g	136.0	3.0	339	4.4	66.0	6.4	3.0
Christmas, Connoisseur, M & S*	1 Slice/60g	216.0	6.0	360	4.1	64.7	9.2	3.3
Christmas, Knightsbridge*	1 Slice/50g	188.0	5.0	377	4.3	65.7	10.8	3.2
Christmas, Rich Fruit, All Iced, Sainsbury's*	1/16 Cake/85g	307.0	8.0	361	4.0	66.4	8.9	1.5
Christmas, Rich Fruit, Free From, Tesco*	1 Serving/100g	301.0	7.0	301	2.9	56.0	7.3	0.9
Christmas, Rich Fruit, Tesco*	1 Serving/75g	256.0	6.0	342	3.9	64.3	7.4	3.1
Classic Lemon Drizzle, M & S*	1/6 Cake/68g	253.0	10.0	375	4.7	55.0	15.3	0.6
Coconut	1 Slice/70g	304.0	17.0	434	6.7	51.2	23.8	2.5
Coconut & Raspberry, M & S*	1 Serving/52g	231.0	14.0	445	5.0	45.5	26.8	2.3
Coconut Delight, Burton's*	1 Cake/21g	89.0	4.0	424	4.0	63.0	16.9	2.0
Coconut Snowball, Bobby's*	1 Cake/18g	80.0	4.0	436	2.2	57.3	22.1	0.0
Coconut Sponge, Mini Classics, Mr Kipling*	1 Cake/38g	155.0	9.0	409	3.7	47.0	22.9	0.9
Coffee & Walnut, Classics, M & S*	1 Serving/71g	308.0	17.0	435	4.3	50.3	24.3	1.6
Coffee & Walnut, Mrs Beeton's*	1 Slice/54g	219.0	13.0	405	3.7	41.4	25.0	0.3
Coffee, Entenmann's*	1 Serving/41g	159.0	7.0	388	4.0	54.7	17.3	0.6
Coffee, Iced, M & S*	1 Slice/33g	135.0	6.0	410	4.4	54.5	19.6	1.6
Colin the Caterpillar, M & S*	1 Slice/60g	234.0	13.0	390	5.3	57.2	21.3	1.3
Cornflake, Chocolate Clusters, Asda*	1 Cake/13.9g	64.0	3.0	460	8.2	65.2	18.5	2.7
Country Farmhouse, Waitrose*	1 Serving/80g	308.0	12.0	385	4.7	57.5	15.1	1.4
Country Slices, Asda*	1 Serving/27g	111.0	5.0	411	3.9	56.0	19.0	2.4
Country Slices, Mr Kipling*	1 Slice/31.8	121.0	5.0	380	4.4	56.7	15.0	1.2
Cream Oysters, M & S*	1 Cake/72g	227.0	15.0	315	3.6	27.5	21.2	3.0
Cream Slices, M & S*	1 Slice/80g	310.0	18.0	387	2.3	45.7	22.9	0.6
Crispy Fruit Slices, Forest Fruit, Go Ahead, McVitie's*	1 Biscuit/14g	58.0	1.0	406	5.5	73.0	9.1	3.7
Date & Walnut Loaf, Sainsbury's*	1/10 Slice/40g	148.0	8.0	371	6.7	40.1	20.4	1.0
Date & Walnut, Slices, Light Choices, Tesco*	1 Slice/25g	72.0	0.0	290	5.6	63.7	1.1	1.1
Date & Walnut, Slices, Weight Watchers*	1 Slice/27g	73.0	0.0	271	3.5	60.6	1.6	4.2
Date & Walnut, Trimlyne*	1 Slice/50g	134.0	2.0	269	5.7	53.8	4.9	1.8
Double Chocolate Ganache, M & S*	1/12 Cake/61g	281.0	17.0	460	5.9	46.1	27.6	2.5
Double Chocolate Wedge, Tesco*	1 Piece/100g	416.0	20.0	416	5.0	53.4	20.3	0.9
Dundee, Co-Op*	1/8 Cake/71g	238.0	8.0	335	5.0	53.0	11.0	2.0
Eccles	1 Cake/45g	214.0	12.0	475	3.9	59.3	26.4	1.6
Eccles, Weight Watchers*	1 Cake/48g	190.0	8.0	396	4.4	57.5	16.5	2.0
Fairy, Holly Lane*	1 Cake/26g	118.0	7.0	460	3.7	52.5	26.1	3.5
Fairy, Lemon Iced, Tesco*	1 Cake/24g	94.0	3.0	393	4.4	63.2	13.6	1.1
Fairy, Mini, Kids, Tesco*	1 Cake/12g	54.0	3.0	435	5.3	53.3	22.3	1.1
Fairy, Mini, Tesco*	1 Cake/13g	53.0	2.0	424	6.1	54.6	20.1	1.3
Fairy, Plain, Sainsbury's*	1 Cake/20g	84.0	4.0	422	4.9	46.4	21.5	1.2
Fairy, Snowman, Christmas, Tesco*	1 Cake/24g	114.0	7.0	471	4.6	49.8	28.1	2.9
Fairy, Strawberry Iced, Tesco*	1 Cake/24g	94.0	3.0	392	4.9	62.9	13.4	1.4

CAKE

	Measure INFO/WEIGHT	per Measure KCAL	per Measure FAT	Nutrition Values per 100g / 100ml KCAL	PROT	CARB	FAT	FIBRE
Fairy, Vanilla Iced, Tesco*	1 Cake/24g	93.0	3.0	388	4.4	65.1	12.2	1.2
Farmhouse Slice, Weight Watchers*	1 Slice/23g	73.0	1.0	317	5.5	64.9	4.0	1.3
Flake, Cadbury*	1 Cake/20.2g	90.0	5.0	445	6.3	54.5	22.3	0.0
Fondant Fancies, Lemon, Waitrose*	1 Cake/40g	176.0	7.0	441	2.5	67.9	17.7	0.6
Fondant Fancies, Sainsbury's*	1 Cake/27g	95.0	2.0	353	2.4	65.7	9.0	0.4
Fondant, Dark Chocolate, Graze*	1 Pack/40g	157.0	6.0	393	3.5	66.2	14.5	0.0
French Fancies, Mr Kipling*	1 Cake/28g	103.0	3.0	369	2.8	68.3	9.4	0.6
Fresh Cream Bramley Apple Sponge, Tesco*	1/6 Slice/43g	130.0	7.0	303	3.6	35.4	16.3	1.0
Fruit, Plain, Average	1 Slice/90g	319.0	12.0	354	5.1	57.9	12.9	0.0
Fruit, Rich, Average	1 Slice/70g	225.0	9.0	322	4.9	50.7	12.5	1.7
Fruit, Rich, Iced	1 Slice/70g	249.0	8.0	356	4.1	62.7	11.4	1.7
Fudge Brownie, The Handmade Flapjack Company*	1 Cake/75g	286.0	9.0	381	4.9	62.8	12.3	0.0
Fudgy Chocolate Slices, COU, M & S*	1 Slice/36g	95.0	1.0	265	4.6	66.4	2.2	2.1
Genoa, Home Bake, McVitie's*	1oz/28g	107.0	4.0	383	4.7	55.9	15.6	1.4
Genoa, Tesco*	1 Serving/50g	162.0	4.0	325	3.6	60.9	7.4	4.0
Ginger Drizzle, Iced, Co-Op*	1/6 Cake/64.5g	226.0	8.0	350	3.0	58.0	12.0	1.0
Ginger Orange, The Handmade Flapjack Company*	1 Cake/75g	289.0	15.0	385	4.3	46.3	20.3	0.0
Glitzy Bag, Birthday, Tesco*	1 Serving/81g	314.0	7.0	388	2.1	75.9	8.5	0.6
Happy Birthday, Sainsbury's*	1 Slice/50g	207.0	8.0	414	2.8	64.5	16.1	0.6
Holly Hedgehog, Tesco*	1 Serving/55g	227.0	8.0	413	2.0	69.0	14.3	0.8
Hot Chocolate Fudge, Sainsbury's*	1/8 Cake/91.2g	343.0	16.0	376	5.1	50.3	17.1	3.5
Iced Madeira, Sainsbury's*	1/8 Cake/47g	182.0	7.0	388	3.6	61.6	14.1	0.7
Jamaica Ginger with Lemon Filling, McVitie's*	1 Cake/33g	143.0	8.0	434	4.0	48.3	25.0	0.8
Jamaica Ginger, McVitie's*	1 Cake/291g	1048.0	31.0	360	3.5	62.2	10.8	1.4
Jammy Strawberry Rolls, Mini, Cadbury*	1 Cake/29g	119.0	5.0	411	4.9	59.8	16.5	0.5
Lemon & Orange, Finest, Tesco*	1 Serving/53g	216.0	11.0	410	4.5	52.4	20.3	1.1
Lemon Bakewell, Mr Kipling*	1 Cake/48g	195.0	7.0	407	2.6	65.0	15.2	0.7
Lemon Buttercream & Lemon Curd, The Cake Shop*	1 Cake/28g	124.0	8.0	444	3.5	43.4	27.8	0.6
Lemon Drizzle, M & S*	1/6 Cake/63g	230.0	9.0	365	4.2	55.8	13.9	1.4
Lemon Iced Madeira, Co-Op*	1 Cake/290g	1131.0	52.0	390	4.0	53.0	18.0	0.6
Lemon Slices, BGTY, Sainsbury's*	1 Slice/26.0g	84.0	0.0	323	3.7	74.0	1.4	1.3
Lemon Slices, Low Fat, Weight Watchers*	1 Slice/26.1g	79.0	1.0	303	3.1	68.1	2.0	2.2
Lemon Slices, Mr Kipling*	1 Slice/29.1g	120.0	5.0	413	4.2	61.9	16.6	0.7
Lemon, Entenmann's*	1 Serving/56g	213.0	9.0	383	3.7	56.9	15.7	1.1
Lemon, French Fancies, Mr Kipling*	1 Fancy/28g	106.0	3.0	378	2.5	69.9	9.8	0.5
Lemon, Half Moon, Bobby's*	1/6 Cake/60g	244.0	11.0	406	4.1	55.7	18.4	0.0
Lemon, Home Bake, McVitie's*	1oz/28g	108.0	5.0	384	4.6	53.9	18.2	1.0
Lemon, Mini, Weight Watchers*	1 Cake/27g	90.0	3.0	333	3.7	66.7	11.1	11.1
Lemon, The Handmade Flapjack Company*	1 Cake/75g	312.0	16.0	416	4.5	50.5	21.8	0.0
Madeira	1 Slice/40g	157.0	7.0	393	5.4	58.4	16.9	0.9
Madeira, All Butter, Sainsbury's*	1 Serving/30g	116.0	6.0	388	5.2	47.4	19.7	0.8
Madeira, Cherry, Tesco*	¼ Cake/100g	342.0	11.0	342	4.3	55.9	11.2	2.6
Madeira, Iced, Tesco*	1/16 Cake/56g	218.0	7.0	389	2.6	67.2	12.2	0.4
Madeira, Lemon Iced, Tesco*	1 Slice/30g	122.0	5.0	407	4.5	57.8	17.5	0.9
Magic Roundabout, Dougal, Tesco*	1 Serving/50g	214.0	8.0	428	2.3	68.7	16.0	0.2
Manor House, Mr Kipling*	1 Serving/69g	277.0	14.0	400	5.3	49.7	20.0	1.4
Marble, Home Bake, McVitie's*	1oz/28g	115.0	5.0	411	3.7	56.9	18.8	0.9
Mini Rolls, Blackforest, Weight Watchers*	1 Cake/24g	89.0	3.0	374	5.3	58.9	14.2	4.4
Mini Rolls, Cadbury*	1 Roll/27g	120.0	6.0	445	4.4	56.4	22.5	1.3
Mini Rolls, Chocolate & Vanilla, Somerfield*	1oz/28g	112.0	4.0	399	5.0	62.0	15.0	0.0
Mini Rolls, Chocolate, Weight Watchers*	1 Roll/26g	87.0	3.0	334	4.6	58.1	13.2	3.7
Mini Rolls, Easter Selection, Cadbury*	1oz/28g	122.0	6.0	434	5.5	55.6	20.6	0.0
Mini Rolls, Juicy Orange, Cadbury*	1 Cake/28g	110.0	5.0	390	5.0	55.0	16.8	0.0

CAKE

	Measure INFO/WEIGHT	per Measure KCAL	per Measure FAT	Nutrition Values per 100g / 100ml KCAL	PROT	CARB	FAT	FIBRE
Mini Rolls, Milk Chocolate Orange, Shapers, Boots*	1 Roll/25g	97.0	3.0	386	4.6	64.0	12.0	2.4
Mini Rolls, Milk Chocolate, Cadbury*	1 Roll/27g	120.0	6.0	445	4.4	56.5	22.2	0.0
Mini Rolls, Rolo, Nestle*	1 Cake/29g	111.0	5.0	388	4.8	49.5	19.0	1.0
Orange & Cranberry, Mini Classics, Mr Kipling*	1 Cake/36g	164.0	7.0	455	4.5	42.2	20.2	0.7
Orange & Ginger, Oat Break, Go Ahead, McVitie's*	1 Cake/35g	121.0	2.0	347	5.2	67.1	6.4	2.6
Orange Marmalade, M & S*	1 Slice/50g	195.0	9.0	390	3.6	53.2	18.3	1.8
Panettone, Bauli*	1 Serving/75g	313.0	15.0	418	5.9	53.5	20.1	0.0
Panettone, M & S*	1/8 Loaf/51g	184.0	7.0	360	6.5	53.4	13.2	2.0
Raisin, Dernys*	1 Cake/45g	175.0	8.0	388	5.0	54.0	17.0	0.0
Raisin, Sainsbury's*	1 Cake/40g	161.0	8.0	403	4.7	53.5	18.9	3.0
Rich Choc' Roll, Cadbury*	1/6 Portion/39g	149.0	6.0	381	4.8	50.2	15.6	1.0
Rock	1 Sm Cake/40g	158.0	7.0	396	5.4	60.5	16.4	1.5
Shrek Birthday, Tesco*	1/16 Cake/72g	248.0	9.0	344	3.3	64.0	12.2	0.5
Snowballs, Sainsbury's*	1 Snowball/18g	80.0	4.0	445	2.5	55.6	23.0	3.6
Snowballs, Tesco*	1 Snowball/18g	79.0	4.0	432	2.5	55.8	22.1	5.4
Sponge	1 Slice/53g	243.0	14.0	459	6.4	52.4	26.3	0.9
Sponge Roll, Chocolate, M & S*	¼ Cake/66g	251.0	12.0	380	3.9	50.5	18.4	1.8
Sponge Roll, Coffee, M & S*	1 Serving/40g	150.0	7.0	375	3.5	51.1	17.3	0.6
Sponge with Butter Icing	1 Slice/65g	318.0	20.0	490	4.5	52.4	30.6	0.6
Sponge, Fatless	1 Slice/53g	156.0	3.0	294	10.1	53.0	6.1	0.9
Sponge, Fresh Cream & Strawberry, Asda*	1/12 Cake/60g	170.0	6.0	284	4.6	44.0	10.0	1.1
Sponge, Iced, M & S*	1 Serving/100g	400.0	17.0	400	3.4	58.4	17.0	1.3
Sponge, Jam Filled	1 Slice/65g	196.0	3.0	302	4.2	64.2	4.9	1.8
Sponge, Victoria, TTD, Sainsbury's*	1 Slice/57g	229.0	11.0	401	5.0	51.8	19.3	1.4
Stem Ginger, 96% Fat Free, Trimlyne*	¼ Cake/62.5g	170.0	2.0	272	4.4	58.1	3.6	1.2
Stem Ginger, Mrs Crimble's*	1 Slice/48g	158.0	1.0	329	2.7	73.3	2.2	2.7
Stollen Slices, Somerfield*	1oz/28g	115.0	5.0	411	7.0	54.0	19.0	0.0
Stollen, Christmas Range, Tesco*	1oz/28g	99.0	4.0	355	5.0	52.9	13.7	1.8
Strawberry Sponge Roll, M & S*	1/6 Cake/49g	160.0	5.0	330	2.8	58.0	9.5	0.8
Sultana & Cherry Slice, Co-Op*	1oz/28g	87.0	3.0	310	3.0	48.0	12.0	2.0
Sultana & Cherry, Tesco*	1 Cake/37g	124.0	4.0	334	4.7	54.4	10.8	2.5
Sultana, Apple & Cranberry, 99% Fat Free, Trimlyne*	1/6 Cake/66.6g	130.0	1.0	195	4.6	45.5	0.9	3.3
Sultana, Fair Trade, Co-Op*	1/8 Cake/45g	155.0	4.0	345	5.0	60.0	9.0	1.0
Summer Fruit Cream, GFY, Asda*	1 Serving/74.0g	165.0	4.0	223	3.6	41.0	4.9	2.5
Summer Strawberry Bakes, Go Ahead, McVitie's*	1 Bar/35g	128.0	3.0	367	2.7	75.1	8.0	1.0
Swiss Roll, Average	1oz/28g	77.0	1.0	276	7.2	55.5	4.4	0.8
Swiss Roll, Chocolate, Individual	1 Roll/26g	88.0	3.0	337	4.3	58.1	11.3	0.0
Swiss Roll, Chocolate, Lyons*	1 Serving/50g	189.0	10.0	379	4.3	47.0	19.3	0.9
Swiss Roll, Chocolate, M & S*	1 Serving/46g	168.0	11.0	365	4.6	32.6	24.2	1.2
Swiss Roll, Chocolate, Mini, Tesco*	1 Roll/22g	87.0	3.0	396	4.6	61.0	14.8	0.0
Swiss Roll, Raspberry & Vanilla, Morrisons*	1 Serving/28g	98.0	3.0	350	4.2	61.8	9.5	0.0
Swiss Roll, Raspberry Jam, Mr Kipling*	1/6 Cake/51.8g	184.0	5.0	355	2.8	63.0	10.2	1.0
Swiss Roll, Raspberry, Lyons*	1 Roll/175g	485.0	2.0	277	5.2	60.6	1.4	0.0
Swiss Roll, Raspberry, Sainsbury's*	1 Serving/35g	105.0	1.0	301	3.5	67.0	2.1	1.1
Syrup & Ginger, Tesco*	1 Serving/32g	134.0	7.0	420	4.5	51.4	21.8	0.7
Tangy Lemon Trickle, M & S*	1 Slice/75g	281.0	14.0	375	4.7	47.4	18.8	1.1
The Ultimate Carrot Passion, Entenmann's*	1 Slice/52g	210.0	13.0	403	4.6	42.4	24.3	1.0
Tiffin, Chocolate, Sainsbury's*	1 Cake/61g	184.0	12.0	301	2.7	29.8	19.0	1.3
Toffee & Pecan Loaf, Safeway*	1/6 Cake/62g	225.0	14.0	363	3.6	35.5	22.9	0.5
Toffee & Pecan Slices, M & S*	1 Slice/36g	160.0	9.0	445	4.7	54.0	23.7	1.3
Toffee Bakewell, Tesco*	1 Cake/49g	203.0	8.0	414	3.9	63.5	16.1	1.4
Toffee Flavour Slices, Low Fat, Weight Watchers*	1 Slice/27g	80.0	1.0	297	4.2	63.9	2.6	3.2
Toffee Fudge, Entenmann's*	1 Serving/65g	274.0	14.0	421	3.4	53.0	21.7	0.5

C

	Measure INFO/WEIGHT	per Measure KCAL	FAT	Nutrition Values per 100g / 100ml KCAL	PROT	CARB	FAT	FIBRE

CAKE

	Measure INFO/WEIGHT	KCAL	FAT	KCAL	PROT	CARB	FAT	FIBRE
Toffee Snap, The Handmade Flapjack Company*	1 Cake/75g	365.0	20.0	487	4.6	62.2	26.1	0.0
Toffee Temptation, Finest, Tesco*	1 Serving/50g	211.0	12.0	423	4.7	49.0	23.1	0.6
Toffee, Iced, Tesco*	1 Serving/35g	132.0	5.0	376	3.3	57.2	14.9	1.6
Toffee, Slices, BGTY, Sainsbury's*	1 Slice/27g	88.0	1.0	327	4.3	71.7	2.5	1.8
Toffee, The Handmade Flapjack Company*,	1 Cake/75g	346.0	19.0	462	5.1	54.0	25.1	0.0
Toffee, Thorntons*	1/6 Cake/70g	302.0	17.0	431	4.6	49.2	24.0	0.8
Triple Chocolate Roll, Cadbury*	1 Serving/40.2g	165.0	7.0	410	4.3	60.1	16.6	1.5
Turkish Delight, Fry's*	1 Cake/26g	96.0	3.0	371	4.5	62.4	10.8	0.5
Vanilla Sponge, Fresh Cream, Sainsbury's*	1 Slice/50g	152.0	5.0	304	7.5	45.6	10.2	0.4
Victoria Sandwich, Classic, Large, M & S*	1/10 Cake/66g	260.0	13.0	395	5.1	49.5	19.6	2.3
Victoria Slices, Mr Kipling*	1 Slice/28.2g	122.0	4.0	432	3.9	68.8	15.7	0.4
Victoria Sponge, Fresh Cream, Value, Tesco*	1 Serving/50g	168.0	9.0	337	4.4	40.7	17.4	0.6
Victoria Sponge, Mini, Mr Kipling*	1 Cake/36.2g	152.0	7.0	420	3.9	58.5	19.0	0.8
Victoria Sponge, Mini, Weight Watchers*	1 Cake/26g	92.0	2.0	354	5.7	64.1	8.3	1.5
Viennese Whirl, Chocolate, Mr Kipling*	1 Whirl/28g	142.0	9.0	507	4.7	52.1	31.1	2.2
Viennese Whirl, Lemon, Mr Kipling*	1 Cake/28g	115.0	4.0	409	4.2	62.2	15.9	0.7
Viennese Whirl, Mr Kipling*	1 Cake/28g	141.0	8.0	504	3.9	59.1	28.0	1.4
Viennese, M & S*	1 Cake/51g	250.0	14.0	495	4.1	58.9	28.0	2.8
Walnut Layer, Somerfield*	¼ Cake/77.5g	295.0	15.0	381	6.0	45.0	20.0	0.0
Walnut, Sandwich, Sainsbury's*	1/8 Cake/48g	182.0	8.0	379	5.4	53.7	17.3	1.3
Welsh, Average	1oz/28g	121.0	5.0	431	5.6	61.8	19.6	1.5
Wild Blueberry & Apple, Bakers Delight*	1oz/28g	99.0	4.0	354	4.6	48.8	15.6	1.5
Winnie the Pooh Birthday, Disney, Nestle*	1 Serving/100g	361.0	11.0	361	2.4	63.3	10.9	0.5
Yorkshire Parkin, Bakers Delight*	1oz/28g	111.0	4.0	395	5.1	60.3	14.8	1.5

CAKE BAR

	Measure INFO/WEIGHT	KCAL	FAT	KCAL	PROT	CARB	FAT	FIBRE
Blueberry, Trimlyne*	1 Cake/50g	141.0	1.0	283	3.9	64.0	2.2	2.2
Bounty, McVitie's*	1 Cake/36g	166.0	9.0	461	5.1	55.2	24.5	0.0
Caramel, Cadbury*	1 Bar/26g	107.0	4.0	411	6.4	57.0	16.8	0.0
Caramel, Weight Watchers*	1 Bar/22.8g	86.0	3.0	377	5.6	58.2	13.5	3.9
Choc Chip, Go Ahead, McVitie's*	1 Cake/28.1g	100.0	3.0	356	6.4	56.9	12.4	1.0
Choc Chip, Mini, Go Ahead, McVitie's*	1 Bar/27g	93.0	3.0	343	5.7	55.3	12.1	0.9
Chocolate & Orange, Go Ahead, McVitie's*	1 Cake/33g	109.0	2.0	330	4.3	64.9	6.0	1.0
Chocolate Chip, HL, Tesco*	1 Serving/37g	109.0	1.0	295	4.8	63.6	2.6	0.6
Chocolate Chip, Mr Kipling*	1 Bar/32g	151.0	8.0	472	5.3	53.5	26.3	1.2
Chocolate Chip, Sainsbury's*	1 Cake/25g	107.0	6.0	430	6.1	51.2	22.3	0.6
Chocolate Dream, Go Ahead, McVitie's*	1 Bar/36g	141.0	5.0	391	4.6	63.2	13.4	0.9
Chocolate, High Lights, Cadbury*	1 Bar/25g	95.0	3.0	380	5.5	58.8	14.0	1.1
Chocolate, Snack Cakes, Penguin, McVitie's*	1 Bar/24g	122.0	7.0	510	4.8	54.6	30.2	1.6
Chocolate, Tesco*	1 Serving/26g	113.0	6.0	435	5.2	51.9	23.0	5.4
Cinder Toffee, Cadbury*	1 Cake Bar/32g	149.0	8.0	465	4.2	53.4	26.2	0.9
Crunchie, Cadbury*	1 Cake/32g	147.0	7.0	460	5.9	58.3	22.6	0.0
Double Chocolate, Free From, Sainsbury's*	1 Cake/50g	196.0	8.0	391	4.2	58.2	15.7	1.0
Dream, Cadbury*	1 Cake/38g	170.0	9.0	450	4.5	57.2	22.6	0.0
Flake, Cadbury*	1 Cake/22g	97.0	5.0	442	6.5	51.8	23.3	0.5
Fruit & Nut Crisp, Go Ahead, McVitie's*	1 Bar/22g	95.0	3.0	430	5.3	71.3	13.7	1.7
Fudge, Cadbury*	1 Pack/52g	220.0	9.0	420	5.7	60.3	17.6	0.0
Galaxy Caramel, McVitie's*	1 Cake/31g	137.0	7.0	441	5.5	57.4	21.1	0.0
Golden Syrup, McVitie's*	1 Cake/33g	127.0	5.0	385	3.6	60.2	14.4	1.2
Jaffa, McVitie's*	1 Bar/25g	97.0	4.0	390	3.2	62.4	14.2	2.4
Jamaica Ginger, McVitie's*	1 Cake/33g	128.0	5.0	388	3.5	60.2	14.7	1.2
Milk Chocolate & Orange, Crispy, Asda*	1 Bar/22g	91.0	2.0	413	4.8	75.6	10.2	2.0
Milk Chocolate, Cadbury*	1 Bar/34.9g	150.0	8.0	430	5.6	53.3	21.7	1.2
Milky Way, McVitie's*	1 Cake/28.2g	144.0	9.0	511	5.0	53.9	30.7	0.0

	Measure INFO/WEIGHT	per Measure KCAL	FAT	Nutrition Values per 100g / 100ml KCAL	PROT	CARB	FAT	FIBRE
CAKE BAR								
Rich Chocolate, Trimlyne*	1 Serving/40g	115.0	2.0	287	5.2	59.2	4.2	2.2
Toffee Cake, High Lights, Cadbury*	1 Bar/25g	95.0	3.0	380	7.6	56.7	14.0	0.9
CAKE MIX								
Carrot Cake, Betty Crocker*	¼ Pack/125g	504.0	8.0	403	5.8	78.9	6.7	1.4
Cheesecake, Original, Made Up, Asda*	1/6 Cake/85g	228.0	10.0	268	4.1	36.0	12.0	1.4
Cheesecake, Strawberry, Real, Green's*	1 Serving/100g	254.0	13.0	253	3.9	30.6	12.8	0.6
Cheesecake, Tesco*	1 Serving/76g	199.0	8.0	262	4.1	38.0	10.4	1.6
Chocolate Brownie, Chocolate Chips, Weight Watchers*	1 Pack/190g	568.0	13.0	299	3.2	55.6	7.1	2.1
Dennis, Green's*	1 Cake/17g	55.0	1.0	319	4.6	57.8	7.7	0.0
Free From, Sainsbury's*	1 Serving/50g	173.0	0.0	346	1.3	84.4	0.3	2.2
Yellow, Super Moist, Betty Crocker*	1 Cake/128.0g	517.0	9.0	404	3.3	81.6	7.4	1.1
CALZONE								
Bolognese, Weight Watchers*	1 Calzone/88g	178.0	3.0	202	11.7	31.2	3.4	4.3
Cheese & Tomato, Weight Watchers*	1 Calzone/88g	191.0	4.0	217	11.3	33.4	4.3	3.4
Ham & Gruyere, Asda*	1 Serving/280g	661.0	22.0	236	10.0	31.0	8.0	2.7
CANAPES								
Aegean Tomato, Finest, Tesco*	1 Canape/15g	45.0	2.0	300	7.2	34.3	14.7	2.1
Caponata, Puff Pastry, Occasions, Sainsbury's*	1 Square/12g	30.0	2.0	249	4.1	22.9	15.7	2.1
Salmon & Dill, Finest, Tesco*	1 Canape/15g	47.0	2.0	315	9.2	32.7	16.1	1.9
Smoked Salmon, Youngs*	1 Canape/10g	21.0	2.0	210	15.9	2.0	15.2	0.7
CANNELLONI								
Beef & Red Wine, Waitrose*	½ Pack/170g	355.0	16.0	209	17.5	13.8	9.4	1.0
Beef, BGTY, Sainsbury's*	1 Pack/300g	249.0	7.0	83	5.5	10.1	2.3	1.7
Beef, Finest, Tesco*	½ Pack/300g	399.0	22.0	133	7.1	9.4	7.4	1.9
Beef, Italian, Sainsbury's*	1 Pack/400g	498.0	26.0	124	5.9	10.5	6.5	1.6
Beef, Italian, Tesco*	1 Pack/400g	520.0	27.0	130	5.3	11.6	6.7	0.9
Beef, Sainsbury's*	1 Pack/400g	372.0	18.0	93	4.4	8.8	4.4	1.6
Beef, TTD, Sainsbury's*	1 Pack/383g	548.0	27.0	143	7.2	12.7	7.0	2.3
Chicken & Pesto, Italian, Sainsbury's*	1 Pack/450g	675.0	34.0	150	6.1	14.4	7.5	1.1
Mediterranean Vegetable, Waitrose*	1 Serving/170g	330.0	15.0	194	9.7	18.7	9.0	1.9
Mushroom, Italian, Sainsbury's*	1 Pack/450g	598.0	31.0	133	5.2	12.5	6.9	0.5
Parmesan & Basil, M & S*	1 Pack/360g	504.0	28.0	140	5.9	11.4	7.9	0.8
Pork, M & S*	1 Pack/400g	460.0	25.0	115	6.2	8.7	6.2	1.1
Ricotta & Spinach, COU, M & S*	1 Pack/400g	320.0	8.0	80	5.3	9.7	2.0	2.8
Ricotta & Spinach, Eat Smart, Morrisons*	1 Pack/400g	328.0	8.0	82	5.2	10.9	2.0	1.6
Ricotta & Spinach, Fresh, Waitrose*	½ Pack/225g	274.0	16.0	122	5.1	8.8	7.3	1.2
Ricotta & Spinach, Perfectly Balanced, Waitrose*	1 Pack/400g	272.0	9.0	68	3.8	7.7	2.3	1.4
Roasted Vegetable, Morrisons*	1 Serving/350g	311.0	9.0	89	3.9	12.5	2.5	2.3
Smoked Salmon & Spinach, Sainsbury's*	1 Pack/450g	598.0	28.0	133	5.7	13.5	6.2	0.4
Spinach & Cheese, Finest, Tesco*	1 Pack/350g	532.0	32.0	152	5.4	12.1	9.1	1.5
Spinach & Ricotta, BGTY, Sainsbury's*	1 Pack/400g	372.0	12.0	93	4.4	12.5	2.9	1.8
Spinach & Ricotta, Finest, Tesco*	1 Serving/120g	276.0	14.0	230	8.4	22.1	11.5	2.1
Spinach & Ricotta, HL, Tesco*	1 Pack/400g	320.0	11.0	80	4.0	10.0	2.8	1.1
Spinach & Ricotta, Italian, Sainsbury's*	1 Pack/400g	476.0	30.0	119	4.8	8.1	7.5	1.7
Spinach & Ricotta, Light Choices, Tesco*	1 Pack/400g	340.0	11.0	85	4.0	10.0	2.8	1.1
Spinach & Ricotta, Waitrose*	1 Pack/400g	460.0	27.0	115	5.1	8.7	6.7	1.3
Spinach & Wild Mushroom, Linda McCartney*	1 Pack/340g	381.0	14.0	112	4.9	14.1	4.0	1.7
Value, Tesco*	1 Serving/250g	320.0	17.0	128	6.6	10.0	6.8	1.4
Vegetarian, Tesco*	1 Pack/400g	552.0	34.0	138	5.3	9.8	8.6	1.5
CAPERS								
Caperberries, Spanish, Waitrose*	1 Serving/55g	9.0	0.0	17	1.1	2.1	0.5	2.5
Capucines, Sainsbury's*	1 Tsp/6g	1.0	0.0	14	1.4	1.3	0.3	2.2
in Brine, Tesco*	1 Tsp/2g	1.0	0.0	29	2.4	3.5	0.6	2.7

	Measure INFO/WEIGHT	per Measure KCAL	FAT	Nutrition Values per 100g / 100ml KCAL	PROT	CARB	FAT	FIBRE
CAPERS								
In Vinegar, Average	1 Tsp/5g	2.0	0.0	34	1.7	3.0	0.6	0.0
CAPPELLETTI								
Goats Cheese & Red Pesto, Waitrose*	½ Pack/125g	374.0	11.0	299	11.6	43.5	8.7	2.2
Parma Ham, Fresh, Waitrose*	½ Pack/125g	367.0	11.0	294	14.1	38.6	9.2	2.2
CAPRI SUN								
Orange	1 Pouch/200ml	90.0	0.0	45	0.0	11.0	0.0	0.0
Orange, 100%, Juice	1 Pouch/200ml	75.0	0.0	38	0.5	9.2	0.0	0.1
CARAMAC								
Nestle*	1 Bar/30g	173.0	11.0	567	5.7	54.7	36.1	0.0
CARAMBOLA								
Average	*1oz/28g*	*9.0*	*0.0*	*32*	*0.5*	*7.3*	*0.3*	*1.3*
CARAMEL								
Egg, Cadbury*	1 Egg/39g	191.0	10.0	490	4.3	58.9	26.1	0.0
CARAWAY								
Seeds, Schwartz*	1 Pack/38g	170.0	8.0	448	23.3	40.9	21.2	0.0
CARDAMOM								
Black, Ground, Average	*1 Tsp/2g*	*6.0*	*0.0*	*311*	*10.8*	*68.5*	*6.7*	*28.0*
Ground, Average	*1 Tsp/2g*	*6.0*	*0.0*	*314*	*10.7*	*53.6*	*7.1*	*28.6*
CAROB POWDER								
Average	*1 Tsp/2g*	*3.0*	*0.0*	*159*	*4.9*	*37.0*	*0.1*	*0.0*
CARP								
Fillet, Raw, Average	1 Av Fillet/218g	244.0	10.0	112	17.5	0.0	4.7	0.0
CARROT & SWEDE								
Diced, for Mashing, Average	*½ Pack/250g*	*57.0*	*1.0*	*23*	*0.6*	*4.7*	*0.3*	*1.9*
Mash, From Supermarket, Average	1 Serving/150g	138.0	7.0	92	1.3	10.4	5.0	1.3
CARROTS								
& Cauliflower, M & S*	1 Serving/335g	74.0	1.0	22	0.6	4.4	0.4	2.3
& Peas, Sainsbury's*	1 Serving/200g	100.0	1.0	50	3.3	8.3	0.5	3.8
Baby, Canned, Average	*1 Can/195g*	*40.0*	*1.0*	*21*	*0.5*	*4.2*	*0.3*	*2.1*
Baby, Fresh, Average	*1 Serving/80g*	*28.0*	*0.0*	*35*	*0.6*	*8.2*	*0.1*	*2.9*
Baby, with Fine Beans, Tesco*	1 Pack/200g	58.0	1.0	29	1.3	4.7	0.5	2.3
Batons, Fresh, Average	*½ Pack/150g*	*41.0*	*0.0*	*27*	*0.6*	*5.7*	*0.3*	*2.6*
Boiled, Average	*1oz/28g*	*6.0*	*0.0*	*22*	*0.6*	*4.4*	*0.3*	*2.5*
Bunched, TTD, Sainsbury's*	1 Serving/100g	30.0	0.0	30	0.7	6.0	0.5	2.4
Canned, Average	*1oz/28g*	*6.0*	*0.0*	*22*	*0.6*	*4.4*	*0.2*	*2.1*
Chantenay, Steamer, Sainsbury's*	½ Pack/125g	60.0	2.0	48	0.5	7.7	1.7	2.2
Chantenay, Tesco*	1oz/28g	7.0	0.0	24	0.6	4.4	0.4	2.3
Raw, Scrubbed, Average	1 Serving/80g	24.0	0.0	30	0.7	6.0	0.5	2.4
Sliced, Canned, Average	*1 Serving/180g*	*36.0*	*0.0*	*20*	*0.7*	*4.1*	*0.1*	*1.5*
Sliced, Fresh, Average	*1 Serving/60g*	*17.0*	*0.0*	*28*	*0.7*	*5.7*	*0.3*	*2.0*
Whole, Raw, Peeled, Average	*1 Carrot/75g*	*21.0*	*0.0*	*29*	*0.6*	*6.3*	*0.3*	*2.2*
CASHEW NUTS								
Bbq, Graze*	1 Pack/26g	142.0	11.0	546	13.9	37.0	41.7	0.0
Black Pepper, Graze*	1 Pack/26g	139.0	11.0	535	14.0	34.5	41.6	0.0
Ca-shew! Bless You, Graze*	1 Punnet/40g	146.0	6.0	365	6.1	57.2	14.5	0.0
Cheese Flavour, Graze*	1 Pack/26g	140.0	11.0	540	15.3	35.7	41.5	0.0
Cracked Black Pepper Cashews, Graze*	1 Punnet/40g	223.0	18.0	558	14.9	29.0	45.0	3.0
Frosted, Graze*	1 Pack /26g	134.0	8.0	516	10.5	53.0	32.2	0.0
Honey, Graze*	½ Pack/13g	67.0	4.0	516	10.5	53.0	32.2	0.0
Hot Chilli, Graze*	1 Box/26g	139.0	11.0	535	14.5	33.6	41.8	0.0
Mexican Chilli, Graze*	1 Pack/26g	140.0	11.0	539	14.3	34.9	41.6	0.0
Plain, Average	*¼ Pack/25g*	*146.0*	*12.0*	*584*	*15.7*	*18.7*	*48.9*	*3.4*
Roasted & Salted, Average	*1 Serving/50g*	*306.0*	*26.0*	*612*	*18.8*	*19.5*	*51.1*	*3.1*

C

	Measure INFO/WEIGHT	per Measure KCAL	FAT	Nutrition Values per 100g / 100ml KCAL	PROT	CARB	FAT	FIBRE
CASHEWS & PEANUTS								
Honey Roasted, Average	*1 Serving/50g*	*289.0*	*21.0*	*579*	*21.6*	*26.6*	*42.9*	*4.2*
Salted, Sainsbury's*	1oz/28g	169.0	14.0	603	24.2	12.7	50.6	6.9
CASSAVA								
Baked, Average	*1oz/28g*	*43.0*	*0.0*	*155*	*0.7*	*40.1*	*0.2*	*1.7*
Boiled in Unsalted Water, Average	*1oz/28g*	*36.0*	*0.0*	*130*	*0.5*	*33.5*	*0.2*	*1.4*
Raw, Average	*1oz/28g*	*40.0*	*0.0*	*142*	*0.6*	*36.8*	*0.2*	*1.6*
Steamed, Average	*1oz/28g*	*40.0*	*0.0*	*142*	*0.6*	*36.8*	*0.2*	*1.6*
CASSEROLE								
Bean, & Lentil, Morrisons*	1 Can/410g	287.0	2.0	70	4.1	12.5	0.4	0.0
Bean, Spicy, BGTY, Sainsbury's*	1 Pack/300g	171.0	3.0	57	3.0	9.1	0.9	4.2
Beef & Melton Red Ale, Roast Potatoes, Weight Watchers*	1 Pack/450g	425.0	9.0	94	6.5	12.6	2.0	1.8
Beef & Red Wine, Weight Watchers*	1 Pack/330g	254.0	9.0	77	4.3	8.6	2.8	0.3
Beef, & Ale, with Dumplings, Sainsbury's*	1 Pack/450g	711.0	33.0	158	7.7	15.4	7.3	0.6
Beef, & Ale, with Mashed Potato, HL, Tesco*	1 Pack/450g	364.0	11.0	81	5.1	10.9	2.5	0.6
Beef, & Onion, Minced, British Classics, Tesco*	1 Pack/340g	367.0	19.0	108	5.0	9.3	5.6	0.8
Beef, & Red Wine, BGTY, Sainsbury's*	1 Pack/300g	192.0	2.0	64	8.0	6.7	0.6	0.9
Beef, Canned, Waitrose*	1 Can/400g	372.0	10.0	93	10.5	7.0	2.5	1.8
Beef, Diet Chef Ltd*	1 Pack/300g	177.0	3.0	59	7.8	4.7	1.0	2.4
Beef, Meal for One, Tesco*	1 Pack/450g	425.0	19.0	94	3.6	10.6	4.2	1.7
Beef, with Dumplings, GFY, Asda*	1 Pack/400g	416.0	9.0	104	11.0	10.0	2.2	0.9
Beef, with Herb Potatoes, Tesco*	1 Serving/475g	503.0	17.0	106	6.8	11.5	3.6	1.6
Chicken & Dumpling, Home Comforts, Weight Watchers*	1 Pack/328g	243.0	7.0	74	5.3	8.3	2.1	0.3
Chicken, & Asparagus, HL, Tesco*	1 Serving/450g	342.0	10.0	76	6.3	8.3	2.3	0.5
Chicken, & Asparagus, in White Wine, Finest, Tesco*	1 Pack/350g	683.0	42.0	195	10.0	11.6	12.1	0.3
Chicken, & Dumplings, HL, Tesco*	1 Pack/450g	441.0	12.0	98	7.4	11.1	2.7	0.6
Chicken, & Dumplings, Sainsbury's*	1 Serving/450g	612.0	32.0	136	6.8	11.0	7.2	0.6
Chicken, & Red Wine, Duchy Originals*	½ Pack/175g	187.0	8.0	107	14.0	5.1	4.3	1.6
Chicken, & Tomato, Asda*	¼ Pack/273g	569.0	41.0	208	16.0	2.2	15.0	0.5
Chicken, & Vegetable, Long Life, Sainsbury's*	1 Pack/300g	186.0	4.0	62	4.6	7.4	1.5	0.8
Chicken, & White Wine, BGTY, Sainsbury's*	1 Serving/300g	216.0	7.0	72	7.2	5.9	2.2	1.3
Chicken, Carrots, Peas & Potatoes, Weight Watchers*	1 Serving/302g	193.0	4.0	64	4.3	8.6	1.4	0.5
Chicken, Diet Chef Ltd*	1 Pack/300g	219.0	3.0	73	9.0	7.2	0.9	2.5
Chicken, Green Isle*	1 Pack/400g	300.0	7.0	75	5.7	9.2	1.7	1.0
Chicken, Leek & Mushroom, Tesco*	1 Pack/350g	381.0	22.0	109	4.5	8.6	6.3	1.0
Chicken, Mediterranean, Tesco*	1 Pack/400g	260.0	9.0	65	6.7	4.5	2.3	0.9
Chicken, Perfectly Balanced, Waitrose*	1 Pack/400g	392.0	14.0	98	6.6	9.8	3.6	1.2
Chicken, with Dumplings, M & S*	½ Pack/227g	261.0	10.0	115	9.7	9.0	4.4	0.9
Ham Hock & Mash, Tesco*	1 Pack/250g	225.0	8.0	90	6.1	9.0	3.2	0.8
Lamb, & Rosemary, Eat Well, M & S*	1 Pack/380g	325.0	11.0	86	7.6	7.0	2.9	2.2
Lamb, BGTY, Sainsbury's*	1 Serving/200g	242.0	9.0	121	20.7	0.1	4.3	0.1
Lamb, COU, M & S*	1 Pack/390g	253.0	7.0	65	5.9	6.7	1.7	1.6
Lamb, with Mint Dumplings, Minced, Sainsbury's*	1 Pack/450g	558.0	31.0	124	5.4	10.4	6.8	1.1
Lamb, With Rosemary Roast Potatoes, Asda*	1 Pack/450g	477.0	22.0	106	8.9	6.9	4.8	1.5
Mediterranean Seafood, HL, Tesco*	1 Pack/344g	292.0	7.0	85	5.8	10.5	2.0	3.2
Minced Beef & Dumplings, Smart Price, Asda*	1 Pack/299g	320.0	13.0	107	4.5	12.7	4.2	2.3
Mushroom, & Onion, Iceland*	1 Pack/400g	272.0	12.0	68	1.3	8.8	3.1	1.9
Pork, Normandy Style, Finest, Tesco*	1 Pack/450g	405.0	22.0	90	7.6	4.1	4.8	2.3
Rabbit, Average	1oz/28g	29.0	1.0	102	11.6	2.6	5.1	0.4
Sausage, & Potato, M & S*	1 Serving/200g	190.0	12.0	95	3.3	7.5	5.9	0.9
Sausage, Pork, Diet Chef Ltd*	1 Pack/300g	303.0	18.0	101	6.6	4.9	6.1	1.4
Steak & Kidney, Mini, Favourites, M & S*	1 Pack/200g	240.0	11.0	120	7.9	9.5	5.4	1.5
Steak, & Ale, Sainsbury's*	1 Pack/300g	288.0	10.0	96	10.6	5.6	3.5	0.4
Steak, & Mushroom with Mustard Mash, Finest, Tesco*	1 Pack/550g	522.0	21.0	95	5.9	9.0	3.9	1.1

C

	Measure	per Measure		Nutrition Values per 100g / 100ml				
	INFO/WEIGHT	KCAL	FAT	KCAL	PROT	CARB	FAT	FIBRE

CASSEROLE

	Measure INFO/WEIGHT	KCAL	FAT	KCAL	PROT	CARB	FAT	FIBRE
Vegetable, & Lentil, Canned, Granose*	1 Can/400g	272.0	8.0	68	3.5	9.0	2.0	3.0
Vegetable, Chunky, M & S*	1 Bag/450g	90.0	1.0	20	0.7	3.4	0.3	1.4
Vegetable, Country, Sainsbury's*	1 Can/400g	300.0	10.0	75	2.2	11.0	2.5	1.1
Vegetable, Tesco*	1 Serving/220g	66.0	1.0	30	0.8	6.1	0.3	1.5
Vegetable, with Herb Dumplings, COU, M & S*	1 Pack/450g	270.0	5.0	60	1.6	10.1	1.2	1.0
Venison, Scottish Wild, & Beaujolais, Tesco*	1 Pack/425g	365.0	9.0	86	11.9	4.9	2.1	0.6

CASSEROLE MIX

Beef & Ale, Colman's*	1 Pack/45g	144.0	1.0	320	9.2	66.3	2.0	2.3
Beef, Authentic, Schwartz*	1 Pack/43g	111.0	0.0	257	7.4	54.5	1.0	0.4
Beef, Colman's*	1 Pack/40g	123.0	1.0	308	7.5	66.0	1.5	2.5
Chicken Chasseur, Asda*	1 Pack/80g	273.0	1.0	341	9.0	74.0	1.0	1.4
Chicken, Authentic, Schwartz*	1 Pack/36g	131.0	2.0	363	10.4	70.7	4.3	2.0
Chicken, Traditional, Colman's*	1 Pack/40g	124.0	1.0	311	5.7	69.4	1.3	1.5
Farmhouse Sausage, Schwartz*	1 Pack/39g	124.0	1.0	317	8.1	64.6	2.9	0.5
Honey Chicken, Colman's*	1 Pack/50g	128.0	1.0	257	3.4	58.3	1.1	1.8
Lamb, Authentic, Schwartz*	1 Pack/35g	116.0	1.0	332	7.7	68.0	3.3	1.3
Liver & Bacon, Colman's*	1 Pack/40g	121.0	1.0	303	10.3	61.6	1.7	4.7
Moroccan Lamb, Schwartz*	1 Pack/35g	124.0	2.0	354	6.2	74.1	5.7	4.5
Peppered Beef, Schwartz*	1 Pack/40g	129.0	2.0	323	7.0	62.9	4.9	7.3
Pork, Colman's*	1 Pack/40g	131.0	1.0	328	6.7	72.0	1.4	2.8
Sausage & Onion, Colman's*	1 Pack/45g	143.0	1.0	318	9.6	64.2	2.6	2.6
Sausage, Classic, Schwartz*	1 Pack/35g	96.0	1.0	275	12.4	50.1	2.7	14.9
Sausage, Colman's*	1 Pack/40g	144.0	1.0	361	8.9	77.7	1.6	1.6
Somerset Pork, Colman's*	1 Pack/45g	144.0	1.0	321	7.1	70.2	1.3	2.2
Somerset Pork, Schwartz*	1 Pack/36g	115.0	1.0	320	9.4	61.9	3.8	7.7
Spicy Chicken, Colman's*	1 Pack/45g	151.0	1.0	336	6.5	73.4	1.8	1.5
Turkey, Colman's*	1 Pack/50g	156.0	1.0	313	5.9	68.0	1.9	3.5

CATFISH

Cooked, Average	1 Fillet/87g	199.0	12.0	229	18.0	8.0	13.3	0.7
Raw, Average	1oz/28g	27.0	1.0	96	17.6	0.0	2.8	0.0

CAULIFLOWER

Boiled, Average	1 Serving/80g	22.0	1.0	28	2.9	2.1	0.9	1.6
Florets, Peas & Carrots, Frozen, Asda*	1 Serving/100g	37.0	1.0	37	3.0	5.0	0.6	2.8
Raw, Average	1 Serving/80g	25.0	1.0	31	3.2	2.7	0.8	1.6

CAULIFLOWER CHEESE

& Bacon, Gastropub, M & S*	1 Pack/300g	318.0	21.0	106	6.3	4.5	7.0	1.0
& Broccoli, Sainsbury's*	1 Serving/130g	83.0	2.0	64	4.8	7.6	1.6	2.7
Birds Eye*	1 Pack/329g	355.0	21.0	108	4.8	7.7	6.4	0.8
Eat Smart, Morrisons*	1 Pack/300g	192.0	6.0	64	4.9	6.7	2.0	1.5
Finest, Tesco*	1 Serving/250g	317.0	21.0	127	6.5	6.1	8.5	0.4
Florets, in a Cheese Sauce, Sainsbury's*	1 Pack/400g	400.0	26.0	100	4.8	5.4	6.6	0.9
Grills, Grassington's Food Co*	1 Grill/92g	157.0	5.0	171	6.1	25.3	5.0	2.6
Grills, Tesco*	1 Grill/92g	207.0	11.0	225	6.5	22.2	11.9	4.0
Iceland*	1 Pack/500g	350.0	14.0	70	3.4	7.9	2.8	1.1
M & S*	1 Serving/150g	150.0	9.0	100	5.5	5.9	6.1	1.1
Made with Half Fat Cheese, HL, Tesco*	1 Pack/500g	285.0	13.0	57	6.5	2.0	2.6	2.2
Made with Semi-Skimmed Milk	1oz/28g	28.0	2.0	100	6.0	5.2	6.4	1.3
Made with Skimmed Milk	1oz/28g	27.0	2.0	97	6.0	5.2	6.0	1.3
Made with Whole Milk	1oz/28g	29.0	2.0	105	6.0	5.2	6.9	1.3
Waitrose*	1 Pack/450g	328.0	22.0	73	4.1	3.3	4.8	1.6
with Crispy Bacon, Finest, Tesco*	1/3 Pack/166g	211.0	14.0	127	6.5	6.1	8.5	0.4

CAVATELLI

Egg, Asda*	1 Serving/100g	203.0	3.0	203	9.0	34.0	3.4	3.0

	Measure INFO/WEIGHT	per Measure KCAL	FAT	Nutrition Values per 100g / 100ml KCAL	PROT	CARB	FAT	FIBRE
CAVATELLI								
King Prawn & Scallop, M & S*	1 Pack/400g	600.0	22.0	150	6.4	18.0	5.6	1.3
CAVIAR								
Average	*1oz/28g*	*26.0*	*1.0*	*92*	*11.9*	*0.5*	*4.7*	*0.0*
CELERIAC								
Boiled in Salted Water, Average	*1oz/28g*	*4.0*	*0.0*	*15*	*0.9*	*1.9*	*0.5*	*3.2*
Raw, Average	*1 Serving/100g*	*42.0*	*0.0*	*42*	*1.5*	*9.2*	*0.3*	*1.8*
CELERY								
Boiled in Salted Water	*1 Serving/50g*	*4.0*	*0.0*	*8*	*0.5*	*0.8*	*0.3*	*1.2*
Raw, Trimmed	*1 Stalk/40g*	*3.0*	*0.0*	*7*	*0.5*	*0.9*	*0.2*	*1.1*
CHAMPAGNE								
Average	*1 Glass/120ml*	*91.0*	*0.0*	*76*	*0.3*	*1.4*	*0.0*	*0.0*
CHANNA MASALA								
Indian, Sainsbury's*	1 Serving/149g	165.0	7.0	111	4.2	12.4	4.9	3.3
M & S*	1 Pack/225g	360.0	24.0	160	5.6	11.2	10.5	8.2
Safeway*	1 Pack/400g	540.0	22.0	135	5.3	16.2	5.4	2.5
CHAPATIS								
Brown Wheat Flour, Waitrose*	1 Chapati/42g	128.0	3.0	305	8.6	49.4	8.0	4.6
Elephant Atta*	1 Chapati/45g	129.0	3.0	287	7.5	53.1	6.4	3.2
Gujarati Style, Safeway*	1 Chapati/40g	111.0	2.0	277	8.1	50.0	4.9	2.8
Indian Style, Asda*	1 Chapati/43g	95.0	0.0	221	8.0	45.0	1.0	2.9
Made with Fat	1 Chapati/60g	197.0	8.0	328	8.1	48.3	12.8	0.0
Made without Fat	1 Chapati/55g	111.0	1.0	202	7.3	43.7	1.0	0.0
Morrisons*	1 Chapati/40g	108.0	3.0	269	8.6	49.8	6.9	0.0
Plain, Wraps, Original, Patak's*	1 Chapati/42g	115.0	3.0	273	9.4	48.8	7.5	0.0
Spicy, Safeway*	1 Chapati/41g	115.0	3.0	280	8.9	47.6	6.6	4.5
Wholemeal, Patak's*	1 Chapati/42g	130.0	4.0	310	11.2	44.9	9.5	9.0
CHARD								
Average	1 Serving/80g	15.0	0.0	19	1.4	3.3	0.2	0.8
Swiss, Boiled in Unsalted Water	*1oz/28g*	*6.0*	*0.0*	*20*	*1.9*	*4.1*	*0.1*	*2.1*
Swiss, Raw	*1oz/28g*	*5.0*	*0.0*	*19*	*1.8*	*3.7*	*0.2*	*1.6*
CHEDDARS								
Baked, Mini, Cheese & Ham Flavour, McVitie's*	1 Bag/30g	160.0	9.0	534	11.0	55.5	29.8	2.0
Baked, Mini, Original, Cheddar Cheese, McVitie's*	1 Bag/30g	155.0	9.0	517	10.8	50.9	30.0	2.5
Baked, Mini, Peperami, McVitie's*	1 Bag/30g	160.0	9.0	532	9.7	55.2	30.2	2.0
Baked, Mini, Tangy Salsa, McVitie's*	1 Bag/50g	266.0	15.0	532	11.0	54.7	29.9	2.1
Branston Pickle, McVitie's*	1 Bag/30g	155.0	9.0	517	9.1	53.1	29.8	2.7
Saucy BBQ, McVitie's*	1 Bag/50g	259.0	15.0	518	9.2	53.4	29.8	2.6
Smokey BBQ, McVitie's*	1 Sm Pack/30g	155.0	9.0	516	9.3	52.8	29.8	2.6
CHEESE								
Babybel, Emmental, Fromageries Bel*	1 Serving/20g	63.0	5.0	316	23.0	1.0	24.5	0.0
Babybel, Mini, Light, Fromageries Bel*	1 Cheese/20g	42.0	2.0	210	25.5	0.2	12.0	0.0
Babybel, Original, Mini, Fromageries Bel*	1 Cheese/20g	61.0	5.0	304	22.0	0.1	24.0	0.0
Babybel, with Cheddar, Mini, Fromageries Bel*	1 Cheese/20g	72.0	6.0	362	23.0	0.2	30.0	0.0
Bavarian, Smoked, Slices, Asda*	1 Slice/18g	50.0	4.0	277	17.0	0.4	23.0	0.0
Bavarian, Smoked, with Ham, Sainsbury's*	1 Serving/30g	89.0	7.0	298	19.4	0.8	24.1	0.0
Bleu d'Auvergne, TTD, Sainsbury's*	1 Serving/100g	322.0	26.0	322	22.0	0.0	26.0	0.0
Blue, Saint Agur*	1 Serving /30g	109.0	10.0	363	16.0	0.2	33.0	0.0
Brie, Average	*1 Serving/25g*	*74.0*	*6.0*	*296*	*19.7*	*0.3*	*24.0*	*0.0*
Brie, Reduced Fat, Average	*1 Serving/50g*	*99.0*	*6.0*	*198*	*23.0*	*0.8*	*11.4*	*0.0*
Caerphilly, Average	*1 Serving/50g*	*187.0*	*16.0*	*374*	*23.0*	*0.1*	*31.3*	*0.0*
Cambazola, Tesco*	1 Serving/30g	127.0	12.0	425	13.5	0.5	41.0	0.0
Camembert, Average	*1 Serving/50g*	*141.0*	*11.0*	*283*	*20.5*	*0.1*	*22.2*	*0.0*
Camembert, Breaded, Average	1 Serving/90g	307.0	21.0	341	16.6	14.2	23.2	0.4

C

C

CHEESE

INFO/WEIGHT	Measure	per Measure		Nutrition Values per 100g / 100ml				
		KCAL	FAT	KCAL	PROT	CARB	FAT	FIBRE
Cheddar, Canadian, Average	*1 Serving/30g*	*123.0*	*10.0*	*409*	*25.0*	*0.1*	*34.3*	*0.0*
Cheddar, Davidstow, Mature, Average	*1 Serving/28g*	*115.0*	*10.0*	*410*	*25.0*	*0.1*	*34.4*	*0.0*
Cheddar, Extra Mature, Average	*1 Serving/30g*	*123.0*	*10.0*	*410*	*25.1*	*0.1*	*34.3*	*0.0*
Cheddar, Grated, Average	*1 Serving/50g*	*206.0*	*17.0*	*413*	*24.4*	*1.5*	*34.3*	*0.0*
Cheddar, Mature, Average	*1 Serving/30g*	*123.0*	*10.0*	*410*	*25.0*	*0.1*	*34.4*	*0.0*
Cheddar, Mature, Grated, Average	*1 Serving/28g*	*113.0*	*9.0*	*404*	*24.7*	*1.6*	*33.2*	*0.0*
Cheddar, Mature, Reduced Fat, Average	*1 Serving/25g*	*68.0*	*4.0*	*271*	*30.0*	*0.1*	*16.7*	*0.0*
Cheddar, Medium, Average	*1 Serving/30g*	*123.0*	*10.0*	*411*	*24.9*	*0.1*	*34.5*	*0.0*
Cheddar, Mild, Average	*1 Serving/30g*	*123.0*	*10.0*	*409*	*25.0*	*0.1*	*34.3*	*0.0*
Cheddar, Reduced Fat, Average	*1 Serving/30g*	*76.0*	*4.0*	*255*	*32.1*	*0.1*	*13.9*	*0.0*
Cheddar, Smoked, Average	*1 Serving/30g*	*123.0*	*10.0*	*411*	*25.2*	*0.1*	*34.4*	*0.0*
Cheddar, West Country Farmhouse, Average	*1 Serving/28g*	*115.0*	*10.0*	*410*	*25.0*	*0.1*	*34.4*	*0.0*
Cheddar, Wexford, Average	*1 Serving/20g*	*82.0*	*7.0*	*410*	*25.0*	*0.1*	*34.4*	*0.0*
Cheestrings, Cheddar, Original, Golden Vale*	1 Stick/21g	69.0	5.0	328	28.0	0.0	24.0	0.0
Cheestrings, Double Cheese Flavour, Golden Vale*	1 Stick/21g	69.0	5.0	328	28.0	0.0	24.0	0.0
Cheshire	*1oz/28g*	*106.0*	*9.0*	*379*	*24.0*	*0.1*	*31.4*	*0.0*
Cottage, Arla*	1 Serving/25g	22.0	1.0	90	12.0	2.0	4.0	0.0
Cottage, Crunchy Vegetable, GFY, Asda*	1 Serving/50g	37.0	1.0	74	11.0	4.5	1.3	0.6
Cottage, Danone*	1 Serving/100g	89.0	4.0	89	11.2	2.3	3.9	0.0
Cottage, Garlic & Herb, Diet, Yoplait*	1 Pot/225g	180.0	4.0	80	12.0	3.9	1.9	0.0
Cottage, Low Fat, 2% Fat, Natural, Average	1 Serving/75g	67.0	1.0	90	13.7	3.6	1.9	0.0
Cottage, Low Fat, Longley Farm*	1oz/28g	32.0	2.0	114	11.5	3.4	6.0	0.0
Cottage, Low Fat, with Onion & Chive, Safeway*	1 Pot/250g	210.0	5.0	84	12.0	4.2	1.9	0.1
Cottage, Natural, Plain, Average	*1oz/28g*	*27.0*	*1.0*	*98*	*11.8*	*3.9*	*3.8*	*0.1*
Cottage, Natural, with Creme Fraiche, Tesco*	½ Pack/125g	131.0	6.0	105	12.1	2.7	4.8	0.6
Cottage, Onion & Chive, Waitrose*	1 Serving/20g	18.0	1.0	91	10.8	4.9	3.1	0.3
Cottage, Onion & Chives, Light Choices, Tesco*	1 Serving/60g	51.0	1.0	85	11.4	4.8	1.5	0.1
Cottage, Pineapple, Perfectly Balanced, Waitrose*	½ Pot/125g	106.0	2.0	85	8.4	9.7	1.4	0.5
Cottage, Plain, Average	*1oz/28g*	*26.0*	*1.0*	*93*	*12.0*	*3.3*	*3.5*	*0.1*
Cottage, Plain, Reduced Fat, Average	*1oz/28g*	*24.0*	*1.0*	*85*	*12.3*	*4.4*	*1.9*	*0.1*
Cottage, Red Pepper, GFY, Asda*	¼ Pot/75g	66.0	2.0	88	11.1	4.3	2.5	0.1
Cottage, Stilton & Celery, BGTY, Sainsbury's*	½ Pot/125g	99.0	3.0	79	10.8	4.0	2.2	1.5
Cottage, Tropical, Westacre*	1 Serving/100g	89.0	1.0	89	13.1	6.4	1.2	1.4
Cottage, Tuna & Sweetcorn, GFY, Asda*	½ Pot/113g	104.0	3.0	92	12.4	5.3	2.4	0.3
Cottage, Virtually Fat Free, Eden Vale*	1oz/28g	22.0	0.0	80	12.9	6.5	0.3	0.0
Cottage, Virtually Fat Free, Longley Farm*	½ Pot/125g	84.0	0.0	67	13.4	3.0	0.1	0.0
Cottage, Virtually Fat Free, Sainsbury's*	1oz/28g	22.0	0.0	80	12.9	6.5	0.3	0.0
Cottage, Whole Milk, Natural, Average	1 Serving/75g	77.0	3.0	103	12.5	2.7	4.5	0.0
Cottage, with Chives, Low Fat, Westacre*	1 Pot/100g	81.0	1.0	81	13.7	3.5	1.4	1.2
Cottage, with Chives, M & S*	1oz/28g	28.0	1.0	100	11.9	3.5	3.9	0.0
Cottage, with Coronation Chicken, BGTY, Sainsbury's*	1oz/28g	25.0	0.0	91	11.3	8.7	1.2	0.1
Cottage, with Cucumber & Mint, COU, M & S*	1 Pot/113g	85.0	2.0	75	11.6	3.1	1.5	0.2
Cottage, with Lime & Coriander, Low Fat, Safeway*	½ Pot/126g	113.0	3.0	90	12.2	5.2	2.0	0.0
Cottage, with Mango & Pineapple, BGTY, Sainsbury's*	½ Pot/125g	112.0	1.0	90	10.7	10.4	0.7	0.2
Cottage, with Mango, COU, M & S*	1 Serving/100g	100.0	1.0	100	10.3	11.0	1.1	0.5
Cottage, with Onion & Chive, GFY, Asda*	1 Serving/50g	42.0	1.0	85	12.0	4.4	1.9	0.1
Cottage, with Onion & Chive, Low Fat, Sainsbury's*	1oz/28g	28.0	1.0	99	11.6	4.4	4.0	0.1
Cottage, with Onion & Chive, M & S*	¼ Pot/65g	88.0	6.0	135	10.4	4.0	8.5	0.1
Cottage, with Peach & Mango, COU, M & S*	1 Pot/113g	96.0	1.0	85	9.1	9.7	1.0	0.4
Cottage, with Pineapple, Asda*	1oz/28g	31.0	1.0	109	10.0	8.0	3.9	0.0
Cottage, with Pineapple, Low Fat, Waitrose*	1 Serving/40g	34.0	1.0	84	10.4	6.7	1.7	0.2
Cottage, with Poached Salmon & Dill, GFY, Asda*	1/3 Pot/75g	64.0	2.0	86	12.0	2.3	2.7	0.6
Cottage, with Prawn Cocktail, BGTY, Sainsbury's*	1oz/28g	25.0	0.0	91	12.3	8.3	0.9	0.1

CHEESE

INFO/WEIGHT	Measure	per Measure		Nutrition Values per 100g / 100ml				
		KCAL	FAT	KCAL	PROT	CARB	FAT	FIBRE
Cottage, with Prawn, GFY, Asda*	1oz/28g	22.0	0.0	79	10.0	6.0	1.7	0.3
Cottage, with Smoked Cheese & Onion, GFY, Asda*	1 Serving/50g	39.0	1.0	78	12.0	3.9	1.6	0.4
Cottage, with Sweet Chilli Chicken, M & S*	1 Serving/200g	190.0	4.0	95	13.8	4.7	2.1	0.5
Cottage, with Tomato & Cracked Black Pepper, Asda*	½ Pot/113g	86.0	2.0	76	10.0	3.1	2.1	1.3
Cottage, with Tuna & Pesto, Asda*	1 Serving/170g	184.0	10.0	108	10.0	3.5	6.0	0.7
Cottage, with Tuna & Sweetcorn, BGTY, Sainsbury's*	1oz/28g	25.0	0.0	91	12.1	8.4	0.9	0.2
Cottage, with Tuna & Sweetcorn, HL, Tesco*	1 Serving/150g	136.0	3.0	91	12.8	4.8	2.1	0.4
Cream, Average	*1 Portion/30g*	*132.0*	*14.0*	*439*	*3.1*	*0.0*	*47.4*	*0.0*
Cream, Garlic & Herbs, Light, Boursin*	1 Portion/20g	28.0	2.0	140	12.0	2.5	9.0	0.0
Cream, Reduced Fat, Average	*1 Serving/20g*	*23.0*	*1.0*	*117*	*13.0*	*4.0*	*5.3*	*0.1*
Cream, with Onion & Chives, Morrisons*	1 Serving/20g	38.0	3.0	190	11.0	3.0	15.0	0.0
Cream, with Pineapple, Asda*	1 Serving/40g	77.0	5.0	193	8.0	11.0	13.0	0.0
Cream, with Red Peppers & Onion, GFY, Asda*	1 Serving/32g	42.0	2.0	130	13.0	6.0	6.0	0.0
Creme de Saint Agur, Saint Agur*	1 Serving/10g	28.0	2.0	285	13.5	2.3	24.7	0.0
Dairylea, Light, Slices, Kraft*	1 Slice/25g	51.0	3.0	205	17.0	8.6	10.5	0.0
Dairylea, Rippers, Straight, Kraft*	1 Ripper/21g	60.0	4.0	285	28.0	1.0	18.5	0.0
Dairylea, Slices, Kraft*	1 Slice/25g	69.0	5.0	275	13.0	8.6	20.5	0.0
Danish Blue, Average	*1 Serving/30g*	*106.0*	*9.0*	*352*	*20.7*	*0.0*	*29.1*	*0.0*
Dolcelatte, Average	*1 Serving/30g*	*110.0*	*10.0*	*366*	*17.8*	*0.4*	*32.3*	*0.4*
Double Gloucester, Average	*1 Serving/30g*	*121.0*	*10.0*	*404*	*24.5*	*0.1*	*34.0*	*0.0*
Double Gloucester, with Onion & Chives, Sainsbury's*	1 Serving/30g	109.0	8.0	365	22.2	5.5	28.2	0.0
Doux De Montagne, Average	*1 Serving/25g*	*88.0*	*7.0*	*352*	*22.9*	*1.5*	*28.3*	*0.0*
Edam, Average	*1 Serving/10g*	*33.0*	*2.0*	*326*	*25.3*	*0.0*	*24.9*	*0.0*
Edam, Dutch, Garlic & Herb Wedge, Asda*	1 Serving/60g	197.0	15.0	329	26.0	0.0	25.0	0.0
Edam, Reduced Fat, Average	*1 Serving/30g*	*69.0*	*3.0*	*230*	*32.4*	*0.1*	*11.1*	*0.0*
Edam, Slices, Average	*1 Slice/30g*	*96.0*	*7.0*	*320*	*25.0*	*0.4*	*24.1*	*0.0*
Emmental, Average	*1 Serving/10g*	*37.0*	*3.0*	*368*	*28.3*	*0.0*	*28.3*	*0.0*
Farmhouse, Reduced Fat, Healthy Range, Average	*1 Serving/30g*	*78.0*	*5.0*	*260*	*30.4*	*0.0*	*15.4*	*0.0*
Feta, Average	*1 Serving/30g*	*79.0*	*6.0*	*262*	*16.3*	*1.0*	*21.5*	*0.0*
Fondue, Original, Fromalp*	1 Pack/400g	888.0	68.0	222	15.0	2.5	17.0	0.0
Fondue, Swiss, Easy Cook, Tesco*	¼ Pack/100g	235.0	17.0	235	15.5	4.0	17.0	0.0
Fontina, Average	*1 Serving/28g*	*109.0*	*9.0*	*389*	*25.0*	*0.0*	*32.1*	*0.0*
for Pizza, Grated, Average	*1 Serving/50g*	*163.0*	*12.0*	*325*	*25.0*	*1.5*	*24.4*	*0.0*
Goats, Average	*1 Tsp/10g*	*26.0*	*2.0*	*262*	*13.8*	*3.8*	*21.2*	*0.0*
Goats, Breaded, Bites, Sainsbury's*	1 Bite/25g	84.0	6.0	337	13.0	15.1	25.0	0.8
Goats, French, Mild, Average	*1 Serving/30g*	*49.0*	*4.0*	*163*	*11.2*	*3.0*	*11.8*	*0.0*
Goats, Premium, Average	*1 Serving/30g*	*98.0*	*8.0*	*327*	*20.5*	*0.6*	*26.1*	*0.0*
Gorgonzola, Average	*1 Serving/30g*	*100.0*	*8.0*	*334*	*20.0*	*0.0*	*27.0*	*0.0*
Gouda, Average	*1 Serving/30g*	*113.0*	*9.0*	*375*	*24.0*	*0.0*	*31.5*	*0.0*
Gruyere	*1oz/28g*	*115.0*	*9.0*	*409*	*27.2*	*0.0*	*33.3*	*0.0*
Halloumi, Average	*1 Serving/80g*	*253.0*	*20.0*	*316*	*20.8*	*1.6*	*24.7*	*0.0*
Italian, Grated, Average	*1 Serving/30g*	*144.0*	*10.0*	*481*	*44.0*	*1.1*	*33.4*	*0.0*
Jarlsberg, Slices, Average	*1 Slice/15g*	*54.0*	*4.0*	*360*	*27.0*	*0.0*	*27.0*	*0.0*
Lactose Free, Arla*	1 Serving/30g	103.0	8.0	344	25.3	1.0	27.0	0.0
Lancashire	*1oz/28g*	*104.0*	*9.0*	*373*	*23.3*	*0.1*	*31.0*	*0.0*
Manchego	*1 Serving/70g*	*339.0*	*31.0*	*485*	*22.2*	*0.1*	*44.0*	*0.0*
Mascarpone, Average	*1 Serving/30g*	*131.0*	*13.0*	*437*	*5.6*	*4.1*	*43.6*	*0.0*
Mature, Farmhouse, Full Flavour, Rosemary Conley*	1 Pack/200g	378.0	10.0	189	36.0	0.1	5.0	0.0
Mature, Full Flavoured, LowLow, Kerry*	1 Serving/30g	91.0	7.0	302	26.0	0.2	22.0	0.0
Mature, Half Fat, Average	1 Av Serving/25g	66.0	4.0	265	29.9	0.4	15.6	0.1
Mature, Reduced Fat, Weight Watchers*	1 Serving/30g	65.0	3.0	217	31.0	0.1	10.3	0.0
Mild, Reduced Fat, Grated, Average	*1 Serving/30g*	*70.0*	*3.0*	*235*	*31.5*	*2.2*	*11.1*	*0.0*
Monterey Jack, Iga*	1 Serving/28g	110.0	9.0	393	25.0	0.0	32.1	0.0

C

	Measure INFO/WEIGHT	per Measure KCAL	FAT	Nutrition Values per 100g / 100ml KCAL	PROT	CARB	FAT	FIBRE

CHEESE

	Measure INFO/WEIGHT	KCAL	FAT	KCAL	PROT	CARB	FAT	FIBRE
Monterey Jack, Shredded, Kraft*	¼ Cup/28g	101.0	8.0	360	22.0	3.6	28.8	0.0
Mozzarella, Average	*1 Serving/50g*	*137.0*	*10.0*	*275*	*21.2*	*1.2*	*20.6*	*0.0*
Mozzarella, Reduced Fat, Average	*1 Serving/50g*	*92.0*	*5.0*	*184*	*21.1*	*1.0*	*10.2*	*0.0*
Ossau-Iraty, Average	*1 Serving/30g*	*120.0*	*10.0*	*400*	*22.3*	*0.2*	*34.0*	*0.0*
Parmesan, Average	*1 Tbsp/10g*	*40.0*	*3.0*	*401*	*35.2*	*0.0*	*29.4*	*0.0*
Philadelphia, for Salad, Kraft*	1 Pot/50g	157.0	15.0	315	6.6	2.6	30.5	0.5
Poivre, Boursin*	1oz/28g	116.0	12.0	414	7.0	2.0	42.0	0.0
Port Salut, M & S*	1oz/28g	90.0	7.0	322	21.0	1.0	26.0	0.0
Quark, Average	*1 Serving/20g*	*13.0*	*0.0*	*66*	*11.9*	*4.0*	*0.2*	*0.0*
Raclette, Richsmonts*	1 Slice/28g	100.0	8.0	357	25.0	0.0	28.6	0.0
Reblochon	*1 Serving/30g*	*95.0*	*8.0*	*318*	*19.7*	*0.0*	*26.6*	*0.0*
Red Leicester, Average	*1 Serving/30g*	*120.0*	*10.0*	*400*	*23.8*	*0.1*	*33.7*	*0.0*
Red Leicester, Reduced Fat, Average	*1 Serving/30g*	*78.0*	*5.0*	*261*	*30.2*	*0.1*	*15.4*	*0.0*
Ricotta, Average	*1 Serving/50g*	*67.0*	*5.0*	*134*	*9.3*	*2.9*	*9.5*	*0.0*
Roquefort, Average	*1oz/28g*	*105.0*	*9.0*	*375*	*19.7*	*0.0*	*32.9*	*0.0*
Roule, French, Sainsbury's*	1 Serving/30g	96.0	9.0	321	8.5	3.0	30.5	0.0
Sage Derby	*1oz/28g*	*113.0*	*9.0*	*402*	*24.2*	*0.1*	*33.0*	*0.0*
Shropshire, Blue, Average	*1 Serving/50g*	*195.0*	*17.0*	*391*	*21.0*	*0.0*	*34.2*	*0.0*
Soft, Blue, Philadelphia, Kraft*	1 Serving/28g	76.0	7.0	270	6.8	3.4	25.5	0.2
Soft, Cracked Pepper, Less Than 5% Fat, M & S*	1 Serving/30g	30.0	1.0	100	11.0	4.2	4.5	0.3
Soft, Creamy, with Shallots & Chives, BGTY, Sainsbury's*	1 Serving/20g	47.0	4.0	235	5.8	2.2	22.5	0.0
Soft, Extra Light, Average	*1 Serving/20g*	*25.0*	*1.0*	*125*	*14.3*	*3.5*	*5.9*	*0.1*
Soft, Full Fat, Average	*1 Serving/50g*	*156.0*	*15.0*	*312*	*8.2*	*1.7*	*30.3*	*0.0*
Soft, Garlic & Herb, Extra Light, Light Choices, Tesco*	1 Serving/38g	49.0	2.0	130	12.3	5.1	6.3	0.3
Soft, Garlic & Herb, M & S*	1oz/28g	58.0	5.0	206	8.5	2.7	18.0	0.0
Soft, Goats Milk	*1oz/28g*	*55.0*	*4.0*	*198*	*13.1*	*1.0*	*15.8*	*0.0*
Soft, Light, Average	*1 Serving/30g*	*54.0*	*4.0*	*179*	*12.1*	*3.2*	*13.1*	*0.0*
Soft, Lighter, Asda*	1 Serving/33g	36.0	1.0	109	14.0	3.7	4.0	0.0
Soft, Medium Fat, Average	*1 Serving/30g*	*62.0*	*5.0*	*207*	*8.4*	*3.0*	*17.9*	*0.0*
Soft, Onion & Chives, Extra Light, Light Choices, Tesco*	1 Serving/30g	37.0	2.0	125	11.7	5.6	6.0	0.2
Soft, Onion & Chives, Less Than 5% Fat, M & S*	1 Serving/30g	30.0	1.0	100	10.7	4.4	4.7	1.2
Soft, Philadelphia, Extra Light, Kraft*	1 Serving/30g	33.0	1.0	111	12.0	5.0	4.7	0.4
Soft, Philadelphia, Garlic & Herb, Light, Kraft*	1 Serving/30g	47.0	3.0	156	8.2	3.9	11.5	0.4
Soft, Philadelphia, Light, Basil, Philadelphia, Kraft*	1 Serving/35g	51.0	4.0	146	8.0	4.0	10.5	0.5
Soft, Philadelphia, Mini Tubs, Cracked Pepper, Kraft*	1 Tub/35g	56.0	5.0	161	7.7	2.5	13.0	0.4
Soft, Philadelphia, Mini Tubs, Extra Light, Kraft*	1 Tub/35g	39.0	2.0	111	11.0	4.8	5.2	0.4
Soft, Philadelphia, Mini Tubs, Light, Kraft*	1 Tub/35g	57.0	5.0	163	7.1	2.9	14.0	0.0
Soft, Philadelphia, Tomato & Basil, Light, Kraft*	1 Tbsp/20g	38.0	3.0	190	7.6	4.3	16.0	0.5
Soft, Philadelphia, with Chives, Light, Kraft*	1 Serving/30g	48.0	4.0	160	8.4	4.2	12.0	0.5
Soft, Philadelphia, with Ham, Light, Kraft*	1oz/28g	52.0	4.0	184	7.9	4.3	15.0	0.2
Soft, White, Lactofree, Arla*	1 Spread/10g	20.0	2.0	197	8.6	3.0	16.5	0.0
Soft, with Black Pepper, Light, Sainsbury's*	½ Pack/100g	205.0	16.0	205	11.0	3.0	16.5	0.0
Soft, with Garlic & Herbs, Full Fat, Deli, Boursin*	1 Serving/28g	84.0	8.0	299	3.5	5.0	29.5	0.0
Soft, with Garlic & Herbs, Medium Fat, Westacre*	1 Serving/30g	56.0	5.0	188	8.0	3.0	16.0	0.1
Soft, with Garlic & Herbs, Sainsbury's*	1 Serving/33g	89.0	9.0	269	6.1	2.7	26.0	0.0
Soft, with Garlic and Herbs, Lighter, Asda*	½ Pack/100g	106.0	4.0	106	11.8	4.3	4.4	0.1
Soya	*1oz/28g*	*89.0*	*8.0*	*319*	*18.3*	*0.0*	*27.3*	*0.0*
Stilton, Average	*1 Serving/30g*	*123.0*	*11.0*	*410*	*22.4*	*0.1*	*35.5*	*0.0*
Stilton, Blue, Average	*1 Serving/30g*	*124.0*	*11.0*	*412*	*22.8*	*0.1*	*35.7*	*0.0*
Stilton, White, & Apricot, M & S*	1oz/28g	94.0	6.0	337	13.8	18.5	23.1	0.0
Stilton, White, & Cranberry, M & S*	1oz/28g	101.0	7.0	362	18.2	15.5	25.3	0.0
Stilton, White, Average	*1oz/28g*	*101.0*	*9.0*	*362*	*19.9*	*0.1*	*31.3*	*0.0*
Stilton, White, with Apricot, Somerfield*	1oz/28g	103.0	8.0	369	16.0	8.0	30.0	0.0

CHEESE	Measure INFO/WEIGHT	per Measure KCAL	per Measure FAT	Nutrition Values per 100g / 100ml KCAL	PROT	CARB	FAT	FIBRE
Stilton, White, with Cranberries, Tesco*	1 Serving/50g	184.0	15.0	368	15.8	9.5	29.7	0.7
Stilton, White, with Mango & Ginger, Tesco*	1/3 Pack/65g	227.0	14.0	350	13.1	25.8	21.6	0.6
Wedge, Leerdammer*	1 Serving/30g	112.0	9.0	373	28.3	0.0	28.6	0.0
Wedges, Camembert, Breaded, Morrisons*	1 Wedge/25g	88.0	6.0	352	15.1	22.9	22.2	2.0
Wensleydale with Cranberries, Sainsbury's*	1 Serving/50g	179.0	14.0	359	20.7	6.4	27.8	0.0
Wensleydale, Average	**1 Serving/25g**	**92.0**	**8.0**	**369**	**22.4**	**0.1**	**31.0**	**0.0**
CHEESE ALTERNATIVE								
Cheezly, Cream, Original Flavour, The Redwood Co*	1 Pack/113g	357.0	34.0	316	5.6	4.8	30.5	0.0
Cheezly, Feta Style, in Oil, The Redwood Co*	1 Serving/25g	119.0	12.0	475	2.5	10.6	47.0	0.0
Cheezly, Grated Cheddar Style, The Redwood Co*	1 Pack/150g	241.0	11.0	161	3.1	21.5	7.5	0.0
Cheezly, Mozzarella Style, The Redwood Co*	1 Portion/25g	69.0	6.0	274	5.4	5.9	25.4	1.0
Cheezly, Nacho Style, The Redwood Co*	1 Serving/25g	42.0	2.0	169	3.3	21.1	7.9	0.0
Cheezly, Sour Cream & Chive Flavour, The Redwood Co*	1 Serving/25g	79.0	8.0	318	5.7	5.1	30.5	0.0
Plain, Better Than Cream Cheese, Tofutti*	2 Tbsp/28g	78.0	5.0	280	3.3	6.7	17.0	0.0
Vegetarian, Average	1 Serving/30g	110.0	8.0	368	28.2	0.0	28.1	0.0
CHEESE ON TOAST								
Average	1oz/28g	106.0	7.0	380	13.8	23.8	26.3	0.7
CHEESE SINGLES								
50% Less Fat, Asda*	1 Slice/20g	38.0	2.0	190	19.0	6.0	10.0	0.0
American, 2% Milk, Kraft*	1 Slice/19g	45.0	3.0	237	21.0	5.3	15.8	0.0
Cheese Food Slices, 50% Less Fat, BGTY, Sainsbury's*	1 Slice/20g	39.0	2.0	195	19.2	7.1	10.0	0.0
Kraft*	1 Single/20g	52.0	4.0	260	13.5	7.6	18.5	0.0
Light Choices, Tesco*	1 Slice/20g	37.0	2.0	185	19.8	4.0	10.0	0.0
CHEESE SPREAD								
60% Less Fat, Asda*	1 Serving/30g	52.0	3.0	174	16.0	7.3	9.0	0.0
Asda*	1 Serving/33g	92.0	8.0	280	9.0	7.0	24.0	0.0
BGTY, Sainsbury's*	1 Serving/25g	28.0	1.0	111	11.0	4.3	5.5	0.4
Cheese & Garlic, Primula*	1 Serving/20g	49.0	4.0	247	15.7	4.3	18.6	0.0
Cheese & Salmon with Dill, Primula*	1 Serving/30g	78.0	6.0	261	17.6	3.8	19.5	0.0
Cheez Whiz, Original, Light, 41% Less Fat, Kraft*	1 Tbsp/15g	31.0	2.0	210	15.7	11.7	11.3	0.0
Cream, Light, Sainsbury's*	1 Serving/50g	93.0	8.0	187	7.8	4.1	15.5	0.3
Dairylea, Light, Tub, Kraft*	1 Serving/30g	44.0	2.0	147	14.5	6.1	7.0	0.0
Dairylea, Tub, Kraft*	1 Serving/25g	60.0	5.0	240	11.0	5.3	19.5	0.0
Flavoured	1oz/28g	72.0	6.0	258	14.2	4.4	20.5	0.0
Garlic & Herbs, Light, Benecol*	1 Serving/20g	35.0	3.0	174	7.8	4.2	14.0	0.7
Kerrygold*	1oz/28g	60.0	4.0	213	11.0	8.5	15.0	0.0
Light, Primula*	1oz/28g	39.0	2.0	141	18.8	4.1	5.5	0.5
Low Fat, Weight Watchers*	1 Serving/50g	56.0	1.0	112	18.1	3.4	2.9	1.2
Mediterranean Soft & Creamy, Extra Light, Asda*	1 Serving/32g	42.0	2.0	130	13.0	6.0	6.0	0.0
Plain, Original, Primula*	1 Serving/30g	68.0	6.0	227	12.9	2.1	18.7	0.6
Soft, Low Fat, M & S*	1 Pack/100g	111.0	4.0	111	13.0	4.2	4.5	0.3
Squeeze, Light, The Laughing Cow, Fromageries Bel*	1 Portion/30g	42.0	2.0	139	12.0	7.0	7.0	5.0
Squeeze, Original, The Laughing Cow, Fromageries Bel*	1 Portion/30g	71.0	6.0	236	9.0	5.0	20.0	0.0
Triangles, 50% Less Fat, Morrisons*	1 Portion/17.5g	29.0	1.0	166	15.0	8.5	8.0	0.0
with Chives, Primula*	1 Serving/30g	76.0	6.0	253	15.0	1.0	21.0	0.0
with Garlic & Herb, Soft, Free From, Sainsbury's*	1 Serving/30g	91.0	9.0	302	2.5	5.5	30.0	0.1
with Ham, Primula*	1 Serving/30g	70.0	6.0	232	13.5	2.1	18.8	0.3
with Shrimp, Primula*	1 Tbsp/15g	38.0	3.0	253	15.0	1.0	21.0	0.0
CHEESE STRAWS								
& Bacon, Party, Tesco*	1 Straw/12.5g	40.0	3.0	321	10.5	23.8	20.4	2.1
Cheddar, M & S*	1 Straw/11g	59.0	4.0	535	14.9	40.1	34.9	2.4
Finest, Tesco*	1 Straw/7g	39.0	3.0	558	13.3	41.5	37.6	1.5
Fudges*	1 Serving/10g	53.0	3.0	534	14.9	40.1	34.9	0.0

C

	Measure INFO/WEIGHT		KCAL	FAT	Nutrition Values per 100g / 100ml				
					KCAL	PROT	CARB	FAT	FIBRE
CHEESE STRAWS									
Homemade or Bakery, Average	1 Straw/41g		173.0	13.0	422	11.9	24.1	30.7	0.7
Selection, Sainsbury's*	1 Straw/7g		41.0	3.0	558	16.6	34.5	39.3	2.8
CHEESE TRIANGLES									
Average	1 Triangle/14g		35.0	3.0	247	10.6	6.6	19.9	0.0
Extra Light, The Laughing Cow, Fromageries Bel*	1 Triangle/17.5g		20.0	1.0	116	15.0	6.5	3.0	0.0
Reduced Fat, Average	1 Triangle/18g		30.0	2.0	170	14.8	7.4	9.0	0.0
CHEESE TWISTS									
All Butter, M & S*	1 Pack/125g		625.0	33.0	500	14.2	50.2	26.7	3.2
Asda*	1 Twist/8g		42.0	2.0	500	14.0	48.0	28.0	5.0
Gruyere, & Poppy Seed, Truly Irresistible, Co-Op*	1 Twist/8g		42.0	2.0	520	13.2	48.8	30.1	2.5
CHEESECAKE									
American Red White & Blueberry, Sainsbury's*	1/6 Cake/83g		264.0	15.0	318	3.8	35.1	18.5	0.4
Apple & Cinnamon, Baked, M & S*	1 Serving/116g		390.0	22.0	335	3.7	39.7	18.9	2.1
Apricot, HL, Tesco*	1 Pot/100g		179.0	2.0	179	4.9	34.7	2.3	1.6
Average	1 Slice/115g		490.0	41.0	426	3.7	24.6	35.5	0.4
Belgian Chocolate, M & S*	1 Slice/100g		385.0	24.0	385	5.3	39.2	23.9	2.5
Blackcurrant Devonshire, McVitie's*	1/6 Cake/67g		193.0	11.0	288	3.8	29.7	17.1	1.7
Blackcurrant Swirl, Heinz*	1/5 Cake/87g		241.0	13.0	277	4.1	30.3	15.4	3.6
Blackcurrant, Perfectly Balanced, Waitrose*	1/6 Cake/99g		212.0	4.0	214	4.0	39.6	3.6	2.4
Blackcurrant, Sainsbury's*	1 Cake/100g		238.0	9.0	238	3.9	34.6	9.3	1.3
Blackcurrant, VLH Kitchens	1 Serving/120g		341.0	20.0	285	3.4	32.0	16.4	0.9
Blackcurrant, Weight Watchers*	1 Cake/103g		191.0	3.0	185	4.6	35.4	2.8	3.5
Blueberry & Lemon Flavour Wedges, Sainsbury's*	1 Serving/80g		262.0	17.0	327	5.1	29.2	21.1	1.2
Blueberry & Vanilla, TTD, Sainsbury's*	1 Serving/95g		353.0	25.0	372	5.4	28.9	26.1	2.1
Caramel Swirl, Cadbury*	1 Slice/91g		373.0	23.0	410	6.0	40.1	25.8	0.0
Cherry, BGTY, Sainsbury's*	1 Serving/91g		181.0	4.0	199	4.6	35.5	4.3	0.5
Cherry, Low Saturated Fat, Waitrose*	1/6 Cake/107.5g		198.0	2.0	184	3.6	37.6	2.1	0.4
Chocolate & Hazelnut, Sara Lee*	1 Serving/65g		224.0	14.0	345	6.5	31.2	21.4	1.2
Chocolate & Vanilla, Reduced Fat, M & S*	1 Serving/114g		319.0	14.0	280	7.0	37.9	12.0	1.5
Chocolate Chip, M & S*	1oz/28g		109.0	7.0	391	5.1	39.7	23.6	0.2
Chocolate Swirl, Deeply Delicious, Heinz*	1/5 Cake/81.5g		221.0	9.0	271	4.6	37.4	11.5	4.7
Chocolate Truffle, HL, Tesco*	1 Slice/96g		250.0	13.0	260	10.3	23.7	13.8	6.5
Chocolate, & Irish Cream Liqueur, Tesco*	1 Serving/93g		385.0	28.0	414	5.0	30.7	30.1	0.8
Chocolate, Baked, Ultimate, Entenmann's*	1 Serving/100g		331.0	19.0	331	5.7	34.2	19.0	2.8
Chocolate, M & S*	1oz/28g		106.0	6.0	380	6.5	40.3	21.5	0.4
Chocolate, Pure Indulgence, Thorntons*	1 Serving/75g		307.0	18.0	410	5.6	44.3	23.4	0.6
Chocolate, Weight Watchers*	1 Cake/95g		143.0	4.0	151	7.5	20.7	4.0	0.7
Citrus, Good Choice, Mini, Iceland*	1 Cake/111g		198.0	5.0	178	3.5	31.6	4.2	0.4
Commercially Prepared	1/6 Cake/80g		257.0	18.0	321	5.5	25.5	22.5	0.4
Devonshire Strawberry, McVitie's*	1/6 Cake/66g		192.0	11.0	291	4.4	31.8	16.2	3.6
Double Chocolate Wedge, Sainsbury's*	1 Serving/75g		327.0	25.0	436	5.7	29.0	33.0	1.7
Fudge, Tesco*	1 Serving/102g		384.0	24.0	376	4.6	37.5	23.1	0.5
Homestyle Chocolate, M & S*	1oz/28g		105.0	6.0	376	6.0	38.0	22.2	0.7
Irish Cream, McVitie's*	¼ Slice/190g		616.0	37.0	324	4.4	33.0	19.4	0.4
Lemon Creamy & Light, M & S*	1/6 Cake/68g		236.0	14.0	350	3.5	32.3	20.4	0.4
Lemon Meringue, Tesco*	1 Slice/94g		352.0	25.0	375	3.8	30.1	26.6	0.3
Lemon, BGTY, Sainsbury's*	1/6 Cake/71g		142.0	3.0	200	4.4	37.0	3.8	0.5
Lemon, Carb Control, Tesco*	1 Serving/85g		269.0	23.0	316	8.6	9.6	27.1	11.1
Lemon, Sainsbury's*	1 Serving/180g		650.0	37.0	361	4.0	39.9	20.6	1.3
Lemon, Swirl, Asda*	1 Pack/125g		445.0	30.0	356	3.1	32.1	23.9	1.8
Lemon, Value, Tesco*	1 Serving/79g		221.0	12.0	281	4.3	32.2	15.0	4.2
Lemon, Weight Watchers*	1 Serving/100g		211.0	5.0	211	6.3	30.1	5.0	1.8
Mandarin, GFY, Asda*	1/6 Cake/92g		178.0	4.0	194	3.6	35.0	4.4	1.2

	Measure INFO/WEIGHT	per Measure KCAL	FAT	Nutrition Values per 100g / 100ml KCAL	PROT	CARB	FAT	FIBRE
CHEESECAKE								
Mandarin, Light Choices, Tesco*	1/6 Cake/92g	170.0	3.0	185	4.1	33.1	3.8	1.5
Mandarin, Morrisons*	1 Serving/135g	335.0	17.0	248	3.8	32.2	12.5	0.8
Mandarin, Weight Watchers*	1 Cake/103g	180.0	3.0	175	4.6	32.9	2.8	1.5
Praline, Asda*	1/8 Cake/62g	226.0	15.0	364	7.0	30.0	24.0	3.2
Raspberry & Strawberry, M & S*	1 Slice/104.6g	340.0	21.0	325	3.9	33.4	20.2	1.2
Raspberry Brulee, M & S*	1 Serving/100g	255.0	13.0	255	5.7	29.7	12.9	2.1
Raspberry Ripple, M & S*	1oz/28g	84.0	4.0	300	5.9	32.8	15.6	0.3
Raspberry Swirl, Heinz*	1 Serving/100g	266.0	14.0	266	3.9	30.1	14.5	2.8
Raspberry, BGTY, Sainsbury's*	1 Pot/94.5g	154.0	2.0	163	6.6	28.2	2.6	2.8
Raspberry, Creamy, Tesco*	1 Serving/100g	365.0	23.0	365	5.9	32.1	23.4	0.9
Raspberry, Low Saturated Fat, Waitrose*	1/6th Cake/108g	187.0	2.0	174	3.6	35.4	2.0	0.4
Raspberry, M & S*	1 Slice/105g	331.0	22.0	315	5.0	32.2	20.5	1.0
Raspberry, Perfectly Balanced, Waitrose*	1 Serving/106g	212.0	4.0	200	4.0	36.2	3.5	1.7
Raspberry, Weight Watchers*	1 Cake/100g	213.0	4.0	213	5.9	29.7	4.3	1.9
Rhubarb Crumble, Sainsbury's*	1 Serving/114g	268.0	11.0	235	3.1	34.8	9.3	2.4
Sticky Toffee, Tesco*	1 Slice/66g	247.0	16.0	375	4.0	35.3	24.2	0.5
Strawberries & Cream, Finest, Tesco*	1 Serving/104g	325.0	22.0	312	4.3	25.3	21.5	0.5
Strawberry Shortcake, Sara Lee*	1/6 Slice/68g	230.0	16.0	337	4.9	27.6	23.0	0.5
Strawberry, Baked New York, Sara Lee*	1 Serving/100g	248.0	10.0	248	4.7	34.9	9.9	0.7
Strawberry, Creamy, Weight Watchers*	1 Cake/105g	187.0	3.0	178	4.7	34.2	2.5	2.2
Strawberry, Finest, Tesco*	1 Slice/113g	383.0	25.0	339	4.8	30.1	22.2	0.9
Strawberry, Fresh, M & S*	¼ Cake/125g	300.0	19.0	240	2.8	23.1	15.4	1.1
Strawberry, Frozen, Sainsbury's*	1/6 Cake/83.5	277.0	14.0	332	4.3	40.4	17.0	2.3
Strawberry, Heinz*	1 Pack/245g	588.0	31.0	240	3.4	28.1	12.7	2.4
Summerfruit, GFY, Asda*	1/6 Cake/92g	175.0	4.0	191	3.7	34.5	4.2	1.4
The Ultimate New York Baked, Entenmann's*	1 Cake/100g	347.0	21.0	347	4.2	35.7	21.3	0.9
Toffee & Banana, M & S*	1oz/28g	88.0	5.0	315	5.0	35.7	16.7	0.2
Toffee & Pecan, Wedge, Sainsbury's*	1 Serving/75g	296.0	22.0	395	5.4	28.1	29.0	3.1
Toffee, American Style, Asda*	1 Serving/75g	269.0	16.0	359	4.5	38.0	21.0	3.8
Toffee, Asda*	1 Cake/87g	295.0	19.0	339	4.3	31.0	22.0	3.5
Toffee, M & S*	1 Serving/105g	357.0	23.0	340	5.2	37.2	21.5	0.9
Vanilla Chocolate, Baked, Slice, Sainsbury's*	1 Slice/90g	349.0	23.0	388	5.7	33.8	25.6	2.7
Vanilla, Tesco*	1 Serving/115g	417.0	28.0	363	5.7	29.4	24.7	0.6
Zesty Lemon, M & S*	1/6 Cake/97g	325.0	19.0	335	4.0	38.7	19.5	2.6
CHEETOS								
Cheese, Walkers*	1 Bag/24g	120.0	6.0	500	6.5	61.0	26.0	1.3
CHERRIES								
Black, Fresh, Average	*1 Serving/80g*	*41.0*	*0.0*	*51*	*0.9*	*11.5*	*0.1*	*1.6*
Black, in Syrup, Average	*1 Serving/242g*	*160.0*	*0.0*	*66*	*0.6*	*16.0*	*0.0*	*0.7*
Dried, Sainsbury's*	1 Tbsp/14g	45.0	0.0	319	3.8	72.4	1.5	6.2
Glace, Average	*1oz/28g*	*79.0*	*0.0*	*280*	*0.3*	*71.2*	*0.1*	*1.1*
Morello, Dried, Graze*	1 Pack/30g	100.0	0.0	335	4.5	82.0	1.5	0.0
Raw, Average	*1oz/28g*	*14.0*	*0.0*	*49*	*0.9*	*11.2*	*0.1*	*1.4*
Stewed, with Sugar, Average	*1oz/28g*	*23.0*	*0.0*	*82*	*0.7*	*21.0*	*0.1*	*0.7*
Stewed, without Sugar, Average	*1oz/28g*	*12.0*	*0.0*	*42*	*0.8*	*10.1*	*0.1*	*0.8*
CHESTNUTS								
Average	*1 Nut/10g*	*17.0*	*0.0*	*170*	*2.0*	*36.6*	*2.7*	*4.1*
CHEWING GUM								
Airwaves, Sugar Free, Wrigleys*	1 Pack/15g	23.0	0.0	155	0.0	62.0	0.0	0.0
Extra, Peppermint, Sugar Free, Wrigleys*	1 Piece/2g	3.0	0.0	155	0.0	39.0	0.0	0.0
Spearmint, Wrigleys*	1 Piece/3g	9.0	0.0	295	0.0	73.0	0.0	0.0
Splash, Raspberry & Peach, Trident*	1 Piece/2g	4.0	0.0	180	1.6	68.5	0.5	0.0

C

CHICK PEAS

	Measure INFO/WEIGHT	per Measure KCAL	FAT	KCAL	PROT	CARB	FAT	FIBRE
Dried, Average	*1 Serving/100g*	*319.0*	*5.0*	*319*	*21.7*	*47.4*	*5.4*	*8.0*
Dried, Boiled, Average	*1 Serving/75g*	*85.0*	*2.0*	*114*	*7.3*	*16.4*	*2.2*	*2.5*
in Salted Water, Canned, Average	*1 Can/179g*	*204.0*	*5.0*	*114*	*7.2*	*14.9*	*2.9*	*4.1*
in Water, Canned, Average	*1 Can/250g*	*282.0*	*7.0*	*113*	*7.2*	*15.3*	*2.6*	*4.8*

CHICKEN

	Measure INFO/WEIGHT	per Measure KCAL	FAT	KCAL	PROT	CARB	FAT	FIBRE
Bites, Tikka, Average	1 Serving/50g	96.0	5.0	193	20.7	3.8	10.5	1.9
Breast, Chargrilled, Lemon & Herb, Bernard Matthews*	1 Serving/100g	154.0	4.0	154	23.7	4.7	4.5	0.0
Breast, Chargrilled, Lime & Coriander, Asda*	1 Breast/159.5g	260.0	11.0	163	25.0	0.1	7.0	1.5
Breast, Chargrilled, Premium, Average	1 Piece/10g	20.0	1.0	197	21.6	1.5	11.2	0.3
Breast, Chargrilled, Sliced, Average	1 Slice/19g	24.0	1.0	124	24.4	0.5	2.7	0.4
Breast, Chinese Style, Cooked, Sliced, Sainsbury's*	½ Pack/65g	96.0	1.0	148	28.3	4.7	1.8	0.1
Breast, Diced, Average	*1 Serving/188g*	*215.0*	*4.0*	*114*	*25.0*	*0.1*	*2.0*	*0.1*
Breast, Eastern Spices, Birds Eye*	1 Portion/175g	308.0	21.0	176	13.5	3.8	11.9	1.5
Breast, Escalope, Pesto Chargrilled, M & S*	1 Serving/100g	135.0	6.0	135	19.6	0.7	6.2	0.6
Breast, Escalope, Plain, Average	*1 Serving/100g*	*110.0*	*2.0*	*110*	*22.3*	*0.7*	*2.2*	*0.5*
Breast, Fillet, Mesquite, KP Snacks*	1 Serving/85g	130.0	7.0	153	20.0	1.2	8.2	0.0
Breast, Fillets, Breaded, Average	1 Fillet/112g	246.0	12.0	220	17.5	14.0	10.4	1.3
Breast, Fillets, Breaded, Lemon & Pepper, Average	1 Fillet/89g	133.0	2.0	150	22.0	10.1	2.3	1.3
Breast, Fillets, Cajun, Average	1 Fillet/93g	124.0	3.0	134	23.6	3.5	2.8	0.3
Breast, Fillets, Chargrilled, Average	1 Serving/100g	120.0	1.0	120	27.3	0.3	1.1	0.3
Breast, Fillets, Korma Style, Average	1 Serving/100g	131.0	3.0	131	27.4	0.8	2.7	0.5
Breast, Fillets, Lemon Parsley, M & S*	½ Pack/145g	232.0	3.0	160	14.3	20.7	2.4	4.3
Breast, Fillets, Mini, Raw, Average	*1oz/28g*	*34.0*	*0.0*	*121*	*26.9*	*0.2*	*1.5*	*0.1*
Breast, Fillets, Organic, Average	*1 Serving/150g*	*153.0*	*1.0*	*102*	*23.9*	*0.0*	*0.7*	*0.0*
Breast, Fillets, Skin On, Free Range, TTD, Sainsbury's*	1 Fillet/162g	235.0	8.0	145	25.7	0.0	4.7	0.0
Breast, Fillets, Skinless & Boneless, Raw, Average	*1 Serving/100g*	*126.0*	*2.0*	*126*	*25.1*	*1.2*	*2.3*	*0.2*
Breast, Grilled, Average	*1 Breast/130g*	*192.0*	*3.0*	*148*	*32.0*	*0.0*	*2.2*	*0.0*
Breast, Joint, Lemon & Tarragon, Finest, Tesco*	1 Serving/175g	247.0	11.0	141	18.8	2.3	6.3	0.2
Breast, Lemon & Pepper, Breaded, Asda*	1 Portion/90g	187.0	8.0	208	15.3	17.7	8.4	1.8
Breast, Lemon Pepper, Cooked, Birds Eye*	1 Piece/100.5g	261.0	14.0	260	15.0	19.0	14.0	0.9
Breast, Meat & Skin, Raw, Average	*1 Serving/145g*	*249.0*	*13.0*	*172*	*20.8*	*0.0*	*9.2*	*0.0*
Breast, Meat & Skin, Weighed with Bone, Raw, Average	*1oz/28g*	*48.0*	*3.0*	*172*	*20.8*	*0.0*	*9.2*	*0.0*
Breast, Meat Only, Fried	*1 Serving/50g*	*93.0*	*2.0*	*187*	*33.4*	*0.5*	*4.7*	*0.0*
Breast, Pieces, Tikka, Average	1 Serving/100g	154.0	3.0	154	28.2	2.7	3.3	0.4
Breast, Roast, Sliced, From Supermarket, Average	*1 Slice/13g*	*17.0*	*0.0*	*139*	*25.0*	*1.8*	*3.5*	*0.2*
Breast, Roast, without Skin, Average	*1oz/28g*	*42.0*	*1.0*	*149*	*25.4*	*1.0*	*4.7*	*0.2*
Breast, Roll, Average	*1 Slice/10g*	*17.0*	*1.0*	*167*	*16.1*	*3.2*	*10.0*	*0.2*
Breast, Short Sliced, Mexican, Sainsbury's*	1 Pack/130g	177.0	3.0	136	26.4	2.5	2.2	0.1
Breast, Slices, Roast, Hot 'n' Spicy, Sainsbury's*	½ Pack/65.2g	90.0	1.0	138	26.7	2.7	2.3	0.4
Breast, Smoked, Sliced, Average	*1 Slice/20g*	*22.0*	*1.0*	*110*	*20.7*	*0.9*	*2.6*	*0.1*
Breast, Southern Fried, Premium, Bernard Matthews*	1 Serving/60g	70.0	2.0	117	19.6	3.1	2.9	0.6
Breast, Strips, Raw, Average	*1 Serving/280g*	*358.0*	*6.0*	*128*	*27.1*	*0.3*	*2.0*	*0.3*
Breast, Tandoori Style, Average	1 Serving/180g	237.0	7.0	131	22.3	2.3	3.7	1.0
Breast, Tikka, Sliced, Average	1oz/28g	34.0	0.0	120	24.9	2.0	1.7	0.6
Chargrills, Garlic, Weight After Cooking, Birds Eye*	1 Chargrill/95g	182.0	10.0	192	19.0	4.0	11.0	0.1
Chargrills, Garlic, Weight Before Cooking, Birds Eye*	1 Chargrill/95g	190.0	11.0	200	20.3	4.2	11.3	0.1
Chargrills, Original, Weight Before Cooking, Birds Eye*	1 Chargrill/95g	156.0	9.0	164	17.5	3.2	9.0	0.1
Chargrills, Weight After Cooking, Baked, Birds Eye*	1 Chargrill/90g	160.0	9.0	178	18.9	3.4	9.7	0.1
Cooked, Sliced, Average	*1 Slice/15g*	*18.0*	*0.0*	*118*	*22.4*	*1.6*	*2.4*	*0.1*
Dippers, Crispy, Average	5 Dippers/93g	231.0	14.0	249	13.2	14.4	15.4	0.6
Drumsticks, & Thighs, Garlic & Herb, Sainsbury's*	1 Serving/120g	184.0	11.0	153	16.6	1.5	8.9	0.1
Drumsticks, BBQ Flavour, Average	1 Serving/200g	348.0	16.0	174	22.6	3.1	8.0	0.4
Drumsticks, Breaded, Fried, Average	1oz/28g	70.0	4.0	248	19.6	9.9	14.6	0.6

CHICKEN

	Measure INFO/WEIGHT	per Measure KCAL	per Measure FAT	Nutrition Values per 100g / 100ml KCAL	PROT	CARB	FAT	FIBRE
Drumsticks, Roast, without Skin, Average	1 Serving/100g	163.0	8.0	163	22.6	0.5	7.8	0.2
Drumsticks, Southern Fried, Sainsbury's*	1 Serving/87g	190.0	9.0	218	20.8	11.2	9.9	0.7
Drumsticks, with Skin, Average	1 Piece/125g	268.0	17.0	215	22.1	1.8	13.3	0.3
Escalope, Breaded, Average	1 Piece/128g	361.0	22.0	282	13.4	19.1	16.9	0.7
Fillet Strips, Barbeque, Birds Eye*	4 Strips/100.6g	180.0	9.0	179	18.9	6.5	8.6	0.2
Fillet Strips, Dijon Mustard, Birds Eye*	4 Strips/113g	155.0	6.0	137	18.9	3.7	5.2	0.1
Fillet Strips, Red Pesto, Birds Eye*	4 Strips/100g	135.0	5.0	135	19.1	3.2	5.1	0.2
Fillet Strips, Tomato & Basil, Birds Eye*	4 Strips/101g	150.0	5.0	149	19.4	5.6	5.4	0.3
Fillet, Thigh, TTD, Sainsbury's*	1 Piece/60g	96.0	4.0	160	26.8	0.0	5.9	0.0
Fillets, Battered, Average	1 Fillet/90g	199.0	10.0	221	16.1	13.3	11.5	0.5
Fillets, Breaded, Average	1 Piece/98g	214.0	10.0	219	14.2	15.9	10.7	1.9
Fillets, Chilli & Mango, Tesco*	1 Serving/100g	130.0	1.0	130	27.1	3.7	0.7	1.0
Fillets, Chinese Style, Average	1oz/28g	37.0	0.0	131	24.4	4.6	1.7	0.5
Fillets, Coronation, BGTY, Sainsbury's*	1 Fillet/100g	136.0	3.0	136	27.1	2.4	2.6	1.0
Fillets, Hickory Barbecue & Chilli, BGTY, Sainsbury's*	1 Fillet/100g	133.0	1.0	133	26.9	3.6	1.2	0.9
Fillets, Hickory Style BBQ, Tesco*	1 Fillet/80g	112.0	2.0	140	28.4	1.5	2.2	0.5
Fillets, Honey & Maple, Roast, Mini, Waitrose*	½ Pack/100g	131.0	0.0	131	23.0	8.6	0.5	1.5
Fillets, Honey & Mustard, Average	1 Serving/100g	138.0	4.0	138	18.4	7.5	3.7	0.8
Fillets, Hot & Spicy, Average	1oz/28g	58.0	3.0	206	16.4	10.5	11.0	1.1
Fillets, Lime & Coriander, Mini, Average	1 Fillet/42g	49.0	1.0	118	24.3	2.6	1.3	0.6
Fillets, Red Thai, Mini, Average	1oz/28g	36.0	1.0	127	21.7	5.4	2.0	0.6
Fillets, Southern Fried, Meat Only, Average	1 Piece/100g	222.0	12.0	222	16.4	12.2	12.0	1.1
Fillets, Sweet Chilli & Lime, Mini, M & S*	1 Serving/50g	77.0	1.0	155	28.3	5.1	2.2	0.0
Fillets, Sweet Chilli, Mini, Sainsbury's*	½ Pack/100g	119.0	1.0	119	21.8	5.4	1.1	0.9
Fillets, Tandoori Style, Mini, Average	1 Serving/100g	127.0	2.0	127	24.7	2.5	2.0	0.3
Fillets, Thai, COU, M & S*	1 Fillet/120g	160.0	2.0	133	19.5	10.4	1.6	1.3
Fillets, Tikka, Average	1 Serving/100g	141.0	5.0	141	22.4	1.7	5.0	1.1
Fillets, Tikka, Mini, Average	1oz/28g	35.0	1.0	124	25.1	1.3	2.1	1.1
Fillets, Tomato & Basil, Mini, Average	1oz/28g	34.0	1.0	123	23.4	2.5	2.1	0.3
Fingers, Average	1 Serving/75g	187.0	10.0	250	13.7	18.7	13.2	1.1
Goujons, Breaded, Average	1 Serving/114g	293.0	17.0	258	15.8	15.2	15.0	1.0
Goujons, Breast, Fresh, Average	1oz/28g	36.0	0.0	127	28.0	0.0	1.6	0.0
Honey Roast, Sliced, Average	1 Slice/13g	15.0	0.0	117	21.5	2.1	2.4	0.1
Leg or Thigh, Hot & Spicy, Average	1oz/28g	50.0	3.0	179	19.4	1.0	10.8	0.4
Leg Portion, Roast, Skin, Without Bone, Average	1 Quarter/120g	244.0	15.0	203	21.6	0.3	12.7	0.2
Leg, Meat Only, Raw, Average	1oz/28g	34.0	1.0	120	20.1	0.0	3.8	0.0
Leg, Meat Only, Raw, with Skin & Bone, Average	1oz/28g	38.0	1.0	134	22.5	0.0	4.3	0.0
Leg, Meat Only, Stewed, with Bone & Skin, Average	1oz/28g	52.0	2.0	185	26.3	0.0	8.1	0.0
Leg, with Skin, Raw, Average	1oz/28g	48.0	3.0	172	19.1	0.0	10.4	0.0
Leg, with Skin, Roasted, Average	1oz/28g	66.0	5.0	234	21.5	0.1	16.4	0.0
Light Meat, Raw	1oz/28g	30.0	0.0	106	24.0	0.0	1.1	0.0
Light Meat, Roasted	1oz/28g	43.0	1.0	153	30.2	0.0	3.6	0.0
Meat & Skin Portions, Deep Fried, Average	1oz/28g	73.0	5.0	259	26.9	0.0	16.8	0.0
Meat & Skin, Raw, Average	1oz/28g	64.0	5.0	230	17.6	0.0	17.7	0.0
Meat & Skin, Roasted, Average	1oz/28g	60.0	4.0	216	22.6	0.0	14.0	0.0
Meat, Roasted, Average	1oz/28g	50.0	2.0	177	27.3	0.0	7.5	0.0
Mince, Average	1oz/28g	39.0	2.0	140	20.9	0.1	6.0	0.2
Nuggets, Battered, Average	1 Nugget/20g	50.0	3.0	251	13.5	16.9	14.4	0.9
Nuggets, Breaded, Average	1 Nugget/14g	37.0	2.0	263	14.8	19.8	13.8	1.9
Peri Peri, Chargrill, Birds Eye*	1 Serving/92g	157.0	8.0	171	16.9	5.2	9.2	0.3
Pieces, Boneless, Breaded, Fried, From Restaurant	1 Piece/17g	51.0	3.0	301	17.0	14.4	19.4	0.0
Soy Braised, M & S*	1 Serving/100g	130.0	7.0	130	13.1	3.4	7.0	0.7
Spatchcock, Poussin, Sainsbury's*	1 Serving/122g	168.0	7.0	138	21.1	0.1	5.4	0.2

	Measure INFO/WEIGHT	per Measure KCAL	FAT	Nutrition Values per 100g / 100ml KCAL	PROT	CARB	FAT	FIBRE

CHICKEN

	Measure INFO/WEIGHT	KCAL	FAT	KCAL	PROT	CARB	FAT	FIBRE
Spatchcock, Salt & Cracked Pepper, Sainsbury's*	1 Serving/122g	168.0	7.0	138	21.1	0.1	5.4	0.2
Steaks, Average	*1 Serving/100g*	*205.0*	*9.0*	*205*	*21.1*	*9.0*	*9.4*	*0.7*
Strips Or Tenders, Chinese Style, Average	1oz/28g	41.0	1.0	145	19.6	7.9	4.1	1.0
Thigh, Meat & Skin, Average	*1 Serving/100g*	*218.0*	*15.0*	*218*	*21.4*	*0.0*	*14.7*	*0.0*
Thigh, Meat & Skin, Casseroled, Average	*1oz/28g*	*65.0*	*5.0*	*233*	*21.5*	*0.0*	*16.3*	*0.0*
Thigh, Meat Only, Diced, Casseroled	*1oz/28g*	*50.0*	*2.0*	*180*	*25.6*	*0.0*	*8.6*	*0.0*
Thigh, Meat Only, Raw, Average	*1 Thigh/90g*	*113.0*	*5.0*	*126*	*19.4*	*0.0*	*5.4*	*0.0*
Thigh, Roast, Average	*1 Serving/100g*	*238.0*	*16.0*	*238*	*23.8*	*0.4*	*15.6*	*0.0*
Vindaloo, Average	1 Serving/410g	787.0	51.0	192	18.5	2.6	12.5	0.3
Wafer Thin, Average	1 Slice/10g	12.0	0.0	120	19.0	2.8	3.6	0.1
Whole, Roast, Average	*1oz/28g*	*59.0*	*4.0*	*211*	*21.2*	*1.5*	*13.4*	*0.2*
Wing Quarter, Meat Only, Casseroled	*1oz/28g*	*46.0*	*2.0*	*164*	*26.9*	*0.0*	*6.3*	*0.0*
Wing, Breaded, Fried, Average	1oz/28g	82.0	5.0	294	18.4	14.0	18.5	0.4
Wing, Meat & Skin, Cooked, Average	*1oz/28g*	*67.0*	*4.0*	*241*	*23.3*	*1.9*	*15.6*	*0.3*
Wings, BBQ Flavour, Average	1oz/28g	61.0	3.0	219	20.3	6.5	12.4	0.6
Wings, Chinese Style, Average	1oz/28g	72.0	4.0	256	24.2	5.1	15.5	0.6
Wings, Hot & Spicy, Average	1oz/28g	65.0	4.0	231	21.8	5.1	13.6	0.8
Wings, Meat & Skin, Raw, Average	*1oz/28g*	*52.0*	*3.0*	*184*	*19.0*	*0.5*	*11.8*	*0.2*

CHICKEN &

	Measure INFO/WEIGHT	KCAL	FAT	KCAL	PROT	CARB	FAT	FIBRE
Apricot Rice, COU, M & S*	1 Pack/400g	360.0	4.0	90	9.4	10.6	0.9	0.7
Asparagus, Baby Potatoes, Creamy, Sainsbury's*	1 Pack/450g	472.0	20.0	105	8.0	8.3	4.4	0.9
Asparagus, BGTY, Sainsbury's*	1 Pack/400g	428.0	6.0	107	9.1	14.5	1.4	0.9
Asparagus, in a Champagne Sauce, Finest, Tesco*	1 Pack/500g	615.0	33.0	123	8.8	7.0	6.7	0.9
Asparagus, Long Grain & Wild Rice, BGTY, Sainsbury's*	1 Pack/451g	555.0	9.0	123	9.2	17.1	2.0	0.8
Bacon, Easy Steam, Tesco*	1 Pack/400g	728.0	36.0	182	11.7	13.6	9.1	0.8
Black Bean Noodles, Sainsbury's*	1 Serving/130g	155.0	1.0	119	4.3	23.9	0.7	0.8
Black Bean, Chinese, Tesco*	1 Pack/350g	381.0	17.0	109	8.9	7.4	4.9	0.7
Black Bean, Safeway*	1 Pack/350g	262.0	6.0	75	10.3	4.4	1.6	2.5
Black Bean, Special Fried Rice, HL, Tesco*	1 Pack/450g	360.0	6.0	80	6.8	9.5	1.4	0.9
Black Bean, with Chinese Rice, COU, M & S*	1 Pack/400g	320.0	10.0	80	7.4	7.6	2.4	1.1
Black Bean, with Rice, HL, Tesco*	1 Pack/450g	463.0	7.0	103	6.9	19.6	1.6	0.6
Broccoli, with Herb Potatoes, Tesco*	1 Pack/475g	499.0	11.0	105	7.8	12.5	2.3	1.5
Cashew Nuts, Asda*	1 Pack/400g	528.0	36.0	132	8.2	4.2	9.1	0.8
Cashew Nuts, Chinese, Cantonese, Sainsbury's*	½ Pack/175g	171.0	9.0	98	8.4	4.9	5.0	1.3
Cashew Nuts, with Egg Fried Rice, HL, Tesco*	1 Pack/450g	441.0	6.0	98	8.9	12.7	1.3	1.3
Chargrilled Vegetable Roll, HL, Tesco*	1 Pack/221g	336.0	6.0	152	10.1	21.8	2.7	2.3
Chips, BBQ, BGTY, Sainsbury's*	1 Pack/381g	423.0	7.0	111	7.9	15.9	1.8	2.5
Chorizo Paella, Go Cook, Asda*	½ Pack/475g	591.0	10.0	124	10.2	15.9	2.2	2.6
Cranberry, Perfectly Balanced, Waitrose*	1 Pack/240g	161.0	1.0	67	11.8	4.1	0.4	1.1
Gravy, COU, M & S*	1 Pack/300g	216.0	4.0	72	7.2	7.8	1.3	1.6
Herb Pasta with Lemon, HL, Tesco*	1 Pack/400g	520.0	8.0	130	8.2	18.8	2.0	1.6
King Prawn Special Fried Rice, Finest, Tesco*	1 Pack/450g	733.0	32.0	163	7.7	17.0	7.1	0.7
Mushroom, Chinese, Sainsbury's*	½ Pack/175g	115.0	3.0	66	7.6	4.4	2.0	0.9
Mushroom, Chinese, Tesco*	1 Pack/460g	474.0	13.0	103	5.7	13.8	2.8	1.0
Mushroom, in White Wine Sauce, GFY, Asda*	1 Pack/400g	272.0	7.0	68	6.0	7.0	1.8	1.2
Mushroom, with Egg Fried Rice, Iceland*	1 Pack/500g	410.0	6.0	82	4.9	13.0	1.2	0.7
Mushroom, with Vegetable Rice, BGTY, Sainsbury's*	1 Pack/400g	376.0	7.0	94	6.4	13.0	1.8	0.9
Peppers, in a Black Bean Sauce, M & S*	1 Pack/320g	256.0	5.0	80	9.4	7.3	1.5	1.2
Peppers, M & S*	1 Serving/240g	264.0	11.0	110	14.7	2.3	4.5	0.6
Pineapple, Chilled, Tesco*	1 Pack/350g	364.0	8.0	104	9.6	11.1	2.4	5.5
Pineapple, with Egg Fried Rice, HL, Tesco*	1 Pack/450g	414.0	3.0	92	6.0	15.4	0.7	0.6
Pineapple, with Egg Fried Rice, Tesco*	1 Pack/450g	450.0	11.0	100	7.6	12.1	2.4	1.2
Pineapple, with Vegetable Rice, M & S*	1 Pack/400g	400.0	8.0	100	7.2	13.0	1.9	1.6

	Measure INFO/WEIGHT	per Measure KCAL	FAT	Nutrition Values per 100g / 100ml KCAL	PROT	CARB	FAT	FIBRE
CHICKEN &								
Stuffing, Roast, HL, Tesco*	1 Serving/17g	19.0	0.0	111	23.3	1.3	1.4	0.2
Tomato & Basil, COU, M & S*	½ Pack/200g	180.0	5.0	90	14.3	3.4	2.3	0.8
CHICKEN ARRABBIATA								
Al Forno, Sainsbury's*	1 Pack/900g	1026.0	22.0	114	6.5	16.4	2.5	1.4
Bistro, Waitrose*	½ Pack/175g	156.0	5.0	89	12.9	2.5	3.0	0.5
Easy Steam, HL, Tesco*	1 Pack/400g	284.0	3.0	71	8.4	7.6	0.8	1.2
GFY, Asda*	1 Pack/447.7g	394.0	3.0	88	5.2	15.1	0.7	1.1
Perfectly Balanced, Waitrose*	1 Serving/240g	211.0	6.0	88	12.4	4.0	2.4	0.6
Weight Watchers, Heinz*	1 Serving/300g	222.0	2.0	74	5.4	11.5	0.6	0.8
CHICKEN BUTTER								
& Rice, Indian, Finest, Tesco*	1 Serving/475g	660.0	28.0	139	7.1	14.0	6.0	1.6
Curry, Fresh, Tesco*	1 Pack/350g	486.0	24.0	139	11.8	7.1	7.0	1.8
Indian, with Pilau Rice, Asda*	1 Pack/500g	770.0	23.0	154	7.0	21.0	4.7	1.3
Rich & Aromatic, Sainsbury's*	1 Pack/400g	592.0	36.0	148	12.1	4.4	9.1	1.2
Tesco*	1 Pack/350g	515.0	33.0	147	11.7	3.7	9.4	0.7
CHICKEN CAJUN								
& Potato Hash, HL, Tesco*	1 Pack/450g	427.0	6.0	95	6.5	14.1	1.4	1.5
Breast, Chargrilled, Iceland*	1 Serving/80g	114.0	1.0	142	27.4	3.9	1.9	0.0
Breast, Morrisons*	½ Pack/180g	328.0	17.0	182	16.6	7.7	9.4	2.0
CHICKEN CANTONESE								
& Rice, Sizzler, Tesco*	1 Serving/450g	639.0	26.0	142	7.7	14.9	5.7	0.9
Breast, Fillets, Sainsbury's*	1 Serving/154g	168.0	2.0	109	20.3	3.6	1.5	0.6
Chinese, Tesco*	½ Pack/175g	196.0	6.0	112	10.3	9.4	3.7	0.4
Honey Pepper, Sainsbury's*	½ Pack/175g	124.0	4.0	71	6.6	6.1	2.2	0.9
Honey, Sesame, Sainsbury's*	1/3 Pack/135g	116.0	4.0	86	9.8	5.5	2.7	0.8
CHICKEN CARIBBEAN								
Fruity, with Rice & Peas, New, BGTY, Sainsbury's*	1 Pack/400g	352.0	4.0	88	6.9	13.1	0.9	2.2
Style, Breasts, COU, M & S*	1 Serving/205g	205.0	3.0	100	14.6	7.3	1.5	1.3
CHICKEN CHASSEUR								
BGTY, Sainsbury's*	1 Pack/320g	243.0	4.0	76	6.8	9.5	1.1	1.0
Breast Fillets, Morrisons*	1 Pack/380g	384.0	11.0	101	15.7	2.9	3.0	0.8
Finest, Tesco*	½ Pack/200g	200.0	6.0	100	14.3	2.4	3.2	1.1
Mix, Colman's*	1 Pack/38g	120.0	0.0	316	8.6	68.2	1.0	3.7
CHICKEN CHILLI								
& Lemongrass, with Egg Noodles, BGTY, Sainsbury's*	1 Pack/450g	499.0	15.0	111	10.0	10.2	3.4	1.2
Sweet, & Egg Fried Rice, HL, Tesco*	1 Serving/450g	446.0	8.0	99	5.7	15.0	1.8	0.4
Sweet, Findus*	1 Pack/350g	420.0	12.0	120	6.0	15.0	3.5	1.5
Sweet, Just Cook, Sainsbury's*	½ Pack/190.5g	200.0	1.0	105	15.2	9.4	0.7	0.5
Sweet, with Noodles, Frozen, HL, Tesco*	1 Pack/450g	472.0	6.0	105	4.9	17.3	1.4	1.4
CHICKEN CHINESE								
& Prawns, Sizzler, House Special, Tesco*	1 Serving/450g	684.0	23.0	152	7.5	18.8	5.2	1.2
Balls, M & S*	1 Ball/16g	45.0	2.0	280	10.8	29.2	13.6	2.1
Battered, with Plum Sauce, Tesco*	1 Pack/350g	647.0	20.0	185	6.7	26.5	5.8	0.8
Crispy Aromatic, Half, Tesco*	1 Serving/233g	524.0	24.0	225	16.3	16.7	10.4	1.2
Fillets, with Sweet Chilli Sauce, Tesco*	1 Serving/350g	591.0	22.0	169	8.8	19.2	6.3	0.7
Stir Fry, Morrisons*	1 Serving/319g	341.0	5.0	107	5.7	17.0	1.7	1.5
Style Sauce, Breast Fillets, Morrisons*	½ Pack/200g	162.0	2.0	81	13.5	4.6	1.0	1.2
with Ginger & Spring Onion, Tesco*	1 Serving/350g	299.0	10.0	85	7.6	7.3	2.9	0.6
CHICKEN CIDER								
COU, M & S*	1 Pack/400g	300.0	9.0	75	7.2	6.7	2.3	0.8
with Colcannon, Perfectly Balanced, Waitrose*	1 Pack/401g	353.0	12.0	88	6.2	8.9	3.1	1.1
CHICKEN CORDON BLEU								
Breast, Fillets, Sainsbury's*	1 Serving/150g	304.0	14.0	203	17.5	11.5	9.5	1.6

C

	Measure INFO/WEIGHT	per Measure KCAL	FAT	Nutrition Values per 100g / 100ml KCAL	PROT	CARB	FAT	FIBRE
CHICKEN CORDON BLEU								
Waitrose*	1 Serving/160g	325.0	15.0	203	20.1	9.1	9.6	2.4
CHICKEN CORONATION								
M & S*	1 Serving/200g	420.0	26.0	210	12.6	10.6	13.2	1.3
CHICKEN DINNER								
Breast, with Pork, Sage & Onion Stuffing, Tesco*	1 Serving/180g	277.0	15.0	154	19.4	0.7	8.2	0.5
Kershaws*	1 Pack/350g	210.0	3.0	60	4.3	8.4	1.0	1.2
Tesco*	1 Serving/400g	388.0	7.0	97	9.2	10.9	1.8	1.2
with Gravy, The Crafty Cook*	1 Serving/320g	330.0	7.0	103	5.6	15.3	2.1	1.9
CHICKEN EN CROUTE								
Asda*	½ Pack/174g	393.0	17.0	226	14.0	20.0	10.0	1.5
Breast, Tesco*	1 Serving/215g	555.0	33.0	258	9.4	20.4	15.4	0.6
Just Cook, Sainsbury's*	1 Serving/180g	481.0	27.0	267	16.8	15.9	15.1	0.4
CHICKEN ESCALOPE								
Creamy Peppercorn, Sainsbury's*	1 Serving/150g	367.0	24.0	245	13.3	11.2	16.3	1.1
Lemon, & Herb, Waitrose*	1 Serving/200g	242.0	6.0	121	22.0	1.0	3.2	0.6
Sour Cream & Chive, Tesco*	1 Piece/143g	390.0	25.0	274	13.3	16.1	17.4	2.0
Spinach & Ricotta, Sainsbury's*	1 Piece/150g	354.0	23.0	236	13.1	11.5	15.3	0.9
Topped with Cheese, Ham & Mushrooms, Asda*	½ Pack/149g	217.0	9.0	145	22.0	0.8	6.0	0.4
CHICKEN FLORENTINE								
Asda*	1 Serving/200g	322.0	18.0	161	18.0	2.1	9.0	0.9
Finest, Tesco*	½ Pack/225g	358.0	19.0	159	11.0	9.7	8.5	1.3
HL, Tesco*	1 Pack/400g	340.0	11.0	85	12.1	3.0	2.7	0.9
CHICKEN GINGER								
& Lemon, with Apricot Rice, BGTY, Sainsbury's*	1 Pack/402g	438.0	6.0	109	9.7	14.5	1.4	0.3
& Plum, with Rice, Perfectly Balanced, Waitrose*	1 Pack/400g	492.0	2.0	123	6.3	23.5	0.5	1.0
& Spring Onion, with Rice, Sharwood's*	1 Pack/375g	347.0	6.0	93	5.1	14.2	1.7	1.7
CHICKEN GLAZED								
Balsamic, HL, Tesco*	1 Pack/400g	288.0	4.0	72	5.1	10.8	0.9	0.9
CHICKEN HARISSA								
BGTY, Sainsbury's*	1 Serving/250g	211.0	3.0	84	10.4	8.0	1.2	1.5
with Cous Cous, Perfectly Balanced, Waitrose*	1 Pack/400g	348.0	8.0	87	7.6	9.5	2.0	1.7
CHICKEN HONEY & MUSTARD								
HL, Tesco*	1 Serving/375g	424.0	9.0	113	5.8	17.3	2.3	1.4
Shapers, Boots*	1 Pack/241g	304.0	6.0	126	7.0	19.0	2.4	1.7
Weight Watchers*	1 Serving/320g	291.0	2.0	91	5.1	16.2	0.7	0.2
with Baby Potatoes, BGTY, Sainsbury's*	1 Pack/450g	391.0	3.0	87	8.5	11.7	0.7	0.8
CHICKEN IN								
Bacon, Mushroom & Red Wine Sauce, Asda*	1 Serving/151g	145.0	4.0	96	16.0	2.2	2.6	0.5
Barbecue Sauce, COU, M & S*	1 Pack/352g	370.0	6.0	105	8.6	13.8	1.6	1.2
Barbeque Sauce, Breasts, COU, M & S*	1 Pack/350g	420.0	7.0	120	8.5	20.6	1.9	0.6
BBQ Sauce, Breast, Sainsbury's*	1 Serving/170g	199.0	1.0	117	14.5	13.1	0.7	1.3
BBQ Sauce, Chargrilled, Breast, GFY, Asda*	1 Serving/166g	214.0	6.0	129	19.0	5.0	3.7	1.0
BBQ Sauce, Weight Watchers*	1 Pack/339g	332.0	12.0	98	5.8	10.8	3.5	0.9
Black Bean Sauce, & Rice, Morrisons*	1 Pack/400g	408.0	9.0	102	3.9	16.4	2.3	1.2
Black Bean Sauce, Canned, BGTY, Sainsbury's*	1 Can/400g	308.0	4.0	77	9.3	7.9	0.9	0.7
Black Bean Sauce, Frozen, BGTY, Sainsbury's*	1 Pack/400g	380.0	4.0	95	4.5	16.6	1.1	0.5
Black Bean Sauce, M & S*	1 Pack/350g	297.0	7.0	85	8.7	8.0	2.0	1.1
Black Bean Sauce, Sainsbury's*	1 Pack/465g	484.0	8.0	104	5.0	17.3	1.7	0.3
Black Bean Sauce, Tinned, Tesco*	1 Serving/200g	164.0	3.0	82	10.0	7.7	1.3	1.1
Black Bean Sauce, Waitrose*	1 Pack/300g	243.0	4.0	81	10.9	6.6	1.2	0.8
Black Bean Sauce, with Egg Fried Rice, GFY, Asda*	1 Serving/416g	320.0	4.0	77	5.0	12.0	1.0	0.9
Black Bean Sauce, with Rice, Asda*	1 Pack/400g	500.0	8.0	125	7.0	20.0	1.9	0.6
Black Bean, with Egg Fried Rice, HL, Tesco*	1 Pack/450g	468.0	4.0	104	6.8	17.1	0.9	0.5

	Measure INFO/WEIGHT	per Measure		Nutrition Values per 100g / 100ml				
		KCAL	FAT	KCAL	PROT	CARB	FAT	FIBRE
CHICKEN IN								
Broccoli & Mushroom, Good Choice, Iceland*	1 Pack/500g	590.0	11.0	118	6.4	18.1	2.2	0.6
Cheese & Bacon, Wrapped, Breast, Tesco*	1 Serving/300g	474.0	23.0	158	20.7	1.2	7.8	0.5
Cheesy Salsa, Fillets, Safeway*	½ Pack/175g	192.0	5.0	110	17.9	2.2	3.0	1.1
Chilli & Lemon Grass with Rice, Sainsbury's*	1 Pack/450g	526.0	11.0	117	6.2	17.4	2.5	0.7
Coconut, Sizzler, HL, Tesco*	1 Pack/350g	280.0	8.0	80	9.8	4.5	2.2	2.1
Creamy Madeira Sauce, HL, Tesco*	1 Pack/400g	320.0	7.0	80	12.8	2.3	1.7	1.0
Creamy Mushroom Sauce, HL, Tesco*	1 Pack/400g	296.0	6.0	74	13.2	1.8	1.5	0.5
Creamy Mustard Sauce, GFY, Asda*	1 Pack/400g	468.0	9.0	117	6.0	18.0	2.3	0.4
Creamy Thai Sauce, Somerfield*	1 Pack/440g	748.0	35.0	170	22.0	2.0	8.0	0.0
Creamy Tikka Style Sauce, Tesco*	1 Breast/190g	215.0	10.0	113	15.1	0.7	5.5	0.8
Creamy Tomato & Mascarpone Sauce, Waitrose*	1 Serving/400g	492.0	23.0	123	7.9	9.9	5.8	0.8
Creamy White Wine Sauce, Sainsbury's*	1 Pack/324g	285.0	12.0	88	8.9	4.7	3.7	1.0
Garlic & Cream Sauce, Breast Fillet, Morrisons*	1 Serving/180g	262.0	16.0	146	14.9	1.8	8.8	0.5
Garlic & Herbs, Breast, Sainsbury's*	1 Serving/200g	316.0	5.0	158	28.3	5.4	2.6	0.1
Ginger & Chilli with Veg Noodles, COU, M & S*	1 Pack/400g	300.0	2.0	75	6.4	10.7	0.6	1.1
Gravy, Breast, Sainsbury's*	1 Box/200g	124.0	1.0	62	11.8	2.9	0.5	0.2
Gravy, Chunky, M & S*	1 Can/489g	465.0	19.0	95	13.6	1.4	3.9	0.8
Honey Mustard & Parsnip Mash, Light Choices, Tesco*	1 Pack/400g	340.0	7.0	85	8.0	9.0	1.7	2.0
Hot Ginger Sauce, with Thai Sticky Rice, Sainsbury's*	1 Pack/450g	603.0	21.0	134	6.8	16.3	4.6	0.5
Leek & Bacon Sauce, with Mash, HL, Tesco*	1 Pack/450g	337.0	8.0	75	6.7	8.0	1.8	1.6
Lemon Sauce with Rice, Sainsbury's*	1 Pack/450g	513.0	7.0	114	8.1	17.0	1.5	0.7
Lime & Coriander Marinade, Chargrilled, Asda*	½ Pack/163g	286.0	15.0	175	23.0	0.5	9.0	0.0
Madeira Sauce, with Mushrooms, Finest, Tesco*	½ Pack/200g	210.0	8.0	105	13.8	2.9	4.1	0.9
Mango Ginger Marinade, Breast, Chargrilled, GFY, Asda*	½ Pack/190g	234.0	2.0	123	17.0	11.0	1.2	0.5
Masala with Spiced Indian Lentils, M & S*	1 Pack/330g	297.0	8.0	90	10.3	6.1	2.5	5.9
Mediterranean Style Sauce, Breasts, BGTY, Sainsbury's*	½ Pack/170g	148.0	3.0	87	14.5	2.7	2.0	0.9
Mexican Salsa, Tesco*	1 Pack/320g	368.0	9.0	115	19.5	3.1	2.7	0.6
Mexican Style Sauce, Tesco*	1 Serving/180g	128.0	1.0	71	13.3	2.6	0.8	0.7
Mushroom & Ham Sauce with Rice, BGTY, Sainsbury's*	1 Pack/450g	580.0	7.0	129	9.7	18.9	1.6	0.3
Mushroom & Red Wine Sauce, Breast Fillets, Morrisons*	1 Serving/177g	184.0	4.0	104	15.7	4.6	2.5	0.7
Mushroom & White Wine Sauce, Fillets, Morrisons*	1 Serving/190g	243.0	10.0	128	18.8	0.9	5.5	0.5
Oyster Sauce, & Mushrooms, Tesco*	1 Pack/350g	252.0	6.0	72	8.0	6.3	1.6	0.7
Peppercorn Sauce, GFY, Asda*	1 Serving/399g	431.0	7.0	108	6.0	17.0	1.8	0.5
Peppers, Fillets, Sainsbury's*	1 Pack/360g	378.0	13.0	105	13.7	4.2	3.7	1.1
Pesto Style Dressing, Asda*	1 Serving/150g	210.0	10.0	140	18.7	1.3	6.7	0.0
Red Pepper Dressing, Tesco*	1 Serving/140g	228.0	13.0	163	19.2	0.1	9.5	0.5
Red Wine & Bacon Sauce, Breast, Somerfield*	1 Breast/150g	130.0	3.0	87	14.0	3.0	2.0	0.0
Red Wine Sauce, Fillets, Safeway*	1 Serving/175g	210.0	7.0	120	17.7	2.9	3.9	0.7
Red Wine, with Mash, Eat Smart, Morrisons*	1 Serving/400g	288.0	5.0	72	9.1	6.1	1.3	1.4
Satay Sauce, Safeway*	1 Serving/250g	362.0	20.0	145	10.5	7.1	8.0	1.4
Shiraz Wine Sauce, Finest, Tesco*	1 Pack/600g	420.0	10.0	70	10.9	2.9	1.6	1.3
Smoky Barbecue Sauce, Breast, Fresh Tastes, Asda*	1 Breast/160g	258.0	6.0	161	21.9	9.6	3.9	0.9
Smoky Barbeque Sauce, Tesco*	1 Serving/185g	229.0	4.0	124	16.3	9.9	2.1	1.0
Spicy Chilli Sauce, Topped with Cheese, Breast, Asda*	½ Pack/190g	241.0	7.0	127	20.0	3.4	3.7	0.0
Sun Dried Tomato & Basil Sauce, Breast, Iceland*	1 Serving/156g	134.0	2.0	86	14.6	3.3	1.6	1.0
Sweet Chilli Sauce, Breast, Fresh Tastes, Asda*	½ Pack/180g	288.0	9.0	160	18.4	10.3	5.0	0.5
Tarragon Sauce, Lean Cuisine*	1 Pack/338g	270.0	7.0	80	4.0	11.0	2.0	1.5
Tomato & Basil Sauce, Breast, Fresh Tastes, Asda*	½ Pack/130g	136.0	3.0	105	19.3	2.3	2.1	0.7
Tomato & Basil Sauce, HL, Tesco*	1 Breast/200g	154.0	2.0	77	12.4	4.2	1.2	0.6
Tomato & Herb Sauce, Breasts, Tesco*	½ Pack/172.5g	155.0	2.0	90	15.0	3.6	1.4	0.5
White Sauce, BGTY, Sainsbury's*	1 Can/200g	162.0	4.0	81	1.2	2.4	2.1	1.1
White Sauce, Canned, Asda*	½ Can/400g	644.0	44.0	161	12.0	3.5	11.0	0.0
White Sauce, Canned, HL, Tesco*	½ Can/200g	180.0	6.0	90	14.3	1.3	2.9	5.4

CHICKEN IN	INFO/WEIGHT	KCAL	FAT	KCAL	PROT	CARB	FAT	FIBRE
White Wine & Asparagus Panzerotti, Asda*	½ Pack/150g	238.0	3.0	159	8.0	28.0	1.7	0.0
White Wine & Mushroom Sauce, Breasts, Asda*	1 Breast/168g	217.0	8.0	129	20.0	1.0	5.0	0.4
White Wine & Mushroom Sauce, M & S*	1 Serving/200g	260.0	14.0	130	15.6	1.6	6.8	1.0
White Wine & Tarragon Sauce, Breasts, Finest, Tesco*	½ Pack/200g	326.0	20.0	163	16.8	1.3	10.1	0.0
White Wine & Tarragon Sauce, Waitrose*	½ Pack/225g	281.0	17.0	125	10.7	3.1	7.7	0.3
White Wine Sauce, Breasts, Tesco*	1 Serving/370g	388.0	14.0	105	16.9	0.8	3.8	0.6
White Wine Sauce, Simple Solutions, Tesco*	½ Pack/200g	198.0	4.0	99	19.3	0.9	2.0	0.5
White Wine Sauce, Wild Rice, Pub Specials, Birds Eye*	1 Pack/450g	335.0	6.0	74	7.1	8.4	1.3	2.1
White Wine Sauce, with Rice, HL, Tesco*	1 Pack/450g	500.0	7.0	111	7.1	17.0	1.6	0.8
White Wine, with Pasta, Perfectly Balanced, Waitrose*	1 Pack/400g	400.0	10.0	100	8.2	12.1	2.5	2.5
Wild Mushroom Sauce, Extra Special, Asda*	1 Serving/225g	319.0	19.0	142	14.2	2.2	8.4	0.3
Zesty Orange Sauce, Breast, Asda*	1 Serving/200g	326.0	14.0	163	16.0	9.0	7.0	0.0
CHICKEN ITALIAN								
Good Choice, Iceland*	1 Pack/400g	388.0	2.0	97	4.7	18.3	0.5	0.6
Style, BGTY, Sainsbury's*	1 Pack/400g	364.0	4.0	91	6.0	14.5	1.1	0.9
Style, Dinner, Asda*	1 Pack/400g	244.0	4.0	61	6.0	7.0	1.0	1.1
Style, Meal, Asda*	1 Pack/408g	241.0	3.0	59	6.0	7.0	0.8	0.8
Style, Sainsbury's*	½ Pack/190g	222.0	8.0	117	16.3	3.9	4.0	0.1
CHICKEN KUNG PO								
Sainsbury's*	½ Pack/175g	131.0	4.0	75	9.2	4.0	2.5	1.0
Waitrose*	1 Pack/350g	318.0	4.0	91	8.2	12.1	1.1	1.2
with Egg Fried Rice, Asda*	1 Pack/450g	688.0	22.0	153	6.0	21.0	5.0	1.0
CHICKEN LEMON								
Balls, Asda*	1 Ball/15g	42.0	3.0	279	14.0	19.0	17.0	1.6
Battered, Cantonese, Sainsbury's*	1 Pack/350g	560.0	20.0	160	10.7	16.6	5.6	0.9
Battered, Chinese Meal for Two, Tesco*	½ Serving/175g	294.0	13.0	168	6.6	18.8	7.4	2.0
Breast, Fillets, BGTY, Sainsbury's*	1 Fillet/113g	195.0	2.0	173	18.4	19.9	2.1	1.9
Cantonese, Sainsbury's*	½ Pack/140g	218.0	9.0	156	11.0	13.9	6.3	0.6
Chinese, Tesco*	1 Serving/350g	563.0	11.0	161	7.0	26.0	3.2	0.3
COU, M & S*	1 Pack/150g	150.0	1.0	100	17.9	5.6	0.9	0.8
Waitrose*	1 Serving/400g	596.0	23.0	149	12.7	11.7	5.8	0.9
with Rice, HL, Tesco*	1 Pack/450g	477.0	12.0	106	5.9	14.4	2.7	0.9
CHICKEN MEXICAN								
Style Sauce, Breast, Tesco*	1 Serving/180g	128.0	1.0	71	13.3	2.6	0.8	0.7
Style, BGTY, Sainsbury's*	1 Serving/260g	255.0	6.0	98	6.9	12.1	2.5	2.2
Style, Combo, Asda*	1 Pack/380g	562.0	17.0	148	21.0	6.0	4.4	2.0
Style, GFY, Asda*	½ Pack/200g	256.0	10.0	128	17.0	3.7	5.0	0.3
CHICKEN MOROCCAN								
Style, with Spicy Cous Cous, BGTY, Sainsbury's*	1 Serving/225g	304.0	4.0	135	9.2	20.6	1.7	0.0
CHICKEN MUSTARD								
with Creme Fraiche Mash, Perfectly Balanced, Waitrose*	1 Pack/400g	408.0	16.0	102	7.2	9.4	4.0	0.8
with Gratin Potatoes, HL, Tesco*	1 Pack/450g	463.0	12.0	103	9.0	10.7	2.7	2.5
CHICKEN ORIENTAL								
& Pineapple, HL, Tesco*	1 Serving/450g	414.0	3.0	92	6.0	15.4	0.7	0.6
with Noodles, SteamFresh, Birds Eye*	1 Pack/400g	336.0	9.0	84	7.1	9.0	2.2	0.3
CHICKEN PAPRIKA								
COU, M & S*	1 Pack/400g	380.0	6.0	95	9.0	11.7	1.6	2.0
with Savoury Rice & Vegetables, BGTY, Sainsbury's*	1 Pack/400g	383.0	2.0	96	7.1	15.5	0.6	1.1
CHICKEN PARMESAN								
Sun Dried Tomato, Fillets, BGTY, Sainsbury's*	½ Pack/100g	138.0	3.0	138	22.1	6.0	2.9	0.5
CHICKEN PEPPER								
Fry, Sainsbury's*	1 Pack/400g	508.0	25.0	127	15.0	2.9	6.2	1.6
Hot, & Hash, HL, Tesco*	1 Pack/450g	396.0	9.0	88	7.0	10.7	1.9	1.0

	Measure INFO/WEIGHT	per Measure KCAL	FAT	Nutrition Values per 100g / 100ml KCAL	PROT	CARB	FAT	FIBRE
CHICKEN PEPPER								
Hot, with Minted Mash, BGTY, Sainsbury's*	1 Serving/450g	333.0	5.0	74	7.3	8.4	1.2	1.3
CHICKEN PIRI PIRI								
Breast, Fillets, Mini, Tesco*	½ Pack/100g	135.0	1.0	135	22.7	7.6	1.1	0.0
GFY, Asda*	1 Pack/400g	360.0	2.0	90	4.7	17.0	0.4	0.5
M & S*	1 Pack/300g	420.0	23.0	140	10.0	7.3	7.7	1.3
CHICKEN RENDANG								
Sainsbury's*	1 Pack/350g	689.0	54.0	197	9.6	5.1	15.3	1.7
CHICKEN ROAST								
in a Pot, Sainsbury's*	1 Pack/450g	477.0	13.0	106	9.6	10.3	2.9	0.7
Meal, Blue Parrot Cafe, Sainsbury's*	1 Pack/285g	259.0	10.0	91	6.9	8.1	3.4	1.5
CHICKEN ROLL								
Value, Tesco*	1 Slice/13g	30.0	2.0	223	15.4	3.9	16.2	0.1
with Pork, Sage & Onion Stuffing, Value, Tesco*	1 Roll/125g	166.0	9.0	133	9.4	7.8	7.1	0.5
CHICKEN STUFFED								
with Moroccan Style Cous Cous, GFY, Asda*	½ Pack/180g	259.0	5.0	144	20.0	10.0	2.7	0.0
with Mushrooms, Finest, Tesco*	1 Serving/150g	177.0	8.0	118	15.9	2.0	5.1	0.6
CHICKEN SUPREME								
BGTY, Sainsbury's*	1 Pack/350g	416.0	5.0	119	9.4	17.2	1.4	0.5
Breast, Sainsbury's*	1 Serving/187g	421.0	30.0	225	20.6	0.3	15.8	0.6
with Rice, Asda*	1 Pack/450g	616.0	31.0	137	15.0	3.4	7.0	1.1
with Rice, Birds Eye*	1 Pack/376g	470.0	10.0	125	6.6	18.8	2.6	0.5
with Rice, Weight Watchers*	1 Pack/300g	255.0	5.0	85	5.6	11.9	1.6	0.5
CHICKEN SZECHUAN								
Chilli & Peppercorn, Sainsbury's*	1 Pack/400g	352.0	16.0	88	9.9	3.2	4.0	0.5
Tesco*	1 Pack/350g	385.0	10.0	110	7.2	13.6	3.0	0.3
with Noodles, Sainsbury's*	1 Pack/450g	423.0	14.0	94	6.0	10.4	3.1	0.9
CHICKEN TAGINE								
with Cous Cous, BGTY, Sainsbury's*	1 Pack/450g	625.0	18.0	139	10.1	15.9	3.9	1.5
CHICKEN TANDOORI								
Finest, Tesco*	1 Pack/450g	495.0	18.0	110	7.4	10.2	4.1	1.3
Fresh Tastes, Asda*	1 Pack/400g	356.0	6.0	89	6.4	12.7	1.4	2.1
GFY, Asda*	1 Pack/400g	324.0	10.0	81	7.5	7.3	2.4	1.7
Masala, & Rice, HL, Tesco*	1 Serving/450g	409.0	8.0	91	6.6	12.9	1.7	0.6
Masala, Sainsbury's*	1 Pack/400g	536.0	27.0	134	13.2	5.0	6.8	0.5
Sizzler, HL, Tesco*	1 Pack/350g	275.0	7.0	79	11.1	3.8	2.0	4.3
Sizzler, Sainsbury's*	1 Pack/400g	536.0	29.0	134	12.8	4.3	7.3	1.7
Sizzler, Tesco*	1 Serving/175g	243.0	12.0	139	10.0	10.0	6.6	1.0
Tesco*	1 Serving/175g	198.0	9.0	113	10.6	6.7	4.9	1.0
with Rice, Easy Steam, Tesco*	1 Pack/400g	484.0	12.0	121	8.7	14.7	3.0	0.7
with Spicy Vegetable Rice, Eat Smart, Safeway*	1 Serving/350g	367.0	8.0	105	9.7	11.1	2.2	7.0
CHICKEN TERIYAKI								
& Noodles, Asda*	½ Pack/340g	445.0	9.0	131	9.0	18.0	2.6	0.9
Asda*	1 Pack/360g	299.0	5.0	83	9.1	8.6	1.4	0.8
Japanese, with Ramen Noodles, Sainsbury's*	1 Pack/450g	481.0	9.0	107	6.5	15.5	2.1	0.8
CHICKEN THAI								
& Siu Mai Dumplings, M & S*	1 Dumpling/21g	35.0	2.0	170	16.0	9.4	7.6	0.8
& Vegetables, Eat Positive, Birds Eye*	1 Packet/400g	412.0	12.0	103	5.9	13.0	3.0	1.0
Chiang Mai, & Noodles, BGTY, Sainsbury's*	1 Pack/448g	484.0	18.0	108	6.9	11.0	4.0	1.7
Green, Fillets, Mini, Sainsbury's*	½ Pack/100g	130.0	2.0	130	27.9	0.9	1.6	0.8
Style Marinade, Breast, Chargrilled, GFY, Asda*	½ Pack/178g	178.0	5.0	100	17.0	1.3	3.0	0.5
Style, with Noodles, Tesco*	1 Pack/400g	332.0	7.0	83	7.5	9.5	1.7	1.0
with Rice, SteamFresh, Birds Eye*	1 Serving/400g	380.0	8.0	95	6.7	12.7	1.9	0.9

	Measure INFO/WEIGHT	per Measure KCAL	FAT	Nutrition Values per 100g / 100ml KCAL	PROT	CARB	FAT	FIBRE
CHICKEN TIKKA								
& Coriander Rice, Weight Watchers*	1 Pack/400g	348.0	2.0	87	6.2	14.3	0.6	1.6
& Cous Cous, Boots*	1 Pack/160g	307.0	18.0	192	6.2	17.0	11.0	1.3
& Lemon Rice, Deli Meal, M & S*	1 Pack/360g	342.0	7.0	95	9.8	10.2	2.0	0.7
BGTY, Sainsbury's*	1 Serving/188g	265.0	3.0	141	10.5	21.2	1.6	0.0
Creamy, Breast, Tesco*	1 Breast/190g	215.0	10.0	113	15.1	0.7	5.5	0.8
Masala & Pilau Rice, Asda*	1 Serving/500g	720.0	20.0	144	6.2	20.7	4.0	0.9
Masala, with Pilau Rice, Hot, Tesco*	1 Pack/550g	797.0	32.0	145	7.4	15.0	5.8	1.4
Masala, with Rice & Naan, Big Dish, Tesco*	1 Pack/600g	960.0	40.0	160	6.7	18.1	6.7	1.2
Pinwheels, BGTY, Sainsbury's*	1 Serving/214g	261.0	5.0	122	9.6	16.0	2.2	0.0
with Basmati Rice, GFY, Asda*	1 Pack/400g	592.0	7.0	148	9.0	24.0	1.8	1.6
with Pilau Rice, GFY, Asda*	1 Pack/450g	382.0	3.0	85	7.0	13.0	0.6	1.8
CHICKEN VINDALOO								
Asda*	1 Pack/411g	649.0	25.0	158	7.0	19.0	6.0	0.0
Sainsbury's*	1 Pack/400g	460.0	17.0	115	14.6	4.8	4.2	0.6
Waitrose*	1 Pack/340g	398.0	18.0	117	10.6	6.4	5.4	1.6
CHICKEN WITH								
a Sea Salt & Black Pepper Crust, Breasts, Asda*	1 Serving/154g	186.0	4.0	121	19.0	5.0	2.8	0.0
a Sticky Honey & Chilli Sauce, Breast, Asda*	1 Serving/175g	247.0	6.0	141	20.0	8.0	3.2	0.0
Asparagus & Rice, BGTY, Sainsbury's*	1 Pack/400g	428.0	6.0	107	9.1	14.5	1.4	0.9
Bacon & Leeks, with Mashed Potato, BGTY, Sainsbury's*	1 Pack/450g	435.0	11.0	97	8.4	10.1	2.5	0.7
Broccoli & Pesto Pasta, BGTY, Sainsbury's*	1 Pack/301g	328.0	5.0	109	10.3	13.2	1.7	2.5
Caesar Melt & Prosciutto, Breast, M & S*	1 Pack/375g	487.0	19.0	130	19.6	1.3	5.0	1.0
Caramelised Peppers, Chargrilled, M & S*	½ Pack/237g	225.0	9.0	95	12.9	2.1	3.8	1.3
Cheddar & Bacon Filling, Breast, Just Cook, Sainsbury's*	1 Serving/180g	346.0	15.0	192	23.2	6.5	8.1	0.1
Cheese & Bacon, Tesco*	½ Pack/175g	262.0	12.0	150	18.9	2.6	6.8	0.4
Cheese & Chive Sauce, Carb Control, Tesco*	1 Serving/400g	400.0	26.0	100	8.4	2.0	6.4	1.6
Cheese Croutons & Onion, Asda*	1 Serving/200g	200.0	6.0	100	16.0	2.0	3.2	0.9
Cheese, Leek & Ham, Breast, Fresh Tastes, Asda*	1 Pack/430g	658.0	31.0	153	18.9	3.4	7.1	0.7
Cherrywood Barbecue Sauce, Simply Cook, Tesco*	1 Serving/147g	165.0	2.0	112	16.6	7.6	1.7	0.4
Chorizo, & Patatas Bravas, COU, M & S*	1 Pack/400g	380.0	9.0	95	7.8	10.8	2.3	1.7
Coriander & Lime, Asda*	1 Serving/105g	122.0	1.0	116	24.0	2.9	0.9	0.2
Cous Cous, Lemon & Herb, Finest, Tesco*	1 Pack/370g	492.0	18.0	133	10.5	11.5	5.0	0.9
Cranberry Stuffing, Breast, Finest, Tesco*	½ Pack/200g	252.0	5.0	126	16.2	9.9	2.4	0.9
Creamy Spinach & Parmesan, M & S*	1 Pack/390g	468.0	17.0	120	10.8	12.3	4.4	2.5
Fusilli & Courgette, Sainsbury's*	1 Pack/450g	675.0	29.0	150	8.6	14.6	6.4	0.5
Garlic & Chilli Balti, Tesco*	1 Pack/400g	320.0	8.0	80	11.0	4.4	1.9	0.8
Garlic & Herbs, Asda*	1 Slice/25g	28.0	0.0	114	23.9	1.1	1.5	0.0
Garlic Mushrooms, Asda*	1 Serving/320g	342.0	16.0	107	13.7	1.7	5.0	2.2
Garlic Mushrooms, Breast, Fresh Tastes, Asda*	½ Pack/160g	226.0	8.0	141	22.6	1.0	5.2	0.5
Garlic Mushrooms, Breast, Simply Cook, Tesco*	½ Pack/125g	170.0	7.0	136	22.0	0.1	5.3	0.1
Garlic Mushrooms, Breast, Tesco*	1 Breast/125g	149.0	6.0	119	19.0	0.2	4.7	0.1
Grapes & Asparagus, Sainsbury's*	½ Pack/200g	240.0	13.0	120	13.3	1.8	6.6	1.0
Gravy & Stuffing, Breasts, Tesco*	½ Pack/173g	257.0	11.0	149	14.4	8.3	6.4	2.2
Gruyere Cheese & Parma Ham, Breast, COOK!, M & S*	1 Breast/194g	349.0	21.0	180	18.0	2.5	11.0	0.9
Hoi Sin Sauce, Ooodles of Noodles, Oriental Express*	1 Pack/425g	399.0	9.0	94	5.3	13.2	2.2	1.7
Honey & Mustard Sauce, Breasts, Simply Cook, Tesco*	½ Pack/219g	230.0	1.0	105	16.3	8.0	0.6	0.3
Honey & Sesame, with Rice, Light Choices, Tesco*	1 Pack/400g	432.0	12.0	108	5.3	14.9	3.0	2.2
Lemon Grass, Thai Greens & Baby Corn, Sainsbury's*	1 Serving/200g	196.0	7.0	98	10.0	6.9	3.4	1.4
Lime & Coriander, Easy, Waitrose*	½ Pack/168g	203.0	8.0	121	18.9	0.7	4.7	0.5
Lime & Tequila, Asda*	1 Serving/150g	193.0	3.0	129	24.0	4.3	1.8	0.5
Lyonnaise Potatoes, M & S*	½ Pack/260g	286.0	8.0	110	12.6	8.0	3.1	0.9
Mango Salsa & Potato Wedges, BGTY, Sainsbury's*	1 Pack/400g	336.0	6.0	84	7.0	10.4	1.6	1.5
Mango, Lime & Coriander, Asda*	1 Pack/400g	416.0	6.0	104	6.6	15.9	1.5	1.4

CHICKEN WITH	Measure INFO/WEIGHT	per Measure KCAL	FAT	Nutrition Values per 100g / 100ml KCAL	PROT	CARB	FAT	FIBRE
Mascarpone, Bacon & Roasted Onions, Finest, Tesco*	1 Serving/200g	312.0	18.0	156	14.5	4.7	8.8	0.5
Mozzarella & Pancetta, Breast, Finest, Tesco*	½ Pack/225g	326.0	14.0	145	14.4	7.9	6.2	1.1
Mozzarella & Pesto Melt, Breasts, COOK!, M & S*	½ Pack/165g	206.0	10.0	125	16.4	1.3	6.2	0.7
Mushroom & Bacon, Fillets, M & S*	½ Pack/188g	225.0	11.0	120	15.5	0.5	6.0	1.7
Mushroom & Tomato Sauce, GFY, Asda*	1 Serving/175g	180.0	4.0	103	19.0	2.0	2.1	2.7
Mushroom Risotto, M & S*	1 Pack/365g	493.0	27.0	135	6.9	10.4	7.4	1.3
Mushroom Sauce & Herby Rice, Fillets, M & S*	1 Pack/380g	475.0	19.0	125	7.7	12.0	5.1	1.3
Pancakes & Plum Sauce, COU, M & S*	1 Pack/245g	257.0	6.0	105	7.9	12.7	2.3	0.3
Pasta, Chianti & Balsamic, BGTY, Sainsbury's*	1 Pack/400g	372.0	8.0	93	9.4	9.5	1.9	1.9
Pesto & Linguine Pasta, Steamfresh Meal, Birds Eye*	1 Pack/400g	440.0	16.0	110	8.5	10.0	4.0	1.3
Plum Sauce, Battered, Tesco*	1 Serving/175g	324.0	10.0	185	6.7	26.5	5.8	0.8
Plum Tomatoes & Basil, Breast, Birds Eye*	1 Serving/172g	200.0	8.0	116	13.3	5.0	4.7	0.6
Pork Stuffing & Chipolatas, Breast Joint, Tesco*	½ Pack/340g	524.0	28.0	154	16.7	3.4	8.2	0.5
Pork Stuffing, Breast, Roast, M & S*	1 Serving/100g	165.0	6.0	165	24.1	3.0	6.5	0.0
Pork, Parsnip Herb Stuffing, Sainsbury's*	1 Serving/100g	181.0	9.0	181	22.9	2.1	9.0	0.7
Pork, Sage & Onion Stuffing, Mini Roasts, Tesco*	1 Serving/240g	353.0	21.0	147	14.7	2.6	8.6	0.2
Potato & Smoked Bacon Topping, M & S*	1 Serving/175g	227.0	8.0	130	17.8	3.2	4.8	1.2
Prosciutio, Dolcelatte & 3 Cheese Sauce, Asda*	½ Pack/195g	355.0	12.0	182	30.0	1.9	6.0	1.2
Rice 'n' Peas, Sainsbury's*	1 Pack/300g	489.0	18.0	163	12.5	14.4	6.1	2.1
Rice, Breast, Chargrilled, Spicy, Asda*	1 Pack/400g	372.0	2.0	93	6.0	16.0	0.6	1.0
Rice, Fiesta, Weight Watchers*	1 Pack/330g	307.0	7.0	93	6.1	12.8	2.0	0.4
Salsa & Potato Wedges, GFY, Asda*	1 Serving/400g	327.0	7.0	82	6.0	10.5	1.7	1.7
Spinach & Pasta, M & S*	1oz/28g	64.0	4.0	228	9.4	14.0	15.0	1.3
Spinach, Honey Mustard, American Style, Asda*	1 Serving/240g	394.0	24.0	164	14.0	4.4	10.0	0.3
Stuffing, Sage & Onion & Chipolatas, Breast Joint, Tesco*	½ Pack/280g	507.0	33.0	181	16.2	2.8	11.7	1.9
Stuffing, TTD, Sainsbury's*	1 Slice/34g	50.0	2.0	148	22.7	1.3	5.8	0.9
Sun Dried Tomato & Basil Butter, Sainsbury's*	1 Breast/185g	363.0	18.0	196	25.0	2.5	9.5	0.2
Sun Dried Tomato & Basil Sauce, Bistro, Waitrose*	½ Pack/175g	254.0	14.0	145	14.2	3.7	8.1	0.3
Sweet Chilli & Garlic, Chinese, Asda*	1 Serving/400g	436.0	2.0	109	8.0	18.0	0.6	2.1
Sweet Chilli Noodles, Eat Smart, Morrisons*	1 Pack/380g	236.0	4.0	62	5.9	7.1	1.1	1.3
Sweet Chilli Sauce & Egg Fried Rice, Tesco*	1 Pack/380g	494.0	10.0	130	7.5	18.2	2.7	1.3
Sweet Potato Mash, Jerk, Super Naturals, Sainsbury's*	1 Pack/400g	284.0	4.0	71	6.1	9.2	1.1	2.2
Tagine, Cous Cous, Perfectly Balanced, Waitrose*	1 Pack/400g	516.0	14.0	129	8.2	16.2	3.5	1.0
Tangy Lemon Sauce, Breasts, Just Cook, Sainsbury's*	1 Serving/164g	244.0	3.0	149	16.2	16.9	1.8	0.1
CHICORY								
Fresh, Raw, Average	**1 Av Head/150g**	**30.0**	**1.0**	**20**	**0.6**	**2.8**	**0.6**	**0.9**
CHILLI								
& Lemongrass Prawns with Noodles, BGTY, Sainsbury's*	1 Pack/400g	328.0	3.0	82	5.0	13.8	0.7	1.3
& Potato Wedges, Sainsbury's*	1 Pack/371g	393.0	15.0	106	7.2	10.1	4.1	2.2
& Potato Wedges, Weight Watchers*	1 Pack/400g	364.0	11.0	91	5.4	11.2	2.8	2.5
& Rice, Birds Eye*	1 Serving/285g	305.0	8.0	107	3.4	17.2	2.7	1.0
& Rice, Frozen, Sainsbury's*	1 Pack/400g	436.0	8.0	109	4.8	18.4	1.9	0.6
& Rice, GFY, Asda*	1 Pack/400g	352.0	2.0	88	5.0	16.0	0.4	1.8
& Wedges, BBQ, HL, Tesco*	1 Pack/420g	391.0	11.0	93	5.4	12.2	2.6	1.9
& Wedges, GFY, Asda*	1 Pack/400g	364.0	10.0	91	7.0	10.1	2.5	2.5
Beef & Mushrooms, GFY, Asda*	1 Pack/400g	364.0	6.0	91	9.1	10.2	1.5	1.2
Beef, & Potato Crush, Weight Watchers*	1 Pack/400g	232.0	6.0	58	5.0	5.9	1.5	3.4
Beef, Asda*	½ Pack/200g	190.0	8.0	95	7.0	8.0	3.9	1.2
Beef, with Potato Wedges, Naturally Good Food, Tesco*	1 Pack/440g	352.0	12.0	80	7.2	6.2	2.8	1.8
Beef, with Rice, Sainsbury's*	1 Serving/300g	360.0	5.0	120	5.6	20.6	1.7	1.1
Bowl, American Style, Sainsbury's*	½ Pack/300g	255.0	10.0	85	8.8	4.6	3.5	2.0
Chicken Grande, Stagg*	1 Serving/205g	168.0	1.0	82	9.7	9.4	0.6	1.6
Con Carne with Rice, GFY, Asda*	1 Serving/400g	456.0	6.0	114	6.0	19.0	1.6	0.9

C

	Measure INFO/WEIGHT	per Measure KCAL	per Measure FAT	Nutrition Values per 100g / 100ml KCAL	PROT	CARB	FAT	FIBRE
CHILLI								
Con Carne with Rice, Organic, Sainsbury's*	1 Pack/400g	472.0	11.0	118	5.0	18.5	2.7	1.8
Con Carne with Rice, Perfectly Balanced, Waitrose*	1 Pack/400g	404.0	7.0	101	5.8	15.3	1.8	1.7
Con Carne, 2 Minute Meals, Sainsbury's*	1 Pouch/200g	146.0	3.0	73	6.0	8.6	1.6	2.7
Con Carne, Baked Bean, Heinz*	1 Can/390g	324.0	6.0	83	7.0	10.3	1.5	2.8
Con Carne, BGTY, Sainsbury's*	1 Serving/400g	384.0	9.0	96	5.3	13.8	2.2	2.8
Con Carne, Canned, Morrisons*	1 Can/392g	368.0	12.0	94	8.8	8.0	3.0	2.4
Con Carne, Diet Chef Ltd*	1 Pack/300g	306.0	14.0	102	8.6	6.2	4.8	4.4
Con Carne, Fluffy White Rice, COU, M & S*	1 Pack/400g	360.0	8.0	90	5.7	12.3	1.9	1.5
Con Carne, From Restaurant, Average	1 Serving/253g	256.0	8.0	101	9.7	8.7	3.3	0.0
Con Carne, M & S*	1 Pack/285g	285.0	11.0	100	8.7	7.4	3.7	2.0
Con Carne, Restaurant, Sainsbury's*	1 Serving/100g	80.0	3.0	80	6.9	7.0	2.7	1.5
Con Carne, with Rice, Birds Eye*	1 Pack/285g	291.0	7.0	102	3.3	16.6	2.5	0.8
Con Carne, with Rice, Weight Watchers*	1 Serving/301g	262.0	3.0	87	4.6	14.7	1.1	0.4
Medium, Uncle Ben's*	1 Jar/500g	305.0	4.0	61	1.8	11.1	0.8	0.0
Mexican Chilli with Potato Wedges, Weight Watchers*	1 Pack/300g	249.0	9.0	83	4.6	9.6	2.9	1.3
Mixed Vegetable, Tesco*	1 Pack/400g	352.0	12.0	88	3.9	11.0	2.9	3.2
Non Carne, Linda McCartney*	1 Pack/340g	275.0	8.0	81	5.8	9.2	2.3	1.7
Spicy Bean & Vegetable, Safeway*	1 Pack/311g	196.0	4.0	63	3.3	9.6	1.3	2.5
Spicy, & Wedges, Healthy Options, Birds Eye*	1 Pack/350g	259.0	6.0	74	4.7	9.7	1.8	1.4
Three Bean, Diet Chef Ltd*	1 Pack/300g	195.0	3.0	65	4.0	10.3	0.9	3.6
Vegetable & Rice, BGTY, Sainsbury's*	1 Pack/450g	409.0	5.0	91	3.5	16.7	1.1	3.5
Vegetable & Rice, Safeway*	1 Pack/500g	530.0	4.0	106	3.4	21.2	0.8	1.7
Vegetable Garden, Stagg*	1 Can/410g	254.0	2.0	62	3.6	10.8	0.5	2.3
Vegetable, Canned, Sainsbury's*	1 Can/400g	368.0	2.0	92	5.1	16.7	0.5	4.9
Vegetable, Chesswood*	½ Can/200g	138.0	1.0	69	3.3	13.3	0.3	2.1
Vegetable, Retail	1oz/28g	20.0	1.0	70	4.0	9.4	2.1	0.0
Vegetable, Tinned, GFY, Asda*	½ Can/200g	140.0	2.0	70	3.5	12.0	0.9	3.5
Vegetarian, with Rice, Tesco*	1 Pack/500g	575.0	13.0	115	4.0	19.0	2.6	1.8
CHINESE LEAF								
Fresh, Raw, Average	***1oz/28g***	***4.0***	***0.0***	***14***	***1.5***	***1.5***	***0.2***	***1.7***
CHIPS								
& Curry Sauce, Tesco*	1 Serving/400g	440.0	20.0	110	2.1	14.1	5.0	1.0
11mm Fresh, Deep Fried, McCain*	1oz/28g	66.0	3.0	235	3.2	31.8	10.6	0.0
14mm Fresh, Deep Fried, McCain*	1oz/28g	59.0	2.0	209	2.7	34.2	6.8	0.0
American Style, Oven, Sainsbury's*	1 Serving/165g	313.0	14.0	190	5.4	23.6	8.3	1.3
American Style, Thin, Oven, Tesco*	1 Serving/125g	210.0	8.0	168	2.7	24.6	6.5	2.1
Beefeater, Deep Fried, McCain*	1oz/28g	71.0	3.0	253	3.3	37.7	9.9	0.0
Beefeater, Oven Baked, McCain*	1oz/28g	55.0	2.0	195	4.0	32.2	5.6	0.0
Chunky Oven, Harry Ramsden's*	1 Serving/150g	184.0	5.0	123	2.8	19.9	3.6	1.6
Chunky, COU, M & S*	1 Serving/150g	157.0	2.0	105	2.1	20.5	1.6	2.3
Chunky, Fresh, Chilled, Finest, Tesco*	1 Pack/450g	607.0	18.0	135	2.1	22.3	4.0	2.7
Chunky, Ready to Bake, M & S*	1 Serving/200g	310.0	8.0	155	2.2	26.8	4.2	2.0
Chunky, Waitrose*	1 Portion/155g	200.0	9.0	129	1.9	17.6	5.7	2.8
Crinkle Cut, M & S*	1 Serving/150g	270.0	8.0	180	3.3	29.5	5.4	2.4
Crinkle Cut, Oven Baked, Aunt Bessie's*	1 Serving/100g	206.0	9.0	206	2.9	28.0	9.2	3.2
Crinkle Cut, Oven, Asda*	1 Serving/100g	134.0	4.0	134	2.0	23.0	3.8	8.0
Fat, with Fluffy Centres, M & S*	1 Serving/200g	210.0	9.0	105	1.6	14.2	4.5	1.8
Fried, Chip Shop, Average	1 Serving/400g	956.0	50.0	239	3.2	30.5	12.4	2.2
Frozen, Crinkle Cut, Aunt Bessie's*	1 Serving/100g	163.0	7.0	163	3.1	21.3	7.3	2.2
Frying, Crinkle Cut, Tesco*	1 Serving/125g	161.0	4.0	129	2.6	22.2	3.3	1.9
Homefries, Chunky, Weighed Baked, McCain*	1 Serving/100g	153.0	3.0	153	3.2	28.0	3.1	2.3
Homefries, Chunky, Weighed Frozen, McCain*	1 Serving/100g	123.0	2.0	123	2.5	22.6	2.5	1.6
Homefries, Crinkle Cut, Weighed Baked, McCain*	1 Serving/100g	197.0	6.0	197	3.0	31.7	6.5	2.5

	Measure INFO/WEIGHT	per Measure KCAL	per Measure FAT	Nutrition Values per 100g / 100ml KCAL	PROT	CARB	FAT	FIBRE
CHIPS								
Homefries, Crinkle Cut, Weighed Frozen, McCain*	1 Serving/100g	197.0	6.0	197	3.0	31.7	6.5	2.5
Homefries, Jacket Oven, McCain*	1 Serving/100g	220.0	7.0	220	3.9	37.9	7.4	0.0
Homefries, Straight Cut, Weighed Baked, McCain*	1 Serving/100g	181.0	6.0	181	3.1	28.1	6.2	2.4
Homefries, Straight Cut, Weighed Frozen, McCain*	1 Serving/100g	134.0	5.0	134	2.2	21.0	4.6	1.7
Homefries, Thin & Crispy, Weighed Frozen, McCain*	1 Serving/100g	143.0	4.0	143	2.6	24.0	4.1	1.5
Homemade, Fried in Oil, Average	1oz/28g	53.0	2.0	189	3.9	30.1	6.7	2.2
Homestyle Oven, Sainsbury's*	1 Serving/125g	206.0	5.0	165	2.4	29.2	4.3	2.1
Just Bake, Low Fat, M & S*	1oz/28g	37.0	1.0	133	2.0	24.7	3.7	1.7
Microwave, Cooked	1oz/28g	62.0	3.0	221	3.6	32.1	9.6	2.9
Oven, 5% Fat, Frozen, McCain*	1 Serving/200g	238.0	6.0	119	1.9	21.0	3.0	1.6
Oven, Best in the World, Iceland*	1 Serving/175g	332.0	12.0	190	3.4	28.9	6.7	3.5
Oven, Chunky, Extra Special, Asda*	1 Serving/125g	237.0	7.0	190	3.4	31.5	5.6	3.2
Oven, Chunky, Ross*	1 Serving/100g	177.0	6.0	177	3.1	26.6	6.5	3.9
Oven, Cooked, Weight Watchers*	1 Serving/100g	150.0	3.0	150	2.8	33.7	3.0	5.9
Oven, Crinkle Cut, 5% Fat, Weighed Baked, McCain*	1 Serving/100g	163.0	4.0	163	3.1	27.9	4.3	3.0
Oven, Crinkle Cut, 5% Fat, Weighed Frozen, McCain*	1 Serving/100g	134.0	4.0	134	2.4	23.2	3.6	2.4
Oven, Crinkle Cut, Sainsbury's*	1 Serving/165g	297.0	9.0	180	3.3	29.5	5.5	2.4
Oven, Frozen, Baked	1oz/28g	45.0	1.0	162	3.2	29.8	4.2	2.0
Oven, Homefries, McCain*	1 Serving/100g	134.0	5.0	134	2.2	21.0	4.6	1.7
Oven, Morrisons*	1 Serving/100g	134.0	4.0	134	2.4	22.2	3.9	0.0
Oven, Organic, Waitrose*	1 Serving/165g	233.0	6.0	141	1.5	25.1	3.8	1.6
Oven, Original, McCain*	1 Serving/100g	158.0	4.0	158	2.5	28.5	3.8	2.3
Oven, Original, Straight Cut, 5% Fat, Cooked, McCain*	1 Serving/100g	172.0	5.0	172	3.4	32.4	4.9	2.3
Oven, Original, Straight Cut, 5% Fat, Frozen, McCain*	1 Serving/100g	138.0	4.0	138	2.5	26.2	4.0	1.9
Oven, Reduced Fat, Waitrose*	1oz/28g	37.0	1.0	133	2.3	24.3	3.0	1.6
Oven, Steak Cut, Waitrose*	1 Serving/165g	218.0	6.0	132	2.7	22.7	3.4	1.7
Oven, Steakhouse, Frozen, Tesco*	1 Serving/125g	165.0	4.0	132	2.7	22.7	3.4	1.7
Oven, Straight Cut, 5% Fat, Sainsbury's*	1 Serving/165g	280.0	8.0	170	3.4	28.0	4.9	2.5
Oven, Straight Cut, Asda*	1 Serving/100g	199.0	5.0	199	3.5	35.0	5.0	3.0
Oven, Straight Cut, Waitrose*	1 Serving/165g	219.0	6.0	133	2.0	23.0	3.7	1.7
Oven, Sweet Potato, Tesco*	1 ¼ Pack/125g	169.0	6.0	135	2.6	18.9	5.2	5.0
Oven, Thick Cut, Frozen, Baked	1oz/28g	44.0	1.0	157	3.2	27.9	4.4	1.8
Oven, Thin & Crispy, Tesco*	1 Portion/100g	205.0	5.0	205	2.7	37.6	4.9	5.8
Oven, Thin Cut, American Style, Asda*	1 Serving/100g	240.0	10.0	240	3.4	34.0	10.0	3.0
Oven, Thin Fries, Morrisons*	1 Serving/100g	161.0	6.0	161	2.9	23.6	6.1	1.2
Steak Cut, Frying, Asda*	1 Serving/97g	181.0	7.0	187	2.9	28.0	7.0	2.8
Straight Cut, Frozen, Fried in Blended Oil	1oz/28g	76.0	4.0	273	4.1	36.0	13.5	2.4
Straight Cut, Frozen, Fried in Corn Oil	1oz/28g	76.0	4.0	273	4.1	36.0	13.5	2.4
Thick Cut, Caterpack, Deep Fried, McCain*	1oz/28g	60.0	3.0	215	3.1	28.8	9.7	0.0
Thick Cut, Frozen, Fried in Corn Oil, Average	1oz/28g	66.0	3.0	234	3.6	34.0	10.2	2.4
Three Way Cook, Skinny, Co-Op*	1 Serving/100g	175.0	7.0	175	2.0	26.0	7.0	3.0
Vending 3/8" Straight Cut, Deep Fried, McCain*	1oz/28g	62.0	3.0	220	3.3	29.6	9.8	0.0
Waffle, Birds Eye*	1 Serving/75g	156.0	8.0	208	2.5	24.3	11.2	2.6
CHIVES								
Fresh, Average	*1 Tsp/2g*	*0.0*	*0.0*	*23*	*2.8*	*1.7*	*0.6*	*1.9*
CHOC ICES								
Average	1 Ice/50g	138.0	9.0	277	3.5	28.1	17.5	0.0
Belgian Milk, Sainsbury's*	1 Ice/80ml	170.0	11.0	212	1.9	21.1	13.4	0.5
Chocolate, Dark, Seriously Creamy, Waitrose*	1 Ice/82g	195.0	13.0	238	2.6	21.6	15.7	1.7
Chocolate, Real Milk, Sainsbury's*	1 Ice/48g	151.0	10.0	312	3.5	30.3	19.7	0.8
Chunky, Wall's Ice Cream*	1 Ice/81g	162.0	11.0	200	2.6	18.9	13.1	0.0
Dark, Sainsbury's*	1 Ice/43g	136.0	10.0	315	3.8	25.5	22.0	0.4
Dark, Tesco*	1 Ice/43g	141.0	9.0	325	2.8	30.2	21.0	0.1

	Measure INFO/WEIGHT		per Measure KCAL FAT		Nutrition Values per 100g / 100ml				
					KCAL	PROT	CARB	FAT	FIBRE
CHOC ICES									
Light, Sainsbury's*	1 Ice/43g		135.0	9.0	313	3.2	27.0	21.4	0.3
Light, Waitrose*	1 Ice/70ml		141.0	10.0	201	1.7	17.0	14.3	0.3
Neapolitan Chocolate, Co-Op*	1 Ice/62g		120.0	8.0	194	2.0	16.9	13.2	0.4
Rum & Raisin, Safeway*	1 Ice/45g		136.0	9.0	303	3.3	28.9	19.3	1.1
Vanilla, Co-Op*	1 Ice/70g		130.0	12.0	186	3.6	3.6	17.1	0.0
White Chocolate, Sainsbury's*	1 Ice/48g		140.0	9.0	292	3.8	27.3	18.6	0.1
White, Real, Tesco*	1 Ice/52g		198.0	14.0	381	4.0	26.9	27.6	1.1
CHOCOLATE									
Advent Calendar, Dairy Milk, Cadbury*	1 Chocolate/4.2g		22.0	1.0	525	7.5	56.6	30.1	0.7
Advent Calendar, Magic of Christmas, Cadbury*	1 Chocolate/9.5g		48.0	3.0	510	7.0	57.7	28.0	0.7
Advent Calendar, Maltesers, Mars*	1 Chocolate/4g		21.0	1.0	537	6.8	57.9	30.9	0.0
Advent Calendar, Milky Bar, Nestle*	1 Chocolate/4g		22.0	1.0	547	7.3	58.4	31.7	0.0
Almond & Honey, Dairy Milk, Cadbury*	1 Sm Bar/54g		281.0	16.0	520	8.0	57.1	28.9	1.0
Animal Bar, Nestle*	1 Bar/19g		97.0	5.0	513	5.8	63.6	26.1	0.0
Baking, Belgian, Milk, for Cakes, Luxury, Sainsbury's*	1 Chunk/8g		44.0	3.0	556	7.6	56.5	33.3	1.5
Baking, Continental, for Home Baking, Luxury, Tesco*	1 Pack/150g		822.0	68.0	548	2.7	27.7	45.1	0.9
Baking, Milk, for Home Baking, Luxury, Tesco*	1 Pack/150g		838.0	54.0	559	7.0	51.4	36.2	1.7
Bar, Apricot & Raisin, Thorntons*	1 Bar/40g		185.0	11.0	462	8.0	46.0	27.3	3.5
Bar, Cappuccino, Thorntons*	1 Bar/38g		201.0	13.0	529	5.2	49.7	34.7	0.5
Bar, Chunky Hazelnut, M & S*	1 Bar/52g		293.0	19.0	563	8.8	48.1	37.3	1.7
Bar, Dark Chocolate, Diabetic, Thorntons*	1 Bar/75g		345.0	27.0	460	5.4	28.5	35.8	8.1
Bar, Dark, 60% Cocoa, with Macadamia, Thorntons*	1 Bar/70g		183.0	13.0	523	6.5	42.3	36.5	12.6
Bar, Dark, Thorntons*	1 Sm Bar/48g		250.0	18.0	521	7.3	39.9	36.9	10.9
Bar, Dark, with Ginger, Thorntons*	1 Bar/100g		509.0	35.0	509	5.8	44.3	35.1	8.8
Bar, Extra Dark, 60% Cocoa, Lindor, Lindt*	1 Bar/150g		900.0	73.0	600	5.0	35.0	49.0	2.0
Bar, Hazel Nut & Cashew, Dairy Milk, Cadbury*	3 Chunks/18g		96.0	6.0	540	8.8	50.6	33.5	1.8
Bar, Jazz Orange, Thorntons*	1 Bar/56g		304.0	18.0	543	6.8	55.7	32.3	1.2
Bar, Milk Chocolate, Diabetic, Thorntons*	½ Bar/37g		174.0	12.0	470	7.3	43.0	33.1	2.2
Bar, Milk, Thorntons*	1 Sm Bar/50g		269.0	16.0	538	7.5	54.8	32.0	1.0
Bar, Twisted, Creme Egg, Cadbury*	1 Bar/45g		210.0	9.0	465	5.2	64.6	20.8	0.5
Bar, Viennese, Continental, Thorntons*	1 Bar/38g		206.0	13.0	542	4.2	53.9	34.2	0.8
Bar, White, Thorntons*	1 Bar/50g		273.0	16.0	547	6.5	59.5	31.3	0.0
Bars, Alpini, Continental, Thorntons*	1 Bar/36g		192.0	11.0	538	6.9	55.3	32.0	2.7
Bars, Bubbles, Galaxy, Mars*	1 Bar/31g		169.0	10.0	544	6.6	56.1	32.5	0.0
Bars, Chocolate, Cherry, Lindt*	1 Bar/100g		470.0	23.0	470	4.5	61.7	22.8	0.0
Bars, Chocolate, Pistacho, Lindt*	1 Bar/100g		585.0	41.0	585	7.1	48.2	40.5	0.0
Bars, Chocolate, Strawberry, Lindt*	1 Bar/100g		470.0	23.0	470	4.5	61.6	22.8	0.0
Bars, Chocoletti, Stracciatella, Lindt*	1 Bar/5.5g		32.0	2.0	590	7.7	49.0	41.0	0.0
Bars, Milk Chocolate, Galaxy, Mars*	1 Bar/46g		250.0	15.0	544	6.6	56.3	32.5	1.5
Bars, Milk Chocolate, Gold, Lindt*	1 Bar/300g		1605.0	93.0	535	6.6	58.7	31.0	0.0
Bars, Milk Chocolate, Hazelnut, Gold, Lindt*	1 Bar/300g		1665.0	108.0	555	7.9	50.7	36.1	0.0
Bars, Milk Chocolate, Hazelnut, Lindt*	1 Bar/100g		570.0	39.0	570	8.5	47.0	38.8	0.0
Bars, Milk Chocolate, Lindt*	1 Bar/100g		535.0	31.0	535	6.6	57.6	31.0	0.0
Bars, Milk Chocolate, Raisin & Hazelnut, Gold, Lindt*	1 Bar/300g		1590.0	95.0	530	6.8	54.7	31.6	0.0
Bars, Milk Chocolate, Raisin & Hazelnut, Lindt*	1 Bar/ 100g		530.0	32.0	530	3.1	54.7	31.6	0.0
Beans, Coffee, Dark, Solid, M & S*	1 Serving/10g		53.0	4.0	532	4.7	42.4	37.6	11.6
Bear, Lindt*	1 Bear/84g		480.0	29.0	572	7.5	57.7	34.6	0.0
Belgian Milk, TTD, Sainsbury's*	1 Piece/10g		55.0	4.0	549	9.6	48.3	35.3	2.0
Black Magic, Nestle*	1oz/28g		128.0	6.0	456	4.4	62.6	20.8	1.6
Breakaway, Nestle*	1 Bar/20g		100.0	5.0	499	6.5	61.1	25.2	0.0
Bubbly, Dairy Milk, Cadbury*	1 Bar/35g		185.0	10.0	525	7.7	56.9	29.7	0.7
Bunny, Easter, Mars*	1 Bunny/29g		155.0	9.0	535	6.2	56.2	31.7	0.0
Bunny, Lindt*	1 Bunny/84g		480.0	29.0	572	7.5	57.5	34.6	0.0

CHOCOLATE

	Measure INFO/WEIGHT	per Measure KCAL	FAT	Nutrition Values per 100g / 100ml KCAL	PROT	CARB	FAT	FIBRE
Cappuccino, Nestle*	1 Serving/20g	109.0	7.0	545	6.1	56.0	32.9	0.0
Caramel, Chunk, Dairy Milk, Cadbury*	1 Chunk/33g	158.0	8.0	480	5.0	63.0	23.0	0.0
Caramel, Dairy Milk, Cadbury*	1 Bar/50g	240.0	12.0	480	4.9	62.1	23.5	0.4
Choco Swing, Kraft*	1 Square/16g	89.0	6.0	555	5.7	54.0	34.5	0.0
Chocolat Noir, Lindt*	1/6 Bar/17g	87.0	5.0	510	6.0	50.0	32.0	0.0
Chomp, Cadbury*	1 Bar/24g	112.0	5.0	465	3.3	67.9	20.0	0.2
Coconut, White, Excellence, Lindt*	1 Square/10g	61.0	4.0	610	6.0	48.0	44.0	0.0
Cool & Delicious, Dairy Milk, Cadbury*	1 Bar/21g	110.0	6.0	525	7.6	56.1	30.1	0.0
Crispies, Chunk, Dairy Milk, Cadbury*	1 Chunk/31g	158.0	8.0	510	7.6	58.6	27.4	0.0
Crispies, Dairy Milk, Cadbury*	1 Bar/49g	250.0	13.0	510	7.6	58.6	27.4	0.0
Crispy, Sainsbury's*	4 Squares/19g	99.0	5.0	521	9.1	56.9	28.5	2.1
Dairy Milk, Cadbury*	1 Bar/49g	255.0	15.0	520	7.5	56.9	29.8	0.6
Dark, 70% Cocoa Solida, Extra Fine, Lindt*	1 Square/10g	54.0	4.0	537	8.0	33.0	41.0	0.0
Dark, 70% Cocoa Solids, Organic, Green & Black's*	1 Sm Bar/35g	193.0	14.0	551	9.3	36.0	41.1	11.5
Dark, 70% Cocoa Solids, Organic, Morrisons*	½ Bar/50g	265.0	21.0	531	7.9	31.6	41.1	11.0
Dark, 85% Cocoa, Excellence, Lindt*	1 Serving/40g	212.0	18.0	530	11.0	19.0	46.0	0.0
Dark, 85% Cocoa, TTD, Sainsbury's*	1 Serving/25g	142.0	13.0	569	9.7	17.0	51.4	14.1
Dark, 99% Cocoa, Excellence, Lindt*	1 serving/25g	132.0	12.0	530	13.0	8.0	50.0	8.0
Dark, Belgian, Luxury Continental, Sainsbury's*	1 Bar/100g	490.0	39.0	490	11.1	24.2	38.7	7.4
Dark, Chilli, Excellence, Lindt*	1 Serving/40g	202.0	13.0	506	5.4	49.0	32.0	0.0
Dark, Classic, Bourneville, Cadbury*	1 99 Cal Bar/18g	87.0	5.0	495	4.0	61.1	26.3	6.0
Dark, Continental, Luxury, Tesco*	1 Bar/100g	571.0	38.0	571	11.3	46.5	37.8	0.1
Dark, Espresso, with Coffee, Organic, Green & Black's*	1 Bar/150g	823.0	62.0	549	9.8	33.8	41.6	11.7
Dark, Luxury Continental, Sainsbury's*	½ Bar/50g	252.0	20.0	504	10.7	25.5	40.0	16.1
Dark, Orange with Slivered Almonds, Excellence, Lindt*	1 Square/10g	50.0	3.0	500	6.0	46.0	30.0	0.0
Dark, Plain, Average	**1oz/28g**	**143.0**	**8.0**	**510**	**5.0**	**63.5**	**28.0**	**2.5**
Dark, Raw Organic, Loving Earth*	1 Av Serving/20g	99.0	8.0	495	9.3	46.4	39.5	0.0
Dark, Rich, Tesco*	1 Serving/20g	98.0	6.0	491	5.8	60.0	30.4	11.5
Dark, Smooth, Bar, Galaxy, Mars*	1 Bar/125g	651.0	42.0	521	6.2	48.0	33.6	9.3
Dark, Special, Hershey*	1 Pack/41g	180.0	12.0	439	4.9	61.0	29.3	7.3
Dark, Whole Nut, Tesco*	1 Serving/13g	67.0	4.0	539	6.1	48.3	35.7	6.5
Dark, with a Soft Mint Centre, Organic, Green & Black's*	1 Bar/100g	478.0	27.0	478	7.4	50.5	27.3	8.6
Dark, with Chilli, Thorntons*	4 Squares/20g	107.0	8.0	533	7.2	36.3	39.5	10.4
Dark, with Hazelnuts & Currant, Organic, Green & Black's*	1 Bar/100g	513.0	33.0	513	7.6	45.4	33.5	9.2
Dark, with Orange & Spices, Maya Gold, Green & Black's*	1 Sm Bar/35g	184.0	12.0	526	7.3	48.2	33.8	8.2
Double Blend, Nestle*	1 Rectangle/11g	61.0	4.0	553	7.3	55.9	33.0	0.0
Double Chocolate, Nestle*	1 Serving/25g	133.0	8.0	532	9.1	49.4	33.1	0.0
Dream, with Real Strawberries, Cadbury*	1 Bar/45.0g	250.0	15.0	555	4.5	59.6	33.1	0.0
Drops, Plain, Sainsbury's*	1 Serving/125g	637.0	34.0	510	5.3	60.1	27.6	4.0
Egg, Double Cream, Nestle*	1 Egg/28.0g	163.0	11.0	582	6.9	49.2	39.7	0.4
Egg, Mars*	1 Egg/38g	183.0	9.0	482	5.3	59.7	24.7	0.0
Freddo, Caramel, Dairy Milk, Cadbury*	1 Bar/19.6g	95.0	5.0	485	5.5	60.2	24.6	0.0
Freddo, Dairy Milk, Cadbury*	1 Freddo/20g	105.0	6.0	525	7.5	57.0	29.8	0.7
Fruit & Nut, Belgian, Waitrose*	1 Serving/50g	254.0	15.0	508	8.6	54.6	29.2	3.4
Fruit & Nut, Dark, Tesco*	4 Squares/25g	123.0	7.0	494	5.8	54.8	27.9	6.5
Fudge, Keto Bar*	1 Serving/65g	250.0	7.0	385	36.9	36.9	10.8	32.3
Ginger, Traidcraft*	1 Bar/50g	212.0	7.0	424	3.9	68.2	14.8	0.0
Hazelnut & Walnut, Dark, Organic, Seeds of Change*	1 Bar/100g	559.0	42.0	559	8.4	37.5	41.7	9.2
Kinder Maxi, Ferrero*	1 Bar/21g	115.0	7.0	550	10.0	51.0	34.0	0.0
Kinder Surprise, Ferrero*	1 Egg/20g	110.0	7.0	550	10.0	51.0	34.0	0.4
Kinder, Bueno Bar, Ferrero*	1 Bar/21.5g	121.0	8.0	563	9.8	46.6	37.5	0.0
Kinder, Riegel, Ferrero*	1 Bar/21g	117.0	7.0	558	10.0	53.0	34.0	0.0
Kitten, Milk Chocolate, Lindt*	1 Kitten/84g	480.0	29.0	572	7.5	57.7	34.6	0.0

CHOCOLATE

	Measure INFO/WEIGHT	per Measure KCAL	FAT	Nutrition Values per 100g / 100ml KCAL	PROT	CARB	FAT	FIBRE
Lait Intense, Experiences, Cote D'or*	3 Squares/100g	575.0	40.0	575	7.2	44.5	40.0	5.0
Light & Whippy, Bite Sized, Sainsbury's*	1 Bar/15.0g	66.0	2.0	439	3.3	69.7	16.3	0.1
Little Bars, Dairy Milk, Cadbury*	1 Bar/20.8g	110.0	6.0	530	7.7	56.6	30.1	0.7
Macadamia Nut. Excellence, Lindt*	1 Bar/100g	560.0	37.0	560	7.0	51.0	37.0	0.0
Milk, & Hazelnut, Bar, Swiss, M & S*	1oz/28g	156.0	10.0	556	6.4	51.9	36.0	3.3
Milk, A Darker Shade of Milk Chocolate, Green & Black's*	1 Sm Bar/35g	183.0	10.0	523	9.9	54.0	29.7	3.7
Milk, Average	*1oz/28g*	*146.0*	*9.0*	*520*	*7.7*	*56.9*	*30.7*	*0.8*
Milk, Bubbly, Swiss, M & S*	1 Serving/40g	218.0	14.0	545	8.0	52.0	34.3	2.5
Milk, Extra Au Lait, Milch Extra, Lindt*	½ Bar/50g	267.0	15.0	535	6.5	57.0	31.0	0.0
Milk, Extra Creamy, Excellence, Lindt*	1 Bar/100g	560.0	37.0	560	6.0	51.1	37.1	0.0
Milk, Extra Fine, Swiss, M & S*	1 Serving/25g	141.0	9.0	565	7.2	50.9	36.7	2.3
Milk, Fair Trade, Tesco*	1 Serving/45g	236.0	13.0	524	7.6	56.7	29.6	2.0
Milk, Fimbles Bar, Kinnerton*	1 Bar/12g	65.0	4.0	539	5.8	57.0	31.8	1.9
Milk, Less Than 99 Calories, M & S*	1 Bar/16g	85.0	5.0	531	7.5	61.2	28.7	0.6
Milk, Lindor, Lindt*	1 Square/11g	68.0	5.0	615	4.7	43.0	47.0	0.0
Milk, Santas, Tesco*	1 Bag/90g	433.0	22.0	481	4.5	61.4	24.2	1.4
Milk, Super Naturals, Sainsbury's*	4 Pieces/40g	85.0	5.0	212	2.4	23.0	12.2	0.9
Milk, Swiss Made, Organic, Traidcraft*	4 Squares/17g	91.0	6.0	550	7.0	50.0	34.0	0.0
Milk, Whole Nut, Tesco*	1 Serving/25g	129.0	8.0	517	8.7	53.4	33.8	9.0
Milk, Winnie the Pooh, Solid Shapes, M & S*	1 Chocolate/6g	32.0	2.0	540	8.1	54.1	32.4	1.3
Milk, with Biscuit Pieces, Asda*	2 Squares/14g	73.0	4.0	521	8.0	57.0	29.0	1.9
Milk, with Honey & Almond Nougat, Swiss, Toblerone*	1 Piece/8g	42.0	2.0	525	5.4	59.0	29.5	2.2
Milk, with Peanut Butter Filling, Ghirardelli*	1 Serving/45g	250.0	17.0	556	8.9	48.9	37.8	2.2
Milk, with Raisins & Hazelnuts, Green & Black's*	1 Bar/100g	556.0	37.0	556	9.2	46.8	36.9	3.2
Milk, with Whole Almonds, Organic, Green & Black's*	1 Bar/100g	578.0	42.0	578	11.8	37.7	42.2	5.2
Mini, Toblerone*	1 Serving/6g	31.0	2.0	525	5.6	57.5	30.0	3.5
Mint Chips, Chunk, Dairy Milk, Cadbury*	1 Chunk/32g	162.0	8.0	505	6.5	61.2	26.1	0.0
Mint Creme, Sainsbury's*	1 Serving/20g	93.0	5.0	467	2.8	62.7	24.5	2.1
Mint Crisp, Sainsbury's*	4 Squares/19g	95.0	5.0	501	5.0	63.7	25.0	3.6
Mountain Bar, Swiss, M & S*	1 Bar/100g	555.0	35.0	555	6.5	55.2	35.3	0.2
Mountain Bar, with Orange, Swiss, M & S*	½ Bar/50g	267.0	16.0	535	8.0	52.2	32.8	3.2
Natural Orange, Excellence, Lindt*	1 Bar/100g	560.0	37.0	560	7.0	50.0	37.0	0.0
Natural Vanilla, Excellence, Lindt*	1 Bar/100g	590.0	40.0	590	6.0	51.0	40.0	0.0
NutRageous, Reese's, Hershey*	1 Bar/51g	260.0	16.0	510	11.8	54.9	31.4	3.9
Nuts About Caramel, Cadbury*	1 Bar/55g	272.0	15.0	495	5.8	56.6	27.4	0.0
Nutty Nougat, Bite Sized, Sainsbury's*	1 Bar/23g	111.0	5.0	481	7.6	59.0	23.8	0.6
Old Jamaica, Cadbury*	1oz/28g	129.0	7.0	460	5.8	56.9	23.3	0.0
Orange Cream, Fry's*	1 Bar/50g	210.0	7.0	420	2.8	72.3	13.7	0.0
Orange, Fair Trade, Divine Foods*	4 Squares/17g	92.0	5.0	541	6.5	57.7	31.5	0.0
Orange, Sainsbury's*	4 Squares/19g	100.0	6.0	531	9.2	54.3	30.7	2.2
Panna Cotta & Raspberry, M & S*	1 Bar/36g	190.0	12.0	528	4.7	51.4	33.6	0.3
Peppermint Cream, Fry's*	1 Bar/51g	217.0	8.0	425	2.6	68.8	15.4	0.0
Praline, M & S*	1 Bar/34g	185.0	12.0	545	7.3	49.6	35.2	3.1
Rafaello, Roche, Ferrero*	1 Sweet/10g	60.0	5.0	600	9.7	35.4	46.6	0.0
Snickers, More Nuts, Snickers*	1 Bar/58g	299.0	17.0	515	10.1	52.8	29.8	0.0
Turkish Delight, Large Bar, Dairy Milk, Cadbury*	1 Square/7.5g	35.0	2.0	470	5.6	63.2	21.4	0.5
Wafer, Dairy Milk, Cadbury*	1 Bar/46g	235.0	13.0	510	7.7	57.0	28.0	0.0
White, Average	*1oz/28g*	*148.0*	*9.0*	*529*	*8.0*	*58.3*	*30.9*	*0.0*
White, Bar, Swiss, M & S*	1oz/28g	152.0	9.0	543	8.0	58.3	30.9	0.0
White, Creamy Vanilla, Green & Black's*	1 Sm Bar/35g	201.0	13.0	573	7.4	53.5	36.6	0.1
White, Crispy, Fair Trade, Co-Op*	½ Bar/50g	277.0	17.0	555	9.0	51.0	35.0	0.1
White, Double Berry, Nestle*	¼ Bar/30g	167.0	10.0	556	6.6	54.9	34.5	0.0
White, Nestle*	4 Pieces/40g	220.0	13.0	550	7.5	55.0	32.5	0.0

CHOCOLATE	Measure INFO/WEIGHT	per Measure KCAL	FAT	KCAL	PROT	CARB	FAT	FIBRE
White, No Added Sugar, Belgian, Boots*	1 Serving/30g	146.0	11.0	488	6.0	47.8	36.0	7.0
White, with Honey & Almond Nougat, Toblerone*	1 Serving/25g	132.0	7.0	530	6.2	60.5	29.0	0.2
White, with Strawberry Pieces, Under 99 Cals, M & S*	1 Bar/16g	86.0	5.0	540	6.6	60.4	30.4	0.3
Whole Nut, Dairy Milk, Cadbury*	1 Bar/49.1g	270.0	17.0	550	8.9	49.5	35.4	1.7
Whole Nut, Sainsbury's*	4 Chunks/25g	141.0	9.0	566	8.5	48.5	37.6	2.6
Whole Nut, Smart Price, Asda*	½ Bar/16g	92.0	6.0	562	8.0	47.0	38.0	3.3
with Almonds, Nestle*	1 Square/20g	109.0	7.0	547	9.2	48.7	35.1	0.1
with Creme Egg, Dairy Milk, Cadbury*	1 Bar/45g	210.0	9.0	470	5.2	64.8	20.9	0.5
with Crunchie Bits, Dairy Milk, Cadbury*	1 Bar/200g	1000.0	49.0	500	6.2	63.3	24.4	0.0
with Shortcake Biscuit, Dairy Milk, Cadbury*	1 Square/6g	31.0	2.0	520	7.5	59.0	28.0	0.0
CHOCOLATE DROPS								
Plain, Asda*	1 Serving/100g	489.0	29.0	489	7.0	50.0	29.0	10.0
White, for Cooking & Decorating, Sainsbury's*	1oz/28g	152.0	9.0	544	6.5	60.3	30.8	0.0
CHOCOLATE NUTS								
Almonds, Dark Chocolate Covered, Bolero*	2 Almonds/3g	15.0	1.0	510	2.6	48.8	33.5	0.0
Peanuts, Assorted, Thorntons*	1 Bag/140g	785.0	57.0	561	13.8	34.8	40.8	3.6
Peanuts, Belgian Coated, M & S*	1 Serving/20g	109.0	8.0	545	14.7	35.6	38.0	5.8
Peanuts, Co-Op*	1oz/28g	153.0	11.0	545	15.0	34.0	39.0	4.0
Peanuts, Milk, Tesco*	1 Bag/227g	1221.0	86.0	538	17.5	31.8	37.9	4.4
CHOCOLATE ORANGE								
Bar, Montana*	1 Serving/25g	131.0	7.0	523	7.0	62.2	27.4	0.0
Crunchball, Terry's*	1 Segment/9g	45.0	2.0	520	6.9	59.8	28.1	2.0
Dark, Terry's*	1 Segment/9g	45.0	3.0	511	4.3	57.0	29.3	6.2
Egg & Spoon, Terry's*	1 Egg/34g	195.0	13.0	575	5.5	51.6	38.0	1.7
Goes Minty, Terry's*	3 Slices/26g	133.0	8.0	510	4.3	57.0	29.5	6.2
Milk, Mini Segments, Terry's*	1 Segment/8g	42.0	2.0	527	7.7	57.9	29.4	2.1
Milk, Terry's*	1 Orange/175g	931.0	52.0	532	7.4	57.8	29.5	2.1
Plain, Terry's*	1 Orange/175g	889.0	51.0	508	3.8	56.8	29.4	6.2
Segsations, Terry's*	1 Segsation/8g	43.0	2.0	520	6.9	58.5	28.5	2.8
White, Terry's*	1 Segment/11g	61.0	3.0	535	6.3	60.9	29.4	0.0
CHOCOLATE RAISINS								
Assorted, Thorntons*	1 Bag/140g	601.0	28.0	429	4.2	58.8	19.7	2.9
Bonds Sweetstars*	1 Serving/28g	109.0	4.0	391	4.7	57.0	16.0	0.0
Californian, Belgian White Chocolate, M & S*	1 Pack/100g	450.0	21.0	450	4.3	60.6	20.9	0.8
Californian, Tesco*	¼ Bag/57g	268.0	12.0	472	5.2	66.2	20.7	1.3
Coated, Californian, M & S*	1 Bag/130g	520.0	19.0	400	4.3	63.2	14.7	1.9
Co-Op*	¼ Pack/50g	205.0	7.0	410	4.0	64.0	15.0	1.0
Jameson's*	1 Serving/23g	96.0	4.0	418	4.7	62.7	16.5	1.4
M & S*	1oz/28g	116.0	4.0	414	4.5	66.5	14.6	1.2
Milk, Asda*	1 Serving/28g	127.0	6.0	452	6.0	62.0	20.0	1.2
Milk, Co-Op*	½ Bag/100g	420.0	17.0	420	5.0	63.0	17.0	6.0
Milk, Sainsbury's*	1oz/28g	117.0	5.0	418	4.7	62.7	16.5	1.4
Milk, Tesco*	1 Lge Bag/227g	933.0	35.0	411	4.8	63.3	15.4	0.9
CHOCOLATE SPREAD								
Average	*1 Tsp/12g*	*68.0*	*5.0*	*569*	*4.1*	*57.1*	*37.6*	*0.0*
with Nuts	*1 Tsp/12g*	*66.0*	*4.0*	*549*	*6.2*	*60.5*	*33.0*	*0.8*
CHOCOLATES								
All Gold, Dark, Terry's*	1 Serving/30g	151.0	9.0	505	4.0	57.5	29.0	4.3
All Gold, Milk, Terry's*	1 Serving/30g	157.0	9.0	525	4.8	58.0	30.5	1.5
Almond Marzipan, Milk Chocolate, Thorntons*	1 Chocolate/13g	60.0	3.0	464	6.6	59.4	22.6	5.6
Almond Mocca Mousse, Thorntons*	1 Chocolate/14g	76.0	5.0	543	8.5	40.7	37.9	2.9
Alpini, Thorntons*	1 Chocolate/13g	70.0	4.0	538	7.0	54.6	32.3	2.3
Assortment, Occasions, Tesco*	1 Chocolate/15g	70.0	3.0	470	4.6	65.8	20.9	0.5

C

CHOCOLATES

Measure INFO/WEIGHT	per Measure KCAL	FAT	KCAL	PROT	CARB	FAT	FIBRE

	Measure INFO/WEIGHT	per Measure KCAL	FAT	KCAL	PROT	CARB	FAT	FIBRE
Big Purple One, Nestle*	1 Chocolate/39g	191.0	10.0	489	5.0	60.2	25.4	0.6
Bittermint, Bendicks*	1 Mint/18g	80.0	3.0	440	4.3	68.9	16.3	2.4
Brandy Liqueurs, Asda*	1 Chocolate/8g	34.0	1.0	409	4.0	60.0	17.0	0.8
Cafe Au Lait, From Continental Selection, Thorntons*	1 Chocolate/16g	77.0	4.0	481	5.3	58.1	25.0	0.6
Cappuccino, From Continental Selection, Thorntons*	1 Chocolate/13g	70.0	5.0	538	5.9	48.5	36.2	0.8
Caramels, Sainsbury's*	1 Sweet/11.6g	57.0	3.0	490	3.5	69.0	22.2	0.2
Celebrations, Mars*	1 Av Sweet/8g	41.0	2.0	512	5.7	61.5	27.0	1.7
Cherry Liqueur, M & S*	1 Chocolate/10g	39.0	2.0	395	2.9	52.8	17.8	4.3
Chocolate Mousse, Thorntons*	1 Chocolate/13g	67.0	5.0	515	7.5	40.0	36.2	3.1
Coffee Creme, Dark, Thorntons*	1 Chocolate/13g	52.0	1.0	400	3.0	71.5	10.8	0.8
Coffee Creme, Milk, Thorntons*	1 Chocolate/13g	52.0	1.0	400	2.8	74.6	10.0	0.8
Coins, Milk, Sainsbury's*	1 Coin/5g	26.0	1.0	502	5.5	58.8	27.1	2.5
Continental, Belgian, Thorntons*	1 Chocolate/13g	67.0	4.0	514	5.8	53.0	30.3	2.9
Continental, Thorntons*	1 Chocolate/15g	76.0	4.0	506	5.6	54.5	29.3	2.7
Country Caramel, Milk, Thorntons*	1 Chocolate/9g	45.0	2.0	500	4.6	62.2	26.7	0.0
Dairy Box, Milk, Nestle*	1 Piece/11g	50.0	2.0	456	4.4	65.9	19.4	0.7
Dark, Elegant, Elizabeth Shaw*	1 Chocolate/8g	38.0	2.0	469	2.9	62.5	23.1	0.0
Dark, Swiss Thins, Lindt*	1 Pack/125g	681.0	46.0	545	4.7	49.2	37.0	0.0
Ferrero Rocher, Ferrero*	1 Chocolate/12.5g	74.0	5.0	593	7.0	49.0	41.0	0.0
Fondant, Chocolate Coated, Usda Average	1 Chocolate/11g	40.0	1.0	366	2.2	80.4	9.3	2.1
Gorgeous, Bendicks*	3 Sweets/15g	82.0	5.0	550	6.6	55.3	33.3	1.1
Italian Collection, Amaretto, M & S*	1 Chocolate/13g	60.0	3.0	480	4.4	59.7	25.1	2.3
Italian Collection, Cappuccino, M & S*	1 Bag/100g	545.0	37.0	545	6.3	46.7	37.0	1.8
Italian Collection, Favourites, M & S*	1 Chocolate/14g	74.0	5.0	530	5.7	50.4	33.7	1.6
Italian Collection, Panna Cotta, M & S*	1 Chocolate/13g	70.0	5.0	545	5.3	49.4	36.4	0.1
Liqueur, Barrels, Cointreau	1 Chocolate/10g	43.0	2.0	435	3.5	57.0	18.0	0.0
Liqueurs, Cognac Truffle, Thorntons*	1 Chocolate/14g	65.0	4.0	464	7.3	40.0	27.1	2.9
Matchmakers, Mint, Nestle*	1 Stick/4g	20.0	1.0	477	4.3	69.7	20.1	0.9
Milk Tray, Cadbury*	1 Chocolate/9g	47.0	2.0	495	4.7	61.5	25.8	0.7
Milk, Biscuit Sticks, Mikado, Kraft*	1 Stick/2.3g	11.0	0.0	475	7.8	67.0	19.8	3.1
Milk, Figures, Hollow, Dairyfine, Aldi*	1 Serving/11g	58.0	3.0	523	5.5	59.9	29.0	3.1
Milk, Shapes, Easter Friends, Tesco*	1 Chocolate/13g	67.0	4.0	540	8.0	52.3	34.2	2.3
Milk, Swiss Thins, Lindt*	1 Pack/125g	687.0	43.0	550	5.8	53.6	34.6	0.0
Mingles, Bendicks*	1 Chocolate/5g	27.0	2.0	540	6.5	54.0	31.3	0.1
Mini Bites, Chunky, Moments, Fox's*	1 Roll/20g	90.0	5.0	450	5.7	52.4	24.6	2.2
Mini Eggs, Cadbury*	1 Egg/3.3g	16.0	1.0	485	4.6	67.8	21.9	1.3
Mini Eggs, Lindor, Lindt*	3 Eggs/15g	90.0	7.0	600	6.7	46.7	46.7	0.0
Mini Eggs, with Soft White Truffle Centre, M & S*	1 Egg/6g	33.0	2.0	550	6.5	56.3	33.9	1.4
Mint Crisp, Bendicks*	1 Mint/8g	38.0	2.0	494	5.2	55.0	29.9	0.0
Mint Crisp, Dark, Elizabeth Shaw*	1 Chocolate/6g	27.0	1.0	458	1.9	68.0	20.7	0.0
Mint Crisp, Milk, Elizabeth Shaw*	1 Chocolate/6g	30.0	1.0	493	4.0	70.9	21.4	0.0
Mint Crisp, Thorntons*	1 Chocolate/7g	34.0	2.0	486	7.7	40.0	31.4	4.3
Mints, Twilight, Terry's*	1 Chocolate/8g	38.0	2.0	475	2.5	56.2	26.2	3.7
Misshapes, Assorted, Cadbury*	1 Chocolate/8g	41.0	2.0	515	5.2	57.5	29.1	0.0
Mistletoe Kisses, Mars*	1 Packet /42g	209.0	11.0	498	5.3	57.0	27.3	0.0
Moments, Thorntons*	1 Chocolate/7g	37.0	2.0	511	5.4	59.9	27.8	1.9
Neapolitans, Terry's*	1oz/28g	146.0	8.0	522	6.0	57.3	29.7	4.1
Orange Crisp, Elizabeth Shaw*	1 Chocolate/6g	29.0	1.0	478	2.9	68.2	21.5	0.0
Peanut Butter Cup, Big Cup, Reese's, Hershey*	1 Cup/39g	210.0	12.0	538	10.3	53.8	30.8	2.6
Peanut Butter Cup, Miniature, Reese's, Hershey*	1 Cup/7g	36.0	2.0	514	10.0	55.7	30.0	4.3
Peanut Butter Cup, Reese's, Hershey*	1 Cup/17g	90.0	5.0	529	11.8	58.8	29.4	5.9
Peanut Butter Cup, White, Mini, Reese's, Hershey*	5 Cups/39g	210.0	12.0	538	12.8	53.8	30.8	2.6
Peppermint Patty, Hershey*	3 Patties/41g	160.0	3.0	390	2.4	80.5	7.3	0.0

CHOCOLATES

INFO/WEIGHT	Measure	per Measure KCAL	FAT	Nutrition Values per 100g / 100ml KCAL	PROT	CARB	FAT	FIBRE
Planets, Mars*	1 Pack/37g	178.0	8.0	481	4.9	65.4	22.4	0.0
Praline, Coffee, Thorntons*	1 Chocolate/7g	37.0	2.0	529	7.0	47.1	34.3	2.9
Praline, Hazelnut, Thorntons*	1 Chocolate/5g	27.0	2.0	540	7.0	48.0	36.0	4.0
Praline, Marzipan, Thorntons*	1 Chocolate/14g	63.0	3.0	450	5.9	58.6	21.4	2.1
Quality Street, Nestle*	1 Av Sweet/8g	39.0	2.0	464	4.0	66.3	20.3	0.8
Rocher, Continental, Thorntons*	1 Chocolate/15g	76.0	5.0	507	6.8	45.3	33.3	2.0
Rocky Road, Clusters, Tesco*	1 Serving/32g	160.0	10.0	500	7.1	51.0	29.7	6.7
Roses, Cadbury*	1 Chocolate/8g	42.0	2.0	495	4.8	62.6	25.3	0.7
Sea Shells, Belgian, Guylian*	1 Shell/11.3g	65.0	4.0	574	8.0	49.0	39.0	0.0
Seashells, Milk & White, Belgian, Waitrose*	1 Serving/15g	77.0	5.0	511	5.0	53.1	31.0	2.8
Snaps, Hazelnut, Cadbury*	1 Curl/4g	20.0	1.0	520	6.8	57.8	28.8	0.0
Snaps, Milk, Cadbury*	1 Snap/3g	15.0	1.0	505	6.3	60.5	27.0	1.0
Snaps, Orange, Cadbury*	1 Snap/3g	15.0	1.0	505	6.3	60.4	27.0	1.0
Speckled Eggs, M & S*	1 Egg/6g	25.0	1.0	440	6.6	63.1	18.2	1.5
Strawberries & Cream, Thorntons*	1 Chocolate/12g	64.0	4.0	533	5.1	54.2	32.5	0.8
Tasters, Dairy Milk, Cadbury*	1 Bag/45g	238.0	14.0	530	7.6	56.4	30.5	0.0
Teddy Bear, Milk Chocolate, Thorntons*	1 Teddy/250g	1357.0	84.0	543	7.6	52.6	33.5	1.0
Toffifee, Storck*	1 Sweet/6g	32.0	2.0	535	6.0	58.0	31.0	0.0
Truffle Filled, Swiss, Balls, Finest, Tesco*	3 Balls/37g	240.0	19.0	640	5.0	40.7	50.8	1.5
Truffle Hearts, Baileys*	1 Chocolate/15g	76.0	4.0	506	5.2	52.6	28.9	1.3
Truffle, Amaretto, Thorntons*	1 Chocolate/14g	66.0	4.0	471	5.5	55.0	25.7	2.9
Truffle, Belgian Milk, Waitrose*	1 Truffle/14g	73.0	5.0	525	5.8	52.9	34.1	1.2
Truffle, Brandy, Thorntons*	1 Chocolate/14g	68.0	4.0	486	6.1	52.1	27.1	0.7
Truffle, Caramel, Thorntons*	1 Chocolate/14g	67.0	4.0	479	4.2	57.9	25.7	2.1
Truffle, Champagne, Premier, Thorntons*	1 Chocolate/17g	88.0	6.0	518	6.9	45.3	32.9	2.4
Truffle, Cherry, Thorntons*	1 Chocolate/14g	58.0	3.0	414	4.2	50.7	21.4	1.4
Truffle, Dark Chocolate, Balls, Lindor, Lindt*	1 Ball/12g	76.0	6.0	630	3.4	38.5	51.4	0.0
Truffle, French Cocoa Dusted, Sainsbury's*	1 Truffle/10g	57.0	4.0	570	4.0	37.0	45.0	0.0
Truffle, Grand Marnier, Thorntons*	1 Chocolate/15g	77.0	5.0	513	7.2	40.7	34.0	4.0
Truffle, Irish Milk Chocolate Cream, Elizabeth Shaw*	1 Chocolate/12g	57.0	3.0	477	3.9	63.4	22.8	0.0
Truffle, Lemon, White, Thorntons*	1 Chocolate/14g	63.0	3.0	450	4.6	64.3	25.0	0.7
Truffle, Milk Chocolate, Balls, Lindor, Lindt*	1 Ball/12g	74.0	6.0	617	4.9	43.1	47.2	0.0
Truffle, Rum, Average	1 Truffle/11g	57.0	4.0	521	6.1	49.7	33.7	1.9
Truffle, Selection, Tesco*	1 Chocolate/14g	75.0	4.0	539	5.1	62.0	29.8	0.5
Truffle, Seville, Thorntons*	1 Chocolate/14g	76.0	5.0	543	7.1	53.6	33.6	1.4
Truffle, Thorntons*	1 Chocolate/7g	33.0	2.0	471	6.0	48.6	27.1	1.4
Truffle, Vanilla, Thorntons*	1 Chocolate/13g	64.0	3.0	492	4.8	57.7	26.9	1.5
Truffle, Viennese, Dark, Thorntons*	1 Chocolate/10g	53.0	4.0	530	5.9	47.0	36.0	3.0
Truffle, Viennese, Milk, Thorntons*	1 Chocolate/10g	56.0	4.0	560	4.9	54.0	36.0	0.0
Truffles, Belgian, Flaked, Tesco*	1 Truffle/14g	80.0	5.0	575	4.4	52.7	38.5	2.3
Valentine, Thorntons*	1 Chocolate/11g	60.0	4.0	542	5.7	52.0	34.5	2.1
Winter Selection, Thorntons*	1 Chocolate/10g	51.0	3.0	506	6.2	51.3	30.6	3.8

CHOCOLATINE

All Butter, Sainsbury's*	1 Serving/58g	241.0	14.0	415	7.9	42.5	23.7	3.3
Mini, Sainsbury's*	1 Serving/30g	120.0	7.0	400	7.7	41.0	23.0	3.3
Sainsbury's*	1 Serving/58g	263.0	16.0	454	8.5	42.3	27.9	2.1

CHOP SUEY

Chicken, with Noodles, Sainsbury's*	1 Pack/300g	300.0	7.0	100	5.7	13.6	2.5	1.2
Chinese, Vegetable, Stir Fry, Sharwood's*	1 Pack/310g	223.0	3.0	72	1.5	13.9	1.1	0.6
Vegetable, M & S*	½ Pack/150g	90.0	6.0	60	2.0	3.1	4.1	2.9

CHORIZO

Iberico, Bellota, TTD, Sainsbury's*	1 Slice/3g	17.0	1.0	498	27.0	1.0	42.9	0.0

	Measure INFO/WEIGHT	per Measure KCAL	FAT	Nutrition Values per 100g / 100ml KCAL	PROT	CARB	FAT	FIBRE
CHOW MEIN								
Beef, Sainsbury's*	1 Pack/450g	499.0	11.0	111	6.6	15.5	2.5	0.8
Cantonese Vegetable Stir Fry, Sainsbury's*	¼ Pack/100g	85.0	4.0	85	2.2	10.6	3.8	1.2
Char Sui, Cantonese, Sainsbury's*	½ Pack/225g	205.0	7.0	91	5.7	10.0	3.1	1.1
Chicken with Vegetable Spring Roll, Oriental Express*	1 Pack/300g	213.0	2.0	71	5.5	12.4	0.6	1.9
Chicken, Ainsley Harriott*	1 Serving/250g	447.0	12.0	179	14.0	21.2	4.7	2.0
Chicken, Chinese Takeaway, Sainsbury's*	1 Pack/316g	338.0	9.0	107	9.1	11.6	2.7	0.7
Chicken, COOK!, M & S*	1 Pack/375g	356.0	8.0	95	7.9	10.5	2.1	1.7
Chicken, COU, M & S*	1 Pack/200g	180.0	5.0	90	9.3	8.1	2.3	1.1
Chicken, Frozen, Sainsbury's*	1 Pack/404g	424.0	12.0	105	6.1	13.4	3.0	0.9
Chicken, Less Than 3% Fat, BGTY, Sainsbury's*	1 Pack/450g	355.0	10.0	79	5.8	8.7	2.3	1.4
Chicken, New Improved Recipe, Sainsbury's*	1 Pack/449g	395.0	9.0	88	5.7	11.7	2.0	1.2
Chicken, New, BGTY, Sainsbury's*	1 Pack/450g	373.0	6.0	83	6.0	11.4	1.4	1.1
Chicken, Waitrose*	1 Serving/400g	384.0	12.0	96	6.0	11.4	2.9	1.3
Pork, Perfectly Balanced, Waitrose*	½ Pack/310g	332.0	3.0	107	7.6	17.2	0.9	1.6
Special, COU, M & S*	1 Pack/400g	320.0	4.0	80	7.4	9.9	1.0	1.0
Special, HL, Tesco*	1 Pack/450g	351.0	5.0	78	6.3	10.6	1.2	0.6
Special, Perfectly Balanced, Waitrose*	1 Pack/400g	316.0	4.0	79	7.4	10.0	1.1	0.9
Stir Fry, Asda*	1 Pack/350g	269.0	17.0	77	2.1	6.0	5.0	0.0
Stir Fry, Tesco*	½ Pack/240g	180.0	3.0	75	2.8	12.0	1.4	1.6
Vegetable, Asda*	1 Pack/400g	520.0	15.0	130	2.4	21.5	3.8	3.0
Vegetable, Take Away, Meal for One, Tesco*	1 Serving/345g	262.0	8.0	76	6.7	7.3	2.2	1.3
Vesta*	1 Pack/433.3g	585.0	10.0	135	5.4	23.1	2.3	2.9
CHRISTMAS PUDDING								
Average	1oz/28g	81.0	3.0	291	4.6	49.5	9.7	1.3
BGTY, Sainsbury's*	1 Serving/114g	302.0	3.0	266	2.8	58.2	2.5	4.6
Rich Fruit, Laced with Brandy, Tesco*	1 Serving/100g	305.0	10.0	305	3.7	50.8	9.7	1.3
Rich Fruit, Tesco*	1 Serving/114g	331.0	7.0	290	2.4	55.0	5.9	0.0
Sticky Toffee, Tesco*	¼ Pudding/114g	372.0	7.0	326	2.5	64.5	6.4	0.8
Toffee Sauce Coated, Morrisons*	1 Pudding/100g	324.0	6.0	324	2.5	64.5	6.4	0.0
Wheat Free, Gluten Free, Tesco*	1oz/28g	84.0	2.0	295	1.9	60.4	7.1	4.5
with Cider, Value, Tesco*	1 Serving/100g	312.0	7.0	312	2.7	59.6	7.0	3.3
CHUTNEY								
Apple & Pear, TTD, Sainsbury's*	1 Serving/20g	38.0	0.0	190	0.6	45.2	0.8	1.7
Apple, Tomato & Sultana, Tesco*	1 Serving/50g	88.0	0.0	176	1.1	42.4	0.2	1.3
Apricot, Sharwood's*	1 Tsp/16g	21.0	0.0	131	0.6	32.0	0.1	2.3
Bengal Spice Mango, Sharwood's*	1 Tsp/5g	12.0	0.0	236	0.5	58.0	0.2	1.2
Caramelised Onion, Sainsbury's*	1 Serving/25g	28.0	0.0	111	1.1	23.5	1.4	1.1
Caramelised Onion, TTD, Sainsbury's*	1 Serving/20g	31.0	0.0	157	0.8	37.3	0.5	2.1
Caramelised Red Onion, Loyd Grossman*	1 Serving/10g	11.0	0.0	111	0.5	27.2	0.0	0.5
Cranberry & Caramelised Red Onion, Baxters*	1 Serving/20g	31.0	0.0	154	0.3	38.0	0.1	0.3
Fruit, Spiced, Baxters*	1 Tsp/16g	23.0	0.0	143	6.0	34.8	0.1	0.0
Indian Appetisers, Pot, Waitrose*	1 Pot/158g	330.0	2.0	209	1.8	47.3	1.4	1.8
Lime & Chilli, Geeta's*	1 Serving/25g	69.0	0.0	277	2.0	64.0	1.4	1.9
Mango & Apple, Sharwood's*	1oz/28g	65.0	0.0	233	0.4	57.6	0.1	1.1
Mango & Ginger, Baxters*	1 Jar/320g	598.0	1.0	187	5.0	45.7	0.2	0.9
Mango & Lime, Sharwood's*	1oz/28g	58.0	0.0	206	0.4	50.5	0.3	0.8
Mango, Green Label, Sharwood's*	1 Tsp/10g	23.0	0.0	234	0.3	57.8	0.2	0.9
Mango, Hot, Patak's*	1 Jar/340g	877.0	1.0	258	0.4	67.1	0.2	0.7
Mango, Indian Takeaway, Asda*	1 Pack/70g	145.0	0.0	207	0.3	50.9	0.2	1.0
Mango, Major Grey, Patak's*	1 Tbsp/15g	38.0	0.0	255	0.4	66.0	0.2	0.7
Mango, Spiced, M & S*	1 Serving/15g	26.0	0.0	175	1.2	42.3	0.4	3.2
Mango, Spicy, Sainsbury's*	1 Tbsp/15g	24.0	0.0	160	0.7	37.0	0.7	1.3
Mango, Tesco*	1 Serving/20g	45.0	0.0	224	0.4	55.5	0.1	1.3

C

	Measure INFO/WEIGHT	per Measure KCAL	FAT	Nutrition Values per 100g / 100ml KCAL	PROT	CARB	FAT	FIBRE
CHUTNEY								
Mango, Waitrose*	1 Serving/20g	43.0	0.0	215	1.0	49.0	1.5	2.0
Peach, Spicy, Waitrose*	1 Serving/20g	43.0	0.0	215	1.0	49.0	1.5	1.5
Ploughman's Plum, The English Provender Co.*	1 Tsp/10g	16.0	0.0	160	1.3	38.1	0.2	1.6
Red Onion & Sherry Vinegar, Sainsbury's*	1 Serving/10g	24.0	0.0	236	0.5	57.1	0.6	1.4
Spicy Fruit, Baxters*	1 Serving/15g	22.0	0.0	146	0.6	35.4	0.2	0.0
Tomato	*1 Heap Tsp/16g*	*20.0*	*0.0*	*128*	*1.2*	*31.0*	*0.2*	*1.3*
Tomato & Red Pepper, Baxters*	1 Jar/312g	512.0	1.0	164	2.0	38.0	0.4	1.5
Tomato, Waitrose*	1 Pot/100g	195.0	0.0	195	1.3	46.8	0.3	0.0
CIDER								
Dry, Average	*1 Pint/568ml*	*205.0*	*0.0*	*36*	*0.0*	*2.6*	*0.0*	*0.0*
Light, Bulmers*	1 Can/500ml	140.0	0.0	28	0.0	0.8	0.0	0.0
Low Alcohol	*1 Pint/568ml*	*97.0*	*0.0*	*17*	*0.0*	*3.6*	*0.0*	*0.0*
Low Carb, Stowford*	1 Bottle/500ml	140.0	0.0	28	0.0	0.2	0.0	0.0
Pear, Average	*1 Serving/200ml*	*86.0*	*0.0*	*43*	*0.0*	*3.6*	*0.0*	*0.0*
Scrumpy, Average	*1 Serving/200ml*	*93.0*	*0.0*	*46*	*0.0*	*2.3*	*0.0*	*0.0*
Sweet, Average	*1 Pint/568ml*	*239.0*	*0.0*	*42*	*0.0*	*4.3*	*0.0*	*0.0*
Vintage	*1 Pint/568ml*	*574.0*	*0.0*	*101*	*0.0*	*7.3*	*0.0*	*0.0*
CINNAMON								
Ground, Average	*1 Tsp/3g*	*8.0*	*0.0*	*261*	*3.9*	*55.5*	*3.2*	*0.0*
Stick, Schwartz*	1 Stick/2g	7.0	0.0	339	4.7	79.3	0.3	0.0
CLAMS								
in Brine, Average	*1oz/28g*	*22.0*	*0.0*	*79*	*16.0*	*2.4*	*0.6*	*0.0*
Raw, Average	*20 Sm/180g*	*133.0*	*2.0*	*74*	*12.8*	*2.6*	*1.0*	*0.0*
CLEMENTINES								
Raw, Weighed with Peel, Average	*1 Med/60g*	*22.0*	*0.0*	*36*	*0.8*	*11.3*	*0.1*	*1.6*
Raw, Weighed without Peel, Average	*1 Med/46g*	*22.0*	*0.0*	*47*	*0.8*	*12.0*	*0.1*	*1.7*
Sweet, TTD, Sainsbury's*	1 Serving/100g	37.0	0.0	37	0.9	8.7	0.1	1.2
COCKLES								
Boiled	*1 Cockle/4g*	*2.0*	*0.0*	*53*	*12.0*	*0.0*	*0.6*	*0.0*
Bottled in Vinegar, Drained	*1oz/28g*	*17.0*	*0.0*	*60*	*13.3*	*0.0*	*0.7*	*0.0*
COCOA BUTTER								
Average	*1oz/28g*	*251.0*	*28.0*	*896*	*0.0*	*0.0*	*99.5*	*0.0*
COCOA POWDER								
Cadbury*	1 Tbsp/16g	52.0	3.0	322	23.1	10.5	20.8	0.0
Dry, Unsweetened, Average	1 Tbsp/5.4g	12.0	1.0	229	19.6	54.3	13.7	33.2
Organic, Green & Black's*	1 Tbsp/15g	52.0	3.0	350	23.6	13.6	22.3	0.0
Valrhona*	1 Tsp/5g	22.0	1.0	450	25.0	45.0	20.0	30.0
COCONUT								
Creamed, Average	*1oz/28g*	*186.0*	*19.0*	*665*	*6.0*	*6.7*	*68.4*	*7.0*
Desiccated, Average	*1oz/28g*	*169.0*	*17.0*	*604*	*5.6*	*6.4*	*62.0*	*13.7*
Fresh, Flesh Only, Average	*1oz/28g*	*98.0*	*10.0*	*351*	*3.2*	*3.7*	*36.0*	*7.3*
Ice, Average	*1oz/28g*	*104.0*	*4.0*	*371*	*1.7*	*66.7*	*12.7*	*2.6*
Milk, Average	*1 Can/400ml*	*698.0*	*70.0*	*174*	*1.4*	*2.9*	*17.4*	*2.9*
Milk, Organic, Tesco*	1/8 Can/49g	85.0	8.0	175	1.8	2.7	17.0	1.3
Milk, Reduced Fat, Amoy*	1 Tin/400ml	504.0	48.0	126	1.0	2.5	12.0	1.0
Milk, Reduced Fat, Asda*	1 Serving/50ml	62.0	5.0	124	1.1	1.7	10.0	0.5
Milk, Reduced Fat, Average	*1 Serving/100g*	*103.0*	*10.0*	*103*	*0.9*	*2.4*	*10.0*	*0.4*
COD								
Baked, Average	*1oz/28g*	*27.0*	*0.0*	*96*	*21.4*	*0.0*	*1.2*	*0.0*
Beer Battered, Crispy, Finest, Tesco*	1 Portion/250g	575.0	35.0	230	12.0	13.4	14.0	1.3
Dried, Salted, Average	*1oz/28g*	*82.0*	*1.0*	*290*	*62.8*	*0.0*	*2.4*	*0.0*
Dried, Salted, Boiled, Average	*1oz/28g*	*39.0*	*0.0*	*138*	*32.5*	*0.0*	*0.9*	*0.0*
Fillets, Battered, Average	1 Serving/90g	158.0	7.0	175	12.5	12.9	8.1	1.0

	Measure INFO/WEIGHT	per Measure KCAL	FAT	Nutrition Values per 100g / 100ml KCAL	PROT	CARB	FAT	FIBRE
COD								
Fillets, Breaded, Average	1 Serving/97g	200.0	9.0	206	13.0	16.7	9.7	1.0
Fillets, Breaded, Chunky, Average	1 Piece/135g	204.0	8.0	151	13.7	10.9	5.9	1.4
Fillets, Breaded, Light, Healthy Range, Average	1 Fillet/135g	209.0	7.0	154	13.6	13.3	5.1	1.2
Fillets, Chunky, Average	*1 Fillet/198g*	*267.0*	*7.0*	*135*	*17.1*	*8.2*	*3.7*	*0.8*
Fillets, Skinless & Boneless, Raw, Average	*1 Portion/92g*	*90.0*	*2.0*	*98*	*17.8*	*2.7*	*1.7*	*0.4*
Fillets, Smoked, Average	*1 Serving/150g*	*151.0*	*2.0*	*101*	*21.6*	*0.0*	*1.6*	*0.0*
Loins, Average	*1 Serving/145g*	*116.0*	*1.0*	*80*	*17.9*	*0.1*	*0.8*	*0.2*
Poached, Average	*1oz/28g*	*26.0*	*0.0*	*94*	*20.9*	*0.0*	*1.1*	*0.0*
Smoked, Raw, Average	*1oz/28g*	*22.0*	*0.0*	*79*	*18.3*	*0.0*	*0.6*	*0.0*
Steaks, Battered, Chip Shop Style, Average	1 Serving/150g	321.0	18.0	214	12.5	14.3	12.0	1.1
Steamed, Average	*1oz/28g*	*23.0*	*0.0*	*83*	*18.6*	*0.0*	*0.9*	*0.0*
COD &								
Cauliflower Bake, Asda*	1 Pack/400g	492.0	28.0	123	9.5	5.5	7.0	1.0
Cauliflower Cheese, Fillets, Iceland*	½ Pack/176g	234.0	14.0	133	12.7	3.3	7.7	1.7
Chips, Oven Baked, Safeway*	1 Pack/250g	522.0	21.0	209	8.4	25.0	8.4	3.5
Parsley Sauce, Frozen, M & S*	1 Pack/184g	156.0	7.0	85	11.1	1.9	3.9	1.0
Salmon, Steam Cuisine, COU, M & S*	1 Pack/400g	340.0	7.0	85	6.8	8.9	1.8	1.2
COD IN								
a Sweet Red Pepper Sauce, Fillets, GFY, Asda*	½ Pack/170g	143.0	3.0	84	15.0	2.3	1.6	0.1
Butter Sauce, Steaks, Birds Eye*	1 Pack/170g	185.0	9.0	109	9.8	5.0	5.5	0.1
Butter Sauce, Steaks, Frozen, Asda*	1 Pouch/152g	163.0	4.0	107	16.0	5.0	2.6	0.8
Butter Sauce, Steaks, Sainsbury's*	1 Serving/170g	184.0	10.0	108	10.5	3.1	5.9	0.3
Cheese Sauce, BGTY, Sainsbury's*	1 Serving/170g	144.0	4.0	85	12.8	3.1	2.4	0.0
Cheese Sauce, Steaks, Birds Eye*	1 Pack/182g	175.0	6.0	96	10.9	5.2	3.5	0.1
Mushroom Sauce, BGTY, Sainsbury's*	1 Serving/170g	112.0	3.0	66	9.9	2.8	1.7	0.1
Parsley Sauce, COU, M & S*	1 Pack/185g	129.0	5.0	70	10.6	1.4	2.5	0.6
Parsley Sauce, Fillets, BGTY, Sainsbury's*	1 Pack/351g	316.0	15.0	90	11.6	1.3	4.3	0.7
Parsley Sauce, Frozen, Morrisons*	1 Serving/170g	131.0	5.0	77	9.6	3.2	2.7	0.5
Parsley Sauce, Portions, Ocean Trader*	1 Serving/120g	112.0	5.0	93	9.4	4.0	3.9	0.1
Parsley Sauce, Steaks, Birds Eye*	1 Steak/172g	155.0	5.0	90	10.5	5.6	2.8	0.1
Parsley Sauce, Steaks, Sainsbury's*	1 Portion/150g	121.0	5.0	81	10.2	3.0	3.1	0.2
Red Pepper Sauce, SteamFresh, Birds Eye*	1 Serving/125g	115.0	2.0	92	14.4	4.7	1.9	0.3
Rich Butter Sauce, Steaks, Ocean Trader*	1 Pouch/150g	136.0	6.0	91	10.3	3.3	4.1	0.1
COD WITH								
a Mediterranean Pepper Sauce, Fillets, Waitrose*	1 Pack/370g	240.0	5.0	65	12.2	1.1	1.3	0.9
a Thai Crust, Perfectly Balanced, Waitrose*	1 Pack/280g	249.0	7.0	89	15.1	1.6	2.5	0.6
Chunky Chips, M & S*	1 Serving/340g	510.0	20.0	150	6.5	17.5	6.0	1.5
Fish Pesto, Fillets, COOK!, M & S*	½ Pack/165g	210.0	5.0	127	16.4	8.4	3.1	4.2
Mediterranean Butter, Sainsbury's*	1 Pack/170g	196.0	9.0	115	17.0	0.1	5.2	0.1
Parma Ham & Sardinian Chick Peas, M & S*	½ Pack/255g	268.0	12.0	105	9.8	5.3	4.9	0.5
Roasted Vegetables, M & S*	1 Serving/280g	238.0	11.0	85	8.0	4.9	3.8	1.7
Salsa & Rosemary Potatoes, BGTY, Sainsbury's*	1 Pack/450g	355.0	4.0	79	4.7	13.1	0.9	1.6
Sunblush Tomato Sauce, GFY, Asda*	½ Pack/177g	117.0	3.0	66	13.0	0.1	1.5	1.0
Sweet Chilli, COU, M & S*	1 Pack/400g	360.0	2.0	90	7.7	13.1	0.5	1.6
Tomato Sauce, Fillets, Asda*	1 Serving/181g	210.0	11.0	116	13.0	2.6	6.0	2.3
Vegetables, Haches, Steaks, Peche Ocean*	1 Serving/200g	184.0	8.0	92	12.0	2.1	3.9	0.0
COFFEE								
Alternative, Wake Up, Whole Earth*	1 Cup/5g	19.0	0.0	377	5.5	88.4	0.2	0.0
Black, Average	1 Mug/270ml	5.0	0.0	2	0.2	0.3	0.0	0.0
Cafe Caramel, Cafe Range, Nescafe*	1 Sachet/17g	72.0	2.0	423	9.2	64.6	14.1	1.3
Cafe Hazelnut, Nescafe*	1 Sachet/17g	73.0	2.0	428	9.3	66.0	14.1	0.0
Cafe Irish Cream, Cafe Range, Nescafe*	1 Sachet/23g	98.0	3.0	425	8.2	65.2	14.1	1.2
Cafe Latte, Dry, Douwe Egberts*	1 Serving/12g	58.0	3.0	480	10.0	60.0	22.0	0.0

	Measure INFO/WEIGHT	per Measure KCAL	FAT	Nutrition Values per 100g / 100ml KCAL	PROT	CARB	FAT	FIBRE
COFFEE								
Cafe Latte, Instant, Maxwell House*	1 Serving/16g	67.0	3.0	420	17.0	45.5	18.9	0.1
Cafe Mocha, Cafe Range, Nescafe*	1 Sachet/22g	92.0	3.0	418	8.5	66.6	13.1	0.0
Cafe Vanilla, Cafe Range, Nescafe*	1 Sachet/18.5g	79.0	3.0	429	9.3	64.6	14.9	1.2
Cappuccino Ice, Made up, Dolce Gusto, Nescafe*	1 Serving/240ml	111.0	3.0	46	1.7	7.2	1.2	0.2
Cappuccino, Cafe Mocha, Dry, Maxwell House*	1 Serving/23g	100.0	2.0	434	4.3	78.2	10.8	0.0
Cappuccino, Cappio, Iced, Kenco*	1 Can/200ml	138.0	6.0	69	3.0	7.0	3.0	0.0
Cappuccino, Cappio, Kenco*	1 Sachet/18g	79.0	2.0	439	11.7	73.9	10.6	0.6
Cappuccino, Decaff, Instant, Made Up, Nescafe*	1 Mug/200ml	68.0	2.0	34	0.9	5.0	1.1	0.0
Cappuccino, Decaff, Nescafe*	1 Sachet/16g	68.0	2.0	428	11.6	62.6	14.6	0.0
Cappuccino, Decaff, Unsweetened, Nescafe*	1 Sachet/16g	70.0	3.0	437	14.5	51.2	19.4	4.3
Cappuccino, Dry, Maxwell House*	1 Mug/15g	52.0	1.0	350	12.0	64.0	9.6	0.4
Cappuccino, for Filter Systems, Kenco*	1 Sachet/6g	22.0	1.0	375	19.0	44.0	13.5	0.0
Cappuccino, Instant, Kenco*	1 Sachet/20g	80.0	3.0	401	13.5	55.7	13.8	0.0
Cappuccino, Instant, Made Up, Maxwell House*	1 Serving/280g	123.0	5.0	44	0.6	5.8	1.9	0.0
Cappuccino, Instant, Unsweetened, Douwe Egberts*	1 Serving/12g	48.0	2.0	400	11.0	53.0	16.0	0.0
Cappuccino, Made up, Dolce Gusto, Nescafe*	1 Serving/240ml	84.0	4.0	35	1.1	4.0	1.5	0.3
Cappuccino, Original Mugsticks, Maxwell House*	1 Serving/18g	73.0	3.0	406	14.4	52.8	15.6	0.0
Cappuccino, Original, Sachets, Nescafe*	1 Sachet/18g	80.0	3.0	444	11.7	60.3	17.4	0.0
Cappuccino, Semi Skimmed Milk, Average	1 Serving/200ml	48.0	2.0	24	1.6	2.6	1.1	0.0
Cappuccino, Skinny, Nescafe*	1 Sachet/16g	51.0	1.0	318	23.6	43.9	4.4	10.6
Cappuccino, Swiss Chocolate, Nescafe*	1 Sachet/20g	81.0	2.0	404	10.5	65.3	11.5	2.9
Cappuccino, to Go, Original, Nescafe*	1 Serving/19g	84.0	3.0	444	11.7	60.3	17.4	0.0
Cappuccino, Unsweetened Taste, Maxwell House*	1 Serving/15g	65.0	3.0	434	17.4	47.6	19.3	0.3
Cappuccino, Unsweetened, Cappio, Kenco*	1 Serving/18g	73.0	2.0	406	12.2	66.7	10.0	0.6
Cappuccino, Unsweetened, Nescafe*	1 Sachet/16g	74.0	4.0	464	15.0	47.3	23.8	0.0
Chococino, Made up, Dolce Gusto, Nescafe*	1 Serving/210g	147.0	5.0	70	2.3	9.4	2.6	0.7
Columbian, Nescafe*	1 Serving/2g	2.0	0.0	111	16.7	11.1	0.0	5.6
Decaffeinated, Gold Blend, Nescafe*	1 Tsp/5g	5.0	0.0	101	14.9	10.0	0.2	8.4
Double Choca Mocha, Cafe Range, Nescafe*	1 Sachet/23g	94.0	3.0	408	9.2	68.0	11.0	2.8
Espresso, Made up, Dolce Gusto, Nescafe*	1 Serving/60ml	1.0	0.0	2	0.1	0.0	0.1	0.3
Frappe Iced, Nestle*	1 Sachet/24g	92.0	1.0	384	15.0	72.0	4.0	0.5
Ice Mocha Drink, Nescafe, Nestle*	1 Bottle/280ml	160.0	3.0	57	1.1	10.5	1.2	0.0
Infusion, Average with Semi-Skimmed Milk	1 Cup/220ml	15.0	0.0	7	0.6	0.7	0.2	0.0
Infusion, Average with Single Cream	1 Cup/220ml	31.0	3.0	14	0.4	0.3	1.2	0.0
Infusion, Average with Whole Milk	1 Cup/220ml	15.0	1.0	7	0.5	0.5	0.4	0.0
Instant, Alta Rica, Nescafe*	1 Tsp/1.8g	2.0	0.0	98	13.8	10.0	0.3	21.0
Instant, Decaffeinated, Nescafe*	1 Tsp/1.8g	2.0	0.0	101	14.9	10.0	0.2	8.4
Instant, Made with Skimmed Milk	1 Serving/270ml	15.0	0.0	6	0.6	0.8	0.0	0.0
Instant, Made with Water & Semi-Skimmed Milk	1 Serving/350ml	24.0	1.0	7	0.4	0.5	0.4	0.0
Instant, Original, Nescafe*	1 Tsp/1.8g	1.0	0.0	63	7.0	9.0	0.2	27.0
Instant, with Skimmed Milk, Costa Rican, Kenco*	1 Mug/300ml	17.0	0.0	6	0.6	0.8	0.0	0.0
Latte Macchiato, Made up, Dolce Gusto, Nescafe*	1 Serving/220g	89.0	4.0	40	1.9	4.1	1.9	0.3
Latte, Instant, Skinny, Douwe Egberts*	1 Serving/12g	35.0	1.0	290	11.0	38.0	11.0	29.0
Latte, Luscious, Options*	1 Serving/14g	62.0	2.0	443	14.3	57.9	17.1	3.6
Latte, Macchiato, Tassimo*	1 Cup/275ml	135.0	8.0	49	2.3	3.6	2.8	0.0
Latte, Nescafe*	1 Sachet/22g	110.0	6.0	498	14.5	45.7	28.5	0.0
Latte, No Sugar, In Cup, From Machine, Kenco*	1 Cup/4.2g	17.0	1.0	400	7.6	44.0	22.0	0.0
Latte, Skinny, Nescafe*	1 Sachet/20g	72.0	1.0	359	24.1	54.3	5.3	1.1
Mocha, Instant, Skinny, Douwe Egberts*	1 Serving/12g	37.0	1.0	308	10.8	40.8	10.8	25.0
Mocha, Made up, Dolce Gusto, Nescafe*	1 Serving/210g	117.0	5.0	56	2.4	6.1	2.4	0.6
COFFEE MATE								
Original, Nestle*	1 Tsp/3.5g	19.0	1.0	547	2.4	56.7	34.4	0.0
Virtually Fat Free, Nestle*	1 Tsp/5g	10.0	0.0	200	1.0	42.0	3.0	0.0

	Measure INFO/WEIGHT	per Measure KCAL	FAT	Nutrition Values per 100g / 100ml KCAL	PROT	CARB	FAT	FIBRE
COFFEE WHITENER								
Half Fat, Co-Op*	1 Tsp/5g	21.0	1.0	430	0.9	78.0	13.0	0.0
Light, Asda*	1 Serving/3g	13.0	0.0	433	0.9	78.0	13.0	0.0
Tesco*	1 Tsp/3g	16.0	1.0	533	1.2	61.3	31.4	0.0
COGNAC								
40% Volume	*1 Shot/35ml*	*78.0*	*0.0*	*222*	*0.0*	*0.0*	*0.0*	*0.0*
COLA								
Average	1 Can/330ml	135.0	0.0	41	0.0	10.9	0.0	0.0
Coke, Cherry, Coca-Cola*	1 Bottle/500ml	225.0	0.0	45	0.0	11.2	0.0	0.0
Coke, Coca-Cola*	1 Can/330ml	142.0	0.0	43	0.0	10.7	0.0	0.0
Coke, Diet, Caffeine Free, Coca-Cola*	1 Can/330ml	1.0	0.0	0	0.0	0.1	0.0	0.0
Coke, Diet, Coca-Cola*	1 Can/330ml	1.0	0.0	0	0.0	0.0	0.0	0.0
Coke, Diet, with Cherry, Coca-Cola*	1 Bottle/500ml	5.0	0.0	1	0.0	0.0	0.0	0.0
Coke, Vanilla, Coca-Cola*	1 Bottle/500ml	215.0	0.0	43	0.0	10.7	0.0	0.0
Coke, with Lemon, Diet, Coca-Cola*	1 Can/330ml	5.0	0.0	1	0.0	0.0	0.0	0.0
Coke, with Vanilla, Diet, Coca-Cola*	1 Glass/200ml	1.0	0.0	0	0.0	0.1	0.0	0.0
Coke, Zero, Coca-Cola*	1 Can/330	2.0	0.0	0	0.0	0.0	0.0	0.0
Diet, Classic, Sainsbury's*	1 Can/330ml	1.0	0.0	0	0.0	0.0	0.0	0.0
Diet, M & S*	1 Can/330ml	3.0	0.0	1	0.0	0.3	0.0	0.0
Diet, Pepsi*	1 Can/330ml	1.0	0.0	0	0.0	0.0	0.0	0.0
Diet, Tesco*	1 Glass/200ml	2.0	0.0	1	0.1	0.1	0.1	0.0
Diet, Virgin Trains*	1 Glass/250ml	1.0	0.0	0	0.1	0.1	0.1	0.0
Max, Pepsi*	1 Can/330ml	2.0	0.0	1	0.1	0.1	0.0	0.0
Pepsi*	1 Can/330ml	145.0	0.0	44	0.0	11.1	0.0	0.0
Pepsi, Twist, Light, Pepsi*	1 Bottle/500ml	4.0	0.0	1	0.0	0.1	0.0	0.0
Pepsi, Twist, Pepsi*	1 Bottle/500ml	235.0	0.0	47	0.0	11.7	0.0	0.0
COLESLAW								
20% Less Fat, Asda*	1 Serving/100g	88.0	6.0	88	1.5	7.0	6.0	1.7
50% Less Fat, Asda*	1oz/28g	17.0	1.0	61	2.1	6.8	2.8	0.9
99% Fat Free, Kraft*	1 Serving/40ml	50.0	0.0	126	1.0	28.9	1.0	0.0
Apple, M & S*	1oz/28g	53.0	5.0	190	1.4	9.2	16.6	1.4
Bryn Wharf Food Co*	1 Serving/90g	109.0	9.0	121	1.4	5.7	10.4	1.8
Cheese, Asda*	1 Serving/100g	242.0	22.0	242	4.8	6.3	22.0	1.6
Cheese, M & S*	1 Serving/57g	185.0	19.0	325	4.2	2.0	33.5	1.7
Cheese, Sainsbury's*	1 Serving/75g	174.0	16.0	232	3.4	5.6	21.8	0.6
Cheese, Supreme, Waitrose*	¼ Pack/87.6g	197.0	18.0	225	4.5	5.0	20.8	1.2
Coronation, Sainsbury's*	¼ Pot/75g	135.0	11.0	180	1.2	11.9	14.2	2.4
COU, M & S*	½ Pack/125g	75.0	3.0	60	1.3	7.4	2.7	1.7
Creamy, GFY, Asda*	1 Serving/100g	163.0	15.0	163	0.7	6.5	14.9	0.8
Creamy, Tesco*	1 Serving/75g	142.0	13.0	190	1.0	5.5	17.8	1.5
Crunchy, Premium, Millcroft*	1 Pack/400g	756.0	70.0	189	0.9	7.3	17.4	1.5
Deli Style, BGTY, Sainsbury's*	1 Serving/75g	64.0	5.0	85	1.5	6.0	6.1	1.7
Deli Style, M & S*	1 Serving/320g	336.0	31.0	105	3.5	1.5	9.7	1.4
Fruity, M & S*	1 Serving/63g	151.0	14.0	240	1.1	8.3	22.7	3.1
Garlic & Herb, Asda*	1 Tbsp/15g	22.0	2.0	147	0.9	5.8	13.3	1.7
Half Fat, Waitrose*	1 Serving/100g	64.0	4.0	64	1.0	4.8	4.5	2.0
Heinz*	1oz/28g	38.0	3.0	135	1.6	9.4	10.2	1.2
Luxury, M & S*	1oz/28g	43.0	4.0	152	1.0	6.0	13.8	1.0
M & S*	1oz/28g	50.0	5.0	180	1.7	6.1	16.5	1.1
Organic, M & S*	1oz/28g	41.0	3.0	145	1.1	7.3	12.4	1.0
Prawn, Asda*	1oz/28g	54.0	5.0	192	2.4	6.6	17.3	1.4
Premium, Co-Op*	1 Serving/50g	160.0	17.0	320	1.0	3.0	34.0	2.0
Reduced Fat, Asda*	1 Pot/250g	217.0	16.0	87	1.5	6.0	6.3	1.6
Reduced Fat, Co-Op*	1 Serving/50g	45.0	3.0	90	0.9	6.0	7.0	2.0

C

	Measure INFO/WEIGHT	per Measure KCAL	per Measure FAT	Nutrition Values per 100g / 100ml KCAL	PROT	CARB	FAT	FIBRE
COLESLAW								
Reduced Fat, M & S*	½ Tub/112.2g	230.0	22.0	205	1.1	5.4	20.0	2.8
Sainsbury's*	1 Serving/75g	103.0	9.0	138	1.4	6.1	12.0	1.7
Supreme, Waitrose*	1oz/28g	53.0	5.0	190	1.8	4.9	18.1	1.7
Tesco*	1 Serving/50g	79.0	7.0	158	2.2	5.2	14.3	1.6
Three Cheese, Finest, Tesco*	1/3 Pack/100g	255.0	23.0	255	6.4	5.8	22.7	1.1
Three Cheese, Safeway*	½ Pot/113g	189.0	16.0	168	4.5	6.2	14.2	1.1
TTD, Sainsbury's*	¼ Pack/75g	218.0	23.0	291	1.5	3.5	30.1	2.8
with Mayonnaise, Retail	1oz/28g	72.0	7.0	258	1.2	4.2	26.4	1.4
with Reduced Calorie Dressing, Retail	1oz/28g	19.0	1.0	67	0.9	6.1	4.5	1.4
COLESLAW MIX								
Average	*1oz/28g*	*8.0*	*0.0*	*30*	*0.8*	*4.9*	*0.8*	*2.0*
COLEY								
Portions, Raw, Average	*1 Serving/92g*	*75.0*	*1.0*	*81*	*18.4*	*0.0*	*0.7*	*0.0*
Steamed, Average	*1oz/28g*	*29.0*	*0.0*	*105*	*23.3*	*0.0*	*1.3*	*0.0*
CONCHIGLIE								
Cooked, Average	*1 Serving/185g*	*247.0*	*2.0*	*133*	*4.8*	*26.6*	*0.8*	*0.5*
Dry Weight, Average	*1 Serving/100g*	*352.0*	*2.0*	*352*	*12.5*	*71.6*	*1.7*	*2.6*
Shells, Dry, Average	*1 Serving/100g*	*345.0*	*1.0*	*345*	*12.3*	*70.4*	*1.5*	*3.0*
Whole Wheat, Dry Weight, Average	*1 Serving/75g*	*237.0*	*1.0*	*316*	*12.6*	*62.0*	*2.0*	*10.7*
CONCHIGLIONI								
Dry, Waitrose*	1 Serving/75g	256.0	1.0	341	12.5	69.8	1.3	3.7
CONSERVE								
Apricot, Average	*1 Tbsp/15g*	*37.0*	*0.0*	*244*	*0.5*	*59.3*	*0.2*	*1.5*
Apricot, Reduced Sugar, Streamline*	1 Tbsp/20g	37.0	0.0	184	0.5	45.0	0.2	0.0
Black Cherry, with Amaretto, Finest, Tesco*	1 Serving/10g	26.0	0.0	261	0.5	64.4	0.1	0.8
Blackcurrant, Average	*1 Tbsp/15g*	*37.0*	*0.0*	*245*	*0.6*	*60.0*	*0.1*	*1.9*
Blueberry, M & S*	1 Tsp/8g	15.0	0.0	206	0.3	51.1	0.1	1.3
Hedgerow, TTD, Sainsbury's*	1 Tbsp/15g	41.0	0.0	276	0.5	68.2	0.1	0.5
Morello Cherry, Waitrose*	1 Tbsp/15g	39.0	0.0	258	0.4	64.2	0.0	1.4
Plum, TTD, Sainsbury's*	1 Tbsp/15g	44.0	0.0	295	0.3	73.1	0.1	0.5
Raspberry, Average	*1 Tbsp/15g*	*37.0*	*0.0*	*249*	*0.6*	*61.0*	*0.3*	*1.3*
Red Cherry, Finest, Tesco*	1 Tbsp/15g	42.0	0.0	277	0.6	67.6	0.1	0.8
Red Cherry, TTD, Sainsbury's*	1 Tbsp/15g	43.0	0.0	283	0.4	70.2	0.1	0.5
Rhubarb & Ginger, M & S*	1 Tbsp/15g	29.0	0.0	194	0.3	47.9	0.1	1.0
Strawberry, 60% Fruit, Reduced Sugar, M & S*	1 Tsp/7g	9.0	0.0	135	0.4	30.1	0.2	1.9
Strawberry, Average	*1 Tbsp/15g*	*37.0*	*0.0*	*250*	*0.4*	*61.6*	*0.1*	*0.5*
CONSOMME								
Average	*1oz/28g*	*3.0*	*0.0*	*12*	*2.9*	*0.1*	*0.0*	*0.0*
COOKIES								
All Butter, Almond, Italian Style, M & S*	1 Cookie/23g	120.0	6.0	515	6.7	59.4	27.6	3.6
All Butter, Ginger Bread, M & S*	1 Cookie/23g	102.0	5.0	445	4.3	57.5	21.8	2.4
All Butter, Italian Style Sorrento Lemon, M & S*	1 Cookie/24g	120.0	6.0	500	4.9	60.4	26.7	2.1
All Butter, Melting Moment, M & S*	1 Cookie/23g	110.0	6.0	470	4.5	51.5	27.5	3.4
All Butter, Sultana, TTD, Sainsbury's*	1 Biscuit/17g	79.0	4.0	476	5.4	62.7	22.6	2.0
Almond, Ose*	1 Cookie/10g	46.0	1.0	456	8.4	74.0	14.0	0.0
Apple & Raisin, Go Ahead, McVitie's*	1 Cookie/15g	66.0	2.0	443	5.3	76.8	12.7	3.4
Apple Crumble, M & S*	1 Cookie/26g	90.0	1.0	345	4.6	76.8	2.0	2.9
Apple Pie, The Biscuit Collection*	1 Cookie/19g	90.0	4.0	474	3.9	65.0	22.1	0.0
Apricot, COU, M & S*	1 Cookie/26g	88.0	1.0	340	5.4	75.0	2.4	2.0
Big Milk Chocolate Chunk, Cookie Coach*	1 Cookie/35g	174.0	9.0	497	6.2	61.4	25.1	0.0
Bites, Weight Watchers*	1 Pack/21g	97.0	4.0	464	5.8	67.0	19.2	4.3
Brazil Nut, Prewett's*	1 Cookie/50g	122.0	7.0	244	2.6	25.2	14.8	1.0
Butter & Sultana, Sainsbury's*	1 Cookie/13g	61.0	3.0	473	4.5	68.4	20.1	1.6

COOKIES

	Measure INFO/WEIGHT	per Measure KCAL	per Measure FAT	Nutrition Values per 100g / 100ml KCAL	PROT	CARB	FAT	FIBRE
Cherry Bakewell, COU, M & S*	1 Cookie/25g	90.0	1.0	355	6.0	77.2	2.5	3.4
Choc Chip & Coconut, Maryland*	1 Cookie/10g	55.0	3.0	512	5.1	62.9	23.7	0.0
Choc Chip & Hazelnut, Maryland*	1 Cookie/11g	55.0	3.0	513	6.3	65.3	25.0	0.0
Choc Chip 'n' Chunk, McVitie's*	1 Cookie/11g	55.0	3.0	498	5.8	59.2	26.4	3.5
Choc Chip, Reduced Fat, Maryland*	1 Cookie/10.7g	51.0	2.0	478	5.9	73.0	18.0	0.0
Choc Chunk, Fabulous Bakin' Boys*	1 Cookie/60g	270.0	13.0	450	5.0	59.0	21.0	3.0
Chocolate & Nut, Organic, Evernat*	1 Cookie/69g	337.0	16.0	489	7.2	64.1	22.6	0.0
Chocolate & Orange, COU, M & S*	1 Cookie/26g	90.0	1.0	350	5.7	77.2	2.6	3.2
Chocolate Chip, Average	1 Cookie/10g	49.0	2.0	489	5.5	64.1	24.7	2.9
Chocolate Chip, BGTY, Sainsbury's*	1 Cookie/17g	72.0	2.0	428	4.5	75.6	11.9	2.5
Chocolate Chip, Carb Check, Heinz*	1 Cookie/20g	91.0	5.0	457	7.2	43.1	24.9	7.2
Chocolate Chip, Mini, Tesco*	1 Bag/30g	148.0	7.0	493	5.4	64.6	23.7	1.7
Chocolate Chip, Organic, Sainsbury's*	1 Cookie/17g	89.0	5.0	530	5.0	61.8	29.2	0.3
Chocolate Chip, Organic, Tesco*	1 Cookie/17g	88.0	5.0	520	4.0	63.3	27.4	2.8
Chocolate Chip, The Decadent, President's Choice*	1 Cookie/16g	79.0	4.0	513	6.1	61.3	26.4	3.5
Chocolate Chip, Weight Watchers*	1 Cookie/11g	49.0	2.0	443	7.6	65.4	17.2	4.6
Chocolate Chunk & Hazelnut, TTD, Sainsbury's*	1 Biscuit/17g	88.0	5.0	528	6.5	54.8	31.4	2.8
Chocolate Chunk, All Butter, COU, M & S*	1 Cookie/23.9g	110.0	4.0	460	5.7	69.1	17.9	2.3
Chocolate Chunk, All Butter, M & S*	1 Cookie/24g	120.0	6.0	500	5.2	62.4	25.2	2.9
Chocolate Chunk, Cadbury*	1 Cookie/22g	119.0	7.0	540	6.5	58.0	31.2	0.0
Chocolate Coated, Wheatfree, Sunstart*	1 Cookie/20.0g	103.0	6.0	516	5.6	54.4	30.7	4.1
Chocolate Fruit & Nut, Extra Special, Asda*	1 Cookie/25g	125.0	7.0	509	6.0	56.0	29.0	2.0
Chocolate Orange, Half Coated, Finest, Tesco*	1 Cookie/22g	107.0	6.0	488	4.9	59.6	25.5	1.2
Chocolate, Belgian, Extra Special, Asda*	1 Cookie/26g	138.0	8.0	535	6.0	58.0	31.0	2.0
Chocolate, Milk, Free From, Tesco*	1 Cookie/20g	100.0	6.0	500	5.6	50.4	30.7	4.1
Chocolate, Quadruple, Sainsbury's*	1 Cookie/20g	117.0	7.0	585	6.0	66.5	33.0	1.5
Chocolate, Triple, Half Coated, Finest, Tesco*	1 Cookie/25g	131.0	7.0	525	5.7	58.7	29.3	2.3
Cocoa, Organic, Bites, No Junk, Organix*	1 Bag/25g	105.0	3.0	421	7.0	69.0	13.0	5.5
Coconut & Raspberry, Gluten Free, Sainsbury's*	1 Cookie/20g	102.0	6.0	511	5.9	56.0	29.3	6.7
Coconut, Gluten-Free, Sainsbury's*	1 Cookie/20g	103.0	6.0	516	5.6	54.4	30.7	4.1
Cranberry & Orange, Finest, Tesco*	1 Cookie/25.5g	125.0	6.0	490	4.1	67.4	22.6	3.2
Cranberry & Orange, Go Ahead, McVitie's*	1 Cookie/17g	77.0	2.0	452	5.3	78.0	13.2	2.4
Danish Butter, Tesco*	1 Cookie/26g	133.0	7.0	516	4.7	66.7	25.6	1.3
Dark Chocolate Chunk & Ginger, The Best, Morrisons*	1 Cookie/25g	126.0	6.0	503	4.6	63.7	25.5	2.8
Dark Treacle, Weight Watchers*	1 Cookie/11g	49.0	2.0	423	5.2	66.7	15.1	1.7
Double Choc Chip, Giant, Paterson's*	1 Cookie/60g	293.0	15.0	489	0.3	61.3	25.3	3.7
Double Choc Chip, Mini, M & S*	1 Cookie/22g	108.0	5.0	490	5.3	63.6	23.7	1.8
Double Choc Chip, Tesco*	1 Cookie/11g	55.0	3.0	500	4.2	65.3	24.7	3.0
Double Choc Chip, Weight Watchers*	1 Biscuit/11g	49.0	2.0	443	7.6	65.4	17.2	4.6
Double Choc, Cadbury*	1 Biscuit/11g	55.0	3.0	485	7.3	64.3	22.2	0.0
Double Choc, Maryland*	1 Cookie/10g	51.0	3.0	510	5.2	64.4	25.7	0.0
Double Chocolate & Walnut, Soft, Tesco*	1 Cookie/25g	116.0	6.0	463	5.8	52.1	25.7	4.7
Double Chocolate Chip, Organic, Waitrose*	1 Cookie/18g	96.0	6.0	535	5.1	58.6	31.0	1.9
Double Chocolate Chip, Traidcraft*	1 Cookie/22g	114.0	6.0	520	5.8	64.1	26.7	2.4
Double Fudge & Chocolate, Sugar Free, Murray*	1 Cookie/12g	47.0	2.0	400	5.7	65.7	20.0	5.7
Fortune, Average	1 Cookie/8g	30.0	0.0	378	4.2	84.0	2.7	1.6
Fudge Brownie American Cream, Sainsbury's*	1 Cookie/12g	60.0	3.0	499	4.8	67.9	23.2	2.2
Fudge Brownie, Maryland*	1 Cookie/11g	56.0	3.0	510	5.8	63.0	25.0	0.0
Ginger, Low Fat, M & S*	1 Cookie/23g	82.0	1.0	358	5.1	74.9	4.3	2.4
Ginger, Safeway*	1 Cookie/22g	106.0	5.0	480	4.7	66.5	22.7	2.4
Hazelnut & Choc Chip 'n' Chunk, McVitie's*	1 Cookie/11g	55.0	3.0	505	6.1	57.8	27.7	3.5
Hazelnut, Gluten Free, Dove's Farm*	1 Cookie/16.5g	80.0	4.0	484	4.5	56.8	26.8	1.8
Lemon & Ginger, Weight Watchers*	1 Biscuit/11g	49.0	2.0	450	6.4	65.0	18.2	5.0

	Measure INFO/WEIGHT	per Measure KCAL	FAT	Nutrition Values per 100g / 100ml KCAL	PROT	CARB	FAT	FIBRE
COOKIES								
Lemon Meringue, COU, M & S*	1 Cookie/25g	89.0	1.0	355	5.6	77.6	2.6	3.0
Milk Chocolate, Classic, Millie's Cookies*	1 Cookie/45g	190.0	10.0	422	5.1	49.3	22.7	1.3
Oat & Cranberry, BGTY, Sainsbury's*	1 Cookie/28g	126.0	5.0	449	6.8	65.0	18.0	5.1
Oat & Raisin, Health Matters*	1 Cookie/8g	33.0	1.0	414	7.0	76.6	8.8	3.3
Oat & Treacle, TTD, Sainsbury's*	1 Biscuit/25g	121.0	6.0	482	5.7	61.8	23.6	3.7
Oat, Giant Jumbo, Paterson's*	1 Cookie/60g	299.0	16.0	499	0.4	58.4	27.0	3.2
Oatflake & Honey, Organic, Sainsbury's*	1 Cookie/17g	82.0	4.0	480	6.3	66.0	21.2	2.6
Oatflake & Raisin, Waitrose*	1 Cookie/17g	80.0	4.0	469	5.8	61.7	22.1	4.7
Oreo, Nabisco*	1 Cookie/11g	52.0	2.0	471	5.9	70.6	20.6	2.9
Pecan & Maple, Mini, Bronte*	1 Pack/100g	509.0	27.0	509	5.4	60.3	27.3	1.6
Quadruple Chocolate, TTD, Sainsbury's*	1 Biscuit/20g	104.0	6.0	518	6.2	59.8	28.2	1.6
Raisin & Cinnamon, Low Fat, M & S*	1 Cookie/22g	78.0	1.0	355	6.2	73.0	4.1	3.2
Raspberry & White Chocolate, Weight Watchers*	1 Cookie/11g	49.0	2.0	443	5.2	71.4	17.2	4.6
Raspberry Spritz, Heaven Scent*	1 Cookie/19g	90.0	6.0	474	5.3	52.6	31.6	0.0
Rolo, Nestle*	1 Cookie/73g	242.0	11.0	331	3.4	46.0	15.2	0.6
Spiced Apple, COU, M & S*	1 Cookie/25g	82.0	1.0	330	5.0	72.8	2.5	2.1
Stem Ginger, BGTY, Sainsbury's*	1 Cookie/17g	73.0	2.0	431	4.5	76.5	11.9	1.7
Stem Ginger, Free From, Sainsbury's*	1 Cookie/17.1g	84.0	5.0	489	6.5	58.0	28.0	6.8
Stem Ginger, Less Than 5% Fat, M & S*	1 Cookie/22g	79.0	1.0	360	6.2	73.9	4.3	3.0
Stem Ginger, Reduced Fat, Waitrose*	1 Cookie/16.7g	75.0	3.0	448	4.5	71.0	16.2	1.6
Stem Ginger, Tesco*	1 Cookie/20g	98.0	5.0	489	4.2	64.0	24.0	2.0
Stem Ginger, TTD, Sainsbury's*	1 Cookie/17g	79.0	4.0	476	5.2	64.3	22.0	2.3
Sultana & Cinnamon, Weight Watchers*	1 Cookie/11.5g	46.0	1.0	398	5.0	67.1	12.1	1.8
Sultana, All Butter, Reduced Fat, M & S*	1 Cookie/17g	70.0	2.0	420	4.9	68.6	14.2	2.6
Sultana, Soft & Chewy, Sainsbury's*	1 Cookie/25g	103.0	3.0	414	4.4	67.8	13.9	2.5
Tennessee American Style, Stiftung & Co*	1 Cookie/19g	96.0	5.0	504	6.0	66.0	24.0	0.0
Toffee, Weight Watchers*	1 Cookie/11.5g	52.0	2.0	456	5.2	71.1	16.8	2.9
White Chocolate & Raspberry, McVitie's*	1 Cookie/17g	87.0	4.0	512	4.7	64.1	25.9	1.8
White Chocolate, Maryland*	1 Cookie/10g	51.0	2.0	512	5.7	64.0	25.0	0.0
White Chocolate, TTD, Sainsbury's*	1 Cookie/25g	126.0	6.0	504	5.5	62.5	25.8	1.2
COQ AU VIN								
Finest, Tesco*	1 Serving/273g	251.0	10.0	92	14.3	0.7	3.6	1.8
HL, Tesco*	½ Pack/200g	172.0	4.0	86	15.2	2.1	1.9	0.4
M & S*	1 Serving/295g	398.0	23.0	135	14.2	1.5	7.7	1.0
Perfectly Balanced, Waitrose*	1 Pack/500g	445.0	15.0	89	12.6	2.7	3.1	0.6
Sainsbury's*	1 Pack/400g	484.0	18.0	121	16.8	3.5	4.4	0.2
with Potatoes, Diet Chef Ltd*	1 Pack/300g	285.0	13.0	95	7.7	6.1	4.4	2.2
CORDIAL								
Elderflower, Made Up, Bottle Green*	1 Glass/200ml	46.0	0.0	23	0.0	5.6	0.0	0.0
Elderflower, Undiluted, Waitrose*	1 Serving/20ml	22.0	0.0	110	0.0	27.5	0.0	0.0
CORIANDER								
Leaves, Dried, Average	**1oz/28g**	**78.0**	**1.0**	**279**	**21.8**	**41.7**	**4.8**	**0.0**
Leaves, Fresh, Average	**1 Bunch/20g**	**5.0**	**0.0**	**23**	**2.1**	**3.7**	**0.5**	**2.8**
Seeds, Ground, Schwartz*	1 Tsp/5g	22.0	1.0	446	14.2	54.9	18.8	0.0
CORN								
Baby, & Asparagus Tips, Tesco*	1 Pack/150g	37.0	1.0	25	2.6	2.5	0.5	1.9
Baby, & Mange Tout, Tesco*	1 Serving/100g	27.0	0.0	27	2.9	3.3	0.2	2.1
Baby, & Sugar Snap Peas, Safeway*	½ Pack/100g	27.0	0.0	27	2.9	3.3	0.2	0.0
Baby, Average	**1 Serving/80g**	**21.0**	**0.0**	**26**	**2.5**	**3.1**	**0.4**	**1.7**
Cobs, Boiled, Weighed with Cob, Average	**1 Ear/200g**	**132.0**	**3.0**	**66**	**2.5**	**11.6**	**1.4**	**1.3**
Creamed Style, Green Giant*	1 Can/418g	238.0	2.0	57	1.2	11.9	0.5	3.0
in Brine, for Stir Fry, Braxted Hall*	1 Can/133g	25.0	0.0	19	1.5	3.0	0.0	1.5

	Measure INFO/WEIGHT	per Measure KCAL	FAT	Nutrition Values per 100g / 100ml KCAL	PROT	CARB	FAT	FIBRE
CORN CAKES								
M & S*	½ Pack/85g	238.0	17.0	280	6.4	19.8	20.0	3.4
Organic, Kallo*	1 Cake/5g	16.0	0.0	340	12.7	74.3	4.1	11.2
Ryvita*	1 Pack/13.1g	48.0	0.0	366	10.0	74.3	3.2	7.2
Slightly Salted, Mrs Crimble's*	1 Pack/27.5g	104.0	1.0	380	7.9	80.0	3.4	5.4
Thick Slices, Orgran*	1 Cake/11g	42.0	0.0	385	13.2	79.0	3.7	14.2
CORN SNACKS								
Crispy, Bugles*	1 Bag/20g	102.0	6.0	508	4.8	60.7	28.0	1.4
Light Bites, Cheese Flavour, Special K, Kellogg's*	1 Packet/28g	116.0	2.0	416	9.0	77.0	8.0	1.0
Light Bites, Tikka Flavour, Special K, Kellogg's*	1 Pack/28g	116.0	2.0	416	7.0	79.0	8.0	1.5
Paprika Flavour, Shapers, Boots*	1 Pack/13g	64.0	4.0	494	8.7	54.0	27.0	2.2
Scampi, Smiths, Walkers*	1 Bag/27g	134.0	7.0	496	13.0	52.5	26.0	0.0
Toasted, Holland & Barrett*	1 Serving/100g	412.0	12.0	412	8.1	69.7	12.1	4.0
CORNED BEEF								
Average	*1 Slice/35g*	*75.0*	*4.0*	*214*	*25.9*	*0.7*	*12.1*	*0.0*
CORNFLAKE NEST								
Crunchy Chocolate, M & S*	1 Nest/15g	70.0	3.0	475	6.3	67.2	20.2	2.2
CORNFLOUR								
Average	*1 Tsp/5g*	*18.0*	*0.0*	*355*	*0.6*	*86.9*	*1.2*	*0.1*
COURGETTE								
& Sweetcorn, Fresh 'n' Ready, Sainsbury's*	1oz/28g	12.0	0.0	42	2.3	6.7	0.9	1.3
Boiled in Unsalted Water, Average	*1oz/28g*	*5.0*	*0.0*	*19*	*2.0*	*2.0*	*0.4*	*1.2*
Fried, Average	*1oz/28g*	*18.0*	*1.0*	*63*	*2.6*	*2.6*	*4.8*	*1.2*
COUS COUS								
& Chargrilled Vegetables, M & S*	1 Serving/200g	200.0	3.0	100	3.9	17.3	1.5	1.6
Alle Spices Mediterraneo, Antony Worrall Thompson's*	½ Pack/100g	352.0	3.0	352	10.7	71.0	2.8	3.8
Chargrilled Red & Yellow Pepper, Tesco*	1 Pack/200g	212.0	4.0	106	4.6	17.8	1.8	0.5
Chargrilled Vegetables & Olive Oil, Delphi*	½ Pot/75g	105.0	3.0	140	3.8	22.5	3.9	1.9
Citrus Kick, Cooked, Ainsley Harriott*	1 Serving/130g	182.0	2.0	140	4.3	27.9	1.2	2.4
Citrus Kick, Dry, Ainsley Harriott*	½ Sachet/50g	184.0	1.0	368	11.6	77.0	2.4	9.2
Cooked, Average	*1 Cup/157g*	*249.0*	*3.0*	*158*	*4.3*	*31.4*	*1.9*	*1.3*
Coriander & Lemon, Sainsbury's*	½ Pack/137g	205.0	6.0	150	4.3	23.4	4.3	2.7
Dry, Average	*1 Serving/50g*	*178.0*	*1.0*	*356*	*13.7*	*72.8*	*1.5*	*2.6*
Garlic & Coriander, Dry, Waitrose*	1 Serving/70g	235.0	3.0	336	11.7	64.2	3.6	6.2
Harissa Style Savoury, Sainsbury's*	1 Serving/260g	434.0	12.0	167	4.7	26.8	4.6	1.3
in Soy Sauce, with Sesame Ginger, Amazing Grains*	½ Sachet/50g	180.0	1.0	360	11.2	73.0	2.6	3.1
Indian Style, Sainsbury's*	½ Pack/143g	204.0	4.0	143	4.5	25.1	2.7	1.0
Israeli & Sardinian, TTD, Sainsbury's*	¼ Pot/55g	69.0	3.0	126	3.2	17.7	4.7	1.6
Lemon & Coriander, Cooked, Tesco*	1 Serving/137g	207.0	3.0	151	4.0	28.3	2.4	2.0
Lemon & Coriander, Dry, Tesco*	1 Pack/110g	375.0	3.0	341	11.0	68.2	2.7	6.1
Mediterranean Style, Cooked, Tesco*	1 Serving/146g	215.0	4.0	147	4.4	26.5	2.6	1.3
Mediterranean Style, Dry, Tesco*	1 Pack/110g	368.0	3.0	335	11.9	65.1	3.0	5.6
Mediterranean Tomato, GFY, Asda*	½ Pack/141g	192.0	1.0	136	5.0	27.0	0.9	1.7
Mint & Coriander Flavour, Dry, Amazing Grains*	1 Sachet/99g	349.0	3.0	353	12.2	70.0	2.7	3.2
Moroccan Medley, Cooked, Ainsley Harriott*	½ Sachet/130g	186.0	2.0	143	5.4	25.4	1.5	2.2
Moroccan Style, Break, GFY, Asda*	1 Pack/150.3g	215.0	3.0	143	5.6	26.1	1.8	1.8
Moroccan Style, Finest, Tesco*	1 Tub/225g	292.0	6.0	130	4.3	22.6	2.5	3.7
Moroccan Style, Fruity, M & S*	1 Serving/200g	370.0	5.0	185	3.4	36.7	2.7	3.4
Moroccan Style, Sainsbury's*	½ Pack/150g	195.0	4.0	130	5.0	21.5	2.7	1.0
Moroccan Sultana & Pine Nuts, Dry, Sammy's*	1 Serving/50g	171.0	1.0	343	12.0	72.0	3.0	6.0
Moroccan, Roast Chicken, Delicious, Shapers, Boots*	1 Pack/250g	247.0	4.0	99	9.2	12.0	1.5	2.6
Mushrooms, Onion, Garlic & Herbs, Dry, Tesco*	½ Pack/50g	166.0	1.0	333	11.3	66.2	2.6	4.9
Plain, Dry Weight, Tesco*	1 Serving/50g	182.0	1.0	365	15.1	73.1	1.1	0.8
Red Pepper & Chilli, Waitrose*	1 Pack/200g	344.0	14.0	172	4.5	23.0	6.9	1.3

	Measure INFO/WEIGHT	per Measure KCAL	per Measure FAT	Nutrition Values per 100g / 100ml KCAL	PROT	CARB	FAT	FIBRE
COUS COUS								
Roast Garlic & Olive Oil, Dry Weight, Sammy's*	1 Serving/50g	169.0	1.0	339	12.0	71.5	3.0	0.0
Roasted Vegetable, Dry, Ainsley Harriott*	½ Sachet/50g	180.0	2.0	360	14.6	66.4	4.0	6.8
Roasted Vegetable, Snack Salad Pot, HL, Tesco*	1 Pack/60g	213.0	2.0	355	15.1	64.6	4.0	4.2
Roasted Vegetables, Waitrose*	1 Serving/200g	328.0	13.0	164	3.9	22.0	6.6	0.9
Spice Fusion, Lyttos*	1 Serving/100g	134.0	1.0	134	4.3	23.9	1.5	3.4
Spice Sensation, Dry, Ainsley Harriott*	½ Sachet/50g	166.0	1.0	332	11.6	66.2	2.4	9.2
Spicy Moroccan Chicken & Veg, COU, M & S*	1 Pack/400g	380.0	7.0	95	9.1	10.3	1.7	1.9
Spicy Vegetable, GFY, Asda*	½ Pack/55g	71.0	1.0	129	4.7	25.0	1.1	2.0
Sun Dried Tomato, & Mediterranean Herbs, Sammy's*	1 Serving/63g	210.0	2.0	333	13.2	70.5	2.9	6.7
Tangy Tomato, Dry, Ainsley Harriott*	½ Sachet/50g	166.0	1.0	332	12.2	67.2	1.6	8.8
Tomato & Basil, Made Up, Tesco*	1 Serving/200g	348.0	17.0	174	3.9	21.0	8.3	3.4
Tomato & Onion, Dry Weight, Waitrose*	1 Pack/110g	376.0	4.0	342	12.6	64.9	3.6	5.1
Tomato & Vegetable, Snack Pack, Dry, Sammy's*	1 Serving/70g	228.0	2.0	326	12.0	67.9	3.5	6.3
with Balsamic Roasted Vegetables, TTD, Sainsbury's*	1/3 Pack/80g	94.0	4.0	117	2.8	14.3	5.4	1.1
Zesty Lemon & Coriander, Dry, Sammy's*	1 Serving/50g	171.0	1.0	342	13.0	74.0	2.8	6.0
CRAB								
Boiled, Meat Only, Average	*1 Tbsp/40g*	*51.0*	*2.0*	*128*	*19.5*	*0.0*	*5.5*	*0.0*
Claws, Asda*	1oz/28g	25.0	0.0	89	11.0	9.0	1.0	0.2
Dressed, Average	*1 Can/43g*	*66.0*	*3.0*	*154*	*16.8*	*4.1*	*7.9*	*0.2*
Meat, in Brine, Average	*½ Can/60g*	*46.0*	*0.0*	*76*	*17.2*	*0.9*	*0.4*	*0.1*
Meat, Raw, Average	*1oz/28g*	*28.0*	*0.0*	*100*	*20.8*	*2.8*	*0.6*	*0.0*
CRAB CAKES								
Goan, M & S*	1 Pack/190g	228.0	8.0	120	8.0	12.9	4.0	1.8
Iceland*	1 Serving/18g	52.0	3.0	288	7.2	25.6	18.0	1.3
Shetland Isles, Dressed, TTD, Sainsbury's*	1 Crab/75g	130.0	8.0	174	12.4	6.0	11.1	0.5
Tesco*	1 Serving/130g	281.0	16.0	216	11.0	15.4	12.3	1.1
Thai, TTD, Sainsbury's*	½ Pack/106g	201.0	9.0	189	9.5	17.8	8.9	1.4
CRAB STICKS								
Average	1 Stick/15g	14.0	0.0	94	9.1	13.9	0.3	0.0
CRACKERBREAD								
High Fibre, Crackerbread, Ryvita*	1 Slice/5.2g	17.0	0.0	325	12.5	62.4	2.8	15.0
Original, Ryvita*	1 Slice/5.5g	21.0	0.0	380	10.3	76.9	3.5	3.5
Rice, Asda*	1 Slice/5g	19.0	0.0	374	9.1	79.4	2.2	1.9
Rice, Ryvita*	1 Slice/5.1g	19.0	0.0	374	9.1	79.4	2.2	1.9
Sainsbury's*	1 Slice/5g	19.0	0.0	380	10.0	80.0	4.0	2.0
Wheat, Original, Ryvita*	1 Slice/5g	19.0	0.0	380	10.3	76.9	3.5	3.5
Wholemeal, Crackerbread, Ryvita*	1 Serving/5g	17.0	0.0	373	11.0	73.2	4.0	6.5
CRACKERS								
Bath Oliver, Jacob's*	1 Cracker/12g	52.0	2.0	432	9.6	67.6	13.7	2.6
Black Olive, M & S*	1 Cracker/4g	20.0	1.0	485	8.3	59.4	23.5	4.3
Blazing BBQ, Jacobites, Jacob's*	1 Pack/9g	41.0	2.0	461	5.2	55.8	24.2	1.7
Bran, Jacob's*	1 Cracker/7g	32.0	1.0	454	9.7	62.8	18.2	3.2
Butter Puff, Sainsbury's*	1 Cracker/10g	54.0	3.0	523	10.4	60.7	26.5	2.5
Chapati Chips, Tikka, Medium Spicy, Patak's*	1 Serving/25g	127.0	7.0	508	8.0	56.0	28.0	4.0
Cheddars, McVitie's*	1 Cracker/4g	22.0	1.0	543	10.0	55.1	31.3	2.6
Cheese Thins, Asda*	1 Cracker/4g	21.0	1.0	532	12.0	49.0	32.0	0.0
Cheese Thins, Cheddar, The Planet Snack Co*	1 Serving/30g	153.0	9.0	509	11.5	50.1	29.2	2.1
Cheese Thins, Mini, Snack Rite*	1 Bag/30g	144.0	7.0	480	12.9	55.9	22.7	2.5
Cheese Thins, Waitrose*	1 Cracker/4g	21.0	1.0	545	11.9	52.6	31.9	2.5
Cheese, Cheddar, Crispies, TTD, Sainsbury's*	1 Thin/4g	21.0	1.0	576	14.2	39.0	40.4	2.2
Cheese, Mini, Heinz*	1 Pack/25g	108.0	4.0	433	9.4	68.6	14.6	0.6
Cheese, Mini, Shapers, Boots*	1 Serving/23g	97.0	3.0	421	9.4	65.0	14.0	4.6
Cheese, Ritz*	1 Cracker/4g	17.0	1.0	486	10.1	55.9	24.7	2.2

CRACKERS

INFO/WEIGHT	Measure KCAL	FAT	KCAL	PROT	CARB	FAT	FIBRE
Chinese, Pop Pan*	1 Cracker/7.5g	40.0	2.0	533	13.3	53.3	33.3	0.0
Chives, Jacob's*	1 Cracker/6g	28.0	1.0	457	9.5	67.5	16.5	2.7
Choice Grain, Jacob's*	1 Cracker/7.5g	32.0	1.0	427	9.0	65.5	14.3	5.4
Corn Thins, Real Foods*	1 Serving/6g	22.0	0.0	378	10.2	81.7	3.0	8.6
Cream, Average	1 Cracker/7g	31.0	1.0	440	9.5	68.3	16.3	2.2
Cream, BGTY, Sainsbury's*	1 Cracker/8g	32.0	1.0	400	10.9	71.7	7.7	3.1
Cream, Choice Grain, Jacob's*	1 Cracker/7g	30.0	1.0	400	9.0	64.5	11.8	7.0
Cream, Light, Jacob's*	1 Cracker/8g	31.0	1.0	388	10.6	72.2	6.3	4.1
Cream, Roasted Onion, Jacob's*	1 Cracker/8g	35.0	1.0	441	10.2	66.8	14.8	2.9
Cream, Sun Dried Tomato Flavour, Jacob's*	1 Cracker/8g	35.0	1.0	434	10.2	66.7	14.0	3.0
Crispy Cheese, M & S*	1 Cracker/4.3g	20.0	1.0	470	9.4	58.1	22.1	3.0
Extra Wheatgerm, Hovis*	1 Serving/6g	27.0	1.0	447	10.2	60.0	18.5	4.4
Garden Herbs, Jacob's*	1 Cracker/6g	28.0	1.0	457	9.5	67.5	16.5	2.7
Glutafin*	1 Serving/11g	52.0	2.0	470	2.4	70.0	20.0	0.7
Harvest Grain, Sainsbury's*	1 Cracker/6g	27.0	1.0	458	8.5	64.5	18.4	4.1
Herb & Onion, 99% Fat Free, Rakusen's*	1 Cracker/5g	18.0	0.0	360	9.1	82.6	1.0	3.9
Herb & Onion, Trufree*	1 Cracker/6g	25.0	1.0	418	2.5	75.0	12.0	10.0
Herb & Spice, Jacob's*	1 Cracker/6g	27.0	1.0	457	9.5	67.5	16.5	2.7
Herbs & Spice Selection, Jacob's*	1 Cracker/6g	27.0	1.0	451	9.5	68.0	15.7	2.7
Japanese Style Rice Mix, Asda*	1 Serving/25g	96.0	0.0	385	6.8	88.0	0.6	0.5
Krackawheat, McVitie's*	1 Cracker/7.4g	33.0	1.0	446	9.7	60.0	18.6	5.8
Light & Crispy, Sainsbury's*	1 Cracker/11g	42.0	1.0	384	11.3	61.0	10.5	13.0
Lightly Salted, Crispy, Sainsbury's*	1 Cracker/5g	25.0	1.0	533	7.8	62.6	27.9	2.1
Lightly Salted, Italian, Jacob's*	1 Cracker/6g	26.0	1.0	429	10.3	67.6	13.0	2.9
Mediterranean, Jacob's*	1 Cracker/6g	27.0	1.0	450	9.7	66.5	16.1	2.7
Mixed Seed, Multi Grain, Asda*	1 Cracker/6g	28.0	1.0	445	11.0	62.0	17.0	4.4
Multigrain, Corn Thins, Real Foods*	1 Cracker/6g	23.0	0.0	388	10.9	71.0	3.7	10.3
Multigrain, Snack Crackers, Special K, Kellogg's*	1 Pack/30g	120.0	3.0	400	10.0	73.3	10.0	6.7
Multigrain, Tesco*	1 Cracker/6g	27.0	1.0	458	8.5	64.5	18.4	4.1
Oat & Wheat, Weight Watchers*	4 Crackers/20g	74.0	0.0	368	8.3	78.9	2.1	3.5
Olive Oil & Oregano, Mediterreaneo, Jacob's*	1 Cracker/6g	25.0	1.0	412	12.4	65.5	11.2	6.0
Oriental, Asda*	1 Serving/30g	115.0	6.0	383	1.7	49.0	20.0	4.3
Passionately Pizza, Jacobites, Jacob's*	1 Pack/150g	708.0	38.0	472	5.7	55.3	25.4	1.7
Pesto, Jacob's*	1 Cracker/6g	27.0	1.0	450	9.7	66.5	16.1	2.7
Poppy & Sesame Seed, Sainsbury's*	1 Cracker/4g	21.0	1.0	530	9.6	58.9	28.4	3.4
Ritz, Original, Jacob's*	1 Cracker/3.3g	17.0	1.0	509	6.9	55.6	28.8	2.0
Rye, Organic, Dove's Farm*	1 Cracker/7g	28.0	1.0	393	7.0	58.4	14.6	8.7
Salt & Black Pepper, Jacob's*	1 Cracker/6g	27.0	1.0	457	9.5	67.5	16.5	2.7
Salted, Ritz, Nabisco*	1 Cracker/3.4g	17.0	1.0	493	7.0	57.5	26.1	2.9
Selection, Finest, Tesco*	1 Serving/30g	136.0	4.0	452	9.6	71.0	14.4	0.0
Sesame & Poppy Thins, Tesco*	1 Cracker/4g	20.0	1.0	485	9.9	57.6	23.5	4.4
Spicy Indonesian Vegetable, Waitrose*	1 Pack/60g	295.0	16.0	492	1.2	60.6	27.2	2.2
Spicy Vegetable, Tesco*	1 Serving/60g	340.0	23.0	566	2.6	52.4	38.4	1.2
Spicy, Trufree*	1 Cracker/6g	25.0	1.0	412	3.8	70.0	13.0	12.5
Sweet Chilli, Thins, Savours, Jacob's*	1 Cracker/4.4g	21.0	1.0	472	8.0	62.3	21.2	3.6
Tempting Tandoori, Jacobites, Jacob's*	1 Pack/150g	711.0	38.0	474	5.7	55.5	25.5	1.7
Thai Spicy Vegetable, Sainsbury's*	1 Pack/50g	231.0	10.0	462	7.2	61.5	20.8	2.6
Tuc, Cheese Sandwich, Jacob's*	1 Cracker/13.6g	72.0	4.0	531	8.4	53.8	31.4	0.0
Tuc, Jacob's*	1 Cracker/5g	24.0	1.0	522	7.0	60.5	28.0	2.9
Tuc, Mini, with Sesame Seeds, Jacob's*	1 Biscuit/2g	10.0	1.0	523	9.7	63.1	25.8	3.9
Unsalted, Tops, Premium Plus, Impress*	1 Cracker/3g	13.0	0.0	448	10.3	75.9	10.3	0.0
Vegetable, Oriental Snack Selection, Sainsbury's*	1 Cracker/20g	42.0	2.0	209	4.5	26.2	9.6	3.4
Veggie, Heinz, Heinz*	1 Pack/25g	110.0	3.0	440	7.0	76.0	12.0	3.6

	Measure INFO/WEIGHT	per Measure KCAL	FAT	Nutrition Values per 100g / 100ml KCAL	PROT	CARB	FAT	FIBRE
CRACKERS								
Waterthins, Wafers, Philemon*	1 Crackers/2g	7.0	0.0	392	10.6	77.9	3.6	5.0
Wheaten, M & S*	1 Cracker/4g	20.0	1.0	450	10.2	57.0	20.2	5.0
Whole Wheat, 100%, Oven Baked, Master Choice*	1 Cracker/4g	17.0	0.0	429	10.0	75.0	9.6	12.1
Wholemeal, Tesco*	1 Cracker/7g	29.0	1.0	414	9.4	60.6	14.9	10.4
Wholewheat, Saiwa*	1 Pack/31g	128.0	4.0	414	12.5	62.9	12.5	7.9
Wholmeal, Organic, Nairn's*	1 Cracker/14g	58.0	2.0	413	9.0	61.4	14.6	8.7
with Onion, Cumin Seed, & Garlic, GFY, Asda*	1 Cracker/6g	22.0	0.0	380	11.0	78.0	2.7	1.7
CRANBERRIES								
Dried, Sweetened, Average	*1 Serving/10g*	*34.0*	*0.0*	*335*	*0.3*	*81.1*	*0.8*	*4.4*
Fresh, Raw	*1oz/28g*	*4.0*	*0.0*	*15*	*0.4*	*3.4*	*0.1*	*3.0*
CRAYFISH								
Raw	*1oz/28g*	*19.0*	*0.0*	*67*	*14.9*	*0.0*	*0.8*	*0.0*
CREAM								
Aerosol, Average	*1oz/28g*	*87.0*	*9.0*	*309*	*1.7*	*6.2*	*30.9*	*0.0*
Aerosol, Reduced Fat, Average	*1 Serving/55ml*	*33.0*	*3.0*	*59*	*0.6*	*1.9*	*5.4*	*0.0*
Brandy, Pourable, with Remy Martin*, Finest, Tesco*	½ Pot/125ml	460.0	35.0	368	2.7	19.8	28.4	0.0
Brandy, Really Thick, Tesco*	1 Sm Pot/250ml	1162.0	98.0	465	1.4	21.3	39.3	0.0
Chantilly, TTD, Sainsbury's*	2 Tbsp/30g	136.0	14.0	455	1.4	6.9	46.8	0.0
Clotted, Fresh, Average	*1 Serving/28g*	*162.0*	*18.0*	*579*	*1.6*	*2.3*	*62.7*	*0.0*
Double, Average	*1 Serving/25ml*	*110.0*	*12.0*	*438*	*1.8*	*2.7*	*46.7*	*0.0*
Double, Reduced Fat, Average	*1 Serving/30g*	*73.0*	*7.0*	*243*	*2.7*	*5.6*	*23.3*	*0.1*
Extra Thick, 99% Real Dairy Cream, Anchor*	1 Serving/12.5g	51.0	5.0	409	1.7	3.9	43.0	0.0
Single, Average	*1 Tbsp/15ml*	*18.0*	*2.0*	*123*	*2.6*	*4.4*	*10.5*	*0.1*
Single, Extra Thick, Average	*1 Serving/38ml*	*72.0*	*7.0*	*192*	*2.7*	*4.1*	*18.4*	*0.0*
Soured, Fresh, Average	*1 Tbsp/15ml*	*29.0*	*3.0*	*191*	*2.7*	*3.9*	*18.4*	*0.0*
Soured, Reduced Fat, Average	*1 fl oz/30ml*	*36.0*	*3.0*	*119*	*5.2*	*6.7*	*8.6*	*0.4*
Strawberry, Light, Real Dairy, Uht, Anchor*	1 Serving/12.5g	25.0	2.0	198	2.6	8.7	17.0	0.0
Thick, Sterilised, Average	*1 Tbsp/15ml*	*35.0*	*3.0*	*233*	*2.6*	*3.6*	*23.1*	*0.0*
Uht, Double, Average	*1 Tbsp/15g*	*41.0*	*4.0*	*274*	*2.2*	*7.3*	*26.3*	*0.0*
Uht, Reduced Fat, Average	*1 Serving/25ml*	*15.0*	*1.0*	*62*	*0.5*	*2.2*	*5.6*	*0.0*
Uht, Single, Average	*1 Tbsp/15ml*	*29.0*	*3.0*	*194*	*2.6*	*4.0*	*18.8*	*0.0*
Whipping, Average	*1 Tbsp/15ml*	*52.0*	*5.0*	*348*	*2.1*	*3.2*	*36.4*	*0.0*
CREAM ALTERNATIVE								
Supreme, Better Than Sour Cream, Tofutti*	2 Tbsp/28g	85.0	5.0	304	3.6	32.1	17.9	0.0
CREAM SODA								
American, with Vanilla, Tesco*	1 Glass/313ml	75.0	0.0	24	0.0	5.9	0.0	0.0
Diet, Sainsbury's*	1 Serving/250ml	2.0	0.0	1	0.0	0.0	0.0	0.0
No Added Sugar, Sainsbury's*	1 Can/330ml	2.0	0.0	0	0.1	0.1	0.1	0.1
Traditional Style, Tesco*	1 Can/330ml	139.0	0.0	42	0.0	10.4	0.0	0.0
CREME BRULEE								
Gastropub, M & S*	1 Brulee/83.8g	285.0	25.0	340	3.1	15.7	29.3	0.7
M & S*	1 Pot/100g	360.0	33.0	360	3.3	13.0	32.6	0.0
Nestle*	1 Serving/100g	305.0	26.0	305	4.0	14.6	25.6	0.0
Somerfield*	1 Pot/100g	316.0	27.0	316	4.0	15.0	27.0	0.0
CREME CARAMEL								
Average	1 Serving/128g	140.0	3.0	109	3.0	20.6	2.2	0.0
CREME EGG								
Cadbury*	1 Egg/39g	174.0	6.0	445	3.0	71.0	16.0	0.0
Minis, Cadbury*	1 Egg/11.2g	50.0	2.0	445	4.1	67.5	16.4	0.4
CREME FRAICHE								
Average	*1 Pot/295g*	*1067.0*	*112.0*	*362*	*2.2*	*2.6*	*38.0*	*0.0*
Cucumber & Mint, Triangles, Sainsbury's*	1 Serving/25g	105.0	2.0	421	11.0	72.3	9.7	2.5
Extra Light, President*	1 Tub/200g	182.0	10.0	91	2.7	8.7	5.0	0.0

	Measure INFO/WEIGHT	per Measure KCAL	FAT	Nutrition Values per 100g / 100ml KCAL	PROT	CARB	FAT	FIBRE
CREME FRAICHE								
Half Fat, Average	*1 Serving/30g*	*54.0*	*5.0*	*181*	*3.1*	*5.5*	*16.2*	*0.0*
Lemon & Rocket, Sainsbury's*	1 Serving/150g	187.0	17.0	125	2.2	3.0	11.5	0.5
CREPES								
Chocolate Filled, Tesco*	1 Crepe/32g	140.0	6.0	437	5.9	62.5	18.1	1.6
Lobster, Finest, Tesco*	1 Serving/160g	250.0	10.0	156	10.7	14.0	6.4	1.2
Mushroom, M & S*	1 Pack/186g	195.0	4.0	105	5.7	17.1	2.4	2.5
CRISPBAKES								
Broccoli & Leek, Asda*	1 Bake/132.2g	263.0	13.0	199	6.3	21.0	10.0	2.0
Bubble & Squeak, M & S*	1 Bake/47g	79.0	4.0	170	2.7	19.6	8.8	1.5
Cheese & Onion, Dalepak*	1 Bake/98.4g	239.0	13.0	243	7.2	24.1	12.8	1.7
Cheese & Onion, M & S*	1 Bake/114g	285.0	18.0	250	6.4	19.4	16.2	1.7
Cheese & Onion, Tesco*	1 Bake/109g	275.0	17.0	252	7.9	19.6	15.8	2.1
Cheese, Spring Onion & Chive, Sainsbury's*	1 Bake/113.5g	287.0	17.0	253	7.1	24.5	14.8	1.7
Dutch, Asda*	1 Bake/8g	31.0	0.0	388	14.7	74.9	3.3	4.2
Dutch, HL, Tesco*	1 Bake/8g	30.0	0.0	385	14.7	74.9	2.7	4.2
Dutch, Sainsbury's*	1 Bake/10g	38.0	0.0	392	14.5	72.3	5.0	5.8
Minced Beef, M & S*	1 Bake/113g	226.0	12.0	200	10.0	15.6	10.9	1.5
Mushroom & Garlic, Ovenbaked, Iceland*	1 Bake/140g	241.0	9.0	172	4.3	23.7	6.7	2.9
Mushroom, Uncooked, Dalepak*	1 Bake/84g	141.0	7.0	168	3.8	18.5	8.8	2.1
Tuna & Sweetcorn, Lakeland*	1 Bake/170g	391.0	20.0	230	11.3	20.1	11.6	0.0
Vegetable, Sainsbury's*	1 Bake/114g	246.0	13.0	216	2.0	26.2	11.4	2.0
CRISPBREAD								
3 Seed, Organic, Gourmet	1 Bread/25g	101.0	5.0	405	15.8	48.8	18.8	14.6
Breaks, with Currants, Oats & Honey, Ryvita*	1 Bread/14.5g	48.0	0.0	332	8.0	69.7	2.3	12.0
Corn, Orgran*	1 Bread/5g	18.0	0.0	360	7.5	83.0	1.8	3.0
Cream, Cheese & Chives, 3% Fat, Minis, Ryvita*	1 Pack/30g	103.0	1.0	342	8.0	71.0	2.9	11.5
Crisp 'n' Light, Wasa*	1 Bread/7g	24.0	0.0	360	12.0	73.0	2.2	5.3
Dark Rye, Morrisons*	1 Bake/13g	39.0	0.0	300	11.5	61.5	3.1	16.9
Dark Rye, Ryvita*	1 Bread/10g	31.0	0.0	311	8.5	65.5	1.7	18.0
Emmental Cheese & Pumpkin Seed, Organic, Dr Karg*	1 Bread/25g	102.0	4.0	408	17.1	50.7	14.9	9.6
Fruit Crunch, Ryvita*	1 Slice/15.5g	57.0	1.0	366	10.9	65.8	6.6	11.1
Garlic & Rosemary, Wholegrain Rye, Ryvita*	1 Bread/12g	39.0	0.0	325	8.3	70.0	1.7	16.7
Gluten Free	1 Serving/8g	25.0	0.0	331	6.4	72.9	1.5	0.0
Light, Ryvita*	1 Bread/5g	19.0	0.0	383	9.8	79.3	3.0	2.6
Mildly Seasoned, Organic, Dr Karg*	1 Bread/25g	100.0	4.0	401	16.0	48.5	15.9	13.8
Minis, Apple, Ryvita*	1 Pack/30g	101.0	1.0	336	6.1	71.9	2.7	12.0
Minis, Caramel, Ryvita*	1 Pack/30g	100.0	1.0	335	6.1	71.7	2.7	11.9
Minis, Garlic & Herb, Ryvita*	1 Bag/30g	103.0	1.0	343	7.9	71.5	2.8	11.5
Minis, Mature Cheddar & Onion, Ryvita*	1 Bag/30g	101.0	1.0	337	9.3	68.2	3.0	11.5
Minis, Salt & Vinegar, Ryvita*	1 Pack/30g	94.0	1.0	312	6.8	64.8	2.8	12.1
Minis, Sweet Chilli, Ryvita*	1 Pack/30g	100.0	1.0	335	7.0	71.0	2.6	11.9
Minis, Worcester Sauce, Ryvita*	1 Pack/30g	102.0	1.0	339	6.9	71.9	2.6	12.0
Multigrain, Ryvita*	1 Bread/11g	36.0	1.0	331	10.0	61.1	5.2	16.7
Multigrain, Wasa*	1 Bread/13g	43.0	0.0	320	12.0	62.0	2.6	14.0
Poppyseed, Wasa*	1 Bread/13g	45.0	1.0	350	13.0	56.0	8.0	14.0
Provita*	1 Bread/6g	26.0	1.0	416	12.5	68.4	9.9	0.0
Pumpkin Seeds & Oats, Ryvita*	1 Bread/12g	43.0	1.0	362	12.5	55.6	9.9	14.5
Rice, & Cracked Pepper, Orgran*	1 Bread/5g	18.0	0.0	388	8.4	81.9	1.8	2.0
Rice, Original, Sakata*	1 Bread/25g	102.0	1.0	410	6.9	88.0	2.6	1.3
Roasted Onion, Organic, Dr Karg*	1 Bread/25g	97.0	4.0	390	15.8	48.5	14.8	12.9
Rounds, Multigrain, Finn Crisp*	1 Bread/12.5g	41.0	1.0	330	13.0	56.0	6.0	18.0
Rounds, Original, Rye, Finn Crisp*	1 Bread/14g	45.0	0.0	320	11.0	60.0	2.7	16.0
Rounds, Wholegrain Wheat, Finn Crisp*	1 Bread/12.5g	45.0	1.0	360	11.0	66.0	5.9	10.0

CRISPBREAD

Measure INFO/WEIGHT	per Measure KCAL	FAT	Nutrition Values per 100g / 100ml KCAL	PROT	CARB	FAT	FIBRE
Rye, Original, Ryvita*	1 Bread/10g	32.0	0.0	317	8.5	66.6	1.7	16.5
Seeded, Spelt, Organic, Dr Karg*	1 Bread/25g	102.0	4.0	408	17.2	44.4	18.0	10.4
Sesame Rye, Ryvita*	1 Bread/10.1g	34.0	1.0	338	10.5	58.3	7.0	17.5
Snacks, Caribbean Chicken, Seasons, Quaker Oats*	1 Pack/28g	118.0	3.0	421	7.9	77.1	8.9	2.1
Snacks, Cheese, Onion & Chive Flavour, Quaker Oats*	1 Pack/28g	118.0	3.0	420	8.3	76.0	9.1	2.4
Snacks, Lime & Coriander, Seasons, Quaker Oats*	1 Pack/28g	115.0	3.0	410	7.5	75.0	9.0	2.3
Spelt, Cheese, Sunflower Seeds, Organic, Dr Karg*	1 Bread/25g	103.0	5.0	411	19.2	42.8	18.1	10.4
Spelt, Muesli, Organic, Dr Karg*	1 Bread/25g	94.0	3.0	375	14.2	54.4	11.2	10.6
Spelt, Sesame, Sunflower, Amisa*	1 Bread/28.5g	85.0	4.0	297	11.7	28.5	15.1	5.0
Sunflower Seeds & Oats, Ryvita*	1 Bread/12g	42.0	1.0	348	10.1	57.2	8.8	16.7
Thin Crisps, Original Taste, Finn Crisp*	1 Bread/6.3g	20.0	0.0	320	11.0	63.0	2.4	19.0
Trufree*	1 Bread/6g	22.0	0.0	370	6.0	82.0	2.0	1.0
Whole Grain, Classic, Organic, Dr Karg*	1 Bread/25g	89.0	4.0	355	13.4	38.2	16.5	10.2
Wholegrain, Classic Three Seed, Organic, Dr Karg*	1 Bread/25g	101.0	4.0	405	15.8	44.8	18.0	14.6
Wholemeal Rye, Organic, Kallo*	1 Bread/10g	31.0	0.0	314	9.7	65.0	1.7	15.4
Wholemeal, Light, Allinson*	1 Bread/5g	17.0	0.0	349	11.7	69.7	2.6	11.0
Wholemeal, Organic, Allinson*	1 Bread/5g	17.0	0.0	336	14.2	66.0	1.7	12.2

CRISPS

Measure INFO/WEIGHT	per Measure KCAL	FAT	Nutrition Values per 100g / 100ml KCAL	PROT	CARB	FAT	FIBRE
American Cheeseburger Flavour, Quarterbacks, Red Mill*	1 Pack/14g	72.0	4.0	512	6.7	54.2	29.8	3.7
Apple, The Fruit Factory*	1 Packet/10g	33.0	0.0	334	1.3	81.1	0.5	12.4
Apple, Thyme & Sage, M & S*	1 Bag/55g	253.0	13.0	460	5.5	55.3	24.3	6.1
Argentinean Flame Grilled Steak, Walkers*	1 Bag/35g	182.0	11.0	520	6.5	50.7	32.4	4.2
Bacon & Cheddar, Baked, Walkers*	1 Pack/37.5g	149.0	3.0	397	6.5	73.7	8.5	4.7
Bacon Crispies, Sainsbury's*	1 Bag/25g	117.0	6.0	468	19.9	45.8	22.8	4.8
Bacon Flavour Rashers, BGTY, Sainsbury's*	1 Pack/10g	34.0	0.0	340	10.8	70.3	1.6	3.5
Bacon Rashers, Blazin, Tesco*	1 Bag/25g	121.0	7.0	485	16.5	45.7	26.3	3.8
Bacon Rashers, COU, M & S*	1 Pack/20g	72.0	1.0	360	9.4	77.5	2.9	3.5
Bacon Rashers, Tesco*	1 Serving/25g	125.0	6.0	500	7.1	59.8	25.5	4.0
Bacon Rice Bites, Asda*	1 Bag/30g	136.0	5.0	452	7.0	70.0	16.0	0.4
Bacon, Shapers, Boots*	1 Bag/23g	99.0	3.0	431	8.0	66.0	15.0	3.0
Baked Bean Flavour, Walkers*	1 Bag/35g	184.0	12.0	525	6.5	50.0	33.0	4.0
Baked, Cheese & Onion, Walkers*	1 Sm Bag/25g	99.0	2.0	396	6.5	73.8	8.3	4.7
Baked, Ready Salted, Walkers*	1 Packet/37.5g	146.0	3.0	390	6.0	74.0	8.0	5.5
Baked, Salt & Vinegar, Walkers*	1 Packet/37.5g	146.0	3.0	390	6.0	73.0	8.0	5.0
Baked, Sour Cream & Chive, Walkers*	1 Packet/37.5g	148.0	3.0	395	7.0	73.0	8.5	5.0
Banging BBQ, Shots, Walkers*	1 Pack/18g	87.0	4.0	485	5.5	60.0	25.0	1.3
Barbecue Beef, Select, Tesco*	1 Pack/25g	134.0	9.0	536	6.4	49.2	34.8	4.4
Barbecue, Handcooked, Tesco*	1 Bag/40g	187.0	10.0	468	6.6	53.8	25.1	5.2
Barbecue, Sunseed Oil, Walkers*	1 Pack/25g	131.0	8.0	525	6.5	50.0	33.0	4.0
BBQ Rib, Sunseed, Walkers*	1 Bag/25g	131.0	8.0	525	6.5	50.0	33.0	4.0
Beef & Horseradish, Extra Special, Asda*	1 Serving/100g	516.0	32.0	516	7.0	50.0	32.0	3.4
Beef & Onion, Potato, M & S*	1 Bag/25g	130.0	8.0	530	6.6	48.2	34.5	5.0
Beef & Onion, Walkers*	1 Bag/35g	184.0	12.0	525	6.5	50.0	33.0	4.0
Beef, Squares, Walkers*	1 Bag/25g	105.0	4.0	420	6.0	59.0	18.0	4.6
Beefy, Smiths, Walkers*	1 Bag/25g	133.0	9.0	531	4.3	45.2	37.0	0.0
Buffalo Mozzarella & Herbs, Walkers*	1 Serving/35g	171.0	9.0	490	6.1	57.0	26.0	4.2
Buffalo Mozzarella Tomato & Basil, Kettle Chips*	1 Serving/50g	238.0	13.0	476	6.7	54.4	25.7	4.9
Builders Breakfast, Walkers*	1 Sm Bag/25g	131.0	8.0	524	5.6	50.8	33.2	4.0
Butter & Chive, COU, M & S*	1 Bag/26g	95.0	0.0	365	7.7	77.3	1.9	4.6
Cajun Squirrel, Walkers*	1 Sm Bag/25g	130.0	8.0	522	5.8	51.2	32.7	4.2
Chargrilled Chicken Crinkles, Shapers, Boots*	1 Bag/20g	96.0	5.0	482	6.6	60.0	24.0	4.0
Chargrilled Steak, Max, Walkers*	1 Bag/55g	289.0	18.0	525	6.5	50.0	33.0	4.0
Cheddar & Onion, Ridge Cut, McCoys*	1oz/28g	144.0	9.0	516	7.0	53.2	30.6	3.9

CRISPS

	Measure INFO/WEIGHT	per Measure KCAL	per Measure FAT	Nutrition Values per 100g / 100ml KCAL	PROT	CARB	FAT	FIBRE
Cheddar & Red Onion Chutney, Sensations, Walkers*	1 Bag/40g	198.0	11.0	495	6.5	54.0	28.0	4.5
Cheddar & Spring Onion, 35% Less Fat, Sainsbury's*	1 Pack/20g	93.0	4.0	463	6.3	62.4	20.9	0.9
Cheddar Cheese & Bacon, Walkers*	1 Bag/25g	131.0	8.0	523	5.9	50.6	33.0	4.1
Cheese & Branston Pickle, Walkers*	1 Bag/34.5g	181.0	11.0	525	6.5	50.0	33.0	4.0
Cheese & Chives, Walkers*	1 Bag/35g	185.0	12.0	530	6.5	50.0	33.0	4.1
Cheese & Onion, BGTY, Sainsbury's*	1 Bag/25g	120.0	6.0	479	7.0	57.0	24.8	5.7
Cheese & Onion, Crinkle Cut, Low Fat, Waitrose*	1 Bag/25g	122.0	6.0	490	7.7	62.6	23.2	4.7
Cheese & Onion, Golden Wonder*	1 Bag/25g	131.0	8.0	524	6.1	49.2	33.6	2.0
Cheese & Onion, KP Snacks*	1 Bag/25g	133.0	9.0	534	6.6	48.7	34.8	4.8
Cheese & Onion, Lights, Walkers*	1 Sm Bag/24g	113.0	5.0	470	7.5	62.0	21.0	5.0
Cheese & Onion, Limbos, Ryvita*	1 Pack/18g	63.0	1.0	352	12.1	69.1	3.0	9.3
Cheese & Onion, M & S*	1 Bag/25g	134.0	9.0	535	5.5	48.8	35.5	5.0
Cheese & Onion, Max, Walkers*	1 Pack/50g	262.0	16.0	525	6.8	52.0	32.0	5.2
Cheese & Onion, Organic, Tesco*	1 Bag/25g	128.0	8.0	514	5.2	49.9	32.6	7.0
Cheese & Onion, Potato Heads, Walkers*	1 Pack/23g	108.0	5.0	470	6.0	60.0	23.0	5.5
Cheese & Onion, Sainsbury's*	1 Bag/25g	132.0	9.0	527	4.6	48.8	34.8	3.9
Cheese & Onion, Squares, Walkers*	1 Bag/25g	107.0	4.0	430	6.5	61.0	18.0	5.5
Cheese & Onion, Sunseed Oil, Walkers*	1 Bag/34.5g	181.0	11.0	525	7.0	50.0	33.0	4.0
Cheese Bites, Weight Watchers*	1 Pack/18g	73.0	1.0	406	13.9	71.1	5.6	2.2
Cheese Curls, Red Mill*	½ Bag/50g	276.0	18.0	553	6.6	50.6	36.0	2.0
Cheese Curls, Shapers, Boots*	1 Pack/14g	68.0	4.0	489	4.5	57.0	27.0	2.7
Cheese Curls, Tesco*	1 Bag/14.4g	75.0	4.0	520	4.5	54.4	31.1	1.9
Cheese Curls, Weight Watchers*	1 Pack/20g	78.0	2.0	392	5.0	73.8	8.6	3.4
Cheese Puffs, Weight Watchers*	1 Pack/18g	75.0	2.0	417	7.8	72.2	10.6	2.2
Cheese Tasters, M & S*	1 Sm Bag/30g	154.0	9.0	515	8.1	55.0	29.3	1.7
Cheese Twirls, Boulevard, Simply Delicious*	1 Pack/25g	137.0	9.0	550	12.1	46.7	35.0	0.0
Cheese XI, Golden Wonder*	1 Bag/30g	155.0	10.0	516	6.2	50.6	32.1	4.2
Cheeses with Onion, Soulmates, Kettle Chips*	1 Pack/40g	195.0	12.0	488	7.7	50.2	29.0	5.4
Chicken, Firecracker, McCoys*	1 Bag/35g	177.0	10.0	506	6.2	54.0	29.5	4.0
Chicken, Oven Roasted with Lemon & Thyme, Walkers*	1 Bag/40g	200.0	11.0	500	6.5	55.0	28.0	4.5
Chicken, Potato Heads, Walkers*	1 Pack/23g	106.0	5.0	460	8.5	58.0	21.0	6.0
Chilli & Chocolate, Walkers*	1 Pack/25g	131.0	8.0	523	6.1	50.1	33.1	4.2
Chilli & Lemon, Walkers*	1 Pack/25g	131.0	8.0	525	6.3	51.0	33.0	3.8
Chinese Sizzling Beef, McCoys*	1 Bag/35g	178.0	11.0	506	6.9	51.8	30.2	4.0
Chinese Spare Rib, Walkers*	1 Bag/25g	131.0	8.0	525	6.5	50.0	33.0	4.0
Cider Vinegar & Sea Salt, Tyrells*	1 Pack/40g	192.0	10.0	481	7.2	60.1	24.6	2.4
Corn Chips, Fritos*	1 Pack/42.5g	240.0	15.0	565	4.7	56.5	35.3	0.0
Coronation Chicken, Walkers*	1 Bag/25g	131.0	8.0	525	6.5	50.0	33.0	4.0
Crinkle Cut, Lower Fat, No Added Salt, Waitrose*	1 Bag/40g	193.0	10.0	483	6.5	58.0	25.0	3.9
Crisps, Superbly Spiced, Cassava, Hale & Hearty*	1 Bag/30g	134.0	7.0	448	3.3	56.1	23.1	6.6
Crispy Duck & Hoi Sin, Walkers*	1 Bag/25g	131.0	8.0	523	5.8	51.5	32.6	4.0
Curls, Cheesy, Asda*	1 Pack/17g	87.0	5.0	511	3.8	59.7	28.6	1.7
D'lites, Cheddar & Red Onion Bites, The Real Crisp Co.*	1 Pack/20g	83.0	2.0	414	2.1	78.8	10.0	2.7
Double Cheddar & Chives, Deli Style, Brannigans*	1oz/28g	148.0	9.0	529	7.6	49.5	33.4	3.8
Double Gloucester & Red Onion, Kettle Chips*	1 Serving/40g	188.0	10.0	471	6.6	55.5	24.7	4.8
Dutch Edam Cheese, Walkers*	1 Bag/25g	131.0	8.0	523	6.1	50.2	33.1	4.0
English Cheddar & Red Onion, Red Sky*	1 Pack/40g	183.0	8.0	457	6.9	60.2	21.0	5.1
English Roast Beef, & Yorkshire Pudding, Walkers*	1 Bag/34.5g	180.0	11.0	522	6.6	50.4	32.7	4.0
Feta Cheese Flavour, Mediterranean, Walkers*	1 Pack/25g	127.0	8.0	510	6.5	49.0	33.0	4.5
Flame Grilled Steak, Ridge Cut, McCoys*	1 Bag/32g	165.0	10.0	516	7.0	53.0	30.7	4.0
Four Cheese & Red Onion, Sensations, Walkers*	1 Bag/40g	194.0	11.0	485	6.5	54.0	27.0	4.5
Garlic & Herbs Creme Fraiche, Kettle Chips*	1 Bag/50g	248.0	14.0	497	6.0	54.7	28.3	4.2
Grilled Chicken Flavour, Golden Lights, Golden Wonder*	1 Bag/21g	93.0	4.0	444	4.4	66.2	18.0	4.3

CRISPS

	Measure INFO/WEIGHT	per Measure KCAL	per Measure FAT	Nutrition Values per 100g / 100ml KCAL	PROT	CARB	FAT	FIBRE
Heinz Tomato Ketchup, Sunseed, Walkers*	1 Bag/34.5g	179.0	11.0	520	6.5	51.0	32.0	4.0
Honey Roast Gammon & English Mustard, Sainsbury's*	1 Serving/50g	236.0	12.0	472	7.2	55.0	24.8	5.0
Honey Roasted Ham, Sensations, Walkers*	1 Bag/40g	196.0	11.0	490	6.5	55.0	27.0	4.0
Hot & Spicy Salami, Tesco*	1 Bag/50g	215.0	18.0	431	26.2	0.7	35.9	0.0
Lamb & Mint, Slow Roasted, Sensations, Walkers*	1 Bag/35g	170.0	9.0	485	6.5	54.0	27.0	4.5
Lamb & Mint, Sunseed Oil, Walkers*	1 Pack/34.5g	181.0	11.0	525	6.5	50.0	33.0	4.0
Lightly Salted, Baked, COU, M & S*	1 Bag/25g	87.0	1.0	350	8.5	76.4	2.3	5.7
Lightly Salted, Crinkle Cut, Low Fat, Waitrose*	1 Pack/35g	163.0	8.0	466	5.2	60.1	22.8	5.1
Lightly Salted, Crinkles, Shapers, Boots*	1 Pack/20g	96.0	5.0	482	6.6	60.0	24.0	4.0
Lightly Salted, Handcooked, Finest, Tesco*	½ Pack/150g	708.0	39.0	472	6.4	52.9	26.1	5.1
Lightly Salted, Hoops, Mini, Weight Watchers*	1 Pack/20g	71.0	0.0	355	4.0	82.0	1.0	3.5
Lightly Salted, Kettle Chips*	1 Serving/50g	241.0	13.0	482	6.3	56.0	25.8	5.1
Lightly Salted, Low Fat, Waitrose*	1 Bag/25g	125.0	6.0	500	7.5	61.3	25.0	4.8
Lightly Salted, Organic, Kettle Chips*	1 Serving/40g	198.0	11.0	495	5.5	54.1	28.5	4.4
Lightly Salted, Potato Bakes, Weight Watchers*	1 Pack/20g	78.0	2.0	392	5.0	72.0	9.0	5.0
Lightly Salted, Reduced Fat, Crinkles, Eat Well, M & S*	1 Pack/30.4g	140.0	7.0	460	6.7	59.4	21.8	4.5
Lincolnshire Sausage, Tyrells*	1 Pack/100g	530.0	28.0	530	8.6	60.8	28.2	3.0
Mango & Chilli, Baked, Walkers*	1 Packet/37.5g	147.0	3.0	392	6.4	74.0	8.0	4.8
Mango Chilli, Kettle Chips*	1 Serving/40g	190.0	10.0	475	6.3	53.9	24.0	6.1
Marmite, Sunseed, Walkers*	1 Bag/34.5g	179.0	11.0	520	6.5	49.0	33.0	4.0
Mature Cheddar & Chive, Kettle Chips*	1 Serving/50g	239.0	13.0	478	8.1	54.4	25.4	5.0
Mature Cheddar & Chive, Tyrells*	1 Bag/40g	194.0	10.0	485	8.4	58.7	25.1	2.4
Mature Cheddar & Red Onion, Kettle Chips*	1 Bag/40g	187.0	10.0	467	7.5	52.2	25.4	6.2
Mature Cheddar & Shallot, Temptations, Tesco*	1/6 Bag/25g	131.0	9.0	524	6.6	47.4	34.2	4.4
Mediterranean Baked Potato, COU, M & S*	1 Pack/25g	90.0	1.0	360	7.6	74.0	2.4	6.8
Mexican Chilli & Cheese, Golden Wonder*	1 Pack/45g	230.0	14.0	511	6.6	50.7	31.3	0.0
Mexican Chilli, Ridge Cut, McCoys*	1 Bag/50g	257.0	15.0	514	6.9	53.0	30.5	4.5
Mexican Lime with a Hint of Chilli, Kettle Chips*	1 Serving/50g	242.0	14.0	484	5.0	54.1	27.5	5.4
Mixed Pepper Flavour Burst, M & S*	1 Bag/55g	286.0	18.0	520	6.0	50.1	33.5	4.0
Naked, Tyrells*	1 Pack/150g	748.0	41.0	499	7.7	56.5	27.5	0.0
New York Cheddar, Kettle Chips*	1 Bag/50g	241.0	13.0	483	6.7	53.9	26.7	4.5
Olive Oil, Mozzarella & Oregano, Walkers*	1 Serving/30g	151.0	9.0	505	6.5	54.0	29.0	4.0
Onion Bhaji, Walkers*	1 Pack/25g	130.0	8.0	522	6.1	50.7	32.7	4.3
Onion Rings, Crunchy, Shapers, Boots*	1 Bag/12g	61.0	3.0	507	2.5	62.0	28.0	2.6
Onion Rings, M & S*	1 Pack/40g	186.0	9.0	465	5.2	62.1	21.5	4.3
Oriental Ribs, Ridge Cut, McCoys*	1 Pack/50g	255.0	15.0	511	7.3	52.7	30.1	4.2
Paprika, Handcooked, Shapers, Boots*	1 Bag/20g	99.0	5.0	493	7.2	62.0	24.0	5.0
Paprika, Max, Walkers*	1 Bag/50g	260.0	16.0	520	6.5	52.0	31.9	5.1
Paprika, Mini Hoops, Shapers, Boots*	1 Bag/13.0g	64.0	4.0	494	8.7	54.0	27.0	2.2
Parsnip & Black Pepper, Sainsbury's*	1 Serving/35g	166.0	11.0	473	3.2	43.6	31.8	15.2
Parsnip, Passions, Snack Rite*	1 Serving/25g	123.0	9.0	494	4.5	34.5	37.6	18.8
Pastrami & Cheese, Crinkle, M & S*	1 Bag/25g	120.0	6.0	485	6.5	61.0	24.0	3.5
Peri Peri Chicken, Nando's*	½ Bag/75g	410.0	20.0	547	5.1	57.4	27.0	3.4
Pickled Onion, Golden Wonder*	1 Bag/25g	131.0	8.0	524	5.6	49.0	34.0	2.0
Pickled Onion, M & S*	1 Bag/20g	70.0	0.0	345	5.0	81.7	1.5	3.7
Pickled Onion, Monster Bites, Sainsbury's*	1 Bag/20g	107.0	7.0	535	5.2	53.5	33.3	1.0
Pickled Onion, Sunseed, Walkers*	1 Bag/34.5g	181.0	11.0	525	6.5	50.0	33.0	4.0
Potato	1oz/28g	148.0	10.0	530	5.7	53.3	34.2	5.3
Potato Chips, Anglesey Sea Salt, Red Sky*	1 Serving/40g	185.0	9.0	463	6.8	59.8	21.8	5.0
Potato Chips, Roasted Red Pepper & Lime, Red Sky*	1 Serving/40g	187.0	9.0	467	6.8	59.5	22.4	4.8
Potato Chips, Sour Cream & Green Herbs, Red Sky*	1 Pack/40g	188.0	9.0	471	6.8	58.4	23.4	4.8
Potato Squares, Ready Salted, Sainsbury's*	1 Bag/50g	192.0	8.0	384	6.5	53.8	15.9	7.8
Potato Thins, Lightly Salted, Light Choices, Tesco*	1 Pack/20g	72.0	0.0	360	5.1	79.5	2.0	4.2

CRISPS

	Measure INFO/WEIGHT	per Measure KCAL	per Measure FAT	Nutrition Values per 100g / 100ml KCAL	PROT	CARB	FAT	FIBRE
Potato Triangles, Ready Salted, Sainsbury's*	½ Pack/50g	243.0	12.0	486	9.4	59.7	23.4	3.4
Potato, Low Fat	1oz/28g	128.0	6.0	458	6.6	63.5	21.5	5.9
Prawn Cocktail, 30% Less Fat, Sainsbury's*	1 Pack/25g	117.0	6.0	470	6.3	58.9	23.6	5.7
Prawn Cocktail, BGTY, Sainsbury's*	1 Bag/25g	118.0	6.0	473	6.3	58.6	23.7	5.7
Prawn Cocktail, Golden Wonder*	1 Bag/25g	130.0	8.0	521	5.8	49.0	33.5	2.0
Prawn Cocktail, KP Snacks*	1 Bag/25g	133.0	9.0	531	5.9	48.4	34.9	4.7
Prawn Cocktail, M & S*	1 Bag/30.1g	155.0	9.0	515	6.2	58.0	28.6	2.2
Prawn Cocktail, Sunseed Oil, Walkers*	1 Bag/34.5g	181.0	11.0	525	6.5	50.0	33.0	4.0
Ready Salted, Golden Wonder*	1 Bag/25g	135.0	9.0	539	5.5	49.9	35.3	2.0
Ready Salted, KP Snacks*	1 Bag/24g	131.0	9.0	545	5.6	47.9	36.8	4.9
Ready Salted, Lower Fat, Sainsbury's*	1 Bag/25g	111.0	5.0	444	7.0	55.0	21.8	5.1
Ready Salted, M & S*	1 Bag/25g	136.0	9.0	545	5.6	47.8	36.6	4.9
Ready Salted, Ridge Cut, McCoys*	1 Bag/49g	257.0	16.0	524	6.6	52.6	31.9	4.1
Ready Salted, Sainsbury's*	1 Bag/25g	134.0	9.0	538	4.3	47.4	36.8	4.1
Ready Salted, Snack Rite*	1 Bag/25g	136.0	9.0	545	4.9	50.3	36.0	0.0
Ready Salted, Squares, Walkers*	1 Pack/25g	109.0	5.0	435	6.5	60.0	19.0	6.0
Ready Salted, Sunseed Oil, Walkers*	1 Bag/34.5g	183.0	12.0	530	6.5	49.0	34.0	4.0
Red Leicester & Spring Onion, Handcooked, M & S*	1 Pack/40g	194.0	11.0	485	6.8	55.0	26.4	5.1
Roast Beef & Mustard, Thick Cut, Brannigans*	1 Bag/40g	203.0	12.0	507	7.6	51.7	30.0	3.7
Roast Beef, KP Snacks*	1 Bag/25g	133.0	9.0	534	6.6	47.5	35.3	4.7
Roast Chicken & Sage Flavour, M & S*	1 Bag/25g	135.0	9.0	540	5.9	50.6	34.6	4.6
Roast Chicken Flavour, BGTY, Sainsbury's*	1 Bag/25g	118.0	6.0	473	6.2	58.9	23.6	5.7
Roast Chicken, 30% Less Fat, Sainsbury's*	1 Pack/25g	115.0	5.0	460	7.4	58.3	21.9	5.2
Roast Chicken, Golden Wonder*	1 Bag/25g	130.0	8.0	522	6.2	48.6	33.6	2.0
Roast Chicken, Highlander*	1 Bag/25g	138.0	10.0	554	5.3	46.0	38.9	5.1
Roast Chicken, Select, Tesco*	1 Bag/25g	134.0	9.0	536	6.6	48.6	35.0	4.4
Roast Chicken, Snack Rite*	1 Bag/25g	131.0	8.0	526	5.3	51.3	33.3	0.0
Roast Chicken, Sunseed Oil, Walkers*	1 Bag/34.5g	181.0	11.0	525	6.5	50.0	33.0	4.0
Roast Ham & Mustard, Ridge Cut, McCoys*	1 Pack/35g	181.0	11.0	518	7.1	53.5	30.6	3.9
Roast Pork & Apple Sauce, Select, Tesco*	1 Bag/25g	136.0	9.0	544	6.5	50.0	35.3	3.7
Roasted Lamb, Moroccan Spices, Sensations, Walkers*	1 Bag/40g	198.0	12.0	495	6.0	53.0	29.0	4.5
Salt & Black Pepper, Handcooked, M & S*	1 Bag/40g	180.0	9.0	450	5.7	55.0	22.9	5.2
Salt & Malt Vinegar, Hunky Dorys*	1 Serving/30g	141.0	9.0	469	6.3	49.3	28.7	0.0
Salt & Malt Vinegar, Ridgecut, McCoys*	1 Sm Bag/32g	164.0	10.0	514	6.7	53.2	30.4	3.9
Salt & Shake, Walkers*	1 Bag/30g	162.0	10.0	540	6.5	50.0	35.0	4.0
Salt & Vinegar Spirals, Shapers, Boots*	1 Pack/15g	71.0	3.0	475	3.1	64.0	23.0	1.7
Salt & Vinegar, BGTY, Sainsbury's*	1 Bag/25g	120.0	6.0	482	6.5	57.3	25.2	5.2
Salt & Vinegar, Crinkle Cut, Low Fat, Waitrose*	1 Bag/25g	121.0	6.0	484	7.1	61.3	23.4	4.5
Salt & Vinegar, Crinkle Cut, Seabrook*	1 Bag/32g	181.0	12.0	569	5.4	54.4	36.7	3.9
Salt & Vinegar, Golden Lights, Golden Wonder*	1 Bag/21g	94.0	4.0	446	4.2	65.7	18.5	3.7
Salt & Vinegar, Golden Wonder*	1 Bag/25g	130.0	8.0	522	5.4	48.5	34.0	2.0
Salt & Vinegar, KP Snacks*	1 Bag/25g	133.0	9.0	532	5.5	48.7	35.0	4.7
Salt & Vinegar, Lights, Walkers*	1 Bag/28g	133.0	6.0	475	7.0	62.0	22.0	4.5
Salt & Vinegar, M & S*	1 Bag/25g	131.0	9.0	525	5.4	48.8	34.5	4.6
Salt & Vinegar, Potato Bakes, Weight Watchers*	1 Bag/20g	81.0	2.0	404	5.3	76.0	8.8	2.3
Salt & Vinegar, Red Mill*	1 Bag/40g	174.0	7.0	436	3.9	65.8	17.5	2.4
Salt & Vinegar, Rough Cuts, Tayto*	1 Bag/30g	152.0	9.0	506	4.6	56.8	30.8	0.0
Salt & Vinegar, Squares, Walkers*	1 Bag/25g	107.0	4.0	430	6.5	61.0	18.0	5.5
Salt & Vinegar, Sunseed Oil, Walkers*	1 Bag/34.5g	181.0	11.0	525	6.5	50.0	33.0	4.0
Salt & Vinegar, Tayto*	1 Bag/35g	184.0	12.0	526	7.6	47.3	34.0	4.5
Salt & Vinegar, Waitrose*	1 Pack/25g	132.0	8.0	529	6.3	50.5	33.8	4.4
Salt & Vinegar, Walkers*	1 Pack/25g	131.0	8.0	524	6.4	50.0	33.2	4.0
Sausage & Tomato Flavour, Golden Wonder*	1 Bag/35g	174.0	11.0	505	6.1	51.3	30.6	4.5

CRISPS

Measure INFO/WEIGHT		per Measure KCAL	FAT	Nutrition Values per 100g / 100ml KCAL	PROT	CARB	FAT	FIBRE
Sea Salt & Balsamic Vinegar, Kettle Chips*	1 Bag/40g	190.0	10.0	476	5.9	56.8	25.0	4.5
Sea Salt & Black Pepper, GFY, Asda*	1 Bag/100g	476.0	24.0	476	6.0	59.0	24.0	6.0
Sea Salt & Black Pepper, Tyrells*	¼ Pack/38g	182.0	9.0	480	7.3	59.9	24.5	2.4
Sea Salt & Cider Vinegar, TTD, Sainsbury's*	1/3 Pack/50g	245.0	14.0	489	5.5	52.7	28.5	6.1
Sea Salt & Cracked Black Pepper, Lights, Walkers*	1 Bag/24g	115.0	5.0	480	7.0	63.0	22.0	5.0
Sea Salt & Cracked Black Pepper, Sensations, Walkers*	1 Bag/40g	196.0	11.0	490	6.5	55.0	27.0	4.0
Sea Salt & Indian Black Pepper, Pipers Crisps*	1 Pack/40g	195.0	12.0	487	6.6	49.9	29.0	0.0
Sea Salt & Malt Vinegar, Sensations, Walkers*	1 Bag/40g	194.0	11.0	485	6.5	54.0	27.0	4.5
Sea Salt with Crushed Black Peppercorns, Kettle Chips*	1 Serving/40g	193.0	11.0	482	6.5	53.8	26.7	4.9
Sea Salt, Golden Lights, Golden Wonder*	1 Bag/21g	94.0	4.0	448	3.9	66.4	18.5	4.4
Sea Salt, Gourmet, TTD, Sainsbury's*	1/3 Pack/50g	249.0	15.0	498	5.7	51.4	30.0	6.4
Sea Salt, Original, Crinkle Cut, Seabrook*	1 Bag/32g	181.0	12.0	569	5.4	54.4	36.7	3.9
Smoked Ham & Pickle, Thick Cut, Brannigans*	1 Bag/40g	203.0	12.0	507	7.0	52.8	29.8	3.8
Smokey Bacon, Crinkle, Shapers, Boots*	1 Pack/20g	96.0	5.0	482	6.6	60.0	24.0	4.0
Smokey Bacon, Seabrook*	1 Bag/32g	181.0	12.0	569	5.4	54.4	36.7	3.9
Smokey Bacon, Select, Tesco*	1 Bag/25g	134.0	9.0	536	6.4	49.0	34.9	4.3
Smoky Bacon, 30% Lower Fat, Sainsbury's*	1 Bag/25g	118.0	6.0	471	6.5	58.4	23.6	5.7
Smoky Bacon, BGTY, Sainsbury's*	1 Bag/25g	118.0	6.0	472	6.5	58.5	23.6	5.7
Smoky Bacon, Golden Wonder*	1 Bag/25g	131.0	8.0	523	5.9	49.1	33.7	2.0
Smoky Bacon, Sainsbury's*	1 Bag/25g	132.0	9.0	529	5.7	49.5	34.2	4.4
Smoky Bacon, Snack Rite*	1 Bag/25g	131.0	8.0	525	5.5	51.2	33.1	4.0
Smoky Bacon, Tayto*	1 Bag/35g	184.0	12.0	526	7.6	47.3	34.0	4.5
Sour Cream & Chive, Crinkle, Reduced Fat, M & S*	1 Bag/40g	178.0	8.0	445	5.6	58.8	20.6	5.6
Sour Cream & Chive, Lights, Walkers*	1 Bag/24g	114.0	5.0	475	7.5	62.0	22.0	5.0
Sour Cream & Chive, Perfectly Balanced, Waitrose*	1 Pack/20g	69.0	1.0	347	4.4	76.3	2.7	5.2
Sour Cream & Chive, Potato Bakes, Weight Watchers*	1 Bag/20g	83.0	2.0	417	3.8	80.7	8.8	3.6
Sour Cream & Chives, Jordans*	1 Bag/30g	125.0	4.0	417	7.3	69.9	12.0	2.7
Sour Cream & Onion, Golden Lights, Golden Wonder*	1 Bag/21g	93.0	4.0	442	4.1	66.0	17.9	4.4
Space Raiders, Cheese, KP Snacks*	1 Bag/16g	76.0	4.0	473	7.1	61.6	22.0	3.1
Space Raiders, Pickled Onion, KP Snacks*	1 Bag/16g	77.0	4.0	480	6.7	61.3	23.3	4.0
Space Raiders, Salt & Vinegar, KP Snacks*	1 Bag/17g	81.0	4.0	478	6.9	61.7	22.6	2.2
Spare Rib Flavour, Chinese, Walkers*	1 Bag/35g	181.0	11.0	525	6.5	50.0	33.0	4.0
Spiced Chilli, McCoys*	1 Bag/35g	175.0	10.0	500	6.1	54.2	28.8	4.2
Spicy Chilli, Sunseed, Walkers*	1 Pack/34.5g	183.0	11.0	530	6.5	51.0	33.0	4.0
Spring Onion Flavour, M & S*	1 Bag/40g	210.0	14.0	525	5.9	48.7	34.3	5.1
Spring Onion Flavour, Tayto*	1 Bag/35g	184.0	12.0	526	7.6	47.3	34.0	4.5
Spring Onion, Seabrook*	1 Bag/32g	182.0	12.0	569	5.4	54.4	36.7	3.9
Steak & Onion, Walkers*	1 Pack/34.5g	179.0	11.0	520	6.5	49.0	33.0	4.0
Strawberry Raisin Snack, Fruitwonders, Golden Wonder*	1 Bag/30g	113.0	4.0	383	3.8	62.9	12.9	0.0
Sun Dried Tomato & Basil, Jonathan Crisp*	1 Pack/35g	176.0	10.0	503	5.6	52.0	29.0	5.4
Sun Dried Tomato & Chilli, Asda*	1 Pack/150g	700.0	34.0	467	7.0	58.0	23.0	4.1
Sunbites, Sweet Chilli, Sun Ripened, Walkers*	1 Bag/25g	117.0	5.0	467	7.3	61.1	21.5	6.6
Sweet Chill, Mexican, Phileas Fogg*	1 Bag/38g	193.0	11.0	507	6.7	54.8	29.0	4.2
Sweet Chilli & Red Peppers, Fusion, Tayto*	1 Bag/28g	140.0	8.0	500	4.9	52.2	29.8	4.6
Sweet Chilli, Crinkle Cut, Weight Watchers*	1 Sm Bag/20g	80.0	2.0	400	4.5	74.5	9.5	4.0
T Bone Steak, Roysters*	1 Pack/28g	148.0	9.0	530	5.2	55.3	32.0	3.0
Tangy Malaysian Chutney, Sensations, Walkers*	1 Bag/24g	116.0	6.0	485	0.9	62.0	26.0	0.0
Thai Curry & Coriander, Tyrells*	1 Pack/50g	261.0	14.0	522	6.1	56.5	27.9	5.4
Thai Sweet Chilli, Sensations, Walkers*	1 Bag/40g	202.0	12.0	505	6.5	54.0	29.0	4.5
Tomato & Basil, Mediterranean, Walkers*	1 Pack/25g	127.0	8.0	510	6.5	49.0	33.0	4.5
Tomato & Herb, Shapers, Boots*	1 Bag/20g	94.0	4.0	468	3.7	66.0	21.0	3.9
Tomato Sauce, Golden Wonder*	1 Bag/25g	130.0	8.0	521	5.7	49.2	33.5	2.0
Tortillas, Nacho Cheese Flavour, Weight Watchers*	1 Pack/18g	78.0	3.0	433	6.1	66.7	16.1	3.9

	Measure INFO/WEIGHT	KCAL	FAT	Nutrition Values per 100g / 100ml KCAL	PROT	CARB	FAT	FIBRE

CRISPS

	Measure INFO/WEIGHT	KCAL	FAT	KCAL	PROT	CARB	FAT	FIBRE
Traditional, Hand Cooked, Finest, Tesco*	1 Bag/150g	708.0	39.0	472	6.4	52.9	26.1	5.1
Turkey & Paxo, Walkers*	1 Bag/35g	181.0	11.0	525	6.4	50.1	33.0	4.1
Unsalted, Potato Heads, Walkers*	1 Serving/23g	106.0	5.0	460	5.0	61.0	22.0	5.0
Wild Chilli, McCoys*	1 Bag/50g	255.0	15.0	510	6.0	53.2	30.3	4.8
Wild Paprika Flavour, Croky*	1 Pack/45g	234.0	13.0	521	6.0	58.0	29.0	0.0
Worcester Sauce Flavour, Hunky Dorys*	1 Bag/45g	211.0	13.0	469	6.3	49.3	28.7	0.0
Worcester Sauce, Sunseed Oil, Walkers*	1 Bag/34.5g	183.0	11.0	530	6.5	52.0	33.0	4.0

CRISPY PANCAKE

Beef Bolognese, Findus*	1 Pancake/65g	104.0	3.0	160	6.5	25.0	4.0	1.0
Chicken, Bacon & Sweetcorn, Findus*	1 Pancake/63g	101.0	3.0	160	5.5	26.0	4.0	1.1
Minced Beef, Findus*	1 Pancake/62g	100.0	2.0	160	6.5	25.0	4.0	1.0
Three Cheeses, Findus*	1 Pancake/62g	118.0	4.0	190	7.0	25.0	6.5	0.9

CROISSANT

All Butter, BGTY, Sainsbury's*	1 Croissant/44g	151.0	7.0	343	9.3	42.7	14.8	1.8
All Butter, Budgens*	1 Croissant/45g	185.0	11.0	412	7.9	39.7	24.6	3.3
All Butter, Finest, Tesco*	1 Croissant/77g	328.0	18.0	426	8.6	44.9	23.6	1.9
All Butter, M & S*	1 Croissant/54g	222.0	13.0	415	7.4	45.2	23.8	1.6
All Butter, Mini, Sainsbury's*	1 Croissant/35g	150.0	9.0	428	9.2	42.6	24.5	1.2
All Butter, Mini, Tesco*	1 Croissant/35g	150.0	8.0	430	9.3	45.2	23.5	2.0
All Butter, Reduced Fat, Tesco*	1 Croissant/52g	164.0	6.0	315	7.5	47.4	10.6	1.8
All Butter, Sainsbury's*	1 Croissant/44g	188.0	11.0	428	9.2	42.6	24.5	1.2
All Butter, Tesco*	1 Croissant/48g	192.0	10.0	400	8.5	41.7	21.6	2.6
Average	1 Croissant/50g	180.0	10.0	360	8.3	38.3	20.3	1.6
Butter, Asda*	1 Croissant/46g	191.0	11.0	416	8.0	42.0	24.0	1.9
Butter, GFY, Asda*	1 Croissant/44g	153.0	7.0	352	6.0	46.0	16.0	2.0
Butter, Morrisons*	1 Croissant/44g	196.0	12.0	446	9.3	38.2	28.4	2.0
Butter, Part Baked, De Graaf*	1 Croissant/45g	170.0	8.0	378	7.3	45.2	18.7	0.0
Cheese & Ham, Delice de France*	1 Serving/91g	225.0	12.0	247	7.0	24.4	13.5	2.5
Flaky Pastry with a Plain Chocolate Filling, Tesco*	1 Croissant/78g	318.0	19.0	408	6.5	41.0	24.3	2.0
Heart Shaped, Breakfast in Bed, M & S*	1 Croissant/54g	230.0	14.0	430	8.2	43.7	25.5	1.2
Homebake, Long Life, Stay Fresh Range, Harvestime*	1 Croissant/44g	159.0	6.0	362	7.6	51.9	13.7	1.9
Low Fat, M & S*	1 Croissant/45g	180.0	9.0	400	8.2	46.0	20.2	1.8
Organic, Tesco*	1 Croissant/45g	195.0	12.0	433	8.2	42.0	25.8	2.2
Reduced Fat, Asda*	1 Croissant/44g	159.0	7.0	361	9.7	47.2	14.8	2.0
Reduced Fat, Sainsbury's*	1 Croissant/44g	173.0	8.0	393	9.8	49.2	17.5	2.2
Wholesome, Sainsbury's*	1 Croissant/44g	192.0	12.0	436	8.8	38.3	27.5	4.0

CROQUETTES

Morrisons*	1 Serving/150g	231.0	8.0	154	3.3	23.1	5.4	1.1
Potato, Birds Eye*	1 Croquette/29g	44.0	2.0	152	2.6	22.6	5.7	1.2
Potato, Chunky, Aunt Bessie's*	1 Serving/41g	62.0	3.0	152	2.3	23.9	6.1	1.8
Potato, Fried in Blended Oil, Average	1 Croquette/80g	171.0	10.0	214	3.7	21.6	13.1	1.3
Potato, Sainsbury's*	1 Croquette/28g	50.0	2.0	180	2.8	22.6	8.6	2.5
Potato, Waitrose*	1 Croquette/30g	47.0	2.0	157	3.0	17.9	8.1	1.5
Vegetable, Sainsbury's*	1 Serving/175g	392.0	21.0	224	5.8	23.3	11.9	2.2

CROUTONS

Cracked Black Pepper & Sea Salt, Safeway*	1 Serving/20g	77.0	2.0	385	11.8	61.6	10.2	4.4
Fresh, M & S*	1 Serving/10g	53.0	3.0	530	11.4	50.0	32.8	3.2
Garlic, Waitrose*	1 Serving/40g	209.0	12.0	522	10.8	52.1	30.0	2.7
Herb & Garlic, La Rochelle*	¼ Pack/18g	106.0	7.0	587	6.9	49.8	40.0	2.1
Herb, Sainsbury's*	1 Serving/15g	64.0	2.0	429	13.4	68.2	11.4	2.8
Italian Salad, Sainsbury's*	1 Pack/40g	204.0	10.0	510	8.5	62.7	25.0	2.5
La Rochelle*	1 Bag/70g	400.0	28.0	572	7.0	49.0	40.0	0.0
Lightly Sea Salted, Asda*	1 Serving/20g	83.0	2.0	414	12.9	69.7	9.3	4.3

	Measure INFO/WEIGHT	per Measure KCAL	FAT	Nutrition Values per 100g / 100ml KCAL	PROT	CARB	FAT	FIBRE
CROUTONS								
Migros*	1 Serving/15g	56.0	0.0	375	14.0	72.0	3.0	3.5
Sun Dried Tomato for Salad, Safeway*	1/5 Packet/15g	59.0	2.0	395	13.3	59.4	11.5	8.8
Sun Dried Tomato, Sainsbury's*	1/4 Pack/15g	75.0	4.0	497	11.7	55.2	25.5	2.5
CRUDITE								
Platter, Sainsbury's*	1 Pack/275g	96.0	1.0	35	1.4	6.6	0.3	1.6
Selection, Prepared, M & S*	1 Serving/250g	75.0	1.0	30	1.4	5.8	0.4	2.0
CRUMBLE								
Apple	1 Pot/240g	497.0	12.0	207	0.9	40.5	5.0	1.1
Apple & Blackberry, Asda*	1 Serving/175g	427.0	16.0	244	2.7	38.0	9.0	1.2
Apple & Blackberry, M & S*	1 Serving/135g	398.0	15.0	295	3.5	44.9	11.2	1.6
Apple & Blackberry, Sainsbury's*	1 Serving/110g	232.0	6.0	211	3.0	37.1	5.6	2.1
Apple & Blackberry, Tesco*	1 Crumble/335g	737.0	32.0	220	2.8	30.7	9.6	2.0
Apple & Custard, Asda*	1 Serving/125g	250.0	9.0	200	2.3	32.0	7.0	0.0
Apple & Toffee, Weight Watchers*	1 Pot/98g	190.0	5.0	194	1.6	36.6	4.6	0.0
Apple with Custard, Green's*	1 Serving/79g	171.0	5.0	216	1.9	37.0	6.7	1.2
Apple with Custard, Individual, Sainsbury's*	1 Pudding/120g	286.0	14.0	238	2.0	31.4	11.6	2.4
Apple, Fresh, Chilled, Tesco*	1/4 Pack/150g	367.0	13.0	245	2.8	38.0	8.9	1.4
Apple, Frozen, Tesco*	1/4 Pack/150g	345.0	16.0	230	2.1	30.7	10.9	3.9
Apple, Iceland*	1 Pie/45g	175.0	7.0	389	4.0	58.4	15.6	2.0
Apple, Sara Lee*	1 Serving/200g	606.0	18.0	303	2.3	53.3	9.0	1.2
Apple, Waitrose*	1 Serving/125g	310.0	3.0	248	2.2	54.5	2.3	1.2
Apple, with Sultanas, Weight Watchers*	1 Dessert/110g	196.0	4.0	178	1.4	34.2	3.9	1.3
Bramley Apple, Favourites, M & S*	1 Serving/140g	390.0	14.0	279	4.6	43.2	9.9	1.2
Bramley Apple, M & S*	1 Serving/149g	387.0	14.0	260	4.3	40.3	9.2	1.1
Bramley Apple, Tesco*	1/3 Pack/155g	378.0	15.0	244	2.8	36.7	9.6	1.8
Cauliflower & Camembert, Sainsbury's*	1 Pack/400g	588.0	43.0	147	5.5	6.9	10.8	0.7
Fish & Prawn, Youngs*	1 Pie/375g	476.0	27.0	127	5.8	9.7	7.2	1.3
Fruit	1oz/28g	55.0	2.0	198	2.0	34.0	6.9	1.7
Fruit, Wholemeal	1oz/28g	54.0	2.0	193	2.6	31.7	7.1	2.7
Gooseberry, M & S*	1 Serving/133g	379.0	14.0	285	3.5	43.3	10.7	1.7
Ocean, Good Choice, Iceland*	1 Pack/340g	377.0	9.0	111	7.2	14.4	2.7	1.1
Ocean, Low Fat, Light & Easy, Youngs*	1/2 Pie/150g	130.0	3.0	87	4.6	12.9	1.9	1.7
Ocean, Low Fat, Ross*	1 Crumble/300g	219.0	2.0	73	5.1	11.4	0.8	0.4
Rhubarb, Farmfoods*	1oz/28g	54.0	1.0	192	2.0	35.0	4.9	2.3
Rhubarb, M & S*	1 Serving/133g	366.0	13.0	275	3.4	42.6	9.9	1.4
Rhubarb, Sainsbury's*	1 Serving/50g	112.0	3.0	224	3.1	40.4	5.6	1.8
Rhubarb, with Custard, Sainsbury's*	1 Serving/120g	288.0	14.0	240	2.4	31.4	11.6	2.3
Salmon, Youngs*	1 Pie/360g	367.0	14.0	102	5.4	11.1	4.0	1.0
CRUMBLE MIX								
Luxury, Tesco*	1/4 Pack/55g	243.0	9.0	441	5.7	67.9	16.3	3.2
CRUMPETS								
Finger, Sainsbury's*	1 Crumpet/30g	55.0	0.0	182	7.0	36.6	0.8	1.8
Fruit, From Bakery, Tesco*	1 Crumpet/73g	161.0	2.0	220	6.2	43.2	2.3	1.1
Kingsmill*	1 Crumpet/55g	99.0	0.0	180	5.8	37.5	0.8	1.7
Less Than 2% Fat, M & S*	1 Crumpet/61g	116.0	1.0	190	8.0	36.9	1.3	2.1
Morning Fresh*	1 Crumpet/20g	36.0	0.0	180	7.3	34.8	1.3	5.2
Mother's Pride*	1 Crumpet/43g	80.0	0.0	185	5.6	38.3	1.0	2.3
Perfectly Balanced, Waitrose*	1 Crumpet/55g	94.0	0.0	171	6.1	36.1	0.3	4.4
Premium, Sainsbury's*	1 Crumpet/50g	95.0	1.0	191	6.1	38.6	1.4	1.7
Soldier, Mother's Pride*	1 Crumpet/30g	58.0	0.0	193	7.8	37.1	1.6	1.6
Square, Spongebob Squarepants*	1 Crumpet/50g	93.0	0.0	186	7.0	37.2	1.0	1.0
Tesco*	1 Crumpet/44g	77.0	1.0	175	5.6	34.5	1.2	3.5
Toasted, Average	1 Crumpet/40g	80.0	0.0	199	6.7	43.4	1.0	2.0

C

	Measure INFO/WEIGHT	per Measure KCAL	FAT	Nutrition Values per 100g / 100ml KCAL	PROT	CARB	FAT	FIBRE
CRUMPETS								
Toaster, Organic, Waitrose*	1 Crumpet/55g	95.0	0.0	172	7.3	34.4	0.6	4.6
TTD, Sainsbury's*	1 Crumpet/65g	124.0	1.0	191	5.9	38.5	1.5	2.3
Waitrose*	1 Crumpet/55g	99.0	1.0	180	7.3	34.8	1.3	5.2
Warburton's*	1 Crumpet/58g	100.0	0.0	172	5.5	36.0	0.7	2.2
CRUNCHERS								
BBQ, Atkins*	1 Bag/28g	100.0	3.0	357	46.4	28.6	10.7	14.3
Nacho Cheese, Atkins*	1 Bag/28g	100.0	3.0	357	46.4	28.6	10.7	10.7
CRUNCHIE								
Blast, Cadbury*	1 Serving/42g	199.0	8.0	480	4.7	69.6	20.1	0.7
Cadbury*	1 Bar/40g	186.0	8.0	465	4.0	69.5	18.9	0.5
Nuggets, Cadbury*	1 Bag/125g	569.0	20.0	455	3.8	73.1	16.4	0.0
Treat Size, Cadbury*	1 Treat Bar/17g	80.0	3.0	470	4.0	71.5	18.4	0.0
CRUNCHY STICKS								
Salt & Vinegar, BGTY, Sainsbury's*	1 Bag/15g	51.0	0.0	340	6.0	80.1	1.5	4.1
Salt & Vinegar, Sainsbury's*	1 Bag/25g	118.0	6.0	474	5.9	58.0	24.3	2.4
Salt & Vinegar, Shapers, Boots*	1 Pack/21g	96.0	4.0	457	5.7	66.7	18.1	2.4
CUCUMBER								
Average	*1 Serving/80g*	*8.0*	*0.0*	*10*	*0.7*	*1.5*	*0.1*	*0.6*
Crunchies, with a Yoghurt & Mint Dip, Shapers, Boots*	1 Serving/110g	35.0	1.0	32	2.1	3.7	0.9	0.8
CUMIN								
Seeds, Ground, Schwartz*	1 Tsp/5g	22.0	1.0	446	19.0	40.3	23.2	0.0
Seeds, Whole, Average	*1 Tsp/2g*	*7.0*	*0.0*	*375*	*17.8*	*44.2*	*22.7*	*10.5*
CUPCAKES								
Assorted, Sainsbury's*	1 Cake/38g	130.0	2.0	341	2.2	69.3	6.1	0.4
Chocolate, 5% Fat, Sainsbury's*	1 Cake/38g	133.0	2.0	349	2.5	74.8	4.4	1.7
Chocolate, BGTY, Sainsbury's*	1 Cake/38g	121.0	2.0	318	2.5	66.5	4.6	0.8
Chocolate, COU, M & S*	1 Cake/45g	130.0	1.0	290	4.6	62.2	2.8	4.3
Chocolate, Fabulous Bakin' Boys*	1 Cupcake/34g	152.0	8.0	448	4.0	54.0	24.0	1.0
Chocolate, Lyons*	1 Cake/39g	125.0	2.0	321	2.4	67.5	4.6	0.8
Chocolate, Mini, Weight Watchers*	1 Cupcake/21g	89.0	4.0	422	6.1	52.0	21.1	1.8
Lemon, COU, M & S*	1 Cupcake/43g	130.0	1.0	305	3.3	68.1	2.1	2.0
Pink, M & S*	1 Cupcake/39g	160.0	3.0	410	2.5	81.3	8.5	0.6
CURACAO								
Average	*1 Pub Shot/35ml*	*109.0*	*0.0*	*311*	*0.0*	*28.3*	*0.0*	*0.0*
CURLY WURLY								
Cadbury*	1 Bar/26g	117.0	5.0	450	3.4	69.4	17.6	0.7
Squirlies, Cadbury*	1 Squirl/3g	13.0	1.0	450	3.9	69.0	17.8	0.0
CURRANTS								
Average	*1oz/28g*	*75.0*	*0.0*	*267*	*2.3*	*67.8*	*0.4*	*1.9*
CURRY								
& Chips, Curry Sauce, Chipped Potatoes, Kershaws*	1 Serving/330g	391.0	8.0	118	10.0	14.0	2.5	2.0
Aubergine	1oz/28g	33.0	3.0	118	1.4	6.2	10.1	1.5
Beef, Hot, Canned, M & S*	1 Can/425g	446.0	22.0	105	12.2	2.8	5.1	1.0
Beef, Sainsbury's*	1 Serving/400g	552.0	33.0	138	10.7	5.4	8.2	0.9
Beef, Smart Price, Asda*	1 Serving/392g	223.0	2.0	57	4.0	9.0	0.5	1.0
Beef, Thai, Finest, Tesco*	1 Serving/500g	770.0	29.0	154	9.0	16.5	5.8	1.2
Beef, with Rice, Asda*	1 Pack/406g	548.0	16.0	135	6.0	19.0	3.9	1.2
Beef, with Rice, Healthy Choice, Asda*	1 Pack/400g	476.0	10.0	119	6.0	18.0	2.6	0.9
Beef, with Rice, Morrisons*	1 Serving/400g	480.0	20.0	120	6.0	12.6	5.0	0.6
Beef, with Rice, Tesco*	1 Pack/400g	456.0	13.0	114	4.5	16.7	3.3	0.6
Beef, with Rice, Weight Watchers*	1 Pack/328g	249.0	3.0	76	4.2	12.5	1.0	0.3
Bombay Butternut Squash Curry, Veg Pot, Innocent*	1 Pot/380g	403.0	10.0	106	3.1	15.4	2.6	4.1
Cabbage	1oz/28g	23.0	1.0	82	1.9	8.1	5.0	2.1

CURRY	Measure INFO/WEIGHT	per Measure KCAL	FAT	Nutrition Values per 100g / 100ml KCAL	PROT	CARB	FAT	FIBRE
Cauliflower & Potato	1oz/28g	17.0	1.0	59	3.4	6.6	2.4	1.8
Chana Dahl, Curry Special*	1 Pack/350g	434.0	23.0	124	6.0	10.5	6.5	5.9
Chick Pea, Whole, Average	1oz/28g	50.0	2.0	179	9.6	21.3	7.5	4.5
Chick Pea, Whole, Basic, Average	1oz/28g	30.0	1.0	108	6.0	14.2	3.6	3.3
Chicken & Vegetable, Big Eat, Heinz*	1 Pot/350g	392.0	18.0	112	5.4	10.9	5.2	4.3
Chicken Biryani, Recipe Mix, Schwartz*	1 Pack/30g	75.0	2.0	249	14.6	58.1	8.1	28.6
Chicken Katsu, City Kitchen, Tesco*	1 Pack/385g	465.0	13.0	121	6.0	16.3	3.4	1.3
Chicken, & Rice, Value, Tesco*	1 Pack/300g	399.0	14.0	133	6.5	16.2	4.7	1.0
Chicken, Canned, Sainsbury's*	1 Serving/100g	136.0	6.0	136	11.1	9.1	6.1	1.0
Chicken, Chinese with Egg Fried Rice, Morrisons*	1 Pack/500g	600.0	15.0	120	5.7	17.4	3.1	0.9
Chicken, Extra Strong, M & S*	1oz/28g	28.0	1.0	100	13.8	2.5	3.9	1.4
Chicken, Green Thai, BGTY, Sainsbury's*	1 Pack/400g	316.0	10.0	79	10.6	3.4	2.6	1.9
Chicken, Green Thai, Birds Eye*	1 Pack/450g	535.0	20.0	119	4.7	15.2	4.4	0.3
Chicken, Green Thai, Breasts, Finest, Tesco*	1 Serving/200g	292.0	16.0	146	16.5	2.0	8.0	0.7
Chicken, Green Thai, Jasmine Rice, Weight Watchers*	1 Pack/320g	291.0	3.0	91	6.1	14.3	1.0	0.5
Chicken, Green Thai, Sainsbury's*	½ Pack/200g	264.0	14.0	132	13.0	4.8	6.8	0.9
Chicken, Kashmiri, Waitrose*	1 Serving/400g	640.0	36.0	160	14.5	5.0	9.1	0.6
Chicken, Medium Hot, M & S*	1 Serving/200g	310.0	14.0	155	7.8	14.3	7.1	0.8
Chicken, Mild, Asda*	½ Can/190g	239.0	11.0	126	11.0	7.0	6.0	0.5
Chicken, Mild, BGTY, Sainsbury's*	1 Serving/200g	184.0	5.0	92	10.0	7.2	2.6	0.5
Chicken, Mild, Iceland*	½ Can/200g	234.0	9.0	117	10.6	8.5	4.5	0.7
Chicken, Mild, Sainsbury's*	1 Can/400g	472.0	28.0	118	10.5	3.5	6.9	1.3
Chicken, Mild, Tinned, Sainsbury's*	1 Serving/200g	214.0	7.0	107	12.7	6.1	3.5	1.1
Chicken, Red Thai, 97% Fat Free, Birds Eye*	1 Pack/366g	425.0	7.0	116	5.7	19.0	1.9	0.5
Chicken, Red Thai, COU, M & S*	1 Pack/400g	420.0	9.0	105	7.1	13.4	2.3	1.4
Chicken, Red Thai, Tesco*	1 Serving/175g	215.0	12.0	123	10.5	5.5	6.6	1.4
Chicken, Red Thai, with Rice, Tesco*	1 Serving/475g	746.0	32.0	157	7.2	16.8	6.8	1.1
Chicken, Reduced Fat, Asda*	1 Pack/400g	476.0	10.0	119	6.0	18.0	2.6	0.9
Chicken, Thai Mango, Sainsbury's*	½ Pack/200g	288.0	18.0	144	11.2	4.8	8.9	1.9
Chicken, Thai Peanut, Sainsbury's*	½ Pack/200g	314.0	19.0	157	12.8	4.9	9.6	1.2
Chicken, Thai, with Rice, Oriental Express*	1 Pack/340g	303.0	4.0	89	4.1	15.3	1.3	1.2
Chicken, Value, Tesco*	1 Pack/300g	399.0	16.0	133	5.5	15.9	5.2	1.7
Chicken, Weight Watchers*	1 Pack/300g	303.0	6.0	101	4.8	16.0	2.0	0.1
Chicken, with Naan Bread, Iceland*	1 Portion/260g	484.0	16.0	186	10.1	22.3	6.3	1.4
Chicken, with Potatoes, Diet Chef Ltd*	1 Pack/300g	291.0	13.0	97	7.5	6.9	4.4	2.8
Chicken, with Rice, Asda*	1 Pack/400g	492.0	12.0	123	6.0	18.0	3.0	1.0
Chicken, with Rice, Dunnes Stores*	1 Pack/375g	400.0	6.0	107	4.2	20.2	1.7	0.8
Chicken, with Rice, Frozen, Sainsbury's*	1 Pack/400g	528.0	10.0	132	6.5	20.8	2.5	1.7
Chicken, with Rice, Frozen, Tesco*	1 Pack/400g	488.0	16.0	122	4.6	17.2	3.9	0.7
Chicken, with Rice, Fruity, HL, Tesco*	1 Pack/450g	495.0	5.0	110	6.5	18.2	1.2	1.2
Chicken, with Rice, Hot, Asda*	1 Pack/400g	476.0	12.0	119	5.0	18.0	3.0	1.0
Chicken, with Rice, Iceland*	1 Pack/500g	566.0	15.0	113	5.2	16.4	3.0	1.2
Chicken, with Rice, Quick Bite, Asda*	1 Serving/300g	294.0	10.0	98	5.0	12.0	3.3	0.5
Chicken, with Rice, Ross*	1 Serving/320g	272.0	4.0	85	3.4	14.7	1.3	0.5
Chicken, with Rice, Tesco*	1 Pack/300g	390.0	13.0	130	4.4	17.5	4.2	1.2
Chicken, with Rice, Weight Watchers*	1 Serving/320g	294.0	4.0	92	5.2	14.5	1.4	0.1
Chicken, with Vegetables, Canned, Value, Tesco*	1 Can/392g	294.0	10.0	75	4.2	7.9	2.6	1.4
Chicken, with Vegetables, Morrisons*	1 Can/392g	392.0	16.0	100	9.0	7.0	4.0	1.0
Chicken, Yellow Thai Style, HL, Tesco*	1 Pack/450g	504.0	12.0	112	9.3	12.6	2.7	0.5
Chinese Chicken, Morrisons*	1 Pack/340g	347.0	16.0	102	10.3	5.0	4.6	0.8
Chinese Chicken, with Rice, GFY, Asda*	1 Pack/400g	444.0	12.0	111	10.7	10.6	2.9	0.5
Chinese Chicken, with Vegetable Rice, M & S*	1 Pack/400g	320.0	8.0	80	7.1	8.4	2.0	1.3
Courgette & Potato	1oz/28g	24.0	1.0	86	1.9	8.7	5.2	1.2

	Measure INFO/WEIGHT	per Measure KCAL	per Measure FAT	Nutrition Values per 100g / 100ml KCAL	PROT	CARB	FAT	FIBRE
CURRY								
Fish, & Vegetable, Bangladeshi, Average	1oz/28g	33.0	2.0	117	9.1	1.4	8.4	0.5
Fish, Bangladeshi, Average	1oz/28g	35.0	2.0	124	12.2	1.5	7.9	0.3
Fish, Red Thai, Waitrose*	1 Pack/500g	275.0	11.0	55	5.2	3.7	2.2	1.0
Gobi Aloo Sag, Retail	1oz/28g	27.0	2.0	95	2.2	7.1	6.9	1.4
Green Thai, & Rice, GFY, Asda*	1 Pack/400g	356.0	8.0	89	7.0	11.0	1.9	1.6
Green Thai, with Sticky Rice, HL, Tesco*	1 Pack/450g	517.0	12.0	115	7.7	14.9	2.7	0.6
Indian Daal, Tasty Veg Pot, Innocent*	1 Pot/380g	308.0	10.0	81	3.9	10.4	2.6	4.4
King Prawn Malay, Waitrose*	1 Pack/350g	364.0	19.0	104	6.6	7.1	5.5	0.9
King Prawn, Coconut & Lime, Sainsbury's*	½ Pack/351g	207.0	9.0	59	3.7	5.4	2.5	1.0
King Prawn, Malay with Rice, Sainsbury's*	1 Pack/400g	608.0	20.0	152	5.0	21.5	5.1	1.4
King Prawn, Red Thai, City Kitchen, Tesco*	1 Pack/385g	460.0	14.0	119	4.5	16.7	3.7	1.0
Lamb, Hot, M & S*	½ Can/213.3g	320.0	20.0	150	14.9	6.0	9.2	2.3
Lamb, Kefthedes, Waitrose*	½ Pack/200g	294.0	18.0	147	9.0	8.0	8.8	2.1
Lamb, with Rice, Birds Eye*	1 Pack/382g	520.0	13.0	136	5.6	20.8	3.4	0.9
Masala Veg Pot, Innocent*	1 Pot/400g	331.0	10.0	87	2.9	11.6	2.5	3.6
Masala, Aubergine, TTD, Sainsbury's*	½ Pack/115g	135.0	11.0	117	2.9	4.1	9.9	5.8
Masala, Vegalicious, Pick Me*	1 Pot/400g	156.0	6.0	39	1.6	4.8	1.5	2.8
Matar Paneer, Peas & Cheese, Ashoka*	½ Pack/150g	183.0	10.0	122	5.3	10.0	6.7	2.0
Potato & Pea	1oz/28g	26.0	1.0	92	2.9	13.0	3.8	2.4
Prawn, & Mushroom	1oz/28g	47.0	4.0	168	7.3	2.5	14.4	1.0
Prawn, King, Goan, M & S*	1 Pack/400g	680.0	44.0	170	5.1	11.6	11.1	1.5
Prawn, with Rice, Asda*	1 Pack/400g	420.0	10.0	105	3.5	17.0	2.6	1.1
Prawn, with Rice, Birds Eye*	1 Pack/375g	442.0	0.0	118	3.5	20.6	0.0	0.0
Prawn, with Rice, Frozen, Sainsbury's*	1 Pack/400g	552.0	8.0	138	3.9	26.4	1.9	2.1
Prawn, with Rice, Iceland*	1 Pack/450g	468.0	14.0	104	3.2	16.4	3.2	1.5
Prawn, with Rice, Light & Easy, Youngs*	1 Pack/310g	248.0	3.0	80	3.3	14.2	1.1	0.9
Red Kidney Bean, Punjabi	1oz/28g	30.0	2.0	106	4.7	10.1	5.6	3.8
Salmon, Green, Waitrose*	1 Pack/401g	581.0	40.0	145	9.1	4.5	10.1	2.7
Thai Chicken, Diet Chef Ltd*	1 Pack/300g	291.0	13.0	97	5.8	9.0	4.2	2.4
Thai Chicken, Solo Slim, Rosemary Conley*	1/100g	79.0	2.0	79	21.6	7.0	2.5	2.3
Vegetable, Diet Chef Ltd*	1 Pack/300g	153.0	4.0	51	2.0	8.0	1.2	2.1
Vegetable, Frozen, Mixed Vegetables, Average	1oz/28g	25.0	2.0	88	2.5	6.9	6.1	0.0
Vegetable, in Sweet Sauce, Average	1 Serving/330g	162.0	7.0	49	1.4	6.7	2.1	1.3
Vegetable, Medium, Tesco*	1 Pack/350g	325.0	22.0	93	2.3	7.1	6.2	1.9
Vegetable, Mild, COU, M & S*	1 Pack/400g	340.0	2.0	85	2.6	17.0	0.5	2.8
Vegetable, Pakistani, Average	1oz/28g	17.0	1.0	60	2.2	8.7	2.6	2.2
Vegetable, Sabzi Tarkari, Patak's*	1 Pack/400g	500.0	31.0	125	2.5	11.1	7.8	2.2
Vegetable, Takeaway, Average	1 Serving/330g	346.0	24.0	105	2.5	7.6	7.4	0.0
Vegetable, with Rice, Retail, Average	1oz/28g	29.0	1.0	102	3.3	16.4	3.0	0.0
Vegetable, with Yoghurt, Average	1oz/28g	17.0	1.0	62	2.6	4.6	4.1	1.4
Vegetable, Yellow Thai, Sainsbury's*	1 Pack/400g	624.0	49.0	156	2.2	9.4	12.2	1.1
Vegetable, Yellow, Tesco*	1 Pack/356g	324.0	17.0	91	1.9	9.9	4.9	1.4
CURRY LEAVES								
Fresh	***1oz/28g***	***27.0***	***0.0***	***97***	***7.9***	***13.3***	***1.3***	***0.0***
CURRY PASTE								
Balti, Asda*	1 Tube/100g	220.0	15.0	220	4.7	17.2	14.7	1.9
Balti, Sharwood's*	¼ Pack/72.5g	328.0	29.0	453	5.0	19.2	39.6	3.1
Balti, Tomato & Coriander, Original, Patak's*	1 Tbsp/15g	58.0	5.0	388	4.0	14.6	34.0	3.7
Bhuna, Tomato & Tamarind, Patak's*	1 Serving/10g	40.0	6.0	397	4.3	17.5	56.2	6.3
Garam Masala, Cinnamon & Ginger, Hot, Patak's*	1 Serving/30g	121.0	11.0	403	3.2	17.9	35.4	0.6
Green Thai, Mild, Sainsbury's*	1 Tbsp/15g	23.0	1.0	156	2.2	14.5	9.9	2.7
Green Thai, Tesco*	1 Tbsp/15g	17.0	1.0	115	2.1	8.7	7.9	3.1
Green, Thai, Asda*	1 Tbsp/25g	28.0	2.0	114	1.6	10.0	8.0	5.0

	Measure INFO/WEIGHT	per Measure KCAL	FAT	Nutrition Values per 100g / 100ml KCAL	PROT	CARB	FAT	FIBRE
CURRY PASTE								
Hot, M & S*	1oz/28g	69.0	5.0	245	4.2	13.4	19.2	3.3
Hot, Sharwood's*	1oz/28g	123.0	11.0	439	5.1	18.6	38.3	2.6
Jalfrezi, Patak's*	1 Serving/30g	96.0	8.0	320	3.7	14.2	26.9	5.6
Korma, Asda*	1 Tube/100g	338.0	23.0	338	5.1	26.6	23.5	1.2
Korma, Coconut & Coriander, Original, Patak's*	1 Serving/30g	124.0	12.0	415	3.5	11.6	39.0	5.2
Madras, Cumin & Chilli, Hot, Patak's*	¼ Jar/70g	202.0	18.0	289	4.7	7.6	25.9	10.8
Medium, Asda*	1 Tsp/5ml/5g	18.0	2.0	364	5.0	14.0	32.0	5.0
Medium, Barts Spices*	1 Serving/30g	88.0	6.0	295	4.5	19.2	21.5	5.5
Medium, Sharwood's*	1oz/28g	122.0	11.0	434	4.5	16.8	38.8	2.7
Mild, Asda*	¼ Jar/46g	206.0	19.0	448	3.8	16.0	41.0	7.0
Mild, Coriander & Cumin, Original, Patak's*	1 Serving/30g	169.0	16.0	562	4.8	16.8	52.5	2.8
Mild, Sharwood's*	1oz/28g	78.0	6.0	279	3.6	17.7	21.5	3.4
Red Thai, M & S*	½ Jar/100g	150.0	11.0	150	1.3	11.9	10.8	2.8
Red Thai, Sainsbury's*	1 Jar/250g	385.0	31.0	154	2.2	8.5	12.4	3.5
Red Thai, Tesco*	1 Tsp/5g	5.0	0.0	110	1.5	8.9	7.3	3.7
Red, Thai, Asda*	1 Tbsp/25g	31.0	2.0	124	1.6	7.0	10.0	5.0
Rogan Josh, Tomato & Paprika, Patak's*	1 Serving/30g	119.0	11.0	397	4.1	12.7	36.7	5.9
Tamarind & Ginger, Original, Patak's*	1 Tbsp/15g	20.0	0.0	133	3.4	23.1	2.0	2.9
Tandoori, Sharwood's*	1oz/28g	64.0	4.0	228	5.9	15.5	15.8	1.9
Tandoori, Tamarind & Ginger, Patak's*	1 Serving/30g	33.0	1.0	110	3.1	20.4	1.8	2.6
Tikka Masala, Coriander & Lemon, Medium, Patak's*	1 Serving/30g	111.0	10.0	369	3.8	16.9	31.8	2.9
Tikka Masala, Sharwood's*	1oz/28g	53.0	4.0	191	3.2	9.9	15.4	2.6
Tikka, Asda*	½ Tube/50g	117.0	8.0	235	4.5	16.1	17.0	1.6
CURRY POWDER								
Average	*1 Tsp/2g*	*6.0*	*0.0*	*325*	*12.7*	*41.8*	*13.8*	*0.0*
CURRY SAUCE								
Asda*	1 Tbsp/15g	62.0	2.0	414	13.0	59.0	14.0	1.3
Balti, Asda*	¼ Jar/125g	155.0	12.0	124	1.6	7.0	10.0	1.7
Chinese Style, Cooking, Asda*	1 Jar/560g	465.0	24.0	83	1.5	9.6	4.3	1.7
Dopiaza, Finest, Tesco*	1 Jar/350g	234.0	10.0	67	1.3	8.5	3.0	3.7
Green Curry, Thai, Stir Fry, Blue Dragon*	1 Sachet/120g	74.0	5.0	62	0.9	5.7	4.0	0.5
Green Thai, Asda*	1 Jar/340g	309.0	27.0	91	0.5	4.3	8.0	0.2
Green Thai, Express, Uncle Ben's*	1 Pack/170g	131.0	10.0	77	1.1	5.4	5.8	0.0
Jalfrezi, Loyd Grossman*	½ Jar/212.5g	270.0	20.0	127	2.1	8.2	9.5	1.2
Jalfrezi, Piri Piri, Finest, Tesco*	1 Serving/175g	145.0	11.0	83	1.2	5.7	6.2	1.5
Jalfrezi, Tesco*	1 Jar/500g	450.0	32.0	90	1.3	6.6	6.5	2.4
Korma, Loyd Grossman*	½ Jar/222g	542.0	38.0	244	3.6	19.1	17.0	0.6
Korma, Uncle Ben's*	1 Jar/500g	630.0	42.0	126	1.4	11.1	8.4	0.0
Madras, Cooking, Asda*	¼ Jar/142g	109.0	6.0	77	1.3	8.0	4.4	1.0
Madras, Cooking, Sharwood's*	1 Tsp/2g	2.0	0.0	86	1.5	6.9	5.8	1.3
Madras, Cooking, Tesco*	1/3 Jar/161g	145.0	9.0	90	1.9	6.9	5.7	2.5
Madras, Cumin & Chilli, Original, in Glass Jar, Patak's*	1 Jar/540g	648.0	38.0	120	2.1	11.9	7.1	1.8
Madras, Indian, Sharwood's*	1 Jar/420g	433.0	26.0	103	1.8	9.7	6.3	1.9
Madras, Sharwood's*	1 Jar/420g	521.0	38.0	124	1.7	8.9	9.1	1.4
Madras, Tesco*	½ Jar/200g	168.0	13.0	84	1.1	5.2	6.5	1.3
Makhani, Sharwood's*	1 Jar/420g	399.0	29.0	95	0.9	7.2	6.9	0.4
Malaysian Rendang, Loyd Grossman*	1 Serving/100g	143.0	10.0	143	2.6	10.4	10.1	1.4
Masala, Red Pepper & Mango, Sainsbury's*	½ Jar/175g	142.0	9.0	81	1.4	7.8	4.9	1.1
Medium, Uncle Ben's*	1 Jar/500g	330.0	10.0	66	0.9	10.9	2.0	0.0
Moglai Pasanda, Asda*	½ Jar/170g	277.0	21.0	163	2.9	10.0	12.3	1.1
Red Curry, Thai, Stir Fry, Blue Dragon*	1 Sachet/120g	112.0	10.0	93	0.9	4.4	8.0	0.5
Rogan Josh, Loyd Grossman*	1 Serving/106g	206.0	17.0	194	2.4	10.5	15.8	1.5
Rogan Josh, Worldwide Sauces*	1 Jar/500g	255.0	1.0	51	1.1	11.0	0.3	0.0

	Measure INFO/WEIGHT	per Measure KCAL	FAT	Nutrition Values per 100g / 100ml KCAL	PROT	CARB	FAT	FIBRE
CURRY SAUCE								
Singapore, Blue Dragon*	1 Sachet/120g	89.0	4.0	74	1.8	9.0	3.4	3.7
Sri Lankan Devil Curry, Sharwood's*	1 Jar/380g	220.0	11.0	58	0.5	7.2	3.0	2.1
Tikka Masala, Cooking, HL, Tesco*	¼ Jar/125g	94.0	4.0	75	2.6	8.2	3.0	1.2
Tikka Masala, COU, M & S*	½ Pack/100g	80.0	3.0	80	4.5	9.9	2.6	1.7
Tikka Masala, Loyd Grossman*	½ Jar/212.5g	438.0	34.0	206	2.6	12.5	16.2	1.0
Tikka, Cooking, Tesco*	1 Std Jar/500g	617.0	42.0	123	1.7	10.1	8.4	2.0
Vindaloo, Hot, Patak's*	1 Jar/540g	643.0	46.0	119	1.7	8.5	8.6	2.1
CUSTARD								
Banana Flavour, Ambrosia*	1 Sm Pot/135g	139.0	4.0	103	2.9	16.1	2.9	0.0
Chocolate Flavour, Ambrosia*	1 Pot/150g	177.0	4.0	118	3.0	20.0	2.9	0.7
Chocolate, COU, M & S*	1 Pot/140g	147.0	3.0	105	3.1	18.6	2.2	1.0
Dairy Free, Sainsbury's*	1 Serving/250g	210.0	4.0	84	3.0	14.2	1.7	0.2
Low Fat, Average	*1/3 Pot/141g*	*116.0*	*2.0*	*82*	*2.9*	*15.0*	*1.2*	*0.0*
Pot, Forest Fruits Flavour, Hot 'n' Fruity, Bird's*	1 Pot/174g	171.0	4.0	98	0.9	18.5	2.4	0.1
Powder	*1 Tsp/5g*	*18.0*	*0.0*	*354*	*0.6*	*92.0*	*0.7*	*0.1*
Ready to Serve, Average	*1 Serving/50g*	*59.0*	*2.0*	*118*	*3.3*	*16.1*	*4.6*	*0.2*
Strawberry Flavoured, Ambrosia*	1 Serving/135g	139.0	4.0	103	2.8	16.7	2.8	0.0
Strawberry Style, Shapers, Boots*	1 Pot/148g	83.0	1.0	56	4.0	8.2	0.8	0.1
Summer, Ambrosia*	1 Pack/500g	490.0	15.0	98	2.7	15.0	3.0	0.0
Toffee Flavour, Ambrosia*	1 Pot/150g	156.0	4.0	104	2.8	17.0	2.8	0.0
Vanilla with Apple Crunch, Ambrosia*	1 Pack/193g	276.0	9.0	143	3.4	22.4	4.5	0.8
Vanilla, COU, M & S*	1 Pot/140g	147.0	3.0	105	4.3	16.6	2.5	0.6
Vanilla, Fresh, Waitrose*	1 Serving/100g	214.0	15.0	214	3.2	15.8	15.3	1.1
Vanilla, TTD, Sainsbury's*	1 Pot/150g	312.0	23.0	208	2.5	14.7	15.5	0.1
with Strawberry Sauce, Ambrosia*	1 Pot/160g	171.0	4.0	107	2.4	19.0	2.4	0.1
CUTLETS								
Nut, Goodlife*	1 Cutlet/88g	283.0	19.0	322	9.1	21.8	22.0	3.4
Nut, Meat Free, Tesco*	1 Cutlet/83g	224.0	14.0	270	8.1	20.5	16.9	4.3
Nut, Retail, Fried in Vegetable Oil, Average	1 Cutlet/90g	260.0	20.0	289	4.8	18.7	22.3	1.7
Nut, Retail, Grilled, Average	1 Cutlet/90g	191.0	12.0	212	5.1	19.9	13.0	1.8
Vegetable & Nut, Asda*	1 Cutlet/88g	296.0	20.0	335	10.0	22.0	23.0	4.6
CUTTLEFISH								
Raw	*1oz/28g*	*20.0*	*0.0*	*71*	*16.1*	*0.0*	*0.7*	*0.0*

	Measure INFO/WEIGHT	per Measure KCAL	FAT	Nutrition Values per 100g / 100ml KCAL		PROT	CARB	FAT	FIBRE
DAB									
Fillets, Lightly Dusted, M & S*	1 Fillet/112g	190.0	10.0	170		12.8	9.7	8.7	0.5
Raw	*1oz/28g*	*21.0*	*0.0*	*74*		*15.7*	*0.0*	*1.2*	*0.0*
DAIRYLEA DUNKERS									
Baked Crisps, Dairylea, Kraft*	1 Pack/45g	101.0	4.0	225		9.2	26.0	9.0	1.1
Jumbo Munch, Dairylea, Kraft*	1 Serving/50g	150.0	9.0	300		7.2	26.5	18.5	1.2
Salt & Vinegar, Dairylea, Kraft*	1 Tub/42g	115.0	8.0	275		6.7	17.5	19.5	0.3
Smokey Bacon, Dairylea, Kraft*	1 Pack/45g	135.0	9.0	300		7.3	24.0	19.5	0.0
with Ritz Crackers, Dairylea, Kraft*	1 Tub/46g	122.0	6.0	265		9.6	25.0	13.9	0.6
DAIRYLEA LUNCHABLES									
Double Cheese, Dairylea, Kraft*	1 Pack/110g	412.0	29.0	375		18.0	17.0	26.0	0.3
Ham & Cheese Pizza, Dairylea, Kraft*	1 Pack/97g	247.0	11.0	255		11.5	26.0	11.0	1.6
Harvest Ham, Dairylea, Kraft*	1 Pack/110g	313.0	19.0	285		16.5	16.5	17.0	0.3
Tasty Chicken, Dairylea, Kraft*	1 Pack/110g	313.0	18.0	285		17.0	17.5	16.5	0.3
DAMSONS									
Raw, Weighed with Stones, Average	*1oz/28g*	*10.0*	*0.0*	*34*		*0.5*	*8.6*	*0.0*	*1.6*
Raw, Weighed without Stones, Average	*1oz/28g*	*11.0*	*0.0*	*38*		*0.5*	*9.6*	*0.0*	*1.8*
DANDELION & BURDOCK									
Fermented Botanical, Fentimans*	1 Bottle/275ml	130.0	0.0	47		0.0	11.3	0.0	0.0
Original, Ben Shaws*	1 Can/440ml	128.0	0.0	29		0.0	7.0	0.0	0.0
DANISH PASTRY									
Apple & Cinnamon, Danish Twist, Entenmann's*	1 Serving/52g	150.0	1.0	288		5.6	62.0	1.9	1.5
Apple & Sultana, Tesco*	1 Pastry/72g	293.0	16.0	407		5.4	45.0	22.8	1.4
Apple, Bar, Sara Lee*	1/6 Bar/70g	160.0	4.0	229		4.3	42.1	5.7	1.7
Apple, Fresh Cream, Sainsbury's*	1 Pastry/67g	248.0	15.0	368		3.1	40.2	21.6	0.4
Average	1 Pastry/110g	411.0	19.0	374		5.8	51.3	17.6	1.6
Cherry & Custard, Bar, Tesco*	1 Bar/350g	910.0	49.0	260		3.5	29.9	14.0	7.7
Cherry, Bar, Sainsbury's*	¼ Bar/88g	220.0	10.0	252		4.2	33.2	11.4	1.7
Custard, Bar, Sara Lee*	¼ Bar/100g	228.0	6.0	228		6.6	36.1	6.4	0.8
Fruit Filled, Average	1 Pastry/94g	335.0	16.0	356		5.1	47.9	16.9	0.0
Pecan, M & S*	1 Serving/67g	287.0	17.0	428		6.2	45.0	26.0	1.3
Toasted Pecan, Danish Twist, Entenmann's*	1 Slice/48g	171.0	8.0	351		7.0	47.2	15.6	1.4
DATES									
Deglet Nour, Graze*	1 Pack/60g	181.0	0.0	301		2.1	72.0	0.5	0.0
Dried, Average	*1 Date/5g*	*14.0*	*0.0*	*272*		*2.8*	*65.4*	*0.4*	*4.2*
Dried, Medjool, Average	*1 Date/20g*	*56.0*	*0.0*	*279*		*2.2*	*69.3*	*0.3*	*4.3*
Fresh, Raw, Yellow, Average	*1 Date/20g*	*23.0*	*0.0*	*115*		*1.4*	*29.1*	*0.1*	*1.6*
Halawi, Tesco*	6 Dates/60g	165.0	0.0	275		2.3	65.5	0.2	4.3
Medjool, Stuffed with Walnuts, Tesco*	2 Dates/40g	98.0	2.0	245		4.4	44.0	5.7	3.4
Medjool, TTD, Sainsbury's*	1 Serving/50g	148.0	0.0	296		1.9	72.0	0.1	6.7
DELI FILLER									
Chicken & Bacon, Co-Op*	1 Pack/200g	420.0	30.0	210		17.6	1.0	14.8	2.6
Chicken, Caesar Style, Sainsbury's*	1 Pack/80g	212.0	18.0	265		14.0	1.0	22.7	2.6
Chinese, Princes*	1 Serving/50g	47.0	1.0	94		3.6	15.6	1.9	0.3
King Prawn & Avocado, M & S*	1 Pack/170g	425.0	39.0	250		9.5	1.4	22.8	0.5
Prawn & Mayonnaise, M & S*	1 Serving/60g	150.0	14.0	250		11.3	1.0	23.0	0.5
Smoked Salmon & Soft Cheese, M & S*	1 Serving/85g	208.0	17.0	245		11.7	3.3	20.4	0.5
DELIGHT									
Blackcurrant, Made Up, Asda*	1 Serving/100g	115.0	4.0	115		3.2	17.0	3.8	0.0
Butterscotch Flavour, No Added Sugar, Tesco*	1 Pack/49g	225.0	10.0	460		4.8	63.3	20.5	0.0
Butterscotch, Dessert, Safeway*	1 Pack/69g	302.0	8.0	438		1.8	81.5	11.6	0.3
Chocolate Flavour, Dry, Tesco*	1 Pack/49g	220.0	9.0	450		6.2	64.2	18.4	2.3
Ravishing Raspberry, Made Up, Asda*	1/3 Pack/100g	112.0	4.0	112		3.2	16.0	3.9	0.0
Strawberry, No Added Sugar, Dry, Tesco*	1 Pack/49g	51.0	2.0	105		3.4	13.7	3.7	0.1

D

	Measure INFO/WEIGHT	per Measure KCAL	per Measure FAT	Nutrition Values per 100g / 100ml KCAL	PROT	CARB	FAT	FIBRE
DELIGHT								
Strawberry, Shapers, Boots*	1 Pot/122g	96.0	1.0	79	4.5	13.0	1.0	0.1
Vanilla, No Added Sugar, Dry, Tesco*	1 Pack/49g	51.0	2.0	105	3.4	13.7	3.7	0.1
DESSERT								
Almond, Naturgreen*	1 Serving/130g	143.0	6.0	110	2.3	14.5	4.8	0.2
Apple Crumble, Sainsbury's*	1 Pot/136g	291.0	10.0	214	3.2	33.0	7.7	2.7
Baked Lemon, COU, M & S*	1 Serving/100g	140.0	2.0	140	6.8	22.0	2.5	0.8
Banoffee Layered, Sainsbury's*	1 Pot/115g	270.0	15.0	235	2.2	27.8	12.8	1.0
Banoffee, Sainsbury's*	1 Pot/140g	360.0	19.0	257	2.7	30.9	13.6	1.3
Banoffee, Shape, Danone*	1 Pot/120g	175.0	3.0	146	3.3	28.0	2.3	0.5
Banoffee, Weight Watchers*	1 Dessert/81g	170.0	4.0	210	4.9	37.7	4.4	1.4
Black Cherry & Chocolate, COU, M & S*	1 Pack/115g	132.0	2.0	115	3.6	22.6	1.4	1.2
Black Cherry, Dragana, Waitrose*	1 Pot/125g	236.0	11.0	189	2.1	24.7	9.1	0.5
Black Forest, Light Choices, Tesco*	1 Pot/145g	188.0	2.0	130	3.2	25.8	1.6	0.9
Bounty, Mars*	1 Pot/110g	253.0	15.0	230	5.3	23.2	13.6	0.0
Butterscotch Flavour Whip, Co-Op*	1 Pack/64g	241.0	0.0	377	0.6	93.4	0.1	0.0
Buttons, Milk Chocolate, Cadbury*	1 Pot/100g	280.0	15.0	280	6.2	30.8	14.9	0.0
Cafe Latte, COU, M & S*	1 Pot/120g	162.0	3.0	135	5.0	24.0	2.2	0.9
Cafe Mocha, COU, M & S*	1 Dessert/115g	155.0	3.0	135	5.5	21.8	2.7	1.0
Cappuccino, BGTY, Sainsbury's*	1 Pot/119g	224.0	10.0	188	3.3	25.2	8.1	0.8
Caramel Crunch, Weight Watchers*	1 Serving/89g	174.0	3.0	196	4.6	37.9	2.9	1.7
Caramel Flavour, Soya, Dairy Free, Organic, Provamel*	1 Pot/125g	122.0	2.0	98	3.0	17.5	1.7	0.6
Caramel Shortcake, Luxury, Weight Watchers*	1 Pot/100ml	103.0	3.0	103	1.9	17.9	3.5	0.8
Caramel, Delights, Shape, Danone*	1 Pot/110g	109.0	3.0	99	3.3	16.3	2.3	0.1
Catalan Cream, Sainsbury's*	1 Pot/95g	375.0	35.0	395	4.2	11.2	37.0	0.1
Cherry & Chocolate, Eat Smart, Safeway*	1 Serving/100g	150.0	3.0	150	3.2	27.5	2.7	0.1
Cherry & Vanilla, BGTY, Sainsbury's*	1 Pot/115g	225.0	8.0	196	1.6	32.6	6.6	1.0
Cherry Rice, M & S*	1 Pot/200g	220.0	4.0	110	2.4	19.7	2.2	0.1
Chocolate & Coconut, COU, M & S*	1 Pot/125g	169.0	3.0	135	3.6	25.6	2.2	0.7
Chocolate & Mallow, Weight Watchers*	1 Pot/150ml	140.0	2.0	93	2.0	18.7	1.2	2.3
Chocolate Brownie, M & S*	¼ Pack/144g	610.0	39.0	425	4.7	39.6	27.5	1.0
Chocolate Dream, Co-Op*	1 Pot/110g	184.0	8.0	167	4.1	22.0	7.0	0.0
Chocolate Duetto, Weight Watchers*	1 Pot/85g	99.0	2.0	117	4.4	18.4	2.8	0.0
Chocolate Flavour, Soya, Dairy Free, Organic, Provamel*	1 Pot/125g	116.0	2.0	93	3.0	16.4	1.6	1.5
Chocolate Fudge Brownie, Tesco*	1 Pot/125g	374.0	17.0	299	4.6	40.2	13.3	1.3
Chocolate Honeycomb Crisp, COU, M & S*	1 Serving/71g	110.0	2.0	155	4.6	27.6	2.9	1.0
Chocolate Marshmallow, Weight Watchers*	1 Serving/50g	97.0	2.0	194	3.2	34.5	4.7	1.3
Chocolate Mint Torte, Weight Watchers*	1 Dessert/88g	174.0	4.0	198	4.7	34.3	4.7	5.2
Chocolate Mocha, BGTY, Sainsbury's*	1 Pot/100g	115.0	3.0	115	3.8	19.2	2.6	2.8
Chocolate Mousse Cake, Weight Watchers*	1 Dessert/75g	148.0	2.0	198	5.9	37.1	2.9	1.0
Chocolate Muffin, COU, M & S*	1 Pot/110g	154.0	3.0	140	6.1	26.1	2.5	1.5
Chocolate Muffin, Tesco*	1 Serving/104g	354.0	21.0	340	3.5	35.5	20.4	2.1
Chocolate Toffee, Weight Watchers*	1 Dessert/89g	177.0	4.0	197	4.3	34.9	4.5	2.2
Chocolate, Campina*	1 Pot/125g	186.0	9.0	149	3.2	18.5	6.9	0.0
Chocolate, Delights, Shape, Danone*	1 Pot/110g	109.0	2.0	99	3.3	16.3	2.2	0.6
Chocolate, M & S*	1 Serving/120g	168.0	3.0	140	5.6	26.4	2.1	1.1
Chocolate, Triple Delight, Weight Watchers*	1 Dessert/110g	183.0	3.0	166	4.9	30.8	2.6	2.6
Chocolate, Weight Watchers*	1 Serving/82g	145.0	2.0	177	5.2	32.3	3.0	2.9
Crazy Chocolate Overload, M & S*	1 Pot/120g	402.0	27.0	335	3.1	30.0	22.5	0.5
Creme Caramel, Sainsbury's*	1 Pot/100g	102.0	1.0	102	2.5	21.1	0.9	0.0
Crunchie, Dairy Milk, Cadbury*	1 Pot/100g	260.0	12.0	260	4.4	33.4	12.2	0.0
Custard, with Caramel, Layers, Ambrosia*	1 Pot/161g	183.0	5.0	114	2.5	19.6	2.9	0.0
Double Chocolate Brownie, Weight Watchers*	1 Pot/86g	163.0	3.0	189	5.1	33.7	3.8	2.4
Double Chocolate Fudge, M & S*	1 Pot/119g	387.0	25.0	325	3.0	30.6	21.4	1.6

DESSERT

	Measure INFO/WEIGHT	per Measure KCAL	per Measure FAT	Nutrition Values per 100g / 100ml KCAL	PROT	CARB	FAT	FIBRE
Dreamy Vanilla, BGTY, Sainsbury's*	1 Serving/58g	146.0	8.0	252	3.5	27.6	14.2	5.3
Flake, Milk Chocolate, Cadbury*	1 Pot/100g	275.0	15.0	275	6.2	29.8	14.6	0.0
Fruit & Nut, Cadbury*	1 Pot/100g	285.0	12.0	285	6.4	36.3	12.5	0.0
Fudge, Cadbury*	1 Pot/90g	216.0	11.0	240	4.1	28.5	12.4	0.0
Galaxy, Mars*	1 Pot/75g	166.0	9.0	221	4.9	22.7	12.3	0.0
Gulabjam Indian, Waitrose*	1 Pot/180g	479.0	15.0	266	4.8	42.9	8.6	0.6
Irish Cream Cafe Latte, COU, M & S*	1 Pot/120g	160.0	3.0	133	5.0	24.0	2.2	0.9
Jaffa Cake, COU, M & S*	1 Serving/120g	138.0	3.0	115	2.4	20.1	2.6	1.0
Lemon & Sultana Sponge, COU, M & S*	1 Pot/130g	169.0	2.0	130	2.8	26.5	1.2	0.5
Lemon Meringue, Weight Watchers*	1 Pot/85g	161.0	0.0	189	2.4	43.1	0.5	0.6
Lemon Mousse Cake, Weight Watchers*	1 Serving/90g	130.0	2.0	144	3.2	26.7	2.7	0.5
Lemon, Sainsbury's*	1 Pot/115g	136.0	2.0	118	2.8	23.2	1.5	0.9
Lemoncillo, Tesco*	1 Pot/100g	273.0	10.0	273	4.2	41.8	9.9	0.8
Mandarin, COU, M & S*	1 Serving/150g	195.0	6.0	130	1.0	22.0	3.8	0.1
Maple & Pecan, American Style, Sainsbury's*	1 Pot/110g	287.0	16.0	261	2.6	30.6	14.2	1.2
Mars, Mars*	1 Pot/110g	214.0	7.0	195	6.0	28.2	6.7	0.7
Millionaire's Shortbread, M & S*	1 Dessert/120g	425.0	26.0	355	2.6	38.3	21.5	1.4
Mint Chocolate Top, Weight Watchers*	1 Pot/75g	160.0	7.0	214	4.0	31.4	9.2	3.5
Mix, Chocolate, Basics, Sainsbury's*	1 Serving/100g	92.0	3.0	92	4.0	11.5	3.3	0.5
Peach & Raspberry, COU, M & S*	1 Pot/90g	135.0	1.0	150	2.6	30.5	1.6	1.0
Pineapple & Passionfruit, M & S*	1 Pot/100g	130.0	4.0	130	0.8	21.7	3.8	0.3
Raspberry & Chardonnay, COU, M & S*	1 Serving/135g	155.0	1.0	115	1.6	25.5	0.5	2.7
Raspberry Flavour Whip, Co-Op*	1 Whip/64g	241.0	0.0	377	1.2	92.5	0.2	0.0
Raspberry Royale, Finest, Tesco*	½ Pack/170g	314.0	16.0	185	1.7	22.8	9.3	1.4
Raspberry with Light Lemon Sponge, Weight Watchers*	1 Dessert/85g	152.0	4.0	178	4.1	30.4	4.4	2.8
Rich Chocolate, Weight Watchers*	1 Pot/70g	62.0	2.0	89	3.5	13.4	2.4	1.4
Rocky Road, Sainsbury's*	1 Pot/110g	328.0	22.0	298	3.6	26.8	19.6	2.1
Rolo, Nestle*	1 Pot/77g	187.0	9.0	243	3.1	30.0	12.3	0.5
Soya, Mocha Flavour, Provamel*	1 Serving/125g	117.0	2.0	94	3.0	16.3	1.8	0.6
Splijies, Vanilla, Tip Top, Nestle*	1 Tube/85g	97.0	3.0	114	4.0	16.1	3.7	0.0
Strawberries & Cream, BFY, Morrisons*	1 Serving/200g	244.0	2.0	122	2.2	26.0	1.1	0.1
Strawberry & Rhubarb, COU, M & S*	1 Pot/110g	104.0	1.0	95	1.5	20.1	0.7	0.9
Strawberry Flavour, Smart Price, Asda*	1 Pot/115g	113.0	3.0	98	2.4	17.0	2.3	0.0
Strawberry Meringue, Iced, Luxury, Weight Watchers*	1 Pot/100ml	86.0	1.0	162	2.4	34.2	1.4	1.0
Strawberry Mousse Cake, Weight Watchers*	1 Serving/90g	124.0	2.0	138	3.0	25.5	2.7	0.5
Strawberry, BGTY, Sainsbury's*	1 Pot/115g	133.0	2.0	116	2.7	23.1	1.4	1.3
Strawberry, HL, Tesco*	1 Pot/122g	94.0	2.0	77	2.7	12.3	1.9	1.1
Strawberry, Value, Tesco*	1 Pot/115g	113.0	3.0	98	2.4	16.9	2.3	0.0
Summer Berry, HL, Tesco*	1 Pot/92.5g	120.0	2.0	130	2.8	24.5	2.3	1.5
Summer Fruits, COU, M & S*	1 Serving/105g	110.0	1.0	105	2.1	21.6	1.1	1.2
Tantalising Toffee Flavour, Weight Watchers*	1 Serving/57g	93.0	3.0	163	2.7	26.2	4.8	0.2
Tantalising Toffee, COU, M & S*	¼ Pot/85g	144.0	2.0	170	3.1	32.8	2.9	0.5
Toffee & Vanilla, Weight Watchers*	1 Pot/67g	107.0	1.0	159	3.1	34.8	0.8	3.9
Toffee Chocolate, Weight Watchers*	1 Pot/100g	197.0	4.0	197	4.3	34.9	4.5	2.2
Toffee Flavour Custard, Ambrosia*	1 Pack/135g	139.0	4.0	103	2.7	16.4	2.9	0.1
Toffee Muffin, COU, M & S*	1 Serving/100g	180.0	2.0	180	3.7	35.8	2.2	0.3
Toffee, with Biscuit Pieces, Iced, Weight Watchers*	1 Pot/57g	93.0	3.0	163	2.7	26.2	4.8	0.2
Triple Chocolate Layered, BGTY, Sainsbury's*	1 Pot/105g	147.0	3.0	140	4.2	24.4	2.8	0.5
Triple Chocolate Truffle, Entenmann's*	1 Serving/100g	304.0	19.0	304	4.5	28.4	19.1	2.2
Triple Chocolate, Delice, Sainsbury's*	1 Serving/105g	399.0	27.0	380	3.8	32.4	26.1	0.7
Vanilla & Raspberry Swirl, Weight Watchers*	1 Serving/100ml	81.0	2.0	81	1.5	13.3	2.2	0.2
Vanilla & Strawberry Compote, Weight Watchers*	1 Pot/57g	81.0	2.0	142	2.5	23.4	3.9	0.2
Vanilla & Toffee, Heavenly Swirls, Tesco*	1 Pot/73g	106.0	2.0	145	2.5	28.1	2.5	0.5

D

	Measure INFO/WEIGHT	per Measure KCAL	FAT	Nutrition Values per 100g / 100ml KCAL	PROT	CARB	FAT	FIBRE
DESSERT								
Vanilla Creamed Rice, Weight Watchers*	1 Pot/100g	108.0	1.0	108	4.2	20.8	0.9	0.4
Vanilla Flavour, Soya, Dairy Free, Organic, Provamel*	1 Pot/125g	114.0	2.0	91	3.0	15.5	1.8	0.6
Vanilla Supreme, Sainsbury's*	1 Pot/95g	116.0	4.0	122	3.0	18.0	4.0	0.0
Vanilla with Strawberries Swirl, Weight Watchers*	1 Pot/57g	46.0	1.0	81	1.5	13.3	2.2	0.2
Vanilla, Exquisa*	1 Serving/100g	103.0	0.0	103	5.2	20.0	0.2	0.0
Vanilla, Luxury, Charolait*	1 Serving/200g	248.0	10.0	124	3.0	16.6	5.1	0.0
White Chocolate & Raspberry, Tesco*	1 Dessert/88g	180.0	9.0	204	3.4	25.0	10.1	3.1
White Chocolate, Delights, Shape, Danone*	1 pot/110g	109.0	3.0	99	3.5	15.9	2.4	0.1
DHAL								
Black Gram, Average	1oz/28g	21.0	1.0	74	4.2	7.0	3.4	1.7
Blackeye Bean, Patak's*	1oz/28g	29.0	1.0	102	3.6	12.4	4.6	1.8
Chick Pea	1oz/28g	42.0	2.0	149	7.4	17.7	6.1	3.8
Lentil, Patak's*	1 Can/283g	156.0	3.0	55	2.8	9.3	1.0	1.0
Lentil, Red Masoor & Tomato with Butter, Average	1oz/28g	26.0	1.0	94	4.0	9.7	4.9	0.9
Lentil, Red Masoor & Vegetable, Average	1oz/28g	31.0	1.0	110	5.8	14.7	3.8	1.8
Lentil, Red Masoor with Vegetable Oil, Average	1oz/28g	48.0	2.0	172	7.6	19.2	7.9	1.8
Lentil, Red Masoor, Punjabi, Average	1oz/28g	39.0	1.0	139	7.2	19.2	4.6	2.0
Lentil, Red Masoorl & Mung Bean, Average	1oz/28g	32.0	2.0	114	4.8	9.9	6.7	1.6
Lentil, Red, Way to Five, Sainsbury's*	½ Pack/273g	254.0	4.0	93	5.5	14.4	1.5	1.4
Lentil, Tesco*	1 Serving/200g	248.0	13.0	124	5.1	10.6	6.6	2.5
Mung Bean, Bengali	1oz/28g	20.0	1.0	73	4.2	7.4	3.3	1.7
Mung Beans, Dried, Boiled in Unsalted Water	1oz/28g	26.0	0.0	92	7.8	15.3	0.4	0.0
Mung Beans, Dried, Raw	1oz/28g	81.0	0.0	291	26.8	46.3	1.1	0.0
Regular, Eastern Essence*	1 Serving/113g	105.0	4.0	93	7.1	19.5	3.5	2.6
Split Peas, Yellow, Chana, Asda*	1 Serving/275g	300.0	19.0	109	2.6	9.0	7.0	1.8
Tarka, Asda*	½ Pack/150g	216.0	12.0	144	6.0	12.0	8.0	6.0
Vegetable Spicy, & Lentil, Solo Slim, Rosemary Conley*	1 Serving/100g	79.0	2.0	79	4.2	11.3	2.0	3.5
DHANSAK								
Chicken with Bagara Rice, Waitrose*	1 Pack/450g	549.0	8.0	122	8.2	18.2	1.8	1.2
Chicken, Ready Meals, M & S*	1oz/28g	50.0	3.0	180	12.4	6.6	11.5	1.6
Vegetable, Sainsbury's*	1 Serving/200g	148.0	6.0	74	3.1	8.9	2.8	2.8
DILL								
Dried	*1 Tsp/1g*	*3.0*	*0.0*	*253*	*19.9*	*42.2*	*4.4*	*13.6*
Fresh, Average	*1 Tbsp/3g*	*1.0*	*0.0*	*25*	*3.7*	*0.9*	*0.8*	*2.5*
DIM SUM								
From Restaurant, Average	1 Piece/12g	50.0	2.0	433	28.9	31.3	20.4	0.0
Steamed, Prawn, M & S*	6 Pieces/120g	222.0	3.0	185	1.1	39.0	2.7	1.5
DIME								
Terry's*	1oz/28g	154.0	9.0	550	4.6	68.5	33.8	0.6
DIP								
Applewood Cheddar & Onion, Fresh, BGTY, Sainsbury's*	½ Pot/85g	85.0	4.0	100	7.3	7.3	4.6	0.5
Aubergine, Fresh, Waitrose*	1 Serving/85g	159.0	13.0	187	2.5	10.5	15.0	1.7
Bean & Cheese, Asda*	1 Serving/50g	78.0	4.0	157	7.0	12.0	9.0	1.7
Blue Cheese, Fresh, Sainsbury's*	1/5 Pot/34g	115.0	12.0	337	3.6	3.1	34.5	0.1
Buffalo Mozzarella, Tomato & Basil, Kettle Chips*	1 Serving/25g	119.0	6.0	476	6.7	54.4	25.7	4.9
Cajun Red Pepper, Sainsbury's*	1 Serving/50g	25.0	1.0	50	1.4	7.0	1.8	1.4
Cheddar & Spring Onion, M & S*	1 Pack/125g	581.0	60.0	465	3.6	4.7	48.3	0.5
Cheese & Chive, 50% Less Fat, Asda*	1 Pot/125g	261.0	21.0	209	4.5	9.0	17.2	0.0
Cheese & Chive, 50% Less Fat, Morrisons*	1 Serving/50g	86.0	6.0	172	8.8	5.2	12.7	0.2
Cheese & Chive, Asda*	1 Serving/43g	190.0	20.0	447	4.9	3.4	46.0	0.0
Cheese & Chive, Fresh, Safeway*	1 Pot/170g	877.0	92.0	516	4.1	3.0	54.2	0.0
Cheese & Chive, Tesco*	¼ Pack/50g	267.0	28.0	535	4.3	4.3	55.1	0.1
Chilli Cheese, Asda*	1 Serving/50g	131.0	11.0	262	8.0	8.0	22.0	1.1

DIP

	INFO/WEIGHT	KCAL	FAT	KCAL	PROT	CARB	FAT	FIBRE
Chilli Cheese, Max, Walkers*	1 Jar/300g	390.0	27.0	130	3.3	9.4	9.1	0.3
Chilli, M & S*	1 Pot/35g	103.0	0.0	295	0.4	73.2	0.2	0.4
Cranberry, Asda*	½ Pot/40g	53.0	1.0	132	0.4	29.0	1.6	0.8
Cucumber & Mint, Fresh, Sainsbury's*	1oz/28g	34.0	3.0	123	4.5	3.7	10.0	0.0
Garlic & Herb, Big Dipper, Morrisons*	¼ Pot/75g	277.0	28.0	370	1.3	6.9	37.5	0.4
Garlic & Herb, Reduced Fat, M & S*	1 Serving/10g	9.0	0.0	95	6.0	8.1	4.0	0.5
Garlic & Herb, Tesco*	¼ Pack/43g	257.0	28.0	604	0.9	3.2	65.4	0.3
Garlic Herb & Rocket, M & S*	1 Serving/25g	104.0	11.0	415	2.4	4.5	43.0	0.5
Hot Salsa, Doritos, Walkers*	1 Jar/300g	87.0	1.0	29	0.9	5.8	0.2	1.6
Mature Cheddar Cheese & Chive, Fresh, Waitrose*	½ Pot/85g	393.0	41.0	462	5.8	2.4	47.7	1.7
Mexican Bean, Doritos, Walkers*	1 Tbsp/20g	18.0	1.0	89	2.7	12.1	3.3	2.4
Mild Salsa, Doritos, Walkers*	1 Tbsp/30g	9.0	0.0	30	0.8	6.0	0.3	1.5
Nacho Cheese, From Tex-Mex Multipack Selection, Tesco*	1 Tub/125g	619.0	62.0	495	5.9	5.8	49.6	0.0
Nacho Cheese, M & S*	1oz/28g	76.0	7.0	270	9.8	3.8	23.7	0.4
Nacho Cheese, Sainsbury's*	1 Serving/50g	243.0	25.0	487	4.8	3.9	50.2	0.0
Onion & Garlic, Classic, Tesco*	1 Serving/30g	133.0	14.0	442	1.7	4.6	46.3	0.2
Onion & Garlic, Fresh, BGTY, Sainsbury's*	1oz/28g	56.0	5.0	201	4.4	4.8	18.2	0.8
Onion & Garlic, GFY, Asda*	1/5 Pot/34g	56.0	5.0	166	2.1	8.0	14.0	0.2
Onion & Garlic, Half Fat, Safeway*	½ Pot/85g	170.0	15.0	200	3.2	7.4	17.2	0.1
Onion & Garlic, Safeway*	¼ Pack/45g	216.0	23.0	480	1.7	4.7	50.4	0.1
Pea, Yogurt & Mint, Sainsbury's*	¼ Pack/50g	119.0	11.0	238	3.4	7.5	21.6	2.1
Peanut, Satay Selection, Occasions, Sainsbury's*	1 Serving/2g	4.0	0.0	186	7.1	13.8	11.4	1.1
Pecorino, Basil & Pine Nut, Fresh, Waitrose*	½ Pot/85g	338.0	34.0	398	5.1	5.1	39.7	0.0
Raita, Indian, Asda*	1 Pot/70g	120.0	11.0	172	2.6	3.6	16.4	0.5
Red Pepper, Sainsbury's*	1 Pot/100g	103.0	4.0	103	2.3	14.6	4.0	0.0
Roast Onion, Garlic & Rocket, Reduced Fat, Waitrose*	1 Serving/25g	50.0	5.0	202	2.7	5.4	18.8	1.5
Salsa, Chunky Tomato, Tesco*	1 Pot/170g	68.0	2.0	40	1.1	5.9	1.3	1.1
Salsa, Chunky, Fresh, Sainsbury's*	1 Serving/100g	51.0	2.0	51	1.1	7.8	1.7	1.2
Salsa, GFY, Asda*	1 Pot/170g	68.0	1.0	40	1.2	8.0	0.4	1.5
Salsa, Less Than 5% Fat, Safeway*	½ Pot/85g	47.0	2.0	55	1.5	6.1	2.4	0.9
Smoked Salmon & Dill, Fresh, Waitrose*	½ Pot/85g	373.0	38.0	439	5.1	4.1	44.7	0.1
Smoked Salmon & Dill, Reduced Fat, Waitrose*	½ Pot/85g	184.0	17.0	217	3.9	6.1	19.7	1.1
Sour Cream & Chive, Doritos, Walkers*	1 Tbsp/20g	52.0	5.0	258	1.9	6.9	24.7	1.9
Sour Cream & Chive, Fresh, Tesco*	½ Pot/75g	305.0	32.0	407	2.1	4.1	42.4	0.0
Sour Cream & Chive, Half Fat, Waitrose*	½ Pot/85g	133.0	10.0	157	5.5	7.6	11.6	0.1
Sour Cream & Chive, Primula*	1oz/28g	97.0	10.0	346	5.0	1.8	35.3	0.0
Sour Cream & Chive, Sainsbury's*	1 Serving/50g	141.0	14.0	282	3.1	5.4	27.5	0.1
Sour Cream & Chives, Mexican Style, Morrisons*	¼ Pack/25g	68.0	7.0	274	2.2	3.4	27.9	0.4
Sour Cream, Tesco*	1 Serving/38g	111.0	11.0	297	3.4	3.9	29.8	0.2
Soured Cream & Chive, 95% Fat Free, M & S*	1oz/28g	25.0	1.0	90	6.5	9.6	2.8	0.5
Soured Cream & Chive, BGTY, Sainsbury's*	1 Serving/170g	253.0	18.0	149	4.2	9.9	10.3	0.1
Soured Cream & Chive, Classic, Tesco*	1 Serving/25g	81.0	8.0	323	1.7	3.2	33.7	0.2
Soured Cream & Chive, for Skins, Tesco*	1 Serving/12g	36.0	4.0	297	3.4	3.9	29.8	0.2
Soured Cream & Chive, HL, Tesco*	1 Serving/31g	45.0	3.0	145	3.8	7.5	10.6	0.2
Soured Cream & Chive, Light Choices, Tesco*	¼ Pot/50g	65.0	4.0	130	4.3	7.4	9.0	0.1
Soured Cream & Chive, Morrisons*	1 Serving/100g	317.0	33.0	317	2.6	3.3	32.6	0.0
Spiced Mango, Ginger & Chilli Salsa, Weight Watchers*	1 Serving/56g	48.0	0.0	85	1.0	19.9	0.2	2.6
Spicy Moroccan, BGTY, Sainsbury's*	½ Pot/85g	56.0	2.0	66	2.1	10.0	2.0	1.7
Sweet & Sour, M & S*	1oz/28g	36.0	0.0	130	0.7	31.4	0.1	0.5
Sweet Chilli Mango, Encona*	1 Tbsp/15ml	22.0	0.0	148	0.4	35.4	0.6	0.0
Sweet Chilli, Chinese Snack Selection, Morrisons*	½ Pot/20g	64.0	0.0	320	0.1	79.4	0.2	0.6
Sweet Chilli, Oriental Selection, Waitrose*	½ Pot/35g	88.0	0.0	250	1.3	59.4	0.8	0.4
Sweet Pepper & Ricotta, Asda*	1 Serving/20g	74.0	7.0	370	1.0	12.0	35.0	0.0

D

	Measure INFO/WEIGHT	per Measure KCAL	per Measure FAT	Nutrition Values per 100g / 100ml KCAL	PROT	CARB	FAT	FIBRE
DIP								
Tangy Barbecue, M & S*	1oz/28g	28.0	0.0	100	1.1	22.2	0.6	0.6
Thousand Island, HL, Tesco*	1 Serving/31g	57.0	5.0	183	2.5	9.6	14.9	0.3
Thousand Island, M & S*	1oz/28g	69.0	6.0	245	2.1	9.4	22.2	0.7
Tomato Ketchup, Asda*	1 Pack/25g	18.0	0.0	71	1.6	16.0	0.1	1.0
Tortilla Chips, Cool Flavour, Big, Morrisons*	½ Pack/100g	453.0	22.0	453	6.4	57.4	22.0	8.1
Yoghurt & Cucumber Mint, Tesco*	1oz/28g	34.0	2.0	121	7.0	7.2	7.1	0.6
DISCOS								
Beef, KP Snacks*	1 Pack/28g	145.0	8.0	518	5.1	58.7	29.3	2.4
Cheese & Onion, KP Snacks*	1 Pack/28g	146.0	8.0	520	5.1	59.1	29.3	2.5
Salt & Vinegar, KP Snacks*	1 Bag/28g	145.0	8.0	517	4.7	58.3	29.5	2.3
DOLLY MIXTURES								
M & S*	1 Pack/115g	431.0	2.0	375	1.8	89.2	1.4	0.0
Sainsbury's*	1 Serving/10g	40.0	0.0	401	1.4	94.4	1.9	0.1
Smart Price, Asda*	1 Sweet/3g	11.0	0.0	380	0.5	91.0	1.6	0.0
Tesco*	1 Pack/100g	376.0	1.0	376	1.6	88.9	1.5	0.0
DOPIAZA								
Chicken, M & S*	1 Pack/350g	402.0	21.0	115	11.5	3.7	6.1	2.5
Chicken, Safeway*	1 Pack/326g	450.0	27.0	138	10.4	5.3	8.4	1.4
Chicken, Sainsbury's*	½ Pack/200g	272.0	16.0	136	13.2	3.1	7.9	0.8
Chicken, Tesco*	1 Pack/350g	448.0	25.0	128	10.8	5.3	7.1	0.6
Chicken, with Pilau Rice, Sharwood's*	1 Pack/375g	472.0	17.0	126	5.3	15.8	4.6	0.8
Chicken, with Pilau Rice, Tesco*	1 Pack/400g	424.0	15.0	106	5.7	12.3	3.8	1.5
Mushroom, Retail	1oz/28g	19.0	2.0	69	1.3	3.7	5.7	1.1
Mushroom, Tesco*	1 Pack/225g	155.0	10.0	69	2.4	5.1	4.4	1.5
Mushroom, Waitrose*	½ Pack/150g	81.0	5.0	54	2.2	4.3	3.1	2.3
DORITOS								
Chargrilled BBQ, Walkers*	1 Bag/35g	170.0	9.0	485	5.5	59.0	25.0	3.5
Cheesy 3d's, Doritos, Walkers*	1 Pack/20g	89.0	3.0	445	7.0	68.0	16.0	3.0
Chilli Heatwave, Walkers*	1 Bag/35g	175.0	9.0	500	7.0	60.0	26.0	3.0
Cool Original, Walkers*	1 Bag/40g	200.0	11.0	500	7.5	58.0	27.0	3.0
Cool Spice 3ds, Walkers*	1 Bag/24g	108.0	4.0	450	8.0	64.0	18.0	4.4
Cool, Ranch Chips, Walkers*	1 Pack/50g	250.0	13.0	504	8.1	64.5	26.2	4.0
Dippas, Hint of Chilli, Dipping Chips, Walkers*	1 Bag/35g	173.0	9.0	495	7.0	61.0	25.0	3.5
Dippas, Hint of Garlic, Dipping Chips, Walkers*	1 Serving/35g	175.0	9.0	500	7.0	61.0	25.0	3.5
Dippas, Hint of Lime, Walkers*	1 Bag/35g	173.0	9.0	495	7.0	60.0	25.0	3.5
Dippas, Lightly Salted, Dipping Chips, Walkers*	1 Serving/35g	178.0	9.0	510	6.5	60.0	27.0	3.0
Latinos, Chargrilled BBQ, Walkers*	1 Serving/35g	170.0	9.0	485	5.5	59.0	25.0	3.5
Latinos, Mexican Grill, Walkers*	1 Serving/35g	170.0	9.0	485	5.5	59.0	25.0	3.5
Latinos, Sour Cream & Sweet Pepper, Walkers*	1 Pack/40g	194.0	10.0	485	5.5	60.0	25.0	3.5
Lightly Salted Dippas, Doritos, Walkers*	1 Serving/40g	204.0	11.0	510	6.5	60.0	27.0	3.0
Mexican Hot, Walkers*	1 Bag/40g	202.0	11.0	505	8.0	57.0	27.0	3.5
Tangy Cheese, Walkers*	1 Bag/40g	200.0	11.0	500	7.0	57.0	27.0	3.0
DOUBLE DECKER								
Cadbury*	1 Bar/60g	276.0	11.0	460	4.4	68.4	18.9	0.6
Snack Size, Cadbury*	1 Bar/36g	165.0	7.0	465	4.8	64.5	20.9	0.0
with Nuts, Cadbury*	1 Bar/60g	291.0	15.0	485	7.9	58.6	24.5	0.0
DOUGH BALLS								
Garlic & Herb, Asda*	4 Balls/48g	173.0	9.0	361	9.2	40.9	17.8	3.6
Garlic, HL, Tesco*	1 Serving/40g	110.0	3.0	274	8.8	42.0	7.9	2.3
Garlic, Tesco*	1 Serving/10g	40.0	2.0	400	7.0	40.0	23.0	1.0
Garlic, Waitrose*	1 Ball/11g	38.0	2.0	347	8.5	41.4	16.4	3.3
Sainsbury's*	1 Ball/12g	41.0	2.0	343	8.4	38.7	17.2	2.2
Supermarket, Pizza Express*	8 Balls/100g	363.0	2.0	363	14.3	72.9	1.7	3.3

	Measure INFO/WEIGHT	per Measure KCAL	FAT	Nutrition Values per 100g / 100ml KCAL	PROT	CARB	FAT	FIBRE
DOUGH BALLS								
with Garlic & Herb Butter, Aldi*	1 Ball/12g	45.0	2.0	365	7.7	46.7	18.2	1.8
DOUGHNUTS								
Apple & Fresh Cream, Sainsbury's*	1 Doughnut/79g	216.0	11.0	273	5.4	30.5	14.4	1.9
Baked, HL, Tesco*	1 Doughnut/67g	166.0	4.0	248	6.4	42.2	5.9	1.4
Chocolate, Somerfield*	1 Doughnut/57g	203.0	9.0	356	7.8	43.8	16.6	1.7
Cream & Jam, Assorted Box, Sainsbury's*	1 Doughnut/71g	229.0	13.0	322	6.2	34.2	17.9	2.2
Cream & Jam, Tesco*	1 Doughnut/90g	288.0	14.0	320	5.4	39.4	15.7	2.0
Custard & Bramley Apple, Sainsbury's*	1 Doughnut/91g	256.0	13.0	282	4.5	34.6	13.9	1.0
Custard Filled, Average	1 Doughnut/75g	268.0	14.0	358	6.2	43.3	19.0	0.0
Custard, Sainsbury's*	1 Doughnut/70g	172.0	7.0	246	5.1	32.3	10.7	2.3
Custard, Tesco*	1 Doughnut/91g	266.0	14.0	292	4.1	33.4	15.8	1.1
Dairy Cream & Jam, Somerfield*	1 Doughnut/80g	296.0	18.0	370	4.6	35.8	23.1	1.3
Dairy Cream Finger, Safeway*	1 Doughnut/98g	342.0	20.0	349	5.5	36.4	20.1	1.8
Finger, Co-Op*	1 Doughnut/82g	299.0	15.0	365	4.0	45.0	18.0	2.0
Jam Filled, Average	1 Doughnut/75g	252.0	11.0	336	5.7	48.8	14.5	0.0
Jam, American Style, Budgens*	1 Doughnut/46g	126.0	3.0	275	7.1	46.5	6.7	0.0
Jam, American Style, Sainsbury's*	1 Doughnut/65g	220.0	21.0	339	4.9	49.6	31.8	3.5
Jam, Fresh Cream, Sweet Fresh, Tesco*	1 Doughnut/74g	248.0	12.0	335	5.5	40.7	16.4	1.9
Jam, M & S*	1 Doughnut/49g	141.0	2.0	287	5.0	57.6	4.0	1.3
Jam, Mini, Somerfield*	1 Doughnut/45g	138.0	4.0	307	6.4	50.1	9.0	1.4
Mini, Sainsbury's*	1 Doughnut/14g	53.0	3.0	379	5.2	47.9	18.9	2.1
Original, Glazed, Krispy Kreme*	1 Doughnut/52g	217.0	13.0	417	6.0	43.0	25.0	4.0
Plain, Ring, Average	1 Doughnut/60g	238.0	13.0	397	6.1	47.2	21.7	0.0
Ring, Iced, Average	1 Doughnut/70g	268.0	12.0	383	4.8	55.1	17.5	0.0
Ring, Waitrose*	1 Cake/107g	396.0	21.0	370	4.2	43.5	19.9	0.7
Strawberry Jam & Cream, Sainsbury's*	1 Doughnut/80g	299.0	19.0	374	5.3	36.2	23.2	1.3
Toffee, Tesco*	1 Doughnut/75g	235.0	9.0	313	8.0	44.2	11.6	1.6
Yum Yums, Glazed, Sweet, Waitrose*	1 Doughnut/45g	172.0	10.0	382	4.0	41.6	22.2	2.0
Yum Yums, M & S*	1 Doughnut/37g	155.0	9.0	420	4.9	45.7	23.9	1.6
Yum Yums, Tesco*	1 Doughnut/61g	232.0	10.0	380	6.1	51.6	16.6	1.7
DOVER SOLE								
Raw, Average	*1oz/28g*	*25.0*	*1.0*	*89*	*18.1*	*0.0*	*1.8*	*0.0*
DR PEPPER*								
Coca-Cola*	1 Bottle/500ml	210.0	0.0	42	0.0	10.9	0.0	0.0
Z, Coca-Cola*	1 Serving/250ml	10.0	0.0	4	0.0	0.0	0.0	0.0
Zero, Coca-Cola*	1 Can/330ml	2.0	0.0	0	0.0	0.0	0.0	0.0
DRAGON FRUIT								
Raw, Edible Portion, Average	1 Serving/100g	41.0	1.0	41	0.7	9.6	0.5	3.6
DRAMBUIE								
39% Volume	*1 Shot/35ml*	*95.0*	*0.0*	*272*	*0.0*	*23.0*	*0.0*	*0.0*
DREAM								
Double Fudge, Cadbury*	1oz/28g	139.0	7.0	495	6.3	61.4	25.2	0.0
Snowbites, Cadbury*	1 Serving/31g	170.0	10.0	545	3.1	59.7	32.7	0.0
White Chocolate, Cadbury*	1 Piece/8g	44.0	3.0	555	4.5	59.7	33.3	0.0
DREAM TOPPING								
Dry, Bird's*	1oz/28g	193.0	16.0	690	6.7	32.5	58.5	0.5
Made Up, Skimmed Milk, Bird's*	1oz/28g	21.0	1.0	75	2.0	4.8	5.3	0.0
Sugar Free, Dry, Bird's*	1oz/28g	195.0	17.0	695	7.3	30.5	60.5	0.5
DRESSING								
Balsamic Bliss, Ainsley Harriott*	1 Tbsp/15g	41.0	3.0	272	0.8	19.3	21.1	0.0
Balsamic Vinegar, Asda*	1 Pack/44ml	121.0	12.0	275	0.9	7.0	27.0	0.0
Balsamic Vinegar, Olives & Herb, COU, M & S*	1 Serving/30g	22.0	1.0	75	0.5	14.3	2.0	0.5
Balsamic, Light Choices, Tesco*	1 Tbsp/14g	12.0	0.0	85	0.3	16.7	1.5	0.2

	Measure INFO/WEIGHT	per Measure KCAL	FAT	Nutrition Values per 100g / 100ml KCAL	PROT	CARB	FAT	FIBRE

DRESSING

	Measure INFO/WEIGHT	KCAL	FAT	KCAL	PROT	CARB	FAT	FIBRE
Balsamic, M & S*	1 Tbsp/15g	73.0	7.0	490	0.3	9.7	48.0	0.5
Balsamic, Sainsbury's*	1 Tbsp/15ml	47.0	4.0	316	0.4	13.8	28.8	0.4
Balsamic, Schwartz*	1 Tbsp/15ml	12.0	0.0	77	0.5	14.2	2.0	0.0
Balsamic, Sweet, Finest, Tesco*	1 Serving/10ml	15.0	0.0	155	0.4	36.9	0.1	0.4
Balsamic, Weight Watchers*	1 Serving/15ml	12.0	0.0	81	0.1	16.0	1.8	0.5
Basil & Pesto, COU, M & S*	1 Serving/50ml	30.0	1.0	60	0.6	8.3	2.2	0.8
Blue Cheese, 60% Less Fat, BGTY, Sainsbury's*	1 Tbsp/15ml	26.0	2.0	172	1.9	7.3	15.1	0.2
Blue Cheese, Fresh, Sainsbury's*	1 Dtsp/10ml	42.0	5.0	423	2.3	0.5	45.7	0.1
Blue Cheese, Hellmann's*	1 Tbsp/15g	69.0	7.0	459	0.7	6.3	47.2	1.1
Blue Cheese, Sainsbury's*	1 Serving/20g	64.0	6.0	321	2.3	10.6	29.9	0.4
Blue Cheese, Salad, Waitrose*	1 Serving/50g	265.0	25.0	530	2.1	17.3	50.3	4.1
Blue Cheese, Tesco*	1 Serving/15ml	75.0	8.0	500	2.5	6.9	51.4	0.2
Caesar Style, GFY, Asda*	1 Sachet/44ml	34.0	1.0	77	5.0	9.0	2.3	0.0
Caesar, 95% Fat Free, Tesco*	1 Tsp/6g	5.0	0.0	88	4.1	8.9	3.7	0.3
Caesar, Asiago, Briannas*	1 Tbsp/15ml	70.0	7.0	467	3.3	3.3	50.0	0.0
Caesar, Chilled, Reduced Fat, Tesco*	1 Tsp/5ml	13.0	1.0	252	6.5	3.1	23.7	0.1
Caesar, Classic, Sainsbury's*	1 Tsp/5ml	22.0	2.0	442	2.7	4.6	45.9	0.5
Caesar, Finest, Tesco*	1 Tbsp/15ml	72.0	8.0	477	1.9	2.8	50.9	0.2
Caesar, Fresh, Asda*	1 Dtsp/10ml	45.0	5.0	454	2.4	3.2	48.0	0.0
Caesar, Fresh, M & S*	1 Tsp/6g	31.0	3.0	525	2.0	1.8	56.4	0.2
Caesar, Fresh, Sainsbury's*	1 Tbsp/15ml	72.0	7.0	477	3.7	3.7	49.7	1.9
Caesar, Hellmann's*	1 Tsp/6g	30.0	3.0	499	2.5	4.5	51.7	0.3
Caesar, Less Than 3% Fat, BGTY, Sainsbury's*	1 Serving/20g	10.0	0.0	48	0.8	7.0	1.9	0.3
Caesar, Light Choices, Tesco*	1 Serving/15g	9.0	0.0	60	1.5	9.5	1.5	0.5
Caesar, Light, Kraft*	1 Serving/15g	14.0	1.0	95	1.7	13.0	3.6	0.2
Caesar, Loyd Grossman*	1 Dtsp/10g	34.0	3.0	342	2.1	7.0	33.9	0.0
Caesar, Luxury, Hellmann's*	1 Tsp/4g	20.0	2.0	498	2.5	4.4	51.7	0.3
Caesar, Original, Cardini's*	1 Serving/10g	55.0	6.0	555	2.3	1.5	60.0	0.2
Caesar, Waitrose*	1 Serving/15ml	72.0	8.0	479	4.5	0.9	50.8	0.2
Citrus Salad, BGTY, Sainsbury's*	1 Tbsp/15ml	13.0	0.0	90	0.3	14.4	3.1	0.3
Classic French, Fresh, M & S*	1 Serving/10ml	51.0	5.0	515	0.6	8.2	53.1	0.2
Classic Italian, Get Dressed, Kraft*	1 Serving/25ml	30.0	3.0	120	0.1	5.6	10.3	0.5
Creme Fraiche, Salad, Kraft*	1 Tbsp/15ml	12.0	0.0	78	0.8	12.5	2.5	0.0
Dijon Honey Mustard, Briannas*	1 Tbsp/15ml	65.0	6.0	433	0.0	20.0	40.0	0.0
Fire Roasted Garlic & Thyme, Tesco*	1 Serving/10ml	45.0	5.0	447	0.9	4.7	47.2	0.0
Fire Roasted Red Pepper, M & S*	1 Serving/30g	13.0	0.0	45	0.5	10.7	0.1	0.9
Fire Roasted Tomato Basil, COU, M & S*	1 Serving/30g	13.0	0.0	45	0.6	8.1	0.9	1.1
French Herb, Mary Berry*	1 Serving/100g	504.0	49.0	504	0.8	14.2	49.3	0.3
French Salad, M & S*	1 Serving/25ml	156.0	17.0	625	0.5	3.8	67.3	0.1
French Style Calorie-Wise Salad, Kraft*	1 Tbsp/15ml	24.0	2.0	160	0.0	18.7	10.7	0.0
French Style, Eat Smart, Safeway*	1 Serving/15ml	22.0	0.0	145	0.7	28.9	2.5	0.7
French, BGTY, Organic, Sainsbury's*	1 Tbsp/15ml	11.0	1.0	71	0.2	8.3	4.1	0.5
French, BGTY, Sainsbury's*	1 Tbsp/15ml	12.0	1.0	79	1.1	8.8	4.4	0.5
French, Chilled, Tesco*	1 Tbsp/15ml	63.0	6.0	421	1.1	15.1	39.6	0.0
French, Cider Vinegar & Mustard, Tesco*	1 Tbsp/15ml	45.0	4.0	300	0.7	9.9	28.1	0.3
French, Classic, Fat Free, Kraft*	1 Tsp/5ml	2.0	0.0	39	0.1	8.7	0.0	0.5
French, Classic, Sainsbury's*	1 Tbsp/15ml	71.0	7.0	473	1.0	5.7	49.6	0.5
French, Classics, M & S*	1 Tbsp/15ml	77.0	8.0	516	0.6	8.2	53.1	0.2
French, COU, M & S*	1/3 Bottle/105g	73.0	3.0	70	0.7	11.5	2.6	0.7
French, Finest, Tesco*	1 Tbsp/15g	55.0	6.0	370	0.4	5.1	38.7	1.0
French, Fresh, Florette*	1 Bottle/175ml	763.0	73.0	436	0.8	14.1	41.8	0.0
French, Fresh, Morrisons*	1 Tbsp/15ml	75.0	7.0	499	1.5	13.6	48.7	0.0
French, Fresh, Organic, Sainsbury's*	1 Tbsp/15ml	45.0	5.0	301	0.4	5.5	31.0	0.4

DRESSING

INFO/WEIGHT	Measure KCAL	per Measure FAT	Nutrition Values per 100g / 100ml KCAL	PROT	CARB	FAT	FIBRE
French, Fresh, Sainsbury's*	1 Tbsp/15ml	64.0	7.0	429	0.6	6.6	44.6	0.6
French, GFY, Asda*	1 Tbsp/15g	7.0	0.0	50	0.7	7.0	2.1	0.1
French, Less Than 3% Fat, M & S*	1 Tbsp/15ml	10.0	0.0	68	0.7	11.5	2.6	0.7
French, Light Choices, Tesco*	1 Serving/20g	10.0	0.0	48	0.8	7.6	1.6	1.1
French, Light, Heinz*	1 Sachet/12g	13.0	1.0	111	0.7	15.4	5.4	0.0
French, Luxury, Hellmann's*	1 Tbsp/15g	45.0	4.0	297	0.4	14.9	25.9	0.3
French, Oil Free, French, Waitrose*	1 Tsp/5ml	4.0	0.0	76	1.5	13.1	2.0	0.6
French, Oil Free, Perfectly Balanced, Waitrose*	1 Serving/15ml	11.0	0.0	72	2.2	12.2	1.6	1.1
French, Organic, M & S*	1 Tbsp/15g	98.0	10.0	655	0.2	7.5	69.4	0.3
French, Organic, Tesco*	1 Tsp/5ml	23.0	2.0	451	0.6	11.0	44.9	0.2
French, Reduced Fat, M & S*	1 Tbsp/15g	10.0	0.0	70	0.7	11.5	2.8	0.7
French, Sainsbury's*	1 Tbsp/15ml	33.0	3.0	219	0.6	9.8	19.1	0.5
French, Tesco*	1 Serving/25ml	110.0	11.0	441	0.7	7.2	44.9	0.2
Garlic & Herb, Perfectly Balanced, Waitrose*	1 Serving/50ml	67.0	1.0	135	0.6	29.9	1.4	0.8
Garlic & Herb, Reduced Calorie, Hellmann's*	1 Tbsp/15ml	35.0	3.0	232	0.6	12.8	19.3	0.4
Garlic & Herb, Tesco*	1 Tbsp/15g	31.0	3.0	210	0.9	5.8	20.2	0.8
Green Thai, Finest, Tesco*	1 Bottle/250ml	940.0	82.0	376	0.3	19.1	32.7	0.3
Healthy Choice, Safeway*	1 Tbsp/15ml	4.0	0.0	29	0.2	6.3	0.3	0.0
Herb & Garlic, Light, 5% Fat, Get Dressed, Kraft*	1 Serving/25ml	29.0	1.0	116	1.3	15.5	5.1	0.2
Herb, Eat Smart, Safeway*	1 Tbsp/15ml	9.0	0.0	60	0.5	9.5	2.0	0.5
Honey & Mustard, BGTY, Sainsbury's*	1 Tbsp/20g	14.0	0.0	71	0.4	16.1	0.5	0.2
Honey & Mustard, Finest, Tesco*	1 Serving/25ml	72.0	6.0	288	1.7	19.6	22.5	0.7
Honey & Mustard, Fresh, M & S*	1 Serving/10ml	43.0	4.0	430	1.7	9.7	42.4	0.5
Honey & Mustard, GFY, Asda*	1 Tbsp/15g	13.0	1.0	89	1.5	13.0	3.4	0.8
Honey & Mustard, Light Choices, Tesco*	1 Tbsp/13.8g	9.0	0.0	65	1.3	11.6	1.1	0.6
Honey & Mustard, M & S*	1 Tbsp/15ml	64.0	6.0	427	1.7	9.7	42.4	0.6
Honey & Mustard, Sainsbury's*	1 Serving/10ml	37.0	3.0	366	1.0	15.4	33.0	0.1
Honey & Mustard, Tesco*	1 Serving/10ml	38.0	4.0	378	0.8	13.1	35.8	0.6
Honey & Mustard, The English Provender Co.*	1 Tbsp/15ml	17.0	0.0	111	2.5	21.8	1.5	1.0
Honey, Orange & Mustard, BGTY, Sainsbury's*	1 Tbsp/15ml	16.0	0.0	105	1.8	18.6	2.5	1.8
Hot Lime & Coconut, BGTY, Sainsbury's*	1 Tbsp/15ml	8.0	0.0	51	0.7	5.7	2.9	1.2
Italian Salad, Hellmann's*	1 Serving/50g	103.0	8.0	206	0.7	12.8	16.7	0.0
Italian, Low Fat, Heinz*	1 Pot/30ml	26.0	2.0	86	0.9	6.3	6.3	2.7
Italian, M & S*	1 Tbsp/15ml	62.0	6.0	415	0.9	8.9	41.5	1.0
Italian, Reduced Calorie, Hellmann's*	1 Serving/25ml	67.0	5.0	269	0.5	19.5	20.8	0.3
Italian, Waistline, 99% Fat Free, Crosse & Blackwell*	1 Tsp/6g	2.0	0.0	39	0.7	7.0	0.9	0.3
Lemon & Cracked Black Pepper, GFY, Asda*	1 Tbsp/15g	9.0	0.0	57	0.2	14.0	0.0	0.3
Lemon & Watercress, COU, M & S*	1 Serving/28g	14.0	1.0	50	0.4	8.5	1.8	0.5
Lemon, Feta & Oregano, M & S*	1 Tbsp/15ml	24.0	2.0	160	1.3	8.2	13.4	0.6
Lime & Coriander, Oil Free, Waitrose*	1 Tsp/5ml	3.0	0.0	65	1.5	11.9	1.3	0.4
Lime & Coriander, Sainsbury's*	1 Tbsp/15ml	61.0	6.0	409	0.4	10.0	40.8	0.5
Lime & Coriander, The English Provender Co.*	1 Serving/50g	28.0	0.0	57	0.3	13.3	0.3	0.0
Mayonnaise Style, 90% Fat Free, Weight Watchers*	1 Tsp/11g	14.0	1.0	125	1.7	8.9	9.2	0.0
Mild Mustard, Low Fat, Weight Watchers*	1 Tbsp/10g	6.0	0.0	63	2.0	5.7	3.6	0.0
Miracle Whip, Kraft*	1 Tbsp/15ml	60.0	6.0	400	0.3	11.0	39.0	0.1
Mustard & Dill, Perfectly Balanced, Waitrose*	1 Tbsp/15ml	24.0	0.0	159	1.1	31.5	3.2	1.1
Oil & Lemon	1 Tbsp/15g	97.0	11.0	647	0.3	2.8	70.6	0.0
Olive Oil & Balsamic Vinegar, Sainsbury's*	1 Serving/25ml	104.0	10.0	415	0.9	9.4	41.8	0.2
Orange & Cracked Pepper, Tesco*	1 Tbsp/15ml	17.0	0.0	114	0.5	27.8	0.1	0.3
Orange & Honey, Luxury, Hellmann's*	1 Serving/15ml	16.0	1.0	110	0.8	17.5	3.5	0.8
Pesto & Balsamic Vinegar, Extra Special, Asda*	1 Tbsp/15g	33.0	3.0	213	0.3	8.6	19.7	0.0
Pesto, Finest, Tesco*	1 Serving/30ml	108.0	11.0	360	3.5	2.9	37.1	0.9
Ranch Style, Asda*	1 Serving/44ml	37.0	2.0	85	3.5	9.0	3.9	0.0

	Measure INFO/WEIGHT			Nutrition Values per 100g / 100ml				
		KCAL	FAT	KCAL	PROT	CARB	FAT	FIBRE
DRESSING								
Raspberry Balsamic Vinegar, The English Provender Co.*	1 Serving/50g	33.0	0.0	67	0.4	15.7	0.1	0.6
Red Pepper, BGTY, Sainsbury's*	1 Bottle/250g	107.0	1.0	43	0.2	9.8	0.3	0.2
Red Pepper, M & S*	1 Tbsp/15ml	58.0	6.0	385	0.6	7.6	39.2	0.5
Rich Poppy Seed, Briannas*	1 Tbsp/15ml	65.0	6.0	433	0.0	20.0	43.3	0.0
Salad Cream Style, Weight Watchers*	1 Tbsp/10g	11.0	0.0	115	1.5	16.2	4.4	0.0
Salad, Caesar, Light, Fry Light*	1 Spray/0.2ml	1.0	0.0	321	0.4	9.2	30.7	0.1
Salad, Catalina, Kraft*	1 Serving/34g	100.0	6.0	294	0.0	29.4	17.6	0.0
Salad, Honey & Mustard, Light, Kraft*	1 Tbsp/15ml	19.0	1.0	126	1.2	19.0	4.6	1.1
Salad, Italian, Light, Kraft*	1 Tbsp/15ml	5.0	0.0	31	0.1	6.8	0.0	0.6
Salad, Italian, Newman's Own*	1 Tbsp/10g	54.0	6.0	545	0.2	1.0	59.8	0.0
Salad, Kickin' Mango, Oil Free, Ainsley Harriott*	1 Tbsp/15ml	14.0	0.0	92	0.1	21.1	0.1	0.0
Salad, Light, Heinz*	1 Serving/10g	24.0	2.0	244	1.8	13.5	19.9	0.0
Salad, Low Fat, Weight Watchers*	1 Tbsp/10g	10.0	0.0	106	1.5	15.4	4.3	0.0
Salad, Mary Berry*	1 Serving/15g	77.0	7.0	513	0.8	28.5	44.0	0.1
Salad, Raspberry Balsamic, GFY, Asda*	1 Tbsp/15ml	6.0	0.0	40	0.7	9.3	0.7	1.3
Salad, Sun Dried Tomato & Chilli, Loyd Grossman*	1 Tsp/5g	18.0	2.0	361	0.9	5.3	37.3	0.9
Salad, Thousand Island, 95% Fat Free, Asda*	1 Tsp/6g	6.0	0.0	99	1.6	12.6	4.7	0.5
Salad, Vinaigrette Style, 95% Fat Free, Asda*	1 Tbsp/15ml	6.0	0.0	42	0.1	10.6	0.0	0.3
Seafood, M & S*	1 Tsp/7g	39.0	4.0	555	0.9	4.9	59.3	0.9
Smoked Garlic & Parmesan, Sainsbury's*	1 Serving/20ml	83.0	8.0	415	3.0	4.0	41.1	0.3
Special Mustard, & Daughter, Mary Berry*	1 Tbsp/15g	75.0	7.0	499	1.5	23.2	46.4	0.4
Sun Dried Tomato, Safeway*	1 Serving/40ml	126.0	11.0	314	1.1	13.8	28.3	0.0
Sun Dried Tomato, Sainsbury's*	1 Serving/15ml	27.0	2.0	179	1.5	10.9	14.4	0.6
Sweet Balsamic & Smoked Garlic, BGTY, Sainsbury's*	1 Serving/20g	10.0	0.0	51	0.2	11.9	0.3	0.2
Sweet Chilli, COU, M & S*	1 Tbsp/15ml	9.0	0.0	60	0.5	14.5	0.5	0.4
Texas Ranch, Frank Cooper*	1 Pot/28g	128.0	13.0	457	1.9	9.4	45.8	0.2
Thai Lime & Coriander, The English Provender Co.*	1 Serving/25g	26.0	0.0	104	1.6	22.3	0.9	1.1
Thousand Island	1 Tsp/6g	19.0	2.0	323	1.1	12.5	30.2	0.4
Thousand Island, BGTY, Sainsbury's*	1 Serving/50g	47.0	4.0	95	0.4	7.3	7.2	0.5
Thousand Island, COU, M & S*	1 Serving/30g	25.0	1.0	85	1.4	14.2	2.6	1.1
Thousand Island, Frank Cooper*	1 Pot/28g	122.0	13.0	437	1.2	7.2	44.8	0.3
Thousand Island, Light, Kraft*	1 Tbsp/15ml	14.0	0.0	94	0.6	21.5	0.2	3.0
Thousand Island, Reduced Calorie	1 Tsp/6g	12.0	1.0	195	0.7	14.7	15.2	0.0
Thousand Island, Tesco*	1 Tbsp/15g	55.0	5.0	360	1.1	19.5	30.5	0.3
Tomato & Herb, Less Than 1% Fat, Asda*	1 Tbsp/15g	6.0	0.0	43	0.7	8.0	0.9	0.4
Tomato & Olive, Eat Smart, Safeway*	1 Tbsp/15ml	15.0	0.0	100	0.7	22.8	0.7	1.8
Tomato & Red Pepper, BGTY, Sainsbury's*	1 Serving/50ml	41.0	2.0	83	1.1	10.0	4.3	0.6
Tomato Basil, Light, Kraft*	1 Serving/15ml	10.0	0.0	68	1.0	14.5	0.4	2.5
True Blue Cheese, Briannas*	2 Tbsp/30ml	120.0	11.0	400	3.3	16.7	36.7	0.0
Vinaigrette, BGTY, Sainsbury's*	1 Dtsp/20g	13.0	0.0	64	1.1	9.3	2.4	2.5
Yoghurt & Mint, Perfectly Balanced, Waitrose*	1 Serving/100ml	130.0	3.0	130	4.6	22.1	2.6	0.7
Yoghurt Mint Cucumber, M & S*	1 Tsp/5ml	6.0	0.0	115	1.0	8.7	8.0	0.0
DRIED FRUIT MIX								
5 Fruits, Ready to Eat, Sundora*	½ Pack/100g	233.0	0.0	233	1.6	58.4	0.4	6.8
Agadoo, Pineapple, Jumbo & Green Raisins, Graze*	1 Pack/40g	110.0	0.0	275	2.1	69.0	0.9	0.0
Albert Heijn*	1 Serving/50g	110.0	0.0	220	2.1	51.0	0.5	0.0
Apple Strudel, Graze*	1 Pack/40g	123.0	0.0	247	2.2	58.7	0.7	5.9
Apple Strudel, Graze*	1 Pack/55g	172.0	0.0	312	2.6	63.5	0.7	0.0
Average	1 Tbsp/25g	67.0	0.0	268	2.3	68.1	0.4	2.2
Banana, Bites, Kiddylicious, Babylicious*	1 Serving/15g	43.0	3.0	285	10.8	43.6	19.3	6.1
Beach Bum, Graze*	1 Pack/35g	130.0	6.0	372	4.2	54.0	16.2	0.0
Beach Bum, Graze*	1 Pack/40g	168.0	3.0	419	2.2	59.8	8.4	0.0
Berry, Whole Foods, Tesco*	1 Serving/25g	66.0	0.0	265	3.3	60.0	0.7	7.5

	Measure INFO/WEIGHT	per Measure KCAL	FAT	Nutrition Values per 100g / 100ml KCAL	PROT	CARB	FAT	FIBRE
DRIED FRUIT MIX								
Caribbean, Dried, Graze*	1 Box/50g	187.0	6.0	374	1.2	67.6	12.8	0.0
Cherish, Graze*	1 Pack/50g	221.0	10.0	443	5.2	52.5	20.0	0.0
Cherry Oranges, Graze*	1 Pack/119g	56.0	0.0	47	1.1	11.8	0.1	1.0
Detox, Graze*	1 Pack/45g	139.0	0.0	309	1.4	72.4	0.8	0.0
Exotic Mix, Sundora*	1 Sm Pack/50g	138.0	1.0	276	2.3	60.6	2.7	3.8
Exotic, Ready to Eat, Sainsbury's*	1/3 Pack/85g	241.0	0.0	284	0.2	70.6	0.1	2.4
Figgy Pop, Graze*	1 Pack/40g	100.0	0.0	251	2.5	61.6	1.1	0.0
Forest Fruit, Dried, Graze*	1 Pack/50g	159.0	0.0	319	1.8	76.0	0.8	0.0
Fruit Crumble, Graze*	1 Pack/50g	199.0	10.0	399	6.0	48.6	20.2	0.0
Fruit Salad, Whitworths*	1 Serving/62g	113.0	0.0	183	2.9	41.8	0.5	6.6
Go Goji Go Go Go, Graze*	1 Punnet/40g	112.0	0.0	279	2.2	69.0	0.8	0.0
Golden Pineapple Rings, Graze*	1 Punnet/20g	53.0	0.0	263	0.6	72.0	0.6	8.1
Italian Stallion, Graze*	1 Punnet/40g	118.0	0.0	296	1.7	71.0	0.9	2.5
Jewel Of The Nile, Graze*	1 Pack/45g	112.0	0.0	248	2.5	61.3	0.8	0.0
Juicy Orange Raisins, Graze*	1 Pack/40g	110.0	0.0	275	2.1	69.0	0.9	0.0
Juicy Sprinkle, Nature's Harvest*	1 Serving/20g	79.0	2.0	397	4.9	71.9	10.0	4.2
Loco In Acapulco, Graze*	1 Pack /30g	123.0	6.0	410	4.0	53.2	21.4	0.0
Medley, Shapers, Boots*	1 Serving/50g	131.0	0.0	262	3.2	61.0	0.6	5.5
Muffin, Dried, Graze*	1 Box/60g	221.0	7.0	368	1.7	65.8	11.3	1.7
Natural, Positively Healthy, The Food Doctor*	1 Serving/50g	164.0	0.0	328	2.4	77.9	0.7	3.6
Pina Colada, Graze*	1 Punnet/20g	69.0	3.0	343	2.1	58.9	12.9	9.2
Pumpkin Pie, Graze*	1 Pack/65g	274.0	11.0	422	11.4	48.2	17.2	0.0
Razcherries, Graze*	1 Pack/50g	163.0	0.0	327	0.5	80.0	0.5	0.0
Rocky Mountain, Graze*	1 Pack/50g	264.0	19.0	529	3.2	38.2	38.6	0.0
Rouge Dried, Graze*	1 Pack/50g	164.0	1.0	328	1.6	77.6	1.4	0.0
Strawberries & Cream, Graze*	1 Pack/70g	303.0	11.0	433	3.7	66.9	16.3	0.0
Strawberry Fields Forever, Graze*	1 Punnet /40g	117.0	0.0	292	1.9	70.9	0.9	2.5
Strawberry, Banana & Cherry, Sunshine Mix, Graze*	1 Pack/50g	78.0	0.0	157	9.7	37.2	0.4	0.0
Sultanas, Currants, Raisins & Citrus Peel, Asda*	1 Serving/100g	283.0	0.0	283	2.6	67.0	0.5	1.7
Super Dried, Graze*	1 Pack/55g	176.0	1.0	320	5.6	76.4	1.6	0.0
Taste of Hawaii, Extra Special, Asda*	1 Serving/100g	314.0	1.0	314	1.7	75.0	0.8	4.4
Taste of New England, Asda*	1 Serving/50g	158.0	1.0	316	2.2	74.0	1.2	5.0
Top Banana, Graze*	1 Serving/40g	115.0	0.0	287	2.6	70.1	0.9	0.0
Trail Mix, Kick Start, Wholefoods, Asda*	1 Serving/50g	193.0	10.0	387	10.9	40.0	20.4	10.7
DRIFTER								
Nestle*	1 Finger/20g	98.0	5.0	488	4.8	62.7	24.2	0.7
DRINK MIX								
Chocolate Orange, Clipper*	1 Pack/28g	98.0	0.0	350	14.6	69.7	1.5	0.0
Chocolate, Finest, Tesco*	1 Serving/200ml	242.0	13.0	121	4.9	10.7	6.4	0.7
Chocolate, Flavia*	1 Serving/18g	64.0	1.0	368	15.6	67.2	4.0	0.0
Milk Chocolate, Instant Break, Cadbury*	4 Tsp/28g	119.0	4.0	425	10.9	64.2	14.0	0.0
DRINKING CHOCOLATE								
Cadbury*	1 Heap Tbsp/16g	64.0	0.0	402	4.4	89.3	2.4	0.0
Dry Powder, Cocodirect*	1 Serving/18g	67.0	2.0	372	8.9	65.1	8.4	0.0
Dry, Asda*	1 Serving/30g	111.0	2.0	370	6.0	73.0	6.0	0.0
Dry, Tesco*	3 Tsp/25g	92.0	1.0	368	6.4	72.6	5.8	4.2
Dry, Waitrose*	3 Tsp/12g	48.0	1.0	403	7.2	79.9	6.1	2.9
Hot Chocolate, Light Choices, Tesco*	1 Cup/11g	38.0	1.0	345	13.8	54.9	7.7	13.1
Made Up with Semi-Skimmed Milk, Average	1 Mug/227ml	129.0	4.0	57	3.5	7.0	1.9	0.2
Made Up with Skimmed Milk, Average	1 Mug/227ml	100.0	1.0	44	3.5	7.0	0.5	0.0
Made Up with Whole Milk, Average	1 Mug/227ml	173.0	10.0	76	3.4	6.8	4.2	0.2
Made Up, BGTY, Sainsbury's*	1 Serving/178g	114.0	0.0	64	3.9	11.4	0.2	0.7
Maxpax, Light, Suchard*	1 Serving/11g	37.0	1.0	355	20.0	56.0	5.5	9.3

D

	Measure INFO/WEIGHT	per Measure KCAL	FAT	Nutrition Values per 100g / 100ml KCAL	PROT	CARB	FAT	FIBRE
DRINKING CHOCOLATE								
Powder, Made Up with Skimmed Milk	1 Mug/227ml	134.0	1.0	59	3.5	10.8	0.6	0.0
Powder, Made Up with Whole Milk	1 Mug/227ml	204.0	9.0	90	3.4	10.6	4.1	0.0
DRIPPING								
Beef	*1oz/28g*	*249.0*	*28.0*	*891*	*0.0*	*0.0*	*99.0*	*0.0*
DUCK								
Breast, Meat Only, Cooked, Average	*1oz/28g*	*48.0*	*2.0*	*172*	*25.3*	*1.8*	*7.0*	*0.0*
Breast, Meat Only, Raw, Average	*1 Serving/160g*	*206.0*	*7.0*	*128*	*22.5*	*0.0*	*4.2*	*0.2*
Fillets, Gressingham, Mini, TTD, Sainsbury's*	½ Pack/90g	127.0	2.0	141	29.0	0.0	2.7	0.6
Leg, Meat & Skin, Average	*1oz/28g*	*80.0*	*6.0*	*286*	*17.2*	*9.5*	*20.0*	*0.4*
Raw, Meat, Fat & Skin	*1oz/28g*	*109.0*	*10.0*	*388*	*13.1*	*0.0*	*37.3*	*0.0*
Roasted, Meat, Fat & Skin	*1oz/28g*	*118.0*	*11.0*	*423*	*20.0*	*0.0*	*38.1*	*0.0*
DUCK &								
Plum Sauce, Roasted, Sainsbury's*	½ Pack/150g	174.0	4.0	116	6.9	16.0	2.5	1.8
DUCK A L' ORANGE								
Roast, M & S*	½ Pack/270g	553.0	42.0	205	12.5	4.1	15.6	0.6
DUCK AROMATIC								
Crispy, Asda*	1/3 Pack/166g	469.0	25.0	283	19.0	18.0	15.0	0.8
Crispy, Half Duck & Pancakes, M & S*	½ Pack/311g	590.0	27.0	190	13.9	14.0	8.6	2.1
Crispy, Half, with Hoisin Sauce & 12 Pancakes, Tesco*	1/6 Pack/70g	162.0	7.0	232	18.3	15.9	10.6	1.1
Crispy, Quarter, with Hoisin Sauce & 6 Pancakes, Tesco*	1/6 Pack/40g	100.0	4.0	250	12.3	25.3	10.6	2.0
Crispy, Whole, with Hoisin Sauce & 18 Pancakes, Tesco*	1/9 Pack/100g	280.0	17.0	280	18.9	12.0	17.2	0.4
with a Plum Sauce, Finest, Tesco*	1 Serving/250g	400.0	14.0	160	16.1	11.3	5.6	4.6
with Plum Sauce, Tesco*	½ Pack/250g	350.0	11.0	140	9.3	15.2	4.6	0.3
DUCK CANTONESE								
Style, Roast, Tesco*	1 Pack/300g	375.0	7.0	125	8.2	17.9	2.3	0.5
DUCK IN								
a Plum Sauce, Crispy, M & S*	1 Pack/325g	569.0	31.0	175	10.7	11.2	9.6	0.9
Chinese Barbecue, Wings, Sainsbury's*	1 Serving/175g	430.0	25.0	246	19.4	9.7	14.3	0.0
Orange Sauce, Legs, Extra Special, Asda*	1oz/28g	39.0	2.0	141	18.0	4.3	5.7	1.3
Oriental Sauce, Iceland*	1 Pack/201g	352.0	23.0	175	12.0	6.3	11.3	1.5
Plum & Chilli Sauce, Legs, Aldi*	½ Pack/200g	342.0	12.0	171	5.7	24.0	5.8	0.6
Plum Sauce, Legs, Asda*	1 Leg/200g	452.0	23.0	226	24.1	6.4	11.5	0.5
Red Wine Sauce, Free Range Fillets, Waitrose*	½ Pack/250g	377.0	19.0	151	16.4	4.1	7.7	2.2
DUCK PEKING								
Crispy, Aromatic, Sainsbury's*	½ Pack/300g	1236.0	111.0	412	19.5	0.6	36.9	0.1
DUCK WITH								
Apple & Calvados Sauce, GFY, Asda*	1 Serving/162g	144.0	4.0	89	13.0	4.2	2.2	1.4
Noodles, Shanghai Roast, Sainsbury's*	1 Pack/450g	580.0	17.0	129	5.6	18.0	3.8	1.2
Pancakes, Shredded, Iceland*	1 Pack/220g	471.0	6.0	214	20.4	27.0	2.7	1.5
Pancakes, with Hoisin Sauce, M & S*	1 Pack/80g	136.0	3.0	170	13.0	19.9	4.0	0.9
DUMPLING MIX								
Farmhouse, Goldenfry Foods Ltd*	1 Serving/35g	152.0	6.0	434	6.5	61.5	18.0	0.0
DUMPLINGS								
Average	1oz/28g	58.0	3.0	208	2.8	24.5	11.7	0.9
Dried Mix, Tesco*	1 Pack/137g	404.0	17.0	295	5.4	39.9	12.2	2.8
Homestyle, Baked Weight, Frozen, Aunt Bessie's*	1 Dumpling/49g	188.0	9.0	384	9.7	44.4	17.6	2.8
Pork & Garlic Chive, Waitrose*	1 Pack/115g	215.0	8.0	187	9.4	20.4	7.0	1.1
Prawn, Cantonese, Crispy, Sainsbury's*	1 Dumpling/11g	27.0	1.0	241	9.3	20.9	13.4	1.1

D

	Measure INFO/WEIGHT	per Measure KCAL	FAT	Nutrition Values per 100g / 100ml KCAL	PROT	CARB	FAT	FIBRE
EASTER EGG								
Aero Bubbles, Nestle*	1 Egg/235g	1264.0	72.0	538	6.6	57.6	30.8	2.2
Caramel, Cadbury*	1 Lg Egg/336g	1764.0	101.0	525	7.5	56.8	30.0	0.7
Chick, Dairy Milk, Cadbury*	1 Chick/185g	980.0	56.0	530	7.5	56.7	30.1	0.7
Chocolate Orange, Terry's*	1 Egg/120g	636.0	37.0	530	7.4	57.0	30.5	2.4
Creme Egg, Cadbury*	½ Shell/60g	315.0	18.0	525	7.5	56.8	30.0	0.0
Crunchie, Cadbury*	1 Egg/120g	630.0	36.0	525	7.5	56.8	30.0	0.7
Dairy Milk, Cadbury*	1 Pack/215g	1129.0	64.0	525	7.5	56.8	30.0	0.7
Dark Chocolate, 70%, Green & Black's*	1 Egg/110g	606.0	45.0	551	9.3	36.0	41.1	0.0
Dark Chocolate, Thorncroft's*	1 Egg/360g	1890.0	135.0	525	6.8	39.4	37.4	9.8
Disney, Nestle*	1 Egg/65g	342.0	19.0	526	6.3	59.7	29.1	0.6
Mars*	1 Serving/63g	281.0	11.0	449	4.2	69.0	17.4	0.0
Milk Chocolate, Nestle*	½ Egg/42g	205.0	10.0	489	5.0	65.2	23.1	0.5
Milk Chocolate, Swiss, Hollow, M & S*	1 Egg/18g	100.0	6.0	555	6.7	53.2	34.8	2.5
Milky Bar, Nestle*	1 Egg/40g	182.0	7.0	454	4.2	70.8	17.2	0.0
Roses, Cadbury*	1 Egg/200g	1050.0	60.0	525	7.5	56.8	30.0	0.7
Smarties, Nestle*	1 Sm Egg/90g	480.0	26.0	533	5.6	61.0	29.0	1.7
Twirl, Cadbury*	1 Egg/200g	1050.0	60.0	525	7.5	56.8	30.0	0.7
White Chocolate, Thorntons*	1 Egg/360g	1958.0	109.0	544	5.5	62.2	30.3	2.1
Wispa, Cadbury*	1 Egg/200g	1050.0	60.0	525	7.5	56.8	30.0	0.7
ECLAIR								
Belgian Chocolate, Weight Watchers*	1 Eclair/30g	81.0	4.0	271	3.9	37.6	11.7	6.6
Chocolate & Fresh Cream, Tempting, Tesco*	1 Eclair/39g	158.0	11.0	405	6.5	29.1	28.8	1.1
Chocolate, 25% Less Fat, Sainsbury's*	1 Eclair/58g	171.0	9.0	295	6.8	31.1	16.0	1.2
Chocolate, Asda*	1 Eclair/33g	144.0	11.0	436	6.7	27.3	33.3	4.8
Chocolate, Cream filled, VLH Kitchens	1 Serving/66g	286.0	19.0	434	7.0	36.4	29.2	1.8
Chocolate, Cream, Fresh, Tesco*	1 Eclair/66g	285.0	20.0	430	6.0	31.1	30.9	1.8
Chocolate, Filled with Pastry Cream, Average	1 Eclair/100g	262.0	16.0	262	6.4	24.2	15.7	0.6
Chocolate, Fresh Cream, M & S*	1 Eclair/43.6g	170.0	12.0	390	6.3	28.4	27.9	2.0
Chocolate, Fresh Cream, Sainsbury's*	1 Eclair/59g	212.0	14.0	360	4.2	32.7	23.6	0.5
Chocolate, Frozen, Morrisons*	1 Eclair/31g	116.0	10.0	374	5.0	18.8	31.0	1.3
Chocolate, HL, Tesco*	1 Serving/77g	192.0	10.0	249	6.8	27.1	12.6	0.9
Double Chocolate, with Fresh Cream, Tesco*	1 Eclair/68.8g	275.0	19.0	400	5.9	33.4	27.0	1.6
EEL								
Cooked Or Smoked, Dry Heat, Average	**1 Serving/100g**	**236.0**	**15.0**	**236**	**23.6**	**0.0**	**14.9**	**0.0**
Jellied, Average	**1oz/28g**	**27.0**	**2.0**	**98**	**8.4**	**0.0**	**7.1**	**0.0**
Raw, Average	**1oz/28g**	**47.0**	**3.0**	**168**	**16.6**	**0.0**	**11.3**	**0.0**
EGG SUBSTITUTE								
99% Real Eggs, The Crafty Cook*	¼ Cup/61g	30.0	0.0	49	10.0	2.0	0.0	0.0
Original, The Crafty Cook*	¼ Cup 1oz/28g	30.0	0.0	107	21.4	3.6	0.0	0.0
EGGS								
Dried, White, Average	**1 Tbsp/14g**	**41.0**	**0.0**	**295**	**73.8**	**0.0**	**0.0**	**0.0**
Dried, Whole, Average	**1oz/28g**	**159.0**	**12.0**	**568**	**48.4**	**0.0**	**41.6**	**0.0**
Duck, Boiled & Salted, Average	1 Egg/75g	148.0	12.0	198	14.6	0.0	15.5	0.0
Duck, Whole, Raw, Average	**1 Egg/75g**	**122.0**	**9.0**	**163**	**14.3**	**0.0**	**11.8**	**0.0**
Free Range, Large, Average	**1 Egg/56g**	**80.0**	**6.0**	**143**	**12.6**	**0.8**	**9.9**	**0.0**
Free Range, Medium, Average	1 Egg/50g	71.0	5.0	143	12.6	0.8	9.9	0.0
Fried, Average	1 Med/60g	107.0	8.0	179	13.6	0.0	13.9	0.0
Goose, Whole, Fresh, Raw, Average	**1 Egg/144g**	**267.0**	**19.0**	**185**	**13.9**	**1.3**	**13.3**	**0.0**
Large, Average	**1 Egg/56g**	**82.0**	**6.0**	**147**	**12.5**	**0.0**	**10.8**	**0.0**
Medium, Average	**1 Egg/50g**	**71.0**	**5.0**	**143**	**12.6**	**0.8**	**9.9**	**0.0**
Medium, Boiled, Average	1 Egg/50g	73.0	5.0	147	12.5	0.0	10.8	0.0
Poached	1 Med/50g	73.0	5.0	147	12.5	0.0	10.8	0.0
Quail, Whole, Raw	**1 Egg/13g**	**20.0**	**1.0**	**151**	**12.9**	**0.0**	**11.1**	**0.0**

	Measure INFO/WEIGHT	per Measure KCAL	per Measure FAT	Nutrition Values per 100g / 100ml KCAL	PROT	CARB	FAT	FIBRE
EGGS								
Scrambled with Milk, Average	1 Egg/60g	154.0	14.0	257	10.9	0.7	23.4	0.0
Scrambled, Average	1 Egg/68g	109.0	8.0	160	13.8	0.0	11.6	0.0
Turkey, Whole, Raw	*1oz/28g*	*46.0*	*3.0*	*165*	*13.7*	*0.0*	*12.2*	*0.0*
Whites Only, Raw, Average	*1 Lg Egg/33g*	*17.0*	*0.0*	*52*	*10.9*	*0.3*	*0.6*	*0.0*
Whites, Liquid, My Protein*	1 White/32g	16.0	0.0	50	11.2	0.0	0.0	0.0
Whole, Raw	*1 Med/57g*	*84.0*	*6.0*	*147*	*12.5*	*0.0*	*10.8*	*0.0*
Yolks, Raw	*1 Av Yolk/14g*	*47.0*	*4.0*	*339*	*16.1*	*0.0*	*30.5*	*0.0*
ELDERBERRIES								
Average	*1oz/28g*	*10.0*	*0.0*	*35*	*0.7*	*7.4*	*0.5*	*0.0*
ELICHE								
Dry Weight, Buitoni*	1 Serving/80g	282.0	2.0	352	11.2	72.6	1.9	0.0
ENCHILADAS								
Beef, Light Choices, Tesco*	1 Pack/400g	412.0	9.0	103	7.0	13.5	2.3	2.2
Chicken, American, HL, Tesco*	1 Serving/240g	353.0	4.0	147	10.4	22.5	1.8	1.2
Chicken, Asda*	1 Serving/500g	690.0	30.0	138	10.0	17.0	6.0	1.0
Chicken, Diner Specials, M & S*	½ Pack/227g	340.0	12.0	150	9.9	15.4	5.3	2.0
Chicken, in a Spicy Salsa & Bean Sauce, Asda*	½ Pack/212g	373.0	17.0	176	10.0	16.0	8.0	0.0
Chicken, Morrisons*	½ Pack/275g	393.0	13.0	143	10.0	15.4	4.6	1.8
Chicken, Perfectly Balanced, Waitrose*	1 Pack/450g	481.0	14.0	107	6.9	12.7	3.2	1.1
Chicken, Value, Tesco*	1 Serving/212g	297.0	8.0	140	7.0	19.3	3.9	1.1
Three Bean, Vegetarian, Tesco*	1 Pack/440g	572.0	25.0	130	4.9	14.1	5.6	3.3
Vegetable & Bean, Eat Smart, Morrisons*	1 Pack/380g	475.0	10.0	125	4.7	20.7	2.6	3.2
Vegetable, GFY, Asda*	1 Pack/350g	399.0	16.0	114	4.4	14.0	4.5	1.3
Vegetable, Morrisons*	1 Pack/400g	468.0	18.0	117	4.5	14.4	4.6	1.8
ENDIVE								
Raw	*1oz/28g*	*4.0*	*0.0*	*13*	*1.8*	*1.0*	*0.2*	*2.0*
ENERGY DRINK								
Blue Bolt, Sainsbury's*	1 Can/250ml	105.0	0.0	42	0.0	10.0	0.0	0.0
Citrus, Isotonic, Umbro*	1 Bottle/500ml	139.0	0.0	28	0.0	6.5	0.0	0.0
Lemon, Active Sport, Tesco*	1 Bottle/500ml	135.0	0.0	27	0.0	6.5	0.0	0.0
Orange, Active Sport, Tesco*	1 Bottle/500ml	135.0	0.0	27	0.0	6.5	0.0	0.0
Original, Rockstar*	1 Can/500ml	290.0	0.0	60	0.4	13.6	0.0	0.0
Powerade, Aqua+*	1 Bottle/500ml	80.0	0.0	16	0.0	3.7	0.0	0.0
Red Devil, Britvic*	1 Can/250ml	160.0	0.0	64	0.4	15.1	0.0	0.0
Red Rooster, Hi Energy Mixer, Cott Beverages Ltd*	1 Can/250ml	112.0	0.0	45	0.6	10.3	0.0	0.0
Redcard, Britvic*	1 Can/330ml	96.0	0.0	29	0.1	7.0	0.0	0.0
V, Frucor Beverages*	1 Can/250ml	112.0	0.0	45	0.0	11.2	0.0	0.0

E

	Measure INFO/WEIGHT	per Measure KCAL	per Measure FAT	Nutrition Values per 100g / 100ml KCAL	PROT	CARB	FAT	FIBRE
FAGGOTS								
in Rich Gravy, Iceland*	1 Faggot/81g	116.0	5.0	143	6.5	15.9	6.4	1.1
Mushy Peas & Mash, Sainsbury's*	1 Pack/450g	576.0	19.0	128	6.0	16.3	4.3	1.6
FAGOTTINI								
Mushroom, Sainsbury's*	½ Pack/155g	339.0	12.0	219	10.2	27.7	7.5	2.7
FAJITA								
Beef, GFY, Asda*	½ Pack/208g	354.0	10.0	170	11.0	21.0	4.7	1.6
Chicken, American Style, Tesco*	1 Pack/275g	388.0	14.0	141	9.5	14.2	5.1	1.0
Chicken, Asda*	½ Pack/225g	371.0	10.0	165	11.0	20.0	4.5	3.5
Chicken, BGTY, Sainsbury's*	1 Pack/172g	256.0	4.0	149	10.8	20.9	2.5	1.7
Chicken, Boots*	1 Pack/223g	448.0	16.0	201	9.1	25.0	7.2	3.9
Chicken, COU, M & S*	1 Pack/230g	287.0	5.0	125	10.0	16.5	2.3	1.5
Chicken, Finest, Tesco*	½ Pack/288g	457.0	20.0	159	9.9	14.4	6.8	2.1
Chicken, GFY, Asda*	½ Pack/225g	233.0	4.0	104	9.3	12.9	1.8	2.0
Chicken, Just Cook, Sainsbury's*	½ Pack/200g	200.0	3.0	100	18.5	3.1	1.5	2.0
Chicken, M & S*	1 Pack/230g	345.0	12.0	150	8.6	17.7	5.3	1.0
Chicken, Mexican, No Mayo, Foo-Go*	1 Pack/198g	360.0	11.0	182	9.6	23.3	5.6	2.4
Chicken, Morrisons*	1 Serving/300g	370.0	15.0	123	7.4	12.2	5.1	1.9
Chicken, Sainsbury's*	½ Pack/275g	396.0	15.0	144	9.5	14.5	5.3	1.9
Chicken, Salt Balanced, COU, M & S*	1 Pack/230g	253.0	5.0	110	9.5	13.2	2.3	1.7
Chicken, Tesco*	½ Pack /275g	382.0	14.0	139	9.2	13.9	5.2	1.9
Chicken, Value, Tesco*	1 Serving/250g	255.0	6.0	102	6.9	13.2	2.4	1.5
Gammon Steaks, Tesco*	1 Serving/250g	367.0	15.0	147	17.5	5.3	6.2	0.0
Meal Kit, Tesco*	1 Serving/100g	210.0	3.0	210	6.1	38.2	3.4	2.1
Tuna, Sainsbury's*	1 Pack/450g	751.0	24.0	167	11.4	18.2	5.4	1.6
Vegetable, Tesco*	1 Fajita/112g	133.0	6.0	119	4.2	14.3	5.0	1.1
FALAFEL								
Asda*	½ Pack/50g	140.0	10.0	281	8.3	18.9	19.1	8.2
Fried in Vegetable Oil, Average	1 Falafel.25g	45.0	3.0	179	6.4	15.6	11.2	3.4
Mini, M & S*	1 Falafel/14g	43.0	3.0	310	7.9	28.1	18.4	2.6
Mini, Sainsbury's*	1 Serving/168g	499.0	30.0	297	8.0	26.8	17.6	3.2
Mix, Asda*	1 Packet/120g	313.0	15.0	261	6.4	30.8	12.5	2.6
Mix, Lebanese Style, Al'fez*	½ Pack/200g	470.0	28.0	235	7.1	26.3	13.8	0.0
Mix, Sainsbury's*	½ Pack/110g	197.0	7.0	179	7.7	23.5	6.0	5.2
Organic, Cauldron Foods*	1 Falafel/25g	51.0	2.0	203	8.4	20.3	9.8	7.2
Vegetarian, Organic, Waitrose*	1 Felafel/25g	55.0	3.0	220	8.0	23.3	10.5	7.6
FANTA								
Apple, Z, Coca-Cola*	1 Can/330ml	13.0	0.0	4	0.0	0.6	0.0	0.0
Fruit Twist, Coca-Cola*	1 Serving/250ml	132.0	0.0	53	0.0	13.0	0.0	0.0
Icy Lemon, Coca-Cola*	1 Can/330mls	165.0	0.0	50	0.0	12.2	0.0	0.0
Icy Lemon, Zero, Coca-Cola*	1 Can/330mls	7.0	0.0	2	0.0	0.2	0.0	0.0
Lemon, Coca-Cola*	1 Can/330ml	165.0	0.0	50	0.0	12.0	0.0	0.0
Light, Coca-Cola*	1 Glass/250ml	5.0	0.0	2	0.0	0.5	0.0	0.0
Orange, Coca-Cola*	1 Serving/251ml	75.0	0.0	30	0.0	7.1	0.0	0.0
Orange, Z, Coca-Cola*	1 Can/330ml	10.0	0.0	3	0.0	0.5	0.0	0.0
Summer Fruits, Z, Coca-Cola*	1 fl oz/30ml	1.0	0.0	3	0.0	0.6	0.0	0.0
FARFALLE								
Bows, Dry, Average	*1 Serving/75g*	*265.0*	*1.0*	*353*	*11.4*	*72.6*	*1.9*	*1.9*
Salmon & Broccoli, Eat Smart, Safeway*	1 Pack/380g	361.0	9.0	95	6.4	11.6	2.4	1.1
FENNEL								
Florence, Boiled in Salted Water	*1oz/28g*	*3.0*	*0.0*	*11*	*0.9*	*1.5*	*0.2*	*2.3*
Florence, Raw, Unprepared	*1 Bulb/250g*	*30.0*	*0.0*	*12*	*0.9*	*1.8*	*0.2*	*2.4*
Florence, Steamed	*1 Serving/80g*	*9.0*	*0.0*	*11*	*9.0*	*1.5*	*0.2*	*2.3*

F

	Measure INFO/WEIGHT	per Measure KCAL	per Measure FAT	Nutrition Values per 100g / 100ml KCAL	PROT	CARB	FAT	FIBRE
FENUGREEK								
Leaves, Raw, Fresh, Average	*1 Serving/80g*	*28.0*	*0.0*	*35*	*4.6*	*4.8*	*0.2*	*1.1*
FETTUCINI								
Cajun Chicken, COU, M & S*	1 Pack/400g	380.0	8.0	95	8.0	10.8	2.0	2.9
Chicken Mushroom, GFY, Asda*	1 Pack/400g	359.0	7.0	90	7.2	11.2	1.7	0.7
Chicken, Cajun, GFY, Asda*	1 Pack/398g	450.0	9.0	113	8.3	14.9	2.2	1.5
Dry Weight, Buitoni*	1 Serving/90g	326.0	2.0	362	12.2	74.4	1.7	0.0
with Tomato & Mushroom, Easy Cook, Napolina*	1 Pack/120g	461.0	9.0	384	11.8	67.9	7.2	0.0
FIG ROLLS								
Asda*	1 Biscuit/19g	71.0	2.0	372	4.8	68.0	9.0	0.0
Go Ahead, McVitie's*	1 Biscuit/15g	55.0	1.0	365	4.2	76.8	4.6	2.9
Jacob's*	1 Biscuit/18g	68.0	2.0	380	4.0	71.4	8.5	3.3
Sainsbury's*	1 Biscuit/19g	70.0	2.0	377	4.8	68.3	9.4	2.6
FIGS								
Dried, Average	*1 Fig/14g*	*32.0*	*0.0*	*232*	*3.6*	*53.2*	*1.1*	*8.6*
In Light Syrup, Asda*	1 Serving/100g	75.0	0.0	75	0.4	18.0	0.1	0.7
Raw, Average	*1 Fig/35g*	*16.0*	*0.0*	*45*	*1.3*	*9.8*	*0.2*	*1.5*
Smyrna, Soft, Dried, Waitrose*	1 Fig/25g	49.0	0.0	197	2.4	44.0	1.3	10.6
FISH								
Balls, Gefilte, M & S*	1 Pack/200g	280.0	8.0	140	14.1	11.9	3.9	1.0
Balls, Steamed	1oz/28g	21.0	0.0	74	11.8	5.5	0.5	0.0
Battered, Portion, Ross*	1 Serving/110g	223.0	12.0	203	10.4	16.1	10.8	0.8
Battered, White, Skinless & Boneless, Farmfoods*	1 Serving/122g	238.0	12.0	195	9.3	16.7	10.1	2.3
Breaded, Asda*	1 Serving/150g	351.0	21.0	234	15.0	12.0	14.0	0.5
Fillet in a Cheese & Chive Sauce, Light & Easy, Youngs*	1 Pack/240g	178.0	6.0	74	10.2	3.0	2.3	1.2
Fillet in Parsley Sauce, Light & Easy, Youngs*	1 Pack/224g	139.0	4.0	62	8.4	2.8	1.9	1.4
Fillet, Dinner, Light & Easy, Youngs*	1 Pack/385g	362.0	16.0	94	6.2	8.2	4.1	1.4
Fillets, Garlic & Herb, Youngs*	1 Fillet/118g	261.0	15.0	222	11.0	16.2	12.6	1.4
Fillets, Lemon & Pepper, Youngs*	1 Fillet/130g	283.0	17.0	218	10.3	15.3	12.9	4.3
Fillets, White, Breaded, Tesco*	1 Piece/95g	198.0	10.0	208	10.6	16.9	10.9	1.0
Fillets, White, Natural, Tesco*	1 Fillet/100g	72.0	1.0	72	16.6	0.0	0.6	0.0
Goujons, Asda*	1 Serving/125g	240.0	8.0	192	12.8	20.8	6.4	0.2
Haddock, Fillets, Lightly Dusted, Seeded, M & S*	1 Fillet/144g	266.0	13.0	185	14.3	12.2	8.7	1.0
Hake Fillets In Tomato & Basil Marinage, Donegal Catch*	1 Fillet/135g	201.0	9.0	149	15.6	6.7	6.6	1.0
in Batter, Light, Iceland*	1 Fillet/120g	230.0	12.0	192	13.6	11.6	10.1	0.7
in Batter, Morrisons*	1 Fish/140g	235.0	8.0	168	14.0	15.0	5.8	0.2
in Batter, Youngs*	1 Serving/100g	315.0	20.0	315	14.9	20.4	19.7	0.8
Medley, SteamFresh, Birds Eye*	1 Bag/170g	170.0	6.0	100	13.0	2.3	3.7	0.1
Portion, Chip Shop, Youngs*	1 Portion/135g	315.0	20.0	233	11.0	15.1	14.6	0.6
Portions, in Oven Crisp Batter, Value, Tesco*	1 Serving/100g	209.0	11.0	209	11.0	16.4	11.0	2.6
River Cobbler, Smoked, Tesco*	1 Fillet /165g	124.0	3.0	75	13.9	0.0	2.1	1.5
Salmon, Fillet, Select, Farm Prime (4 Pack), Waitrose*	1 Pack/550g	979.0	58.0	178	20.2	0.0	10.5	0.0
Seaside Shapes, Birds Eye*	2 Pieces/80g	197.0	11.0	246	11.0	19.0	14.0	1.1
Steaks, Chip Shop, Youngs*	1 Serving/100g	198.0	10.0	198	11.0	14.9	10.4	0.9
Steaks, Skinless & Boneless, Youngs*	1 Serving/105g	224.0	12.0	214	10.5	16.6	11.8	0.8
White, Breaded, Fillets, Ocean Pure*	1 Fillet/112.5g	276.0	11.0	245	20.8	16.9	10.2	1.2
White, Smoked, Average	1 Serving/100g	108.0	1.0	108	23.4	0.0	0.9	0.0
FISH & CHIPS								
Cod, Asda*	1 Serving/280g	450.0	14.0	161	8.0	21.0	5.0	1.1
Cod, HL, Tesco*	1 Pack/400g	492.0	7.0	123	5.3	21.4	1.8	1.7
Ross*	1 Serving/250g	415.0	19.0	166	6.2	18.1	7.6	1.6
Tesco*	1 Serving/300g	489.0	19.0	163	5.5	21.2	6.2	1.6
FISH BAKE								
Cheese & Leek, HL, Tesco*	1 Pack/400g	340.0	8.0	85	11.0	5.8	2.0	0.8

	Measure INFO/WEIGHT	per Measure KCAL	FAT	Nutrition Values per 100g / 100ml KCAL	PROT	CARB	FAT	FIBRE
FISH BAKE								
Haddock & Prawn, COU, M & S*	1 Pack/340g	289.0	10.0	85	7.3	7.3	2.8	0.4
Italiano, Birds Eye*	1 Pack/400g	404.0	16.0	101	12.0	3.9	4.1	0.4
Mediterranean, HL, Tesco*	½ Pack/200g	158.0	3.0	79	10.3	5.9	1.6	1.4
Vegetable Tuscany, Birds Eye*	1 Pack/380g	391.0	14.0	103	10.6	7.1	3.6	0.4
FISH CAKES								
Breaded, Sainsbury's*	1 Cake/42g	75.0	3.0	179	10.0	16.2	8.1	0.7
Bubbly Batter, Youngs*	1 Cake/44g	109.0	7.0	247	7.1	20.5	15.1	1.4
Captain's Coins, Mini, Captain Birds Eye, Birds Eye*	1 Cake/20g	38.0	2.0	188	9.5	18.7	8.3	1.1
Cod & Parsley, Waitrose*	1 Cake/85g	147.0	6.0	173	9.2	16.9	7.6	1.1
Cod, & Pancetta, Cafe Culture, M & S*	1 Cake/85g	166.0	13.0	195	9.2	7.2	15.5	2.0
Cod, Big Time, Birds Eye*	1 Cake/114g	223.0	12.0	196	8.3	17.8	10.2	1.0
Cod, Birds Eye*	1 Cake/51g	95.0	4.0	186	11.3	15.9	8.6	1.0
Cod, Cheese & Chive, Finest, Tesco*	1 Cake/100g	212.0	11.0	212	9.7	18.3	11.5	1.7
Cod, Chunky, Breaded, Chilled, Youngs*	1 Cake/90g	192.0	12.0	213	9.5	14.9	12.8	1.2
Cod, Fresh, Asda*	1 Cake/75g	164.0	8.0	219	7.0	23.0	11.0	1.6
Cod, Homemade, Average	1 Cake/50g	120.0	8.0	241	9.3	14.4	16.6	0.7
Cod, in Crunch Crumb, Birds Eye*	1 Cake/49.5g	93.0	4.0	187	11.4	16.0	8.6	1.0
Cod, King Prawn & Pancetta, Extra Special, Asda*	1 Cake/115g	202.0	8.0	176	11.0	17.8	6.7	15.0
Cod, Line Caught, Sainsbury's*	1 Cake/90g	161.0	7.0	179	10.4	17.1	7.7	1.3
Cod, Tesco*	1 Cake/90g	202.0	9.0	224	8.9	23.8	10.4	0.2
Crab, & Prawn, Thai, Tesco*	1 Cake/115g	269.0	17.0	234	8.8	17.4	14.4	1.2
Fried in Blended Oil	1 Cake/50g	109.0	7.0	218	8.6	16.8	13.4	0.0
Frozen, Average	1 Cake/85g	112.0	3.0	132	8.6	16.7	3.9	0.0
Grilled, Average	1 Cake/50g	77.0	2.0	154	9.9	19.7	4.5	0.0
Haddock in Breadcrumbs, Sainsbury's*	1 Cake/88g	158.0	6.0	179	10.8	18.2	7.0	1.4
Haddock, Asda*	1 Cake/88g	181.0	9.0	206	8.0	21.0	10.0	1.5
Haddock, Breaded, Asda*	1 Cake/90g	187.0	8.0	208	10.0	22.8	8.5	1.2
Haddock, Sainsbury's*	1 Cake/83g	166.0	7.0	199	11.4	20.1	8.1	1.8
Haddock, Smoked, & Spinach, TTD, Sainsbury's*	½ Pack/107g	213.0	12.0	199	10.3	14.8	10.9	1.2
Haddock, Smoked, Asda*	1 Cake/90g	185.0	9.0	206	10.0	19.0	10.0	1.4
Haddock, Smoked, Frozen, Waitrose*	1 Cake/85g	186.0	10.0	219	9.6	17.8	12.1	0.8
Haddock, Smoked, M & S*	1 Cake/85g	153.0	8.0	180	10.6	13.4	9.4	2.6
Haddock, Smoked, Sainsbury's*	1 Cake/63g	127.0	6.0	201	11.0	17.8	9.5	2.1
Halibut Cod Loin, Finest, Tesco*	1 Cake/115g	213.0	8.0	185	8.8	21.3	7.2	1.4
Salmon, & Asparagus, Finest, Tesco*	1 Cake/115g	300.0	18.0	261	10.7	19.6	15.5	0.4
Salmon, & Broccoli, Morrisons*	1 Cake/60g	126.0	7.0	210	9.8	17.2	11.9	1.3
Salmon, & Dill, Waitrose*	1 Cake/85g	206.0	12.0	242	11.5	17.5	14.0	1.8
Salmon, & Tarragon, Waitrose*	1 Cake/85g	179.0	10.0	211	11.9	14.3	11.8	2.2
Salmon, Asda*	1 Cake/86g	215.0	12.0	250	8.0	23.0	14.0	1.4
Salmon, Chunky, Sainsbury's*	1 Cake/84g	192.0	11.0	228	13.2	15.8	12.5	2.9
Salmon, Homemade, Average	1 Cake/50g	136.0	10.0	273	10.4	14.4	19.7	0.7
Salmon, in Crunch Crumb, Birds Eye*	1 Cake/49.5g	107.0	6.0	216	9.7	15.0	13.0	1.4
Salmon, M & S*	1 Cake/86g	180.0	11.0	210	9.1	15.1	12.7	1.7
Salmon, Melting Middle, M & S*	1 Pack/290g	551.0	30.0	190	9.1	14.3	10.5	1.5
Salmon, Sainsbury's*	1 Cake/88g	171.0	8.0	194	12.6	16.5	8.6	1.6
Salmon, VLH Kitchens	1 Serving/56g	156.0	11.0	278	10.5	14.4	20.0	0.6
Smart Price, Asda*	1 Cake/42g	78.0	3.0	188	7.0	22.0	8.0	0.9
Thai Style, Sainsbury's*	1 Cake/49g	69.0	2.0	141	12.0	13.8	4.2	1.7
Thai, Finest, Tesco*	1 Cake/65g	149.0	9.0	230	7.5	20.3	13.2	1.6
Thai, Frozen, Sainsbury's*	1 Cake/15g	28.0	1.0	187	21.3	9.3	7.3	0.7
Tuna, & Red Pepper, Waitrose*	1 Cake/85g	175.0	10.0	206	9.5	15.4	11.8	1.6
Tuna, Asda*	1 Cake/75g	185.0	10.0	247	14.9	16.5	13.5	1.4
Tuna, Lime & Coriander, BGTY, Sainsbury's*	1 Cake/90.9g	200.0	11.0	220	10.7	17.7	11.8	2.6

F

	Measure INFO/WEIGHT	per Measure KCAL	per Measure FAT	Nutrition Values per 100g / 100ml KCAL	PROT	CARB	FAT	FIBRE
FISH CAKES								
Tuna, Sainsbury's*	1 Cake/90g	183.0	7.0	203	13.7	18.4	8.3	2.1
Tuna, Tesco*	1 Cake/90g	222.0	9.0	247	12.8	25.4	10.5	0.2
FISH FINGERS								
Chip Shop, Youngs*	1 Finger/30g	75.0	5.0	251	9.3	16.6	16.4	1.2
Cod, 100% Cod Fillet, Tesco*	1 Finger/30g	53.0	2.0	177	12.4	14.9	7.5	1.4
Cod, Chunky, Tesco*	1 Finger/40g	70.0	3.0	175	12.3	14.3	7.6	1.6
Cod, Fillet, Asda*	1 Finger/31g	66.0	3.0	214	13.0	18.0	10.0	0.0
Cod, Fillet, Chunky, M & S*	1 Finger/40g	70.0	2.0	175	12.0	17.2	6.0	1.0
Cod, Fillet, Iceland*	1 Finger/30g	61.0	2.0	205	13.0	19.5	8.3	1.4
Cod, Fillet, Waitrose*	1 Finger/30g	55.0	2.0	183	11.9	16.9	7.5	0.7
Cod, Fried in Blended Oil, Average	1 Finger/28g	67.0	4.0	238	13.2	15.5	14.1	0.6
Cod, Frozen, Average	1 Finger/28g	48.0	2.0	170	11.6	14.2	7.8	0.6
Cod, Grilled, Average	1 Finger/28g	56.0	2.0	200	14.3	16.6	8.9	0.7
Cod, Morrisons*	1 Finger/30g	54.0	2.0	180	11.7	16.4	7.5	1.1
Cod, Sainsbury's*	1 Finger/28g	53.0	2.0	190	12.5	17.7	7.7	1.0
Economy, Sainsbury's*	1 Finger/26g	51.0	2.0	198	12.6	17.7	8.5	1.3
Free From, Sainsbury's*	1 Finger/30g	56.0	2.0	188	11.4	18.0	7.8	0.7
Haddock, Fillet, Asda*	1 Finger/30g	61.0	3.0	205	14.0	17.0	9.0	0.0
Haddock, in Crispy Batter, Birds Eye*	1 Finger/30g	56.0	2.0	188	14.3	15.1	7.8	0.7
Haddock, in Crunchy Crumb, Morrisons*	1 Finger/30g	57.0	2.0	190	13.1	16.3	8.0	1.1
Hoki, Fillet, Birds Eye*	1 Finger/30g	58.0	3.0	193	12.6	15.6	8.9	0.7
in Batter, Crispy, Jumbo, Morrisons*	1 Finger/71g	146.0	9.0	205	11.3	12.2	12.5	0.6
Omega 3, Tesco*	1 Finger/30g	58.0	2.0	195	12.7	16.3	8.3	1.6
Salmon, Birds Eye*	1 Finger/28g	63.0	3.0	225	13.2	21.7	9.5	0.9
FISH IN								
Butter Sauce, Steaks, Ross*	1 Serving/150g	126.0	6.0	84	9.1	3.2	3.9	0.1
Butter Sauce, Steaks, Youngs*	1 Steak/150g	115.0	4.0	77	10.2	2.8	2.8	0.8
Parsley Sauce, Steaks, Ross*	1 Serving/150g	123.0	6.0	82	9.1	3.1	3.7	0.1
FISH WITH								
Mushrooms, Carrots & Broccoli, Parcel, Birds Eye*	1 Pack/250g	235.0	14.0	94	7.9	3.1	5.6	0.8
FIVE SPICE								
Powder, Sharwood's*	1 Tsp/2g	3.0	0.0	172	12.2	11.6	8.6	23.4
FLAKE								
Cadbury*	1 Bar/32g	170.0	10.0	530	8.1	55.6	30.8	0.7
Dipped, Cadbury*	1 Bar/41g	215.0	13.0	530	7.6	56.1	30.8	0.8
Luxury, Cadbury*	1 Bar/45g	240.0	14.0	533	7.3	57.8	30.2	0.0
Praline, Cadbury*	1 Bar/38g	201.0	13.0	535	7.7	49.5	34.3	0.0
Snow, Cadbury*	1 Bar/36g	198.0	11.0	550	7.2	60.1	30.9	0.0
FLAN								
Cauliflower Cheese, Safeway*	1 Sm Flan/150g	420.0	25.0	280	7.3	25.0	16.5	2.0
Cauliflower, Cheese & Broccoli, Hot, Sainsbury's*	¼ Flan/100g	303.0	20.0	303	6.4	24.7	19.8	1.2
Cheese & Onion, M & S*	1oz/28g	81.0	5.0	290	6.1	25.1	18.7	1.4
Cheese & Potato, Hot, Tesco*	¼ Flan/100g	282.0	20.0	282	6.0	20.0	19.7	2.3
Chicken & Smoked Bacon, Hot, Sainsbury's*	¼ Flan/100g	293.0	18.0	293	10.2	21.5	18.5	1.2
Mediterranean Vegetable, Co-Op*	¼ Flan/88g	188.0	10.0	215	4.0	22.0	12.0	3.0
Parsnip, Broccoli & Gruyere, Safeway*	½ Flan/200g	534.0	33.0	267	7.0	23.0	16.4	2.8
Pastry, with Fruit	1oz/28g	33.0	1.0	118	1.4	19.3	4.4	0.7
Potato, Cheddar & Onion, Safeway*	1 Serving/150g	420.0	25.0	280	6.4	25.6	16.7	2.7
Smoked Ham Cheese & Leek, Safeway*	½ Flan/200g	520.0	33.0	260	8.0	20.0	16.4	2.0
Sponge with Fruit	1oz/28g	31.0	0.0	112	2.8	23.3	1.5	0.6
FLAN CASE								
Sponge, Average	**1oz/28g**	**90.0**	**2.0**	**320**	**7.0**	**62.5**	**5.4**	**0.7**

FLAPJACK

	Measure INFO/WEIGHT	per Measure KCAL	FAT	Nutrition Values per 100g / 100ml KCAL	PROT	CARB	FAT	FIBRE
90% Fat Free, Cookie Coach*	1 Flapjack/75g	287.0	7.0	383	7.0	66.2	9.9	0.0
All Butter, Blackcurrant Jam, M & S*	1 Serving/65g	279.0	12.0	430	4.8	60.5	18.6	2.2
All Butter, Organic, Sainsbury's*	1 Serving/35g	156.0	8.0	446	5.3	54.5	23.0	2.7
All Butter, Sainsbury's*	1 Flapjack/35g	156.0	8.0	446	5.7	54.5	22.8	2.7
All Butter, Squares, M & S*	1 Flapjack/34g	150.0	7.0	441	6.2	56.2	21.2	4.4
All Butter, Waitrose*	1 Flapjack/34g	126.0	9.0	376	3.8	52.4	26.8	1.2
Apple & Raisin, Lite, Crazy Jack*	1 Flapjack70g	227.0	1.0	324	9.8	72.0	2.1	0.0
Apple & Raspberry, Fox's*	1 Flapjack/26g	105.0	5.0	403	4.8	52.5	19.4	3.7
Apple & Sultana, Mr Kipling*	1 Flapjack/27g	123.0	6.0	456	4.6	59.0	22.4	3.6
Apricot & Raisin, Waitrose*	1 Flapjack/38g	143.0	4.0	376	4.7	64.3	11.1	5.8
Apricot, The Handmade Flapjack Company*	1 Flapjack/90g	321.0	5.0	357	5.5	71.6	5.3	0.0
Average	1 Sm/50g	242.0	13.0	484	4.5	60.4	26.6	2.7
Banana, The Handmade Flapjack Company*	1 Flapjack/90g	379.0	13.0	421	5.3	67.2	14.6	0.0
Black Cherry, Blackfriars*	1 Serving/110g	529.0	25.0	481	5.0	63.0	23.0	0.0
Brazil Nut Cluster, The Handmade Flapjack Company*	1 Flapjack/90g	353.0	9.0	392	6.6	68.7	10.1	0.0
Cappuccino, Blackfriars*	1 Flapjack/110g	481.0	27.0	437	5.0	61.0	25.0	0.0
Caramel Bake, The Handmade Flapjack Company*	1 Flapjack/90g	375.0	13.0	417	6.0	65.6	14.5	0.0
Cherry & Coconut, Blackfriars*	1 Flapjack/110g	489.0	23.0	445	5.0	58.0	21.0	0.0
Cherry & Sultana, Cookie Coach*	1 Pack/90g	373.0	16.0	414	6.2	58.2	17.3	0.0
Chocolate & Hazelnut, M & S*	1 Flapjack/71g	330.0	18.0	465	7.3	55.6	25.5	3.8
Chocolate Chip, Boots*	1 Flapjack/75g	313.0	11.0	417	5.6	65.0	15.0	3.5
Chocolate Chip, Happy Shopper*	1 Flapjack/35g	163.0	8.0	467	5.7	58.7	23.3	0.0
Chocolate Chunk, Boots*	1 Slice/75g	351.0	19.0	468	5.7	55.0	25.0	3.0
Chocolate Dipped, M & S*	1 Flapjack/96g	442.0	22.0	460	6.1	61.3	22.4	3.0
Chocolate Special, The Handmade Flapjack Company*	1 Flapjack/90g	392.0	18.0	436	5.7	58.7	19.8	0.0
Chocolate, McVitie's*	1 Flapjack/85g	422.0	23.0	496	6.6	56.6	27.1	3.2
Chocolate, The Handmade Flapjack Company*	1 Flapjack/90g	391.0	18.0	435	6.0	58.6	19.5	0.0
Chunky Chocolate, M & S*	1 FlapJack/80g	348.0	15.0	435	5.8	59.9	18.9	2.2
Cranberry, Apple & Raisin, Light Choices, Tesco*	1 Flapjack/30g	97.0	2.0	325	5.7	63.1	5.6	5.7
Crazy Raizin, Fabulous Bakin' Boys*	1 Pack/90g	378.0	15.0	420	6.0	60.0	17.0	4.0
Date & Walnut, The Handmade Flapjack Company*	1 Flapjack/90g	360.0	13.0	400	6.1	60.2	14.9	0.0
Fingers, GFY, Asda*	1 Finger/37g	129.0	4.0	350	5.0	60.0	10.0	3.5
Fruit & Nut, Organic, Evernat*	1oz/28g	136.0	7.0	484	4.5	60.4	26.6	0.0
Fruit with Raisins, Boots*	1 Pack/75g	329.0	16.0	439	5.4	57.0	21.0	3.5
Fruit, GFY, Asda*	1 Flapjack/45g	173.0	4.0	384	6.0	72.0	8.0	3.4
Fruit, Mr Kipling*	1 Flapjack/75g	306.0	14.0	408	4.8	56.7	18.1	3.0
Fruit, Tesco*	1 Flapjack/33g	136.0	5.0	412	5.7	62.0	15.7	4.0
Fruit, Weight Watchers*	1 Serving/30g	106.0	2.0	353	6.0	68.3	6.3	4.7
Fruity, Waitrose*	1 Serving/50g	199.0	7.0	398	6.1	62.9	13.5	3.9
Golden Oaty Fingers, Tesco*	1 Finger/25g	112.0	5.0	450	5.7	59.6	21.1	3.4
Golden Oaty, Fingers, Fabulous Bakin' Boys*	1 Finger/28g	126.0	6.0	450	5.7	59.6	21.1	3.4
Hob Nobs, Milk Chocolate, McVitie's*	1 Flapjack/35g	159.0	8.0	454	5.7	59.4	21.4	4.0
Mighty Oat, Fabulous Bakin' Boys*	1 Bar/85g	365.0	17.0	430	6.0	58.0	20.0	3.0
Milk Chocolate Digestive, McVitie's*	1 Flapjack/65g	293.0	14.0	451	5.4	59.7	21.2	3.4
Mixed Fruit, Fabulous Bakin' Boys*	1 Serving/90g	350.0	9.0	389	5.5	71.0	10.5	4.0
Oat & Syrup, Oatjacks, McVitie's*	1 Bar/34g	153.0	7.0	450	5.3	57.6	22.0	5.0
Oats, Butter & Syrup, McVitie's*	1 Bar/78.5g	356.0	18.0	454	4.9	57.9	22.5	3.7
Organic, Wholebake*	1 Bar/90g	388.0	19.0	431	6.0	59.4	20.8	0.0
Plain, The Handmade Flapjack Company*	1 Flapjack/90g	398.0	19.0	442	5.4	57.1	21.3	0.0
Really Raspberry, Fabulous Bakin' Boys*	1 Flapjack/90g	378.0	16.0	420	6.0	60.0	18.0	0.0
Snickers, McVitie's*	1 Flapjack/65g	315.0	19.0	484	7.9	49.0	28.5	6.0
Sultana, Tesco*	1 Flapjack/50g	173.0	10.0	346	5.0	36.2	20.1	3.7
Toffee, Finest, Tesco*	1 Flapjack/35g	156.0	7.0	446	4.9	63.6	19.1	1.3

	Measure INFO/WEIGHT	per Measure KCAL	FAT	Nutrition Values per 100g / 100ml KCAL	PROT	CARB	FAT	FIBRE
FLAPJACK								
Tropical Mix, Reduced Fat, Fabulous Bakin' Boys*	1 Flapjack/90g	346.0	11.0	385	6.0	63.0	12.0	3.0
with Sultanas, Tesco*	1 Flapjack/49g	217.0	10.0	442	5.3	57.9	21.0	3.7
Yoghurt Flavour, Blackfriars*	1 Bar/110g	521.0	26.0	474	7.0	58.0	24.0	0.0
FLATBREAD								
BBQ Chicken, Improved, Shapers, Boots*	1 Pack/165g	268.0	4.0	162	10.0	25.0	2.3	1.2
BBQ Style Chicken, Shapers, Boots*	1 Serving/108g	187.0	5.0	173	10.0	23.0	4.6	2.8
Cajun Style Chicken, GFY, Asda*	1 Wrap/176g	231.0	2.0	131	9.0	21.0	1.2	0.9
Chargrilled Chicken, COU, M & S*	1 Pack/163g	245.0	3.0	150	10.8	23.0	1.9	5.2
Cheese & Tomato, Tesco*	¼ Pack/56g	134.0	4.0	240	8.7	36.1	6.6	2.7
Chicken & Mango Salad, Sainsbury's*	1 Pack/100g	251.0	2.0	251	16.9	40.4	2.5	2.5
Chicken Caesar, Shapers, Boots*	1 Serving/160g	254.0	3.0	159	13.0	22.0	2.1	2.0
Chinese Chicken, Shapers, Boots*	1 Pack/159g	274.0	2.0	172	11.0	29.0	1.3	1.8
Feta Cheese, Shapers, Boots*	1 Pack/166g	255.0	6.0	154	6.7	23.0	3.9	1.4
Greek Feta Salad, Boots*	1 Pack/158g	241.0	6.0	153	6.4	24.0	3.6	1.2
Greek Style Salad, Waitrose*	1 Pack/172g	280.0	8.0	163	7.4	22.3	4.9	3.3
Italian Chicken, Improved, Shapers, Boots*	1 Pack/151g	263.0	7.0	174	11.0	22.0	4.5	1.8
Italian Chicken, Shapers, Boots*	1 Pack/168g	266.0	6.0	158	10.0	22.0	3.3	1.3
King Prawn Tikka, Waitrose*	1 Pack/165g	257.0	3.0	156	9.4	25.1	2.0	1.5
Mediterranean Chicken, Ginsters*	1 Pack/168g	302.0	7.0	180	10.6	25.5	4.0	0.0
Mediterranean Tuna, Ginsters*	1 Pack/167g	297.0	6.0	178	10.3	25.6	3.8	0.0
Mexican Style Chicken, Safeway*	1 Pack/150g	247.0	3.0	165	11.6	24.7	2.1	1.9
Peking Duck, Less Than 3% Fat, Shapers, Boots*	1 Pack/156g	246.0	4.0	158	7.2	27.0	2.4	1.9
Prawn Korma, Shapers, Boots*	1 Pack/169.0g	267.0	7.0	158	8.8	22.0	3.9	1.3
Ranchers Chicken, Shapers, Boots*	1 Pack/194g	303.0	4.0	156	12.0	22.0	2.2	1.5
Salsa Chicken, Shapers, Boots*	1 Pack/191g	328.0	8.0	172	11.0	22.0	4.4	1.6
Spicy Chicken & Salsa, HL, Tesco*	1 Serving/183g	251.0	3.0	137	10.1	21.1	1.4	1.2
Spicy Chicken, Shapers, Boots*	1 Pack/181g	292.0	5.0	161	11.0	23.0	2.5	0.0
Spicy Mexican, New, Shapers, Boots*	1 Pack/184g	281.0	5.0	153	8.0	24.0	2.7	1.9
Sticky BBQ Style Chicken, Shapers, Boots*	1 Pack/158g	274.0	7.0	173	10.0	23.0	4.6	2.8
Vegetable & Salsa, HL, Tesco*	1 Serving/193g	263.0	3.0	136	7.9	22.2	1.8	1.2
FLAXSEED								
Milled, Organic, Linwoods*	2 Dtsp/30g	153.0	14.0	510	21.9	1.7	46.2	28.9
FLOUR								
Arrowroot, Average	*1oz/28g*	*100.0*	*0.0*	*357*	*0.3*	*88.1*	*0.1*	*3.4*
Bread, Brown, Strong, Average	*1 Serving/100g*	*311.0*	*2.0*	*311*	*14.0*	*61.0*	*1.8*	*6.4*
Bread, White, Strong, Average	*1oz/28g*	*94.0*	*0.0*	*336*	*11.8*	*68.4*	*1.5*	*3.4*
Brown, Chapati, Average	*1 Tbsp/20g*	*67.0*	*0.0*	*333*	*11.5*	*73.7*	*1.2*	*0.0*
Brown, Wheat	*1oz/28g*	*90.0*	*1.0*	*323*	*12.6*	*68.5*	*1.8*	*6.4*
Chick Pea	*1oz/28g*	*88.0*	*2.0*	*313*	*19.7*	*49.6*	*5.4*	*10.7*
Gram, Stoneground, Dove's Farm*	1 Serving/100g	336.0	5.0	336	12.8	60.0	5.0	9.7
Millet	*1oz/28g*	*99.0*	*0.0*	*354*	*5.8*	*75.4*	*1.7*	*0.0*
Plain, Average	*1oz/28g*	*98.0*	*0.0*	*349*	*10.3*	*73.8*	*1.5*	*2.2*
Potato	*1oz/28g*	*92.0*	*0.0*	*328*	*9.1*	*75.6*	*0.9*	*5.7*
Rice	*1 Tsp/5g*	*18.0*	*0.0*	*366*	*6.4*	*80.1*	*0.8*	*2.0*
Rye, Whole	*1oz/28g*	*94.0*	*1.0*	*335*	*8.2*	*75.9*	*2.0*	*11.7*
Sauce, Dry, Sainsbury's*	1 Serving/20g	69.0	0.0	343	9.8	73.0	1.3	3.0
Soya, Full Fat, Average	*1oz/28g*	*118.0*	*6.0*	*421*	*37.9*	*19.7*	*21.7*	*11.6*
Soya, Low Fat, Average	*1oz/28g*	*99.0*	*2.0*	*352*	*45.3*	*28.2*	*7.2*	*13.5*
Speciality Gluten Free, Dove's Farm*	1 Serving/100g	353.0	2.0	353	4.7	85.2	1.8	2.7
Spelt, Average	*1 Serving/57g*	*216.0*	*2.0*	*381*	*14.3*	*74.5*	*2.9*	*6.3*
Strong, Wholemeal, Average	*1 Serving/100g*	*315.0*	*2.0*	*315*	*13.2*	*60.5*	*2.2*	*9.0*
White, Average	*1oz/28g*	*89.0*	*0.0*	*319*	*9.8*	*66.8*	*1.0*	*2.9*
White, Chapati, Average	*1 Tbsp/20g*	*67.0*	*0.0*	*335*	*9.8*	*77.6*	*0.5*	*0.0*

F

	Measure INFO/WEIGHT	per Measure KCAL	FAT	Nutrition Values per 100g / 100ml KCAL	PROT	CARB	FAT	FIBRE
FLOUR								
White, Self Raising, Average	*1oz/28g*	*94.0*	*0.0*	*336*	*9.9*	*71.8*	*1.3*	*2.9*
White, Wheat, Average	*1oz/28g*	*95.0*	*0.0*	*341*	*10.4*	*76.5*	*1.3*	*3.1*
Wholemeal, Average	*1oz/28g*	*87.0*	*1.0*	*312*	*12.6*	*61.9*	*2.2*	*9.0*
Wholemeal, Self Raising, Tesco*	1oz/28g	89.0	1.0	317	11.5	62.9	2.2	9.0
FLYING SAUCERS								
Asda*	1 Bag/23g	82.0	1.0	355	0.1	83.0	2.5	0.8
Co-Op*	1 Sweet/1g	4.0	0.0	370	0.5	90.0	1.0	0.6
FLYTE								
Mars*	Bar/23g	99.0	3.0	441	3.4	74.8	14.2	0.0
Snacksize, Mars*	1 Bar/23g	98.0	3.0	436	3.8	72.5	14.5	0.0
FOOL								
Apricot, BGTY, Sainsbury's*	1 Pot/113g	95.0	3.0	84	3.6	11.4	2.6	0.5
Blackcurrant, BGTY, Sainsbury's*	1 Pot/113g	89.0	3.0	79	3.5	10.4	2.6	0.6
Fruit	1oz/28g	46.0	3.0	163	1.0	20.2	9.3	1.2
Fruit, BFY, Morrisons*	1 Pot/114g	96.0	4.0	84	3.4	10.1	3.4	0.3
Gooseberry, BFY, Morrisons*	1 Pot/114g	99.0	4.0	87	3.4	10.7	3.4	0.4
Gooseberry, Fruit, BGTY, Sainsbury's*	1 Pot/121g	93.0	3.0	77	2.9	10.0	2.8	0.8
Gooseberry, Perfectly Balanced, Waitrose*	1 Pot/113g	125.0	3.0	111	3.6	18.3	2.6	0.7
Gooseberry, Sainsbury's*	1 Pot/113g	214.0	13.0	189	2.6	19.1	11.4	1.1
Gooseberry, Tesco*	1 Pot/112.5g	225.0	14.0	200	3.0	17.8	12.5	0.7
Lemon, BFY, Morrisons*	1 Pot/114g	96.0	4.0	84	3.4	10.1	3.4	0.3
Lemon, Fruit, BGTY, Sainsbury's*	1 Pot/113g	94.0	4.0	83	3.4	9.7	3.4	0.3
Raspberry, Fruit, Tesco*	1 Pot/113g	234.0	13.0	207	2.6	23.6	11.3	0.3
Rhubarb, Fruit, BGTY, Sainsbury's*	1 Pot/120g	91.0	3.0	76	3.5	9.5	2.6	0.3
Rhubarb, Fruit, Waitrose*	1 Pot/114g	182.0	13.0	160	2.7	11.9	11.3	0.3
Rhubarb, Perfectly Balanced, Waitrose*	1 Pot/113g	101.0	3.0	89	3.5	13.0	2.6	0.3
Rhubarb, Sainsbury's*	1 Pot/113g	180.0	13.0	159	2.6	11.5	11.4	0.4
Strawberry, Fruit, BGTY, Sainsbury's*	1 Pot/120g	100.0	3.0	83	3.7	11.1	2.6	0.8
Strawberry, GFY, Asda*	1 Pot/114g	95.0	3.0	83	3.8	11.0	2.6	0.8
Strawberry, Perfectly Balanced, Waitrose*	1 Pot/113g	110.0	3.0	97	3.5	14.9	2.6	0.4
Strawberry, Real Fruit, Safeway*	1 Pot/114g	197.0	13.0	173	2.7	15.4	11.2	0.3
FRANKFURTERS								
Average	*1 Sausage/42g*	*123.0*	*11.0*	*292*	*12.0*	*1.3*	*26.6*	*0.0*
FRANKFURTERS VEGETARIAN								
Asda*	1 Sausage/27g	54.0	3.0	199	18.0	3.5	12.5	2.5
Tivall*	1 Sausage/30g	73.0	5.0	244	18.0	7.0	16.0	3.0
FRAZZLES								
Bacon, Smith's, Walkers*	1 Bag/23g	112.0	5.0	485	6.5	62.0	23.0	1.3
FRENCH FRIES								
Cheese & Onion, Walkers*	1 Pack/22g	95.0	4.0	430	5.0	66.0	16.0	5.0
Ready Salted, Walkers*	1 Bag/22g	93.0	4.0	425	5.0	65.0	16.0	5.0
Salt & Vinegar, BGTY, Sainsbury's*	1 Bag/15g	51.0	0.0	340	6.0	80.1	1.5	4.1
Salt & Vinegar, Walkers*	1 Bag/22g	95.0	4.0	430	5.0	66.0	16.0	5.0
Worcester Sauce, Walkers*	1 Bag/22g	93.0	4.0	425	4.5	64.0	17.0	4.1
FRENCH TOAST								
Asda*	1 Toast/8g	30.0	0.0	381	10.0	74.0	5.0	4.0
Co-Op*	1 Toast/8g	31.0	0.0	385	10.0	72.0	6.0	5.0
Morrisons*	1 Toast/8g	31.0	1.0	393	11.0	72.5	6.6	3.0
Sainsbury's*	1 Toast/8g	31.0	1.0	382	10.0	72.0	6.6	5.0
Tesco*	1 Toast/100g	393.0	7.0	393	11.0	72.5	6.6	3.0
FRIES								
9/16" Straight Cut Home, Deep Fried, McCain*	1oz/28g	65.0	3.0	233	3.2	32.7	9.9	0.0
9/16" Straight Cut Home, Oven Baked, McCain*	1oz/28g	53.0	2.0	188	3.2	31.5	5.5	0.0

F

INFO/WEIGHT	Measure	per Measure KCAL	FAT	Nutrition Values per 100g / 100ml KCAL	PROT	CARB	FAT	FIBRE

FRIES

	Measure INFO/WEIGHT	per Measure KCAL	FAT	KCAL	PROT	CARB	FAT	FIBRE
American Style, Frozen, Thin, Tesco*	1 Serving/125g	207.0	10.0	166	2.2	21.1	8.1	1.9
American Style, Slim, Iceland*	1 Serving/100g	187.0	6.0	187	2.4	30.6	6.1	2.4
American, Oven, Asda*	1 Serving/180g	432.0	18.0	240	3.4	34.0	10.0	3.0
American, Somerfield*	1 Serving/100g	165.0	5.0	165	2.1	28.0	5.0	4.6
Crispy French, Weighed Deep Fried, McCain*	1 Serving/100g	193.0	8.0	193	1.9	27.4	8.5	0.9
Curly, Cajun, Weighed Frozen, McCain*	1 Portion/100g	156.0	9.0	156	1.6	17.7	8.7	1.8
Curly, Southern Style, Tesco*	1 Serving/50g	124.0	4.0	248	3.8	41.7	7.3	3.8
Curly, Twisters, Frozen, Conagra Foods*	1 Serving/150g	273.0	14.0	182	2.5	22.0	9.3	2.2
Extra Chunky, Oven Baked, Homefries, McCain*	1 Serving/200g	306.0	6.0	153	3.2	28.0	3.1	2.3
King Size, Salted, Burger King*	1 Bag/174g	489.0	23.0	281	2.9	37.4	13.2	3.4
Medium, Salted, Burger King*	1 Bag/116g	326.0	16.0	281	2.8	37.3	13.4	3.5
Oven, American Style, Asda*	1 Serving/180g	407.0	14.0	226	3.9	34.6	8.0	4.0
Oven, Straight Cut, Morrisons*	1 Serving/100g	149.0	4.0	149	2.8	24.6	4.3	2.6
Seasoned, Conagra Foods*	1 Serving/150g	247.0	12.0	165	2.4	20.8	8.0	1.9
Small, Salted, Burger King*	1 Bag/74g	229.0	11.0	310	2.7	41.8	14.8	2.7
Southern, Oven Cook, Baked, Potato Winners, McCain*	1 Serving/100g	232.0	8.0	232	3.6	35.7	8.3	2.4
Southern, Oven Cook, Frozen, Potato Winners, McCain*	1 Serving/100g	176.0	7.0	176	2.4	26.5	6.7	1.6

FRISPS

Tangy Salt & Vinegar, KP Snacks*	1 Bag/30g	160.0	10.0	532	5.0	52.6	33.5	2.9
Tasty Cheese & Onion, KP Snacks*	1 Bag/28g	150.0	9.0	537	5.5	53.2	33.6	3.2

FROG

Legs, Raw, Meat Only	*1oz/28g*	*20.0*	*0.0*	*73*	*16.4*	*0.0*	*0.3*	*0.0*

FROMAGE FRAIS

0% Fat, Vitalinea, Danone*	1 Tbsp/28g	14.0	0.0	50	7.4	4.7	0.1	0.0
Apple Pie, Low Fat, Sainsbury's*	1 Pot/90g	108.0	2.0	120	6.7	17.3	2.6	0.3
Apple Strudel, Safeway*	1 Pot/100g	116.0	3.0	116	6.6	14.8	3.4	0.7
Apricot, Layered, Weight Watchers*	1 Pot/100g	58.0	0.0	58	5.4	8.1	0.1	1.6
Bakewell Tart Flavour, BGTY, Sainsbury's*	1 Pot/100g	54.0	0.0	54	7.6	5.5	0.2	1.1
Banana, Organic, Yeo Valley*	1 Pot/90g	118.0	5.0	131	6.6	12.6	6.0	0.2
Banoffee Pie Flavour, Low Fat, Safeway*	1 Pot/100g	135.0	4.0	135	6.8	17.6	4.1	0.2
Black Cherry, Asda*	1 Pot/100g	113.0	5.0	113	4.1	13.0	5.0	0.0
Black Cherry, GFY, Asda*	1 Pot/100g	54.0	0.0	54	6.0	7.0	0.2	0.0
Blackberry, Layered, Weight Watchers*	1 Pot/100g	64.0	0.0	64	5.3	10.4	0.2	1.0
Blackcurrant, GFY, Asda*	1 Pot/100g	43.0	0.0	43	6.0	4.2	0.2	0.0
Cherries & Chocolate, Finest, Tesco*	1 Serving/165g	299.0	15.0	181	5.4	20.1	8.8	0.7
Cherry Pie Flavour, BGTY, Sainsbury's*	1 Pot/100g	54.0	0.0	54	7.6	5.5	0.2	1.1
Cherry, 0% Fat, Vitalinea, Danone*	1 Serving/150g	88.0	0.0	59	6.1	8.0	0.1	1.6
Chocolate Fudge, Smooth & Creamy, Tesco*	1 Pot/100g	136.0	6.0	136	6.7	13.3	6.2	0.2
COU, M & S*	1 Pot/100g	48.0	0.0	48	7.8	4.5	0.1	0.5
Exotic Fruits, Eat Smart, Safeway*	1 Pot/100g	60.0	0.0	60	7.9	6.6	0.2	0.4
Fabby, Loved By Kids, M & S*	1 Pot/43g	45:0	2.0	105	6.2	12.3	3.7	0.0
Fat Free, Average	*1oz/28g*	*16.0*	*0.0*	*58*	*7.7*	*6.8*	*0.2*	*0.0*
Fruit on the Bottom, BFY, Morrisons*	1 Pot/100g	66.0	0.0	66	5.6	10.6	0.1	0.0
Kids, Yeo Valley*	1 Serving/90g	111.0	5.0	123	6.6	12.6	5.3	0.0
Lemon Pie, Low Fat, Sainsbury's*	1 Pot/90g	108.0	2.0	120	6.7	17.3	2.7	0.2
Lemon Sponge Flavour, BGTY, Sainsbury's*	1 Pot/100g	52.0	0.0	52	7.6	5.0	0.2	1.1
Lemon, COU, M & S*	1 Serving/100g	60.0	0.0	60	7.0	7.3	0.2	0.6
Mandarin & Orange, Tesco*	1 Pot/100g	75.0	3.0	75	6.5	5.6	3.0	2.3
Mango & Papaya, HL, Tesco*	1 Pot/100g	55.0	0.0	55	6.2	7.0	0.2	0.1
Morello Cherries, Perfectly Balanced, Waitrose*	½ Pot/250ml	260.0	5.0	104	2.5	19.1	1.9	1.8
Munch Bunch, Nestle*	1 Pot/42g	44.0	1.0	105	6.7	12.6	3.0	0.0
Natural, Creamy, Co-Op*	1 Pot/200g	204.0	15.0	102	6.1	2.9	7.3	0.0
Natural, HL, Tesco*	1 Serving/65g	30.0	0.0	46	7.8	3.3	0.2	0.0

FROMAGE FRAIS

	Measure INFO/WEIGHT	per Measure KCAL	per Measure FAT	Nutrition Values per 100g / 100ml KCAL	PROT	CARB	FAT	FIBRE
Natural, Plain, Fat Free, Normandy, BGTY, Sainsbury's*	1 Serving/30g	15.0	0.0	49	8.0	4.2	0.1	0.0
Natural, Virtually Fat Free, French, Waitrose*	1 Tub/500g	260.0	1.0	52	7.3	5.0	0.3	0.0
Normandy, Light Choices, Tesco*	1 Serving/100g	46.0	0.0	46	7.8	3.3	0.2	0.0
Normandy, Sainsbury's*	1 Serving/25g	29.0	2.0	116	7.7	3.4	8.1	0.0
Organic, Vrai*	1 Serving/100g	83.0	4.0	83	8.1	4.5	3.6	0.0
Peach, BGTY, Sainsbury's*	1 Pot/100g	53.0	0.0	53	7.2	5.5	0.2	0.5
Peach, Layered, Weight Watchers*	1 Pot/100g	57.0	0.0	57	5.4	7.9	0.1	1.2
Petit Dessert, Co-Op*	1 Pot/60g	74.0	3.0	123	6.3	14.5	4.4	0.0
Pineapple & Passion Fruit, HL, Tesco*	1 Pot/100g	55.0	0.0	55	6.2	7.1	0.2	0.1
Pineapple, Eat Smart, Safeway*	1 Pot/100g	60.0	0.0	60	7.9	6.3	0.2	0.3
Plain, Average	*1oz/28g*	*32.0*	*2.0*	*113*	*6.8*	*5.7*	*7.1*	*0.0*
Raspberry & Redcurrant, BGTY, Sainsbury's*	1 Pot/100g	51.0	0.0	51	7.4	5.4	0.1	1.6
Raspberry, COU, M & S*	1 Pot/100g	60.0	0.0	60	7.0	8.1	0.2	0.5
Raspberry, GFY, Asda*	1 Pot/100g	43.0	0.0	43	6.0	4.2	0.2	0.0
Raspberry, Healthy Choice, Asda*	1 Pot/100g	41.0	0.0	41	6.0	3.8	0.2	0.0
Raspberry, Layered, Weight Watchers*	1 Pot/100g	51.0	0.0	51	5.5	6.3	0.1	1.1
Raspberry, Little Stars, Muller*	1 Pot/60g	66.0	2.0	110	5.0	12.7	4.0	0.4
Raspberry, Low Fat, Sainsbury's*	1 Pot/90g	96.0	2.0	107	5.8	15.1	2.6	0.1
Raspberry, Organic, Yeo Valley*	1 Pot/100g	127.0	6.0	127	6.1	11.1	6.5	0.4
Real Fruit, Tesco*	1 Pot/100g	54.0	0.0	54	5.6	7.6	0.1	0.1
Red Cherry, Tesco*	1 Pot/100g	75.0	3.0	75	6.5	5.5	3.0	2.3
Rhubarb & Crumble, Low Fat, Sainsbury's*	1 Pot/90g	96.0	2.0	107	6.7	14.1	2.6	0.4
Strawberry & Raspberry, Organic, Yeo Valley*	1 Pot/90g	118.0	5.0	131	6.3	12.9	6.0	0.2
Strawberry Cheesecake, Dessert Selection, Sainsbury's*	1 Pot/90g	95.0	2.0	106	5.8	15.3	2.5	0.1
Strawberry Tart, Sainsbury's*	1 Pot/100g	54.0	0.0	54	7.6	5.5	0.2	1.1
Strawberry, 0% Fat, Vitalinea, Danone*	1 Serving/150g	82.0	0.0	55	6.0	7.4	0.1	1.6
Strawberry, 99.9% Fat Free, Onken*	1 Serving/50g	45.0	0.0	91	6.9	15.3	0.1	0.0
Strawberry, Balanced Lifestyle, Aldi*	1 Serving/100g	52.0	0.0	52	5.4	7.1	0.2	0.7
Strawberry, COU, M & S*	1 Pot/100g	60.0	0.0	60	6.5	8.0	0.2	0.5
Strawberry, GFY, Asda*	1 Pot/100g	58.0	0.0	58	6.0	8.0	0.2	0.0
Strawberry, Healthy Choice, Asda*	1 Pot/100g	41.0	0.0	41	6.0	3.7	0.2	0.0
Strawberry, Langley Farm*	1 Pot/125g	189.0	10.0	151	7.0	13.3	7.8	0.0
Strawberry, Layered, Weight Watchers*	1 Pot/100g	50.0	0.0	50	5.4	6.2	0.1	0.8
Strawberry, Low Fat, St Ivel*	1 Pot/100g	69.0	1.0	69	6.9	6.8	1.2	0.0
Strawberry, Organic, Yeo Valley*	1 Pot/90g	116.0	5.0	129	6.3	12.5	6.0	0.2
Strawberry, Tesco*	1 Pot/100g	75.0	3.0	75	6.5	5.5	3.0	2.5
Strawberry, Thomas the Tank Engine, Yoplait*	1 Pot/50g	50.0	1.0	101	6.8	15.4	1.3	0.0
Toffee & Pecan Pie, Smooth & Creamy, Tesco*	1 Pot/100g	148.0	7.0	148	6.9	14.8	6.8	0.2
Toffee, BGTY, Sainsbury's*	1 Pot/100g	60.0	0.0	60	7.2	7.0	0.3	0.2
Tropical Fruit, COU, M & S*	1 Pot/100g	60.0	0.0	60	6.5	8.4	0.2	0.5
Vanilla, Danone*	1 Serving/200g	274.0	8.0	137	5.3	19.6	4.1	0.0
Virtually Fat Free, Tesco*	1 Pot/100g	56.0	0.0	56	5.6	8.2	0.1	0.0
Wildlife, Strawberry, Raspberry Or Peach, Yoplait*	1 Pot/50g	46.0	1.0	93	7.1	13.2	1.3	0.2
with Cereal, Shape Rise, Danone*	1 Serving/165g	205.0	2.0	124	6.5	23.9	1.3	0.5
with Real Fruit Puree, Nestle*	1 Serving/50g	65.0	1.0	130	7.1	18.9	2.7	0.2

FROZEN DESSERT

	Measure INFO/WEIGHT	per Measure KCAL	per Measure FAT	Nutrition Values per 100g / 100ml KCAL	PROT	CARB	FAT	FIBRE
Banoffee, HL, Tesco*	1 Serving/60g	92.0	2.0	153	2.5	29.9	2.6	0.6
Neapolitan, GFY, Asda*	1 Serving/100g	64.0	2.0	64	1.2	10.0	2.1	0.1
Toffee, BGTY, Sainsbury's*	1 Pot/74g	96.0	1.0	130	3.3	26.0	1.4	4.2
Vanilla Choc Fudge, Non Dairy Soya, Tofutti*	1 Tub/500ml	825.0	45.0	165	1.6	20.0	9.0	0.4
Vanilla, BGTY, Sainsbury's*	1 Serving/75g	89.0	2.0	119	3.0	19.9	3.0	3.7
Vanilla, Too Good to Be True, Wall's Ice Cream*	1 Serving/50ml	35.0	0.0	70	2.0	14.9	0.4	0.1

	Measure INFO/WEIGHT	per Measure KCAL	FAT	Nutrition Values per 100g / 100ml KCAL	PROT	CARB	FAT	FIBRE
FROZEN YOGHURT								
Black Cherry, M & S*	1 Pot/125g	164.0	1.0	131	3.1	27.1	1.1	0.5
Raspberry, Handmade Farmhouse, Sainsbury's*	1 Serving/100g	132.0	4.0	132	2.7	21.8	3.8	2.2
Raspberry, Orchard Maid*	1 Serving/80ml	89.0	2.0	111	2.8	19.9	2.1	0.0
Strawberry, Organic, Yeo Valley*	1 Serving/100g	140.0	3.0	140	4.8	23.5	3.0	0.1
Strawberry, Tesco*	1 Pot/60g	82.0	1.0	136	2.6	26.5	2.2	0.8
Vanilla, Less Than 5% Fat, Tesco*	1 Pot/120g	179.0	3.0	149	8.1	23.8	2.4	0.7
FRUIT								
Berry Medley, Freshly Prepared, M & S*	1 Pack/180g	90.0	0.0	50	0.7	10.9	0.2	2.9
Bites, Apple & Grape, Food Explorers, Waitrose*	1 Pack/80g	44.0	0.0	55	0.4	13.2	0.1	1.4
Bites, Raspberry, Mini, HL, Tesco*	1 Bag/25g	87.0	1.0	350	4.5	76.8	2.7	4.4
Black Forest, Frozen, Tesco*	1 Serving/80g	37.0	0.0	46	0.7	10.5	0.1	1.7
Black Forest, Shearway*	1oz/28g	12.0	0.0	44	0.7	9.9	0.1	0.0
Blueberries, Shearway*	1 Serving/80g	41.0	0.0	51	0.4	12.2	0.6	0.0
Citrus Selection, Fresh, Sainsbury's*	1 Pack/240g	79.0	0.0	33	0.9	7.1	0.1	1.6
Collection, Freshly Prepared, M & S*	1 Pack/400g	180.0	1.0	45	0.6	10.3	0.2	1.3
Deluxe, Fresh, Rindless, Shapers, Boots*	1 Pack/168g	64.0	0.0	38	0.7	8.3	0.2	0.7
Exotic, M & S*	1 Pack/425g	212.0	1.0	50	0.7	11.8	0.3	0.0
Fingers, Sunmaid*	1 Pack/50g	162.0	2.0	325	3.5	68.3	4.3	4.3
Frozen, Garden, M & S*	1 Serving/30g	7.0	0.0	25	0.7	4.6	0.2	1.8
Grapefruit & Orange Segments, Breakfast, Del Monte*	1 Can/411g	193.0	0.0	47	1.0	10.2	0.1	1.0
Juicy Twist, Tesco*	1 Pack/170g	71.0	0.0	42	0.4	9.6	0.2	1.2
Mango, Slices, in Juice, SPC Nature's Finest*	1 Pot/400g	224.0	1.0	56	5.0	12.3	0.2	1.5
Melon, Kiwi, & Strawberry, Fully Prepared, Sainsbury's*	1 Pack/245g	73.0	0.0	30	0.8	6.3	0.2	1.3
Mixed, Fresh, 5 a Day, Tesco*	1 Pack/400g	136.0	1.0	34	0.8	7.4	0.2	1.4
Mixed, Fresh, Tesco*	1 Pack/200g	70.0	0.0	35	0.8	7.4	0.2	1.4
Mixed, Fruitime, Pieces, Tesco*	1 Can/140g	84.0	0.0	60	0.4	14.0	0.0	1.0
Mixed, Pieces, in Orange Jelly, Fruitini, Del Monte*	1 Can/140g	94.0	0.0	67	0.3	15.8	0.1	0.0
Mixed, Tropical, Fruit Express, Del Monte*	1 Pot/185g	89.0	0.0	48	0.2	11.2	0.1	1.2
Mixed, Vine, Crazy Jack*	1 Serving/10g	31.0	0.0	309	2.8	74.0	0.3	4.7
Pieces, Mixed in Fruit Juice, Fruitini, Del Monte*	1 Serving/120g	61.0	0.0	51	0.4	12.0	0.1	0.5
Pineapple, Grape & Kiwi, Asda*	1 Serving/200g	98.0	1.0	49	0.6	11.0	0.3	1.7
Pure, Just Apple, Heinz*	1 Jar/128g	60.0	0.0	47	0.4	11.2	0.1	1.8
Snack Pack, Fresh, Sainsbury's*	1 Serving/120g	54.0	0.0	45	0.1	11.0	0.1	1.3
Snack, Apple & Grape, Blue Parrot Cafe, Sainsbury's*	1 Pack/80g	42.0	0.0	53	0.4	12.5	0.1	2.1
to Go, Del Monte*	1 Can/113g	80.0	0.0	71	0.0	17.7	0.0	0.0
Tropical, in Juice, Dole*	1 Pot/113g	59.0	0.0	52	0.3	14.2	0.0	1.8
Tropical, Tesco*	1 Pack/180g	85.0	0.0	47	0.6	10.8	0.2	1.9
FRUIT & NUT MIX								
Almond, Raisin & Berry, Sainsbury's*	1 Bag/50g	188.0	7.0	377	6.1	57.6	14.3	4.2
Born In The USA, Graze*	1 Pack/50g	285.0	22.0	570	10.6	33.8	43.8	0.0
Bounty Hunter, Graze*	1 Punnet/43g	206.0	13.0	479	4.6	46.0	30.6	0.0
Cacao Vine, Graze*	1 Punnet/45g	187.0	9.0	416	8.5	51.4	20.8	0.0
Checkmate, Graze*	1 Punnet/45g	185.0	11.0	412	9.6	41.8	23.9	6.1
Cheeky Monkey, Graze*	1 Punnet/30g	130.0	6.0	435	6.4	54.7	21.2	0.0
Cinnamon & Prailine, Christmas, Finest, Tesco*	¼ Pot/106g	470.0	27.0	442	8.2	45.9	25.1	11.5
Dried, Bear Necessities, Graze*	1 Pack/35g	126.0	8.0	361	4.6	34.9	23.2	0.0
Exotic, Waitrose*	1 Serving/50g	207.0	9.0	414	9.0	54.6	17.7	4.6
Fajita, Graze*	1 Box/55g	255.0	17.0	463	15.1	38.0	30.9	0.0
Fruit Squash, Graze*	1 Pack/45g	157.0	4.0	350	5.8	62.2	8.4	0.0
Grandma's Apple Crumble, Graze*	1 Punnet/40g	154.0	8.0	385	0.0	48.9	19.6	4.0
Himalayas & Beyond, Graze*	1 Pack/45g	196.0	12.0	435	6.9	48.4	26.4	0.0
Johnny Come Lately, Graze*	1 Pack/65g	262.0	15.0	403	10.0	41.4	22.8	0.0
Jungle Fever, Graze*	1 Pack/30g	135.0	8.0	449	7.4	42.3	27.8	6.8

	Measure INFO/WEIGHT	per Measure KCAL	FAT	Nutrition Values per 100g / 100ml KCAL	PROT	CARB	FAT	FIBRE
FRUIT & NUT MIX								
Lost, Coconut, Banana & Raisins, Graze*	1 Punnet/48g	183.0	9.0	382	3.5	51.0	19.2	0.0
Love Mix, Graze*	1 Pack/55g	155.0	1.0	281	4.6	70.0	1.1	0.0
Luxury, Asda*	1 Serving/50g	225.0	15.0	451	9.0	33.5	30.5	7.4
M & S*	1 Serving/30g	135.0	8.0	450	12.4	44.3	25.3	6.0
Mixed, Unsalted, Tesco*	1 Serving/25g	112.0	5.0	449	12.6	58.1	18.5	12.2
New World, Graze*	1 Serving/50g	206.0	12.0	413	16.8	45.2	23.4	0.0
Organic, Waitrose*	1 Pack/100g	489.0	33.0	489	15.0	33.8	32.6	5.4
Papaya & Cranberry, Sainsbury's*	1 Serving/75g	300.0	11.0	400	4.1	63.1	14.6	7.3
Rock The Casbah, Graze*	1 Pack/60g	284.0	18.0	473	10.0	39.7	30.3	0.0
Swallows & Amazons, Graze*	1 Pack/60g	252.0	12.0	420	6.3	56.3	19.7	0.0
Trail Mix, Average	1oz/28g	121.0	8.0	432	9.1	37.2	28.5	4.3
Tropical Praline, Graze*	1 Punnet/35g	121.0	4.0	347	4.2	59.2	12.1	2.0
Ying & Yang, Graze*	1 Pack/60g	296.0	19.0	493	6.8	41.2	32.5	0.0
FRUIT COCKTAIL								
Fresh & Ready, Sainsbury's*	1 Pack/300g	117.0	0.0	39	0.6	9.0	0.1	1.2
Fresh, Morrisons*	1oz/28g	12.0	0.0	44	0.6	11.3	0.2	1.0
in Apple Juice, Asda*	1/3 Can/80g	40.0	0.0	50	0.3	12.0	0.1	1.6
in Fruit Juice, Heinz*	1 Pot/125g	77.0	0.0	62	0.5	15.0	0.0	1.0
in Fruit Juice, Morrisons*	1 Can/140g	64.0	0.0	46	0.4	11.0	0.0	0.0
in Fruit Juice, Sainsbury's*	1 Serving/198g	97.0	0.0	49	0.3	11.9	0.1	1.3
in Fruit Juice, Waitrose*	1 Can/142g	71.0	0.0	50	0.4	12.0	0.0	1.0
in Juice, Del Monte*	1 Can/415g	203.0	0.0	49	0.4	11.2	0.1	0.0
in Light Syrup, Makes Sense, Somerfield*	1/2 Can/205g	127.0	0.0	62	0.4	15.0	0.0	1.0
in Light Syrup, Princes*	1 Serving/206g	64.0	0.0	31	0.4	7.3	0.0	1.0
in Light Syrup, Sainsbury's*	1/2 Can/125g	72.0	0.0	58	0.4	14.0	0.1	1.3
in Pear Juice, Kwik Save*	1 Can/411g	189.0	0.0	46	0.5	11.0	0.0	1.0
in Syrup, Del Monte*	1 Can/420g	315.0	0.0	75	0.4	18.0	0.1	0.0
in Syrup, Morrisons*	1/2 Can/205g	129.0	0.0	63	0.3	14.9	0.1	0.0
in Syrup, Smart Price, Asda*	1 Can/411g	173.0	0.0	42	0.3	10.0	0.1	1.6
in Syrup, Tesco*	1 Serving/135g	85.0	0.0	63	0.4	15.0	0.0	1.0
No Added Sugar, Asda*	1 Serving/134g	67.0	0.0	50	0.3	12.0	0.1	1.6
Tropical, Asda*	1/2 Can/135g	81.0	0.0	60	0.0	15.0	0.0	1.6
Tropical, Heinz*	1 Pot/113g	61.0	0.0	54	0.5	13.0	0.0	1.0
Tropical, in Juice, Morrisons*	1 Serving/100g	56.0	0.0	56	0.0	14.0	0.0	0.0
Tropical, in Syrup, Sainsbury's*	1/2 Can/130g	95.0	0.0	73	0.5	17.6	0.1	1.4
Tropical, Morrisons*	1/2 Can/212g	144.0	0.0	68	0.0	17.0	0.0	0.0
FRUIT COMPOTE								
& Vanilla Sponge, Weight Watchers*	1 Pack/140g	202.0	3.0	144	2.2	29.0	2.1	1.8
Apple, Strawberry & Blackberry, Organic, Yeo Valley*	1/2 Pot/112g	73.0	0.0	65	0.5	15.5	0.1	1.9
Apricot & Prune, Yeo Valley*	1 Pot/225g	207.0	0.0	92	0.6	22.3	0.1	1.6
Black Cherry & Creme Fraiche, Extra Special, Asda*	1 Pot/118g	188.0	9.0	159	1.7	20.0	8.0	0.8
Hartley's*	1 Serving/95g	63.0	0.0	66	0.8	15.5	0.1	2.4
Orchard Fruits, GFY, Asda*	1 Pot/180g	113.0	0.0	63	0.5	15.0	0.1	0.0
Spiced, Tesco*	1 Serving/112g	122.0	1.0	109	1.7	24.4	0.5	3.1
Strawberry & Raspberry, M & S*	1 Serving/80g	72.0	0.0	90	0.7	23.5	0.1	2.3
Summerfruit, M & S*	1/4 Pot/125g	119.0	1.0	95	0.9	22.7	0.6	0.8
FRUIT DRINK								
Alive Tropical Torrent, Coca-Cola*	1 Glass/200ml	88.0	0.0	44	0.0	11.0	0.0	0.0
Infusion, Peach, Lime & Ginger, M & S*	1 Serving/250ml	87.0	0.0	35	0.0	8.5	0.0	0.0
Lemon & Lime, Diet, Carbonated, M & S*	1 Glass/250ml	5.0	0.0	2	0.0	0.2	0.0	0.0
FRUIT FILLING								
Apricot, Sainsbury's*	1 Can/400g	316.0	0.0	79	0.5	19.1	0.1	0.9
Black Cherry, Tesco*	1 Serving/100g	110.0	0.0	110	0.4	26.9	0.1	0.4

F

	Measure INFO/WEIGHT	per Measure KCAL	FAT	Nutrition Values per 100g / 100ml KCAL	PROT	CARB	FAT	FIBRE
FRUIT FILLING								
Bramley Apple, Morton*	1 Serving/198g	168.0	0.0	85	0.2	21.1	0.1	0.0
Cherry & Amaretto, Asda*	¼ Pack/100g	105.0	0.0	105	0.9	23.0	0.2	0.0
Red Cherry, Morton*	1 Serving/70g	69.0	0.0	98	0.4	23.9	0.0	0.0
FRUIT GUMS								
Fruit Salad, Tesco*	6 Sweets/30g	100.0	0.0	335	8.3	73.4	0.5	0.3
No Added Sugar, Boots*	1 Sweet/2g	1.0	0.0	88	0.0	22.0	0.0	0.0
Rowntree's*	1 Tube/49.4g	170.0	0.0	344	4.8	81.3	0.2	0.0
Sugar Free, Sainsbury's*	1 Serving/30g	63.0	0.0	209	7.7	71.3	0.2	0.1
FRUIT MEDLEY								
Citrus, Somerfield*	1 Serving/81g	25.0	0.0	31	0.6	6.9	0.1	0.4
Dried, Tropical, Soft, Waitrose*	1 Serving/30g	85.0	0.0	283	0.2	70.6	0.0	2.5
Exotic, Co-Op*	1 Serving/120g	54.0	0.0	45	0.6	10.0	0.2	0.0
Exotic, Julian Graves*	1 Serving/50g	156.0	1.0	313	2.9	72.8	1.1	5.5
Fresh, Tesco*	1 Pack/200g	86.0	0.0	43	0.4	10.0	0.1	1.1
in Fresh Orange Juice, Co-Op*	1 Serving/140g	49.0	0.0	35	0.5	9.0	0.0	0.0
Mango, Melon, Kiwi & Blueberry, Fresh, M & S*	1 Pack/260g	104.0	1.0	40	0.7	9.1	0.3	1.6
Melon & Grape, Somerfield*	1 Serving/200g	70.0	0.0	35	0.5	8.0	0.1	0.7
Mixed, Fruit Harvest, Whitworths*	1 Pack/50g	165.0	0.0	331	1.8	79.4	0.7	4.8
Nectarine, Mango & Blueberry, Fresh, M & S*	1 Pack/245g	122.0	0.0	50	1.0	11.1	0.2	2.1
Pineapple, Papaya & Mango, Waitrose*	1 Pack/550g	297.0	1.0	54	0.6	12.8	0.1	1.1
Raisin, Fruit Harvest, Whitworths*	1 Pack/50g	157.0	1.0	315	1.8	74.4	1.3	4.3
Shapers, Boots*	1 Pack/140g	55.0	0.0	39	0.7	8.6	0.2	1.0
FRUIT MIX								
Berry, Sainsbury's*	1 Serving/20g	64.0	0.0	319	1.0	78.1	1.9	5.5
Luxury, Sainsbury's*	1 Serving/30g	78.0	0.0	261	1.8	62.3	0.5	2.7
Mango & Cranberry, Way to Five, Sainsbury's*	1 Serving/50g	165.0	0.0	331	1.8	79.4	0.7	4.8
Melon, Strawberry & Grape, Sainsbury's*	1 Pack/180g	58.0	0.0	32	0.5	7.0	0.2	0.4
Pineapple, Melon, Mango, Tesco*	1 Pack/440g	242.0	1.0	55	1.1	11.4	0.2	1.3
Raisins & Apricots, Great Stuff, Asda*	1 Pack/39.9g	112.0	0.0	281	2.6	66.9	0.3	6.0
Summer Fruits, British, Frozen, Waitrose*	1 Pack/380g	99.0	1.0	26	1.0	5.2	0.2	5.5
Tropical, Fresh, Waitrose*	1 Pack/240g	122.0	0.0	51	0.6	11.6	0.2	1.9
FRUIT PUREE								
Apple & Blueberry, Organic, Clearspring*	1 Tub/100g	76.0	0.0	76	0.4	17.8	0.3	0.0
Apple, & Blueberry, Organix*	1 Pot/100g	54.0	1.0	54	0.4	11.6	0.6	2.5
Apple, & Peach, Organix*	1 Pot/100g	49.0	0.0	49	0.6	11.0	0.3	2.1
Banana, Apple, & Apricot, Organix*	1 Pot/100g	68.0	0.0	68	0.8	15.4	0.4	2.0
FRUIT SALAD								
Autumn, Fresh, M & S*	½ Pack/160g	64.0	0.0	40	0.7	9.4	0.1	2.9
Berry, Asda*	1 Pack/250g	115.0	0.0	46	0.6	10.7	0.1	0.0
Berry, Seasonal, Asda*	1 Pack/300g	93.0	0.0	31	0.6	7.0	0.1	2.1
Chunky, in Fruit Juice, Canned, John West*	1 Can/411g	193.0	1.0	47	0.4	11.0	0.2	0.8
Citrus, Asda*	1 Serving/265g	88.0	0.0	33	0.9	7.2	0.1	1.5
Citrus, Fresh, M & S*	½ Pack/225g	79.0	0.0	35	0.9	7.7	0.1	1.5
Classic, Fresh, Sainsbury's*	1 Pack/400g	148.0	1.0	37	0.6	8.6	0.2	1.8
Classic, Shapers, Boots*	1 Pack/200g	75.0	0.0	37	0.7	8.5	0.1	1.3
Exotic, Fresh, Tesco*	1 Serving/225g	85.0	0.0	38	0.7	8.4	0.2	1.5
Exotic, Fully Prepared, Sainsbury's*	1 Serving/200g	74.0	0.0	37	0.6	8.3	0.2	1.3
Exotic, Morrisons*	1 Serving/150g	78.0	0.0	52	0.6	12.2	0.2	0.0
Exotic, Waitrose*	1 Pack/300g	126.0	1.0	42	0.6	9.5	0.2	1.1
Exotic, with Melon, Mango, Kiwi Fruit & Grapes, Asda*	1 Pot/300g	141.0	1.0	47	0.6	10.5	0.3	1.4
Fresh for You, Tesco*	1 Pack/160g	59.0	0.0	37	0.6	8.2	0.2	1.1
Fresh, Morrisons*	1 Tub/350g	150.0	0.0	43	0.7	9.9	0.1	0.0
Fresh, Sweet, Ripe & Moist, Tesco*	1 Serving/750g	345.0	1.0	46	0.7	10.6	0.1	1.6

	Measure INFO/WEIGHT	per Measure KCAL	FAT	Nutrition Values per 100g / 100ml KCAL	PROT	CARB	FAT	FIBRE
FRUIT SALAD								
Fresh, Tesco*	1 Pack/200g	84.0	0.0	42	0.7	9.3	0.2	1.5
Fresh, Washed, Ready to Eat, Tesco*	1 Pack/200g	92.0	0.0	46	0.7	10.6	0.1	1.6
Freshly Prepared, M & S*	1 Pack/350g	140.0	1.0	40	0.5	9.3	0.2	1.0
Frozen, Basics, Sainsbury's*	1 Serving/100g	38.0	0.0	38	0.5	8.8	0.1	1.1
Fruit, Mediterranean Style, Shapers, Boots*	1 Pack/142g	61.0	0.0	43	0.6	10.0	0.1	1.5
Golden, Fresh, Asda*	1 Pot/147g	69.0	0.0	47	0.6	11.0	0.1	1.6
Grapefruit & Orange, Fresh, M & S*	1 Serving/250g	87.0	0.0	35	0.9	7.4	0.1	1.6
Green, M & S*	1 Pack/400g	200.0	1.0	50	0.6	10.9	0.2	1.2
Homemade, Unsweetened, Average	1 Serving/140g	77.0	0.0	55	0.7	13.8	0.1	1.5
Juicy Melon, Pineapple & Grapes, Asda*	1 Pot/300g	111.0	0.0	37	0.5	8.4	0.1	0.9
Kiwi, Pineapple & Grape, Fresh Tastes, Asda*	1 Pack/200g	84.0	1.0	42	0.7	9.1	0.3	1.8
Layered, Rainbow, M & S*	1 Pack/350g	140.0	1.0	40	0.5	9.3	0.2	1.0
Layered, Tropical Rainbow, Freshly Prepared, M & S*	1 Pack/375g	206.0	1.0	55	0.7	12.6	0.3	1.7
Luxury, Fresh, Tesco*	1 Serving/400g	164.0	1.0	41	0.7	9.2	0.2	1.6
Luxury, Frozen, Boylans*	1 Serving/100g	54.0	0.0	54	0.7	12.7	0.2	0.0
Luxury, Frozen, Tesco*	½ Pack/250g	115.0	0.0	46	0.7	10.7	0.1	1.3
Luxury, M & S*	1oz/28g	11.0	0.0	40	0.6	9.2	0.1	1.1
Mango, Kiwi, Blueberry & Pomegranate, Fresh, M & S*	1 Pack/350g	210.0	1.0	60	0.9	13.4	0.3	2.4
Melon & Grapes, Shapers, Boots*	1 Pack/220g	75.0	0.0	34	0.6	7.7	0.1	0.8
Melon & Red Grape, Freshly Prepared, M & S*	1 Pack/450g	157.0	0.0	35	0.5	8.4	0.1	0.7
Melon, Kiwi, Strawberry, Way to Five, Sainsbury's*	1 Pack/245g	73.0	0.0	30	0.8	6.3	0.2	1.3
Melon, Pineapple & Grapes, Fresh, Tesco*	1 Pack/300g	120.0	0.0	40	0.5	9.2	0.1	1.0
Mixed, Fresh, Sainsbury's*	1 Pack/200g	84.0	0.0	42	0.7	9.4	0.2	1.9
Mixed, Tesco*	1 Pack/225g	85.0	0.0	38	0.7	8.3	0.2	1.3
Oranges, Apple, Pineapple & Grapes, Fresh, Asda*	1 Pack/260g	120.0	0.0	46	0.6	10.5	0.1	2.1
Peaches & Pears, Fruit Express, Del Monte*	1 Serving/185g	87.0	0.0	47	0.4	10.8	0.1	0.9
Pineapple, Apple & Strawberries, Tesco*	1 Pack/190g	80.0	0.0	42	0.4	9.8	0.1	1.4
Pineapple, Apple, Melon & Grape, Shapers, Boots*	1 Serving/100g	49.0	0.0	49	0.4	10.5	0.1	1.2
Pineapple, Mandarin & Grapefruit, Asda*	1 Serving/200g	86.0	0.0	43	0.6	10.0	0.1	0.0
Pineapple, Mango & Passion Fruit, Prepared, M & S*	1 Pack/400g	200.0	1.0	50	0.7	10.8	0.2	1.8
Rainbow, Asda*	1 Pack/350g	140.0	1.0	40	0.6	8.8	0.3	1.4
Rainbow, Fresh, Tesco*	1 Tub/270g	105.0	1.0	39	0.5	8.8	0.2	0.9
Seasonal, Fresh, Asda*	1 Pack/125g	55.0	0.0	44	0.5	10.4	0.1	1.2
Seasonal, M & S*	1 Serving/200g	100.0	0.0	50	0.5	11.8	0.2	2.1
Shapers, Boots*	1 Pack/140g	55.0	0.0	39	0.7	8.6	0.2	1.0
Summer, Red, Fresh, M & S*	1 Pack/400g	160.0	1.0	40	0.0	10.0	0.2	1.2
Summer, Sainsbury's*	1 Pack/240g	84.0	0.0	35	0.7	7.8	0.2	1.3
Sunshine, Fresh, M & S*	1 Serving/200g	70.0	0.0	35	0.0	8.3	0.1	1.3
Tropical, Australian Gold*	1 Pot/130g	92.0	0.0	71	0.6	17.2	0.1	0.0
Tropical, Fresh, Asda*	1 Pack/400g	164.0	1.0	41	0.7	9.0	0.2	1.8
Tropical, Fruit Snacks, Frozen, Sainsbury's*	1 Serving/175g	79.0	0.0	45	0.7	10.4	0.1	1.6
Tropical, in Light Syrup, Passion Fruit Juice, Tesco*	½ Can/216g	130.0	0.0	60	0.3	14.1	0.1	1.1
Tutti Frutti, Freshly Prepared, Tesco*	1 Lg Pack/300g	132.0	1.0	44	0.7	9.8	0.2	1.7
Virgin Trains*	1 Serving/140g	56.0	0.0	40	0.4	10.0	0.1	0.8
Weight Watchers*	1 Serving/135g	50.0	0.0	37	0.2	9.0	0.1	0.7
FRUIT SELECTION								
Fresh, M & S*	1 Pack/400g	180.0	1.0	45	0.6	10.1	0.2	1.3
New, Shapers, Boots*	1 Pack/160g	72.0	0.0	45	0.6	11.0	0.1	1.8
Shapers, Boots*	1 Pack/235g	96.0	0.0	41	0.5	9.2	0.2	0.8
Summerfruit, M & S*	1 Portion/80g	20.0	0.0	25	1.0	5.3	0.2	5.4
FRUIT SHOOT								
Apple & Blackcurrant, Robinson's*	1 Bottle/200ml	10.0	0.0	5	0.1	0.8	0.0	0.0
Apple, Low Sugar, Robinson's*	1 Bottle/200ml	14.0	0.0	7	0.0	1.2	0.0	0.0

	Measure INFO/WEIGHT	per Measure KCAL	FAT	Nutrition Values per 100g / 100ml KCAL	PROT	CARB	FAT	FIBRE
FRUIT SHOOT								
Orange, Pure, Robinson's*	1 Bottle/250ml	115.0	0.0	46	0.5	9.9	0.1	0.2
FRUIT SPREAD								
Apricot, Pure, Organic, Whole Earth*	1 Serving/20g	33.0	0.0	167	0.8	40.0	0.4	0.9
Blackcurrant, Carb Check, Heinz*	1 Tbsp/15g	8.0	0.0	54	0.5	12.8	0.1	2.7
Blackcurrant, Weight Watchers*	1 Tsp/6g	6.0	0.0	106	0.2	26.3	0.0	0.9
Cherries & Berries, Organic, Meridian Foods*	1 Tbsp/15g	16.0	0.0	109	0.5	26.0	0.3	1.1
Cherry & Berry, Meridian Foods*	1 Serving/10g	14.0	0.0	138	0.7	33.7	0.6	3.2
High, Blueberry, St Dalfour*	1 Tsp/15g	34.0	0.0	228	0.5	56.0	0.2	2.2
Raspberry, Weight Watchers*	1 Tsp/6g	7.0	0.0	111	0.4	27.1	0.1	0.9
Seville Orange, Weight Watchers*	1 Tsp/15g	17.0	0.0	111	0.2	27.5	0.0	0.3
Strawberry, Carb Check, Heinz*	1 Tbsp/15g	8.0	0.0	56	0.3	13.6	0.0	0.5
Strawberry, Weight Watchers*	1 Tbsp/15g	23.0	0.0	156	0.7	39.8	0.1	1.8
FU YUNG								
Egg, Average	1oz/28g	67.0	6.0	239	9.9	2.2	20.6	1.3
FUDGE								
All Butter, Finest, Tesco*	1 Sweet/10g	43.0	1.0	429	1.3	73.4	14.5	0.0
Butter Tablet, Thorntons*	1oz/28g	116.0	3.0	414	0.9	77.6	11.1	0.0
Butter, Milk, Thorntons*	1 Sweet/13g	60.0	2.0	462	3.7	68.5	19.2	0.0
Cadbury*	1 Bar/25g	109.0	4.0	440	2.4	73.0	15.1	0.5
Cherry & Almond, Thorntons*	1 Bag/100g	464.0	19.0	464	3.2	70.5	19.1	0.4
Chocolate, Average	1 Sweet/30g	132.0	4.0	441	3.3	81.1	13.7	0.0
Chocolate, Thorntons*	1 Bag/100g	459.0	19.0	459	3.1	69.0	19.1	0.6
Clotted Cream, M & S*	1oz/28g	133.0	6.0	474	1.7	67.6	22.1	0.0
Clotted Cream, Sainsbury's*	1 Sweet/8g	35.0	1.0	430	1.9	81.5	10.7	0.7
Dairy, Co-Op*	1 Sweet/9g	39.0	1.0	430	2.0	76.0	13.0	0.0
Devon, Somerfield*	1 Pack/250g	1060.0	28.0	424	2.0	78.9	11.1	0.0
Double Chocolate Bar, M & S*	1 Bar/43g	202.0	9.0	470	4.2	66.9	21.0	0.7
Pure Indulgence, Thorntons*	1 Bar/45g	210.0	10.0	466	1.8	65.9	21.9	0.0
Vanilla, Bar, Diabetic, Thorntons*	1 Bar/34g	156.0	6.0	460	3.3	69.2	18.8	0.6
Vanilla, Bar, M & S*	1 Bar/43g	205.0	10.0	476	3.7	63.0	23.3	0.4
Vanilla, Thorntons*	1 Bag/100g	465.0	22.0	465	1.8	65.9	21.9	0.0
Vanilla, Whipped, M & S*	1 Serving/43g	210.0	10.0	490	3.8	65.4	23.9	0.3
FUSE								
Cadbury*	1 Bar/49g	238.0	12.0	485	7.6	58.2	24.8	0.0
FUSILLI								
Carb Check, Heinz*	1 Serving/75g	219.0	2.0	292	52.7	15.2	2.3	20.8
Cooked, Average	*1 Serving/210g*	*248.0*	*1.0*	*118*	*4.1*	*23.8*	*0.6*	*1.1*
Dry, Average	*1 Serving/90g*	*316.0*	*1.0*	*351*	*12.3*	*72.0*	*1.6*	*2.2*
Fresh, Cooked, Average	*1 Serving/200g*	*329.0*	*4.0*	*164*	*6.4*	*30.6*	*1.8*	*1.7*
Fresh, Dry, Average	*1 Serving/75g*	*208.0*	*2.0*	*277*	*10.9*	*53.4*	*2.7*	*2.1*
Tomato, Weight Watchers*	1 Can/388g	198.0	2.0	51	1.9	10.1	0.4	0.8
Tricolore, Dry, Average	*1 Serving/75g*	*264.0*	*1.0*	*351*	*12.2*	*71.8*	*1.7*	*2.7*
Whole Wheat, Dry Weight, Average	*1 Serving/90g*	*290.0*	*2.0*	*322*	*13.1*	*62.3*	*2.3*	*9.0*

F

	Measure INFO/WEIGHT	per Measure KCAL	FAT	Nutrition Values per 100g / 100ml KCAL	PROT	CARB	FAT	FIBRE
GALAXY								
Amicelli, Mars*	1 Serving/13g	66.0	4.0	507	6.2	59.7	27.1	0.0
Caramel Crunch, Promises, Mars*	1 Bar/100g	540.0	32.0	540	6.1	57.5	31.8	0.0
Caramel, Mars*	1 Bar/49g	254.0	13.0	518	5.8	64.2	26.4	0.0
Cookie Crumble, Mars*	1 Bar/119g	651.0	40.0	547	6.2	55.6	33.3	1.8
Fruit & Hazelnut, Milk, Mars*	1 Bar/47g	235.0	13.0	501	7.1	55.2	28.0	0.0
Hazelnut, Mars*	1 Piece/6g	37.0	2.0	582	7.8	49.4	39.2	0.0
Hazelnut, Roast, Promises, Mars*	1 Bar/100g	544.0	33.0	544	6.4	55.6	32.9	0.0
Liaison, Mars*	1 Bar/48g	233.0	12.0	485	5.4	60.3	24.7	0.0
Rich Coffee, Promises, Mars*	1 Bar/100g	535.0	33.0	535	5.7	54.4	32.8	0.0
Swirls, Mars*	1 Bag/150g	747.0	40.0	498	4.9	60.2	26.5	0.0
GAMMON								
Breaded, Average	1oz/28g	34.0	1.0	120	22.5	1.0	3.0	0.0
Dry Cured, Ready to Roast, M & S*	½ Joint/255g	255.0	4.0	100	20.5	0.5	1.5	0.5
Honey & Mustard, Average	½ Pack/190g	294.0	14.0	155	19.1	3.6	7.1	0.1
Joint, Applewood Smoked, Tesco*	1 Serving/100g	152.0	9.0	152	17.5	0.2	9.0	0.0
Joint, Boiled, Average	*1 Serving/60g*	*122.0*	*7.0*	*204*	*23.3*	*0.0*	*12.3*	*0.0*
Joint, Raw, Average	*1 Serving/100g*	*138.0*	*7.0*	*138*	*17.5*	*0.0*	*7.5*	*0.0*
Joint, Unsmoked, Tesco*	2 Slices/150g	247.0	16.0	165	16.8	0.2	10.4	0.0
Roast, Toby Carvery*	1 Serving/100g	193.0	9.0	193	25.9	1.0	9.5	0.0
Steaks, Average	*1 Steak/97g*	*157.0*	*7.0*	*161*	*23.3*	*0.4*	*7.4*	*0.0*
Steaks, Honey Roast, Average	*1 Steak/100g*	*142.0*	*5.0*	*142*	*21.5*	*2.3*	*5.3*	*0.0*
Steaks, Smoked, Average	*1 Steak/110g*	*150.0*	*6.0*	*137*	*22.7*	*0.1*	*5.0*	*0.1*
Unsmoked, Dry Cured, TTD, Sainsbury's*	1 Serving/100g	214.0	11.0	214	27.7	0.5	11.2	0.8
GAMMON &								
Parsley Sauce, Steak, Tesco*	½ Pack/140g	217.0	7.0	155	23.7	2.9	5.2	0.5
Pineapple, Roast, Dinner, Iceland*	1 Pack/400g	360.0	6.0	90	6.2	12.7	1.6	1.7
GAMMON IN								
Creamy Cheddar Sauce, Steaks, Fresh Tastes, Asda*	½ Pack/143g	270.0	14.0	189	19.1	5.4	10.1	1.5
GAMMON WITH								
Cheese Sauce & Crumb, Steaks, Simply Cook, Tesco*	½ Pack/156g	218.0	12.0	140	14.2	3.1	7.7	1.0
Orange Glaze, Christmas, Joint, Finest, Tesco*	1/10 Joint/150g	214.0	10.0	143	17.6	2.4	7.0	0.0
Pineapple, Steaks, Asda*	½ Pack/195g	253.0	3.0	130	17.8	11.5	1.4	0.7
Three Cheese & Mustard Crust, Joint, Asda*	1 Serving/270g	351.0	12.0	130	21.7	1.2	4.3	0.0
GARAM MASALA								
Dry, Ground, Average	*1 Tbsp/15g*	*57.0*	*2.0*	*379*	*15.6*	*45.2*	*15.1*	*0.0*
GARGANELLI								
Egg, Dry, Waitrose*	1 Serving/125g	450.0	5.0	360	13.5	66.9	4.2	3.5
GARLIC								
Minced, Nishaan*	1 Tsp/5g	5.0	0.0	97	6.0	16.2	0.9	0.0
Powder, Average	*1 Tsp/3g*	*7.0*	*0.0*	*246*	*18.7*	*42.7*	*1.2*	*9.9*
Raw, Average	*1 Clove/3g*	*4.0*	*0.0*	*149*	*6.4*	*33.1*	*0.5*	*2.1*
Very Lazy, The English Provender Co.*	1 Tsp/3g	3.0	0.0	111	6.0	20.9	0.4	3.0
GARLIC PUREE								
Average	*1 Tbsp/18g*	*68.0*	*6.0*	*380*	*3.5*	*16.9*	*33.6*	*0.0*
GATEAU								
Au Fromage Blanc, Ligne Et Plaisir*	1 Serving/80g	128.0	2.0	160	8.0	26.0	2.6	0.0
Black Forest, 500g Size, Tesco*	1 Cake/500g	1125.0	55.0	225	4.0	27.1	11.0	1.8
Black Forest, Sara Lee*	1 Serving/80g	221.0	10.0	276	3.6	37.9	12.3	1.2
Blackforest, Sainsbury's*	1/8 Cake/63g	163.0	11.0	259	3.9	27.7	17.1	3.5
Chocolate Layer, M & S*	1 Serving/86g	278.0	16.0	323	4.2	35.9	18.3	0.9
Chocolate, Asda*	1 Serving/100g	176.0	10.0	176	2.4	19.0	10.0	0.4
Chocolate, Swirl, Tesco*	1 Serving/83g	230.0	13.0	277	3.8	29.3	16.0	0.2
Coffee, Tesco*	1 Serving/100g	300.0	17.0	300	4.2	32.5	17.0	0.6

G

	Measure INFO/WEIGHT	per Measure KCAL	FAT	Nutrition Values per 100g / 100ml KCAL	PROT	CARB	FAT	FIBRE
GATEAU								
Double Chocolate, Light, Sara Lee*	1/5 Cake/59g	139.0	3.0	237	5.7	43.3	4.6	2.0
Double Chocolate, Sara Lee*	1oz/28g	93.0	5.0	331	5.6	41.3	16.5	0.9
Double Strawberry, Sara Lee*	1/8 Cake/199g	533.0	24.0	268	3.2	36.2	12.2	0.6
Lemon & Lime, M & S*	1 Serving/100g	295.0	16.0	295	3.2	35.0	15.6	0.3
Orange & Lemon, Iceland*	1 Serving/90g	220.0	10.0	245	2.6	33.8	11.0	0.3
Strawberry, Co-Op*	1 Serving/77g	222.0	13.0	288	5.1	29.2	16.7	1.0
Strawberry, Family Size, Tesco*	1 Serving/84g	197.0	11.0	235	2.9	25.2	13.6	0.6
Swiss, Cadbury*	1/6/60g	228.0	10.0	380	5.2	52.0	16.8	0.9
Triple Chocolate, Heinz*	¼ Cake/85g	209.0	9.0	245	5.1	31.2	11.1	2.4
GELATINE								
Average	*1oz/28g*	*95.0*	*0.0*	*338*	*84.4*	*0.0*	*0.0*	*0.0*
GEMELLI								
Durum Wheat, Tesco*	1 Serving/100g	354.0	2.0	354	13.2	68.5	2.0	2.9
GHEE								
Butter	*1oz/28g*	*251.0*	*28.0*	*898*	*0.0*	*0.0*	*99.8*	*0.0*
Palm	*1oz/28g*	*251.0*	*28.0*	*897*	*0.0*	*0.0*	*99.7*	*0.0*
Vegetable	*1oz/28g*	*251.0*	*28.0*	*895*	*0.0*	*0.0*	*99.4*	*0.0*
GHERKINS								
Pickled, Average	*1 Gherkin/36g*	*5.0*	*0.0*	*14*	*0.9*	*2.5*	*0.1*	*1.2*
GIN								
& Tonic, Premixed, Canned, Gordons*	1 Can/250ml	213.0	0.0	85	0.0	6.7	0.0	0.0
37.5% Volume	*1 Shot/35ml*	*72.0*	*0.0*	*207*	*0.0*	*0.0*	*0.0*	*0.0*
40% Volume	*1 Shot/35ml*	*78.0*	*0.0*	*222*	*0.0*	*0.0*	*0.0*	*0.0*
GINGER								
Chunks, Crystallised, Julian Graves*	1 Serving/10g	34.0	0.0	340	0.0	88.0	0.0	0.0
Crystalised, Graze*	1 Pack/25g	61.0	0.0	243	2.9	58.0	0.3	0.0
Crystallised, Suma*	1 Serving/30g	104.0	0.0	348	0.2	82.0	0.1	0.3
Ground, Average	*1 Tsp/2g*	*5.0*	*0.0*	*258*	*7.4*	*60.0*	*3.3*	*0.0*
Root, Raw, Pared, Average	*1 Tsp/2g*	*2.0*	*0.0*	*86*	*2.0*	*19.1*	*0.8*	*2.1*
Root, Raw, Unprepared, Average	*1oz/28g*	*22.0*	*0.0*	*80*	*1.8*	*17.8*	*0.7*	*2.0*
Stem, in Sugar Syrup, Sainsbury's*	1oz/28g	76.0	0.0	271	0.2	67.3	0.1	1.4
GINGER ALE								
1870, Siver Spring*	1 Serving/100ml	18.0	0.0	18	0.0	4.2	0.0	0.0
American, Finest, Tesco*	1 Serving/150ml	68.0	0.0	45	0.0	11.0	0.0	0.0
American, Low Calorie, Tesco*	1 fl oz/30ml	0.0	0.0	1	0.0	0.0	0.0	0.0
American, Tesco*	1 Glass/250ml	57.0	0.0	23	0.0	5.5	0.0	0.0
Dry	1 Glass/250ml	37.0	0.0	15	0.0	3.9	0.0	0.0
GINGER BEER								
Alcoholic, Crabbies*	1 Bottle/500ml	254.0	0.0	51	0.0	7.1	0.0	0.0
Asda*	1 Can/330ml	144.0	0.0	44	0.0	10.9	0.0	0.0
Classic, Schweppes*	1 Can/330ml	115.0	0.0	35	0.0	8.4	0.0	0.0
D & G Old Jamaican*	1 Can/330ml	211.0	0.0	64	0.0	16.0	0.0	0.0
Light, Waitrose*	1 Glass/250ml	2.0	0.0	1	0.0	0.0	0.1	0.1
Sainsbury's*	1 Can/330ml	69.0	0.0	21	0.0	5.1	0.0	0.0
Tesco*	1 Serving/200ml	70.0	0.0	35	0.1	8.2	0.1	0.0
Traditional Style, Tesco*	1 Can/330ml	218.0	0.0	66	0.0	16.1	0.0	0.0
GINGERBREAD								
Average	1oz/28g	106.0	4.0	379	5.7	64.7	12.6	1.2
Men, Mini, M & S*	1 Biscuit/17g	78.0	3.0	470	6.2	63.9	18.6	1.7
Men, Mini, Sainsbury's*	1 Biscuit/12g	56.0	1.0	463	5.7	83.4	11.8	1.5
GNOCCHI								
Aldi*	1 Serving/100g	160.0	0.0	160	3.8	35.6	0.3	0.0
Di Patate, Italfresco*	½ Pack/200g	296.0	0.0	148	3.3	33.2	0.2	0.0

G

	Measure INFO/WEIGHT	per Measure KCAL	FAT	Nutrition Values per 100g / 100ml KCAL	PROT	CARB	FAT	FIBRE
GNOCCHI								
Fresh, Italian, Chilled, Sainsbury's*	¼ Pack/125g	190.0	0.0	152	3.8	33.6	0.3	1.4
Potato, Average	*1 Serving/150g*	*199.0*	*0.0*	*133*	*0.0*	*33.2*	*0.0*	*0.0*
GOAT								
Raw	*1oz/28g*	*31.0*	*1.0*	*109*	*20.6*	*0.0*	*2.3*	*0.0*
GOJI BERRIES								
Average	*1 Serving/100g*	*287.0*	*1.0*	*287*	*6.6*	*65.1*	*0.7*	*6.8*
GOOSE								
Leg, with Skin, Fire Roasted	*1 Leg/174g*	*482.0*	*30.0*	*277*	*28.8*	*0.0*	*17.1*	*0.0*
Leg, with Skin, Raw	*1 Leg/265g*	*943.0*	*84.0*	*356*	*16.3*	*0.0*	*31.8*	*0.0*
Meat & Skin, Roasted	*1 Half/774g*	*2361.0*	*170.0*	*305*	*25.2*	*0.0*	*21.9*	*0.0*
Meat Only, Roasted	*1oz/28g*	*89.0*	*6.0*	*319*	*29.3*	*0.0*	*22.4*	*0.0*
Meat, Fat & Skin, Raw	*1oz/28g*	*101.0*	*9.0*	*361*	*16.5*	*0.0*	*32.8*	*0.0*
Meat, Raw	*1 Portion/185g*	*298.0*	*13.0*	*161*	*23.0*	*0.0*	*7.0*	*0.0*
Meat, Roasted	*1 Portion/143g*	*340.0*	*19.0*	*238*	*29.0*	*0.0*	*13.0*	*0.0*
GOOSEBERRIES								
Dessert, Raw	*1oz/28g*	*11.0*	*0.0*	*40*	*0.7*	*9.2*	*0.3*	*2.4*
Stewed with Sugar	*1oz/25g*	*13.0*	*0.0*	*54*	*0.7*	*12.9*	*0.3*	*4.2*
Stewed without Sugar	*1oz/25g*	*4.0*	*0.0*	*16*	*0.9*	*2.5*	*0.3*	*4.4*
GOULASH								
Beef, Bistro Range, Tesco*	1 Pack/450g	544.0	15.0	121	7.9	14.6	3.4	0.6
Beef, Finest, Tesco*	½ Pack/300g	297.0	9.0	99	11.6	6.2	3.1	0.6
Beef, Weight Watchers*	1 Pack/330g	241.0	6.0	73	4.8	9.5	1.7	0.6
Beef, with Tagliatelle, COU, M & S*	1 Pack/360g	414.0	8.0	115	8.5	14.5	2.3	1.0
GRANOLA								
Nibbles, Apple Crumble, We Are Bear*	1 Serving/30g	99.0	1.0	329	13.0	76.0	4.9	14.0
Nibbles, Tropical Crunch, We Are Bear*	1 Pack/30g	99.0	1.0	329	13.0	76.0	4.9	15.5
Summer Fruits, Pomegranate Infused, M & S*	1 Serving/50g	200.0	6.0	400	8.6	63.2	12.7	5.8
GRAPEFRUIT								
in Juice, Average	*1oz/28g*	*13.0*	*0.0*	*46*	*0.5*	*10.6*	*0.0*	*0.4*
in Syrup, Average	*1oz/28g*	*19.0*	*0.0*	*69*	*0.5*	*16.8*	*0.1*	*0.5*
Raw, Weighed with Skin & Seeds, Average	*1 Lge/340g*	*109.0*	*0.0*	*32*	*0.6*	*8.1*	*0.1*	*1.1*
Ruby Red, in Juice, Average	*1 Serving/135g*	*54.0*	*0.0*	*40*	*0.5*	*9.3*	*0.0*	*0.5*
GRAPES								
Green, Average	*1oz/28g*	*17.0*	*0.0*	*61*	*0.4*	*15.2*	*0.1*	*0.7*
Red & Green Selection, Average	*1 Serving/80g*	*50.0*	*0.0*	*62*	*0.4*	*15.2*	*0.1*	*0.8*
Red, Average	*1 Serving/80g*	*53.0*	*0.0*	*67*	*0.4*	*16.5*	*0.1*	*0.7*
GRATIN								
Cauliflower, Findus*	1 Pack/400g	340.0	20.0	85	3.5	7.0	5.0	0.0
Leek & Carrot, Findus*	1 Pack/400g	440.0	26.0	110	3.5	9.5	6.5	0.0
Potato, Creamy, M & S*	½ Pack/225g	360.0	25.0	160	2.2	11.9	11.1	0.9
Potato, HL, Tesco*	1 Serving/225g	169.0	5.0	75	2.3	11.4	2.2	0.6
Potato, Sainsbury's*	½ Pack/225	448.0	34.0	199	4.4	11.4	15.1	1.0
Spinach & Mushroom, Safeway*	1 Packet/520g	728.0	44.0	140	4.8	10.3	8.4	1.5
Vegetable, Somerfield*	1 Pack/300g	417.0	39.0	139	1.0	5.0	13.0	0.0
GRAVY								
Beef, Aunt Bessie's*	1 Serving/100g	73.0	5.0	73	1.0	5.3	5.3	0.5
Beef, Fresh, Sainsbury's*	1 Serving/83ml	47.0	3.0	56	2.4	4.5	3.2	0.6
Beef, Fresh, Signature, TTD, Sainsbury's*	¼ Pot/123g	38.0	1.0	31	1.9	3.7	0.9	0.6
Beef, Heat & Serve, Morrisons*	1 Serving/150g	27.0	0.0	18	0.3	3.9	0.3	0.5
Beef, Home Style, Savoury, Heinz*	¼ Cup/60g	30.0	1.0	50	1.7	6.7	1.7	0.0
Beef, Rich, Ready to Heat, Schwartz*	½ Pack/100g	31.0	2.0	31	0.8	3.4	1.6	0.5
Beef, with Winter Berry & Shallot, Made Up, Oxo*	1 Serving/105ml	24.0	0.0	23	0.6	4.3	0.3	0.1
Chicken, Granules For, Dry Weight, Bisto*	1 Serving/20g	80.0	3.0	400	1.9	62.5	15.8	0.2

G

	Measure INFO/WEIGHT	per Measure KCAL	FAT	Nutrition Values per 100g / 100ml KCAL	PROT	CARB	FAT	FIBRE
GRAVY								
Chicken, Rich, Ready to Heat, Schwartz*	½ Pack/100g	27.0	1.0	27	0.8	3.3	1.2	0.5
Chips & Onion, Asda*	1 Pack/358g	329.0	9.0	92	2.1	15.0	2.6	1.2
Favourite, Granules, Made Up, Bisto*	1 Serving/50ml	14.0	1.0	28	0.2	4.2	1.2	0.0
Granules for Chicken, Made Up, Smart Price, Asda*	1 Serving/100ml	34.0	2.0	34	0.2	3.0	2.3	0.1
Granules for Meat, Made Up, Asda*	1 Serving/100ml	38.0	2.0	38	0.6	4.0	2.4	0.1
Granules for Meat, Made Up, Sainsbury's*	1 Serving/100ml	37.0	2.0	37	0.4	3.5	2.4	0.1
Granules for Vegetarian Dishes, Dry Weight, Bisto*	1 Serving/28g	100.0	4.0	356	2.7	56.0	13.3	4.5
Granules, Beef, Dry, Tesco*	1 Serving/6g	29.0	2.0	480	5.5	36.4	34.7	1.5
Granules, Beef, Made Up, Tesco*	1 Serving/140ml	48.0	4.0	35	0.3	2.6	2.5	0.1
Granules, Chicken, Dry, Oxo*	1oz/28g	83.0	1.0	296	11.1	54.2	4.9	0.7
Granules, Chicken, Made Up, Oxo*	1 fl oz/30ml	5.0	0.0	18	0.7	3.3	0.3	0.0
Granules, Dry, Bisto*	1 Serving/10g	38.0	2.0	384	3.1	56.4	16.2	1.5
Granules, Dry, Value, Tesco*	1oz/28g	111.0	5.0	397	3.2	54.4	18.5	1.0
Granules, Instant, Dry	**1oz/28g**	**129.0**	**9.0**	**462**	**4.4**	**40.6**	**32.5**	**0.0**
Granules, Instant, Made Up	**1oz/28g**	**10.0**	**1.0**	**34**	**0.3**	**3.0**	**2.4**	**0.0**
Granules, Lamb, Hint of Mint, Made Up, Oxo*	1 Serving/100ml	25.0	0.0	25	0.7	4.3	0.5	0.0
Granules, Made Up, Bisto*	1 Serving/50ml	15.0	1.0	30	0.2	4.2	1.4	0.2
Granules, Made Up, Oxo*	1 Serving/150ml	28.0	0.0	19	0.6	3.4	0.3	0.0
Granules, Onion, Dry, Morrisons*	1 Serving/25g	124.0	9.0	495	3.4	44.0	34.7	0.0
Granules, Onion, Dry, Oxo*	1oz/28g	92.0	1.0	328	8.2	62.3	4.8	0.8
Granules, Onion, Made Up, Oxo*	1 fl oz/30ml	6.0	0.0	20	0.5	3.7	0.3	0.0
Granules, Original, Dry, Oxo*	1oz/28g	88.0	1.0	313	10.2	57.2	4.8	1.0
Granules, Vegetable, Dry, Oxo*	1oz/28g	88.0	1.0	316	8.4	59.5	4.9	0.9
Granules, Vegetable, Dry, Tesco*	½ Pint/20g	94.0	7.0	470	3.8	38.5	33.4	3.7
Onion, Fresh, Asda*	1/6 Pot/77g	30.0	2.0	39	1.7	3.3	2.1	0.4
Onion, Granules For, Dry Weight, Bisto*	4 Tsp/20g	78.0	3.0	391	2.4	62.3	14.7	2.3
Onion, Granules, Made Up, Bisto*	1 Serving/50ml	14.0	0.0	28	0.2	5.6	0.6	0.0
Onion, Rich, M & S*	½ Pack/150g	60.0	2.0	40	2.0	5.9	1.2	0.3
Onion, Rich, Ready to Heat, Schwartz*	½ Sachet/100g	24.0	1.0	24	0.4	4.3	0.6	0.5
Paste, Beef, Antony Worrall Thompson's*	1 Portion/31g	104.0	6.0	334	11.8	30.3	18.4	0.6
Paste, Onion, Antony Worrall Thompson's*	1 Tsp/10g	26.0	0.0	262	7.0	48.7	4.4	1.4
Poultry, Fresh, Signature, TTD, Sainsbury's*	¼ Pot/126g	58.0	2.0	46	3.1	4.9	1.6	0.6
Powder, Gluten Free, Dry, Allergycare*	1 Tbsp/10g	26.0	0.0	260	0.3	63.8	0.4	0.0
Powder, Made Up, Sainsbury's*	1 Serving/100ml	15.0	0.0	15	0.4	3.2	0.1	0.1
Powder, Vegetarian, Organic, Marigold*	1 Serving/22g	79.0	2.0	361	10.6	61.5	7.7	1.3
Roast Beef, Best, in Glass Jar, Made Up, Bisto*	1 Serving/50ml	13.0	0.0	26	0.4	5.4	0.4	0.2
Roast Lamb, Bisto*	1 Serving/20g	60.0	1.0	302	3.4	62.3	4.3	0.0
Roast Pork, Best, in Glass Jar, Dry Weight, Bisto*	4 Tsp/20g	63.0	1.0	314	4.3	64.1	4.5	0.0
Turkey, Granules For, Dry Weight, Bisto*	4 Tsp/20g	75.0	3.0	377	2.4	57.2	15.5	1.0
Turkey, Granules, Made Up, Bisto*	1 Serving/50ml	14.0	1.0	28	0.2	4.0	1.2	0.2
Turkey, Rich, Ready to Heat, Schwartz*	1 Pack/200g	62.0	2.0	31	1.9	3.1	1.2	0.5
Vegetable, Granules For, Dry Weight, Bisto*	1 Tsp/4g	15.0	1.0	380	2.1	63.0	13.3	4.5
Vegetable, Granules For, Made Up, Bisto*	1 Serving/50ml	14.0	0.0	28	0.2	5.6	0.4	0.2
GREENGAGES								
Raw, Average	**1 Fruit/66g**	**26.0**	**0.0**	**39**	**0.7**	**9.4**	**0.1**	**2.0**
GREENS								
Spring, Boiled, Average	**1 Serving/80g**	**16.0**	**1.0**	**20**	**1.9**	**1.6**	**0.7**	**2.6**
Spring, Raw, Average	**1 Serving/80g**	**26.0**	**1.0**	**33**	**3.0**	**3.1**	**1.0**	**3.4**
Spring, Sliced, Fresh, Tesco*	1 Serving/100g	33.0	1.0	33	0.0	2.7	1.0	2.6
GRILLS								
Bacon & Cheese, Tesco*	1 Grill/78g	222.0	15.0	284	15.0	13.4	18.9	1.2
Cheese & Bacon, Danepak*	1 Grill/85g	241.0	16.0	284	15.0	13.4	18.9	1.2
Tikka, Organic, Waitrose*	1 Grill/100g	185.0	9.0	185	6.9	18.5	9.3	3.4

G

	Measure INFO/WEIGHT	per Measure KCAL	FAT	Nutrition Values per 100g / 100ml KCAL	PROT	CARB	FAT	FIBRE
GRILLS								
Vegetable, Dalepak*	1 Grill/83g	125.0	4.0	151	4.0	22.5	5.0	1.6
Vegetable, Mediterranean, Cauldron Foods*	1 Grill/88g	145.0	10.0	166	5.3	15.8	11.9	6.5
Vegetable, Ross*	1 Grill/114g	252.0	13.0	221	4.3	25.5	11.3	0.9
Vegetable, Tesco*	1 Grill/72g	129.0	7.0	179	4.2	18.0	10.0	2.2
Vegetarian, Mushroom & Oregano, Organic, Waitrose*	1 Grill/100g	200.0	10.0	200	7.9	19.5	10.0	4.3
GRILLSTICKS								
Lamb, Minty, Morrisons*	1 Grillstick/65g	192.0	13.0	296	14.9	5.7	20.0	0.3
GRITS								
Enriched White Hominy, Old Fashioned, Quaker Oats*	¼ Cup/41g	140.0	1.0	341	7.3	78.0	1.2	4.9
GROUSE								
Meat Only, Roasted	*1oz/28g*	*36.0*	*1.0*	*128*	*27.6*	*0.0*	*2.0*	*0.0*
GUACAMOLE								
Average	1 Tbsp/17g	22.0	2.0	128	1.4	2.2	12.7	2.5
Avocado, Reduced Fat, The Fresh Dip Company*	1 Serving/113g	128.0	10.0	113	2.5	6.1	8.7	2.3
Chunky, M & S*	1 Pot/170g	221.0	19.0	130	1.5	5.1	11.3	1.7
Chunky, Sainsbury's*	½ Pot/65g	120.0	12.0	185	1.6	3.2	18.4	3.8
Doritos, Walkers*	1 Tbsp/20g	32.0	3.0	159	1.2	2.6	16.0	0.1
Fresh, Sainsbury's*	1oz/28g	59.0	6.0	210	1.8	5.3	20.2	2.5
Fresh, VLH Kitchens	1 Serving/17g	27.0	3.0	158	1.5	3.0	14.6	2.5
Fresh, Waitrose*	½ Pack/100g	190.0	18.0	190	1.9	4.1	18.4	2.5
GFY, Asda*	1 Pack/113g	144.0	12.0	127	2.8	4.3	11.0	2.2
Mexican Style, Dip Selection, Morrisons*	½ Pack/50g	102.0	10.0	204	1.5	3.7	20.4	0.9
Reduced Fat, Sainsbury's*	½ Pot/65g	87.0	8.0	134	1.5	3.5	12.6	4.0
Reduced Fat, Tesco*	1 Pack/200g	280.0	23.0	140	2.7	5.7	11.4	3.0
Reduced Fat, Waitrose*	1 Serving/25g	31.0	3.0	126	2.9	5.7	10.1	2.3
GUAVA								
Canned, in Syrup	*1oz/28g*	*17.0*	*0.0*	*60*	*0.4*	*15.7*	*0.0*	*3.0*
Raw, Flesh Only, Average	*1 Fruit/55g*	*37.0*	*1.0*	*68*	*3.0*	*14.0*	*1.0*	*5.0*
GUINEA FOWL								
Boned & Stuffed, Fresh, Fayrefield Foods*	1 Serving/325g	650.0	39.0	200	19.1	3.3	12.1	0.5
Fresh, Free Range, Waitrose*	1 Portion/193g	258.0	12.0	134	19.5	0.0	6.2	0.3
GUMBO								
Cajun Vegetable, Sainsbury's*	1 Serving/450g	265.0	11.0	59	1.4	7.7	2.5	1.5
Louisiana Chicken, Perfectly Balanced, Waitrose*	1 Serving/235g	207.0	7.0	88	12.2	3.5	2.8	1.3

G

HADDOCK

Fillet, Smoked, in Mustard & Dill, The Saucy Fish Co.*	2 Fillets/270g		262.0	10.0	97	15.5	0.1	3.6	0.0
Fillets, Battered, Average	1oz/28g		64.0	3.0	228	13.4	16.3	12.2	1.1
Fillets, in Breadcrumbs, Average	1oz/28g		57.0	3.0	203	13.5	14.9	9.9	1.2
Fillets, Raw, Average	*1oz/28g*		*22.0*	*0.0*	*80*	*18.0*	*0.2*	*0.8*	*0.0*
Fillets, Smoked, Cooked, Average	*1 Pack/300g*		*337.0*	*8.0*	*112*	*21.9*	*0.4*	*2.6*	*0.1*
Fillets, Smoked, Raw, Average	*1 Pack/227g*		*194.0*	*1.0*	*86*	*20.3*	*0.1*	*0.5*	*0.2*
Goujons, Batter, Crispy, M & S*	1 Serving/100g		250.0	14.0	250	11.7	18.5	14.1	0.8
Loins, Beer Battered, Chunky, TTD, Sainsbury's*	1 Fillet/93g		177.0	9.0	191	15.8	10.5	9.5	2.3
Loins, Skinless, Frozen, TTD, Sainsbury's*	1 Serving/100g		116.0	0.0	116	28.5	0.1	0.2	0.1
Loins, TTD, Sainsbury's*	1 Serving/100g		108.0	1.0	108	25.5	0.0	0.7	0.0

HADDOCK EN CROUTE

Youngs*	1 Serving/170g		432.0	29.0	254	8.0	17.1	16.9	4.3

HADDOCK IN

Butter Sauce, Steaks, Youngs*	1 Serving/150g		133.0	6.0	89	9.9	4.0	3.7	0.5
Cheese & Chive Sauce, Fillets, Go Cook, Asda*	1 Pack/360g		400.0	19.0	111	14.8	1.5	5.3	0.2
Cheese & Chive Sauce, Smoked Fillets, Seafresh*	1 Serving/170g		201.0	10.0	118	14.7	1.2	6.1	0.1
Cheese & Leek Sauce, Fillets, SteamFresh, Birds Eye*	1 Serving/190g		165.0	7.0	87	11.0	2.4	3.7	0.2
Fillets, In Cheese Sauce, Fresh Tastes, Asda*	½ Pack/180g		212.0	10.0	118	16.2	1.3	5.3	0.6
Smoked Leek & Cheese Sauce, Asda*	½ Pack/200g		232.0	10.0	116	14.0	3.7	5.0	1.5
Tomato Herb Sauce, Fillets, BGTY, Sainsbury's*	½ Pack/165g		150.0	5.0	91	12.9	3.6	2.8	0.1
Watercress Sauce, GFY, Asda*	1 Pack/400g		268.0	7.0	67	6.0	7.0	1.7	1.4

HADDOCK WITH

a Rich Cheese Crust, Smoked, Sainsbury's*	1 Serving/199g		295.0	19.0	148	13.0	2.5	9.5	0.9
Broccoli & Cheese, Lakeland*	1 Serving/150g		280.0	10.0	187	10.4	20.6	7.0	0.0
Cheese & Chive Sauce, Atlantic, Youngs*	½ Pack/180g		184.0	9.0	102	13.0	1.7	4.8	0.2
Creme Fraiche & Chive Sauce, Smoked, Tesco*	1 Serving/150g		154.0	5.0	103	16.8	2.1	3.1	0.3

HAGGIS

Neeps & Tatties, M & S*	1 Pack/300g		330.0	14.0	110	3.8	12.3	4.8	0.8
Traditional, Average	*1 Serving/454g*		*1119.0*	*67.0*	*246*	*12.3*	*17.2*	*14.6*	*1.0*
Vegetarian, McSween*	1 Serving/100g		216.0	10.0	216	6.6	26.8	10.2	2.4

HAKE

Fillets, Herby Mediterranean Glaze, Sensations, Youngs*	½ Pack/120g		106.0	3.0	88	16.8	0.4	2.2	0.0
Fillets, in Breadcrumbs, Average	1oz/28g		66.0	4.0	234	12.9	15.9	13.3	1.0
Goujons, Average	1 Serving/150g		345.0	18.0	230	12.4	18.6	11.9	1.3
Raw, Average	*1oz/28g*		*29.0*	*1.0*	*102*	*20.4*	*0.0*	*2.2*	*0.0*
with Tomato & Chilli Salsa, Just Cook, Sainsbury's*	½ Pack/180g		112.0	2.0	62	11.4	2.2	0.9	0.0

HALIBUT

Cooked, Average	*1oz/28g*		*38.0*	*1.0*	*135*	*24.6*	*0.4*	*4.0*	*0.0*
Raw	*1oz/28g*		*29.0*	*1.0*	*103*	*21.5*	*0.0*	*1.9*	*0.0*

HALVA

Average	*1oz/28g*		*107.0*	*4.0*	*381*	*1.8*	*68.0*	*13.2*	*0.0*

HAM

Applewood Smoked, Average	*1 Slice/28g*		*31.0*	*1.0*	*112*	*21.2*	*0.5*	*2.7*	*0.2*
Baked, Average	*1 Slice/74g*		*106.0*	*4.0*	*143*	*21.1*	*1.8*	*5.8*	*0.3*
Boiled, Average	*1 Pack/113g*		*154.0*	*6.0*	*136*	*20.6*	*0.6*	*5.7*	*0.0*
Breaded, Average	*1 Slice/37g*		*57.0*	*2.0*	*155*	*23.1*	*1.8*	*6.3*	*1.6*
Breaded, Dry Cured, Average	*1 Slice/33g*		*47.0*	*2.0*	*142*	*22.1*	*1.4*	*5.4*	*0.0*
Brunswick, Average	*1 Slice/20g*		*32.0*	*2.0*	*160*	*19.5*	*0.6*	*8.8*	*0.0*
Cooked, Sliced, Average	*1 Serving/50g*		*57.0*	*2.0*	*115*	*19.1*	*0.9*	*3.9*	*0.1*
Crumbed, Sliced, Average	*1 Slice/28g*		*33.0*	*1.0*	*117*	*21.5*	*0.9*	*3.1*	*0.0*
Danish, Average	*1 Slice/11g*		*14.0*	*1.0*	*125*	*18.4*	*1.0*	*5.3*	*0.0*
Danish, Lean, Average	*1 Slice/15g*		*14.0*	*0.0*	*92*	*17.8*	*1.0*	*1.8*	*0.0*
Dry Cured, Average	*1 Slice/18g*		*26.0*	*1.0*	*144*	*22.4*	*1.0*	*5.5*	*0.2*

	Measure INFO/WEIGHT	per Measure KCAL	FAT	Nutrition Values per 100g / 100ml KCAL	PROT	CARB	FAT	FIBRE
HAM								
Extra Lean, Average	1 Slice/11g	10.0	0.0	90	18.0	1.4	1.4	0.0
Gammon, Breaded, Average	1 Serving/25g	31.0	1.0	122	22.0	1.5	3.1	0.0
Gammon, Dry Cured, Sliced, Average	1 Slice/33g	43.0	1.0	131	22.9	0.4	4.2	0.0
Gammon, Honey Roast, Average	1 Serving/60g	81.0	3.0	134	22.4	0.4	4.7	0.0
Gammon, Smoked, Average	1 Slice/43g	59.0	2.0	137	22.3	0.7	4.9	0.2
German Black Forest, Average	½ Pack/35g	93.0	6.0	267	27.2	1.3	17.0	0.5
Honey & Mustard, Average	1oz/28g	39.0	1.0	140	20.8	4.6	4.3	0.0
Honey Roast, Average	1 Slice/20g	25.0	1.0	123	20.3	1.5	3.8	0.1
Honey Roast, Dry Cured, Average	1 Slice/33g	46.0	1.0	140	22.7	2.3	4.4	0.2
Honey Roast, Lean, Average	1 Serving/25g	28.0	1.0	111	18.1	2.7	3.1	0.0
Honey Roast, Wafer Thin, Average	1 Slice/10g	11.0	0.0	113	17.4	3.7	3.2	0.3
Honey Roast, Wafer Thin, Premium, Average	1 Slice/10g	15.0	1.0	149	22.0	1.6	6.0	0.0
Lean, Average	1 Slice/18g	19.0	0.0	104	19.5	1.1	2.4	0.3
Oak Smoked, Average	1 Slice/20g	26.0	1.0	130	21.0	1.0	4.7	0.3
Parma, Average	1 Slice/10g	21.0	1.0	213	29.3	0.0	10.6	0.0
Parma, Premium, Average	1 Slice/14g	36.0	2.0	258	27.9	0.3	16.1	0.0
Peppered, Average	1 Slice/12g	13.0	0.0	109	18.5	2.0	2.7	0.0
Peppered, Dry Cured, Average	1 Slice/31g	43.0	1.0	140	23.1	1.3	4.7	0.2
Prosciutto, Average	1 Slice/12g	27.0	1.0	226	28.7	0.0	12.3	0.3
Serrano, Average	1 Slice/20g	46.0	2.0	230	30.5	0.4	11.8	0.0
Smoked, Average	1Slice/18g	21.0	1.0	117	19.7	0.9	3.7	0.0
Smoked, Dry Cured, Average	1 Slice/28g	38.0	1.0	137	23.0	1.4	4.4	0.1
Smoked, Wafer Thin, Average	1 Serving/40g	41.0	1.0	102	17.7	1.2	2.9	0.2
Thick Cut, Average	1 Slice/74g	94.0	3.0	127	22.4	0.6	3.9	0.1
Tinned, Average	½ Can/100g	136.0	9.0	136	12.2	2.0	8.7	0.0
Tinned, Lean, Average	½ Can/100g	94.0	2.0	94	18.1	0.2	2.3	0.4
Wafer Thin, Average	1 Slice/10g	10.0	0.0	101	17.9	1.4	2.6	0.1
Wiltshire, Average	1oz/28g	41.0	2.0	147	23.1	0.0	6.0	0.0
Wiltshire, Breaded, Average	1oz/28g	41.0	1.0	145	23.9	1.0	5.0	0.0
HARE								
Raw, Lean Only, Average	1oz/28g	35.0	1.0	125	23.5	0.2	3.5	0.0
Stewed, Lean Only, Average	1oz/28g	48.0	2.0	170	29.5	0.2	5.5	0.0
HARIBO*								
American Hard Gums, Haribo*	1 Pack/175g	630.0	3.0	360	0.3	85.5	1.9	0.2
Cola Bottles, Haribo*	1 Sm Pack/16g	56.0	0.0	348	7.7	78.9	0.2	0.3
Dinosaurs, Haribo*	1oz/28g	95.0	0.0	340	6.3	78.3	0.2	0.5
Dolly Mixtures, Haribo*	1 Pack/175g	719.0	8.0	411	1.8	90.2	4.8	0.2
Fantasy Mix, Haribo*	1 Pack/100g	344.0	0.0	344	6.6	79.0	0.2	0.3
Fried Eggs/eggstras, Haribo*	1oz/28g	96.0	0.0	344	6.6	79.0	0.2	0.0
Gold Bears, Haribo*	1 Pack/100g	348.0	0.0	348	7.7	78.9	0.2	0.3
Horror Mix, Haribo*	1 Pack/100g	344.0	0.0	344	6.6	79.0	0.2	0.3
Jelly Babies, Haribo*	1oz/28g	97.0	0.0	348	4.5	82.1	0.2	0.5
Kiddies Super Mix, Haribo*	1 Pack/100g	344.0	0.0	344	6.6	79.0	0.2	0.3
Magic Mix, Haribo*	1oz/28g	102.0	1.0	366	5.4	82.0	1.9	0.3
Maoam Stripes, Haribo*	1 Chew/7g	27.0	0.0	384	1.2	81.7	6.1	0.3
Mega Roulette, Haribo*	1oz/28g	97.0	0.0	348	7.7	78.9	0.2	0.3
Micro Mix, Haribo*	1oz/28g	106.0	1.0	379	4.7	84.5	2.5	0.4
Milky Mix, Haribo*	1 Pack/175g	607.0	0.0	347	7.1	79.6	0.2	0.4
Mint Imperials, Haribo*	1 Pack/175g	695.0	1.0	397	0.4	98.8	0.5	0.1
Peaches, Haribo*	1oz/28g	98.0	0.0	350	4.3	82.1	0.0	0.0
Pontefract Cakes, Haribo*	1 Pack/200g	612.0	3.0	306	5.3	68.2	1.3	5.6
Shrimps, Haribo*	1oz/28g	99.0	0.0	352	6.1	81.5	0.2	0.1
Snakes, Haribo*	1 Snake/8g	28.0	0.0	348	7.7	78.9	0.2	0.3

H

	Measure INFO/WEIGHT	per Measure KCAL	FAT	Nutrition Values per 100g / 100ml KCAL	PROT	CARB	FAT	FIBRE
HARIBO*								
Star Mix, Haribo*	1 Mini Pack/16g	55.0	0.0	344	6.6	79.0	0.2	0.3
Starmix, Haribo*	1 Pack/100g	344.0	0.0	344	6.6	79.0	0.2	0.3
Tangfastics, Haribo*	1 Pack/100g	359.0	2.0	359	6.3	78.3	2.3	0.5
Tropifruit, Haribo*	1oz/28g	97.0	0.0	348	4.5	82.1	0.2	0.5
HARISSA PASTE								
Average	1 Tsp/5g	6.0	0.0	123	2.9	12.9	6.7	2.8
Moroccan Style, Al'fez*	1 Tsp/10g	19.0	1.0	190	4.0	18.2	11.2	3.4
HASH								
Barbecue Beef, COU, M & S*	1 Pack/400g	360.0	2.0	90	7.0	14.0	0.4	1.4
Corned Beef, Apetito*	1 Pack/380g	423.0	24.0	111	3.8	10.3	6.2	1.3
Corned Beef, Asda*	1 Pack/400g	416.0	14.0	104	6.0	12.0	3.6	1.1
Corned Beef, Chilled, Co-Op*	1 Pack/300g	345.0	18.0	115	9.0	5.0	6.0	1.0
Corned Beef, Frozen, Tesco*	1 Serving/400g	348.0	10.0	87	5.7	10.3	2.6	0.7
Corned Beef, M & S*	½ Pack/321g	385.0	20.0	120	8.1	7.4	6.3	1.3
Corned Beef, Tesco*	1 Serving/400g	416.0	10.0	104	5.3	14.8	2.6	1.7
HASH BROWNS								
Birds Eye*	1 Serving/63g	126.0	7.0	200	2.0	21.9	11.6	1.6
Farmfoods*	1oz/28g	35.0	1.0	124	2.1	18.2	4.7	2.1
Potato, Iceland*	1 Piece/33g	75.0	4.0	227	2.2	27.1	12.2	2.6
Ross*	1 Piece/46g	84.0	4.0	183	2.0	23.9	8.7	2.0
Tesco*	1oz/28g	43.0	2.0	154	2.4	20.0	7.2	1.7
HAZELNUTS								
Chopped, Average	*1 Serving/10g*	*67.0*	*6.0*	*665*	*16.7*	*5.6*	*64.0*	*6.5*
Whole, Average	*10 Whole/10g*	*65.0*	*6.0*	*655*	*15.3*	*5.8*	*63.5*	*6.5*
HEART								
Lambs, Average	*1 Heart/75g*	*91.0*	*4.0*	*122*	*16.0*	*1.0*	*6.0*	*0.0*
Ox, Raw	*1oz/28g*	*29.0*	*1.0*	*104*	*18.2*	*0.0*	*3.5*	*0.0*
Ox, Stewed	*1oz/28g*	*44.0*	*1.0*	*157*	*27.8*	*0.0*	*5.1*	*0.0*
Pig, Raw	*1oz/28g*	*27.0*	*1.0*	*97*	*17.1*	*0.0*	*3.2*	*0.0*
Pig, Stewed	*1oz/28g*	*45.0*	*2.0*	*162*	*25.1*	*0.0*	*6.8*	*0.0*
HERMESETAS								
Powdered, Hermes*	1 Tsp/0.78	3.0	0.0	387	1.0	96.8	0.0	0.0
The Classic Sweetener, Hermes*	1 Tablet/0.5g	0.0	0.0	294	14.2	59.3	0.0	0.0
HEROES								
Dairy Milk, Whole Nut, Cadbury*	1 Chocolate/11g	60.0	4.0	545	9.1	48.2	35.2	0.0
Fudge, Cadbury*	1 Sweet/10g	43.0	1.0	435	2.5	72.7	14.9	0.0
HERRING								
Canned, in Tomato Sauce, Average	1oz/28g	57.0	4.0	204	11.9	4.1	15.5	0.1
Dried, Salted, Average	*1oz/28g*	*47.0*	*2.0*	*168*	*25.3*	*0.0*	*7.4*	*0.0*
Fillets, in Mustard & Dill Sauce, John West*	1 Can/190g	332.0	27.0	175	9.4	2.9	14.0	0.1
Fillets, in Olive Oil, Succulent, Princes*	1 Serving/50g	107.0	7.0	215	20.0	0.0	15.0	0.0
Fillets, Raw, Average	*1 Herring/100g*	*185.0*	*13.0*	*185*	*18.4*	*0.0*	*12.6*	*0.0*
Grilled, Average	*1oz/28g*	*51.0*	*3.0*	*181*	*20.1*	*0.0*	*11.2*	*0.0*
in Horseradish Sauce, John West*	1oz/28g	64.0	5.0	230	13.0	4.0	18.0	0.0
Pickled, Average	1oz/28g	73.0	5.0	262	14.2	9.6	18.0	0.0
Pickled, in Mustard Sauce, Abba*	1 Serving/58g	149.0	11.0	260	7.0	16.0	19.0	0.0
Rollmop, with Onion, Asda*	1 Rollmop/65g	89.0	3.0	137	13.2	10.3	4.8	0.8
Rollmops, Tesco*	1 Rollmop/65g	110.0	5.0	170	12.0	10.4	8.4	0.4
Smoked, Pepper, in Oil, Glyngøre*	1 Can/130g	338.0	25.0	260	21.0	0.0	19.0	0.0
HIGH LIGHTS								
Caffe Latte, Made Up, Cadbury*	1 Serving/200g	40.0	1.0	20	1.0	2.5	0.7	0.0
Choc Mint, Made Up, Cadbury*	1 Serving/200ml	40.0	1.0	20	1.0	2.5	0.7	0.3
Chocolate Orange, Made Up, Cadbury*	1 Serving/200ml	40.0	1.0	20	1.0	2.3	0.7	0.3

H

	Measure INFO/WEIGHT	KCAL	FAT	Nutrition Values per 100g / 100ml				
				KCAL	PROT	CARB	FAT	FIBRE
HIGH LIGHTS								
Chocolate, Dairy Fudge, Dry Weight, Cadbury*	1 Serving/11g	40.0	1.0	363	17.0	50.0	10.0	0.0
Dairy Fudge, Made Up, Cadbury*	1 Serving/200ml	40.0	1.0	20	1.0	2.8	0.5	0.2
Dark Chocolate, Cadbury*	1 Sachet/11g	35.0	1.0	315	23.1	37.3	8.1	0.0
Dark Chocolate, Made Up, Cadbury*	1 Serving/200ml	35.0	1.0	17	1.2	2.0	0.4	0.0
Espresso, Made Up, Cadbury*	1 Serving/200ml	35.0	1.0	17	1.2	1.9	0.4	0.0
Fudge, Made Up, Cadbury*	1 Serving/200ml	40.0	1.0	20	0.9	2.5	0.5	0.0
Hot Chocolate Drink, Instant, Dry Weight, Cadbury*	1 Sachet/11g	38.0	1.0	350	16.6	42.0	12.8	3.0
Hot Chocolate Drink, Instant, Made Up, Cadbury*	1 Cup/200ml	40.0	1.0	20	1.0	2.5	0.7	0.3
Instant Hot Chocolate, Cadbury*	1 Sachet/22g	80.0	3.0	364	17.3	44.5	12.7	0.0
Mint, Cadbury*	1 Serving/200ml	40.0	1.0	20	1.0	2.5	0.7	0.0
Toffee Flavour, Made Up, Cadbury*	1 Serving/200ml	40.0	1.0	20	1.0	2.6	0.7	0.0
Wafer - Orange, Cadbury*	1 Serving/19g	80.0	3.0	430	5.2	70.6	14.3	1.4
HOKI								
Grilled	*1oz/28g*	*34.0*	*1.0*	*121*	*24.1*	*0.0*	*2.7*	*0.0*
in Breadcrumbs, Average	1 Piece/156g	298.0	14.0	191	14.5	13.9	8.9	1.2
Raw	*1oz/28g*	*24.0*	*1.0*	*85*	*16.9*	*0.0*	*1.9*	*0.0*
Steaks, in Batter, Crispy, Birds Eye*	1 Steak/123g	320.0	17.0	260	12.4	21.3	13.9	0.8
HONEY								
Acacia Blossom, Sainsbury's*	1 Serving/24g	81.0	0.0	339	0.1	84.7	0.1	0.3
Australian Eucalyptus, Finest, Tesco*	1 Tsp/4g	12.0	0.0	307	0.4	76.4	0.0	0.0
Clover, Canadian, TTD, Sainsbury's*	1 Tbsp/15g	50.0	0.0	336	0.2	83.6	0.1	0.1
Florida Orange, Extra Special, Asda*	1 Tbsp/15g	50.0	0.0	334	0.5	83.0	0.0	0.1
Greek, Waitrose*	1 Tsp/6g	18.0	0.0	307	0.4	76.4	0.0	0.0
Pure, Clear, Average	*1 Tbsp/20g*	*63.0*	*0.0*	*314*	*0.3*	*79.1*	*0.0*	*0.0*
Pure, Set, Average	*1 Tbsp/20g*	*62.0*	*0.0*	*312*	*0.4*	*77.6*	*0.0*	*0.0*
Scottish Heather, Waitrose*	1 Serving/20g	61.0	0.0	307	0.4	76.4	0.0	0.0
Spanish Orange Blossom, Sainsbury's*	1 Tbsp/15g	51.0	0.0	339	0.1	84.7	0.0	0.3
HOOCH*								
Vodka, (Calculated Estimate), Hooch*	1 Bottle/330ml	244.0	0.0	74	0.3	5.1	0.0	0.0
HORLICKS								
Malted Drink, Extra Light, Instant, Dry Weight, Horlicks*	1 Serving/11g	35.0	1.0	319	8.4	57.4	6.2	10.5
Malted Drink, Light, Dry Weight, Horlicks*	1 Serving/32g	116.0	1.0	364	14.8	72.2	3.8	1.9
Malted Drink, Light, Made Up, Horlicks*	1 Mug/200ml	116.0	1.0	58	2.3	11.5	0.6	0.3
Powder, Made Up with Semi-Skimmed Milk	1 Mug/227ml	184.0	4.0	81	4.3	12.9	1.9	0.0
Powder, Made Up with Skimmed Milk	1 Mug/227ml	159.0	1.0	70	4.3	12.9	0.5	0.0
Powder, Made Up with Whole Milk	1 Mug/227ml	225.0	9.0	99	4.2	12.7	3.9	0.0
HORSE								
Meat, Raw, Average	*1 Serving/110g*	*146.0*	*5.0*	*133*	*21.4*	*0.0*	*4.6*	*0.0*
HORSERADISH								
Prepared, Average	*1 Tsp/5g*	*3.0*	*0.0*	*62*	*4.5*	*11.0*	*0.3*	*6.2*
HOT CHOCOLATE								
Balanced Lifestyle, Camelot*	1 Sachet/11g	40.0	2.0	363	18.5	40.6	14.1	0.5
Cadbury*	1 Serving/12g	44.0	1.0	370	6.3	73.3	5.9	0.0
Caramel, Whittards of Chelsea*	1 Serving/20g	71.0	1.0	355	7.5	64.5	7.5	13.0
Chococino, Dulce Gusto, Nescafe*	1 Serving/34g	149.0	5.0	437	14.6	58.6	16.1	4.6
Chocolate Break, Dry, Tesco*	1 Serving/21g	110.0	6.0	524	7.9	58.9	28.5	1.7
Dreamtime, Whittards of Chelsea*	5 Tsps/20g	72.0	1.0	361	6.6	72.4	5.1	8.7
Drink, Organic, Green & Black's*	1 Tsp/4g	13.0	0.0	374	9.1	63.5	9.3	0.1
Dry Weight, Tassimo, Suchard*	1 Cup/27g	88.0	2.0	325	3.2	58.0	8.9	2.6
Galaxy, Mars*	1 Sachet/28g	115.0	3.0	411	7.0	68.7	12.1	0.0
Impress*	1 Serving/25g	90.0	1.0	360	5.6	76.0	3.6	6.0
Instant Break, Cadbury*	1 Sachet/28g	119.0	4.0	425	10.9	64.2	14.0	0.0
Instant, BGTY, Made Up, Sainsbury's*	1 Sachet/28g	16.0	0.0	56	2.1	10.6	0.6	0.3

	Measure INFO/WEIGHT	per Measure KCAL	FAT	Nutrition Values per 100g / 100ml KCAL	PROT	CARB	FAT	FIBRE
HOT CHOCOLATE								
Instant, Skinny Cow*	1 Sachet/10g	37.0	1.0	370	19.7	39.3	14.6	0.0
Instant, Tesco*	1 Serving/32g	155.0	10.0	485	10.5	38.1	32.3	5.0
Luxury, Skinny, Whittards of Chelsea*	1 Serving/28g	92.0	1.0	328	12.9	67.1	2.8	13.5
Made Up, Tassimo, Suchard*	1 Serving/280ml	88.0	2.0	31	0.3	5.5	0.9	0.2
Maltesers, Malt Drink, Instant, Made Up, Mars*	1 Serving/220ml	104.0	3.0	47	0.9	7.7	1.4	0.0
Slim Fast*	1 Serving/59g	203.0	3.0	347	22.2	53.8	4.8	8.4
Toffee Flavour, Good Intentions, Somerfield*	1 Serving/34g	130.0	2.0	381	7.4	77.0	4.8	2.6
Velvet, Cadbury*	1 Serving/28g	136.0	7.0	487	8.6	57.8	24.6	2.0
HOT DOG								
Feasters, Eat Well, M & S*	1 Sausage/140g	326.0	11.0	233	11.0	29.1	8.1	1.6
Sausage, American Style, Average	1 Sausage/75g	180.0	14.0	241	11.6	6.2	19.0	0.0
Sausage, Average	1 Sausage/23g	40.0	3.0	175	10.8	4.3	12.8	0.3
HOT DOG VEGETARIAN								
Meat Free, Sainsbury's*	1 Sausage/30g	71.0	5.0	237	18.0	7.6	15.0	1.0
Tesco*	1 Sausage/30g	66.0	4.0	220	18.0	2.7	15.0	2.0
HOT POT								
Beef & Vegetable, Weight Watchers*	1 Pack/300g	228.0	7.0	76	4.0	10.2	2.2	0.9
Beef, Apetito*	1 Pack/340g	303.0	10.0	89	5.1	10.3	3.1	1.3
Beef, Healthy Options, Birds Eye*	1 Pack/350g	294.0	7.0	84	4.5	12.0	2.0	1.2
Beef, Minced, Sainsbury's*	1 Pack/450g	463.0	22.0	103	5.3	9.5	4.9	2.2
Beef, Ross*	1 Pack/322g	254.0	11.0	79	2.5	9.4	3.5	0.4
Beef, Weight Watchers*	1 Pack/320g	209.0	7.0	65	3.5	8.1	2.1	1.3
Chicken & Cider, Ready Meals, Waitrose*	1 Pack/400g	500.0	20.0	125	6.8	12.9	5.1	1.1
Chicken & Mushroom, HL, Tesco*	1 Serving/450g	369.0	7.0	82	6.3	11.8	1.5	0.5
Chicken, Chunky, Weight Watchers*	1 Pack/320g	275.0	9.0	86	4.7	10.4	2.8	0.6
Chicken, Eat Smart, Morrisons*	1 Pack/400g	308.0	6.0	77	4.5	11.1	1.5	1.7
Chicken, Frozen, Asda*	1 Pack/400g	300.0	6.0	75	5.5	9.9	1.5	0.8
Chicken, GFY, Asda*	1 Serving/400g	256.0	5.0	64	4.8	8.2	1.3	1.4
Chicken, Light Choices, Tesco*	1 Pack/450g	315.0	7.0	70	4.1	9.6	1.6	1.2
Chicken, Low Fat, Solo Slim, Rosemary Conley*	1/100g	81.0	3.0	81	6.7	7.1	2.9	2.5
Chicken, Sainsbury's*	1 Pack/400g	340.0	11.0	85	5.2	9.8	2.7	1.3
Chicken, Traditional, Pro Cuisine*	1 Pack/400g	208.0	4.0	52	5.8	5.2	0.9	0.0
Chunky Vegetable & Tomato, Big Eat, Heinz*	1 Pot/355g	213.0	1.0	60	2.5	11.7	0.4	4.1
Lamb & Vegetable, Asda*	1 Pot/500g	240.0	2.0	48	4.0	7.0	0.4	0.0
Lamb Shank, Extra Special, Asda*	1 Pack/450g	508.0	20.0	113	10.2	7.8	4.5	1.3
Lamb, Diet Chef Ltd*	1 Pack/300g	276.0	5.0	92	8.9	10.1	1.8	3.0
Lamb, Heinz*	1 Pack/340g	337.0	11.0	99	4.9	12.7	3.1	1.7
Lamb, Low Fat, Solo Slim, Rosemary Conley*	1/100g	92.0	2.0	92	8.9	10.1	1.8	3.0
Lamb, Minced, Mini Classics, Asda*	1 Pack/300g	222.0	10.0	74	5.3	5.4	3.5	3.3
Lamb, Organic, Great Stuff, Asda*	1 Pack/300g	327.0	10.0	109	8.0	11.6	3.4	1.1
Lancashire, M & S*	1 Pack/454g	431.0	15.0	95	10.1	6.7	3.3	1.0
Lancashire, Sainsbury's*	½ Pack/225g	220.0	9.0	98	6.1	9.5	3.9	1.0
Liver & Bacon, Tesco*	1 Pack/550g	693.0	31.0	126	6.4	12.3	5.7	1.5
Minced Beef & Vegetable, COU, M & S*	1 Pack/400g	380.0	7.0	95	10.3	9.0	1.7	2.4
Minced Beef, Frozen, Tesco*	1 Pack/450g	337.0	11.0	75	4.0	9.1	2.5	1.4
Minced Beef, Smart Price, Asda*	1 Pack/300g	199.0	4.0	66	3.7	10.0	1.3	0.4
Roast, Vegetable, with Gravy, Hometown Buffet*	1 Serving/113g	50.0	0.0	44	0.9	11.5	0.4	1.8
Sausage with Baked Beans, Heinz*	1 Can/340g	354.0	11.0	104	4.6	14.3	3.2	2.4
Sausage, Aunt Bessie's*	¼ Pack/200g	212.0	9.0	106	3.6	12.6	4.6	1.9
Sausage, Smart Price, Asda*	1 Pack/300g	239.0	7.0	80	3.7	11.0	2.3	0.4
Vegetable, Tesco*	1 Serving/450g	432.0	22.0	96	1.7	11.2	4.9	3.5
HOUMOUS								
Balsamic Caramelised Red Onion, Extra Special, Asda*	½ Pack/50g	146.0	11.0	293	6.8	18.2	21.4	1.0

	Measure INFO/WEIGHT	per Measure KCAL	FAT	Nutrition Values per 100g / 100ml KCAL	PROT	CARB	FAT	FIBRE
HOUMOUS								
Caramelised Onion, Tesco*	¼ Pack/50g	125.0	10.0	250	5.5	13.0	19.4	4.2
Chilli & Red Pepper, Topped, Tesco*	½ Pack/100g	281.0	25.0	281	7.1	6.6	25.1	8.1
Feta, Fresh, Sainsbury's*	1 Serving/100g	292.0	27.0	292	8.0	3.5	27.4	6.7
Fresh, Sainsbury's*	1 Serving/50g	156.0	14.0	312	7.3	8.9	27.5	2.2
Fresh, Waitrose*	1 Serving/75g	219.0	20.0	292	7.2	6.3	26.4	7.6
Garlic & Pesto, Asda*	1 Serving/34g	107.0	9.0	314	8.0	12.0	26.0	0.0
Jalapeno, Sainsbury's*	¼ Pot/50g	148.0	13.0	296	6.4	7.2	26.8	5.7
Lemon & Coriander, BGTY, Sainsbury's*	½ Tub/100g	145.0	9.0	145	6.3	9.7	9.0	5.9
Lemon & Coriander, Sainsbury's*	¼ Tub/50g	145.0	13.0	291	7.0	9.1	25.1	6.0
Mediterranean Deli, M & S*	¼ Pack/70g	203.0	18.0	290	7.8	8.0	25.3	6.5
Mixed Olive, Sainsbury's*	¼ Pot/50g	134.0	12.0	268	6.7	8.4	23.1	7.7
Moroccan Style, Sainsbury's*	¼ Pot/50g	113.0	10.0	227	5.5	7.3	19.5	6.6
Moroccan, Tesco*	¼ Pot/50g	144.0	13.0	289	6.8	8.1	25.5	7.3
Olive & Sundried Tomato, Tesco*	1 Serving/50g	117.0	10.0	235	6.5	8.0	19.5	7.4
Olive & Tomato, Mixed, Sainsbury's*	¼ Tub/50g	136.0	13.0	272	6.0	5.3	25.2	7.4
Organic, M & S*	¼ Pack/25g	82.0	7.0	330	6.9	9.1	29.7	3.3
Organic, Sainsbury's*	¼ Pot/43g	139.0	12.0	326	6.8	10.7	28.4	3.5
Pesto Style Houmous, Sainsbury's*	1 Spread/25g	85.0	7.0	339	7.9	10.8	29.4	5.7
Red Pepper Pesto, Tesco*	¼ Pot/50g	137.0	11.0	275	7.4	9.7	22.6	5.7
Red Pepper, Reduced Fat, Tesco*	1 Pot/60g	159.0	11.0	265	7.2	17.4	18.3	4.8
Reduced Fat, Average	1 Serving/30g	72.0	5.0	241	9.2	13.3	16.8	3.6
Roasted Aubergine, M & S*	½ Pot/85g	132.0	10.0	155	4.9	6.9	12.1	5.1
Roasted Red Pepper, 50% Less Fat, Tesco*	½ Pot/85g	156.0	11.0	184	7.3	10.9	12.4	9.5
Roasted Red Pepper, BGTY, Sainsbury's*	¼ Tub/50g	64.0	3.0	129	4.9	11.9	6.9	5.3
Roasted Red Pepper, Sainsbury's*	½ Pot/85g	253.0	23.0	297	7.0	7.4	26.6	3.5
Roasted Red Pepper, Tesco*	1 Serving/75g	255.0	22.0	340	7.1	11.1	29.7	2.4
Roasted Red Pepper, VLH Kitchens	1 Serving/17g	31.0	1.0	183	6.5	15.6	8.4	6.2
Roasted Vegetable, Fresh, Sainsbury's*	¼ Pot/50g	144.0	14.0	287	5.9	4.9	27.1	7.8
Sea Salt & Cracked Black Pepper, Tesco*	¼ Pot/50g	147.0	14.0	295	7.0	4.8	27.2	9.5
Spicy Red Pepper, With Crudite Dippers, M & S*	1 Pack/130g	123.0	8.0	95	3.3	7.1	6.1	3.4
Sun Dried Tomato, Chunky, Tesco*	½ Pot/95g	322.0	27.0	339	6.7	14.0	28.4	3.3
Sweet Chilli, Tesco*	¼ Pot/50g	145.0	11.0	290	8.1	15.0	21.9	5.1
Three Bean, Reduced Fat, BGTY, Sainsbury's*	¼ Tub/50g	91.0	6.0	183	7.3	11.4	12.0	6.0
with Extra Virgin Olive Oil, Tesco*	1 Pack/190g	564.0	46.0	297	7.9	11.7	24.3	5.1
Zorba Delicacies Ltd*	1 Serving/50g	156.0	13.0	313	7.6	10.7	26.6	3.0
HULA HOOPS								
Bacon & Ketchup Flavour, KP Snacks*	1 Bag/27g	140.0	8.0	517	3.4	56.3	30.9	2.0
BBQ Beef, 55% Less Saturated Fat, KP Snacks*	1 Pack/34g	174.0	10.0	512	3.4	60.5	28.5	1.7
Cheese & Onion 55% Less Saturated Fat, KP Snacks*	1 Bag/34g	175.0	10.0	515	3.6	61.0	28.5	1.9
Chilli Salsa, Tortilla, KP Snacks*	1 Bag /25g	123.0	7.0	494	4.9	57.2	27.3	5.3
Minis, Original, KP Snacks*	1 Tub/140g	752.0	49.0	537	3.0	52.9	34.8	1.7
Multigrain, KP Snacks*	1 Pack/23g	113.0	6.0	491	5.6	60.0	25.6	4.3
Original, 55% Less Saturated Fat, KP Snacks*	1 Bag/34g	175.0	10.0	515	3.2	61.6	28.4	1.8
Original, KP Snacks*	1 Bag/25g	128.0	7.0	514	3.2	61.5	28.4	1.8
Roast Chicken, 50% Less Saturated Fat, KP Snacks*	1 Bag/34g	175.0	10.0	514	3.4	61.0	28.5	1.7
Salt & Vinegar, 50% Less Saturated Fat, KP Snacks*	1 Pack/25g	128.0	7.0	513	3.2	61.0	28.4	1.7
Sizzling Bacon, KP Snacks*	1 Bag/34g	175.0	10.0	514	3.4	60.9	28.5	1.7

H

ICE CREAM

	Measure INFO/WEIGHT	per Measure KCAL	FAT	Nutrition Values per 100g / 100ml KCAL	PROT	CARB	FAT	FIBRE
After Dinner Bites, Vanilla, Magnum, Wall's Ice Cream*	1 Serving/29g	100.0	7.0	344	3.4	31.0	23.0	1.4
After Eight, Nestle*	1 Serving/55g	114.0	5.0	207	3.6	27.1	9.4	0.3
Almond Indulgence, Sainsbury's*	1 Serving/120g	286.0	19.0	238	2.8	21.4	15.7	0.6
Baked Alaska, Ben & Jerry's*	1 Serving/100g	260.0	15.0	260	4.0	29.0	15.0	0.1
Bananas Foster, Haagen-Dazs*	1 Serving/125ml	260.0	15.0	208	3.2	22.4	12.0	0.0
Banoffee Fudge, Sainsbury's*	1/8 Pot/67g	119.0	4.0	178	2.8	28.7	5.9	0.2
Banoffee, Haagen-Dazs*	1 Serving/120ml	274.0	16.0	228	4.0	23.0	13.0	0.0
Bourbon Biscuit, Asda*	1 Dessert/37g	120.0	5.0	324	5.9	48.6	12.2	1.6
Brandy, Luxurious, M & S*	1 Serving/100g	228.0	13.0	228	3.8	19.1	13.3	0.2
Caramel & Cinnamon Waffle, Carte d'Or*	2 Scoops/55g	121.0	6.0	220	3.0	27.0	11.0	0.0
Caramel Chew Chew, Ben & Jerry's*	1 Serving/100g	270.0	16.0	270	3.0	29.0	16.0	0.0
Caramel Craze, Organic, Tesco*	1 Serving/100g	253.0	15.0	253	3.3	25.5	15.3	0.0
Caramel, Carte d'Or*	2 Boules/50g	106.0	4.0	212	2.6	30.8	8.7	0.0
Cheeky Choc, Brownie, Skinny Cow*	1 Tub/500ml	590.0	5.0	118	3.0	23.9	1.1	4.1
Cheesecake Brownie, Ben & Jerry's*	1 Serving 100g	260.0	16.0	260	4.0	26.0	16.0	0.0
Cherry Garcia, Ben & Jerry's*	1 Serving/100g	250.0	15.0	250	3.0	26.0	15.0	0.0
Chilli Red, Purbeck*	1 Serving/50g	99.0	6.0	198	4.8	18.7	11.5	0.0
Choc Chip, Haagen-Dazs*	1oz/28g	80.0	5.0	286	4.7	24.8	18.7	0.0
Chocolate & Caramel, Stick, Slim Fast*	1 Ice Cream/55g	87.0	2.0	159	4.1	26.3	4.2	2.2
Chocolate & Orange, Organic, Green & Black's*	1 Serving/100g	248.0	14.0	248	5.0	25.3	14.1	0.1
Chocolate Brownie with Walnuts, Haagen-Dazs*	1 Cup/101g	223.0	16.0	221	4.4	21.0	16.2	0.0
Chocolate Chip, Baskin Robbins*	1 Serving/75g	170.0	10.0	227	4.0	24.0	13.3	0.0
Chocolate Flavour, Soft Scoop, Sainsbury's*	1 Serving/70g	122.0	5.0	174	3.1	23.6	7.5	0.3
Chocolate Fudge Brownie, Ben & Jerry's*	1 Serving/50g	130.0	6.0	260	4.0	32.0	13.0	1.5
Chocolate Fudge Swirl, Haagen-Dazs*	1oz/28g	77.0	5.0	275	4.6	25.6	17.2	0.0
Chocolate Honeycomb, COU, M & S*	1 Serving/100ml	150.0	3.0	150	3.5	31.5	2.6	0.7
Chocolate Macadamia, Ben & Jerry's*	1 Serving/100g	260.0	18.0	260	4.0	22.0	18.0	0.8
Chocolate Midnight Cookies, Haagen-Dazs*	1oz/28g	81.0	5.0	289	4.9	28.7	17.2	0.0
Chocolate Ripple, Perfectly Balanced, Waitrose*	1 Serving/125ml	205.0	3.0	164	4.8	30.5	2.5	4.1
Chocolate Sandwich, Skinny Cow*	1 Portion/36g	101.0	3.0	280	6.0	46.0	7.9	2.9
Chocolate, COU, M & S*	1 Serving/140g	231.0	4.0	165	3.9	35.0	2.9	0.8
Chocolate, Haagen-Dazs*	1 Serving/120ml	269.0	18.0	224	4.0	19.0	15.0	0.0
Chocolate, Organic, Green & Black's*	1 Serving/125g	310.0	18.0	248	5.0	25.3	14.1	1.1
Chocolate, Rich, Organic, Sainsbury's*	1 Serving/100g	213.0	12.0	213	4.4	22.6	11.7	1.2
Chocolate, Soft Scoop, Tesco*	1 Serving/50g	93.0	4.0	186	3.2	25.1	8.1	0.3
Chocolate, Swirl Pot, Skinny Cow*	1 Pot/100ml	98.0	1.0	98	2.9	20.2	0.6	2.7
Chocolate, Weight Watchers*	1 Serving/100ml	140.0	1.0	140	4.3	28.7	1.2	0.0
Chocolatino, Tesco*	1 Serving/56g	115.0	4.0	205	3.4	31.4	6.8	1.8
Chunky Monkey, Ben & Jerry's*	1 Serving/100g	290.0	17.0	290	4.0	27.0	17.0	1.0
Chunky Monkey, Fairtrade, Ben & Jerry's*	1 Serving/100g	290.0	17.0	290	4.0	27.0	17.0	1.0
Coconut, Carte d'Or*	1 Serving/100ml	125.0	7.0	125	1.8	14.0	7.1	0.5
Coffee, Haagen-Dazs*	1 Serving/120ml	271.0	18.0	226	4.1	17.9	15.3	0.0
Coffee, Waitrose*	1/4 Tub/125ml	292.0	16.0	234	3.6	25.4	13.1	0.0
Completely Mintal, Skinny Cow*	1 Serving/100ml	142.0	1.0	142	4.1	28.4	1.3	3.4
Cookie Dough, Ben & Jerry's*	1 Serving/100g	270.0	14.0	270	4.0	31.0	14.0	0.0
Cookies & Cream, Haagen-Dazs*	1 Pot/100ml	226.0	15.0	226	4.0	19.5	14.7	0.0
Cornish Clotted, M & S*	1 Pot/90g	207.0	13.0	230	2.8	21.8	14.5	0.1
Cornish Dairy, Waitrose*	1 Serving/125ml	161.0	8.0	129	2.3	14.6	6.8	0.0
Cornish Vanilla, Soft Scoop, M & S*	1oz/28g	56.0	3.0	199	3.9	21.8	10.7	0.2
Cornish, Vanilla, Kelly's*	1 Carton/125g	265.0	15.0	212	3.8	22.4	11.9	0.2
Crema Di Mascarpone, Carte d'Or*	1 Serving/100g	207.0	9.0	207	2.8	29.0	8.9	0.0
Dairy Cornish, Tesco*	1 Serving/49g	112.0	6.0	228	3.2	24.7	12.3	0.1
Dairy Milk, Orange, Cadbury*	1 Serving/120ml	259.0	14.0	216	3.5	26.0	11.6	0.0

ICE CREAM

INFO/WEIGHT	Measure per Measure KCAL	FAT	Nutrition Values per 100g / 100ml KCAL	PROT	CARB	FAT	FIBRE

	Measure INFO/WEIGHT	per Measure KCAL	FAT	KCAL	PROT	CARB	FAT	FIBRE
Dairy, Flavoured	1oz/28g	50.0	2.0	179	3.5	24.7	8.0	0.0
Dark Toffee, Organic, Green & Black's*	¼ Pot/125ml	192.0	10.0	154	2.8	18.1	7.9	0.1
Date & Almond Cream, Haagen-Dazs*	1 Serving/120ml	254.0	16.0	212	5.0	19.0	13.0	0.0
Demon Chocolate, M & S*	1 Serving/79g	208.0	9.0	263	3.7	37.1	11.1	0.6
Double Chocolate, Nestle*	1 Serving/78g	248.0	14.0	320	4.8	33.7	18.4	0.0
Farmhouse Toffee, TTD, Sainsbury's*	¼ Pot/100g	293.0	19.0	293	3.2	28.3	18.6	0.6
Fig & Orange Blossom Honey, Waitrose*	1 Serving/100g	219.0	12.0	219	3.9	24.3	11.8	0.4
Fruit & Fresh Tropical, Carte d'Or*	1 Serving/83g	154.0	7.0	185	2.5	24.5	8.5	0.0
Fun-Illa, Skinny Cow*	1 Serving/100ml	97.0	2.0	97	3.1	17.6	1.6	2.4
Get Fruit, Tropical, Solero*	1 Serving/125ml	162.0	5.0	130	1.6	20.6	4.4	0.4
Greek Yoghurt & Honey, Carte d'Or*	1 Serving/55g	114.0	5.0	207	2.7	29.0	8.8	0.0
Half Baked, Ben & Jerry's*	1 Serving/100g	270.0	13.0	270	5.0	32.0	13.0	1.0
Heavenly Vanilla, Cadbury*	1 Serving/250ml	355.0	23.0	142	2.5	12.8	9.3	0.0
Knickerbocker Glory	1oz/28g	31.0	1.0	112	1.5	16.4	5.0	0.2
Lavazza, Carte d'Or*	1 Serving/55g	120.0	5.0	218	3.5	29.0	9.9	0.0
Lemon & White Chocolate, Crackpots, Iceland*	1 Serving/100g	202.0	8.0	202	1.7	29.9	8.4	0.3
Lemon Cream, Dairy, Sainsbury's*	1 Serving/100g	199.0	9.0	199	3.0	25.9	9.3	0.1
Lemon Curd Swirl, Duchy Originals*	¼ Pot/101g	247.0	14.0	245	3.7	25.8	14.1	0.0
Lemon Pie, Haagen-Dazs*	1oz/28g	73.0	5.0	261	3.9	24.5	16.3	0.0
Lemon, Haagen-Dazs*	1 Serving/120ml	144.0	0.0	120	0.3	29.3	0.2	0.0
Less Than 5% Fat, Asda*	1 Scoop/40g	56.0	2.0	139	2.7	22.0	4.5	0.0
Log, Mint Chocolate, Sainsbury's*	1 Serving/51g	100.0	5.0	197	3.0	23.8	10.0	0.2
Lychee Cream & Ginger, Haagen-Dazs*	1 Serving/120ml	258.0	13.0	215	3.6	26.1	10.6	0.0
Macadamia Nut, Baskin Robbins*	1 Serving/113g	270.0	18.0	239	4.4	22.1	15.9	0.9
Madly Deeply, Skinny Cow*	1 Serving/100g	149.0	2.0	149	4.2	28.3	2.2	3.4
Mango, 98% Fat Free, Bulla*	1 Serving/70g	94.0	1.0	134	4.2	25.4	1.6	0.0
Maple & Walnut, American, Sainsbury's*	1/8 Pot/68g	121.0	5.0	179	3.1	25.6	7.2	0.2
Maple Brazil, Thorntons*	1oz/28g	66.0	4.0	236	4.1	24.4	13.6	0.0
Marshallow, Weight Watchers*	½ Tub/138g	268.0	6.0	194	3.2	34.5	4.7	1.3
Mince Pie, Finest, Tesco*	¼ Pack/188g	476.0	22.0	254	3.9	33.0	11.8	1.1
Mint & Chocolate, Sainsbury's*	1 Serving/71g	137.0	7.0	192	3.4	23.5	9.4	0.4
Mint Choc Chip, Organic, Iceland*	1oz/28g	55.0	2.0	197	4.7	25.8	8.3	0.0
Mint Chocolate Chip, Baskin Robbins*	1 Scoop/113g	270.0	16.0	239	4.4	24.8	14.2	0.9
Mint Crisp, Nestle*	1 Serving/75ml	232.0	16.0	309	2.9	25.5	21.9	0.9
Mint Crunch, Dairy Milk, Cadbury*	1 Serving/60ml	162.0	13.0	270	3.0	29.0	22.2	0.0
Mint Ripple, Good Choice, Iceland*	1 Scoop/50g	58.0	1.0	117	3.0	21.7	2.1	0.1
Mint, Majestic Luxury, Iceland*	1 Serving/80g	269.0	15.0	337	3.8	39.3	18.3	1.3
Mint, Thorntons*	1oz/28g	66.0	4.0	237	4.0	25.0	13.4	0.0
Mocha Coffee Indulgence, Sainsbury's*	¼ Pot/82g	178.0	11.0	217	3.2	22.1	12.9	0.1
Muddy Pigs, Wall's Ice Cream*	1 Serving/150ml	150.0	7.0	100	1.7	12.1	4.9	0.3
Neapolitan, Brick, Tesco*	1 Serving/50g	81.0	3.0	163	3.3	21.9	6.9	0.4
Neapolitan, Iceland*	1oz/28g	46.0	2.0	164	3.0	21.3	7.4	0.0
Neapolitan, Organic, Iceland*	1oz/28g	55.0	2.0	196	4.2	26.4	8.2	0.0
Neapolitan, Soft Scoop, M & S*	1/8 Tub/62.5g	100.0	5.0	160	2.7	21.3	7.4	0.3
Neapolitan, Soft Scoop, Sainsbury's*	1 Serving/75g	124.0	5.0	165	2.8	22.8	6.9	0.2
Non-Dairy, Mixes	1oz/28g	51.0	2.0	182	4.1	25.1	7.9	0.0
Non-Dairy, Reduced Calorie	1oz/28g	33.0	2.0	119	3.4	13.7	6.0	0.0
Panna Cotta, Haagen-Dazs*	1 Serving/120ml	248.0	16.0	207	3.4	18.4	13.3	0.0
Peach Melba, Soft Scoop, M & S*	1oz/28g	46.0	2.0	165	2.8	21.4	7.6	0.3
Phish Food, Ben & Jerry's*	1 Serving/100g	260.0	13.0	260	3.5	35.0	13.0	0.1
Picnic, Cadbury*	1 Cone/125ml	258.0	12.0	207	3.4	28.9	9.4	0.3
Pistachio, Haagen-Dazs*	1 Serving/120ml	276.0	19.0	230	4.4	17.7	15.7	0.0
Praline & Chocolate, Thorntons*	1oz/28g	87.0	6.0	309	4.6	21.3	22.9	0.6

ICE CREAM

	INFO/WEIGHT	KCAL	FAT	KCAL	PROT	CARB	FAT	FIBRE
Praline, Green & Black's*	1 Sm Pot/100g	191.0	11.0	191	3.5	20.0	10.8	0.9
Pralines & Cream, Haagen-Dazs*	1 Pot/500ml	1210.0	75.0	242	3.7	22.9	15.1	0.0
Raspberries, Clotted Cream, Waitrose*	1 Tub/500ml	790.0	39.0	158	2.9	18.9	7.9	0.1
Raspberry Ripple Brick, Tesco*	1 Serving/48g	71.0	3.0	148	2.6	20.8	6.0	0.2
Raspberry Ripple, Dairy, Waitrose*	1 Serving/186ml	195.0	10.0	105	1.9	12.3	5.4	0.0
Raspberry Ripple, Soft Scoop, Sainsbury's*	1 Serving/75g	127.0	5.0	170	2.6	24.2	7.0	0.3
Raspberry, Haagen-Dazs*	1 Serving/120ml	127.0	0.0	106	0.2	25.9	0.2	0.0
Raspberry, Swirl Pot, Skinny Cow*	1 Pot/100ml	86.0	0.0	86	2.5	18.4	0.3	2.2
Really Creamy Chocolate, Asda*	1 Serving/100g	227.0	11.0	227	4.1	28.0	11.0	0.4
Really Creamy Toffee, Asda*	1 Serving/120ml	146.0	6.0	122	1.7	17.5	5.0	0.1
Rocky Road, M & S*	1 Tub/500g	1475.0	88.0	295	4.2	29.5	17.7	1.2
Rocky Road, Sainsbury's*	1/8 Pot/67g	137.0	5.0	205	3.8	30.9	7.3	1.0
Rolo, Nestle*	½ Tub/500ml	1180.0	52.0	236	3.4	31.9	10.5	0.2
Rum & Raisin, Haagen-Dazs*	1 Serving/120ml	264.0	18.0	220	3.4	18.6	14.7	0.0
Rum & Raisin, TTD, Sainsbury's*	¼ Pot/100g	220.0	10.0	220	3.8	27.7	10.4	1.0
Screwball, Asda*	1 Screwball/60g	122.0	6.0	203	3.3	25.0	10.0	1.5
Screwball, Tesco*	1 Screwball/61g	116.0	5.0	190	2.9	25.2	8.6	0.3
Smarties Ice Cream Pot, Nestle*	1 Pot/69g	151.0	6.0	218	4.4	33.6	8.2	0.0
Smarties, Nestle*	1 Serving/50g	125.0	6.0	250	3.6	32.3	11.9	0.2
Spagnola, Carte d'Or*	1 Serving/100g	187.0	6.0	187	2.0	32.0	5.7	0.0
Sticky Toffee, Cream O' Galloway*	1 Serving/30g	80.0	4.0	266	4.7	28.7	14.7	0.0
Strawberry & Cream, Mivvi, Nestle*	1 Serving/60g	118.0	5.0	196	2.6	29.4	7.6	0.1
Strawberry & Cream, Organic, Sainsbury's*	1 Serving/100g	193.0	10.0	193	3.6	22.6	9.8	0.4
Strawberry & Yoghurt Delice, Carte d'Or*	1 Portion/54.3g	95.0	2.0	175	1.5	34.0	3.6	0.0
Strawberry Cheesecake, Ben & Jerry's*	1 Serving 100g	240.0	14.0	240	3.0	27.0	14.0	0.0
Strawberry Cheesecake, Co-Op*	1/6 Pot/86g	163.0	6.0	190	3.0	29.0	7.0	0.2
Strawberry, Fromage Frais, Asda*	1 Pot/46g	87.0	3.0	190	3.7	28.0	7.0	0.3
Strawberry, Get Fruit, Solero*	1 Serving/100ml	120.0	4.0	120	1.5	18.8	4.5	1.3
Strawberry, Haagen-Dazs*	1oz/28g	67.0	4.0	241	4.0	21.5	15.5	0.0
Strawberry, Soft Scoop, Tesco*	1 Serving/45.8g	78.0	3.0	170	2.8	23.1	7.4	0.1
Strawberry, Swirl Pot, Skinny Cow*	1 Pot/100ml	89.0	0.0	89	2.5	19.0	0.3	2.2
Strawberry, Thorntons*	1oz/28g	52.0	3.0	185	3.2	22.5	9.3	0.1
Strawberry, Weight Watchers*	1 Pot/57g	81.0	2.0	142	2.5	23.4	3.9	0.2
Terry's Chocolate Orange, Carte d'Or*	1 Serving/100g	182.0	7.0	182	2.8	27.0	7.1	0.0
Tiramisu, COU, M & S*	¼ Tub/86g	120.0	2.0	140	2.1	26.4	2.9	3.0
Tiramisu, Haagen-Dazs*	1 Serving/120ml	303.0	20.0	253	3.8	22.7	16.3	0.0
Toblerone, Carte d'Or*	1 Serving/100g	211.0	9.0	211	3.7	29.0	9.1	0.0
Toffee & Biscuit, Weight Watchers*	1 Pot/100ml	93.0	3.0	93	1.5	14.9	2.7	0.1
Toffee & Vanilla, Sainsbury's*	1 Serving/71g	146.0	7.0	205	3.1	26.7	9.5	0.1
Toffee Creme, Haagen-Dazs*	1oz/28g	74.0	4.0	265	4.5	26.7	15.6	0.0
Toffee Fudge, Soft Scoop, Asda*	1 Serving/50g	92.0	3.0	185	2.6	28.0	7.0	0.0
Toffee Ripple, Tesco*	1 Serving/100g	173.0	7.0	173	2.7	24.4	7.2	0.1
Toffee, Deliciously Dairy, Co-Op*	1oz/28g	45.0	2.0	160	3.0	21.0	7.0	0.2
Toffee, Swirl Pot, Skinny Cow*	1 Pot/66g	92.0	0.0	140	3.8	29.8	0.6	4.5
Toffee, Thorntons*	1oz/28g	61.0	3.0	218	4.1	24.5	11.6	0.0
Traditional Cornish Blackberry, M & S*	1oz/28g	61.0	3.0	218	2.3	28.0	10.8	0.3
Traditional Cornish Strawberry, M & S*	1oz/28g	64.0	3.0	229	2.3	29.7	11.2	0.2
Triple Chocolate Centenary, Cadbury*	1 Serving/100ml	255.0	16.0	255	2.5	27.1	15.6	0.0
Triple Chocolate, Carte d'Or*	1 Serving/58g	122.0	6.0	210	3.7	27.0	9.8	0.0
Triple Chocolate, Dairy, Sainsbury's*	1/8 Litre/67g	123.0	4.0	184	3.5	27.6	6.6	1.0
Truffle Berry Fling, Skinny Cow*	1 Serving/100g	156.0	2.0	156	4.0	30.5	2.0	3.3
Vanilla & Chocolate Swirl, Safeway*	1 Serving/125g	250.0	11.0	200	3.3	26.2	9.1	0.1
Vanilla & Cinnamon, Finest, Tesco*	1 Serving/50g	114.0	7.0	229	3.9	20.2	14.7	0.4

ICE CREAM

	Measure INFO/WEIGHT	per Measure KCAL	FAT	Nutrition Values per 100g / 100ml KCAL	PROT	CARB	FAT	FIBRE
Vanilla & Strawberry, Swirl, Safeway*	1 Serving/100g	190.0	7.0	190	2.9	27.0	7.5	0.2
Vanilla & Strawberry, Weight Watchers*	1 Serving/100ml	81.0	2.0	81	1.4	13.3	2.2	0.1
Vanilla Bean, Light, Deluxe*	1 Serving/64g	110.0	3.0	172	4.7	26.6	3.9	0.0
Vanilla Bean, Purbeck*	1 Serving/100g	198.0	11.0	198	4.8	18.7	11.5	0.0
Vanilla Caramel Brownie, Haagen-Dazs*	1 Serving/150g	410.0	25.0	273	4.5	26.8	16.5	0.0
Vanilla Choc Fudge, Haagen-Dazs*	1oz/28g	75.0	5.0	267	4.3	23.5	17.2	0.0
Vanilla Chocolate, Taste Sensation, Frosty's, Aldi*	1 Pot/73.3g	164.0	7.0	224	2.1	32.4	9.6	0.7
Vanilla Flavour, Soft Scoop, Sainsbury's*	1 Serving/71g	96.0	4.0	136	2.9	18.8	5.5	0.2
Vanilla Flavour, Soft VLH Kitchens	1 Serving/100g	235.0	15.0	235	4.0	22.1	15.0	0.2
Vanilla, Ben & Jerry's*	1 Mini Tub/116g	267.0	17.0	230	4.0	20.0	15.0	0.1
Vanilla, Carte d'Or*	1 Serving/50g	105.0	5.0	210	3.0	26.0	9.5	0.0
Vanilla, COU, M & S*	¼ Pot/79g	111.0	2.0	140	1.7	25.9	2.8	0.8
Vanilla, Dairy, Average	1 Scoop/40g	80.0	4.0	201	3.5	23.6	11.0	0.7
Vanilla, Fairtrade, Ben & Jerry's*	1 Serving/100g	230.0	15.0	230	4.0	20.0	15.0	0.1
Vanilla, Haagen-Dazs*	1oz/28g	70.0	5.0	250	4.5	19.7	17.1	0.0
Vanilla, Light Soft Scoop, 25% Less Fat, Morrisons*	1 Scoop/50g	75.0	2.0	150	2.9	23.2	5.0	0.2
Vanilla, Light, Carte d'Or*	1 Serving/100g	136.0	4.0	136	2.4	22.0	4.4	4.0
Vanilla, Low Fat, Weight Watchers*	1 Scoop/125ml	75.0	2.0	60	1.1	9.7	1.7	0.1
Vanilla, Non-Dairy, Average	1 Serving/60g	107.0	5.0	178	3.2	23.1	8.7	0.0
Vanilla, Organic, Sainsbury's*	1 Serving/85g	176.0	10.0	207	4.3	20.5	12.0	0.1
Vanilla, Organic, Waitrose*	1 Serving/125g	177.0	11.0	142	2.7	12.4	9.0	0.0
Vanilla, Pecan, Haagen-Dazs*	1 Serving/120ml	316.0	24.0	263	4.3	17.1	19.6	0.0
Vanilla, Really Creamy, Asda*	1 Serving/50g	98.0	5.0	196	3.5	23.0	10.0	0.1
Vanilla, Soft Scoop, BGTY, Sainsbury's*	1 Serving/75g	88.0	1.0	117	3.1	22.2	1.7	0.2
Vanilla, Soft Scoop, GFY, Asda*	1 Serving/100g	116.0	2.0	116	3.1	22.0	1.7	0.2
Vanilla, Soft Scoop, Light, Wall's*, Wall's Ice Cream*	1 Scoop/50ml	31.0	1.0	62	1.3	7.0	2.6	0.9
Vanilla, Soft Slice, Wall's Ice Cream*	1 Serving/100ml	90.0	4.0	90	1.4	11.2	4.4	0.1
Vanilla, Soft, Non Milk Fat, Waitrose*	1 Serving/125ml	77.0	3.0	62	1.3	8.0	2.7	0.1
Vanilla, Toffe Crunch, Fairtrade, Ben & Jerry's*	1 Serving/100g	280.0	16.0	280	4.0	29.0	16.0	0.5
Vanilla, Toffee Crunch, Ben & Jerry's*	1 Tub/407g	1099.0	65.0	270	4.0	29.0	16.0	0.5
Vanilla, Too Good to Be True, Wall's Ice Cream*	1 Serving/50ml	35.0	0.0	70	2.0	14.9	0.4	0.1
Vanilla, TTD, Sainsbury's*	¼ Pot/100g	246.0	17.0	246	5.2	18.2	16.9	0.0
Vanilla, with Strawberry Swirl, Mini Tub, Weight Watchers*	1 Mini Tub/57g	81.0	2.0	142	2.5	23.4	3.9	0.2
Vanilla, with Vanilla Pods, Sainsbury's*	1 Serving/100g	195.0	10.0	195	3.5	22.5	10.1	0.1
Viennetta, Biscuit Caramel, Wall's Ice Cream*	1/6 Serving/58g	183.0	12.0	315	3.3	27.8	20.9	0.0
Viennetta, Cappuccino, Wall's Ice Cream*	1 Serving/75g	191.0	13.0	255	3.5	22.0	17.0	0.0
Viennetta, Chocolate, Wall's Ice Cream*	¼ Pot/80g	200.0	12.0	250	4.1	24.0	15.2	0.0
Viennetta, Forest Fruit, Wall's Ice Cream*	1 Serving/98g	265.0	16.0	270	3.4	27.2	16.2	0.0
Viennetta, Mint, Wall's Ice Cream*	1 Serving/80g	204.0	13.0	255	3.4	23.0	16.6	0.0
Viennetta, Selection Brownie, Wall's Ice Cream*	1 Serving/70g	194.0	11.0	277	4.2	28.5	16.2	0.0
Viennetta, Strawberry, Wall's Ice Cream*	1 Serving/80g	204.0	13.0	255	3.4	22.1	16.8	0.0
Voluptuous Vanilla, COU, M & S*	1 Pot/400g	520.0	10.0	130	4.6	22.0	2.6	0.6
Walnut & Maple, Waitrose*	1 Serving/60g	68.0	2.0	114	1.8	18.2	3.8	0.0
Zesty Lemon Meringue, COU, M & S*	¼ Pot/73g	120.0	2.0	165	2.6	33.0	2.5	0.5

ICE CREAM BAR

Bailey's, Haagen-Dazs*	1oz/28g	86.0	6.0	307	4.1	24.8	21.2	0.0
Bounty, 100 Ml Bar, Mars*	1 Bar/100ml	278.0	18.0	278	3.4	24.7	18.5	0.7
Choc Chip, Haagen-Dazs*	1oz/28g	90.0	6.0	320	4.3	27.4	21.5	0.0
Chocolate Covered	1oz/28g	90.0	7.0	320	5.0	24.0	23.3	0.0
Dairy Milk, Caramel, Cadbury*	1 Bar/60ml	175.0	10.0	290	3.6	30.2	17.1	0.0
Dairy Milk, Fruit & Nut, Cadbury*	1 Bar/90ml	243.0	15.0	270	3.5	26.1	17.0	0.0
Dairy Milk, Fudge, Cadbury*	1 Bar/60g	165.0	10.0	275	3.0	27.6	17.2	0.0
Dream, Cadbury*	1 Serving/118g	260.0	14.0	220	3.6	26.0	11.9	0.0

	Measure INFO/WEIGHT	per Measure KCAL	per Measure FAT	Nutrition Values per 100g / 100ml KCAL	PROT	CARB	FAT	FIBRE
ICE CREAM BAR								
Galaxy, Mars*	1 Bar/54g	184.0	12.0	341	3.8	30.7	22.5	0.6
Lion, Nestle*	1 Bar/45g	166.0	10.0	370	4.2	39.1	21.9	1.0
Maltesers, Mars*	1 Bar/45ml	113.0	7.0	252	2.9	25.0	15.6	0.7
Mars, Mars*	1 Bar/63g	177.0	10.0	283	3.6	30.1	16.4	0.0
Rage, Chocolate with Caramel Sauce, Treats*	1 Bar/60g	177.0	10.0	295	3.3	30.9	17.5	0.0
Red Fruits, Solero*	1 Bar/80g	99.0	2.0	124	1.6	25.0	2.7	0.0
Snickers, Mars*	1 Bar/67g	250.0	15.0	373	6.0	37.3	22.4	0.0
Toffee Cream, Haagen-Dazs*	1oz/28g	97.0	6.0	345	4.0	31.0	22.0	0.0
Toffee Crunch, English, Weight Watchers*	1 Bar/40g	110.0	6.0	275	2.5	32.5	15.0	5.0
Twix, Mars*	1 Serving/44g	228.0	14.0	524	6.9	52.9	32.2	0.0
Vanilla & Raspberry, Weight Watchers*	1 Serving/100g	81.0	0.0	81	2.0	23.0	0.3	0.0
Yorkie, Nestle*	1 Bar/40g	144.0	9.0	359	4.8	36.5	21.6	0.0
ICE CREAM CONE								
After Eight, Nestle*	1 Cone/100ml	174.0	8.0	174	2.4	23.0	8.0	0.9
Average	1 Cone/75g	139.0	6.0	186	3.5	25.5	8.5	0.0
Blackcurrant, GFY, Asda*	1 Cone/67g	162.0	6.0	241	3.0	37.0	9.0	0.1
Carousel Wafer Company*	1 Cone/5g	19.0	0.0	392	9.8	78.6	4.2	0.0
Chocolate & Caramel, Skinny Cow*	1 Cone/110ml	121.0	3.0	110	2.5	19.3	2.5	2.7
Chocolate & Nut, Co-Op*	1 Cone/110g	307.0	17.0	279	3.9	31.0	15.5	0.6
Chocolate & Vanilla, Good Choice, Iceland*	1 Cone/110ml	161.0	7.0	146	2.7	22.9	6.5	0.8
Chocolate Flavour, Somerfield*	1 Cone/110ml	329.0	16.0	299	4.0	38.0	15.0	0.0
Chocolate, M & S*	1oz/28g	94.0	6.0	335	4.0	28.0	23.0	2.3
Chocolate, Mini, Cornetto, Wall's Ice Cream*	1 Cone/19g	69.0	4.0	363	4.2	34.2	23.2	0.0
Chocolate, Vanilla & Hazelnut, Sainsbury's*	1 Cone/62g	190.0	10.0	306	4.5	33.9	16.9	0.6
Cone, Haagen-Dazs*	1oz/28g	85.0	6.0	303	4.7	25.5	20.3	0.0
Cornetto, Classico, Mini, Wall's Ice Cream*	1 Cone/19g	67.0	4.0	353	4.2	32.6	23.2	0.0
Cornetto, Frutti Disc, Wall's Ice Cream*	1 Cone/80g	200.0	9.0	250	2.5	35.0	11.0	0.0
Cornetto, GFY, Asda*	1 Cone/67g	162.0	6.0	241	3.0	37.0	9.0	0.1
Cornetto, Mint, Wall's Ice Cream*	1 Cone/75g	225.0	13.0	300	3.7	32.0	18.0	1.1
Cornetto, Wall's Ice Cream*	1 Cone/75g	195.0	10.0	260	3.7	34.5	12.9	0.0
Creme Egg, Cadbury*	1 Cone/115ml	270.0	13.0	235	2.9	29.3	11.6	0.0
Dairy Milk, Mint, Cadbury*	1 Cone/115mll	190.0	9.0	165	2.4	21.5	7.7	0.0
Extreme Raspberry, Cornetto, Nestle*	1 Cone/88g	220.0	9.0	250	2.5	36.0	10.0	0.2
Flake 99, Cadbury*	1 Cone/125ml	244.0	12.0	195	2.6	23.2	10.0	0.0
Flake 99, Strawberry, Cadbury*	1 Serving/125g	250.0	11.0	200	2.6	27.3	8.7	0.0
Raspberry & Vanilla, Refreshing, Skinny Cow*	1 Cone/110ml	122.0	3.0	111	1.7	20.4	2.5	1.5
Smarties, Nestle*	1 Cone/100g	177.0	8.0	177	2.4	23.6	8.1	0.7
Sticky Toffee, Farmfoods*	1 Cone/120ml	326.0	15.0	272	3.2	36.0	12.8	2.0
Strawberry & Vanilla, Asda*	1 Cone/115ml	193.0	9.0	168	1.8	22.6	7.8	0.1
Strawberry & Vanilla, HL, Tesco*	1 Serving/69g	149.0	4.0	216	3.4	36.4	6.3	1.4
Strawberry & Vanilla, Iceland*	1 Serving/70g	182.0	8.0	260	3.3	37.5	10.8	0.7
Strawberry & Vanilla, M & S*	1oz/28g	81.0	5.0	290	4.2	30.9	16.5	0.7
Strawberry & Vanilla, Sainsbury's*	1 Cone/70g	171.0	7.0	243	3.4	35.6	9.7	1.0
Strawberry & Vanilla, Tesco*	1 Cone/70g	194.0	9.0	277	3.0	35.9	13.5	0.3
Strawberry, BGTY, Sainsbury's*	1 Cone/69g	151.0	4.0	219	2.6	37.5	6.5	1.3
Strawberry, M & S*	1oz/28g	74.0	4.0	263	3.5	31.1	14.0	0.4
Strawberry, Somerfield*	1 Cone/110g	299.0	12.0	272	3.0	40.0	11.0	0.0
Tropical, GFY, Asda*	1 Cone/100g	135.0	5.0	135	2.6	20.0	5.0	0.3
ICE CREAM ROLL								
Arctic, Average	1 Serving/70g	140.0	5.0	200	4.1	33.3	6.6	0.0
Mini, Cadbury*	1 Roll/45ml	99.0	6.0	220	3.4	24.3	13.1	0.0
ICE CREAM SANDWICH								
Mint, Skinny Cow*	1 Sandwich/71g	140.0	2.0	197	4.2	39.4	2.8	1.4

	Measure INFO/WEIGHT	per Measure KCAL	FAT	Nutrition Values per 100g / 100ml KCAL	PROT	CARB	FAT	FIBRE
ICE CREAM SANDWICH								
Wich, Ben & Jerry's*	1 Pack/117g	398.0	20.0	340	4.0	44.0	17.0	1.0
ICE CREAM STICK								
Berry Blast, Smoothie, Skinny Cow*	1 Stick/110ml	71.0	0.0	65	0.9	15.1	0.1	1.9
Chocolate Cookies, Haagen-Dazs*	1 Stick/43g	162.0	11.0	376	4.9	31.8	25.4	0.0
Cookies 'n' Cream, Skinny Cow*	1 Stick/67g	89.0	1.0	133	4.8	25.3	1.5	3.6
Mint Double Chocolate, Skinny Cow*	1 Stick/110ml	94.0	2.0	85	2.7	15.1	1.6	2.4
Strawberries & Cream, Skinny Cow*	1 Stick/110ml	82.0	1.0	75	2.8	13.6	0.9	2.3
Toffee, Skinny Cow*	1 Stick/72g	87.0	0.0	121	3.9	25.2	0.5	4.2
Triple Chocolate, Skinny Cow*	1 Stick/68g	87.0	1.0	128	4.3	22.8	2.2	2.8
Vanilla Macadamia, Haagen-Dazs*	1 Stick/42g	161.0	12.0	383	4.6	28.7	27.7	0.0
ICE LOLLY								
Assorted, Iceland*	1 Lolly/51g	33.0	0.0	65	0.0	16.2	0.0	0.0
Assorted, Safeway*	1 Lolly/31ml	26.0	0.0	85	0.0	20.9	0.0	0.1
Berry Burst, Sainsbury's*	1 Serving/90ml	93.0	2.0	103	1.1	20.8	1.8	0.7
Blackcurrant Split, Iceland*	1 Lolly/75g	61.0	2.0	81	1.1	12.0	3.2	0.1
Blackcurrant, Dairy Split, Sainsbury's*	1 Lolly/73ml	88.0	3.0	121	1.8	20.4	3.6	0.1
Blackcurrant, Ribena*	1 Lolly/55ml	43.0	0.0	79	0.0	19.2	0.0	0.0
Bournville, Cadbury*	1 Lolly/110g	269.0	17.0	245	2.5	23.2	15.6	0.0
Calippo Shots, Cool Lemon, Wall's Ice Cream*	1oz/28g	8.0	0.0	28	0.1	3.9	1.3	0.0
Calippo Shots, Twisted Berry, Wall's Ice Cream*	1oz/28g	8.0	0.0	28	0.1	4.2	1.2	0.0
Calippo, Lemon Lime, Mini, Wall's Ice Cream*	1 Lolly/80g	68.0	0.0	85	0.0	21.0	0.0	0.2
Calippo, Orange, Mini, Wall's Ice Cream*	1 Lolly/77.8g	70.0	0.0	90	0.0	21.9	0.0	0.2
Calippo, Strawberry Tropical, Wall's Ice Cream*	1 Lolly/105g	89.0	0.0	85	0.1	21.0	0.1	0.0
Choc & Almond, Mini, Tesco*	1 Lolly/31g	103.0	7.0	331	4.4	24.8	23.8	0.9
Choc Lime Split, Morrisons*	1 Lolly/73ml	120.0	6.0	164	1.6	20.4	8.4	0.1
Chocolate & Vanilla, Sainsbury's*	1 Lolly/40g	143.0	10.0	357	3.7	28.7	25.3	2.2
Chocolate, Mini Milk, Milk Time, Wall's Ice Cream*	1 Lolly/23g	31.0	1.0	135	4.3	22.0	3.1	1.0
Chocolate, Plain, Mini, Tesco*	1 Lolly/31g	94.0	7.0	304	3.1	24.8	21.4	1.2
Chocolate, Pooh Stick, Nestle*	1 Lolly/40g	36.0	1.0	89	2.1	12.9	3.6	0.0
Cider Refresher, Treats*	1 Lolly/70ml	54.0	0.0	77	0.0	19.2	0.0	0.0
Cola Lickers, Farmfoods*	1 Lolly/56ml	38.0	0.0	68	0.0	17.0	0.0	0.0
Creamy Tropical Sorbet, Sticks, Waitrose*	1 Lolly/85g	100.0	2.0	118	1.9	22.9	2.1	0.8
Elderflower, Tubes, Frozen, M & S*	1oz/28g	23.0	0.0	82	0.1	20.5	0.1	0.2
Exotic Fruit, Mini, HL, Tesco*	1 Lolly/31g	41.0	1.0	131	1.0	26.4	2.0	1.0
Exotic Split, Bars, M & S*	1oz/28g	36.0	1.0	127	2.5	25.0	1.9	0.4
Fab, Nestle*	1 Lolly/57g	78.0	3.0	136	0.5	22.8	4.7	0.2
Fab, Orange, Nestle*	1 Lolly/58g	81.0	3.0	140	0.6	24.0	4.7	0.0
Feast, Chocolate, Mini, Wall's Ice Cream*	1 Lolly/52g	165.0	12.0	318	3.3	24.0	23.0	0.0
Feast, Ice Cream, Original, Wall's Ice Cream*	1 Lolly/92ml	294.0	22.0	320	3.2	23.8	23.5	0.0
Feast, Toffee, Mini, Wall's Ice Cream*	1 Lolly/52g	163.0	12.0	313	3.0	24.0	23.0	0.0
Feast, Wall's Ice Cream*	1 Lolly/92ml	276.0	20.0	300	3.2	22.0	22.0	0.0
Fruit Flavour, Assorted, Basics, Sainsbury's*	1 Lolly/50g	33.0	0.0	66	0.0	16.5	0.0	0.0
Fruit Fusion, Mini, Farmfoods*	1 Lolly/45ml	36.0	0.0	79	0.2	19.2	0.1	0.2
Fruit Ices, Made with Orange Juice, Del Monte*	1 Lolly/75ml	79.0	0.0	105	0.5	25.7	0.0	0.0
Fruit Luxury, Mini, Co-Op*	1 Lolly/45g	58.0	3.0	130	2.0	18.0	6.0	0.2
Fruit Pastilles, Rowntree's*	1 Lolly/65ml	61.0	0.0	94	0.1	23.2	0.0	0.0
Fruit Split, Asda*	1 Lolly/74g	85.0	3.0	115	1.7	19.0	3.6	0.0
Fruit Split, Assorted, Co-Op*	1 Lolly/73g	80.0	2.0	110	1.0	20.0	3.0	0.1
Fruit Split, BFY, Morrisons*	1 Lolly/73g	50.0	1.0	69	1.6	13.9	0.7	0.1
Fruit Split, Waitrose*	1 Lolly/73g	91.0	3.0	124	2.5	21.7	3.6	0.4
Fruit Splits, Assorted, Somerfield*	1 Lolly/73ml	74.0	2.0	102	0.0	18.0	3.0	0.0
Fruit Splits, Treats*	1 Lolly/75ml	77.0	3.0	103	1.4	17.6	4.1	0.0
Fruit, Assorted, Basics, Somerfield*	1 Lolly/56ml	32.0	0.0	58	0.0	15.0	0.0	0.0

I

ICE LOLLY

	Measure INFO/WEIGHT	per Measure		Nutrition Values per 100g / 100ml				
		KCAL	FAT	KCAL	PROT	CARB	FAT	FIBRE
Fruit, Assorted, Waitrose*	1 Lolly/73g	59.0	0.0	81	0.0	20.0	0.0	0.1
Fruit, Red, Tesco*	1 Lolly/31.5g	40.0	1.0	128	1.8	25.6	2.0	0.6
Fruity 'n' Freezy, Asda*	1 Lolly/30ml	24.0	0.0	80	0.1	20.0	0.0	0.0
Funny Foot, Wall's Ice Cream*	1 Lolly	83.0	5.0	102	2.0	12.5	6.0	0.0
Ice Lolly, Twister, Choc, Wall's Ice Cream*	1 Mini Lolly/27g	40.0	2.0	150	3.5	22.0	6.0	0.9
Icicles, All Flavours, Freezepops, Calypso*	1 Lolly/50ml	1.0	0.0	1	0.0	0.3	0.0	0.0
Kiwi Burst, Pineapple Sorbet in Kiwi Ice, Sainsbury's*	1 Serving/90ml	76.0	0.0	84	0.1	20.7	0.1	0.4
Lemon & Lime, Mini Bar, M & S*	1 Lolly/50g	47.0	0.0	95	0.1	23.6	0.1	0.2
Lemon & Lime, Rocket Split, De Roma*	1 Lolly/60ml	65.0	3.0	108	1.0	16.0	4.3	0.2
Lemonade & Cola, Morrisons*	1 Lolly/55ml	36.0	0.0	65	0.0	16.2	0.0	0.0
Lemonade Sparkle, Wall's Ice Cream*	1 Lolly/55g	40.0	0.0	73	0.0	18.2	0.0	0.0
Mango & Lemon, BGTY, Sainsbury's*	1 Lolly/72g	84.0	0.0	116	0.3	28.1	0.3	0.5
Mango & Passion Fruit Bursts, Sainsbury's*	1 Lolly/89ml	75.0	0.0	84	0.2	20.4	0.1	0.0
Mango & Passion Fruit Smoothie, Waitrose*	1 Lolly/73g	60.0	0.0	82	0.7	18.9	0.4	0.7
Mega Truffle, Nestle*	1 Lolly/71g	217.0	14.0	305	3.2	28.0	20.1	0.8
Milk Chocolate & Crisped Wheat, Co-Op*	1 Lolly/110g	258.0	13.0	235	3.0	28.0	12.0	0.7
Milk Flavour, Farmfoods*	1 Lolly/50ml	91.0	5.0	182	2.8	20.1	10.1	0.1
Milk, Blue Parrot Cafe, Sainsbury's*	1 Lolly/30ml	34.0	1.0	113	2.7	18.0	3.3	0.3
Mint Chocolate, Tesco*	1 Lolly/70g	234.0	14.0	334	3.6	35.4	19.8	1.2
Morrisons*	1 Lolly/100g	30.0	0.0	30	0.0	7.4	0.0	0.0
Nobbly Bobbly, Nestle*	1 Lolly/70ml	158.0	8.0	226	2.3	27.6	11.7	0.3
Orange & Lemon Splits, Farmfoods*	1 Lolly/56ml	69.0	2.0	124	1.6	19.8	4.3	0.2
Orange Juice, Asda*	1 Lolly/70g	58.0	0.0	83	0.7	20.0	0.0	0.0
Orange Juice, Bar, M & S*	1 Lolly/75g	64.0	0.0	86	0.5	21.0	0.0	0.1
Orange Juice, Co-Op*	1 Lolly/73g	51.0	0.0	70	0.4	17.0	0.1	0.1
Orange Juice, Farmfoods*	1 Lolly/79g	74.0	0.0	94	0.1	23.4	0.0	0.3
Orange Juice, Freshly Squeezed, Finest, Tesco*	1 Lolly/80ml	89.0	0.0	111	0.7	27.0	0.0	0.0
Orange Juice, Freshly Squeezed, Waitrose*	1 Lolly/73g	88.0	0.0	120	0.6	29.7	0.1	0.0
Orange Juice, Milfina*	1 Lolly/79g	69.0	0.0	87	0.5	23.3	0.0	0.0
Orange Juice, Morrisons*	1 Lolly/55ml	46.0	0.0	84	0.0	20.0	0.0	0.0
Orange Juice, Tropicana*	1 Lolly/50g	42.0	0.0	85	0.5	20.7	0.0	0.0
Orange Maid, Nestle*	1 Lolly/73ml	66.0	0.0	91	0.5	21.6	0.0	0.0
Orange 'n' Cream, Tropicana*	1 Lolly/65g	83.0	3.0	129	1.4	20.5	4.5	0.3
Orange, Real Fruit Juice, Sainsbury's*	1 Lolly/73ml	49.0	0.0	67	0.2	16.5	0.1	0.1
Orange, Real Juice, Sainsbury's*	1 Lolly/72ml	63.0	0.0	88	0.7	21.0	0.1	0.1
Orange, Real Juice, Tesco*	1 Lolly/32g	25.0	0.0	78	0.6	18.7	0.0	0.3
Orange, Ribena*	1 Lolly/110ml	95.0	0.0	86	0.1	21.4	0.0	0.0
Orange, Tesco*	1 Lolly/77g	53.0	0.0	68	0.2	16.8	0.0	0.3
Orange, Water, Iceland*	1 Lolly/75g	73.0	0.0	98	0.2	24.4	0.0	0.2
Pineapple, Dairy Split, Sainsbury's*	1 Lolly/72ml	84.0	3.0	116	1.8	19.0	3.6	0.1
Pineapple, Real Fruit Juice, Sainsbury's*	1 Lolly/73ml	55.0	0.0	76	0.1	19.0	0.1	0.1
Polar Snappers, Double, Farmfoods*	1 Lolly/60ml	40.0	0.0	66	0.0	16.5	0.0	0.0
Raspberry & Apple, Sainsbury's*	1 Lolly/57ml	39.0	0.0	68	0.1	17.1	0.1	0.1
Raspberry, Real Fruit Juice, Sainsbury's*	1 Lolly/72g	62.0	0.0	86	0.3	21.0	0.1	0.1
Raspberry, Rocket Split, De Roma*	1 Lolly/60ml	65.0	3.0	108	1.0	16.2	4.3	0.2
Raspberry, Smoothie, Iced, Del Monte*	1 Lolly/90ml	96.0	0.0	107	0.1	26.4	0.1	0.0
Real Fruit Juice, Rocket, Blue Parrot Cafe, Sainsbury's*	1 Lolly/58ml	45.0	0.0	77	0.2	19.1	0.0	0.1
Real Fruit, Dairy Split, Sainsbury's*	1 Lolly/73ml	100.0	3.0	137	2.1	22.8	4.2	0.1
Real Orange, Kids, Tesco*	1 Lolly/32g	25.0	0.0	78	0.6	18.7	0.0	0.3
Refresher, Bassett's*	1 Lolly/40g	47.0	1.0	117	2.2	22.2	2.2	0.3
Rocket, Sainsbury's*	1 Lolly/58g	42.0	0.0	72	0.1	17.8	0.1	0.1
Scooby-Doo, Freezepops, Calypso*	1 Lolly/50ml	14.0	0.0	28	0.0	7.0	0.0	0.0
Skinny Dippers Minis, Caramel & Chocolate, Skinny Cow*	1 Lolly/38ml	62.0	2.0	162	3.4	24.3	5.0	3.3

	Measure INFO/WEIGHT	per Measure KCAL	FAT	Nutrition Values per 100g / 100ml KCAL	PROT	CARB	FAT	FIBRE
ICE LOLLY								
Solero, Exotic, Wall's Ice Cream*	1 Lolly/82g	99.0	2.0	121	1.6	21.9	2.8	0.5
Solero, Orange Fresh, Wall's Ice Cream*	1 Lolly/96g	78.0	0.0	81	0.2	20.0	0.0	0.0
Solero, Red Fruits, Wall's Ice Cream*	1 Lolly/95g	99.0	2.0	104	1.3	21.0	2.2	0.0
Strawberries 'n' Cream, Tropicana*	1 Lolly/50g	58.0	1.0	117	1.6	25.0	1.2	0.0
Strawberry & Banana, Smoothies, Sainsbury's*	1 Lolly/60g	100.0	3.0	166	1.5	28.0	5.3	0.2
Strawberry & Vanilla, 99% Fat Free, So-Lo, Iceland*	1 Lolly/92g	98.0	0.0	107	2.3	23.5	0.4	2.2
Strawberry Fruit, Double, Del Monte*	1 Lolly/76g	84.0	2.0	111	1.8	20.1	2.6	0.0
Strawberry Split, Co-Op*	1 Lolly/71g	75.0	2.0	105	1.0	17.0	3.0	0.1
Strawberry, Dairy Split, Sainsbury's*	1 Lolly/73ml	86.0	3.0	118	1.7	19.8	3.6	0.1
Strawberry, Mini Milk, Milk Time, Wall's Ice Cream*	1 Lolly/23g	30.0	1.0	131	4.0	22.0	2.9	0.5
Tip Top, Calypso*	1 Lolly/20ml	6.0	0.0	30	0.1	7.1	0.1	0.0
Traffic Light, Co-Op*	1 Lolly/52g	55.0	0.0	105	0.4	25.0	0.8	0.0
Tropical Fruit Sorbet, Waitrose*	1 Lolly/110g	90.0	2.0	82	1.5	14.5	2.0	0.2
Tropical Fruit, Starburst, Mars*	1 Lolly/93ml	94.0	0.0	101	0.3	24.8	0.1	0.0
Tropical, Mmmm, Tesco*	1 Lolly/73g	109.0	3.0	150	1.2	26.6	4.3	0.4
Twister, Wall's Ice Cream*	1 Lolly/80ml	76.0	2.0	95	0.6	18.4	1.9	0.0
Vanilla, Mini Milk, Milk Time, Wall's Ice Cream*	1 Lolly/23g	29.0	1.0	127	3.8	21.0	2.9	0.3
Vanilla, Pooh Stick, Nestle*	1 Lolly/40g	34.0	1.0	86	1.9	12.9	3.5	0.0
Vimto Soft Drinks*	1 Lolly/73ml	84.0	3.0	115	1.3	18.2	4.1	0.1
Wonka Super Sour Tastic, Nestle*	1 Lolly/60ml	84.0	2.0	140	0.0	26.1	3.6	0.0
Zoom, Nestle*	1 Lolly/58ml	54.0	0.0	93	0.9	20.6	0.7	0.0
ICED DESSERT								
Berrylicious Overload, COU, M & S*	1 Tub/119.2g	155.0	2.0	130	3.0	24.5	2.0	3.0
Cafe Latte, BGTY, Sainsbury's*	1 Serving/75g	104.0	3.0	139	2.9	23.7	3.6	3.3
Chocolate & Mallow, GFY, Asda*	1 Pot/150ml	142.0	2.0	95	2.0	19.0	1.2	2.3
Chocolate Mint Crisp, COU, M & S*	¼ Pot/85g	115.0	2.0	135	5.4	21.9	2.9	1.0
Chocolate, Honeycomb Pieces, Weight Watchers*	1 Pot/58g	92.0	2.0	159	3.1	26.2	4.3	0.8
Greek Style, Yoghurt, Tesco*	1 Serving/56g	90.0	2.0	160	2.6	29.7	3.3	1.4
Raspberry Swirl, Weight Watchers*	1 Scoop/60g	74.0	1.0	124	1.7	23.4	2.5	0.3
Strawberry Swirl, Weight Watchers*	1 Pot/100ml	92.0	2.0	92	1.1	18.1	1.7	0.5
Summer Fruits, Yoghurt, BGTY, Sainsbury's*	¼ Pot/85g	105.0	1.0	124	3.3	25.6	0.9	0.5
Toffee & Walnut, Free From, Sainsbury's*	¼ Tub/81g	203.0	10.0	251	3.3	31.6	12.4	0.3
Toffee Flavoured, Dairy, BGTY, Sainsbury's*	1 Serving/70g	103.0	3.0	147	2.7	24.0	4.5	0.2
Vanilla & Chocolate, HL, Tesco*	1 Pot/73g	104.0	2.0	143	3.0	26.9	2.6	0.7
Vanilla, Dairy, BGTY, Sainsbury's*	1 Serving/65g	78.0	1.0	120	3.0	23.6	1.5	0.6
Vanilla, Non Dairy, Soft, Swedish Glace*	1 Serving/100g	200.0	10.0	200	2.5	25.0	10.0	1.0
INDIAN MEAL								
Banquet, for One, COU, M & S*	1 Pack/500g	400.0	6.0	80	6.7	10.2	1.2	3.1
for One, Asda*	1 Pack/550g	834.0	25.0	152	6.7	20.9	4.6	1.4
for One, Eat Smart, Safeway*	1 Serving/600g	690.0	16.0	115	6.5	16.2	2.6	2.0
for One, GFY, Asda*	1 Serving/495g	643.0	23.0	130	8.0	14.0	4.7	1.0
for One, Vegetarian, Asda*	1 Pack/499g	789.0	45.0	158	3.2	16.0	9.0	1.4
for Two, Hot, Takeaway, Tesco*	1 Pack/825g	1215.0	61.0	147	6.6	13.6	7.3	1.9
for Two, Menu, Tesco*	1 Serving/537g	811.0	34.0	151	6.3	17.0	6.4	0.8
for Two, Peshwari Naan, Finest, Tesco*	½ Pack/200g	612.0	18.0	306	8.3	48.3	8.9	5.2
INDIAN MENU								
COU, M & S*	1 Pack/550g	412.0	7.0	75	8.4	7.5	1.2	2.1
INDIAN SELECTION								
Snack, Safeway*	1 Serving/170g	347.0	16.0	204	4.0	25.8	9.4	1.9
INSTANT WHIP								
Chocolate Flavour, Dry, Bird's*	1oz/28g	109.0	2.0	390	3.8	80.5	5.9	0.7
Strawberry Flavour, Dry, Bird's*	1oz/28g	112.0	2.0	400	2.5	85.0	5.4	0.4

	Measure INFO/WEIGHT	per Measure KCAL	FAT	Nutrition Values per 100g / 100ml KCAL	PROT	CARB	FAT	FIBRE
JACKFRUIT								
Raw, Average, Flesh Only	*1 Portion/162g*	*155.0*	*1.0*	*95*	*1.5*	*24.4*	*0.3*	*1.6*
Raw, Average, Weighed with Skin & Seeds	*1oz/28g*	*26.0*	*0.0*	*94*	*1.5*	*24.0*	*0.3*	*1.6*
JALFREZI								
Chicken, & Pilau Rice, Sainsbury's*	1 Pack/500g	600.0	20.0	120	6.9	13.9	4.1	1.5
Chicken, & Rice, Serves 1, Tesco*	1 Serving/475g	589.0	38.0	124	7.4	5.7	8.0	1.6
Chicken, Asda*	1 Pack/340g	415.0	20.0	122	10.0	7.0	6.0	1.6
Chicken, Finest, Tesco*	1 Pack/350g	402.0	16.0	115	10.4	6.9	4.7	1.2
Chicken, GFY, Asda*	1 Pack/350g	238.0	3.0	68	9.0	6.0	0.9	1.8
Chicken, Hot & Spicy, Sainsbury's*	½ Pack/200g	228.0	11.0	114	12.8	2.9	5.7	1.0
Chicken, Indian Takeaway, Tesco*	1 Serving/350g	245.0	9.0	70	7.4	4.3	2.5	1.8
Chicken, Medium, GFY, Asda*	1 Pack/644g	972.0	28.0	151	6.0	22.0	4.3	0.9
Chicken, with Basmati Rice, Weight Watchers*	1 Pack/330g	238.0	2.0	72	5.0	11.8	0.5	0.5
Chicken, with Pilau Rice, BGTY, Sainsbury's*	1 Pack/400g	337.0	4.0	84	7.1	11.5	1.1	1.9
Chicken, with Pilau Rice, GFY, Asda*	1 Pack/446g	495.0	11.0	111	8.0	14.0	2.5	1.2
Chicken, with Pilau Rice, Tesco*	1 Pack/460g	506.0	17.0	110	5.3	13.6	3.8	0.9
Chicken, with Rice, COU, M & S*	1 Pack/400g	320.0	4.0	80	9.2	8.3	1.1	1.2
Chicken, with Rice, Tesco*	1 Pack/550g	731.0	26.0	133	5.5	17.0	4.8	1.0
Meal for One, M & S*	1 Serving/500g	700.0	35.0	140	6.1	13.4	7.0	3.0
Vegetable, Eastern Indian, Sainsbury's*	1 Pack/400g	208.0	14.0	52	3.4	2.0	3.4	1.7
Vegetable, Take Away Menu for 1, BGTY, Sainsbury's*	1 Pack/148g	43.0	0.0	29	1.8	5.4	0.0	2.3
Vegetable, Waitrose*	1 Pack/400g	256.0	16.0	64	2.2	4.7	4.0	3.7
Vegetable, with Rice, Birds Eye*	1 Pack/350g	353.0	4.0	101	2.5	20.2	1.1	1.0
JAM								
Apricot, Average	*1 Tbsp/15g*	*37.0*	*0.0*	*248*	*0.2*	*61.6*	*0.0*	*1.5*
Apricot, Reduced Sugar, Average	*1 Serving/20g*	*37.0*	*0.0*	*186*	*0.4*	*46.0*	*0.3*	*0.4*
Black Cherry, Average	*1 Tbsp/15g*	*37.0*	*0.0*	*247*	*0.4*	*61.2*	*0.3*	*0.4*
Blackberry, Extra Special, Asda*	1 Tbsp/15g	29.0	0.0	190	0.9	45.0	0.7	0.0
Blackcurrant, Average	*1 Tbsp/15g*	*38.0*	*0.0*	*250*	*0.2*	*62.3*	*0.0*	*1.0*
Blackcurrant, Reduced Sugar, Average	*1 Tsp/6g*	*10.0*	*0.0*	*178*	*0.4*	*44.4*	*0.1*	*1.0*
Blueberry & Blackberry, Baxters*	1 Tsp/15g	38.0	0.0	252	0.0	63.0	0.0	1.2
Blueberry, Best, Hartley's*	1 Tsp/20g	49.0	0.0	244	0.3	60.6	0.1	0.0
Blueberry, St Dalfour*	1 Serving/20g	46.0	0.0	228	0.5	56.0	0.2	2.2
Country Berries, Luxury, Baxters*	1 Tsp/15g	38.0	0.0	252	0.0	63.0	0.0	1.1
Damson, Extra Fruit, Best, Hartley's*	1 Tsp/5g	12.0	0.0	244	0.2	60.8	0.0	0.0
Golden Peach, Rhapsodie De Fruit, St Dalfour*	1 Tsp/10g	23.0	0.0	227	0.5	56.0	0.1	1.3
Kiwi & Gooseberry, 66% Fruit, Asda*	1 Serving/30g	56.0	0.0	187	0.5	45.0	0.5	0.0
Mixed Fruit, Average	*1 Tbsp/15g*	*38.0*	*0.0*	*252*	*0.3*	*63.5*	*0.0*	*0.5*
Plum, Tesco*	1 Serving/50g	130.0	0.0	261	0.2	64.4	0.0	0.6
Raspberry, Average	*1 Tbsp/15g*	*36.0*	*0.0*	*239*	*0.6*	*58.6*	*0.1*	*0.9*
Raspberry, Reduced Sugar, Average	*1 Tsp/6g*	*10.0*	*0.0*	*160*	*0.5*	*39.3*	*0.2*	*0.6*
Raspberry, Seedless, Average	*1 Tsp/10g*	*26.0*	*0.0*	*257*	*0.4*	*63.6*	*0.0*	*0.3*
Rhubarb & Ginger, Baxters*	1 Tsp/15g	31.0	0.0	210	0.0	53.0	0.0	0.6
Strawberry & Redcurrant, Reduced Sugar, Streamline*	1 Tbsp/15g	29.0	0.0	192	0.4	46.8	0.3	0.0
Strawberry & Vanilla, Best, Hartley's*	1 Tsp/5g	12.0	0.0	244	0.4	60.6	0.0	0.0
Strawberry, Average	*1 Tsp/10g*	*25.0*	*0.0*	*253*	*0.3*	*62.7*	*0.0*	*0.6*
Strawberry, Reduced Sugar, Average	*1 Tbsp/15g*	*28.0*	*0.0*	*187*	*0.4*	*45.8*	*0.3*	*0.2*
Wild Blackberry Jelly, Baxters*	1 Tsp/15g	31.0	0.0	210	0.0	53.0	0.0	1.2
JAMBALAYA								
American Style, Tesco*	1 Serving/275g	432.0	19.0	157	7.7	16.0	7.0	0.5
Cajun Chicken, BGTY, Sainsbury's*	1 Pack/400g	364.0	6.0	91	7.7	11.9	1.4	1.1
Chicken, Spicy, Eat Smart, Morrisons*	1 Pack/400g	384.0	5.0	96	7.4	13.9	1.2	2.7
COU, M & S*	1 Pack/400g	340.0	8.0	85	6.5	10.8	2.0	0.9
GFY, Asda*	1 Pack/450g	387.0	3.0	86	6.0	14.0	0.7	2.7

J

	Measure INFO/WEIGHT	per Measure KCAL	FAT	Nutrition Values per 100g / 100ml KCAL	PROT	CARB	FAT	FIBRE
JAMBALAYA								
M & S*	1 Pack/480g	552.0	17.0	115	5.8	14.6	3.5	1.2
Tesco*	1 Pack/550g	764.0	36.0	139	6.9	13.1	6.6	1.1
JELLY								
Apple & Watermelon, Low Calorie, Hartley's*	1 Serving/175g	5.0	0.0	3	0.0	0.3	0.0	0.3
Blackberry, Unprepared, Morrisons*	1 Serving/20g	52.0	0.0	261	0.3	65.0	0.0	0.0
Blackcurrant, Made Up, Rowntree's*	¼ Jelly/140ml	100.0	0.0	71	1.4	16.4	0.1	0.0
Blackcurrant, Made Up, Sainsbury's*	¼ Jelly/150g	97.0	0.0	65	1.2	15.1	0.0	0.0
Blackcurrant, Sugar Free, Unprepared, Rowntree's*	1 Pack/24g	73.0	0.0	305	50.0	25.0	0.0	25.0
Blackcurrant, Tesco*	1 Serving/100g	84.0	0.0	84	0.2	20.5	0.1	0.4
Bramble, Tesco*	1 Serving/100g	257.0	0.0	257	0.3	63.7	0.1	1.3
Crystals, Orange & Peach, Sugar Free, Weight Watchers*	½ Pack/204g	14.0	0.0	7	0.0	1.4	0.1	0.0
Crystals, Orange, Sugar Free, Bird's*	1 Sachet/12g	39.0	0.0	335	62.5	6.4	0.9	0.0
Crystals, Strawberry, Made Up, Tesco*	1 Serving/145g	9.0	0.0	6	1.3	0.3	0.0	0.0
Exotic Fruit, M & S*	1 Pot/175g	140.0	0.0	80	0.1	18.9	0.2	0.9
Fresh Fruit, M & S*	1 Pot/175g	131.0	0.0	75	0.2	18.4	0.1	0.3
Fruit Cocktail, M & S*	1oz/28g	31.0	1.0	110	0.4	16.4	4.7	0.3
Fruitini, Del Monte*	1 Serving/120g	78.0	0.0	65	0.3	15.3	0.1	0.5
Lemon & Lime, Sugar Free, Unprepared, Rowntree's*	1oz/28g	85.0	0.0	305	4.5	60.7	0.0	0.0
Lemon, Unprepared, Co-Op*	1 Pack/135g	412.0	0.0	305	5.0	71.0	0.0	0.0
Lime Flavour, Unprepared, Waitrose*	1 Square/11g	33.0	0.0	296	4.5	69.5	0.0	0.0
Lime, Made Up, Rowntree's*	¼ Jelly/140ml	100.0	0.0	71	1.3	16.3	0.1	0.0
Lime, Unprepared, Co-Op*	1 Pack/135g	397.0	0.0	294	5.5	68.1	0.0	1.0
Made Up with Water, Average	*1oz/28g*	*17.0*	*0.0*	*61*	*1.2*	*15.1*	*0.0*	*0.0*
Mandarin & Pineapple, Sainsbury's*	1 Pot/125g	95.0	0.0	76	0.2	18.9	0.1	1.2
Mandarin, Aroma, M & S*	1oz/28g	17.0	0.0	60	0.2	14.6	0.0	0.4
Mixed Berry, WT5, Sainsbury's*	1 Serving/160g	112.0	0.0	70	0.7	16.3	0.2	1.5
Orange Flavour, Unprepared, Somerfield*	1 Pack/128g	379.0	0.0	296	5.0	69.0	0.0	0.0
Orange, Quickset, Unprepared, Rowntree's*	1oz/28g	95.0	0.0	340	0.0	84.0	0.0	3.0
Orange, Sugar Free, Crystals, Dry Weight, Hartley's*	1 Pack/26g	66.0	0.0	254	57.4	6.1	0.0	0.0
Orange, Sugar Free, Made Up, Hartley's*	1 Serving/140ml	8.0	0.0	6	1.4	0.1	0.0	0.0
Orange, Sugar Free, Rowntree's*	1 Serving/140ml	8.0	0.0	6	1.4	0.1	0.0	0.0
Orange, Sugar Free, Unprepared, Asda*	1 Serving/12g	36.0	0.0	303	63.6	12.0	0.1	0.2
Orange, Unprepared, Rowntree's*	1 Square/11g	33.0	0.0	296	4.4	69.6	0.0	0.0
Pineapple, with Pineapple Pieces, Tesco*	1 Serving/120g	96.0	0.0	80	1.2	18.6	0.1	0.7
Raspberry & Rose, Aroma, M & S*	1oz/28g	14.0	0.0	50	0.2	11.9	0.2	0.4
Raspberry Flavour, Sugar Free, Made Up, Rowntree's*	1 Serving/140ml	9.0	0.0	6	1.4	0.1	0.0	0.0
Raspberry Flavour, Tesco*	1 Serving/34g	22.0	0.0	64	1.0	15.0	0.0	0.1
Raspberry Flavoured, with Raspberries, M & S*	1 Sm Pot/175g	105.0	1.0	60	0.2	14.0	0.3	1.5
Raspberry, Crystals, Vegetarian, Just Wholefoods*	1 Packet/85g	293.0	0.0	345	0.5	85.7	0.0	0.0
Raspberry, Unprepared, Co-Op*	1 Pack/135g	402.0	0.0	298	5.5	68.9	0.0	0.0
Raspberry, Unprepared, Rowntree's*	1 Serving/135g	405.0	1.0	300	5.6	67.3	0.4	0.0
Redcurrant, Average	*1oz/28g*	*70.0*	*0.0*	*250*	*0.1*	*64.4*	*0.0*	*0.0*
Strawberry & Raspberry, Sainsbury's*	½ Pot/280g	230.0	0.0	82	0.2	20.2	0.0	1.2
Strawberry Flavour, Sugar Free, Made Up, Rowntree's*	1 Serving/140ml	10.0	0.0	7	1.5	0.1	0.0	0.0
Strawberry Flavour, Sugar Free, Unprepared, Rowntree's*	1oz/28g	84.0	0.0	300	64.9	3.0	0.0	0.0
Strawberry, No Added Sugar, Hartley's*	1 Pot/115g	3.0	0.0	3	0.0	0.4	0.0	0.3
Strawberry, Sugar Free, Crystals, Dry Weight, Hartley's*	1 Sachet/26g	73.0	0.0	280	56.8	13.1	0.0	0.0
Strawberry, Unprepared, Co-Op*	1 Pack/135g	402.0	0.0	298	5.5	69.1	0.0	0.0
Sugar Free, Dry, Tesco*	1 Pack/12.5g	36.0	0.0	285	55.4	15.6	0.0	0.2
Summer Fruits, Unprepared, Co-Op*	1 Pack/135g	401.0	0.0	297	5.5	68.7	0.0	0.0
Tangerine, Unprepared, Rowntree's*	1 Serving/33g	99.0	0.0	300	5.6	67.3	0.4	0.0
Tropical Fruit, Way to Five, Sainsbury's*	1 Serving/160g	144.0	2.0	90	0.3	19.9	1.0	0.9
Unprepared, Hartley's*	1 Serving/31g	92.0	0.0	296	5.1	68.9	0.0	0.0

J

	Measure INFO/WEIGHT	KCAL	FAT	Nutrition Values per 100g / 100ml				
		per Measure		KCAL	PROT	CARB	FAT	FIBRE
JELLY BABIES								
Bassett's*	1 Baby/6g	20.0	0.0	335	4.0	79.5	0.0	0.0
M & S*	1 Pack/125g	417.0	0.0	334	5.2	78.0	0.0	0.0
Mini, Rowntree's*	1 Small Bag/35g	128.0	0.0	366	4.6	86.9	0.0	0.0
Mini, Waitrose*	1 Bag/125g	370.0	0.0	296	4.3	68.7	0.4	0.0
Sainsbury's*	1 Serving/70g	247.0	0.0	353	4.1	82.5	0.7	0.3
JELLY BEANS								
Asda*	1 Bag/100g	364.0	0.0	364	0.1	90.0	0.4	0.2
Jelly Belly*	35 Beans/40g	140.0	0.0	350	0.0	90.0	0.0	0.0
M & S*	1 Bag/113g	407.0	0.0	360	0.1	89.6	0.0	0.0
No Added Sugar, Jelly Belly*	1 Serving/40g	80.0	0.0	200	0.0	50.0	0.0	20.0
Rowntree's*	1 Pack/35g	128.0	0.0	367	0.0	91.8	0.0	0.0
JELLY BEARS								
Co-Op*	1 Sweet/3g	10.0	0.0	325	6.0	76.0	0.1	0.0
JELLY TOTS								
Rowntree's*	1 Pack/42g	145.0	0.0	346	0.1	86.5	0.0	0.0
JERKY								
Beef, Peppered, Jack Link's*	1 Serving/28g	80.0	1.0	286	53.6	14.3	1.8	0.0
Shiitake Mushroom, Hot & Spicy, Primal Strips*	1 Pack/28g	108.0	4.0	386	21.4	42.9	14.3	21.4
Soy, Cajun Chick'n, Vegan, Tasty Eats*	1 Pack/28g	90.0	3.0	321	42.9	14.3	10.7	7.1
JUICE								
100% Vegetable, V8*	1 Bottle/354ml	67.0	1.0	19	0.8	3.2	0.3	0.5
Apple & Cranberry, Average	*1 Glass/250ml*	*114.0*	*0.0*	*45*	*0.1*	*10.1*	*0.0*	*0.0*
Apple & Elderflower, Copella*	1 Glass/250ml	107.0	0.0	43	0.4	10.2	0.1	0.0
Apple & Mango, Average	*1 Glass/200ml*	*108.0*	*0.0*	*54*	*0.3*	*12.6*	*0.0*	*0.1*
Apple & Orange, Fresh Up*	1 Serving/250ml	105.0	0.0	42	0.0	10.3	0.0	0.0
Apple & Pomegranate, Pommy, Sparky*	1 Serving/250ml	125.0	0.0	50	0.4	10.0	0.2	0.5
Apple & Raspberry, Average	*1 Serving/200ml*	*89.0*	*0.0*	*44*	*0.4*	*10.1*	*0.0*	*0.1*
Apple & Rhubarb, Caxton Vale*	1 Glass/250ml	115.0	1.0	46	0.2	9.7	0.4	0.0
Apple, Concentrate, Average	*1 Tbsp/15ml*	*45.0*	*0.0*	*302*	*0.0*	*73.5*	*0.1*	*0.0*
Apple, Pure, Average	*1 Glass/100ml*	*47.0*	*0.0*	*47*	*0.1*	*11.2*	*0.0*	*0.0*
Apple, Pure, Organic, Average	*1 Serving/200ml*	*92.0*	*0.0*	*46*	*0.0*	*11.1*	*0.0*	*0.0*
Apple, Raspberry, & Grape, Pressed, Sainsbury's*	1 Serving/200ml	92.0	0.0	46	0.3	11.2	0.1	0.5
Apple, Red Grape & Blueberry, Pure, Blends, Del Monte*	1 Serving/250ml	125.0	0.0	50	0.6	11.5	0.0	0.0
Beetroot, Organic, James White*	1 Glass/250ml	105.0	0.0	42	0.9	9.3	0.1	0.0
Berry Tasty, Smoothie, Nak'd*	1 Bottle/450ml	243.0	0.0	54	0.4	12.1	0.0	0.0
Breakfast, Sainsbury's*	1 Serving/200ml	94.0	0.0	47	0.7	11.3	0.0	0.3
Carrot, Average	*1 Glass/200ml*	*48.0*	*0.0*	*24*	*0.5*	*5.7*	*0.1*	*0.0*
Cherry, Original, Cherrygood*	1 Serving/250ml	112.0	0.0	45	0.0	10.5	0.1	0.0
Citrus Fruit & Veg, V8*	1 Serving/150ml	55.0	0.0	37	0.3	8.4	0.2	0.0
Clementine, Morrisons*	1 Serving/100ml	48.0	0.0	48	0.5	10.9	0.1	0.1
Coconut, Foco*	1 Can/520ml	182.0	1.0	35	0.1	8.2	0.2	0.0
Cranberry, Average	*1 Bottle/250ml*	*139.0*	*0.0*	*56*	*0.1*	*13.4*	*0.1*	*0.3*
Exotic Fruit, Pure, Del Monte*	1 Glass/200ml	96.0	0.0	48	0.3	11.3	0.0	0.0
Exotic Fruit, Waitrose*	1 Glass/175ml	87.0	0.0	50	0.4	11.6	0.0	0.0
Fibre, Tropicana*	1 Serving/200ml	130.0	0.0	65	0.4	15.8	0.0	3.4
Froot Refresh, Orange & Passion Fruit, Minute Maid*	1 Bottle/330ml	79.0	0.0	24	0.0	6.0	0.0	0.0
Froot Refresh, Red Grape & Raspberry, Minute Maid*	1 Bottle/330ml	99.0	0.0	30	0.0	7.3	0.0	0.0
Go!, Tropicana*	1 Bottle/200ml	80.0	0.0	40	0.3	9.7	0.0	0.0
Gold Pineapple & Mango, Del Monte*	1 Serving/200ml	104.0	0.0	52	0.4	12.0	0.0	0.0
Grape & Peach, Don Simon*	1 Serving/200ml	94.0	0.0	47	0.4	11.3	0.0	0.0
Grape & Raspberry, Pressed, M & S*	1 Carton/330ml	181.0	0.0	55	0.4	12.9	0.1	0.1
Grape, Purple, Light, Welch's*	1 Serving/100ml	27.0	0.0	27	0.2	6.1	0.3	0.3
Grape, Purple, Welch's*	1 Serving/200ml	136.0	0.0	68	0.1	16.5	0.0	0.0

J

	Measure INFO/WEIGHT	per Measure KCAL	FAT	Nutrition Values per 100g / 100ml KCAL	PROT	CARB	FAT	FIBRE
JUICE								
Grape, Red, Average	**1 Serving/100ml**	**62.0**	**0.0**	**62**	**0.1**	**15.1**	**0.0**	**0.0**
Grape, White, Average	**1 Can/160ml**	**95.0**	**0.0**	**59**	**0.2**	**14.3**	**0.1**	**0.1**
Grapefruit, Low Calorie, Natreen*	1 Glass/100ml	18.0	0.0	18	0.5	3.3	0.5	0.0
Grapefruit, Pink, Average	**1 Glass/200ml**	**81.0**	**0.0**	**40**	**0.6**	**9.0**	**0.0**	**0.2**
Grapefruit, Pure, Average	**1 Glass/200ml**	**77.0**	**0.0**	**38**	**0.5**	**8.5**	**0.1**	**0.1**
Juice and Water, Apple, Tropicana Kids, Tropicana*	1 Bottle/200ml	70.0	0.0	35	0.0	8.7	0.0	0.0
Lemon, Fresh, Average	**1 Juiced/35.5ml**	**2.0**	**0.0**	**7**	**0.3**	**1.6**	**0.0**	**0.1**
Lime, Fresh, Average	**1 Tsp/5ml**	**0.0**	**0.0**	**9**	**0.4**	**1.6**	**0.1**	**0.1**
Mango, Canned	**1 Glass/200ml**	**78.0**	**0.0**	**39**	**0.1**	**9.8**	**0.2**	**0.0**
Mango, Peach, Papaya, Pure, Premium, Tropicana*	1 Glass/200ml	88.0	0.0	44	0.5	9.8	0.0	0.1
Multivitamin, Fruit, Vitafit*	1 Glass/200ml	106.0	0.0	53	1.0	12.0	0.0	0.5
Orange & Banana, Pure, Average	**1 Glass/150ml**	**79.0**	**0.0**	**53**	**0.7**	**12.1**	**0.1**	**0.2**
Orange & Grapefruit, Average	**1 Glass/200ml**	**84.0**	**0.0**	**42**	**0.7**	**9.2**	**0.1**	**0.4**
Orange & Kiwi Fruit, Tropicana*	1 Serving/175ml	90.0	0.0	51	0.5	12.0	0.0	0.0
Orange & Mango, Average	**1 Bottle/375ml**	**176.0**	**0.0**	**47**	**0.5**	**10.7**	**0.1**	**0.2**
Orange & Pineapple, Average	**1 Glass/120ml**	**56.0**	**1.0**	**46**	**0.4**	**10.5**	**0.5**	**0.5**
Orange & Raspberry, Average	**1 fl oz/30ml**	**15.0**	**0.0**	**50**	**0.6**	**11.4**	**0.1**	**0.2**
Orange & Strawberry, Average	**1 Serving/125ml**	**64.0**	**0.0**	**51**	**0.6**	**10.9**	**0.4**	**0.8**
Orange Banana & Grapefruit, M & S*	1 Serving/250ml	125.0	0.0	50	0.8	11.5	0.2	0.3
Orange with Carrot Puree, M & S*	1 Bottle/500ml	200.0	1.0	40	0.6	8.0	0.3	0.3
Orange with Cranberry Juice, M & S*	1 Bottle/250ml	137.0	1.0	55	0.5	14.0	0.5	1.0
Orange, Apple & Mango, Calypso*	1 Carton/200ml	92.0	0.0	46	0.0	11.0	0.2	0.1
Orange, C, No Added Sugar, Libby's*	1 Serving/250ml	32.0	0.0	13	0.1	2.7	0.0	0.0
Orange, Freshly Squeezed, Average	1 Serving/200ml	66.0	0.0	33	0.6	8.1	0.0	1.0
Orange, Mango & Passionfruit, Pure Squeezed, Waitrose*	1 Serving/250ml	130.0	1.0	52	0.6	10.9	0.3	0.3
Orange, No Bits, Innocent*	1 Glass/250ml	120.0	0.0	48	0.8	10.9	0.0	0.2
Orange, No Pulp, with Calcium, Napolina*	1 Serving/240ml	110.0	0.0	46	0.8	10.8	0.0	0.0
Orange, Pulp Free, Napolina*	1 Serving/264ml	110.0	0.0	42	0.8	9.9	0.0	0.0
Orange, Pure, Smooth, Average	**1 Glass/200ml**	**88.0**	**0.0**	**44**	**0.7**	**9.8**	**0.0**	**0.2**
Orange, Pure, with Bits, Average	**1 Glass/200ml**	**90.0**	**0.0**	**45**	**0.6**	**10.2**	**0.1**	**0.1**
Orange, Red, Average	**1 Glass/250ml**	**115.0**	**0.0**	**46**	**0.4**	**10.7**	**0.0**	**0.2**
Orange, Sparkling, 55, Britvic*	1 Bottle/275ml	135.0	0.0	49	0.3	11.3	0.1	0.1
Orange, with Raspberry & Zinc,100% Pure, Minute Maid*	¼ Bottle/250ml	82.0	0.0	33	0.5	8.2	0.0	0.0
Passion Fruit, Average	**1 Glass/200ml**	**94.0**	**0.0**	**47**	**0.8**	**10.7**	**0.1**	**0.0**
Peach, Mango & Passion Fruit, Sainsbury's*	1 Glass/200ml	92.0	0.0	46	0.3	10.3	0.1	0.5
Pear, Pure, Heinz*	1 Serving/100ml	41.0	0.0	41	0.1	9.8	0.1	0.0
Pear, with a Hint of Ginger, Pressed, M & S*	1 Glass/250ml	125.0	0.0	50	0.3	11.7	0.1	0.0
Pineapple & Coconut, Sainsbury's*	1 Glass/250ml	152.0	3.0	61	0.5	11.6	1.4	0.1
Pineapple & Coconut, Waitrose*	1 Serving/250ml	125.0	1.0	50	0.2	11.5	0.3	0.2
Pineapple and Guava, Tropicana*	1 Glass/200ml	106.0	0.0	53	0.3	12.3	0.0	1.2
Pineapple Mango Crush, Just Juice*	1 Glass/250ml	107.0	0.0	43	0.0	10.6	0.0	0.0
Pineapple, Average	**1 Glass/200ml**	**100.0**	**0.0**	**50**	**0.3**	**11.7**	**0.1**	**0.1**
Pomegranate and Blueberry, Sainsbury's*	1oz/28g	14.0	0.0	49	0.0	11.7	0.0	0.1
Pomegranate, Grape & Apple, Tropicana*	1 Bottle/330ml	211.0	0.0	64	0.2	15.5	0.0	0.6
Pomegranate, Pomegreat*	1 Glass/200ml	88.0	0.0	44	0.1	11.1	0.0	0.0
Prune, Average	**1 Glass/200ml**	**123.0**	**0.0**	**61**	**0.6**	**15.3**	**0.1**	**1.8**
Raspberry Cooler, with Mint, Sainsbury's*	1 Serving/250ml	62.0	0.0	25	0.1	6.0	0.1	0.1
Sweet Carrot & Orange, Shapers, Boots*	1 Serving/250ml	100.0	0.0	40	0.9	8.8	0.2	0.4
Tomato, Average	**1 Glass/200ml**	**40.0**	**0.0**	**20**	**0.7**	**4.0**	**0.0**	**0.4**
Tomato, Princes*	1 Serving/100g	16.0	0.0	16	0.8	3.1	0.0	0.6
Tropical Fruit, Plenty*	1 Glass/200ml	120.0	0.0	60	0.5	13.7	0.1	0.0
Tropical, Pure, Sainsbury's*	1 Glass/200ml	104.0	0.0	52	0.5	12.0	0.1	0.1
Tropical, Tropics, Tropicana*	1 Serving/250ml	112.0	0.0	45	0.4	11.0	0.0	0.0

J

	Measure INFO/WEIGHT	per Measure KCAL	FAT	Nutrition Values per 100g / 100ml KCAL	PROT	CARB	FAT	FIBRE
JUICE								
Vegetable, Organic, Evernat*	1 Glass/200ml	36.0	0.0	18	0.9	3.5	0.1	0.2
JUICE DRINK								
Apple & Blueberry, The Feel Good Drinks Co*	1 Serving/375ml	163.0	0.0	43	0.1	10.6	0.1	0.0
Apple & Cranberry, Safeway*	1 Serving/250ml	125.0	0.0	50	0.0	12.1	0.0	0.0
Apple & Elderflower, Tesco*	1 Serving/200ml	76.0	0.0	38	0.0	9.4	0.0	0.0
Apple & Raspberry, Dr Gillian McKeith*	1 Bottle/200ml	86.0	0.0	43	0.1	10.6	0.0	0.0
Apple & Raspberry, Sainsbury's*	1 Serving/200ml	112.0	0.0	56	0.1	13.8	0.1	0.1
Apple & Strawberry, Sainsbury's*	1 Serving/250ml	13.0	0.0	5	0.0	1.0	0.0	0.0
Apple, Cranberry, & Blueberry, Waitrose*	1 Serving/150ml	75.0	0.0	50	0.1	11.9	0.0	0.1
Apple, Libby's*	1 Serving/100ml	43.0	0.0	43	0.0	10.3	0.0	0.0
Apple, No Added Sugar, Asda*	1 Glass/200ml	10.0	0.0	5	0.0	1.0	0.0	0.0
Berry & Elderberry, Fusion, Oasis*	1 Bottle/375ml	11.0	0.0	3	0.0	0.4	0.0	0.0
Blackcurrant & Apple, Oasis*	1 Serving/500ml	140.0	0.0	28	0.0	6.8	0.0	0.0
Blackcurrant & Raspberry, with Soya, Adez*	1 Glass/250ml	82.0	1.0	33	1.1	6.3	0.4	0.3
Blackcurrant, 45% High, No Added Sugar, Asda*	1 Serving/25ml	2.0	0.0	7	0.0	1.4	0.0	0.0
Blackcurrant, CVit*	1 Glass/200ml	4.0	0.0	2	0.0	0.2	0.0	0.0
Blackcurrant, Purity*	1 Bottle/500ml	265.0	0.0	53	0.0	13.2	0.0	0.0
Blueberry, BGTY, Sainsbury's*	1 Serving/250ml	15.0	0.0	6	0.1	1.0	0.0	0.0
Cherry, No Added Sugar, Sainsbury's*	1 Carton/250ml	25.0	0.0	10	0.2	1.9	0.0	0.0
Citrus Burst, 5 Alive*	1 Carton/250ml	125.0	0.0	50	0.0	12.8	0.0	0.0
Citrus, Sainsbury's*	1 Serving/200ml	102.0	0.0	51	0.3	12.3	0.1	0.2
Cranberry & Apple, Ocean Spray*	1 Glass/200ml	92.0	0.0	46	0.0	11.1	0.0	0.0
Cranberry & Blackberry, Ocean Spray*	1 Glass/250ml	120.0	0.0	48	0.1	11.3	0.1	0.2
Cranberry & Blackcurrant, Ocean Spray*	1 Bottle/500ml	265.0	0.0	53	0.2	12.7	0.0	0.0
Cranberry & Blueberry, Ocean Spray*	1 Serving/100ml	48.0	0.0	48	0.0	11.6	0.0	0.0
Cranberry & Mango, Light, Ocean Spray*	1 Glass/250ml	22.0	0.0	9	0.0	2.0	0.0	0.1
Cranberry & Orange, No Added Sugar, Sainsbury's*	1 Glass/250ml	15.0	0.0	6	0.1	1.2	0.1	0.1
Cranberry & Pomegranate, Ocean Spray*	1 Glass/250ml	120.0	0.0	48	0.0	11.5	0.0	0.0
Cranberry & Raspberry, Ocean Spray*	1 Glass/200ml	104.0	0.0	52	0.0	12.6	0.0	0.0
Cranberry & Raspberry, Sainsbury's*	1 Serving/250ml	105.0	0.0	42	0.1	9.9	0.0	0.0
Cranberry & Raspberry, Tesco*	1 Serving/200ml	96.0	0.0	48	0.0	11.6	0.0	0.0
Cranberry, Classic, Ocean Spray*	1 Bottle/500ml	245.0	0.0	49	0.1	11.7	0.1	0.1
Cranberry, Grape & Apple, Ocean Spray*	1 Glass/200ml	108.0	0.0	54	0.1	12.9	0.0	0.0
Cranberry, Juice Burst, Purity*	1 Bottle/500ml	245.0	0.0	49	0.0	12.0	0.0	0.0
Cranberry, Light, Classic, Ocean Spray*	1 Glass/200ml	16.0	0.0	8	0.0	1.4	0.0	0.0
Cranberry, M & S*	1 Serving/100ml	60.0	0.0	60	0.1	14.3	0.0	0.0
Cranberry, Original, Concentrated, Ocean Spray*	1 Serving/15ml	27.0	0.0	183	0.2	44.1	0.0	0.0
Cranberry, Solevita*	1 Serving/200ml	98.0	0.0	49	0.5	11.7	0.0	0.0
Cranberry, Tropical, Ocean Spray*	1 Glass/200ml	96.0	0.0	48	0.1	11.5	0.0	0.0
Cranberry, Waitrose*	1 Serving/250ml	145.0	0.0	58	0.1	13.9	0.0	0.1
Exotic, Tesco*	1 Serving/250ml	127.0	0.0	51	0.1	12.3	0.0	0.0
Fruit Cocktail, Sainsbury's*	1 Glass/200ml	90.0	0.0	45	0.2	10.6	0.0	0.1
Grape & Elderflower, White, Sparkling, Schloer*	1 Glass/200ml	74.0	0.0	37	0.0	9.2	0.0	0.0
Grape, Apple & Raspberry, Asda*	1 Glass/200ml	90.0	0.0	45	0.2	11.0	0.0	0.0
Grape, Apple & Raspberry, Co-Op*	1 Serving/150ml	75.0	0.0	50	0.4	12.0	0.0	0.1
Grape, Red, Sparkling, Schloer*	1 Glass/200ml	84.0	0.0	42	0.0	10.4	0.0	0.0
Grape, White, Sparkling, Schloer*	1 Serving/120ml	59.0	0.0	49	0.0	11.6	0.0	0.0
Grapefruit & Cranberry, M & S*	1 Serving/250ml	125.0	0.0	50	0.2	11.9	0.1	0.0
Grapefruit & Lime, Quest, M & S*	1 Bottle/330ml	53.0	0.0	16	0.0	4.0	0.0	0.0
Guava Exotic, Rubicon*	1 Carton/288ml	150.0	0.0	52	0.2	12.9	0.1	0.0
J20, Apple & Mango, Britvic*	1 Bottle/275ml	118.0	0.0	43	0.1	10.0	0.0	0.2
J20, Apple & Raspberry, Britvic*	1 Bottle/275ml	146.0	0.0	53	0.1	12.0	0.1	0.0
J20, Orange & Passion Fruit, Britvic*	1 Bottle/275ml	132.0	0.0	48	0.1	11.3	0.1	0.0

J

	Measure INFO/WEIGHT	per Measure KCAL	FAT	Nutrition Values per 100g / 100ml KCAL	PROT	CARB	FAT	FIBRE
JUICE DRINK								
Lemon & Lime, Light, Oasis*	1 Bottle/250ml	6.0	0.0	3	0.0	0.2	0.0	0.0
Lemon & Mandarin, Diet, Quest, M & S*	1 Bottle/330ml	13.0	0.0	4	0.0	1.0	0.0	0.0
Lemon, The Feel Good Drinks Co*	1 Bottle/171ml	78.0	0.0	46	0.1	10.8	0.1	0.0
Lemonade, Asda*	1 Glass/200ml	88.0	0.0	44	0.1	11.0	0.0	0.0
Mango & Passionfruit, Shot, Big Shotz*	1 Shot/120ml	67.0	0.0	56	0.0	12.1	0.4	3.4
Mango, Rubicon*	1 Serving/100ml	54.0	0.0	54	0.1	13.1	0.1	0.0
Mango, Sparkling, Rubicon*	1 Can/330ml	172.0	0.0	52	0.0	12.8	0.0	0.0
Mega Green, Smucker's*	1 Serving/473ml	236.0	0.0	50	0.0	12.5	0.0	0.0
Orange, Caprisun*	1 Pouch/200ml	89.0	0.0	45	0.0	10.8	0.0	0.0
Orange, Carrot & Lemon, Pago*	1 Serving/200g	90.0	0.0	45	0.2	10.5	0.1	0.0
Orange, Fruitish, Spar*	1 Carton/330ml	13.0	0.0	4	0.1	0.8	0.1	0.0
Orange, Juice Burst, Purity*	1 Bottle/500ml	220.0	0.0	44	1.0	10.2	0.0	0.0
Orange, Mango & Lime, Fruit Crush, Shapers, Boots*	1 Bottle/330ml	150.0	1.0	45	0.4	10.6	0.2	0.4
Orange, Morrisons*	1 Serving/250ml	12.0	0.0	5	0.1	0.9	0.1	0.1
Orange, No Added Sugar, Tesco*	1 fl oz/30ml	1.0	0.0	4	0.0	0.7	0.0	0.0
Orange, Sainsbury's*	1 Serving/250ml	17.0	0.0	7	0.1	1.4	0.1	0.1
Orange, Value, Tesco*	1 Glass/250ml	32.0	0.0	13	0.0	3.3	0.0	0.0
Passion Fruit, Exotic, Rubicon*	1 Serving/200ml	110.0	0.0	55	0.1	13.6	0.0	0.0
Peach & Passionfruit Fruit, Sunmagic*	1 Serving/330ml	172.0	0.0	52	0.3	13.0	0.0	0.1
Peach, Fruit Float, Frubob*	1 Can/250ml	150.0	0.0	60	0.2	14.8	0.0	0.0
Peach, Passion Fruit, Extra Light, Oasis*	1 Bottle/500ml	17.0	0.0	3	0.0	0.6	0.0	0.0
Pear, Partially Made with Concentrate, Tesco*	1 Glass/200ml	110.0	0.0	55	0.0	12.4	0.0	0.2
Pineapple & Grapefruit, Shapers, Boots*	1 Bottle/500ml	10.0	0.0	2	0.1	0.2	0.1	0.0
Pineapple, Mango & Passionfruit, Sainsbury's*	1 Serving/200ml	74.0	0.0	37	0.1	8.7	0.0	0.2
Pink Grapefruit, Juice Burst, Purity*	1 Bottle/500ml	210.0	0.0	42	0.4	10.0	0.0	0.0
Pomegranate & Blueberry, Weight Watchers*	1 Bottle/500ml	15.0	0.0	3	0.0	0.5	0.0	0.0
Pomegranate & Raspberry, Still, Shapers, Boots*	1 Bottle/500ml	45.0	0.0	9	0.0	2.0	0.0	0.0
Pomegranate, Rubicon*	1 Can/330mll	108.0	0.0	54	0.0	13.5	0.0	0.0
Raspberry & Pear, Tesco*	1 Serving/250ml	117.0	0.0	47	0.0	11.3	0.0	0.0
Spirit, Lemon & Grapefruit, Tropicana*	1 Bottle/400ml	184.0	0.0	46	0.3	10.4	0.0	0.6
Summer Fruits, Fresh, Tesco*	1 Glass/250ml	112.0	0.0	45	0.1	10.8	0.1	0.3
Summer Fruits, Oasis*	1 Bottle/500ml	90.0	0.0	18	0.0	4.2	0.0	0.0
Tropical Fruit, Tesco*	1 Glass/250ml	117.0	0.0	47	0.0	11.4	0.0	0.0
Tropical Fruit, Waitrose*	1 Glass/250ml	117.0	0.0	47	0.2	11.2	0.0	0.0
Tropical Hit, 5 Alive*	1 Carton/250ml	92.0	0.0	37	0.0	9.3	0.0	0.0
White Cranberry & Grape, Oceanspray*	1 Serving/100ml	48.0	0.0	48	0.0	11.6	0.0	0.0
White Cranberry & Lychee, Ocean Spray*	1 Glass/200ml	86.0	0.0	43	0.0	11.5	0.0	0.0
White Grape & Peach, Sainsbury's*	1 Glass/250ml	95.0	0.0	38	0.2	9.0	0.1	0.1
JUNIPER								
Berries, Dried, Average	1 Tsp/2g	6.0	0.0	292	4.0	33.0	16.0	0.0

J

	Measure INFO/WEIGHT	per Measure KCAL	FAT	Nutrition Values per 100g / 100ml KCAL	PROT	CARB	FAT	FIBRE
KALE								
Curly, Boiled in Salted Water, Average	*1 Serving/60g*	*14.0*	*1.0*	*24*	*2.4*	*1.0*	*1.1*	*2.8*
Curly, Raw, Average	*1 Serving/90g*	*30.0*	*1.0*	*33*	*3.4*	*1.4*	*1.6*	*3.1*
KANGAROO								
Raw, Average	*1 Serving/200g*	*196.0*	*2.0*	*98*	*22.0*	*1.0*	*1.0*	*0.0*
Steak, Grilled, Average	*1 Fillet/150g*	*198.0*	*2.0*	*132*	*30.0*	*0.0*	*1.2*	*0.0*
KEBAB								
BBQ Pork, Sainsbury's*	1 Serving/90g	65.0	2.0	72	11.0	1.4	2.4	0.9
Beef & Pepper Kofta, Waitrose*	1 Kebab/138g	223.0	14.0	162	14.8	2.9	10.1	0.6
Beef with Sweet Chilli Seasoning, Sainsbury's*	1 Kebab/61g	151.0	8.0	248	24.1	8.5	13.1	0.8
Beef, Hot & Spicy, Tesco*	1 Kebab/41g	111.0	8.0	270	15.7	4.4	20.6	1.6
Beef, Kofta, Uncooked, Tesco*	1 Kebab/72.5g	163.0	13.0	225	14.0	3.2	17.3	1.2
Cajun Salmon, Tesco*	1 Kebab/75g	100.0	3.0	133	19.8	3.9	4.2	1.3
Chicken & Pineapple, Aldi*	1 Kebab/85g	89.0	3.0	105	13.9	5.3	3.1	0.0
Chicken & Sausage, with Teriyaki Sauce, Asda*	1 Serving/110g	257.0	15.0	234	17.0	10.0	14.0	1.0
Chicken Tikka, Breast, Safeway*	1 Kebab/88g	127.0	1.0	145	23.8	9.8	1.0	0.7
Chicken Tikka, with Red Pepper & Pineapple, Tesco*	1 Kebab/80g	92.0	2.0	115	16.5	6.7	2.4	0.5
Chicken, Barbecue, Sainsbury's*	1 Pack/200g	238.0	3.0	119	24.4	1.5	1.7	1.8
Chicken, Breast, Mediterranean, Sainsbury's*	1 Kebab/65g	73.0	2.0	113	16.5	4.6	3.2	0.6
Chicken, Breast, Salsa, Sainsbury's*	1 Kebab/80g	94.0	1.0	117	20.1	6.5	1.1	0.6
Chicken, Breast, Sweet, Oriental, COU, M & S*	½ Pack/200g	220.0	2.0	110	20.8	4.3	1.0	0.1
Chicken, Caribbean, Iceland*	1 Kebab/44g	36.0	0.0	82	12.0	8.0	0.2	0.5
Chicken, Chilli & Lime, Breast Fillet, Sainsbury's*	1 Kebab/77g	120.0	1.0	156	29.9	6.2	0.9	0.3
Chicken, Citrus Tikka, Mini, Sainsbury's*	1 Serving/48g	72.0	1.0	151	30.3	2.7	2.3	0.2
Chicken, Fillet, Mini, with a Tikka Marinade, Sainsbury's*	1 Kebab/25g	41.0	1.0	164	33.4	0.6	3.1	0.1
Chicken, Honey & Mustard, M & S*	1oz/28g	41.0	1.0	145	16.7	8.2	4.8	1.0
Chicken, Mini Fillet, M & S*	1 Serving/150g	210.0	9.0	140	20.2	2.0	5.8	0.3
Chicken, Red Pepper, Mini, Sainsbury's*	1 Kebab/52g	79.0	1.0	152	30.1	3.5	2.0	0.2
Chicken, Shish, Average	1 Kebab/250g	312.0	5.0	125	25.7	0.9	2.1	0.1
Chicken, Sweet Chilli, Perfectly Balanced, Waitrose*	1 Kebab/83g	111.0	1.0	135	28.6	1.7	1.1	0.5
Chicken, Thigh, Sticky Barbecue, M & S*	1 Kebab/100g	160.0	7.0	160	15.6	7.4	7.5	0.8
Chicken, Thin Sliced, Heat 'n' Eat, Asda*	½ Pack/50g	92.0	6.0	184	15.0	3.9	12.0	1.1
Chicken, with Sweet Chilli Sauce, Finest, Tesco*	½ Pack/175g	241.0	1.0	138	17.9	14.7	0.8	1.2
Chicken, with Sweet Chilli Sauce, M & S*	1 Serving/165g	228.0	1.0	138	17.9	14.7	0.8	1.2
Chinese Salmon, Iceland*	1 Kebab/75g	115.0	3.0	153	23.8	4.1	4.6	1.6
Citrus Tikka Chicken Breast, Sainsbury's*	1 Kebab/61g	79.0	0.0	129	25.6	5.4	0.5	0.9
Doner, Heat 'n' Eat Thin Sliced, Asda*	1 Pack/100g	196.0	11.0	196	16.7	8.4	10.6	1.7
Green Thai Chicken, Waitrose*	1 Serving/180g	223.0	7.0	124	20.5	1.4	4.0	1.4
Halloumi & Vegetable, Waitrose*	1 Kebab/127g	235.0	22.0	185	5.6	2.2	17.0	2.4
Honey & Mustard Chicken, Sainsbury's*	1 Serving/50g	65.0	1.0	131	24.5	4.3	1.8	0.0
Lamb Kofta with a Mint & Coriander Raita, Safeway*	1 Pack/290g	632.0	38.0	218	16.9	8.4	13.0	1.2
Lamb Kofta, Indian Style, Waitrose*	1 Kebab/125g	266.0	20.0	213	12.3	5.5	15.8	1.6
Lamb Shami with a Mint Raita Dip, M & S*	½ Pack/90g	189.0	12.0	210	12.8	9.7	13.4	3.5
Lamb, Greek Style, Sainsbury's*	1 Serving/70g	196.0	15.0	282	16.1	4.9	22.0	1.8
Lamb, Kofta, Citrus Tikka, Sainsbury's*	1 Kebab/84g	199.0	12.0	235	18.1	9.8	13.7	2.6
Lamb, Shish, Sainsbury's*	1 Kebab/85g	178.0	11.0	210	19.7	2.8	13.3	0.7
Lamb, Shish, Waitrose*	1 Kebab/56g	114.0	7.0	203	15.3	6.8	12.7	1.1
Lamb, Shoulder, M & S*	½ Pack/250g	312.0	11.0	125	20.4	0.9	4.3	1.7
Lamb, with Halloumi Cheese & Olives, Waitrose*	1 Kebab/75g	123.0	6.0	164	20.0	2.4	8.3	0.2
Lamb, with Mint, Tesco*	1 Serving/80g	192.0	13.0	240	16.0	5.5	16.7	0.4
Lemon & Ginger Chicken, Delicatezze, Waitrose*	1 Kebab/25g	50.0	3.0	201	24.5	0.3	11.3	2.7
Mango & Lime Chicken, Perfectly Balanced, Waitrose*	1 Kebab/82.5g	103.0	1.0	125	26.0	1.2	1.6	1.1
Mango Salsa Chicken Breast, Sainsbury's*	1 Kebab/60g	85.0	1.0	142	26.3	5.5	1.6	0.6
Pork & Pepper, BBQ, Sainsbury's*	1 Kebab/41g	65.0	2.0	158	24.1	3.1	5.4	1.9

K

	Measure INFO/WEIGHT	per Measure KCAL	per Measure FAT	Nutrition Values per 100g / 100ml KCAL	PROT	CARB	FAT	FIBRE
KEBAB								
Pork & Pepper, Co-Op*	1 Kebab/74g	78.0	3.0	105	17.0	1.0	4.0	0.5
Salmon, Hot & Spicy, Tesco*	1 Kebab/75g	88.0	2.0	118	22.0	1.1	2.9	0.0
Shish in Pitta Bread with Salad	1 Kebab/250g	387.0	10.0	155	13.5	17.2	4.1	1.0
Shish with Onions & Peppers	1oz/28g	59.0	5.0	212	12.9	3.9	16.2	1.2
Spicy Tomato Creole King Prawn, M & S*	1 Pack/240g	240.0	8.0	100	14.3	2.9	3.3	0.7
Sweetcorn, Tesco*	1 Kebab/130g	74.0	1.0	57	2.0	9.9	1.0	0.9
Tandoori, M & S*	1oz/28g	34.0	1.0	120	23.3	1.0	2.5	0.0
Thai Style Chicken, Eat Smart, Safeway*	1 Kebab/85g	85.0	1.0	100	15.3	6.4	1.3	1.4
Tiger Prawn, Asda*	1oz/28g	17.0	0.0	59	14.6	0.0	0.1	0.0
Tikka, Mini, M & S*	1 Kebab/11g	23.0	1.0	205	18.4	4.0	12.7	0.6
Tomato & Basil Chicken, Eat Smart, Safeway*	1 Kebab/72g	82.0	2.0	115	18.0	5.0	2.1	1.5
Turkey, with Chinese Style Dressing, Sainsbury's*	1 Kebab/53.5g	84.0	3.0	157	21.4	6.4	5.1	1.7
Vegetable, Asda*	1 Kebab/40g	25.0	2.0	63	1.8	4.5	4.3	2.4
Vegetable, Sainsbury's*	1 Kebab/100g	36.0	0.0	36	1.5	6.4	0.5	1.2
Vegetable, Tesco*	1 Kebab/120g	47.0	1.0	39	1.7	6.8	0.6	1.1
KEDGEREE								
Average	1oz/28g	48.0	2.0	171	15.9	7.8	8.7	0.1
Seafood Masala, Perfectly Balanced, Waitrose*	1 Pack/400g	380.0	4.0	95	7.5	13.9	1.0	0.6
Smoked Haddock, Big Dish, M & S*	1 Pack/450g	585.0	22.0	130	8.5	13.0	5.0	1.9
KETCHUP								
BBQ, Heinz*	1 Serving/10g	14.0	0.0	137	1.3	31.3	0.3	0.3
Mild Chilli, Twisted, Heinz*	1 Tbsp/15g	16.0	0.0	108	1.0	24.9	0.2	0.7
Tomato, Average	*1 Tsp/5g*	*6.0*	*0.0*	*120*	*1.5*	*28.1*	*0.2*	*0.8*
Tomato, Reduced Sugar, Average	*1 Tbsp/10g*	*9.0*	*0.0*	*87*	*2.0*	*16.9*	*1.2*	*0.9*
Wicked Orange, Heinz*	1 Serving/11g	12.0	0.0	108	1.0	24.7	0.1	0.6
KIDNEY								
Lamb, Raw, Average	*1oz/28g*	*44.0*	*2.0*	*156*	*21.5*	*0.0*	*7.7*	*0.0*
Ox, Raw	*1oz/28g*	*25.0*	*1.0*	*88*	*17.2*	*0.0*	*2.1*	*0.0*
Ox, Stewed	*1oz/28g*	*39.0*	*1.0*	*138*	*24.5*	*0.0*	*4.4*	*0.0*
Pig, Fried	*1oz/28g*	*57.0*	*3.0*	*202*	*29.2*	*0.0*	*9.5*	*0.0*
Pig, Raw	*1oz/28g*	*24.0*	*1.0*	*86*	*15.5*	*0.0*	*2.7*	*0.0*
Pig, Stewed	*1oz/28g*	*43.0*	*2.0*	*153*	*24.4*	*0.0*	*6.1*	*0.0*
Pork, Braised, in Gravy, Pek*	1 Can/198g	133.0	4.0	67	10.7	2.0	1.8	0.0
Veal, Raw, Average	1 Serving/100g	99.0	3.0	99	15.8	0.8	3.1	0.0
KIEV								
Cheese & Herb, Mini, Bernard Matthews*	1 Kiev/23g	46.0	2.0	199	15.7	12.1	9.8	0.0
Cheese & Mushroom Chicken, Somerfield*	½ Pack/142g	294.0	16.0	207	14.0	15.0	11.0	0.0
Chicken Breast, Garlic Butter, Sun Valley*	1 Kiev/141g	436.0	33.0	309	13.2	11.8	23.2	0.9
Chicken Breast, Garlic, Frozen, Tesco*	1 Kiev/141g	430.0	35.0	305	13.0	6.9	24.6	1.3
Chicken, Bernard Matthews*	1 Kiev/125g	374.0	28.0	299	10.6	13.9	22.3	2.7
Chicken, Breast, Hand Filled, Birds Eye*	1 Kiev/172g	330.0	17.0	192	15.5	9.9	10.0	2.0
Chicken, Cheesy Bean, Asda*	1 Kiev/94g	202.0	10.0	215	12.0	17.0	11.0	1.9
Chicken, Creamy Garlic, Chilled, Tesco*	½ Pack/143g	285.0	17.0	200	12.9	9.7	12.0	1.3
Chicken, Creamy Pepper, Safeway*	1 Kiev/133g	306.0	20.0	230	11.9	11.1	15.4	1.1
Chicken, Creamy Peppercorn, Sun Valley*	1 Kiev/140g	382.0	26.0	273	13.3	13.5	18.5	0.0
Chicken, Finest, Tesco*	1 Kiev/237g	503.0	27.0	212	19.5	8.2	11.2	2.6
Chicken, Garlic & Herb, Sainsbury's*	1 Kiev/134g	319.0	20.0	239	15.0	11.7	14.7	1.3
Chicken, Garlic & Mushroom, Sainsbury's*	1 Kiev/142g	346.0	19.0	243	16.2	14.5	13.4	1.4
Chicken, Garlic & Parsley, BGTY, Sainsbury's*	1 Kiev/142g	324.0	18.0	228	15.9	12.3	12.8	1.0
Chicken, Garlic & Parsley, Sainsbury's*	1 Kiev/120g	365.0	26.0	304	11.1	17.1	21.3	0.8
Chicken, Garlic Butter, HL, Tesco*	1 Kiev/143g	285.0	16.0	200	14.3	9.9	11.5	0.6
Chicken, Garlic, 25% Less Fat, GFY, Asda*	1 Kiev/134g	296.0	16.0	221	17.0	11.9	11.7	0.5
Chicken, Garlic, 25% Reduced Fat, Tesco*	1 Kiev/130g	299.0	19.0	230	13.7	11.5	14.3	0.7

K

	Measure INFO/WEIGHT	per Measure KCAL	FAT	Nutrition Values per 100g / 100ml KCAL	PROT	CARB	FAT	FIBRE
KIEV								
Chicken, Garlic, Fresh, Reduced Fat, Morrisons*	1 Kiev/141g	350.0	26.0	248	13.2	8.0	18.1	0.7
Chicken, Garlic, M & S*	1 Kiev/150g	370.0	25.0	247	15.6	8.2	16.5	2.9
Chicken, Garlic, Morrisons*	1 Kiev/122g	289.0	19.0	237	14.3	9.8	15.7	0.0
Chicken, Garlic, Whole Breast, Asda*	1 Pack/290g	638.0	38.0	220	15.2	10.4	13.1	0.0
Chicken, Good Choice, Iceland*	1 Kiev/120g	366.0	27.0	305	12.7	12.6	22.7	0.8
Chicken, Ham & Cheese, BGTY, Sainsbury's*	1 Kiev/132g	264.0	10.0	200	13.2	19.5	7.7	0.8
Chicken, Ham, & Cheese, Tesco*	1 Serving/143g	307.0	19.0	215	14.4	9.3	13.0	1.3
Chicken, in Crispy Breadcrumbs, Sainsbury's*	1 Kiev/117g	310.0	22.0	266	12.8	10.6	19.2	1.1
Chicken, Italian Style, Sainsbury's*	1 Kiev/135g	341.0	22.0	253	14.3	12.8	16.1	1.3
Chicken, Maitre Jean-Pierre*	1 Kiev/140g	385.0	27.0	275	13.3	12.7	19.1	0.8
Chicken, Roast Garlic & Parsley, Sainsbury's*	1 Kiev/143g	369.0	21.0	258	14.5	16.5	14.9	0.8
Chicken, Tesco*	1oz/28g	86.0	7.0	307	11.4	7.6	25.7	1.6
Chicken, Tomato & Mozzarella, Tesco*	1 Kiev/143g	285.0	17.0	200	13.4	9.0	12.2	1.4
Chicken, White Wine & Mushroom, Tesco*	1 Serving/145g	281.0	14.0	194	16.7	10.3	9.5	0.5
Cod & Parsley, Safeway*	1 Kiev/160g	310.0	15.0	194	10.6	17.0	9.2	0.0
Garlic, Meat Free, Tesco*	1 Kiev/125g	244.0	11.0	195	15.0	12.5	9.0	2.6
Lemon Butter Chicken, Somerfield*	½ Pack/142g	409.0	30.0	288	12.0	12.0	21.0	0.0
Salmon, Fillet, Tesco*	1 Kiev/160g	376.0	20.0	235	13.3	18.0	12.2	2.5
Tikka Chicken, Asda*	1 Kiev/134g	274.0	15.0	205	12.8	13.5	11.1	0.6
Turkey, Mini, Baked, Bernard Matthews*	1 Kiev/23g	50.0	3.0	221	17.5	11.2	11.8	1.1
KIEV VEGETARIAN								
Cheesy Garlic, Meat Free, Sainsbury's*	1 Kiev/123g	274.0	15.0	223	13.8	14.3	12.3	3.5
Garlic Butter, Tivall*	1 Kiev/125g	366.0	26.0	293	15.1	10.8	21.0	2.6
Garlic, Meat Free, Asda*	1 Kiev/125g	239.0	11.0	191	15.0	12.5	9.0	2.6
Garlic, Safeway*	1 Kiev/142g	423.0	26.0	298	13.2	20.3	18.2	0.7
Vegetable, M & S*	1 Kiev/155g	325.0	21.0	210	4.6	17.8	13.4	2.5
KIPPER								
Baked, Average	*1oz/28g*	*57.0*	*3.0*	*205*	*25.5*	*0.0*	*11.4*	*0.0*
Fillets, in Brine, John West*	1 Can/140g	269.0	17.0	192	21.0	0.0	12.0	0.0
Fillets, in Sunflower Oil, John West*	1 Can/140g	321.0	24.0	229	19.0	0.0	17.0	0.0
Fillets, Raw, Average	*1 Serving/200g*	*451.0*	*34.0*	*226*	*17.0*	*0.0*	*17.1*	*0.0*
Fillets, with Butter, Farmfoods*	1oz/28g	64.0	5.0	229	17.5	0.0	17.7	0.0
Fillets, with Butter, Scottish, Somerfield*	1 Serving/100g	178.0	12.0	178	16.5	0.0	12.4	0.0
Grilled, Average	*1oz/28g*	*71.0*	*5.0*	*255*	*20.1*	*0.0*	*19.4*	*0.0*
Smoked, Average	*1 Serving/150g*	*322.0*	*23.0*	*214*	*18.9*	*0.0*	*15.3*	*0.0*
KIT KAT								
2 Finger, Nestle*	2 Fingers/21g	107.0	5.0	510	6.4	62.8	25.6	2.3
4 Finger, Nestle*	4 Fingers/46g	233.0	12.0	512	6.3	62.6	25.9	1.1
Caramac, 4 Finger, Nestle*	4 Fingers/49g	259.0	14.0	532	5.9	61.9	29.0	0.6
Chunky, Nestle*	1 Bar/50hg	259.0	14.0	518	5.2	60.9	28.2	1.0
Chunky, Peanut, Nestle*	1 Bar/50g	268.0	16.0	537	8.4	54.9	31.5	0.0
Chunky, Snack Size, Nestle*	1 Bar/26g	133.0	7.0	513	6.6	60.4	27.2	1.1
Editions, Mango & Passionfruit, Nestle*	1 Bar/45g	225.0	11.0	499	4.7	69.0	23.4	0.0
Editions, Red Berry, Chunky, Nestle*	1 Bar/45g	223.0	10.0	496	4.5	69.5	23.3	0.0
Editions, Seville Orange, Nestle*	1 Bar/45g	223.0	10.0	496	4.6	69.3	23.0	0.8
Kubes, Nestle*	1 Pack/50g	257.0	14.0	515	5.9	60.9	27.5	1.0
Kubes, Orange, Nestle*	4 Kubes/13g	66.0	4.0	514	5.7	61.1	27.4	1.0
Lemon & Yoghurt, Nestle*	1 Pack/45g	240.0	13.0	533	7.3	58.0	29.8	0.4
Low Carb, 2 Finger, Nestle*	2 Fingers/21g	92.0	7.0	438	9.2	28.3	31.3	1.3
Low Carb, 4 Finger, Nestle*	1 Finger/11g	46.0	3.0	438	9.2	28.3	31.3	1.3
Mini, Nestle*	1 Bar/15g	75.0	4.0	502	7.5	59.4	26.0	0.0
Mint, 4 Finger, Nestle*	4 Fingers/48g	244.0	13.0	508	6.0	61.5	26.4	1.1
Orange, 2 Finger, Nestle*	2 Fingers/21g	107.0	6.0	507	5.5	61.7	26.5	0.0

K

	Measure INFO/WEIGHT	per Measure KCAL	per Measure FAT	Nutrition Values per 100g / 100ml KCAL	PROT	CARB	FAT	FIBRE
KIT KAT								
Senses, Nestle*	1 Bar/31g	165.0	10.0	531	7.5	56.3	30.7	0.0
White, Chunky, Nestle*	1 Bar/53g	276.0	15.0	521	8.3	60.3	27.5	0.7
KIWI FRUIT								
Fresh, Raw, Average	*1 Med Kiwi/60g*	*29.0*	*0.0*	*49*	*1.1*	*10.6*	*0.5*	*1.9*
Weighed with Skin, Average	*1 Kiwi/60g*	*25.0*	*0.0*	*42*	*1.0*	*9.1*	*0.4*	*1.6*
KOHLRABI								
Boiled in Salted Water	*1oz/28g*	*5.0*	*0.0*	*18*	*1.2*	*3.1*	*0.2*	*1.9*
Raw	*1oz/28g*	*6.0*	*0.0*	*23*	*1.6*	*3.7*	*0.2*	*2.2*
KORMA								
Chicken, & Basmati Rice, Tesco*	1 Pot/350g	588.0	33.0	168	4.3	16.9	9.3	2.3
Chicken, & Pilau Rice, BGTY, Sainsbury's*	1 Pack/400g	404.0	5.0	101	8.0	14.3	1.3	0.6
Chicken, & Pilau Rice, GFY, Asda*	1 Pack/400g	600.0	24.0	150	8.0	16.0	6.0	1.3
Chicken, & Pilau Rice, Indian, Asda*	1 Pack/456g	643.0	23.0	141	8.0	16.0	5.0	2.4
Chicken, & Pilau Rice, Morrisons*	1 Pack/450g	889.0	48.0	198	9.4	15.9	10.7	1.4
Chicken, & Pilau Rice, Tesco*	1 Serving/460g	722.0	45.0	157	5.6	11.5	9.8	1.3
Chicken, & Rice, 95% Fat Free, Birds Eye*	1 Pack/370g	444.0	7.0	120	6.2	19.6	1.9	1.1
Chicken, & Rice, Healthy Living, Co-Op*	1 Pack/400g	480.0	8.0	120	8.0	17.0	2.0	1.0
Chicken, & Rice, Indian Meal for Two, Sainsbury's*	1 Pack/500g	785.0	40.0	157	6.8	14.3	8.1	3.1
Chicken, & Rice, Light Choices, Tesco*	1 Pack/450g	495.0	9.0	110	7.2	16.0	2.0	0.8
Chicken, & Rice, Organic, Tesco*	1 Pack/450g	922.0	48.0	205	6.0	21.5	10.6	0.4
Chicken, & Rice, World Flavours*	1 Pack/500g	705.0	23.0	141	8.7	16.0	4.7	0.0
Chicken, & White Rice, BGTY, Frozen, Sainsbury's*	1 Pack/375g	341.0	4.0	91	5.6	14.9	1.0	0.5
Chicken, & Yellow Pilau Rice, Chilled, Tesco*	1 Pack/550g	698.0	21.0	127	8.2	15.0	3.8	1.2
Chicken, Fresh, Chilled, Tesco*	1 Pack/350g	819.0	61.0	234	13.1	6.3	17.4	2.3
Chicken, HL, Tesco*	1 Pack/350g	371.0	4.0	106	7.7	15.9	1.2	0.8
Chicken, Indian Meal for 2, Finest, Tesco*	½ Pack/200g	348.0	24.0	174	10.3	6.2	12.0	2.5
Chicken, Indian Takeaway for One, Sainsbury's*	1 Serving/300g	498.0	31.0	166	13.0	5.3	10.3	1.6
Chicken, Indian Takeaway, Iceland*	1 Pack/400g	656.0	44.0	164	11.8	4.5	11.0	1.4
Chicken, Indian, Take Away, Tesco*	½ Pack/175g	222.0	13.0	127	9.0	5.5	7.7	1.8
Chicken, Less Than 3% Fat, Birds Eye*	1 Pack/358g	440.0	7.0	123	6.5	20.4	1.9	0.8
Chicken, Less Than 3% Fat, Frozen, GFY, Asda*	1 Pack/401g	405.0	7.0	101	5.3	16.2	1.7	1.2
Chicken, Morrisons*	1 Pack/350g	707.0	47.0	202	13.6	7.0	13.3	0.7
Chicken, Plumrose*	1 Can/392g	431.0	22.0	110	8.0	6.9	5.6	0.0
Chicken, Tesco*	1 Pack/350g	619.0	41.0	177	10.8	6.8	11.8	0.6
Chicken, Tinned, Asda*	½ Can/197g	321.0	22.0	163	8.0	8.0	11.0	2.3
Chicken, Waitrose*	1 Pack/400g	680.0	47.0	170	13.7	2.4	11.7	1.9
Chicken, with Basmati Rice, Eat Smart, Safeway*	1 Pack/380g	399.0	7.0	105	7.0	13.8	1.9	1.5
Chicken, with Coriander & Rice, Slim Fast*	1 Pack/375g	394.0	3.0	105	5.7	18.6	0.9	0.7
Chicken, with Peshwari Coriander Rice, Finest, Tesco*	1 Pack/550g	907.0	48.0	165	7.5	13.9	8.8	0.9
Chicken, with Pilau Rice, Asda*	1 Serving/350g	735.0	49.0	210	12.0	9.0	14.0	2.0
Chicken, with Pilau Rice, Perfectly Balanced, Waitrose*	1 Pack/400g	452.0	7.0	113	8.9	15.4	1.7	1.3
Creamy, with Pilau Rice, Safeway*	1 Pack/400g	560.0	23.0	140	5.2	15.8	5.7	2.3
Vegetable & Rice, Tesco*	1 Pack/450g	621.0	27.0	138	2.9	18.3	5.9	1.6
Vegetable with Rice, Eat Smart, Safeway*	1 Pack/400g	412.0	9.0	103	3.1	17.5	2.3	1.6
Vegetable, Ready to Cook, Fresh, Sainsbury's*	½ Pack/255g	263.0	17.0	103	2.8	7.7	6.8	2.1
Vegetable, Sainsbury's*	1 Serving/200g	302.0	25.0	151	2.7	6.6	12.6	2.2
KUMQUATS								
Canned, in Syrup	*1oz/28g*	*39.0*	*0.0*	*138*	*0.4*	*35.4*	*0.5*	*1.7*
Raw	*1oz/28g*	*12.0*	*0.0*	*43*	*0.9*	*9.3*	*0.5*	*3.8*

K

	Measure INFO/WEIGHT	per Measure KCAL	per Measure FAT	Nutrition Values per 100g / 100ml KCAL	PROT	CARB	FAT	FIBRE
LACES								
Apple Flavour, Tesco*	5 Laces/15g	52.0	0.0	347	3.6	74.8	3.2	2.1
Strawberry, Fizzy, Somerfield*	1 Pack/100g	380.0	2.0	380	3.0	86.0	2.0	0.0
Strawberry, Sainsbury's*	1 Serving/25g	94.0	1.0	377	3.3	76.3	4.6	0.1
Strawberry, Tesco*	1 Serving/75g	260.0	2.0	347	3.6	74.8	3.2	2.1
LAGER								
5%, Heineken*	1 Bottle/250ml	110.0	0.0	44	0.4	3.4	0.0	0.0
Alcohol Free, Becks*	1 Serving/275ml	55.0	0.0	20	0.7	5.0	0.0	0.0
Amstel, Heineken*	1 Pint/568ml	227.0	0.0	40	0.5	3.0	0.0	0.0
Average	1 Pint/568ml	233.0	0.0	41	0.3	3.1	0.0	0.0
Becks*	1 Can/275ml	113.0	0.0	41	0.0	3.0	0.0	0.0
Blanc, Kronenbourg*	½ pt/284ml	119.0	0.0	42	0.0	3.3	0.0	0.0
C2, Carling*	½ Pint/284ml	80.0	0.0	28	0.0	3.5	0.0	0.0
Can, Carlsberg*	1 Can/440ml	141.0	0.0	32	0.0	2.0	0.0	0.0
Draught, Carling*	1 Pint/568ml	189.0	0.0	33	0.0	1.4	0.0	0.0
Edge, Carlsberg*	1 Can/300ml	126.0	0.0	42	0.0	4.3	0.0	0.0
Export, Carlsberg*	1 Can/440ml	185.0	0.0	42	0.3	2.8	0.0	0.3
Export, Foster's*	1 Pint/568ml	210.0	0.0	37	0.0	2.2	0.0	0.0
Foster's*	1 Pint/568ml	227.0	0.0	40	0.0	3.1	0.0	0.0
German, Low Alcohol, Sainsbury's*	1 Bottle/330ml	92.0	0.0	28	0.4	5.9	0.1	0.1
Grolsch*	1 Can/330ml	145.0	0.0	44	0.0	2.2	0.0	0.0
Heineken, Heineken*	1 Pint/568ml	256.0	0.0	45	0.5	3.0	0.0	0.0
Kaliber, Guinness*	1 Can/440ml	110.0	0.0	25	0.2	6.0	0.0	0.0
Light, Coors*	1 Pint/500ml	160.0	0.0	32	0.3	1.7	0.0	0.0
Light, Corona*	1 Bottle/330ml	105.0	0.0	32	1.5	0.0	0.0	0.0
Light, Michelob*	1 Serving/340ml	113.0	0.0	33	0.3	2.0	0.0	0.0
Lite, Carlsberg*	1 Bottle/330ml	89.0	0.0	27	0.1	0.5	0.0	0.0
Low Alcohol	1 Can/440ml	44.0	0.0	10	0.2	1.5	0.0	0.0
Pils, Holsten*	1 Can/440ml	167.0	0.0	38	0.3	2.4	0.0	0.0
Premier, Kronenbourg*	½pt/284ml	136.0	0.0	48	0.0	0.0	0.0	0.0
Premium	1 Can/440ml	260.0	0.0	59	0.3	2.4	0.0	0.0
Premium, French, Biere Speciale, Tesco*	1 Serving/250ml	105.0	0.0	42	0.3	3.3	0.0	0.0
Shandy, Traditional Style, Asda*	1 Serving/200ml	44.0	0.0	22	0.0	4.6	0.0	0.0
Stella Artois*	1 Can/550ml	247.0	0.0	45	1.2	2.9	0.0	0.0
Ultra Low Carb, Michelob*	1 Bottle/275ml	88.0	0.0	32	0.2	0.9	0.0	0.0
LAMB								
Chops, Average	*1oz/28g*	*65.0*	*5.0*	*231*	*20.5*	*0.4*	*16.3*	*0.0*
Chops, Minted, Average	*1 Chop/100g*	*260.0*	*15.0*	*260*	*25.9*	*5.1*	*15.1*	*0.3*
Cutlets, Neck, Raw, Lean & Fat, Weighed with Bone	*1 Pack 210g*	*485.0*	*43.0*	*231*	*11.9*	*0.0*	*20.4*	*0.0*
Cutlets, TTD, Sainsbury's*	1 Serving/100g	238.0	14.0	238	28.5	0.0	13.8	0.0
Diced, From Supermarket, Healthy Range, Average	*½ Pack/200g*	*277.0*	*9.0*	*138*	*24.6*	*0.1*	*4.5*	*0.0*
Escalope, Asda*	1 Serving/100g	173.0	5.0	173	32.0	0.0	5.0	0.0
Escalope, British, HL, Tesco*	1 Piece/95g	104.0	3.0	110	20.1	0.0	3.3	0.0
Fillet, Indian, Somerfield*	1 Pack/300g	570.0	36.0	190	17.0	4.0	12.0	0.0
Grill Steak, Average	*1oz/28g*	*70.0*	*5.0*	*250*	*20.2*	*4.4*	*16.9*	*0.4*
Grill Steak, Prime, Average	*1 Steak/63g*	*197.0*	*16.0*	*312*	*18.5*	*2.0*	*25.5*	*0.1*
Grill Steak, Rosemary & Mint, Tesco*	1 Steak/62g	172.0	11.0	277	24.4	5.6	17.6	1.8
Leg, Joint, Raw, Average	*1 Joint/510g*	*858.0*	*46.0*	*168*	*20.9*	*1.4*	*8.9*	*0.2*
Leg, Roasted, Lean & Fat, Average	*1oz/28g*	*66.0*	*4.0*	*237*	*28.6*	*0.0*	*13.6*	*0.0*
Leg, Roasted, Lean, Average	*1oz/28g*	*58.0*	*3.0*	*206*	*29.9*	*0.0*	*9.6*	*0.0*
Mince, Average	*1oz/28g*	*58.0*	*4.0*	*207*	*17.6*	*0.5*	*14.8*	*0.0*
Mince, Extra Lean, Sainsbury's*	1 Serving/225g	324.0	12.0	144	24.1	0.0	5.3	0.1
Rack, Raw, Lean & Fat	*1oz/28g*	*79.0*	*7.0*	*283*	*17.3*	*0.0*	*23.8*	*0.0*
Rack, Raw, Lean Only, Weighed with Bone	*1 oz / 28g*	*48.0*	*3.0*	*169*	*20.0*	*0.0*	*9.2*	*0.0*

L

	Measure INFO/WEIGHT	per Measure KCAL	per Measure FAT	Nutrition Values per 100g / 100ml KCAL	PROT	CARB	FAT	FIBRE
LAMB								
Rack, Roasted, Lean	*1oz/28g*	*63.0*	*4.0*	*225*	*27.1*	*0.0*	*13.0*	*0.0*
Rack, Roasted, Lean & Fat	*1oz/28g*	*102.0*	*8.0*	*363*	*23.0*	*0.0*	*30.1*	*0.0*
Shank, Tuscan, Somerfield*	½ Shank/200g	350.0	17.0	175	19.0	5.2	8.7	1.5
Shoulder, Cooked, Lean & Fat	*1oz/28g*	*84.0*	*6.0*	*301*	*24.4*	*0.0*	*22.5*	*0.0*
Shoulder, Fillet, Average	*1oz/28g*	*66.0*	*5.0*	*235*	*17.6*	*0.0*	*18.3*	*0.0*
Shoulder, Raw, Average	*1oz/28g*	*70.0*	*6.0*	*248*	*16.7*	*0.0*	*20.2*	*0.0*
Shoulder, Roasted, Whole, Lean	*1oz/28g*	*61.0*	*3.0*	*218*	*27.2*	*0.0*	*12.1*	*0.0*
Steak, Leg, Raw, Average	*1 Steak/150g*	*169.0*	*5.0*	*112*	*20.0*	*0.0*	*3.6*	*0.0*
Steak, Minted, Average	*1 Steak/125g*	*212.0*	*9.0*	*170*	*22.7*	*3.4*	*7.2*	*0.9*
Steak, Raw, Average	*1 Steak/140g*	*190.0*	*8.0*	*136*	*21.7*	*0.2*	*5.4*	*0.0*
Stewing, Raw, Lean & Fat	*1oz/28g*	*57.0*	*4.0*	*203*	*22.5*	*0.0*	*12.6*	*0.0*
Stewing, Stewed, Lean	*1oz/28g*	*67.0*	*4.0*	*240*	*26.6*	*0.0*	*14.8*	*0.0*
Stewing, Stewed, Lean & Fat	*1oz/28g*	*78.0*	*6.0*	*279*	*24.4*	*0.0*	*20.1*	*0.0*
Trimmed Fat, Raw, Average	1 Serving/100g	518.0	52.0	518	13.3	0.0	51.6	0.0
LAMB IN								
a Pot, Sainsbury's*	1 Pack/450g	553.0	17.0	123	7.6	14.6	3.8	0.7
Garlic & Rosemary Gravy, Shank, Asda*	1 Shank/280g	451.0	23.0	161	19.8	1.7	8.3	0.5
Gravy, Minted, Roast, M & S*	1 Pack/200g	140.0	3.0	70	6.8	6.6	1.5	0.9
Gravy, Roast, Birds Eye*	1 Pack/239g	160.0	5.0	67	8.1	3.8	2.2	0.1
Mint Gravy, Sliced, Sainsbury's*	1 Pack/125g	134.0	5.0	107	15.3	2.9	3.8	0.8
Minted Gravy, Shank, Iceland*	1 Shank/350g	651.0	45.0	186	15.0	2.4	12.9	0.5
Rich Minted Gravy, Shank, Morrisons*	1 Pack/400g	612.0	26.0	153	18.8	5.2	6.6	0.0
LAMB MEDITERRANEAN								
Shanks, Finest, Tesco*	1 Serving/404g	671.0	36.0	166	15.0	6.6	8.8	2.0
LAMB MOROCCAN								
with Cous Cous, Perfectly Balanced, Waitrose*	1 Pack/400g	390.0	5.0	97	7.7	13.6	1.3	2.2
LAMB TAGINE								
Moroccan Style, with Couscous, COU, M & S*	1 Pack/400g	340.0	6.0	85	8.9	8.3	1.4	1.6
LAMB WITH								
Carrot & Swede Mash, Braised, Eat Smart, Morrisons*	1 Pack/400g	304.0	9.0	76	5.2	8.2	2.3	1.5
Cous Cous, Moroccan Style, Tesco*	1 Pack/550g	710.0	15.0	129	6.6	19.6	2.7	1.3
Gravy, Joint, Tesco*	1 Serving/225g	277.0	13.0	123	14.9	2.8	5.8	0.0
Honey Roast Vegetables, Extra Special, Asda*	1 Pack/400g	400.0	15.0	100	9.9	6.7	3.7	2.5
Mango & Mint Sauce, Boneless Joint, Asda*	1 Serving/100g	302.0	22.0	302	26.0	0.0	22.0	1.4
Mango & Mint, Shoulder Chops, Waitrose*	1 Chop/250g	555.0	40.0	222	16.7	2.3	16.2	0.5
Mint & Balsamic Vinegar Crust, Rump, Waitrose*	1 Serving/166g	259.0	12.0	156	18.1	5.0	7.1	0.0
Mint Butter, Leg Steaks, Waitrose*	1 Serving/155g	270.0	16.0	174	19.6	0.4	10.5	0.0
Mint Glaze & Redcurrant Sauce, Steaks, Leg, Asda*	½ Pack/145g	247.0	9.0	170	18.0	11.0	6.0	0.5
Mint Gravy, Joint, Tesco*	1 Serving/100g	88.0	2.0	88	16.6	1.8	1.7	0.1
Mint Gravy, Leg Chops, Tesco*	1 Serving/175g	213.0	10.0	122	15.0	3.2	5.6	1.7
Mint Gravy, Shanks, Frozen, Tesco*	1 Shank/200g	420.0	26.0	210	20.1	1.6	13.2	0.7
Mint, Leg Chops, Morrisons*	2 Chops/350g	857.0	45.0	245	29.4	2.4	12.9	0.9
Redcurrant & Rosemary Sauce, Chops, Leg, Tesco*	1 Pack/325g	604.0	36.0	186	17.6	4.0	11.1	0.5
Roasted Vegetables, Shank, M & S*	½ Pack/420g	660.0	31.0	157	14.9	8.3	7.3	0.7
Rosemary Gravy, Shank, Sainsbury's*	1 Serving/200g	204.0	8.0	102	13.2	3.1	4.1	0.3
Rosemary, Joint, Tesco*	1 Serving/125g	250.0	18.0	200	17.5	0.8	14.1	0.5
Sticky Plum & Orange Glaze, Joint, Waitrose*	1 Serving/100g	164.0	8.0	164	13.4	9.8	7.9	3.1
Sweet Mint Dressing, Joint, Tesco*	1 Serving/50g	96.0	6.0	193	19.9	1.8	11.8	0.6
LARD								
Average	*1oz/28g*	*249.0*	*28.0*	*891*	*0.0*	*0.0*	*99.0*	*0.0*
LASAGNE								
Al Forno, Beef, M & S*	1 Pack/400g	640.0	38.0	160	8.2	10.7	9.5	2.8
Al Forno, TTD, Sainsbury's*	1 Pack/383g	571.0	30.0	149	8.6	10.9	7.9	2.1

L

LASAGNE

	Measure INFO/WEIGHT	per Measure KCAL	FAT	Nutrition Values per 100g / 100ml KCAL	PROT	CARB	FAT	FIBRE
Alla Bolognese, Weight Watchers*	1 Pack/350g	416.0	9.0	119	8.0	16.0	2.5	0.0
Asparagus, M & S*	1 Pack/360g	432.0	22.0	120	4.3	11.9	6.1	1.1
Balsamic Onion & Chicken, M & S*	1 Pack/375g	562.0	25.0	150	9.5	12.5	6.7	1.5
Beef & Chunky Vegetable, HL, Tesco*	1 Pack/340g	354.0	10.0	104	5.9	13.8	2.8	1.2
Beef & Red Wine, & Seasoned Wedges, Weight Watchers*	1 Pack/400g	400.0	13.0	100	5.1	12.5	3.3	0.2
Beef, BGTY, Sainsbury's*	1 Pack/400g	352.0	8.0	88	7.8	9.8	2.0	1.4
Beef, Frozen, GFY, Asda*	1 Pack/400g	380.0	10.0	95	6.0	12.0	2.6	0.7
Beef, Frozen, Tesco*	1 Pack/450g	607.0	25.0	135	7.5	12.6	5.6	0.8
Beef, Frozen, Weight Watchers*	1 Pack/300g	252.0	7.0	84	5.4	10.2	2.4	0.3
Beef, HL, Tesco*	1 Pack/450g	450.0	10.0	100	6.7	12.6	2.3	1.4
Beef, Italian, Sainsbury's*	½ Pack/350g	493.0	27.0	141	7.5	10.3	7.7	2.0
Beef, Ready Meals, Waitrose*	1 Pack/ 400g	444.0	21.0	111	5.8	10.4	5.1	0.8
Beef, with Fresh Pasta, Birds Eye*	1 Pack/400g	396.0	9.0	99	7.3	12.2	2.3	0.5
BFY, Morrisons*	1 Pack/350g	339.0	14.0	97	7.1	8.6	4.0	0.2
Bolognese, & Vegetable, Weight Watchers*	1 Pack/300g	279.0	8.0	93	5.0	12.4	2.6	0.0
Bolognese, Trattorie Alfredo*	1 Serving/125g	204.0	11.0	163	9.0	13.0	9.0	0.0
Chicken, Italian, Sainsbury's*	1 Pack/450g	549.0	19.0	122	8.4	12.6	4.2	0.5
Chicken, Light Choices, Tesco*	1 Pack/400g	344.0	7.0	86	7.1	10.5	1.7	1.8
Chicken, Mushroom & Asparagus, Finest, Tesco*	½ Pack/300g	360.0	16.0	120	7.6	10.2	5.4	0.8
Chicken, Ready Meals, Waitrose*	1 Pack/300g	411.0	20.0	137	6.3	13.0	6.6	0.9
Classic, Deep Filled, M & S*	1 Pack/400g	760.0	48.0	190	10.0	11.2	11.9	0.6
Creamy Ricotta & Vegetable, HL, Tesco*	1 Pack/384g	407.0	11.0	106	5.5	14.6	2.8	3.6
Extra Special, Asda*	½ Pack/291g	416.0	20.0	143	7.0	13.0	7.0	0.3
Family, M & S*	¼ Pack/225g	281.0	14.0	125	10.3	6.9	6.2	1.1
Fresh, Findus*	1 Pack/350g	402.0	16.0	115	6.2	11.7	4.5	0.0
Frozen, Safeway*	1 Serving/400g	455.0	18.0	114	6.0	11.8	4.6	0.2
Italian, Family, Asda*	¼ Pack/185g	306.0	18.0	166	8.0	11.0	10.0	1.7
Italian, Fresh, Chilled, Sainsbury's*	1 Pack/400g	480.0	22.0	120	10.1	7.5	5.5	1.4
Layered, Asda*	1 Pack/300g	444.0	24.0	148	5.0	14.0	8.0	0.3
Less Than 5% Fat, BFY, Morrisons*	½ Pack/350g	227.0	9.0	65	5.9	8.2	2.5	0.7
Light Choices, Tesco*	1 Pack/430g	396.0	11.0	92	5.8	11.3	2.6	1.6
Low Saturated Fat, Waitrose*	1 Pack/400g	312.0	6.0	78	4.7	11.4	1.5	0.4
M & S*	1/3 Pack/333g	466.0	25.0	140	8.5	10.4	7.4	0.9
Mediterranean Vegetable, COU, M & S*	1 Pack/360g	306.0	10.0	85	3.4	11.5	2.7	1.4
Minced Beef, Great Stuff, Asda*	1 Pack/300g	333.0	13.0	111	6.2	11.7	4.4	1.3
Mushroom & Spinach, Waitrose*	1 Pack/400g	373.0	14.0	93	3.1	12.3	3.5	1.3
Roasted Mushrooms, Safeway*	1 Serving/400g	440.0	20.0	110	3.9	11.2	5.0	1.4
Roasted Vegetable, GFY, Asda*	1 Pack/425g	306.0	7.0	72	3.3	10.9	1.7	1.6
Salmon, King Prawn & Spinach, Finest, Tesco*	1 Pack/400g	600.0	30.0	150	10.6	9.6	7.4	0.8
Sheets, Boiled, Average	**1 Sheet/20g**	**20.0**	**0.0**	**100**	**3.0**	**22.0**	**0.6**	**0.9**
Sheets, Dry, Average	**1 Sheet/20g**	**70.0**	**0.0**	**349**	**11.9**	**72.1**	**1.5**	**2.9**
Sheets, Fresh, Dry, Average	**1 Sheet/21g**	**56.0**	**0.0**	**271**	**10.9**	**52.7**	**2.1**	**1.9**
Sheets, Verdi, Dry, Average	**1 Sheet/20g**	**71.0**	**0.0**	**355**	**12.6**	**71.1**	**2.2**	**2.7**
Smoked Salmon & Asparagus, Sainsbury's*	1 Pack/350g	665.0	37.0	190	7.9	15.6	10.7	0.7
Spinach & Cheese, Italian, Sainsbury's*	1 Pack/450g	666.0	31.0	148	6.0	15.5	6.8	0.5
Spinach & Ricotta, Finest, Tesco*	1 Pack/350g	584.0	37.0	167	6.1	11.7	10.6	1.2
Vegetable, BGTY, Sainsbury's*	1 Pack/346g	277.0	7.0	80	4.6	11.0	2.0	3.1
Vegetable, Italian Roasted, Asda*	1 Serving/200g	234.0	14.0	117	2.6	11.0	7.0	0.7
Vegetable, Italian Three Layer, Sainsbury's*	1 Pack/450g	553.0	23.0	123	4.8	14.3	5.2	0.5
Vegetable, Italian, Frozen, Cooked, Sainsbury's*	1 Pack/378g	442.0	19.0	117	4.6	13.5	5.0	1.1
Vegetable, Light Choices, Tesco*	1 Pack/400g	320.0	6.0	80	4.0	12.1	1.6	1.9
Vegetable, Low Saturated Fat, Waitrose*	1 Pack/400g	340.0	12.0	85	2.9	11.9	2.9	0.9
Vegetable, Weight Watchers*	1 Pack/330g	251.0	6.0	76	3.6	11.8	1.7	0.7

L

	Measure INFO/WEIGHT	per Measure KCAL	FAT	Nutrition Values per 100g / 100ml KCAL	PROT	CARB	FAT	FIBRE
LASAGNE VEGETARIAN								
Linda McCartney*	1 Pack/360g	451.0	20.0	125	6.3	12.4	5.6	1.4
Tesco*	1 Pack/450g	630.0	35.0	140	6.0	11.6	7.7	1.6
LAVERBREAD								
Average	*1oz/28g*	*15.0*	*1.0*	*52*	*3.2*	*1.6*	*3.7*	*0.0*
LEEKS								
Boiled, Average	*1oz/28g*	*6.0*	*0.0*	*21*	*1.2*	*2.6*	*0.7*	*1.7*
Creamed, Frozen, Waitrose*	1 Serving/225g	115.0	5.0	51	1.8	5.5	2.4	0.0
Raw, Unprepared, Average	*1oz/28g*	*11.0*	*0.0*	*39*	*2.8*	*5.1*	*0.9*	*3.9*
LEMON								
Fresh, Raw, Average	*1 Slice/5g*	*0.0*	*0.0*	*7*	*0.3*	*1.6*	*0.0*	*1.7*
Peel, Raw, Average	*1 Tbsp/6g*	*3.0*	*0.0*	*47*	*1.5*	*16.0*	*0.3*	*10.6*
LEMON CURD								
Average	*1 Tbsp/15g*	*44.0*	*1.0*	*294*	*0.7*	*62.9*	*4.7*	*0.1*
Luxury, Average	*1 Tsp/7g*	*23.0*	*1.0*	*326*	*2.8*	*59.7*	*8.4*	*0.1*
LEMON SOLE								
Fillets, Raw, Average	*1 Serving/220g*	*180.0*	*3.0*	*82*	*17.3*	*0.2*	*1.3*	*0.3*
Goujons, Average	1 Serving/150g	359.0	18.0	239	13.9	18.5	12.2	1.0
Grilled, Average	*1oz/28g*	*27.0*	*0.0*	*97*	*20.2*	*0.0*	*1.7*	*0.0*
in Breadcrumbs, Average	1 Fillet/142g	322.0	17.0	228	13.7	15.7	12.3	1.0
in White Wine, & Herb Butter, Fillets, M & S*	1 Pack/220g	385.0	28.0	175	15.1	0.1	12.6	0.0
Steamed, Average	*1oz/28g*	*25.0*	*0.0*	*91*	*20.6*	*0.0*	*0.9*	*0.0*
with Lemon Mayonnaise, Goujons, Finest, Tesco*	1 Pack/230g	713.0	52.0	310	10.6	15.6	22.8	1.0
LEMONADE								
7-Up, Light, Britvic*	1 Can/330ml	4.0	0.0	1	0.1	0.2	0.0	0.0
7up, Zero, Britvic*	1 Can/330ml	6.0	0.0	2	0.1	0.1	0.0	0.0
Asda*	1 Glass/250ml	82.0	0.0	33	0.0	8.0	0.0	0.0
Average	1 Glass/250ml	52.0	0.0	21	0.1	5.0	0.1	0.1
Cloudy, Diet, Sainsbury's*	1 Can/330ml	7.0	0.0	2	0.1	0.2	0.1	0.3
Cloudy, Diet, Tesco*	1 Serving/200ml	6.0	0.0	3	0.0	0.8	0.0	0.0
Cloudy, Sainsbury's*	1 Glass/250ml	117.0	0.0	47	0.1	12.0	0.1	0.1
Cloudy, Shapers, Boots*	1 Bottle/500ml	15.0	0.0	3	0.0	0.3	0.0	0.0
Cloudy, Waitrose*	1 Glass/250ml	125.0	0.0	50	0.0	12.2	0.0	0.0
Diet, Premium, Tesco*	1 Glass/250ml	7.0	0.0	3	0.0	0.4	0.0	0.0
Diet, Traditional Style, Tesco*	1 Glass/200ml	6.0	0.0	3	0.0	0.8	0.0	0.0
Lime, Safeway*	1 Can/144ml	63.0	0.0	44	0.0	10.6	0.0	0.0
Low Calorie, Smart Price, Asda*	1 Glass/250ml	1.0	0.0	0	0.0	0.1	0.0	0.0
Minute Maid*	1 Bottle/500ml	10.0	0.0	2	0.0	0.6	0.0	0.0
Organic, Tesco*	1 Can/142ml	61.0	0.0	43	0.0	10.6	0.0	0.0
Premium, Freeway*	1 Glass/250ml	42.0	0.0	17	0.0	4.2	0.0	0.0
R White*	1 Glass/250ml	65.0	0.0	26	0.1	6.2	0.0	0.0
Sainsbury's*	1 Glass/250ml	52.0	0.0	21	0.1	4.9	0.1	0.1
Schweppes*	1 Glass/250ml	45.0	0.0	18	0.0	4.2	0.0	0.0
Sicilian, Sainsbury's*	1 Glass/200ml	98.0	0.0	49	0.1	11.5	0.1	0.1
Sicilian, TTD, Sainsbury's*	1/3 Bottle/247ml	84.0	0.0	34	0.1	8.1	0.1	0.0
Sparkling, Morrisons*	1 Glass/250ml	63.0	0.0	25	0.0	6.1	0.0	0.0
Sparkling, with Spanish Lemon Juice, Waitrose*	1 Glass/250ml	85.0	0.0	34	0.0	8.3	0.0	0.0
Still, Freshly Squeezed, M & S*	½ Bottle/250ml	100.0	0.0	40	0.1	9.0	0.2	0.5
SunJuice*	1 Glass/250ml	113.0	0.0	45	0.1	12.7	0.0	0.0
Tesco*	1 Glass/200ml	30.0	0.0	15	0.0	3.6	0.0	0.0
Traditional Style, Tesco*	1 Glass/200ml	100.0	0.0	50	0.0	12.3	0.0	0.0
TTD, Sainsbury's*	1 Serving/248ml	159.0	0.0	64	0.1	14.8	0.0	0.2
LEMONCELLO								
Asda*	1 Serving/100g	217.0	10.0	217	4.7	27.0	10.0	0.2

L

	Measure INFO/WEIGHT	per Measure KCAL	FAT	Nutrition Values per 100g / 100ml KCAL	PROT	CARB	FAT	FIBRE
LEMONGRASS								
Stalks, Tesco*	1 Stalk/13g	12.0	0.0	99	1.8	25.3	0.5	0.0
LENTILS								
Black Beluga, Ready to Eat, Merchant Gourmet*	1 Serving/62.5g	92.0	1.0	147	10.9	20.5	1.2	5.2
Green & Brown, Dried, Boiled in Salted Water, Average	*1 Tbsp/30g*	*31.0*	*0.0*	*105*	*8.8*	*16.9*	*0.7*	*3.8*
Green Or Brown, Dried, Average	*1 Serving/50g*	*150.0*	*1.0*	*301*	*22.8*	*49.8*	*1.5*	*9.6*
Green Or Brown, in Water, Tinned, Average	*½ Can/132g*	*131.0*	*1.0*	*99*	*8.1*	*15.4*	*0.6*	*3.8*
Puy, Green, Dry, Average	1 Serving/100g	306.0	1.0	306	24.7	49.5	1.4	10.3
Red, Boiled in Unsalted Water, Average	*1oz/28g*	*28.0*	*0.0*	*101*	*7.6*	*17.5*	*0.4*	*2.6*
Red, Dried, Average	*1oz/28g*	*88.0*	*0.0*	*315*	*23.8*	*53.8*	*1.3*	*4.9*
LETTUCE								
Cos, Sweet, Baby, Somerfield*	1 Pack/600g	90.0	3.0	15	0.8	1.7	0.5	0.9
Crest, Sainsbury's*	1 Serving/80g	11.0	0.0	14	0.8	1.7	0.5	0.0
Curly Leaf, Sainsbury's*	1 Serving/80g	11.0	0.0	14	0.8	1.7	0.5	0.0
Iceberg, Average	*1 Serving/80g*	*11.0*	*0.0*	*13*	*0.8*	*1.8*	*0.3*	*0.5*
Lamb's, Average	*1 Serving/80g*	*12.0*	*0.0*	*14*	*1.3*	*1.5*	*0.2*	*0.9*
Leafy, Tesco*	1 Serving/80g	11.0	0.0	14	1.2	1.5	0.4	1.9
Radicchio, Red, Raw, Average	*1 Med/220g*	*29.0*	*0.0*	*13*	*1.4*	*1.6*	*0.1*	*3.0*
Romaine, Average	*1 Serving/80g*	*12.0*	*0.0*	*15*	*0.9*	*1.7*	*0.5*	*0.7*
Romaine, Hearts, Average	*1 Serving/80g*	*12.0*	*0.0*	*15*	*0.9*	*1.7*	*0.5*	*1.0*
LILT								
Fruit Crush, Coca-Cola*	1 Can/330ml	66.0	0.0	20	0.0	4.6	0.0	0.0
Fruit Crush, Zero, Coca-Cola*	1 Can/330ml	12.0	0.0	3	0.0	0.3	0.0	0.0
Z, Coca-Cola*	1 Can/330ml	10.0	0.0	3	0.0	0.4	0.0	0.0
LIME								
Peel, Raw	*1 Tbsp/6g*	*3.0*	*0.0*	*47*	*1.5*	*16.0*	*0.3*	*10.6*
Raw, Flesh Only, Average	*1 Lime/71g*	*18.0*	*0.0*	*25*	*0.6*	*8.8*	*0.2*	*2.3*
Raw, Weighed with Peel & Seeds, Average	*1 Lime/85g*	*25.0*	*0.0*	*30*	*0.7*	*10.5*	*0.2*	*2.8*
LINGUINE								
Crab & Chilli, Waitrose*	1 Pack/350g	770.0	45.0	220	7.7	18.0	12.9	1.8
Crab, Rocket & Chilli, Italian, Finest, Tesco*	1 Pack/350g	717.0	36.0	205	6.5	20.7	10.4	1.7
Dry, Average	*1 Serving/100g*	*352.0*	*2.0*	*352*	*13.1*	*70.0*	*2.2*	*2.8*
Fresh, Dry, Average	*1 Pack/250g*	*681.0*	*6.0*	*272*	*12.3*	*51.7*	*2.6*	*4.0*
Garlic & Basil, Asda*	1 Serving/75g	108.0	0.0	144	5.4	29.5	0.5	2.5
Pomodoro, M & S*	1 Pack/300g	360.0	10.0	120	4.1	17.6	3.5	1.2
Prawn King & Roasted Garlic, Light Choices, Tesco*	1 Pack/400g	340.0	5.0	85	5.6	11.9	1.3	1.5
Salmon & Prawn, Iceland*	1 Meal/450g	540.0	20.0	120	4.5	15.8	4.4	1.5
Smoked Salmon, Sainsbury's*	1 Serving/400g	586.0	29.0	146	6.2	14.2	7.2	1.2
Sun Dried Tomato & Egg, Asda*	1 Serving/200g	324.0	5.0	162	7.0	28.0	2.4	3.9
Tomato & Mushroom, Perfectly Balanced, Waitrose*	1 Pack/350g	294.0	13.0	84	2.2	10.6	3.8	1.0
Vegetable & Ham, BGTY, Sainsbury's*	1 Pack/450g	409.0	13.0	91	4.4	11.7	3.0	0.9
with Chicken & Basil Dressing, HL, Tesco*	1 Pack/359g	503.0	15.0	140	8.6	16.6	4.3	2.2
with Prawns & Scallops, BGTY, Sainsbury's*	1 Pack/400g	320.0	2.0	80	6.2	12.7	0.5	0.8
with Salmon, Hot Smoked, GFY, Asda*	1 Pack/400g	348.0	9.0	87	6.0	10.6	2.3	1.6
LINGUINI								
Asparagus & Ricotta, Sainsbury's*	1 Serving/400g	524.0	23.0	131	3.8	15.8	5.8	2.5
LINSEEDS								
Average	*1 Tsp/5g*	*23.0*	*2.0*	*464*	*21.7*	*18.5*	*33.5*	*26.3*
LION BAR								
Mini, Nestle*	1 Bar/16g	80.0	4.0	486	4.6	67.7	21.7	0.0
Nestle*	1 Bar/43g	206.0	9.0	478	6.5	64.6	21.6	0.0
Peanut, Nestle*	1 Bar/49g	256.0	15.0	522	7.1	56.9	29.6	0.0
LIQUEURS								
Amaretto, Average	*1 Shot/25ml*	*97.0*	*0.0*	*388*	*0.0*	*60.0*	*0.0*	*0.0*

L

	Measure INFO/WEIGHT	per Measure KCAL	FAT	Nutrition Values per 100g / 100ml KCAL	PROT	CARB	FAT	FIBRE
LIQUEURS								
Cointreau, Specialite De France	1 Serving/37ml	80.0	0.0	215	0.0	0.0	0.0	0.0
Cream, Average	1 Shot/25ml	81.0	4.0	325	0.0	22.8	16.1	0.0
*Grand Marnier**	1 Shot/35ml	94.0	0.0	268	0.0	22.9	0.0	0.0
High Strength, Average	1 Shot/25ml	78.0	0.0	314	0.0	24.4	0.0	0.0
Kirsch, Average	1 Shot/25ml	67.0	0.0	267	0.0	20.0	0.0	0.0
LIQUORICE								
Allsorts, Average	1 Sm Bag/56g	195.0	3.0	349	3.7	76.7	5.2	2.0
Allsorts, Bassett's*	1 Pack/225g	792.0	10.0	352	2.3	75.5	4.5	1.6
Allsorts, Fruit, Bassett's*	1 Serving/50g	160.0	0.0	320	1.8	76.9	0.4	0.0
Assorted, Filled, Panda*	1 Sweet/4g	15.0	0.0	385	3.7	68.0	11.0	0.0
Bars, Panda*	1 Bar/32g	99.0	0.0	308	3.7	72.0	0.4	0.9
Catherine Wheels, Barratt*	1 Wheel/22g	65.0	0.0	290	3.8	67.2	0.3	0.7
Catherine Wheels, Sainsbury's*	1 Wheel/17g	49.0	0.0	286	3.8	67.2	0.3	0.7
Comfits, M & S*	1oz/28g	100.0	0.0	357	2.4	86.2	0.3	0.7
Log, Raspberry, Choc, RJ's Licorice Ltd*	1 Log/45.1g	178.0	5.0	395	3.9	74.0	10.0	0.9
Organic, Laidback Liquorice*	1 Bar/28g	90.0	0.0	320	4.7	75.0	1.0	3.0
Panda*	1 Bar/32g	109.0	0.0	340	3.8	78.0	0.5	0.0
Piglets, Black, Old Fashioned, Route 29 Napa Inc*	1 Sweet/1.5g	5.0	0.0	325	2.5	70.0	2.5	0.0
Piglets, Red, Old Fashioned, Route 29 Napa Inc*	1 Sweet/1.5g	5.0	0.0	325	0.0	72.5	1.2	0.0
Red, Fresh, 98% Fat Free, RJ's Licorice Ltd*	1oz/28g	96.0	0.0	342	3.0	75.0	1.7	0.0
Shapes, Average	1oz/28g	78.0	0.0	278	5.5	65.0	1.4	1.9
Soft Eating, Australia, Darrell Lea*	1 Piece/20g	68.0	0.0	338	2.8	76.1	1.9	0.0
Sweets, Blackcurrant, Tesco*	1 Sweet/8g	32.0	0.0	410	0.0	92.3	3.8	0.0
Twists, Tesco*	1 Serving/63g	186.0	0.0	297	2.7	71.0	0.3	0.7
LIVER								
Calves, Fried	1oz/28g	49.0	3.0	176	22.3	0.0	9.6	0.0
Calves, Raw	1oz/28g	29.0	1.0	104	18.3	0.0	3.4	0.0
Calves, with Fresh Sage Butter, M & S*	1 Serving/117g	210.0	12.0	180	12.8	10.1	10.7	1.5
Calves, with Garlic Butter, M & S*	1oz/28g	56.0	4.0	200	13.3	7.3	13.5	0.4
Chicken, Cooked, Simmered, Average	1 Serving/100g	167.0	7.0	167	24.5	0.9	6.5	0.0
Chicken, Fried, Average	1oz/28g	47.0	2.0	169	22.1	0.0	8.9	0.0
Chicken, Raw, Average	1oz/28g	26.0	1.0	92	17.7	0.0	2.3	0.0
Lamb's, Braised, Average	1 Serving/100g	220.0	9.0	220	30.6	2.5	8.8	0.0
Lamb's, Fried, Average	1oz/28g	66.0	4.0	237	30.1	0.0	12.9	0.0
Lamb's, Raw, Average	1 Serving/125g	171.0	8.0	137	20.3	0.0	6.2	0.0
Ox, Raw	1oz/28g	43.0	2.0	155	21.1	0.0	7.8	0.0
Ox, Stewed	1oz/28g	55.0	3.0	198	24.8	3.6	9.5	0.0
Pig's, Raw	1oz/28g	32.0	1.0	113	21.3	0.0	3.1	0.0
Pig's, Stewed	1 Serving/70g	132.0	6.0	189	25.6	3.6	8.1	0.0
LIVER & BACON								
Meal for One, M & S*	1 Pack/452g	430.0	17.0	95	7.0	8.0	3.7	1.2
with Creamy Mash, GFY, Asda*	1 Pack/386g	282.0	5.0	73	5.5	9.6	1.4	2.2
with Fresh Mashed Potato, Waitrose*	1 Pack/400g	416.0	17.0	104	7.3	9.0	4.3	1.3
with Mash, British Classics, Tesco*	1 Pack/500g	575.0	23.0	115	6.6	10.6	4.7	1.0
LIVER & ONIONS								
British Classics, Tesco*	1 Pack/250g	265.0	12.0	106	9.7	5.9	4.8	0.5
Finest, Tesco*	½ Pack/225g	349.0	19.0	155	15.6	3.7	8.3	1.6
M & S*	1 Serving/200g	250.0	12.0	125	7.6	10.5	6.0	0.9
LIVER SAUSAGE								
Average	1 Slice/10g	22.0	2.0	216	15.3	4.4	15.2	0.2
LOBSTER								
Boiled, Average	1oz/28g	29.0	0.0	103	22.1	0.0	1.6	0.0
Breaded Squat, & Lemon Mayonnaise Dip, Finest, Tesco*	1 Pack/210g	380.0	19.0	181	6.3	18.4	9.1	0.1

L

	Measure INFO/WEIGHT	per Measure KCAL	FAT	Nutrition Values per 100g / 100ml KCAL	PROT	CARB	FAT	FIBRE
LOBSTER								
Breaded, Mini, Sainsbury's*	1 Serving/100g	204.0	10.0	204	8.7	18.8	10.1	1.4
Dressed, John West*	1 Can/43g	45.0	2.0	105	13.0	2.0	5.0	0.0
Dressed, M & S*	1oz/28g	76.0	7.0	273	14.3	0.8	23.6	0.1
Half, M & S*	1oz/28g	66.0	5.0	235	12.1	2.4	19.6	0.2
Squat, Tails, Youngs*	½ Pack/125g	246.0	11.0	197	9.8	20.1	8.6	1.1
Thermidor, Finest, Tesco*	½ Pack/140g	381.0	25.0	272	15.3	12.1	18.0	1.0
Thermidor, M & S*	1 Serving/140g	287.0	19.0	205	10.7	9.7	13.7	0.0
LOGANBERRIES								
Raw	*1oz/28g*	*5.0*	*0.0*	*17*	*1.1*	*3.4*	*0.0*	*2.5*
LOLLIPOPS								
Assorted Flavours, Asda*	1 Lolly/7g	27.0	0.0	380	0.0	95.0	0.0	0.0
Blackcurrant, Sugar Free, Rowntree's*	1 Lolly/15g	35.0	0.0	233	0.1	89.4	0.0	0.0
Chocolate Lolly, M & S*	1 Lolly/45g	247.0	16.0	550	6.8	54.0	35.1	2.7
Chupa Chups*	1 Lolly/18g	44.0	0.0	247	0.0	96.5	1.3	0.0
Cremosa, Sugar Free, Chupa Chups*	1 Lolly/10g	27.0	1.0	275	0.2	92.5	5.4	0.0
Cuore Di Frutta, Chupa Chups*	1 Lolly/10g	25.0	0.0	247	0.0	96.5	1.3	0.0
No Added Sugar, Tesco*	1 Lolly/32g	26.0	0.0	80	0.1	20.0	0.0	0.1
Orange, Sugar Free, Rowntree's*	1 Lolly/15g	35.0	0.0	235	0.1	89.5	0.0	0.6
Sugar Free, Simpkins*	1 Lolly/15g	51.0	0.0	340	0.0	88.0	0.0	0.0
Super Sour, Tesco*	1 Lolly/8g	32.0	0.0	385	0.1	95.6	0.2	0.5
LONGANS								
Canned, in Syrup, Drained	*1oz/28g*	*19.0*	*0.0*	*67*	*0.4*	*17.1*	*0.3*	*0.0*
LOQUATS								
Raw	*1oz/28g*	*8.0*	*0.0*	*28*	*0.7*	*6.3*	*0.2*	*0.0*
LOZENGES								
Original Extra Strong Lozenge, Fisherman's Friend*	1 Lozenge/1g	4.0	0.0	382	0.3	94.9	0.0	0.5
Original, Victory V*	1 Lozenge/3g	9.0	0.0	350	0.0	91.0	0.0	0.0
LUCOZADE								
Apple, Energy Drink, GlaxoSmithKline UK Limited*	1 Bottle/380ml	262.0	0.0	69	0.0	17.1	0.0	0.0
Citrus Clear, Energy, GlaxoSmithKline UK Limited*	1 Bottle/380ml	266.0	0.0	70	0.1	17.0	0.0	0.0
Citrus Fruits, Hydro Active, Sport, Lucozade*	1 Bottle/500ml	50.0	0.0	10	0.0	2.0	0.0	0.0
Orange Energy Drink, GlaxoSmithKline UK Limited*	1 Bottle/500ml	350.0	0.0	70	0.0	17.2	0.0	0.0
Original, GlaxoSmithKline UK Limited*	1 Bottle/345ml	252.0	0.0	73	0.0	17.9	0.0	0.0
Raspberry Sport Body Fuel, GlaxoSmithKline UK Limited*	1 Bottle/500ml	140.0	0.0	28	0.0	6.4	0.0	0.0
Summer Berries, Sport, Lite, GlaxoSmithKline UK Limited*	1 Serving/200ml	20.0	0.0	10	0.0	2.0	0.0	0.0
Tropical, GlaxoSmithKline UK Limited*	1 Bottle/380ml	266.0	0.0	70	0.0	17.2	0.0	0.0
LUNCHEON MEAT								
Pork, Average	*1oz/28g*	*81.0*	*7.0*	*288*	*13.3*	*4.0*	*24.3*	*0.0*
LYCHEES								
Fresh, Raw, Flesh Only	*1oz/28g*	*16.0*	*0.0*	*58*	*0.9*	*14.3*	*0.1*	*0.7*
in Juice, Amoy*	1oz/28g	13.0	0.0	46	0.4	10.9	0.0	0.0
in Syrup, Average	*1oz/28g*	*19.0*	*0.0*	*69*	*0.4*	*17.7*	*0.0*	*0.4*
Raw, Weighed with Skin & Stone	*1oz/28g*	*10.0*	*0.0*	*36*	*0.5*	*8.9*	*0.1*	*0.4*

L

INFO/WEIGHT	Measure per Measure		Nutrition Values per 100g / 100ml				
	KCAL	FAT	KCAL	PROT	CARB	FAT	FIBRE
M&M'S							
Mars*	1 Pack/20g	97.0	4.0	485	5.0	68.0	21.5	0.0
Mini, Mars*	1 Sm Pack/36g	176.0	8.0	489	6.3	63.6	23.2	0.0
Peanut Butter, Mars*	1 Pack/42g	230.0	12.0	548	9.5	57.1	28.6	4.8
Peanut, Mars*	1 Pack/45g	228.0	11.0	506	9.4	60.1	25.4	2.7
MACADAMIA NUTS							
Plain, Average	*1 Pack/100g*	*750.0*	*78.0*	*750*	*7.9*	*4.8*	*77.6*	*5.3*
Roasted, Salted, Average	*6 Nuts/10g*	*75.0*	*8.0*	*748*	*7.9*	*4.8*	*77.6*	*5.3*
MACARONI							
Dry, Average	*1oz/28g*	*99.0*	*0.0*	*354*	*11.9*	*73.5*	*1.7*	*2.6*
MACARONI CHEESE							
& Spinach, TTD, Sainsbury's*	1 Pack/500g	1025.0	57.0	205	6.5	18.9	11.5	1.3
Average	1 Serving/300g	534.0	32.0	178	7.3	13.6	10.8	0.5
Canned	1oz/28g	39.0	2.0	138	4.5	16.4	6.5	0.4
Canned, Sainsbury's*	1 Can/400g	480.0	24.0	120	4.4	12.0	6.0	0.3
Chilled, GFY, Asda*	1 Pack/443g	469.0	13.0	106	6.0	14.0	2.9	1.6
COU, M & S*	1 Pack/360g	360.0	9.0	100	5.8	13.9	2.4	1.2
Finest, Tesco*	1 Serving/500g	1055.0	53.0	211	8.3	20.6	10.6	0.7
Four Cheese, Extra Special, Asda*	1 Pack/400g	664.0	31.0	166	7.7	16.4	7.7	1.1
HL, Tesco*	1 Serving/385g	443.0	5.0	115	9.3	15.9	1.2	1.0
Italian, Sainsbury's*	½ Pack/225g	360.0	16.0	160	6.9	17.3	7.0	1.5
Italian, Tesco*	1 Pack/420g	830.0	41.0	198	9.2	18.2	9.7	1.2
Kids, Sainsbury's*	1 Pack/300g	336.0	7.0	112	4.6	17.9	2.4	1.7
Light Choices, Tesco*	1 Pack/385g	465.0	7.0	121	7.0	18.7	1.9	1.5
Made With Fresh Pasta, Findus*	1 Pack/360g	360.0	7.0	100	5.0	16.0	2.0	0.5
Morrisons, Canned, Morrisons*	1 Can/410g	279.0	6.0	68	5.1	8.8	1.4	1.0
Red Leicester, Heinz*	1 Can/400g	332.0	11.0	83	3.5	11.1	2.7	0.3
Smart Price, Asda*	1 Can/410g	291.0	6.0	71	2.6	11.8	1.5	0.4
MACAROONS							
Butterscotch, Picard*	1 Macaroon/20g	85.0	4.0	424	9.7	55.1	18.2	0.0
Coconut, Sainsbury's*	1 Macaroon/33g	146.0	6.0	441	4.7	63.7	18.6	0.8
Coconut, Tesco*	1 Macaroon/33g	140.0	6.0	425	4.4	59.0	18.6	5.7
French, Average	1 Serving/60g	225.0	11.0	375	6.7	46.7	18.3	3.3
MACKEREL							
Atlantic, Raw, Average	*1 Fillet/75g*	*154.0*	*10.0*	*205*	*18.6*	*0.0*	*13.9*	*0.0*
Fillets, Honey Roast Smoked, Sainsbury's*	1 Serving/100g	349.0	27.0	349	21.5	4.5	27.3	12.4
Fillets, in a Hot Chilli Dressing, Princes*	1 Pack/125g	370.0	34.0	296	13.3	0.0	27.0	0.0
Fillets, in Brine, Average	*1 Can/88g*	*206.0*	*15.0*	*234*	*19.4*	*0.0*	*17.4*	*0.0*
Fillets, in Curry Sauce, John West*	1 Can/125g	275.0	21.0	220	14.2	3.5	16.6	0.2
Fillets, in Green Peppercorn Sauce, John West*	1 Can/125g	329.0	26.0	263	14.0	4.5	21.0	0.1
Fillets, in Hot Smoked Peppered, Asda*	1 Fillet/100g	341.0	28.0	341	19.0	3.3	28.0	0.6
Fillets, in Mustard Sauce, Average	1 Can/125g	274.0	19.0	219	14.1	5.4	15.5	0.0
Fillets, in Olive Oil, Average	1 Serving/50g	149.0	12.0	297	18.5	1.0	24.3	0.0
Fillets, in Spicy Tomato Sauce, Average	1oz/28g	56.0	4.0	199	14.3	3.8	14.0	0.0
Fillets, in Sunflower Oil, Average	1 Can/94g	262.0	21.0	279	20.2	0.2	21.9	0.2
Fillets, in Tomato Sauce, Average	1 Can/125g	251.0	18.0	200	14.3	2.7	14.7	0.0
Fillets, in White Wine & Spices, Connetable*	1 Can/120g	169.0	10.0	141	15.5	1.2	8.2	0.0
Fillets, Red Pepper & Onion, Smoked, Asda*	1 Serving/90g	319.0	28.0	354	18.0	0.8	31.0	1.2
Fillets, Smoked, Average	*1oz/28g*	*94.0*	*8.0*	*335*	*19.7*	*0.5*	*28.2*	*0.3*
Fried in Blended Oil	*1oz/28g*	*76.0*	*5.0*	*272*	*24.0*	*0.0*	*19.5*	*0.0*
Grilled	*1oz/28g*	*67.0*	*5.0*	*239*	*20.8*	*0.0*	*17.3*	*0.0*
Raw, with Skin, Weighed with Bone, Average	*1oz/28g*	*67.0*	*5.0*	*238*	*19.9*	*0.0*	*17.6*	*0.0*
Roasted, With Piri-piri, Tesco*	1 Fillet/80g	240.0	19.0	300	20.7	0.0	23.8	1.0
Smoked, Lemon & Parsley, Morrisons*	½ Pack/100g	282.0	20.0	282	20.9	4.6	20.0	1.0

	Measure INFO/WEIGHT	per Measure KCAL	FAT	Nutrition Values per 100g / 100ml KCAL	PROT	CARB	FAT	FIBRE
MACKEREL								
Smoked, Peppered, Average	*1oz/28g*	*87.0*	*7.0*	*309*	*20.4*	*0.3*	*25.2*	*0.2*
MADRAS								
Beef, Canned, BGTY, Sainsbury's*	1 Can/400g	344.0	14.0	86	9.5	4.0	3.6	0.9
Beef, Tesco*	1 Pack/460g	616.0	38.0	134	10.6	4.5	8.2	1.2
Beef, Weight Watchers*	1 Pack/320g	317.0	5.0	99	5.6	15.8	1.5	0.3
Chicken, & Pilau Rice, Asda*	1 Pack/400g	588.0	28.0	147	8.0	13.0	7.0	1.7
Chicken, & Rice, Hot & Spicy, Sainsbury's*	1 Pack/500g	670.0	25.0	134	7.1	14.9	5.1	2.2
Chicken, Asda*	1 Serving/350g	430.0	31.0	123	7.0	3.6	9.0	2.3
Chicken, Frozen, GFY, Asda*	1 Pack/400g	448.0	5.0	112	5.6	19.4	1.3	1.2
Chicken, Iceland*	1 Pack/400g	376.0	19.0	94	7.7	4.9	4.8	1.1
Chicken, Indian Take Away, Tesco*	1 Serving/175g	254.0	18.0	145	8.2	4.8	10.1	1.7
Chicken, Indian, Tesco*	1 Pack/350g	518.0	31.0	148	11.3	5.6	8.9	1.9
Chicken, Morrisons*	1 Pack/350g	448.0	30.0	128	9.6	2.8	8.7	2.4
Chicken, Sainsbury's*	1 Pack/400g	468.0	27.0	117	11.7	2.2	6.8	2.8
Chicken, Tesco*	1 Pack/350g	325.0	14.0	93	10.6	3.6	4.1	0.6
Chicken, Waitrose*	1 Pack/400g	672.0	42.0	168	14.6	3.7	10.5	1.8
MAGNUM								
Almond, Wall's Ice Cream*	1 Bar/86g	275.0	18.0	320	5.0	30.0	21.0	0.0
Caramel & Almond, Temptation, Wall's Ice Cream*	1 Lolly/68g	239.0	15.0	351	5.4	34.0	22.0	0.0
Caramel & Nuts Bar, Wall's Ice Cream*	1 Bar/60g	132.0	9.0	220	4.0	19.0	15.0	0.0
Classic, Mini, Wall's*	1 Lolly/50g	170.0	11.0	340	4.0	30.0	22.0	0.0
Classic, Wall's Ice Cream*	1 Lolly/86g	261.0	16.0	303	3.8	29.0	19.0	0.0
Double Chocolate, Wall's Ice Cream*	1 Bar/92g	346.0	22.0	378	4.5	36.0	24.0	0.0
Gluttony, Wall's Ice Cream*	1 Lolly/110ml	425.0	29.0	386	4.5	32.7	26.4	0.0
Greed, Wall's Ice Cream*	1 Bar/110ml	307.0	18.0	279	3.6	29.1	16.4	0.0
White, Wall's Ice Cream*	1 Lolly/87g	256.0	15.0	296	3.8	32.0	17.0	0.0
MAKHANI								
Chicken Tikka & Pilau Rice, BGTY, Sainsbury's*	1 Pack/400g	448.0	4.0	112	8.3	17.5	1.0	1.9
Chicken Tikka, BGTY, Sainsbury's*	1 Pack/251g	186.0	5.0	74	11.3	3.0	1.9	1.7
Chicken Tikka, Waitrose*	1 Pack/400g	560.0	30.0	140	14.0	3.8	7.6	2.1
Chicken, Sainsbury's*	½ Pack/199g	313.0	21.0	157	12.2	2.9	10.7	2.5
King Prawns, Finest, Tesco*	1 Pack/350g	514.0	39.0	147	6.0	6.0	11.1	1.3
Paneer, Ashoka*	½ Pouch/150g	283.0	23.0	189	4.7	8.0	15.3	1.0
MALT DRINK								
Non-alcoholic, Supermalt*	1 Bottle/330g	210.0	0.0	64	0.8	15.1	0.0	0.0
MALTESERS								
MaltEaster, Chocolate Bunny, Mars*	1 Bunny/29g	157.0	9.0	541	6.9	57.0	31.7	0.0
Mars*	1 Reg Bag/37g	187.0	9.0	505	7.9	62.8	24.6	0.9
White Chocolate, Mars*	1 Pack/37g	186.0	9.0	504	7.9	61.0	25.4	0.0
MANDARIN ORANGES								
Broken, Segments in Fruit Juice, Basics, Sainsbury's*	½ Can/149g	51.0	0.0	34	0.7	7.7	0.0	0.3
in Juice, Average	*1oz/28g*	*11.0*	*0.0*	*39*	*0.7*	*9.0*	*0.0*	*0.5*
in Light Syrup, Average	*1 Can/298g*	*201.0*	*0.0*	*67*	*0.5*	*15.9*	*0.0*	*0.1*
in Orange Gel, Del Monte*	1 Can/128g	60.0	0.0	47	0.0	10.9	0.0	0.0
Weighed with Peel, Average	*1 Sm/50g*	*18.0*	*0.0*	*36*	*0.9*	*8.3*	*0.1*	*1.2*
MANGE TOUT								
& Sugar Snap Peas, Tesco*	1 Pack/150g	102.0	1.0	68	7.0	9.2	0.4	3.8
Boiled in Salted Water	*1oz/28g*	*7.0*	*0.0*	*26*	*3.2*	*3.3*	*0.1*	*2.2*
Raw, Average	*1 Serving/80g*	*26.0*	*0.0*	*32*	*3.6*	*4.2*	*0.2*	*1.1*
Stir-Fried in Blended Oil	*1oz/28g*	*20.0*	*1.0*	*71*	*3.8*	*3.5*	*4.8*	*2.4*
MANGO								
& Melon, Sliced, Shapers, Boots*	1 Pack/80g	33.0	0.0	41	0.7	9.2	0.2	1.8
Dried, Average	*1 Serving/50g*	*173.0*	*0.0*	*347*	*1.4*	*83.1*	*1.0*	*4.9*

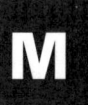

	Measure INFO/WEIGHT	per Measure KCAL	per Measure FAT	Nutrition Values per 100g / 100ml KCAL	PROT	CARB	FAT	FIBRE
MANGO								
Dried, With Chilli, King Henry's*	1 Bag /120g	300.0	0.0	250	0.0	62.5	0.0	1.0
in Syrup, Average	*1oz/28g*	*22.0*	*0.0*	*80*	*0.3*	*20.5*	*0.0*	*0.9*
Pieces in Juice, Natures Finest*	1 Pot/220g	123.0	0.0	56	0.5	12.3	0.2	1.5
Pineapple & Passionfruit, M & S*	1 Pack/400g	200.0	1.0	50	0.6	10.9	0.2	1.7
Ripe, Raw, Weighed with Skin & Stone, Average	*1 Mango/225g*	*88.0*	*0.0*	*39*	*0.5*	*9.6*	*0.1*	*1.8*
Ripe, Raw, Without Peel & Stone, Flesh Only, Average	*1 Mango/207g*	*135.0*	*1.0*	*65*	*0.5*	*17.0*	*0.3*	*1.8*
MANGOSTEEN								
Canned, in Syrup, Drained, Average	*1 Cup/196g*	*143.0*	*1.0*	*73*	*0.4*	*17.9*	*0.6*	*1.8*
Raw, Fresh, Average	*1 Serving/80g*	*50.0*	*0.0*	*63*	*0.6*	*15.6*	*0.6*	*5.1*
MARGARINE								
Average	*1 Thin Spread/7g*	*51.0*	*6.0*	*726*	*0.1*	*0.5*	*81.0*	*0.0*
Butter Style, Average	*1 Thin Spread/7g*	*44.0*	*5.0*	*627*	*0.7*	*1.1*	*68.9*	*0.0*
for Baking, Average	*1 Thin Spread/7g*	*42.0*	*5.0*	*607*	*0.2*	*0.4*	*67.2*	*0.0*
No Salt, Flora*	1 Thin Spread/7g	37.0	4.0	531	0.0	0.0	59.0	0.0
Omega 3 Plus, Flora*	1 Thin Spread/7g	24.0	3.0	350	0.1	3.0	38.0	0.0
Pro Activ, Extra Light, Flora*	1 Thin Spread/7g	15.0	2.0	218	0.1	2.9	23.0	0.2
Pro Activ, Light, Flora*	1 Thin Spread/7g	23.0	2.0	331	0.1	4.0	35.0	0.0
Pro Activ, with Olive Oil, Flora*	1 Thin Spread/7g	23.0	2.0	331	0.1	4.0	35.0	0.0
Reduced Fat, Average	*1 Thin Spread/7g*	*25.0*	*3.0*	*356*	*0.5*	*3.0*	*38.0*	*0.0*
Soya, Granose*	1 Thin Spread/7g	52.0	6.0	745	0.1	0.1	82.0	0.0
Vegetarian, Kosher, Rakusen's*	1 Pack/250g	1800.0	200.0	720	0.0	0.0	80.0	0.0
White, Flora*	1 Thin Spread/7g	60.0	7.0	855	0.0	0.0	95.0	0.0
MARINADE								
Barbecue, COU, M & S*	1 Serving/35g	52.0	0.0	150	1.2	35.5	0.2	1.0
Barbecue, in Minutes, Knorr*	1 Pack/110g	337.0	1.0	306	6.2	66.4	1.3	3.4
Barbeque, Sticky, Sainsbury's*	¼ Jar/77g	112.0	3.0	145	0.8	26.7	3.6	1.0
Cajun Spice, The English Provender Co.*	1 Serving/50g	93.0	7.0	187	1.3	15.3	13.4	1.6
Chinese, Classic, Sharwood's*	1oz/28g	32.0	1.0	113	1.8	16.1	4.8	1.0
Hickory Dickory Smokey, Ainsley Harriott*	1 Pot/300ml	360.0	0.0	120	0.6	28.1	0.1	0.0
Hot & Spicy Barbecue, M & S*	1 Serving/18g	23.0	0.0	130	1.0	31.1	0.3	0.8
Lemon & Rosemary, Nando's*	1fl oz/30ml	44.0	4.0	147	1.0	11.8	13.0	0.2
Lime & Coriander with Peri Peri, Nando's*	1 Tsp/5g	9.0	1.0	182	0.0	13.1	16.6	0.2
Peri Peri, Hot, Nando's*	1 Serving/40g	36.0	2.0	89	0.0	10.9	4.8	0.1
Sticky BBQ, Eat Well, M & S*	1 Bottle/250ml	400.0	1.0	160	0.7	37.8	0.5	1.0
Sun Dried Tomato & Basil with Peri-Peri, Nando's*	1 Bottle/270g	319.0	26.0	118	0.1	15.3	9.5	0.8
Tequila Chilli Lime, M & S*	1 Serving/75ml	116.0	1.0	155	0.6	34.0	1.6	0.5
Thai Coconut, Coriander & Lime, Lea & Perrins*	1oz/28g	45.0	2.0	159	1.3	25.7	6.1	0.0
Tomato & Herb, Lea & Perrins*	1oz/28g	28.0	0.0	100	1.2	24.1	0.5	0.0
Tomato, Basil & Parmesan, M & S*	1 Serving/50g	37.0	1.0	75	2.1	10.1	2.5	1.5
White Wine, Garlic & Pepper, Lea & Perrins*	1oz/28g	28.0	0.0	99	0.0	23.7	0.7	0.0
MARJORAM								
Dried	*1 Tsp/1g*	*2.0*	*0.0*	*271*	*12.7*	*42.5*	*7.0*	*0.0*
MARLIN								
Smoked, H. Forman & Son*	1 Pack/200g	240.0	0.0	120	29.8	0.0	0.1	0.0
Steaks, Chargrilled, Sainsbury's*	1 Steak/240g	367.0	15.0	153	23.6	0.8	6.1	0.6
Steaks, Raw, Sainsbury's*	1 Steak/110g	109.0	0.0	99	24.3	0.0	0.2	0.0
MARMALADE								
3 Fruit, Thick Cut, Waitrose*	1 Tsp/15g	39.0	0.0	262	0.4	64.8	0.1	0.7
Blood Orange, Grandessa*	1 Serving/15g	36.0	0.0	240	0.4	59.0	0.1	0.7
Blood Orange, TTD, Sainsbury's*	1 Tbsp/15g	40.0	0.0	264	0.3	65.7	0.0	0.8
Christmas Orange & Whisky, M & S*	1oz/28g	67.0	0.0	240	0.3	59.5	0.2	1.9
Citrus Shred, Robertson*	1 Tsp/5g	13.0	0.0	253	0.2	63.0	0.0	0.0
Five Fruit, Tesco*	1 Serving/10g	28.0	0.0	278	0.2	68.2	0.1	0.9

M

	Measure INFO/WEIGHT	per Measure KCAL	FAT	Nutrition Values per 100g / 100ml KCAL	PROT	CARB	FAT	FIBRE
MARMALADE								
Fresh Fruit, Three Fruits, TTD, Sainsbury's*	1 Tbsp/15g	40.0	0.0	268	0.3	66.7	0.0	0.8
Grapefruit & Cranberry, M & S*	1 Tsp/15g	36.0	0.0	240	0.3	60.3	0.0	1.5
Grapefruit, Fine Cut, Duerr's*	1 Tsp/15g	39.0	0.0	261	0.2	65.0	0.0	0.0
Lemon & Lime, Average	*1 Tbsp/20g*	*53.0*	*0.0*	*267*	*0.1*	*66.3*	*0.1*	*0.4*
Lemon Jelly, No Peel, Tesco*	1 Tsp/15g	39.0	0.0	263	0.1	65.0	0.0	0.4
Lemon, Fine Cut, Tesco*	1 Serving/15g	39.0	0.0	257	0.2	64.0	0.0	0.5
Lemon, with Shred, Average	*1 Serving/20g*	*49.0*	*0.0*	*247*	*0.1*	*61.6*	*0.0*	*0.6*
Lime, with Shred, Average	*1 Tbsp/15g*	*39.0*	*0.0*	*261*	*0.1*	*65.0*	*0.1*	*0.3*
Orange & Ginger, Average	*1 Tbsp/15g*	*40.0*	*0.0*	*264*	*0.2*	*65.7*	*0.1*	*0.3*
Orange & Lemon, Reduced Sugar, Zest*	1 Tsp/6g	12.0	0.0	195	0.3	47.1	0.2	0.0
Orange & Tangerine, Tiptree, Wilkin & Sons*	1 Tsp/15g	40.0	0.0	268	0.0	67.0	0.0	0.0
Orange, Lemon & Grapefruit, Baxters*	1 Tsp/15g	38.0	0.0	252	0.0	63.0	0.0	0.1
Orange, Reduced Sugar, Average	*1 Tbsp/15g*	*26.0*	*0.0*	*170*	*0.4*	*42.0*	*0.1*	*0.6*
Orange, Reduced Sugar, Thin Cut, Streamline*	1 Serving/10g	18.0	0.0	178	0.5	43.0	0.3	0.0
Orange, Shredless, Average	*1 Tsp/10g*	*26.0*	*0.0*	*261*	*0.2*	*65.0*	*0.0*	*0.1*
Orange, Sweet, Fresh Fruit, TTD, Sainsbury's*	1 Tbsp/15g	39.0	0.0	261	0.5	64.4	0.1	1.1
Orange, with Drambuie, Finest, Tesco*	1 Serving/10g	33.0	0.0	329	0.3	82.0	0.0	0.7
Orange, with Shred, Average	*1 Tbsp/15g*	*39.0*	*0.0*	*263*	*0.2*	*65.2*	*0.0*	*0.3*
Pink Grapefruit, Thin Cut, Waitrose*	1 Serving/10g	26.0	0.0	261	0.2	65.0	0.0	0.4
Seville, Thick Cut, Organic, Fair Trade, Tesco*	1 Tbsp/15.1g	37.0	0.0	245	0.3	60.3	0.1	0.7
Three Fruit, Diabetic, Thursday Cottage*	1 Serving/5g	8.0	0.0	154	0.4	38.0	0.0	1.0
Three Fruit, Finest, Tesco*	1 Serving/15g	39.0	0.0	262	0.5	63.6	0.2	1.6
Three Fruits, Fresh Fruit, Sainsbury's*	1 Tsp/15g	37.0	0.0	250	0.0	61.3	0.0	0.0
MARMITE*								
Yeast Extract, Marmite*	1 Tsp/9g	23.0	0.0	252	38.7	24.1	0.1	3.4
MARROW								
Boiled, Average	*1oz/28g*	*3.0*	*0.0*	*9*	*0.4*	*1.6*	*0.2*	*0.6*
Raw	*1oz/28g*	*3.0*	*0.0*	*12*	*0.5*	*2.2*	*0.2*	*0.5*
MARS								
Bar, 5 Little Ones, Mars*	1 Piece/8g	38.0	1.0	477	4.5	73.6	18.3	0.0
Bar, Duo, Mars*	1 Bar/42g	191.0	8.0	450	4.4	67.5	18.0	1.2
Bar, Funsize, Mars*	1 Bar/18g	80.0	3.0	446	3.5	70.1	16.8	1.1
Bar, Mars*	1 Std Bar/62g	280.0	11.0	448	4.1	68.1	17.6	11.0
Bar, Medium, 58g, Mars*	1 Serving/58g	263.0	10.0	453	4.6	67.9	18.1	0.0
Delight, Mars*	1 Bar/19.9g	110.0	7.0	552	4.5	57.8	33.6	1.3
MARSHMALLOWS								
Average	1 Mallow/5g	16.0	0.0	327	3.9	83.1	0.0	0.0
Haribo*	1 Mallow/5g	16.0	0.0	330	3.0	80.0	0.0	0.0
Raspberry & Cream, Sainsbury's*	1 Mallow/7g	23.0	0.0	330	4.1	78.5	0.0	0.5
MARZIPAN								
Bar, Chocolate, Plain, Thorntons*	1 Bar/46g	206.0	8.0	448	5.2	69.1	17.4	2.0
Dark Chocolate, Thorntons*	1 Serving/46g	207.0	8.0	451	5.2	69.4	17.4	2.1
Plain, Average	*1oz/28g*	*115.0*	*4.0*	*412*	*5.8*	*67.5*	*14.1*	*1.7*
MASALA								
Chicken, Tandoori, M & S*	½ Pack/175g	210.0	12.0	120	11.3	4.3	6.6	4.5
Prawn, & Rice, Tesco*	1 Pack/475g	655.0	25.0	138	5.2	17.9	5.2	1.2
Prawn, King, Waitrose*	1 Pack/350g	385.0	26.0	110	7.1	3.8	7.4	1.8
Vegetable, Sainsbury's*	1 Pack/400g	388.0	30.0	97	2.1	5.2	7.5	2.5
Vegetable, Waitrose*	1 Serving/400g	288.0	19.0	72	2.2	4.9	4.8	2.5
Vegetable, with Rice, Feeling Great, Findus*	1 Pack/350g	350.0	7.0	100	3.0	18.0	2.0	1.7
MASH								
Davidstow Cheddar, Extra Special, Asda*	1 Serving/225g	292.0	17.0	130	5.3	10.4	7.5	2.6
Parsnip & Parmesan, Finest, Tesco*	½ Packet/250g	245.0	12.0	98	1.6	11.9	4.9	2.4

	Measure INFO/WEIGHT	per Measure KCAL	per Measure FAT	Nutrition Values per 100g / 100ml KCAL	PROT	CARB	FAT	FIBRE
MASH								
Root Vegetable, Finest, Tesco*	½ Pack/250g	225.0	12.0	90	1.1	9.1	5.0	3.4
Root, Asda*	½ Pack/200g	142.0	8.0	71	0.7	8.0	4.0	3.1
Winter Root, Sainsbury's*	1 Serving/140g	157.0	2.0	112	2.7	22.0	1.5	0.9
MAYONNAISE								
50% Less Fat, GFY, Asda*	1 Tbsp/10g	32.0	3.0	322	0.8	10.0	31.0	0.0
60% Less Fat, BGTY, Sainsbury's*	1 Tbsp/15ml	42.0	4.0	277	0.4	7.3	27.3	0.0
Aioli, Finest, Tesco*	1 Tsp/5g	20.0	2.0	408	0.8	8.5	41.2	0.0
Average	***1 Tsp/11g***	***80.0***	***9.0***	***724***	***1.9***	***0.2***	***79.3***	***0.0***
Beolive Roasted Garlic Flavour, Vandemooetele*	1 Serving/15ml	46.0	4.0	305	1.3	11.3	28.2	0.0
Deli, Caramelised Onion, Heinz*	1 Serving/20g	110.0	11.0	548	1.4	5.9	57.5	0.1
Deli, Moroccan, Heinz*	1 Tbsp/15g	80.0	8.0	532	0.9	4.6	56.5	0.1
Deli, Roasted Garlic, Heinz*	1 Tbsp/15g	81.0	8.0	537	1.1	5.5	56.6	0.0
Deli, Sundried Tomato, Heinz*	1 Tbsp/15g	88.0	9.0	589	1.3	4.9	62.5	0.0
Extra Light, Asda*	1 Tbsp/10ml	12.0	1.0	119	0.7	13.1	7.1	0.2
Extra Light, Heinz*	1 Tbsp/12ml	9.0	1.0	75	0.6	11.4	3.0	0.6
Extra Light, Now Only 3% Fat, Hellmann's*	1 Serving/16g	12.0	0.0	73	0.6	11.0	3.0	0.6
Extra Light, Sainsbury's*	1 Tbsp/15ml	17.0	1.0	115	0.7	11.9	7.0	0.0
Extra Light, Tesco*	1 Serving/45ml	40.0	2.0	90	0.6	10.2	4.7	0.0
Extra Light, Weight Watchers*	1 Serving/15g	15.0	1.0	97	1.1	9.6	5.9	3.2
Finest, Tesco*	1 Dtsp/22g	155.0	17.0	703	1.1	1.5	77.0	0.0
French Style, BGTY, Sainsbury's*	1 Tbsp/15ml	55.0	6.0	366	0.6	7.5	36.9	0.0
Garlic & Herb, M & S*	1 Tsp/6g	43.0	5.0	712	3.4	2.4	76.9	0.9
Garlic & Herb, Reduced Calorie, Hellmann's*	1 Serving/25ml	58.0	5.0	233	0.7	13.1	19.3	0.4
Garlic Flavoured, Frank Cooper*	1 Tsp/6g	28.0	3.0	460	2.2	8.8	46.2	0.1
Garlic, Waitrose*	1 Tsp/6g	21.0	2.0	346	0.6	8.6	34.3	0.0
Heinz*	1 Tbsp/15g	99.0	11.0	663	0.9	3.0	71.8	0.0
Lemon, Waitrose*	1 Tsp/8ml	56.0	6.0	694	1.2	1.3	76.0	5.4
Light Dijon, Benedicta*	1 Tbsp/15g	44.0	4.0	292	0.7	6.7	29.2	0.0
Light, BGTY, Sainsbury's*	1 Tsp/11g	33.0	3.0	296	0.5	7.2	29.3	0.0
Light, Hellmann's*	1 Serving/10g	30.0	3.0	298	0.7	6.5	29.8	0.1
Light, Knorr*	1 Tbsp/15g	50.0	5.0	333	0.0	6.7	33.3	0.0
Light, Kraft*	1 Serving/25g	61.0	5.0	245	0.6	15.0	20.0	0.0
Light, Reduced Calorie, Hellmann's*	1 Tsp/10g	30.0	3.0	297	0.7	6.5	29.8	0.0
Light, Reduced Fat, Heinz*	1 Tbsp/15g	42.0	4.0	279	1.1	7.7	26.8	0.5
Light, Squeezable, Hellmann's*	1 Tbsp/15g	44.0	4.0	293	0.7	6.4	29.4	0.0
Low Fat, Belolive*	1 Serving/15ml	45.0	4.0	298	0.8	11.1	29.0	0.0
Mild Dijon Mustard, Frank Cooper*	1 Pot/28g	114.0	11.0	406	3.3	9.3	39.5	0.1
Mustard, Safeway*	1 Tbsp/15ml	105.0	11.0	703	1.4	2.1	76.5	0.0
Organic, Evernat*	1 Tsp/11g	83.0	9.0	752	1.3	2.8	81.0	0.0
Organic, Whole Foods*	1 Tbsp/14g	100.0	11.0	714	0.0	7.1	78.6	0.0
Real, Best Foods*	1 Tbsp/13g	90.0	10.0	692	0.0	0.0	76.9	0.0
Real, Hellmann's*	1 Tsp/11g	79.0	9.0	722	1.1	1.3	79.1	0.0
Real, The Big Squeeze, Hellmann's*	1 Tbsp/15ml	101.0	11.0	676	1.0	1.2	74.0	0.0
Reduced Calorie, Average	***1 Tsp/11g***	***32.0***	***3.0***	***288***	***1.0***	***8.2***	***28.1***	***0.0***
Vegetarian, Tesco*	1 Tsp/12g	89.0	10.0	738	1.5	0.8	81.0	0.0
with Coarse Ground Mustard, French, Sainsbury's*	1 Serving/15ml	93.0	10.0	618	0.8	1.7	67.3	0.3
with Dijon Mustard, Hellmann's*	1 Tbsp/15ml	31.0	3.0	210	2.9	5.1	19.7	0.0
MEAL REPLACEMENT								
Bars, Chocolate & Hazelnut, Tesco*	1 Bar/65g	250.0	7.0	385	24.2	41.0	11.0	6.3
Crispy, Raspberry, Meal Bar, Tesco*	1 Bar/60g	216.0	7.0	360	22.3	42.1	11.2	7.6
Ny-Tro Pro-40, Cool Vanilla, AST Sports Science*	1 Sachet/72g	250.0	1.0	347	55.6	30.6	2.1	2.8
Shake, Chocolate, Advantage, Atkins*	1 Serving/34g	121.0	4.0	361	49.0	8.1	12.5	15.5
Shake, Chocolate, Ready to Drink, Advantage, Atkins*	1 Carton/330ml	172.0	9.0	52	6.0	0.6	2.8	1.2

	Measure INFO/WEIGHT	per Measure KCAL	FAT	Nutrition Values per 100g / 100ml KCAL	PROT	CARB	FAT	FIBRE
MEAL REPLACEMENT								
Shake, Herbalife*	1 Serving/250ml	245.0	6.0	98	10.0	8.8	2.6	1.0
Shake, Neways*	1 Serving/39g	142.0	4.0	364	46.0	34.0	9.0	15.4
Shake, Vanilla, Ready to Drink, Advantage, Atkins*	1 Carton/330ml	175.0	9.0	53	6.2	0.6	2.7	0.9
Strawberry, High Protein, Energy Meal, Spiru-tein*	1 Serving/34g	99.0	0.0	291	41.2	32.3	0.0	2.9
Ultra Slim, Chocolate, Meal Bar, Tesco*	1 Bar/60g	219.0	7.0	365	28.5	37.3	11.1	8.2
Ultra Slim, Ready to Drink, Strawberry, Tesco*	1 Carton/330ml	231.0	3.0	70	4.2	10.5	0.9	1.5
Ultra Slim, Ready to Drink, Vanilla, Tesco*	1 Carton/330ml	224.0	3.0	68	4.2	10.5	0.9	1.5
Ultra-Slim, Ready to Drink, Chocolate, Tesco*	1 Carton/330ml	214.0	4.0	65	4.0	9.8	1.1	1.3
MEAT LOAF								
Beef & Pork, Co-Op*	¼ Loaf/114g	313.0	25.0	275	13.0	7.0	22.0	1.0
Iceland*	1 Serving/150g	331.0	24.0	221	10.8	9.3	15.7	0.9
in Onion Gravy, M & S*	¼ Pack/140g	203.0	12.0	145	11.3	6.3	8.5	1.2
Turkey & Bacon, Tesco*	1 Serving/225g	400.0	22.0	178	14.7	7.4	9.9	1.1
MEATBALLS								
& Mashed Potato, Tesco*	1 Pack/450g	526.0	30.0	117	4.0	10.4	6.6	1.0
Aberdeen Angus in Sauce, Perfectly Balanced, Waitrose*	½ Pack/240g	228.0	7.0	95	10.5	6.5	3.0	1.1
Aberdeen Angus, Fresh, Chilled, Waitrose*	1 Meatball/36g	92.0	7.0	256	18.0	1.5	19.8	0.0
Aberdeen Angus, with Herb Potatoes, Finest, Tesco*	1 Serving/393g	471.0	24.0	120	6.0	9.1	6.0	2.0
Beef, Aberdeen Angus, 12 Pack, Waitrose*	1 Meatball/36g	93.0	7.0	259	18.0	2.3	19.8	0.1
Beef, British, With Italian Herbs, Finest, Tesco*	1oz/28g	63.0	5.0	225	15.4	2.1	16.8	1.7
Beef, in Tomato Sauce, Diet Chef Ltd*	1 Pack/300g	408.0	19.0	136	11.3	8.7	6.2	2.7
Beef, Sainsbury's*	1 Meatball/29g	75.0	5.0	257	21.7	3.4	17.4	0.8
Beef, Tesco*	3 Meatballs/53g	140.0	11.0	265	15.0	2.9	21.5	0.9
Beef, TTD, Sainsbury's*	1 Meatball/35g	73.0	5.0	208	16.7	1.5	15.0	0.1
Chicken, in Tomato Sauce, Average	1 Can/392g	580.0	33.0	148	7.7	10.4	8.4	0.0
Greek, M & S*	1 Serving/350g	402.0	19.0	115	7.7	9.1	5.4	1.5
in Bolognese Sauce, Fray Bentos*	½ Can/204g	188.0	6.0	92	4.8	11.6	2.9	0.7
in Gravy, Campbell's*	½ Can/205g	164.0	5.0	80	5.6	8.6	2.6	0.0
in Gravy, Fray Bentos*	1 Meatball/21g	17.0	1.0	79	4.6	8.7	2.9	0.6
in Onion Gravy, Tesco*	½ Pack/200g	310.0	17.0	155	8.4	11.3	8.5	0.8
in Rich Gravy, Westlers*	½ Can/200g	170.0	7.0	85	4.1	9.5	3.4	0.4
in Sherry Sauce, Tapas, Waitrose*	1 Serving/185g	272.0	7.0	147	18.8	5.9	4.0	1.2
in Tomato & Basil Sauce, Go Cook, Asda*	½ Pack/270g	526.0	38.0	195	12.4	4.4	14.2	2.4
in Tomato Sauce, Canned, Average	1 Can/410g	387.0	15.0	94	5.6	9.8	3.7	0.0
in Tomato Sauce, Fray Bentos*	½ Can/206g	183.0	6.0	89	4.7	11.1	2.9	0.7
in Tomato Sauce, Tapas, Waitrose*	1 Pack/185g	285.0	17.0	154	10.8	7.2	9.1	1.3
Lamb, Asda*	1 Pack/340g	928.0	71.0	273	16.0	5.1	21.0	0.6
Lemon Chicken, with Rice, BGTY, Sainsbury's*	1 Pack/400g	388.0	8.0	97	6.8	12.8	2.1	1.4
Mighty, in Tomato Sauce, Westlers*	1 Can/400g	424.0	19.0	106	5.8	10.2	4.7	0.0
Pork & Beef, Swedish Style, Tesco*	1 Meatball/14g	34.0	2.0	245	14.3	6.5	17.7	2.0
Pork, Diet Chef Ltd*	1 Pack/300g	273.0	5.0	91	9.4	9.4	1.7	3.2
Roman-Style with Basil Mash, COU, M & S*	1 Pack/430g	344.0	9.0	80	3.7	10.9	2.2	1.9
Spicy, Deli Melt, Sainsbury's*	1 Pack/200g	338.0	21.0	169	12.7	5.5	10.7	2.9
Spicy, M & S*	1 Pack/400g	540.0	24.0	135	8.8	12.0	6.0	1.4
Swedish, Average	¼ Pack/88g	198.0	14.0	224	14.0	7.4	15.7	1.3
Turkey, GFY, Asda*	½ Pack/330g	333.0	12.0	101	10.0	7.0	3.7	0.0
with Paprika-Spiced Potatoes, Extra Special, Asda*	1 Pack/450g	589.0	24.0	131	6.5	13.4	5.3	2.0
with Spicy Tomato Sauce, Just Cook, Sainsbury's*	½ Pack/169.7g	246.0	12.0	145	14.8	5.7	7.0	0.9
MEATBALLS VEGETARIAN								
Swedish Style, Sainsbury's*	1 Ball/27g	53.0	3.0	194	21.5	5.5	9.5	4.0
with Penne, Tesco*	1 Serving/460g	414.0	11.0	90	5.9	11.4	2.3	2.1
MEDLAR								
Raw, Flesh Only	*1 Fruit/28g*	*11.0*	*0.0*	*40*	*0.5*	*10.6*	*0.4*	*10.0*

	Measure INFO/WEIGHT	per Measure KCAL	FAT	Nutrition Values per 100g / 100ml KCAL	PROT	CARB	FAT	FIBRE
MELBA TOAST								
Average	1 Serving/3g	13.0	0.0	396	12.0	76.0	4.9	4.6
Dutch, Light Choices, Tesco*	1 Pack/20g	75.0	0.0	375	13.1	75.0	2.4	4.6
Original, Van Der Meulen*	1 Slice/3g	12.0	0.0	399	12.8	80.5	2.9	3.9
Thinly Sliced Toasted Wheat Bread, Sainsbury's*	1 Slice/3g	12.0	0.0	374	13.1	75.1	2.4	4.6
Wholegrain, HL, Tesco*	1 Pack/20g	62.0	1.0	310	16.8	63.8	4.9	8.9
with Sesame, Tesco*	1 Slice/3g	11.0	0.0	370	12.8	61.7	8.0	3.8
MELON								
& Blueberry, Snack Pot, Great Stuff, Asda*	1 Pack/80g	25.0	0.0	31	0.6	6.8	0.1	1.2
Cantaloupe, Flesh Only, Average	*½ Melon/255g*	*87.0*	*0.0*	*34*	*0.8*	*8.2*	*0.2*	*0.9*
Cantaloupe, Weighed with Rind, Average	*1 Slice/100g*	*35.0*	*0.0*	*35*	*0.8*	*8.3*	*0.3*	*0.8*
Galia, Average	*1 Serving/240g*	*60.0*	*0.0*	*25*	*0.7*	*5.7*	*0.0*	*0.2*
Honeydew, Raw, Flesh Only, Average	*1oz/28g*	*8.0*	*0.0*	*29*	*0.7*	*6.9*	*0.1*	*0.5*
Medley, Average	1 Pack/240g	66.0	0.0	27	0.6	6.0	0.1	0.5
Pineapple & Strawberry, Fully Prepared, Sainsbury's*	1 Serving/245g	86.0	0.0	35	0.6	7.8	0.1	0.9
MELT								
Cheese, Chilli, Fresh, Asda*	1 Melt/29g	87.0	5.0	301	6.0	31.0	17.0	0.0
Cheesy Fish, Youngs*	1 Pack/340g	418.0	22.0	123	7.6	8.3	6.6	0.9
Chilli with Spicy Potato Wedges, Asda*	1 Pack/450g	540.0	20.0	120	8.0	12.0	4.4	1.2
Salmon & Broccoli Wedge, From Heinz, Weight Watchers*	1 Pack/320g	298.0	11.0	93	5.1	10.6	3.3	1.1
Sausage & Bean, Iceland*	1 Pack/400g	588.0	23.0	147	6.5	17.1	5.8	1.6
Tuna, Go Large, Asda*	1 Melt/175g	509.0	26.0	291	12.0	27.0	15.0	0.0
Tuna, Iceland*	1 Pack/400g	424.0	17.0	106	6.0	11.3	4.2	0.7
Tuna, M & S*	1 Pack/218g	621.0	37.0	285	13.0	20.1	17.0	1.0
Vegetable & Potato, Asda*	1 Serving/100g	451.0	23.0	451	17.0	44.0	23.0	6.2
MERINGUE								
Average	*1 Meringue/8g*	*30.0*	*0.0*	*379*	*5.3*	*95.4*	*0.0*	*0.0*
Belgian Chocolate, Mini, Extra Special, Asda*	1 Meringue/6g	28.0	1.0	459	6.0	75.0	15.0	0.7
Bombe, Raspberry & Vanilla, M & S*	1 Bombe/100g	155.0	2.0	155	3.4	33.3	1.8	2.6
Chocolate, Waitrose*	1 Meringue/77g	341.0	11.0	444	2.6	75.3	14.7	0.5
Coffee Fresh Cream, Asda*	1 Meringue/28g	109.0	5.0	396	3.8	57.0	17.0	0.3
Cream, Fresh, Sainsbury's*	1 Meringue/35g	142.0	5.0	407	3.5	65.4	14.6	0.5
Lemon, Morrisons*	1 Serving/120g	295.0	14.0	246	2.5	32.0	12.0	0.5
Nests, M & S*	1 Nest/12g	47.0	0.0	390	6.1	91.6	0.0	0.0
Nests, Sainsbury's*	1 Nest/13.3g	52.0	0.0	392	4.2	93.6	0.1	0.1
Nests, Tropical Fruit, Sainsbury's*	1 Nest/95g	234.0	7.0	246	2.0	42.0	7.8	2.4
Raspberry, M & S*	1 Serving/105g	215.0	14.0	205	1.8	20.6	13.1	3.1
Shells, Sainsbury's*	2 Shells/24g	93.0	0.0	387	3.9	92.8	0.0	0.0
Strawberry, COU, M & S*	1 Meringue/5g	20.0	0.0	385	6.4	90.0	0.1	1.4
Strawberry, Mini, Extra Special, Asda*	1 Meringue/4g	15.0	0.0	387	5.0	91.0	0.3	0.5
Toffee, COU, M & S*	1 Mini/5g	20.0	0.0	395	5.0	95.3	1.7	0.7
Toffee, M & S*	1 Meringue/30g	124.0	6.0	415	4.1	52.2	20.9	0.8
Tropical, M & S*	1 Serving/53g	212.0	14.0	400	3.1	37.0	26.9	0.0
MIDGET GEMS								
M & S*	1 Bag/113g	367.0	0.0	325	6.3	75.1	0.1	0.0
Smart Price, Asda*	1 Pack/178g	586.0	0.0	329	6.0	76.0	0.1	0.0
MILK								
Condensed, Semi Skimmed, Sweetened	*1oz/28g*	*75.0*	*0.0*	*267*	*10.0*	*60.0*	*0.2*	*0.0*
Condensed, Skimmed, Unsweetened, Average	*1oz/28g*	*30.0*	*1.0*	*108*	*7.5*	*10.5*	*4.0*	*0.0*
Condensed, Whole, Sweetened, Average	*1oz/28g*	*93.0*	*3.0*	*333*	*8.5*	*55.5*	*10.1*	*0.0*
Dried, Skimmed, Average	*1oz/28g*	*99.0*	*0.0*	*355*	*35.4*	*52.3*	*0.9*	*0.0*
Dried, Whole, Average	*1oz/28g*	*137.0*	*7.0*	*490*	*26.3*	*39.4*	*26.3*	*0.0*
Evaporated, Average	*1 Serving/85g*	*136.0*	*8.0*	*160*	*8.2*	*11.6*	*9.0*	*0.0*
Evaporated, Reduced Fat, Average	*1oz/28g*	*33.0*	*1.0*	*118*	*7.4*	*10.5*	*5.2*	*0.0*

MILK

	Measure INFO/WEIGHT	per Measure KCAL	FAT	Nutrition Values per 100g / 100ml KCAL	PROT	CARB	FAT	FIBRE
Goats, Pasteurised	*1 fl oz/30ml*	*18.0*	*1.0*	*60*	*3.1*	*4.4*	*3.5*	*0.0*
Goats, Semi-Skimmed, St Helen's Farm*	1 Serving/250ml	109.0	4.0	44	3.0	4.3	1.6	0.0
Low Fat, Calcia Extra Calcium, Unigate*	1 fl oz/30ml	13.0	0.0	45	4.3	6.3	0.5	0.0
Powder, Instant, Skimmed, Basics, Sainsbury's*	1 Serving/60g	209.0	0.0	349	35.6	50.4	0.6	0.0
Semi Skimmed, Advance, with Omega 3, St Ivel*	1 Glass/250ml	122.0	4.0	49	3.4	5.0	1.7	0.0
Semi Skimmed, Average	*1 fl oz/30ml*	*15.0*	*1.0*	*49*	*3.4*	*5.0*	*1.7*	*0.0*
Semi Skimmed, Long Life, Average	*1 fl oz/30ml*	*15.0*	*1.0*	*49*	*3.4*	*5.0*	*1.7*	*0.0*
Semi Skimmed, Low Lactose, Lactofree, Arla*	1 Glass/125ml	56.0	2.0	45	3.4	5.0	1.5	0.0
Semi Skimmed, Low Lactose, UHT, Lactofree, Arla*	1 Serving/100ml	38.0	2.0	38	3.2	2.6	1.7	0.0
Skimmed, Average	*1 fl oz/30ml*	*10.0*	*0.0*	*34*	*3.3*	*5.0*	*0.1*	*0.0*
Skimmed, Uht, Average	*1 fl oz/30ml*	*10.0*	*0.0*	*34*	*3.3*	*5.0*	*0.1*	*0.0*
Whole, Average	*1 Glass/200ml*	*134.0*	*8.0*	*67*	*3.3*	*4.7*	*3.9*	*0.0*
MILK DRINK								
Banana Flavour, Sterilised, Low Fat, Gulp*	1 Bottle/500ml	315.0	5.0	63	3.8	9.7	1.0	0.0
Chocolate Sterilised Skimmed, Happy Shopper*	1 Bottle/500ml	295.0	1.0	59	3.6	10.4	0.3	0.0
Chocolate, Break Time, Arla*	1 Bottle/500ml	290.0	1.0	58	3.6	10.2	0.3	0.0
Chocolate, Spar*	1 Serving/500ml	290.0	1.0	58	3.6	10.2	0.3	0.0
Chocolatte, Cafe Met*	1 Bottle/290ml	174.0	4.0	60	3.7	9.1	1.4	0.3
Colombian Coffee Flavoured, Waitrose*	1 Serving/250ml	232.0	9.0	93	4.3	10.5	3.8	0.0
Extra Choc, Mars*	1 Bottle/330g	280.0	7.0	85	3.1	13.7	2.0	0.0
Family Fuel, Mars*	1 Serving/200ml	172.0	4.0	86	3.1	13.7	2.0	0.0
Mocalatte, Cafe Met*	1 Bottle/290ml	159.0	4.0	55	2.9	8.0	1.3	0.0
No Added Sugar, Mars*	1 Serving/200ml	108.0	3.0	54	3.4	6.2	1.7	0.5
Original, Mars*	1 Serving/330g	284.0	7.0	86	3.1	13.7	2.1	0.0
Refuel, Mars*	1 Bottle/388ml	299.0	6.0	77	3.1	13.5	1.5	0.0
Semi Skimmed, Cholesterol Lowering, Pro Activ, Flora*	1 Serving/250ml	125.0	4.0	50	3.6	4.8	1.8	0.0
Strawberry Flavoured, Tesco*	1 Serving/500ml	370.0	8.0	74	4.4	10.4	1.6	0.3
MILK SHAKE								
Banana Flavour, Frijj*	1 Bottle/500ml	310.0	4.0	62	3.4	10.1	0.8	0.0
Banana Flavour, Shapers, Boots*	1 Bottle/250ml	201.0	2.0	80	5.6	12.8	0.8	1.9
Banana, Diet Chef Ltd*	1 Drink/330ml	225.0	3.0	68	4.2	10.5	0.9	1.5
Banana, Yazoo, Campina*	1 Bottle/200ml	130.0	3.0	65	3.1	10.3	1.3	0.0
Chocolate Flavour, BGTY, Sainsbury's*	1 Bottle/500ml	290.0	2.0	58	5.3	8.0	0.5	0.9
Chocolate Flavoured, Fresh, Thick, Frijj*	1 Bottle/500ml	350.0	5.0	70	3.5	11.7	1.0	0.0
Chocolate, Asda*	1 Serving/250ml	197.0	9.0	79	4.4	7.0	3.7	0.4
Chocolate, Diet Chef Ltd*	1 Carton/330ml	214.0	4.0	65	3.9	9.8	1.1	1.3
Chocolate, Extreme, Frijj*	1 Bottle/500g	425.0	10.0	85	3.9	12.7	2.1	0.0
Latte Coffee, Diet Chef Ltd*	1 Drink/330ml	225.0	3.0	68	4.2	10.5	0.9	1.5
Measure Up, Asda*	1 Glass/250ml	200.0	2.0	80	6.0	12.0	1.0	2.4
Mount Caramel, Frijj*	1 Bottle/500ml	360.0	4.0	72	3.4	12.7	0.9	0.0
Powder, Made Up with Semi-Skimmed Milk	1 Serving/250ml	172.0	4.0	69	3.2	11.3	1.6	0.0
Powder, Made Up with Whole Milk	1 Serving/250ml	217.0	9.0	87	3.1	11.1	3.7	0.0
Strawberry Flavour, Thick, Low Fat, Frijj*	1 Bottle/250ml	155.0	2.0	62	3.4	10.1	0.8	0.0
Strawberry, Diet Chef Ltd*	1 Drink/330g	225.0	3.0	68	4.2	10.5	0.9	1.5
Strawberry, Yazoo, Campina*	1 Bottle/500ml	325.0	6.0	65	3.1	10.3	1.2	0.0
Vanilla Flavour, BGTY, Sainsbury's*	1 Bottle/500ml	230.0	0.0	46	5.3	5.9	0.1	0.4
Vanilla, Diet Chef Ltd*	1 Pack/330ml	225.0	3.0	68	4.2	10.5	0.9	1.5
Vanilla, Frijj*	1 Bottle/500ml	320.0	4.0	64	3.4	10.7	0.8	0.0
MILKY BAR								
Buttons, Nestle*	1 Std Pack/30g	164.0	10.0	547	7.3	58.4	31.7	0.0
Choo, Nestle*	1 Bar/25g	116.0	4.0	464	4.2	73.1	17.2	0.0
Chunky, Nestle*	¼ Bar/37.8g	207.0	12.0	547·	7.3	58.4	31.7	0.0
Crunchies, Nestle*	1 Pack/30g	168.0	10.0	560	7.0	54.9	34.7	0.0

	Measure INFO/WEIGHT	per Measure KCAL	FAT	Nutrition Values per 100g / 100ml KCAL	PROT	CARB	FAT	FIBRE
MILKY BAR								
Eggs, Mini, Nestle*	1 Pack/100g	500.0	23.0	500	4.2	68.4	23.3	0.0
Funsize (17g), Mars*	1 Bar/17g	75.0	3.0	449	3.8	71.8	16.3	0.6
Munchies, Nestle*	1 Serving/70g	392.0	24.0	560	7.0	54.9	34.7	0.1
Nestle*	1 Sm Bar/12.5g	68.0	4.0	547	7.3	58.4	31.7	0.0
MILKY WAY								
Fun Size, Mars*	1 Bar/17g	75.0	3.0	447	3.8	71.6	16.2	0.0
Funsize (15.5g), Mars*	1 Bar/15.5g	70.0	3.0	450	3.9	71.6	16.3	0.6
Magic Stars, Mars*	1 Bag/33g	184.0	11.0	559	6.3	55.3	34.7	0.0
Mars*	1 Single Bar/26g	118.0	4.0	455	3.7	72.4	15.9	0.6
Medium, Mars*	1 Med Bar/48g	218.0	8.0	454	3.5	72.0	16.9	0.6
MINCEMEAT								
Average	*1oz/28g*	*77.0*	*1.0*	*274*	*0.6*	*62.1*	*4.3*	*1.3*
Organic, Waitrose*	1oz/28g	81.0	1.0	290	0.9	65.8	2.6	2.0
Traditional, Robertson*	1 Tbsp/17g	49.0	1.0	286	0.6	62.5	3.4	2.5
Traditional, Sainsbury's*	1 Tbsp/23g	65.0	1.0	282	0.9	62.4	3.2	1.4
with Cherries, Almonds & Brandy, Tesco*	¼ Jar/103g	295.0	5.0	287	1.4	58.8	4.9	1.4
MINSTRELS								
Galaxy, Mars*	1 Serving/100g	503.0	22.0	503	5.2	70.3	22.3	1.1
MINT								
Dried, Average	*1 Tsp/5g*	*14.0*	*0.0*	*279*	*24.8*	*34.6*	*4.6*	*0.0*
Fresh, Average	*2 Tbsp/3.2g*	*1.0*	*0.0*	*43*	*3.8*	*5.3*	*0.7*	*0.0*
MINTS								
After Dinner, Dark, Elizabeth Shaw*	1 Sweet/9g	42.0	2.0	469	2.8	62.5	23.1	0.0
After Dinner, Sainsbury's*	1 Mint/7g	32.0	1.0	456	4.1	62.1	21.2	4.1
After Dinner, Tesco*	1oz/28g	132.0	5.0	471	5.0	70.0	19.0	0.0
After Eight, Dark Chocolate, Nestle*	1 Sweet/7g	32.0	1.0	461	5.0	63.0	12.9	2.0
After Eight, Orange, Nestle*	1 Sweet/7g	29.0	1.0	417	2.5	72.6	12.9	1.1
After Eight, Straws, Nestle*	1 Sweet/4.6g	24.0	1.0	526	5.1	56.6	31.0	4.0
Butter Mintoes, M & S*	1 Sweet/9g	35.0	1.0	391	0.0	84.0	6.8	0.0
Butter Mintoes, Tesco*	1 Sweet/7g	24.0	0.0	349	0.0	71.3	7.1	0.0
Clear, Co-Op*	1 Sweet/6g	24.0	0.0	395	0.0	98.0	0.0	0.0
Cream, Luxury, Thorntons*	1 Sweet/13g	62.0	3.0	477	4.2	62.3	23.8	2.3
Creams, Bassett's*	1 Sweet/11g	40.0	0.0	365	0.0	91.8	0.0	0.0
Curiously Strong, M & S*	1 Sweet/1g	4.0	0.0	390	0.4	97.5	0.0	0.0
Everton, Co-Op*	1 Sweet/6g	25.0	0.0	410	0.6	92.0	4.0	0.0
Extra Strong, Peppermint, Trebor*	1 Roll/46g	180.0	0.0	395	0.4	98.1	0.2	0.0
Extra Strong, Spearmint, Trebor*	1 Pack/44g	174.0	0.0	395	0.4	98.7	0.0	0.0
Extra, Peppermint Coolburst, Wrigleys*	1 Pack/22g	53.0	0.0	240	0.0	98.0	1.0	0.0
Extra, Spearmint, Wrigleys*	1 Sweet/1.1g	3.0	0.0	244	0.0	98.0	1.0	0.0
Extra, Wrigleys*	1 Sweet/1.1g	3.0	0.0	240	0.0	64.0	1.0	0.0
Glacier, Fox's*	1 Sweet/5g	19.0	0.0	386	0.0	96.4	0.0	0.0
Humbugs, Co-Op*	1 Sweet/8g	34.0	1.0	425	0.6	89.9	7.0	0.0
Humbugs, M & S*	1 Sweet/9g	37.0	0.0	407	0.6	91.1	4.4	0.0
Humbugs, Thorntons*	1 Sweet/9g	31.0	0.0	340	1.0	87.8	4.4	0.0
Imperials, Co-Op*	1 Sweet/3g	12.0	0.0	395	0.3	98.0	0.2	0.0
Imperials, M & S*	1 Sweet/3g	12.0	0.0	391	0.0	97.8	0.0	0.0
Imperials, Sainsbury's*	1 Sweet/2.6g	10.0	0.0	374	0.0	92.1	0.0	0.0
Imperials, Tesco*	1 Sweet/3g	12.0	0.0	397	0.6	98.7	0.0	0.0
Mento, Sugar Free, Mentos*	1 Sweet/2g	5.0	0.0	260	1.0	87.0	5.5	0.0
Mighty, 24-7, Sugar Free, Trebor*	1 Sweet/0.1g	0.0	0.0	277	0.0	94.7	0.0	0.0
Mint Assortment, M & S*	1 Sweet/7g	26.0	0.0	375	0.4	78.2	6.9	0.0
Mint Favourites, Bassett's*	1 Sweet/6g	22.0	0.0	367	0.9	77.4	5.9	0.0
Peppermints, Strong, Altoids*	1 Sweet/1g	3.0	0.0	385	0.5	96.0	0.0	0.0

M

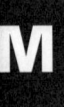

M

	Measure INFO/WEIGHT	per Measure KCAL	FAT	Nutrition Values per 100g / 100ml KCAL	PROT	CARB	FAT	FIBRE
MINTS								
Smooth, Weight Watchers*	1 Tube/25g	58.0	0.0	231	0.2	61.6	0.0	0.0
Soft, Trebor*	1 Pack/48g	182.0	0.0	380	0.0	94.9	0.0	0.0
Softmints, Peppermint, Trebor*	1 Pack/48g	170.0	0.0	355	0.0	88.9	0.0	0.0
Softmints, Spearmint, Trebor*	1 Pack/45g	170.0	0.0	375	0.0	94.3	0.0	0.0
Thins, Chocolate, Waitrose*	1 Thin/5g	27.0	1.0	509	4.2	69.6	23.8	0.2
Thins, Plain Chocolate, Safeway*	1 Thin/10g	48.0	2.0	480	2.3	67.5	22.3	0.7
MIRIN								
Rice Wine, Sweetened, Average	*1 Tbsp/15ml*	*35.0*	*0.0*	*231*	*0.2*	*41.6*	*0.0*	*0.0*
MISO								
Average	*1oz/28g*	*57.0*	*2.0*	*203*	*13.3*	*23.5*	*6.2*	*0.0*
MIXED HERBS								
Average	*1 Tsp/5g*	*13.0*	*0.0*	*260*	*12.9*	*37.5*	*8.5*	*6.7*
Herbes De Provence, Dried, Schwartz*	1 Tsp/2g	7.0	0.0	364	12.9	65.0	5.8	0.0
MIXED SPICE								
Rub, Moroccan, Schwartz*	1 Serving/3g	9.0	0.0	309	15.0	36.4	11.4	19.5
Schwartz*	1 Tsp/2g	8.0	0.0	390	10.4	65.8	9.5	2.0
MIXED VEGETABLES								
& Mung Bean Sprouts, with Asian Seasoning, Dawnfield*	1 Bag/750g	412.0	21.0	55	2.5	5.0	2.8	0.0
Baby Corn, Mange Tout & Baby Carrots, Tesco*	1 Pack/220g	64.0	1.0	29	2.3	4.3	0.4	2.2
Baby, Iceland*	1 Serving/100g	20.0	0.0	20	1.2	3.9	0.0	2.7
Baby, Steam, Fresh, Tesco*	1 Pack/160g	72.0	1.0	45	2.7	6.7	0.8	3.8
Bag, M & S*	1 Serving/200g	70.0	1.0	35	2.9	5.6	0.2	0.0
Broccoli & Cauliflower Florets, Baby Carrots, Asda*	1 Serving/113g	28.0	1.0	25	2.2	2.6	0.6	2.4
Canned, Drained, Co-Op*	½ Can/100g	45.0	0.0	45	2.0	9.0	0.1	2.0
Canned, Drained, Sainsbury's*	1 Can/200g	114.0	1.0	57	3.0	10.6	0.3	2.3
Canned, Re-Heated, Drained	1oz/28g	11.0	0.0	38	1.9	6.1	0.8	1.7
Carrot Batons, Cauliflower & Broccoli, Steamed, Asda*	1 Bag/120g	28.0	1.0	23	1.8	2.6	0.6	3.1
Carrot, Cauliflower, & Broccoli, Fresh, Tesco*	1 Serving/80g	26.0	0.0	32	2.6	3.9	0.2	2.8
Carrots, Broccoli & Sweetcorn, Easy Steam, Sainsbury's*	1 Pack/120g	67.0	1.0	56	2.6	8.7	1.2	2.0
Carrots, Broccoli & Sweetcorn, Steam Veg, Tesco*	1 Sachet/160g	80.0	2.0	50	2.5	7.5	1.1	3.0
Carrots, Cauliflower & Broccoli, Waitrose*	1 Serving/100g	35.0	1.0	35	2.4	4.9	0.6	2.9
Casserole Selection, Somerfield*	1 Pack/600g	174.0	2.0	29	1.0	5.7	0.3	1.4
Casserole, Co-Op*	1 Serving/100g	40.0	0.0	40	1.2	7.5	0.3	2.1
Casserole, Frozen, Morrisons*	1 Serving/150g	21.0	0.0	14	0.5	2.8	0.2	1.5
Casserole, Frozen, Tesco*	1 Serving/100g	26.0	0.0	26	0.8	4.8	0.4	2.0
Casserole, Ready to Cook, Sainsbury's*	½ Pack/240g	74.0	1.0	31	0.9	6.2	0.3	1.4
Casserole, Tesco*	1 Pack/440g	176.0	1.0	40	1.2	8.0	0.3	2.3
Casserole, with Baby Potatoes, Fresh, M & S*	½ Pack/350g	140.0	1.0	40	1.2	7.8	0.3	2.1
Cauliflower, Carrots, Green Beans, SteamFresh, Birds Eye*	1 Bag/120g	40.0	1.0	33	2.0	5.0	0.5	2.2
Chef's Style, Ready Prepared, M & S*	1 Pack/240g	72.0	1.0	30	2.6	4.5	0.5	2.9
Chinese, Stir Fry, Amoy*	1 Serving/110g	27.0	0.0	25	1.8	3.7	0.3	0.0
Chunky, Frozen, Sainsbury's*	1 Serving/85g	31.0	1.0	37	2.9	4.7	0.7	3.1
Corn Baby, Fine Beans & Baby Carrots, Tesco*	1 Pack/250g	67.0	1.0	27	1.7	4.0	0.5	2.2
Country Selection, Budgens*	1 Serving/113g	27.0	0.0	24	1.6	3.6	0.4	2.9
Crunchy, Tesco*	1 Pack/210g	63.0	1.0	30	1.7	5.0	0.4	2.4
Farmhouse, Four Seasons*	1 Serving/100g	26.0	1.0	26	2.2	2.7	0.7	0.0
Farmhouse, Frozen, Four Seasons, Aldi*	1oz/28g	10.0	0.0	34	2.8	4.3	0.7	0.0
Farmhouse, Frozen, Waitrose*	1 Serving/90g	22.0	1.0	25	1.9	3.1	0.6	2.4
Fresh, Asda*	1oz/28g	7.0	0.0	26	1.9	3.0	0.7	1.0
Freshly Frozen, Asda*	1 Serving/80g	42.0	1.0	52	3.2	8.0	0.8	3.0
Freshly Frozen, Iceland*	1 Serving/100g	54.0	1.0	54	3.3	8.3	0.8	3.7
Frozen, Aldi*	1 Serving/100g	34.0	1.0	34	2.8	4.3	0.7	0.0
Frozen, Boiled in Salted Water	1oz/28g	12.0	0.0	42	3.3	6.6	0.5	0.0

	Measure INFO/WEIGHT	per Measure KCAL	FAT	Nutrition Values per 100g / 100ml KCAL	PROT	CARB	FAT	FIBRE
MIXED VEGETABLES								
Frozen, Safeway*	1 Serving/120g	70.0	1.0	58	3.0	9.4	0.9	3.4
Frozen, SuperValu*	1 Serving/70g	22.0	0.0	31	1.7	5.1	0.4	0.0
Frozen, Waitrose*	1 Serving/80g	43.0	1.0	54	3.1	8.7	0.8	3.5
Green, Microwave, Aldi*	1 Serving/300g	189.0	9.0	63	3.5	5.6	3.0	4.1
in Salt Water, Tesco*	1/3 Can/65g	34.0	0.0	53	2.6	9.2	0.6	2.7
in Salted Water, Canned, Asda*	1 Serving/65g	31.0	0.0	48	2.6	9.0	0.2	1.7
in Salted Water, Nisa Heritage*	1 Serving/100g	39.0	1.0	39	1.9	6.1	0.8	1.7
Layered, Classics, M & S*	½ Pack/160g	112.0	6.0	70	1.2	7.3	3.9	1.2
Organic, Waitrose*	1oz/28g	19.0	0.0	69	4.4	10.0	1.3	2.7
Oriental, M & S*	1 Serving/250g	50.0	1.0	20	1.6	3.4	0.3	1.6
Peas, Carrots, & Baby Leeks, Prepared, Tesco*	½ Pack/130g	57.0	1.0	44	3.1	5.8	0.9	3.5
Potatoes, Broad Beans & Peas, M & S*	1 Pack/245g	147.0	3.0	60	2.9	12.9	1.3	3.4
Premium, Frozen, Somerfield*	1 Serving/100g	53.0	1.0	53	3.2	7.9	1.0	2.7
Ready to Roast, Asda*	½ Pack/362g	315.0	12.0	87	1.6	13.0	3.2	2.4
Red Peppers & Courgette, Tesco*	1 Pack/250g	67.0	1.0	27	1.7	3.8	0.5	2.0
Roast, Four Seasons*	1 Serving/187g	79.0	0.0	42	1.2	8.8	0.2	0.0
Sainsbury's*	1 Serving/230g	55.0	1.0	24	2.1	2.5	0.6	0.0
Seasonal Selection, Tesco*	1 Serving/100g	37.0	0.0	37	1.1	7.2	0.4	2.2
Special, Freshly Frozen, Morrisons*	1 Serving/100g	48.0	1.0	48	3.2	7.2	0.8	0.0
Special, Sainsbury's*	1 Serving/120g	68.0	1.0	57	3.2	8.9	1.0	2.9
Summer, Tesco*	1 Pack/167g	55.0	1.0	33	2.6	4.5	0.5	2.8
Supreme, Frozen, Somerfield*	1 Serving/90g	22.0	0.0	25	1.9	4.3	0.0	3.1
Tenderstem Broccoli, Carrots & Mange Tout, M & S*	½ Pack/100g	35.0	0.0	35	2.9	5.6	0.2	2.1
Thai Style, in a Herb Marinade, Straight to Wok, Amoy*	1 Pouch/400g	74.0	1.0	19	0.7	3.5	0.2	0.0
MIXER								
Russchian, Schweppes*	1 Bottle/500ml	125.0	0.0	25	0.0	6.0	0.0	0.0
MOLASSES								
Average	*1 Tbsp/20g*	*53.0*	*0.0*	*266*	*0.0*	*68.8*	*0.1*	*0.0*
MONKEY NUTS								
Average	*1oz/28g*	*158.0*	*13.0*	*565*	*25.5*	*8.2*	*47.9*	*6.3*
MONKFISH								
Grilled	*1oz/28g*	*27.0*	*0.0*	*96*	*22.7*	*0.0*	*0.6*	*0.0*
Raw	*1oz/28g*	*18.0*	*0.0*	*66*	*15.7*	*0.0*	*0.4*	*0.0*
MONSTER MUNCH								
Flamin' Hot, Walkers*	1 Std Bag/22g	108.0	5.0	490	7.0	59.0	25.0	1.5
Pickled Onion, Walkers*	1 Std Bag/22g	108.0	5.0	490	6.0	60.0	25.0	1.7
Roast Beef, Walkers*	1 Std Bag/22g	108.0	5.0	490	7.0	59.0	25.0	1.7
Spicy, Walkers*	1 Std Bag/25g	125.0	7.0	500	5.0	55.0	29.0	1.3
MORNAY								
Broccoli, Somerfield*	1 Pack/400g	372.0	25.0	93	3.5	5.9	6.2	0.5
Cod, Fillets, Sainsbury's*	1 Serving/153g	236.0	14.0	154	15.2	2.2	9.4	0.9
Cod, Nutritionally Balanced, M & S*	1 Pack/400g	320.0	10.0	80	6.8	7.2	2.6	1.6
Cod, Sainsbury's*	1 Serving/180g	277.0	17.0	154	15.2	2.2	9.4	0.9
Cod, with Mashed Potato, Carrots & Broccoli, Sainsbury's*	½ Pack/200g	144.0	3.0	72	6.9	7.4	1.7	1.6
Haddock, COU, M & S*	½ Pack/194g	165.0	4.0	85	14.5	2.6	2.0	0.6
Haddock, Perfectly Balanced, Waitrose*	1 Pack/360g	310.0	5.0	86	16.6	1.6	1.5	0.5
Haddock, with Leek Mash, Eat Smart, Safeway*	1 Pack/370g	307.0	9.0	83	7.1	7.9	2.5	1.0
Haddock, Youngs*	½ Pack/190g	236.0	15.0	124	12.1	1.3	7.8	0.6
Salmon, with Broccoli, Weight Watchers*	1 Pack/290g	261.0	5.0	90	9.6	9.0	1.7	0.7
Spinach, Waitrose*	½ Pack/125g	112.0	9.0	90	3.3	3.6	6.9	1.6
MOUSSAKA								
Aubergine & Lentil, Asda*	1 Pack/451g	370.0	17.0	82	3.9	8.1	3.8	2.9
Beef, BGTY, Sainsbury's*	1 Pack/400g	300.0	10.0	75	6.1	6.8	2.6	1.2

	Measure INFO/WEIGHT	per Measure KCAL	FAT	Nutrition Values per 100g / 100ml KCAL	PROT	CARB	FAT	FIBRE
MOUSSAKA								
Beef, GFY, Asda*	1 Pack/400g	300.0	8.0	75	7.0	7.0	2.1	0.7
Beef, Good Intentions, Somerfield*	1 Pack/400g	364.0	15.0	91	7.1	7.2	3.7	3.3
Beef, HL, Tesco*	1 Pack/450g	396.0	12.0	88	5.0	10.9	2.7	0.8
Cafe Culture, M & S*	1 Serving/375g	619.0	39.0	165	9.2	7.8	10.5	0.8
COU, M & S*	1 Pack/340g	272.0	10.0	80	5.3	8.5	2.9	1.4
Eat Smart, Safeway*	1 Pack/400g	380.0	10.0	95	5.2	12.6	2.6	1.2
Lamb, Eat Smart, Safeway*	1 Pack/380g	304.0	10.0	80	6.8	6.4	2.7	1.3
Lamb, Finest, Tesco*	1 Pack/349g	510.0	38.0	146	5.8	6.2	10.9	3.4
Lamb, Light Choices, Tesco*	1 Pack/350g	259.0	7.0	74	5.3	8.5	2.1	2.6
Lamb, Sainsbury's*	1 Pack/329g	497.0	32.0	151	8.4	7.2	9.8	1.0
Light Choices, Tesco*	1 Pack/350g	259.0	7.0	74	5.3	8.5	2.1	2.6
Low Saturated Fat, Waitrose*	1 Pack/350g	304.0	11.0	87	6.3	8.4	3.1	3.1
Ready Meals, Waitrose*	1 Pack/300g	492.0	29.0	164	8.2	10.9	9.7	1.7
TTD, Sainsbury's*	1 Pack/399g	546.0	36.0	137	8.1	5.8	9.0	0.6
Vegetable, Ready Meals, Waitrose*	1oz/28g	38.0	2.0	134	3.7	12.3	7.8	2.3
Vegetable, Roasted, Safeway*	1 Pack/365g	365.0	21.0	100	3.7	7.9	5.7	2.9
Vegetarian, COU, M & S*	1 Pack/400g	280.0	11.0	70	2.7	9.1	2.7	2.4
Vegetarian, Tesco*	1 Pack/300g	489.0	31.0	163	6.4	11.0	10.4	0.9
MOUSSE								
Aero Chocolate, Nestle*	1 Pot/58g	101.0	3.0	174	4.8	27.3	5.1	1.1
Aero Twist Cappuccino & Chocolate, Nestle*	1 Pot/75g	135.0	8.0	180	4.2	16.8	10.8	0.2
Apricot, Lite, Onken*	1 Pot/150g	156.0	2.0	104	4.6	18.0	1.5	0.3
Banoffee, COU, M & S*	1 Pot/70g	101.0	1.0	145	2.9	28.8	2.1	1.5
Belgian Chocolate & Vanilla, Weight Watchers*	1 Pot/80g	106.0	2.0	132	4.4	22.2	2.8	0.9
Belgian Chocolate, Finest, Tesco*	1 Pot/120g	360.0	23.0	300	5.1	26.6	18.9	1.1
Black Cherry, Lite, Onken*	1 Pot/150g	156.0	2.0	104	4.6	17.9	1.5	0.2
Blackcurrant, HL, Tesco*	1 Pot/113g	80.0	3.0	71	3.7	8.3	2.6	1.8
Blackcurrant, Onken*	1 Pot/150g	210.0	10.0	140	5.2	14.6	6.8	0.0
Cadbury's Light Chocolate, St Ivel*	1 Pot/64g	79.0	2.0	123	6.2	17.3	3.2	0.0
Caramel, Meringue, Cadbury*	1 Pot/65g	181.0	7.0	277	4.6	42.4	10.3	1.0
Caramelised Orange, COU, M & S*	1 Pot/70g	91.0	1.0	130	2.8	26.3	1.7	3.4
Chocolate	1 Pot/60g	83.0	3.0	139	4.0	19.9	5.4	0.0
Chocolate & Hazelnut, Creamy, Dr Oetker*	1 Pot/115g	158.0	7.0	137	3.3	17.6	6.0	0.6
Chocolate & Hazelnut, Onken*	1 Pot/125g	171.0	7.0	137	3.3	17.8	6.0	0.0
Chocolate & Mint, COU, M & S*	1 Pot/70g	84.0	2.0	120	6.2	18.7	2.5	1.0
Chocolate & Orange, COU, M & S*	1 Pot/70g	77.0	2.0	110	5.9	16.0	2.6	0.9
Chocolate Orange, Low Fat, Cadbury*	1 Pot/100g	110.0	3.0	110	5.6	15.1	3.0	0.0
Chocolate with Vanilla Layer, Cadbury*	1 Pot/100g	162.0	6.0	162	4.8	21.9	6.1	0.0
Chocolate, Asda*	1 Pot/61g	134.0	6.0	219	3.7	26.0	10.0	1.0
Chocolate, Basics, Sainsbury's*	1 Pot/62.5g	94.0	4.0	150	5.1	18.9	6.0	0.0
Chocolate, BGTY, Sainsbury's*	1 Pot/63g	83.0	2.0	133	4.9	21.8	2.9	0.5
Chocolate, Cadbury*	1 Pot/55g	107.0	5.0	195	6.1	24.6	8.2	0.0
Chocolate, COU, M & S*	1 Pot/70.4g	84.0	2.0	120	5.2	20.3	2.7	1.0
Chocolate, Eat Smart, Safeway*	1 Pot/62g	81.0	2.0	130	4.1	21.5	2.7	1.1
Chocolate, Finest, Tesco*	1 Pot/82g	321.0	26.0	391	3.7	21.7	32.2	0.0
Chocolate, GFY, Asda*	1 Pot/60g	70.0	2.0	117	4.8	17.9	2.9	3.5
Chocolate, Good Choice, Iceland*	1 Pot/62.0g	85.0	2.0	137	5.4	22.7	2.7	0.0
Chocolate, Iceland*	1 Pot/62g	113.0	4.0	183	4.0	26.3	6.9	0.0
Chocolate, Italian Style, Tesco*	1 Pot/90g	243.0	12.0	270	5.0	32.8	13.2	2.4
Chocolate, Light Choices, Light Choices, Tesco*	1 Pot/62.5g	91.0	2.0	145	4.3	25.3	2.7	0.5
Chocolate, Light, Cadbury*	1 Pot/55g	60.0	2.0	110	4.6	14.2	3.4	0.0
Chocolate, Low Fat, Danette, Danone*	1 Pot/60g	73.0	1.0	121	5.1	20.8	1.9	1.5
Chocolate, Minty, Bubbly, Dessert, Aero, Nestle*	1 Pot/58g	108.0	6.0	186	4.6	18.9	10.2	0.3

MOUSSE

	Measure INFO/WEIGHT	per Measure KCAL	FAT	Nutrition Values per 100g / 100ml KCAL	PROT	CARB	FAT	FIBRE
Chocolate, Organic, Evernat*	1oz/28g	83.0	5.0	296	10.1	21.1	19.1	0.0
Chocolate, Safeway*	1 Pot/62g	127.0	6.0	205	4.0	25.3	9.8	1.1
Chocolate, Sainsbury's*	1 Pot/62.5g	119.0	5.0	190	4.7	23.8	8.5	1.0
Chocolate, Shapers, Boots*	1 Pot/70g	97.0	2.0	138	5.3	23.0	2.7	1.7
Chocolate, Somerfield*	1 Pot/60g	115.0	5.0	192	4.3	24.5	8.5	0.0
Chocolate, Tesco*	1 Pot/60g	120.0	5.0	200	3.6	27.6	8.4	0.9
Chocolate, White, Bubbly, Dessert, Aero, Nestle*	1 Pot/58g	108.0	6.0	187	4.5	19.1	10.1	0.3
Chocolate, with Mini Chunks of, Dairy Milk, Cadbury*	1 Pot/100g	215.0	10.0	215	6.1	25.7	9.9	0.0
Creamy Strawberry, Boots*	1 Pot/90g	59.0	3.0	66	3.9	6.4	2.8	0.3
Dream, Cadbury*	1 Pot/53g	100.0	4.0	189	6.0	22.0	8.0	0.0
Fruit Juice, Shape, Danone*	1 Pot/100g	115.0	3.0	115	3.5	18.5	2.8	0.0
Layered Lemon, Co-Op*	1 Pot/100g	140.0	3.0	140	3.0	24.0	3.0	0.2
Layered Strawberry, Co-Op*	1 Pot/100g	120.0	3.0	120	3.0	19.0	3.0	0.2
Lemon Fruit Juice, Shape, Danone*	1 Pot/100g	116.0	3.0	116	3.5	18.6	2.8	0.0
Lemon, Classic, Onken*	1 Pot/150g	210.0	9.0	140	5.1	15.8	6.3	0.0
Lemon, COU, M & S*	1 Pot/70g	80.0	2.0	115	2.9	19.4	3.5	3.5
Lemon, Dessert, Sainsbury's*	1 Pot/62.5g	114.0	6.0	182	3.6	20.7	9.4	0.6
Lemon, Eat Smart, Safeway*	1 Pot/70g	94.0	2.0	135	3.4	23.5	2.7	0.4
Lemon, GFY, Asda*	1 Pot/63g	57.0	2.0	92	3.6	13.0	2.8	1.7
Lemon, HL, Tesco*	1 Pot/113g	94.0	3.0	83	3.6	11.3	2.6	0.2
Lemon, Less Than 3% Fat, BGTY, Sainsbury's*	1 Pot/62g	70.0	2.0	113	4.5	17.6	2.8	0.3
Lemon, Lite, Onken*	1 Pot/150g	156.0	2.0	104	4.6	17.2	1.5	0.1
Lemon, Low Fat, Morrisons*	1 Pot/62.5g	99.0	6.0	158	3.7	15.4	9.3	0.3
Lemon, Perfectly Balanced, Waitrose*	1 Pot/95g	150.0	3.0	158	3.1	30.2	2.7	0.1
Lemon, Somerfield*	1 Pot/63g	113.0	6.0	181	3.5	20.7	9.4	0.6
Lemon, Tesco*	1 Pot/60g	67.0	2.0	111	3.4	18.2	2.7	0.0
Mars, Eden Vale*	1 Pot/110g	214.0	7.0	195	6.0	28.2	6.7	0.7
Milk Chocolate, M & S*	1 Pot/90g	180.0	8.0	200	5.3	24.8	8.7	1.5
Orange & Nectarine, Shape, Danone*	1 Pot/100g	47.0	2.0	47	3.0	4.9	1.9	0.0
Orange Fruit Juice, Shape, Danone*	1 Pot/100g	76.0	1.0	76	3.7	13.8	0.7	0.0
Orange, Mango & Lime, Onken*	1 Pot/150g	207.0	9.0	138	5.1	15.3	6.3	0.1
Peach & Passion Fruit, Perfectly Balanced, Waitrose*	1 Pot/95g	118.0	3.0	124	3.5	21.2	2.8	0.5
Peach, Onken*	1 Pot/150g	204.0	9.0	136	5.1	15.1	6.3	0.2
Peach, Shape, Danone*	1 Pot/100g	43.0	2.0	43	3.0	3.9	1.8	0.1
Pineapple, COU, M & S*	1 Pot/70g	84.0	2.0	120	3.3	20.7	2.4	3.5
Pineapple, Lite, Onken*	1 Pot/150g	162.0	2.0	108	4.6	19.0	1.5	0.2
Pineapple, Shape, Danone*	1 Pot/100g	43.0	2.0	43	2.9	3.8	1.8	0.1
Plain Chocolate, Low Fat, Nestle*	1 Pot/120g	71.0	1.0	59	2.4	10.4	0.7	0.0
Raspberry & Cranberry, Luxury, Weight Watchers*	1 Pot/80g	62.0	1.0	78	3.8	13.0	1.2	1.0
Raspberry Ripple, Value, Tesco*	1 Pot/47g	70.0	3.0	149	2.1	21.3	6.1	0.1
Raspberry, Lite, Onken*	1 Pot/150g	156.0	2.0	104	4.6	17.3	1.5	0.1
Rhubarb & Vanilla, Onken*	1 Pot/150g	210.0	9.0	140	5.0	15.8	6.3	0.2
Rhubarb, COU, M & S*	1 Pot/70g	87.0	1.0	125	2.9	25.7	2.1	4.2
Rhubarb, Lite, Onken*	1 Pot/150g	154.0	2.0	103	4.6	17.8	1.5	0.3
Strawberry & Vanilla, Weight Watchers*	1 Pot/80g	87.0	2.0	109	3.7	18.1	2.4	0.4
Strawberry Fruity, Organic, Sainsbury's*	1 Pot/125g	129.0	4.0	103	6.2	15.7	3.0	3.6
Strawberry, Asda*	1 Pot/64g	107.0	6.0	167	3.5	18.0	9.0	0.2
Strawberry, BGTY, Sainsbury's*	1 Pot/63g	63.0	2.0	101	3.4	15.0	2.8	0.2
Strawberry, Eat Smart, Safeway*	1 Pot/70g	94.0	2.0	135	3.2	24.4	2.7	0.5
Strawberry, HL, Tesco*	1 Pot/114g	90.0	3.0	79	3.8	10.2	2.6	0.8
Strawberry, Light, Muller*	1 Pot/150g	147.0	1.0	98	4.3	19.4	0.4	0.0
Strawberry, Lite, Onken*	1 Pot/150g	151.0	2.0	101	4.6	17.2	1.5	0.1
Strawberry, Low Fat, Waitrose*	1 Pot/95g	112.0	3.0	118	3.2	20.0	2.8	0.6

M

MOUSSE

INFO/WEIGHT	Measure	per Measure KCAL	FAT	Nutrition Values per 100g / 100ml KCAL	PROT	CARB	FAT	FIBRE
Strawberry, Morrisons*	1 Pot/63g	106.0	6.0	170	3.5	17.6	9.5	0.2
Strawberry, Safeway*	1 Pot/63g	106.0	6.0	168	3.5	17.3	9.4	0.1
Strawberry, Sainsbury's*	1 Pot/63g	106.0	6.0	168	3.4	17.5	9.4	0.1
Strawberry, Shape, Danone*	1 Pot/100g	44.0	2.0	44	3.0	4.0	1.8	0.0
Strawberry, Tesco*	1 Pot/63g	106.0	6.0	169	3.5	17.9	9.3	0.2
Summer Fruits, Light, Muller*	1 Pot/149g	143.0	1.0	96	4.3	18.7	0.4	0.0
Toffee, M & S*	1 Pot/90g	180.0	7.0	200	4.5	27.6	8.0	0.6
Tropical, Eat Smart, Safeway*	1 Pot/90g	121.0	2.0	135	3.3	24.5	2.3	3.2
White Chocolate, Finest, Tesco*	1 Pot/92g	436.0	34.0	474	3.9	30.2	37.5	0.0

MUFFIN

INFO/WEIGHT	Measure	per Measure KCAL	FAT	Nutrition Values per 100g / 100ml KCAL	PROT	CARB	FAT	FIBRE
All Butter, M & S*	1 Muffin/64.8g	175.0	5.0	270	10.3	40.8	7.3	2.1
Apple, Sultana & Cinnamon, GFY, Asda*	1 Muffin/50g	134.0	2.0	268	6.0	53.0	3.5	3.9
Banana & Walnut, The Handmade Flapjack Company*	1 Muffin/135g	520.0	31.0	385	5.3	40.5	22.7	0.0
Berry Burst, Asda*	1 Muffin/60g	139.0	1.0	232	6.2	46.7	2.3	1.7
Blueberry Buster, McVitie's*	1 Muffin/95g	408.0	22.0	429	4.3	49.9	23.6	1.1
Blueberry Mega, The Handmade Flapjack Company*	1 Muffin/135g	562.0	31.0	416	5.1	47.8	22.8	0.0
Blueberry, & Redcurrant, BGTY, Sainsbury's*	1 Muffin/65g	159.0	2.0	245	5.0	50.0	2.5	3.1
Blueberry, American Style, Aldi*	1 Muffin/85g	344.0	17.0	405	4.3	51.2	20.3	0.0
Blueberry, American Style, Sainsbury's*	1 Muffin/72g	256.0	13.0	355	5.1	42.7	18.2	1.9
Blueberry, Asda*	1 Muffin/77g	273.0	13.0	353	5.0	45.0	17.0	1.3
Blueberry, Big, Asda*	1 Muffin/105g	342.0	11.0	326	7.5	49.8	10.7	2.3
Blueberry, Budgens*	1 Muffin/100g	385.0	20.0	385	4.9	45.6	20.3	1.3
Blueberry, GFY, Asda*	1 Muffin/59g	146.0	1.0	249	6.0	51.0	2.3	3.0
Blueberry, Low Fat, David Powell*	1 Muffin/100g	246.0	4.0	246	6.0	47.9	3.8	0.0
Blueberry, M & S*	1 Muffin/75g	255.0	13.0	340	4.9	41.9	16.8	1.3
Blueberry, Mini, Sainsbury's*	1 Muffin/28g	82.0	2.0	293	6.3	48.9	8.1	1.9
Blueberry, Mini, Tesco*	1 Muffin/28g	104.0	5.0	370	5.6	43.5	19.3	1.2
Blueberry, Perfectly Balanced, Waitrose*	1 Muffin/100g	225.0	2.0	225	4.6	46.5	2.2	1.8
Blueberry, Tesco*	1 Muffin/73g	248.0	12.0	340	4.7	41.0	17.1	1.9
Blueberry, The Handmade Flapjack Company*	1 Muffin/135g	479.0	27.0	355	4.7	39.9	19.7	0.0
Blueberry, Waitrose*	1 Muffin/65g	239.0	9.0	367	4.7	55.2	14.2	1.7
Blueberry, Weight Watchers*	1 Muffin/65g	172.0	4.0	265	6.4	46.9	5.7	2.6
Blueberry, Wild Canadian, Fabulous Bakin' Boys*	1 Muffin/40g	140.0	8.0	349	4.0	39.0	20.0	1.0
Bran & Sultana, Weight Watchers*	1 Muffin/60g	144.0	1.0	240	4.5	50.7	2.1	2.3
Bran, Average	1 Muffin/57g	155.0	4.0	272	7.8	45.6	7.7	7.7
Cappuccino Mega, The Handmade Flapjack Company*	1 Muffin/135g	653.0	40.0	484	14.0	48.4	29.6	0.0
Caramel, Cadbury*	1 Muffin/116g	535.0	30.0	461	5.9	50.8	26.1	0.0
Carrot Cake, Entenmann's*	1 Muffin/105g	344.0	16.0	328	5.1	45.8	15.1	3.0
Carrot Cakelet, The Handmade Flapjack Company*	1 Muffin/135g	479.0	24.0	355	4.0	45.1	17.7	0.0
Carrot, Asda*	1 Muffin/59g	138.0	1.0	233	6.0	47.0	2.3	1.6
Cheese, Tesco*	1 Muffin/67g	150.0	2.0	224	13.0	36.4	2.9	3.0
Cherry Bakewell, Mr Kipling*	1 Muffin/100g	355.0	20.0	355	5.0	55.0	19.6	1.4
Cherry Mega, The Handmade Flapjack Company*	1 Muffin/135g	506.0	27.0	375	4.4	44.8	19.8	0.0
Cherry, Cheeky, Fabulous Bakin' Boys*	1 Muffin/118g	446.0	21.0	378	5.5	51.0	17.8	0.7
Cherry, The Handmade Flapjack Company*	1 Muffin/135g	499.0	27.0	370	4.6	43.8	19.7	0.0
Choc Chip, Mini, Weight Watchers*	1 Muffin/15g	47.0	1.0	312	6.6	52.1	8.6	3.1
Chocolate Chip, American Style, Sainsbury's*	1 Muffin/72g	284.0	14.0	395	5.0	48.8	20.0	2.1
Chocolate Chip, BGTY, Sainsbury's*	1 Muffin/75g	282.0	12.0	376	5.2	51.8	16.4	1.6
Chocolate Chip, Blackfriars*	1 Muffin/50g	217.0	11.0	435	6.0	51.0	23.0	4.0
Chocolate Chip, Mini, Asda*	1 Muffin/22g	77.0	3.0	349	7.0	51.0	13.0	2.1
Chocolate Chip, Mini, BGTY, Sainsbury's*	1 Muffin/28g	91.0	2.0	324	6.5	55.1	8.7	1.6
Chocolate Chip, Plain, Tesco*	1 Muffin/72g	270.0	13.0	375	5.0	48.1	17.6	1.4
Chocolate Indulgence, McVitie's*	1 Muffin/75g	253.0	7.0	338	5.8	57.9	9.2	1.3

MUFFIN

	Measure INFO/WEIGHT	per Measure KCAL	FAT	Nutrition Values per 100g / 100ml KCAL	PROT	CARB	FAT	FIBRE
Chocolate, Dairy Cream, Safeway*	1 Muffin/110g	429.0	29.0	391	7.3	31.9	26.1	3.1
Chocolate, Galaxy, McVitie's*	1 Muffin/88g	319.0	17.0	364	5.0	44.5	19.5	0.0
Chocolate, HL, Tesco*	1 Muffin/71g	204.0	6.0	288	5.5	46.9	8.7	5.5
Chocolate, The Handmade Flapjack Company*	1 Muffin/135g	526.0	31.0	390	5.3	41.5	22.8	0.0
Chunky Chocolate Chip, McVitie's*	1 Muffin/94g	393.0	20.0	418	5.3	50.6	21.6	0.8
Cinnamon & Sultana, Morrisons*	1 Muffin/75g	169.0	1.0	226	8.7	44.1	1.6	4.5
Cranberry & White Chocolate, Sainsbury's*	1 Muffin/72g	253.0	13.0	352	5.7	40.7	18.5	1.5
Dairy Cream Lemon, Safeway*	1 Muffin/110g	409.0	22.0	372	4.4	44.5	19.6	0.0
Deeply Fruity, Belgian Chocolate & Forest Fruits, Waitrose*	1 Muffin/125g	451.0	23.0	361	5.4	43.3	18.4	0.5
Double Berry Burst, Entenmann's*	1 Muffin/59g	140.0	1.0	238	4.6	50.1	2.1	1.6
Double Choc Chip, Weight Watchers*	1 Muffin/65g	189.0	5.0	291	6.8	47.2	8.3	3.6
Double Chocolate Chip, American Style, Sainsbury's*	1 Muffin/72g	276.0	15.0	384	5.2	45.0	20.3	2.9
Double Chocolate Chip, Co-Op*	1 Muffin/60g	246.0	13.0	410	6.0	49.0	21.0	3.0
Double Chocolate Chip, Mini, Asda*	1 Muffin/19g	76.0	4.0	400	7.4	48.5	19.6	2.7
Double Chocolate Chip, Mini, Weight Watchers*	1 Muffin/15g	45.0	1.0	300	7.0	48.5	8.7	3.5
Double Chocolate Chip, Tesco*	1 Muffin/100g	360.0	18.0	360	6.1	44.9	17.9	5.4
Double Chocolate, 95% Fat Free, Entenmann's*	1 Muffin/58g	152.0	3.0	262	2.6	52.3	4.7	1.8
Double Chocolate, Chocolate Chip, Mini, Tesco*	1 Muffin/28g	116.0	6.0	414	6.3	45.7	23.0	1.4
Double Chocolate, Free From, Tesco*	1 Muffin/70g	281.0	13.0	402	4.7	54.8	18.2	1.7
Double Chocolate, Mini, M & S*	1 Muffin/32g	133.0	7.0	416	5.4	49.8	21.7	1.1
Double Chocolate, Somerfield*	1 Muffin/70g	297.0	16.0	425	6.8	46.5	23.5	0.0
English	1 Muffin/57g	120.0	1.0	211	7.0	43.9	1.8	1.8
English, Butter, Tesco*	1 Muffin/67g	170.0	4.0	253	11.2	39.8	5.4	2.0
English, Kingsmill*	1 Muffin/75g	168.0	1.0	224	9.8	42.3	1.7	2.2
English, M & S*	1 Muffin/60g	135.0	1.0	225	11.2	43.7	1.9	2.9
English, Plain, Oakrun Bakery*	1 Muffin/57g	139.0	1.0	244	8.4	47.4	1.8	1.4
English, Tesco*	1 Muffin/72g	171.0	2.0	237	11.2	41.7	3.2	2.8
Family, Irwin's Bakery*	1 Muffin/40g	116.0	2.0	291	8.9	50.0	6.2	0.0
Finger, Double Chocolate, Bakers Delight*	1 Muffin/25g	104.0	5.0	416	5.8	56.9	18.4	1.7
Iceland*	1 Muffin/76g	173.0	1.0	228	8.6	44.5	1.7	2.0
Lemon & Blueberry, Tesco*	1 Muffin/110g	411.0	23.0	374	4.0	42.4	20.9	1.1
Lemon & Poppy Seed, Entenmann's*	1 Muffin/105g	417.0	20.0	397	5.6	52.8	19.3	2.5
Lemon & Poppy Seed, M & S*	1 Muffin/72g	281.0	14.0	390	6.3	46.1	19.8	1.5
Lemon & Sultana, BGTY, Sainsbury's*	1 Muffin/75g	211.0	3.0	281	4.5	55.6	4.5	1.4
Lemon, Boots*	1 Muffin/110g	423.0	21.0	385	3.6	50.0	19.0	1.3
Mini, Tesco*	1 Muffin/28g	120.0	6.0	428	6.4	50.0	22.6	1.2
Mixed Fruit, Low Fat, Abbey Bakery*	1 Muffin/35g	93.0	2.0	267	4.5	55.6	4.5	1.4
Morning Sunrise, Ryvita*	1 Muffin/110g	330.0	10.0	300	4.5	49.1	9.1	1.8
Muesli, Sainsbury's*	1 Muffin/113g	447.0	26.0	396	6.5	41.5	22.7	1.4
Oven Bottom, Aldi*	1 Muffin/68g	173.0	1.0	255	10.0	50.4	1.5	2.2
Oven Bottom, Asda*	1 Muffin/68g	173.0	1.0	255	10.0	50.4	1.5	2.2
Oven Bottom, Mini, Morrisons*	1 Muffin/42g	107.0	1.0	255	10.0	50.4	1.5	2.2
Oven Bottom, Tesco*	1 Muffin/68g	173.0	1.0	255	10.0	50.4	1.5	2.2
Oven Bottom, Warburton's*	1 Muffin/69g	175.0	2.0	253	10.9	45.8	2.9	0.0
Plain, Co-Op*	1 Muffin/60g	135.0	1.0	225	11.2	41.3	1.9	2.4
Plain, Morrisons*	1 Muffin/70g	140.0	1.0	200	8.0	41.4	1.1	0.0
Plain, Prepared From Recipe, Average	1 Muffin/57g	169.0	6.0	296	6.9	41.4	11.4	2.7
Raspberry Cream, Sainsbury's*	1 Muffin/90g	314.0	20.0	349	3.9	33.8	22.0	1.3
Raspberry Injected, The Handmade Flapjack Company*	1 Muffin/135g	564.0	27.0	418	4.5	54.7	20.2	0.0
Raspberry, Perfectly Balanced, Waitrose*	1 Muffin/101g	220.0	2.0	219	4.7	45.4	2.1	3.7
Rolo, Nestle*	1 Muffin/80g	289.0	14.0	361	5.4	44.3	18.0	0.8
Saltana, The Handmade Flapjack Company*	1 Muffin/135g	499.0	26.0	370	4.7	44.8	19.3	0.0
Sausage, Egg & Cheese, American Style, Tesco*	1 Muffin/155g	383.0	20.0	247	12.2	19.9	13.2	1.0

M

	Measure INFO/WEIGHT	per Measure KCAL	FAT	Nutrition Values per 100g / 100ml KCAL	PROT	CARB	FAT	FIBRE
MUFFIN								
Somerfield*	1 Muffin/60g	130.0	1.0	216	12.2	39.3	1.6	1.9
Spiced Fruit, Co-Op*	1 Muffin/60g	159.0	1.0	265	11.0	52.0	2.0	3.0
Strawberry Cakelet, The Handmade Flapjack Company*	1 Muffin/135g	526.0	30.0	390	4.5	43.6	21.9	0.0
Sunblest*	1 Muffin/72g	166.0	1.0	230	9.6	43.9	1.8	2.2
Toasting, Warburton's*	1 Muffin/64g	138.0	1.0	216	8.9	41.4	1.6	2.9
Toffee & Pecan, Finest, Tesco*	1 Muffin/127g	551.0	29.0	434	5.4	51.8	22.8	0.9
Toffee Choo Choo, Tesco*	1 Muffin/95g	402.0	21.0	423	6.4	49.1	22.4	1.0
Toffee Mega, The Handmade Flapjack Company*	1 Muffin/135g	567.0	35.0	420	4.5	43.2	25.7	0.0
Toffee Temptation, McVitie's*	1 Muffin/86g	297.0	8.0	347	4.7	60.8	9.5	0.8
Toffee, GFY, Asda*	1 Muffin/90g	151.0	2.0	168	2.1	34.0	2.6	0.0
Toffee, The Handmade Flapjack Company*	1 Muffin/135g	533.0	32.0	395	4.4	41.2	23.4	0.0
Triple Chocolate, Triumph, Fabulous Bakin' Boys*	1 Muffin/40g	160.0	10.0	400	4.5	42.0	24.0	0.0
Truly Madly Chocolate, Fabulous Bakin' Boys*	1 Muffin/105g	405.0	23.0	386	5.0	41.0	22.0	2.0
Vanilla & Choc Chip, GFY, Asda*	1 Muffin/59g	152.0	1.0	260	7.0	53.0	2.2	1.6
White Chocolate & Strawberry Filled, Tesco*	1 Muffin/102.5g	415.0	20.0	405	5.2	51.3	19.8	1.3
White Chocolate Chunk Lemon, Mini, M & S*	1 Muffin/28g	130.0	7.0	464	6.4	55.4	23.9	2.1
White, All Butter, Sainsbury's*	1 Muffin/67g	173.0	4.0	258	10.6	39.6	6.3	3.6
White, Asda*	1 Muffin/66.7g	148.0	1.0	222	11.0	40.0	2.0	2.5
White, Finest, Tesco*	1 Muffin/70g	159.0	1.0	227	8.4	45.7	1.2	2.1
White, M & S*	1 Muffin/60g	135.0	1.0	225	11.2	43.7	1.9	2.9
White, Safeway*	1 Muffin/63g	142.0	1.0	226	10.3	43.2	1.3	2.0
White, Tesco*	1 Muffin/72g	173.0	2.0	240	11.3	41.6	3.2	2.8
Wholemeal, Tesco*	1 Muffin/65g	130.0	1.0	200	12.6	32.9	2.0	5.7
MUFFIN MIX								
Banana Nut, Betty Crocker*	1 Serving/30g	130.0	5.0	433	6.7	70.0	16.7	0.0
MULBERRIES								
Raw	*1oz/28g*	*10.0*	*0.0*	*36*	*1.3*	*8.1*	*0.0*	*0.0*
MULLET								
Grey, Grilled	*1oz/28g*	*42.0*	*1.0*	*150*	*25.7*	*0.0*	*5.2*	*0.0*
Grey, Raw	*1oz/28g*	*32.0*	*1.0*	*115*	*19.8*	*0.0*	*4.0*	*0.0*
Red, Grilled	*1oz/28g*	*34.0*	*1.0*	*121*	*20.4*	*0.0*	*4.4*	*0.0*
Red, Raw, Weighed Whole	*1oz/28g*	*31.0*	*1.0*	*109*	*18.7*	*0.0*	*3.8*	*0.0*
MUNCHIES								
Mint, Nestle*	1 Pack/62g	267.0	10.0	432	3.8	67.5	16.4	0.0
Original, Tube, Nestle*	1 Pack/54.7g	272.0	13.0	498	4.1	65.6	24.4	0.5
MUSHROOMS								
Breaded, Average	*1oz/28g*	*42.0*	*2.0*	*151*	*4.3*	*20.8*	*5.7*	*0.6*
Breaded, Garlic, Average	1 Serving/50g	92.0	5.0	183	5.2	18.7	9.7	1.7
Buna Shimeji, Livesey Brothers*	½ Pack/75g	29.0	0.0	39	2.7	5.9	0.4	1.2
Button, Average	*1 Serving/50g*	*7.0*	*0.0*	*15*	*2.3*	*0.5*	*0.4*	*1.2*
Chargrilled & Truffle Sauce, The Best, Safeway*	1 Pot/350g	385.0	27.0	110	3.4	5.8	7.6	0.8
Cheesey, Stuffed, Asda*	1 Serving/290g	322.0	17.0	111	4.3	10.0	6.0	0.0
Chestnut, Average	*1 Med/5g*	*1.0*	*0.0*	*13*	*1.8*	*0.4*	*0.5*	*0.5*
Chinese, Dried, Raw	*1oz/28g*	*80.0*	*1.0*	*284*	*10.0*	*59.9*	*1.8*	*0.0*
Closed Cup, Average	*1oz/28g*	*5.0*	*0.0*	*18*	*2.9*	*0.4*	*0.5*	*0.5*
Common, Boiled in Salted Water, Average	*1oz/28g*	*3.0*	*0.0*	*11*	*1.8*	*0.4*	*0.3*	*1.1*
Common, Fried, Average	*1oz/28g*	*44.0*	*5.0*	*157*	*2.4*	*0.3*	*16.2*	*1.5*
Common, Raw, Average	*1 Serving/80g*	*10.0*	*0.0*	*13*	*1.9*	*0.3*	*0.5*	*1.1*
Creamed, Average	*1oz/28g*	*23.0*	*2.0*	*82*	*1.3*	*6.8*	*5.5*	*0.5*
Crispy, M & S*	1 Serving/130g	390.0	33.0	300	4.2	12.5	25.7	1.8
Dried	*1oz/28g*	*45.0*	*2.0*	*159*	*21.8*	*4.8*	*6.0*	*13.3*
Enoki, Average	*1 Serving/80g*	*34.0*	*0.0*	*42*	*3.0*	*7.0*	*0.0*	*3.0*
Flat, Large, Average	*1 Mushroom/52g*	*10.0*	*0.0*	*19*	*3.3*	*0.5*	*0.5*	*0.7*

	Measure INFO/WEIGHT	per Measure KCAL	FAT	Nutrition Values per 100g / 100ml KCAL	PROT	CARB	FAT	FIBRE
MUSHROOMS								
Garlic, Average	½ Pack/150g	159.0	14.0	106	2.1	3.7	9.3	1.7
Giant, with Tomatoes & Mozzarella, M & S*	1 Serving/145g	217.0	16.0	150	6.3	7.1	10.9	5.5
Hon Shimeji, Sainsbury's*	1 Serving/80g	18.0	0.0	22	4.0	3.9	0.5	1.1
Medley, Asda*	½ Pack/100g	89.0	8.0	89	3.2	1.4	7.8	2.8
Oyster, Average	*1 Serving/80g*	*12.0*	*0.0*	*15*	*1.6*	*1.6*	*0.2*	*1.3*
Porcini, Dried, Asda*	1 Bag/25g	65.0	1.0	260	30.4	24.1	4.7	17.5
Porcini, Wild, Dried, Merchant Gourmet*	1 Pack/25g	66.0	1.0	265	27.9	30.6	3.4	18.7
Shiitake, Cooked	*1oz/28g*	*15.0*	*0.0*	*55*	*1.6*	*12.3*	*0.2*	*0.0*
Shiitake, Dried, Raw	*1oz/28g*	*83.0*	*0.0*	*296*	*9.6*	*63.9*	*1.0*	*0.0*
Shiitake, TTD, Sainsbury's*	1 Serving/100g	40.0	0.0	40	5.5	3.4	0.5	4.9
Sliced, Average	*1oz/28g*	*3.0*	*0.0*	*12*	*1.8*	*0.4*	*0.3*	*1.1*
Straw, Canned, Drained	*1oz/28g*	*4.0*	*0.0*	*15*	*2.1*	*1.2*	*0.2*	*0.0*
Stuffed, Ready to Eat, Morrisons*	1oz/28g	29.0	1.0	104	3.5	10.8	4.1	2.6
Stuffed, Ready to Roast, Waitrose*	1 Serving/125g	94.0	5.0	75	3.9	6.5	3.7	1.5
Stuffed, with Cheese, Parsley, & Butter, Sainsbury's*	½ Pack/110g	246.0	24.0	224	4.1	2.3	22.0	2.6
MUSSELS								
Boiled, Flesh Only, Average	1 Mussel/1.9g	2.0	0.0	104	16.7	3.5	2.7	0.0
Boiled, Weighed in Shell, Average	*1 Mussel/7g*	*7.0*	*0.0*	*104*	*16.7*	*3.5*	*2.7*	*0.0*
Pickled, Drained, Average	*1oz/28g*	*31.0*	*1.0*	*112*	*20.0*	*1.5*	*2.2*	*0.0*
Raw, Weighed in Shell, Average	*1oz/28g*	*24.0*	*1.0*	*87*	*12.7*	*3.6*	*2.5*	*0.2*
MUSSELS IN								
Creamy Garlic Butter Sauce, Bantry Bay*	1 Serving/225g	198.0	8.0	88	9.0	5.2	3.5	0.6
Garlic Butter Sauce, Average	½ Pack/225g	179.0	11.0	79	6.3	1.9	5.1	0.1
Garlic Butter Sauce, Cooked, Scottish, Sainsbury's*	1 Pack/500g	465.0	17.0	93	9.6	5.8	3.5	0.0
Seasoned White Wine Sauce, Bantry Bay*	1 Serving/450g	270.0	9.0	60	6.3	4.1	2.0	0.1
Thai Sauce, Scottish, Waitrose*	1 Serving/250g	135.0	6.0	54	5.4	2.6	2.5	0.6
White Wine Cream Sauce, Cooked, Scottish, Morrisons*	½ Pack/250g	222.0	9.0	89	8.0	5.8	3.7	0.0
White Wine Sauce, Sainsbury's*	½ Pack/250g	221.0	9.0	88	8.0	5.8	3.7	0.0
MUSSELS WITH								
Tomato & Garlic, Fresh, M & S*	1 Serving/650g	455.0	10.0	70	7.9	6.5	1.6	0.1
MUSTARD								
American, Average	*1 Tsp/5g*	*5.0*	*0.0*	*102*	*4.4*	*10.5*	*5.0*	*2.5*
Cajun, Colman's*	1 Tsp/6g	11.0	0.0	187	7.0	23.0	6.5	2.7
Coarse Grain, Average	*1 Tsp/5g*	*7.0*	*0.0*	*141*	*7.7*	*8.4*	*8.3*	*5.9*
Dijon, Average	*1 Tsp/5g*	*8.0*	*1.0*	*163*	*7.4*	*7.7*	*11.3*	*1.1*
English, Average	*1 Tsp/5g*	*9.0*	*0.0*	*173*	*6.8*	*19.2*	*7.6*	*1.2*
English, with Chillies, Sainsbury's*	1 Tsp/5g	10.0	1.0	204	8.3	18.1	10.9	6.4
French, Average	*1 Tsp/5g*	*5.0*	*0.0*	*105*	*5.4*	*8.1*	*5.6*	*1.8*
German Style, Sainsbury's*	1 Serving/10g	9.0	1.0	92	5.5	2.8	6.5	0.0
Honey, Colman's*	1 Tsp/6g	12.0	0.0	208	7.4	24.0	8.2	0.0
Peppercorn, Colman's*	1 Tsp/6g	11.0	1.0	182	8.8	12.0	10.0	4.9
Powder, Average	*1 Tsp/3g*	*15.0*	*1.0*	*452*	*28.9*	*20.7*	*28.7*	*0.0*
Powder, Made Up, Average	*1oz/28g*	*63.0*	*4.0*	*226*	*14.5*	*10.4*	*14.4*	*0.0*
Smooth, Average	*1 Tsp/8g*	*11.0*	*1.0*	*139*	*7.1*	*9.7*	*8.2*	*0.0*
Sweet Peppers, Colman's*	1 Tsp/6g	13.0	1.0	218	7.9	20.0	11.0	4.9
Tarragon, Tesco*	1 Tbsp/15ml	59.0	6.0	396	0.9	8.6	39.8	0.2
Whole Grain, Average	*1 Tsp/8g*	*11.0*	*1.0*	*140*	*8.2*	*4.2*	*10.2*	*4.9*
Whole Grain, with Green Peppercorns, Finest, Tesco*	1 Serving/20g	41.0	2.0	205	7.9	22.0	9.5	3.3
Yellow, Prepared	*1 Tbsp/15ml*	*11.0*	*1.0*	*73*	*4.0*	*6.0*	*4.0*	*0.0*
MUSTARD CRESS								
Raw	*1oz/28g*	*4.0*	*0.0*	*13*	*1.6*	*0.4*	*0.6*	*1.1*

	Measure INFO/WEIGHT	per Measure KCAL	per Measure FAT	Nutrition Values per 100g / 100ml KCAL	PROT	CARB	FAT	FIBRE
NACHOS								
American Chilli Beef, Asda*	1 Serving/200g	208.0	10.0	104	10.0	4.7	5.0	0.8
Cheesy, with Salsa & Soured Cream, Sainsbury's*	½ Pack/170g	449.0	27.0	264	8.8	21.5	15.8	1.4
Chicken, Safeway*	½ Pack/170g	352.0	19.0	207	10.3	15.7	11.4	1.8
Chilli, Sainsbury's*	½ Pack/250g	695.0	32.0	278	10.9	29.5	12.9	1.3
Kit, Old El Paso*	½ Pack/260g	598.0	26.0	230	4.0	31.0	10.0	0.0
NASI GORENG								
Indonesian, Asda*	1 Pack/360g	778.0	23.0	216	7.4	32.3	6.3	1.3
NECTARINES								
Weighed with Stone, Fresh, Raw, Average	*1 Med/140g*	*53.0*	*0.0*	*38*	*1.3*	*8.5*	*0.1*	*1.1*
NESQUIK								
Chocolate Flavour, Powder, Dry Weight, Nesquik, Nestle*	1 Serving/15g	56.0	0.0	372	3.0	82.9	3.1	6.5
Strawberry Flavour, Powder, Dry Weight, Nesquik, Nestle*	1 Serving/15g	59.0	0.0	393	0.0	98.1	0.0	0.0
Strawberry Milk, Fresh, Nesquik, Nestle*	1 Glass/250g	175.0	4.0	70	3.3	10.4	1.6	0.3
NIK NAKS								
Cream 'n' Cheesy, Golden Wonder*	1 Bag/34g	195.0	13.0	575	5.2	52.7	38.1	0.2
Nice 'n' Spicy, KP Snacks*	1 Bag/30g	171.0	12.0	571	4.6	51.6	38.4	1.6
Rib 'n' Saucy, Golden Wonder*	1 Bag/34g	194.0	13.0	571	4.5	53.7	37.6	0.5
Scampi & Lemon, Golden Wonder*	1 Bag/25g	141.0	10.0	564	5.2	49.6	38.4	3.2
Scampi 'n' Lemon, Golden Wonder*	1 Bag/34g	195.0	13.0	573	4.9	53.1	37.5	0.1
NOODLE BOWL								
Chilli Beef, HL, Tesco*	1 Pack/400g	368.0	6.0	92	4.5	15.4	1.4	1.1
Chilli Beef, Tesco*	1 Serving/475g	456.0	8.0	96	7.2	13.2	1.6	1.1
Chow Mein, Chicken, Uncle Ben's*	1 Pack/330g	307.0	5.0	93	6.1	13.5	1.4	0.0
Coconut & Coriander Chicken, Oriental, Finest, Tesco*	1 Pack/450g	562.0	23.0	125	8.3	10.8	5.2	2.1
King Prawn, Hot & Sour, Finest, Tesco*	1 Pack/400g	260.0	6.0	65	4.4	8.6	1.4	1.7
Szechuan Style Prawn, Tesco*	1 Pack/400g	376.0	1.0	94	5.5	17.3	0.3	0.9
NOODLE BOX								
Cantonese Chow Mein, Sharwood's*	1 Pack/350g	465.0	10.0	133	3.8	22.9	2.9	1.5
Hong Kong Sweet & Sour, Sharwood's*	1 Pack/350g	409.0	5.0	117	3.7	22.6	1.3	1.8
Thai Red Curry, Sharwood's*	1 Pack/350g	444.0	11.0	127	3.9	20.9	3.1	1.6
NOODLES								
Barbecue Beef, Instant, Asda*	1 Pack/333g	420.0	16.0	126	2.6	18.0	4.8	0.0
Beef Flavour, Instant, Prepared, Heinz*	1 Pack/384g	257.0	0.0	67	2.1	14.4	0.1	0.6
Beef, Oriental, GFY, Asda*	1 Pack/400g	372.0	7.0	93	7.4	12.1	1.7	1.7
Buckwheat, Cold, Famima*	1 Pack/295g	163.0	3.0	55	4.7	9.5	1.0	0.7
Char Sui, Cantonese, Sainsbury's*	1 Pack/450g	378.0	7.0	84	6.8	10.5	1.6	1.5
Chicken & Coconut & Lime, Simply Fuller Longer, M & S*	1 Pack/390g	448.0	18.0	115	8.7	10.0	4.5	1.6
Chicken & Red Thai, Easy Steam, Tesco*	1 Serving/400g	556.0	28.0	139	10.3	8.6	7.1	1.1
Chicken Curry Flavour, Instant, Sainsbury's*	1 Pack/85g	167.0	6.0	196	4.6	27.9	7.3	0.8
Chicken Flavour, 3 Minute, Dry, Blue Dragon*	1 Pack/85g	403.0	18.0	475	9.3	61.2	21.4	0.0
Chicken Flavour, Dry, Eldorado*	1 Pack/85g	360.0	13.0	423	14.0	61.0	15.0	0.0
Chicken Flavour, Dry, Princes*	1 Pack/85g	395.0	16.0	465	10.0	63.8	18.8	0.0
Chicken Flavour, Instant, Made Up, Tesco*	½ Pack/168g	285.0	11.0	170	4.1	23.7	6.3	1.5
Chicken Flavour, Instant, Sainsbury's*	1 Pack/335g	549.0	21.0	164	4.4	22.3	6.4	1.3
Chicken Flavour, Value, Made Up, Tesco*	1 Serving/265g	450.0	17.0	170	4.1	23.7	6.3	1.5
Chicken, Chinese Style, GFY, Asda*	1 Pack/393g	295.0	7.0	75	6.0	9.0	1.7	0.6
Chicken, Chinese, Asda*	1 Pot/302g	305.0	4.0	101	6.0	16.0	1.4	0.8
Chicken, Dry Weight, Heinz*	1 Pack/85g	257.0	0.0	302	9.5	65.3	0.4	2.7
Chicken, Instant, Less Than 1% Fat, Prepared, Heinz*	1 Pack/385g	258.0	0.0	67	2.1	14.4	0.1	0.6
Chicken, Instant, Weight Watchers*	1 Pack/385g	269.0	0.0	70	2.3	14.9	0.1	0.6
Chilli Beef, Finest, Tesco*	1 Pack/450g	486.0	9.0	108	7.7	15.2	1.9	0.9
Chilli Chicken, GFY, Asda*	1 Pack/415g	461.0	3.0	111	6.0	20.0	0.8	1.0
Chilli Chicken, Sweet, Sainsbury's*	1 Pack/200g	202.0	3.0	101	6.6	15.5	1.4	0.8

NOODLES

	Measure INFO/WEIGHT	per Measure KCAL	FAT	Nutrition Values per 100g / 100ml KCAL	PROT	CARB	FAT	FIBRE
Chilli Chicken, Tesco*	1 Pack/385g	545.0	16.0	142	6.4	19.5	4.1	1.4
Chilli Infused, Blue Dragon*	1 Serving/150g	286.0	1.0	191	6.1	33.6	0.7	0.3
Chinese, Stir Fry, Sainsbury's*	1 Serving/100g	185.0	5.0	185	6.0	29.5	4.8	1.5
Chow Mein Flavour, Dry, Princes*	1 Pack/85g	396.0	16.0	466	10.1	64.6	18.6	0.0
Chow Mein Flavour, Instant, Morrisons*	1 Pack/85g	162.0	6.0	191	4.8	29.9	6.5	1.6
Chow Mein, Dry Weight, Snack in a Pot, HL, Tesco*	1 Pot/56g	202.0	1.0	360	13.4	72.2	1.4	5.0
Chow Mein, Instant, Made Up, Tesco*	1 Pack/168g	255.0	8.0	152	3.8	23.0	5.0	1.2
Chow Mein, Sainsbury's*	1 Pack/125g	136.0	2.0	109	3.9	19.2	1.8	0.8
Chow Mein, Snack In A Pot, Light Choices, Tesco*	1 Pot/235g	235.0	1.0	100	3.7	19.4	0.5	1.8
Crab Flavour, Dry, 3 Minute, Blue Dragon*	1 Pack/85g	393.0	16.0	463	9.9	62.6	19.2	0.0
Crispy, Dry, Blue Dragon*	1 Box/125g	437.0	1.0	350	2.4	84.0	0.5	0.0
Curry Flavour, Instant, From Heinz, Weight Watchers*	1 Pack/385g	266.0	0.0	69	2.2	14.8	0.1	0.6
Curry Flavour, Instant, Sainsbury's*	1 Pack/335g	412.0	15.0	123	2.6	17.8	4.6	0.1
Curry Flavour, Instant, Value, Made Up, Tesco*	1 Pack/65g	83.0	2.0	127	3.1	20.3	3.7	0.8
Curry, Instant, Dry, Heinz*	1 Serving/85g	261.0	0.0	307	9.5	66.4	0.4	2.7
Egg Fried, Cantonese, Safeway*	1oz/28g	29.0	1.0	104	3.4	10.7	5.3	1.1
Egg, & Bean Sprouts, Cooked, Tesco*	1 Pack/250g	237.0	5.0	95	4.4	14.6	2.1	1.5
Egg, Asda*	1 Pack/184g	213.0	13.0	116	2.3	11.0	7.0	0.6
Egg, Boiled	*1oz/28g*	*17.0*	*0.0*	*62*	*2.2*	*13.0*	*0.5*	*0.6*
Egg, Cooked, Somerfield*	½ Pack/150g	189.0	8.0	126	3.2	16.0	5.5	0.6
Egg, Dry	*1 Block/62.5g*	*244.0*	*5.0*	*391*	*12.1*	*71.7*	*8.2*	*2.9*
Egg, Fine Thread, Dry, M & S*	1 Serving/63g	220.0	1.0	350	14.3	71.6	0.9	5.1
Egg, Fine, Blue Dragon*	1 Serving/100g	171.0	1.0	171	5.5	35.0	0.9	0.0
Egg, Fine, Dry Weight, Sharwood's*	1 Block/63g	216.0	1.0	346	12.0	70.0	2.1	2.5
Egg, Fine, Fresh, M & S*	1 Pack/275g	330.0	6.0	120	4.4	20.7	2.2	1.5
Egg, Fine, Waitrose*	¼ Pack/62.5g	221.0	2.0	353	15.0	67.3	2.6	3.8
Egg, Free Range, Asda*	1 Serving/125g	205.0	5.0	164	5.1	27.0	3.9	1.8
Egg, Free Range, Morrisons*	1 Pack/300g	372.0	9.0	124	4.9	19.7	2.9	1.3
Egg, Fresh, Just Stir Fry, Sainsbury's*	½ Pack/192g	314.0	7.0	163	5.0	28.1	3.4	1.8
Egg, Fresh, Tesco*	1 Serving/150g	102.0	2.0	68	2.8	11.8	1.3	0.6
Egg, M & S*	½ Pack/110g	165.0	2.0	150	4.9	28.3	1.7	2.8
Egg, Medium, Asda*	1 Serving/83.3g	125.0	1.0	150	4.8	31.0	0.8	1.3
Egg, Medium, Dry, Blue Dragon*	1 Serving/81g	288.0	1.0	356	13.8	70.0	1.7	3.4
Egg, Medium, Dry, Sharwood's*	1 Serving/63g	216.0	1.0	346	12.0	70.0	2.1	2.5
Egg, Medium, Sainsbury's*	1 Serving/122g	168.0	1.0	138	5.7	26.9	0.8	1.0
Egg, Ramen, Fresh, The Original Noodle Company*	1 Serving/63g	186.0	2.0	298	11.3	57.0	2.7	0.0
Egg, Raw, Medium, Waitrose*	¼ Pack/63g	221.0	2.0	353	15.0	67.3	2.6	3.8
Egg, Stir Fry, Fresh, Tesco*	½ A Pack/205g	287.0	4.0	140	4.9	25.3	1.9	2.0
Egg, Thick, Dry Weight, Sharwood's*	1 Serving/63g	214.0	1.0	342	10.8	71.0	1.7	2.5
Egg, Thread, Cooked Weight, Sharwood's*	1oz/28g	30.0	0.0	107	3.6	21.8	0.6	1.1
Egg, Tossed in Sesame Oil, Asda*	½ Pack/150g	174.0	10.0	116	2.3	11.0	7.0	0.6
Fried, Average	*1oz/28g*	*43.0*	*3.0*	*153*	*1.9*	*11.3*	*11.5*	*0.5*
Garlic, Chilli & Ginger, Tesco*	1 Serving/350g	507.0	11.0	145	4.8	24.1	3.2	2.6
Instant, Dry, Sainsbury's*	1 Pack/100g	392.0	14.0	392	9.4	57.0	14.0	0.2
Instant, Express, Dry, Blue Dragon*	1 Serving/75g	337.0	13.0	450	10.0	65.0	17.0	2.0
Instant, Fat Free, Koka*	1 Piece/80g	143.0	0.0	179	6.2	38.5	0.0	1.0
Instant, Vegetable Flavour, Made Up, Indo Mie*	1 Pack/348.6g	373.0	16.0	107	2.6	14.0	4.5	0.8
Japanese Udon, Sainsbury's*	1 Serving/150g	210.0	3.0	140	3.9	27.1	1.8	1.2
King Prawn, Japanese, Box, M & S*	1 Pack/300g	330.0	8.0	110	5.8	16.0	2.7	1.6
Medium, Traditional, Straight to Wok, Amoy*	1 Serving/150g	243.0	2.0	162	4.3	34.3	1.5	1.3
Nest, Medium, Cooked, Waitrose*	1 Nest/63g	88.0	0.0	139	5.0	28.6	0.5	0.6
Oriental, Chinese, Tesco*	1 Pack/200g	184.0	5.0	92	2.8	14.7	2.5	1.0
Oriental, Snack Pot, Dry, HL, Tesco*	1 Pot/57g	210.0	1.0	369	14.0	74.4	1.7	2.0

NOODLES

INFO/WEIGHT	Measure	per Measure KCAL	per Measure FAT	Nutrition Values per 100g / 100ml KCAL	PROT	CARB	FAT	FIBRE
Oriental, Snack Pot, Made Up, HL, Tesco*	1 Serving/238g	221.0	1.0	93	3.1	19.4	0.3	0.6
Pasta, 100% Hard Durum Wheat, Dry, Goody*	1 Serving/100g	362.0	2.0	362	12.5	73.0	1.7	0.0
Peking Duck, Shapers, Boots*	1 Pack/280g	395.0	4.0	141	7.2	25.0	1.4	1.8
Plain, Boiled	*1oz/28g*	*17.0*	*0.0*	*62*	*2.4*	*13.0*	*0.4*	*0.7*
Plain, Dry	*1oz/28g*	*109.0*	*2.0*	*388*	*11.7*	*76.1*	*6.2*	*2.9*
Prawn Satay, Safeway*	1 Serving/400g	460.0	18.0	115	5.3	12.4	4.6	1.8
Prawn, Instant, Made Up, Tesco*	1 Serving/168g	251.0	9.0	150	3.8	21.9	5.2	1.3
Ramen, with Chilli Beef, M & S*	1 Pack/484g	532.0	17.0	110	8.1	11.9	3.6	0.8
Ramen, with Wakame, The Original Noodle Company*	½ Pack/124g	304.0	1.0	245	7.4	51.8	0.8	1.8
Rice, Brown, 100%, Organic, King Soba*	1 Pack/83g	252.0	2.0	303	6.0	64.4	2.4	0.0
Rice, Cooked	1 Cup/176g	192.0	0.0	109	0.9	24.9	0.2	1.0
Rice, Cooked, Sharwood's*	1 Serving/200g	239.0	1.0	119	2.0	27.1	0.3	0.7
Rice, Dry, Amoy*	1oz/28g	101.0	0.0	361	6.5	86.6	1.0	0.0
Rice, Dry, Blue Dragon*	1 Serving/30g	113.0	0.0	376	7.0	84.0	0.0	0.0
Rice, Medium, Blue Dragon*	1 Serving/63g	235.0	0.0	376	7.0	84.0	0.0	0.0
Rice, Oriental, Thai, Stir Fry, Dry Weight, Sharwood's*	1 Serving/63g	226.0	1.0	361	6.5	86.8	1.0	2.4
Rice, Stir Fry, Tesco*	½ Pack/190g	304.0	11.0	160	2.0	24.8	5.7	1.0
Rice, Thick, Thai, Dry, M & S*	1 Serving/100g	355.0	1.0	355	6.5	80.6	0.7	1.4
Rice, With Spring Onions, Fresh Tastes, Asda*	½ Pack/188g	248.0	4.0	132	2.2	25.9	2.2	1.4
Savoury Vegetable, COU, M & S*	1 Pack/450g	270.0	3.0	60	2.9	11.5	0.6	1.2
Shanghai Beef, COU, M & S*	1 Pack/400g	380.0	6.0	95	6.8	13.1	1.6	1.5
Singapore Spicy, Safeway*	1 Serving/225g	270.0	10.0	120	6.0	14.2	4.3	1.7
Singapore Style, Asda*	1 Pack/400g	688.0	32.0	172	7.0	18.0	8.0	1.0
Singapore, Light Choices, Tesco*	1 Pack/450g	337.0	8.0	75	4.8	9.8	1.7	1.2
Singapore, Morrisons*	1 Serving/400g	480.0	27.0	120	4.8	11.6	6.7	1.6
Singapore, Sainsbury's*	1 Pack/400g	368.0	7.0	92	7.5	11.6	1.7	0.9
Singapore, Somerfield*	1 Pot/300g	261.0	3.0	87	5.0	15.0	1.0	0.0
Singapore, Waitrose*	1 Pack/400g	476.0	18.0	119	7.3	12.6	4.4	2.1
Special, Chinese Takeaway, Iceland*	1 Pack/340g	422.0	11.0	124	6.5	17.2	3.2	0.6
Spicy Curry Flavour, Dry, Princes*	1 Pack/85g	395.0	16.0	465	9.6	64.1	18.8	0.0
Spicy Thai, Instant, Heinz*	1 Pack/385g	262.0	0.0	68	2.1	14.6	0.1	0.6
Stir Fry, Tesco*	1 Serving/150g	202.0	4.0	135	5.3	23.0	2.4	1.5
Straight to Wok, Medium, Amoy*	1 Pack/150g	240.0	2.0	160	5.8	31.7	1.5	0.0
Straight to Wok, Rice, Amoy*	1 Pack/150g	174.0	0.0	116	1.6	27.4	0.1	0.0
Straight to Wok, Singapore, Amoy*	1 Serving/150g	232.0	4.0	155	4.8	28.4	2.8	0.0
Straight to Wok, Thread, Fine, Amoy*	1 Pack/150g	237.0	4.0	158	5.0	28.7	2.6	0.0
Straight to Wok, Udon, Amoy*	1 Pack/150g	211.0	2.0	141	4.4	28.8	1.3	0.0
Super, Bacon Flavour, Dry Weight, Batchelors*	1 Packet/100g	526.0	24.0	526	9.4	69.2	23.6	1.6
Super, Barbecue Beef, Made Up, Batchelors*	1 Serving/100g	156.0	7.0	156	3.2	20.9	6.7	1.1
Super, Barbecue Beef, to Go, 98% Fat Free, Batchelors*	1 Pack/380g	308.0	1.0	81	2.4	17.5	0.2	0.6
Super, Cheese & Ham, Made Up, Batchelors*	1 Serving/100g	171.0	7.0	171	3.4	22.9	7.3	0.6
Super, Chicken & Ham, Dry Weight, Batchelors*	1 Pack/100g	472.0	20.0	472	9.4	63.2	20.2	1.5
Super, Chicken & Herb, Low Fat, Dry Weight, Batchelors*	½ Pack/43g	161.0	1.0	379	12.2	78.3	1.9	2.3
Super, Chicken & Herb, Low Fat, Made Up, Batchelors*	1 Pack/170g	322.0	2.0	189	6.1	39.2	0.9	1.2
Super, Chicken Flavour, Dry Weight, Batchelors*	1 Serving/100g	449.0	19.0	449	8.7	60.3	19.2	2.5
Super, Chicken Flavour, Made Up, Batchelors*	1 Serving/100g	170.0	7.0	170	3.3	22.9	7.3	0.9
Super, Chow Mein Flavour, Made Up, Batchelors*	½ Pack/150g	262.0	12.0	175	3.0	23.0	7.9	0.4
Super, Mild Curry Flavour, Made Up, Batchelors*	1 Serving/100g	157.0	7.0	157	3.2	20.9	6.7	1.0
Super, Mild Curry, Dry Weight, Batchelors*	½ Pack/50g	260.0	12.0	520	9.4	67.8	23.4	1.4
Super, Mushroom Flavour, Made Up, Batchelors*	1 Serving/100g	157.0	7.0	157	3.2	20.9	6.8	1.0
Super, Roast Chicken, to Go, 98% Fat Free, Batchelors*	1 Serving/380g	308.0	1.0	81	2.6	17.2	0.2	0.5
Super, Southern Fried Chicken, Made Up, Batchelors*	1 Serving/100g	171.0	7.0	171	3.3	23.2	7.2	0.5
Super, Spicy Balti, Made Up, Batchelors*	1 Serving/100g	166.0	7.0	166	3.0	21.5	7.5	1.1

	Measure INFO/WEIGHT	per Measure KCAL	FAT	Nutrition Values per 100g / 100ml KCAL	PROT	CARB	FAT	FIBRE
NOODLES								
Super, Spicy Salsa, Dry Weight, Batchelors*	1 Pack/105g	474.0	20.0	451	7.0	63.8	18.6	1.7
Super, Sweet Thai Chilli Flavour, 98% Fat Free, Batchelors*	1 Pack/270g	292.0	1.0	108	3.3	22.8	0.4	0.9
Super, Sweet Thai Chilli, Dry Weight, Batchelors*	1 Pack/85g	292.0	1.0	343	10.6	72.5	1.2	3.0
Sweet & Sour, BGTY, Sainsbury's*	1 Serving/100g	112.0	3.0	112	2.3	18.6	3.1	0.0
Sweet Chilli, Wok, Findus*	1 Pack/300g	300.0	1.0	100	3.0	20.0	0.5	0.0
Szechuan Beef Flavour, Dry, Blue Dragon*	½ Pack/100g	350.0	1.0	350	10.5	72.3	1.2	0.0
Thai Chicken, Takeaway, Somerfield*	1 Pack/300g	426.0	17.0	142	7.8	16.0	5.6	0.8
Thai Style, Asda*	1 Pot/238g	226.0	1.0	95	3.0	20.0	0.3	0.8
Thai Style, Sainsbury's*	1 Pack/340g	381.0	8.0	112	3.3	19.4	2.3	0.7
Thai, Spicy, Stir Fry, HL, Tesco*	½ Pack/250g	220.0	5.0	88	4.1	12.9	2.2	1.7
Thai, Waitrose*	1 Pack/300g	357.0	6.0	119	6.8	18.4	2.1	1.7
Tiger Prawn, Stir Fry, Tesco*	1 Pack/400g	596.0	15.0	149	6.0	23.0	3.7	2.7
Udon Japanese, & Dashi Soup Stock, Yutaka*	1 Pack/230g	290.0	1.0	126	3.0	26.8	0.5	0.0
Whole Wheat, Dry, Blue Dragon*	1 Serving/65g	208.0	1.0	320	12.5	63.0	2.0	8.0
with Sweet Chilli Chicken, COU, M & S*	1oz/28g	34.0	1.0	120	6.6	17.8	2.7	1.3
with Sweet Chilli Chicken, Tesco*	1 Pack/405g	445.0	7.0	110	5.3	18.5	1.7	1.0
Yaki Udan, Chicken & Prawn, M & S*	1 Pack/395g	434.0	14.0	110	8.1	11.9	3.6	0.8
NOUGAT								
Almond & Cherry, M & S*	1 Sweet/7g	28.0	1.0	405	4.5	76.0	9.1	1.1
Average	1 Sm Bar/28g	108.0	2.0	384	4.4	77.3	8.5	0.9
Bassetts & Beyond, Cadbury*	1oz/28g	105.0	1.0	375	4.0	82.0	4.0	0.0
Raspberry & Orange Hazelnut, Thorntons*	1 Sweet/9g	39.0	2.0	433	4.8	60.0	20.0	2.2
Soft, Bar, Bassett's*	1 Bar/25g	94.0	1.0	375	4.0	82.0	4.0	0.0
NUT CLUSTERS								
Almond, Sweet, Pecan, and Peanut, Red Sky*	1 Serving/30g	182.0	14.0	607	17.9	32.1	46.4	7.1
Peanut, Red Sky*	1 Serving/30g	182.0	14.0	607	21.4	32.1	46.4	7.1
NUT MIX								
Americas, Graze*	1 Pack/50g	333.0	31.0	667	16.0	11.8	61.6	5.6
Ancient Forest, Graze*	1 Med Pack/35g	229.0	21.0	654	17.4	10.8	60.2	0.0
Black Forest, Graze*	1 Pack/55g	258.0	14.0	470	6.6	54.4	25.1	0.0
Fantasy Forest, Graze*	1 Pack/55g	302.0	24.0	549	7.5	31.1	43.6	0.0
Fiery Almonds, Graze*	1 Punnet/35g	206.0	18.0	588	21.9	8.2	51.6	11.4
Honey Monster, Graze*	1 Med Pack/50g	279.0	20.0	559	10.8	45.2	40.8	0.0
Island, Graze*	1 Pack/55g	354.0	33.0	643	15.1	10.5	60.0	0.0
Sweet & Sour, Graze*	1 Pack/40g	222.0	17.0	556	19.1	23.7	43.4	0.0
NUT ROAST								
Asda*	1 Roast/230g	389.0	16.0	169	8.7	23.2	7.1	5.6
Average	1 Serving/200g	704.0	51.0	352	13.3	18.3	25.7	4.2
Courgette & Spiced Tomato, Cauldron Foods*	1 Serving/100g	208.0	12.0	208	11.7	12.5	12.3	4.9
Leek, Cheese & Mushroom, Organic, Cauldron Foods*	½ Pack/143g	343.0	21.0	240	13.2	13.2	14.9	4.1
Lentil, Average	*1oz/28g*	*62.0*	*3.0*	*222*	*10.6*	*18.8*	*12.1*	*3.8*
Tomato & Courgette, Vegetarian, Organic, Waitrose*	½ Pack/142g	295.0	17.0	208	11.7	12.5	12.3	4.9
NUTMEG								
Ground, Average	*1 Tsp/3g*	*16.0*	*1.0*	*525*	*5.8*	*45.3*	*36.3*	*0.0*
NUTS								
Assortment, Eat Well, M & S*	1 Pack/70g	441.0	41.0	630	16.7	8.5	58.9	5.3
Bento Mix, Graze*	1 Portion/30g	141.0	7.0	469	17.9	50.1	22.1	3.7
Cashews, Salsa Tossed, Graze*	1 Pack/40g	220.0	17.0	549	14.7	29.4	43.5	0.0
Clusters, Sweet Tomato Salsa, Sensations, Walkers*	1 Serving/35g	187.0	13.0	535	14.0	36.0	37.0	5.0
Fire, Graze*	1 Pack /50g	264.0	19.0	528	16.6	37.0	37.8	0.0
Honey Roasted, M & S*	1oz/28g	175.0	15.0	625	18.1	20.5	52.2	5.1
Luxury Assortment, Tesco*	1 Serving/10g	68.0	6.0	676	17.5	6.1	64.6	5.0
Luxury, Organic, M & S*	1oz/28g	179.0	16.0	640	21.1	11.6	56.6	6.1

	Measure INFO/WEIGHT	per Measure KCAL	per Measure FAT	Nutrition Values per 100g / 100ml KCAL	PROT	CARB	FAT	FIBRE

NUTS

	Measure INFO/WEIGHT	KCAL	FAT	KCAL	PROT	CARB	FAT	FIBRE
Mixed	1 Pack/40g	243.0	22.0	607	22.9	7.9	54.1	6.0
Mixed, Americas, Graze*	1 Punnet/40g	263.0	26.0	658	15.5	5.2	64.0	0.0
Mixed, Ancient Forest, Graze*	1 Pack/35g	226.0	22.0	645	16.9	5.7	61.9	0.0
Mixed, Chopped, Safeway*	1 Serving/2g	12.0	1.0	588	22.0	10.3	51.0	5.9
Mixed, Chopped, Sainsbury's*	1 Serving/100g	605.0	51.0	605	27.1	9.6	50.9	6.0
Mixed, Chopped, Tesco*	1 Serving/25g	149.0	13.0	595	23.5	10.5	50.6	6.0
Mixed, Delicious, Boots*	1 Pack/37.5g	235.0	22.0	628	18.0	6.1	59.0	10.0
Mixed, Honey Roasted, Waitrose*	1 Serving/50g	291.0	22.0	583	17.1	27.5	45.0	5.3
Mixed, Luxury, Unsalted, Somerfield*	1oz/28g	186.0	17.0	663	18.0	10.0	61.0	0.0
Mixed, Natural, Asda*	1 Snack/30g	197.0	19.0	656	18.0	4.3	62.7	7.4
Mixed, Natural, Luxury, Tesco*	1oz/28g	179.0	16.0	639	22.6	6.9	57.9	5.6
Mixed, Nature's Harvest*	1 Serving/25g	145.0	13.0	581	17.5	7.7	53.4	6.3
Mixed, Organic, Waitrose*	1oz/28g	179.0	17.0	640	19.3	7.7	59.1	8.4
Mixed, Roast, Salted, Somerfield*	1oz/28g	175.0	15.0	625	24.0	11.0	54.0	0.0
Mixed, Roasted, Salted, Waitrose*	1 Pack/200g	1252.0	117.0	626	13.7	11.3	58.4	4.4
Mixed, Roasted, Waitrose*	1 Serving/25g	165.0	16.0	662	15.2	6.2	64.0	8.2
Mixed, Unsalted, Sainsbury's*	1 Serving/50g	311.0	29.0	622	18.5	7.2	57.7	8.7
Natural Assortment, Tesco*	1 Serving/50g	338.0	32.0	676	17.5	6.1	64.6	5.0
Natural, Mixed, Waitrose*	1 Serving/50g	324.0	31.0	648	17.7	6.8	61.1	8.2
Oak Smoke Flavour Selection, Finest, Tesco*	1 Serving/25g	158.0	14.0	633	21.4	11.2	55.8	6.3
Omega Booster Seeds, Graze*	1 Punnet/45g	243.0	20.0	540	22.8	16.2	44.7	6.4
Peanuts & Cashews, Honey Roast, Tesco*	1 Serving/25g	145.0	11.0	579	21.6	26.6	42.9	4.2
Peri-Peri, Nando's*	1 Serving/75g	193.0	18.0	257	8.0	4.0	24.0	0.0
Pine, Tesco*	1 Pack/100g	699.0	69.0	699	16.5	4.0	68.6	1.9
Roast Salted, Luxury, KP Snacks*	1oz/28g	181.0	16.0	646	21.9	10.1	57.6	5.9
Roasted, Salted, Assortment, Luxury, Tesco*	1 Serving/25g	161.0	14.0	643	21.1	9.4	57.9	8.1
Salted, Selection, Sainsbury's*	1 Serving/30g	190.0	17.0	634	20.6	9.7	56.9	8.2
Soya, Dry Roasted, The Food Doctor*	1 Serving/50g	203.0	11.0	406	37.5	15.9	21.4	16.1
Unsalted, Selection, Sainsbury's*	1 Serving/75g	491.0	48.0	655	14.7	5.0	64.0	6.7

NUTS & RAISINS

	Measure INFO/WEIGHT	KCAL	FAT	KCAL	PROT	CARB	FAT	FIBRE
Mixed, Average	1 Serving/30g	144.0	10.0	481	14.1	31.5	34.1	4.5
Mixed, KP Snacks*	1 Serving/50g	273.0	20.0	546	21.4	24.4	40.3	5.2
Mixed, Natural, Waitrose*	1 Serving/50g	250.0	18.0	501	19.0	26.8	35.3	5.7
Mixed, Nature's Harvest*	1 Serving/50g	231.0	17.0	463	12.4	32.9	33.7	3.4
Mixed, Safeway*	1 Serving/50g	263.0	18.0	527	18.6	30.7	36.7	4.8
Mixed, Somerfield*	1oz/28g	159.0	13.0	568	18.0	24.0	45.0	0.0
Mixed, Tesco*	1 Serving/25g	115.0	7.0	450	18.6	32.6	26.8	12.5

	Measure INFO/WEIGHT	per Measure KCAL	FAT	Nutrition Values per 100g / 100ml KCAL	PROT	CARB	FAT	FIBRE
OAT BAKES								
Cheese, Nairn's*	1 Bag/30g	127.0	4.0	423	14.7	60.7	13.7	6.3
Mediterranean Tomato and Herb, Nairn's*	1 Bag/30g	129.0	5.0	431	8.1	64.2	15.8	8.3
Sweet Chilli, Nairn's*	1 Bag/30g	128.0	4.0	426	8.1	68.4	13.3	7.2
OAT CAKES								
Bran, Paterson's*	1 Cake/13g	52.0	2.0	416	10.0	58.5	15.8	9.5
Cheese, Nairn's*	1 Cake/9g	42.0	2.0	471	13.2	43.3	27.2	6.8
Fine Milled, Nairn's*	1 Cake/7.8g	35.0	2.0	449	10.5	52.6	21.8	8.6
Herb and Pumpkin Seed, Nairn's*	1 Cake/10g	43.0	2.0	426	12.2	46.8	21.1	13.0
Highland, Organic, Sainsbury's*	1 Cake/13g	57.0	2.0	456	10.2	59.8	19.5	5.5
Highland, Walkers*	1 Cake/12g	54.0	2.0	451	10.3	56.0	20.6	6.7
Oatmeal, Rough, Nairn's*	1 Cake/11g	45.0	2.0	421	10.6	52.8	18.6	10.5
Oatmeal, Rough, Organic, Nairn's*	1 Cake/10.3g	43.0	2.0	418	10.2	57.7	16.3	7.5
Organic, The Village Bakery*	1 Cake/13g	56.0	3.0	452	10.9	54.5	21.3	5.6
Retail, Average	1 Cake/13g	57.0	2.0	441	10.0	63.0	18.3	0.0
Rough Scottish, Sainsbury's*	1 Cake/11g	51.0	2.0	462	12.3	59.9	19.3	6.5
Rough with Bran, Walkers*	1 Cake/13g	55.0	2.0	424	11.0	57.1	16.8	8.1
Rough, Sainsbury's*	1 Cake/11g	45.0	2.0	426	11.7	65.2	16.9	8.6
Rough, Scottish, Tesco*	1 Cake/10.3g	45.0	2.0	435	11.4	55.3	18.4	8.0
Rough, with Olive Oil, Paterson's*	1 Cake/12.5g	54.0	2.0	431	10.6	58.4	17.2	8.1
Scottish, Organic, Waitrose*	1 Cake/13g	58.0	3.0	447	11.2	57.0	19.4	6.6
Scottish, Rough, Waitrose*	1 Cake/12.5g	55.0	2.0	438	10.4	57.4	18.5	8.0
Traditional, M & S*	1 Cake/11g	49.0	2.0	445	11.0	59.3	18.3	6.6
with Cracked Black Pepper, Walkers*	1 Cake/10g	41.0	2.0	433	10.4	55.0	19.0	8.5
OAT DRINK								
Healthy Oat, Enriched, Oatly*	1 Serving/250ml	112.0	4.0	45	1.0	6.5	1.5	0.8
Healthy Oat, Organic, Oatly*	1 Serving/250ml	87.0	2.0	35	1.0	6.5	0.7	0.8
OATMEAL								
Raw	*1oz/28g*	*112.0*	*2.0*	*401*	*12.4*	*72.8*	*8.7*	*6.8*
OCEAN								
Pinks, Asda*	1oz/28g	24.0	0.0	86	10.0	10.0	0.7	0.2
Prawnies, Mini, Asda*	1 Prawnie/11g	9.0	0.0	84	11.0	8.0	0.9	0.5
Snacks, Sainsbury's*	1 Stick/16g	18.0	0.0	113	7.0	21.0	0.1	0.1
Sticks, Average	1 Stick/16g	17.0	0.0	109	7.1	19.8	0.1	0.1
OCTOPUS								
Chunks, in Olive Oil, Palacio De Oriente*	1 Tin/111g	148.0	4.0	133	21.6	4.5	3.6	0.0
Raw	*1oz/28g*	*23.0*	*0.0*	*83*	*17.9*	*0.0*	*1.3*	*0.0*
OIL								
Again & Again, No Cholesterol, Anglia*	1 Tbsp/15ml	124.0	14.0	828	0.0	0.0	92.0	0.0
Almond, Average	1 Tbsp/14g	120.0	14.0	884	0.0	0.0	100.0	0.0
Avocado, Olivado*	1 Tsp/5ml	40.0	4.0	802	0.0	0.0	88.0	0.0
Black Truffle, Grapeseed, Cuisine Perel*	1 Tsp/5ml	43.0	5.0	857	0.0	7.1	100.0	0.0
Chilli, Average	*1 Tsp/5ml*	*41.0*	*5.0*	*823*	*0.0*	*0.0*	*91.5*	*0.0*
Chinese Stir Fry, Asda*	1 Tbsp/15ml	123.0	14.0	823	0.0	0.0	91.4	0.0
Coconut, Average	*1 Tsp/5ml*	*45.0*	*5.0*	*899*	*0.0*	*0.0*	*99.9*	*0.0*
Cod Liver, Average	*1 Capsule/1g*	*9.0*	*1.0*	*900*	*0.0*	*0.0*	*100.0*	*0.0*
Corn, Average	*1 Tsp/5ml*	*43.0*	*5.0*	*864*	*0.0*	*0.0*	*95.9*	*0.0*
Dipping, Herb, Italian Style, Finest, Tesco*	1 Serving/5g	44.0	5.0	877	0.4	0.9	96.9	0.4
Dipping, with Balsamic Vinegar, Finest, Tesco*	1 Tsp/5ml	33.0	4.0	668	0.0	4.4	71.7	0.0
Evening Primrose, Average	*1 Serving/1g*	*9.0*	*1.0*	*900*	*0.0*	*0.0*	*100.0*	*0.0*
Fish, Average	*1 Serving/1g*	*9.0*	*1.0*	*900*	*0.0*	*0.0*	*100.0*	*0.0*
Fish, Omega 3, Capsule, Holland & Barrett*	1 Capsule/1g	10.0	1.0	1000	0.1	0.1	100.0	0.1
Flax Seed, Average	*1 Tbsp/15ml*	*124.0*	*14.0*	*829*	*0.0*	*0.0*	*92.5*	*0.0*
Fry Light, Bodyline*	1 Spray/0.25ml	1.0	0.0	522	0.0	0.0	55.2	0.0

O

	Measure INFO/WEIGHT	per Measure KCAL	FAT	Nutrition Values per 100g / 100ml KCAL	PROT	CARB	FAT	FIBRE
OIL								
Grapeseed, Average	*1 Tsp/5ml*	*43.0*	*5.0*	*865*	*0.0*	*0.0*	*96.1*	*0.0*
Groundnut, Average	*1 Serving/25ml*	*206.0*	*23.0*	*824*	*0.0*	*0.0*	*91.8*	*0.0*
Hazelnut, Average	*1 Tsp/5ml*	*45.0*	*5.0*	*899*	*0.0*	*0.0*	*99.9*	*0.0*
Linseed, Organic, Biona*	1 Serving/10ml	84.0	9.0	837	0.0	0.0	93.0	0.0
Macadamia Nut, Oz Tukka*	1 Tsp/5ml	40.0	5.0	805	0.0	0.0	91.0	0.0
Olive, Average	*1 Tsp/5ml*	*43.0*	*5.0*	*855*	*0.0*	*0.0*	*94.9*	*0.0*
Olive, Basil Infused, Tesco*	1 Serving/20ml	180.0	20.0	900	0.0	0.0	100.0	0.0
Olive, Extra Virgin, Average	*1 Tsp/5ml*	*42.0*	*5.0*	*848*	*0.0*	*0.0*	*94.5*	*0.0*
Olive, Extra Virgin, Mist Spray, Belolive*	1 Serving/5ml	25.0	3.0	500	0.0	0.0	55.0	0.0
Olive, Extra Virgin, Only 1 Cal, Spray, Fry Light*	1 Spray/0.2ml	1.0	0.0	498	0.0	0.0	55.2	0.0
Olive, Garlic, Average	*1 Tbsp/15ml*	*127.0*	*14.0*	*848*	*0.0*	*0.0*	*94.3*	*0.0*
Olive, Lemon Flavoured, Sainsbury's*	1 Tbsp/15ml	123.0	14.0	823	0.1	0.0	91.4	0.1
Olive, Mild, Average	*1 Tbsp/15ml*	*129.0*	*14.0*	*861*	*0.0*	*0.0*	*95.7*	*0.0*
Omega, Organic, Clearspring*	1 Tbsp/15ml	124.0	14.0	828	0.0	0.0	92.0	0.0
Palm, Average	*1 Tsp/5ml*	*45.0*	*5.0*	*899*	*0.0*	*0.0*	*99.9*	*0.0*
Peanut, Average	*1 Tsp/5ml*	*45.0*	*5.0*	*899*	*0.0*	*0.0*	*99.9*	*0.0*
Rapeseed, Average	*1 Tbsp/15ml*	*130.0*	*14.0*	*863*	*0.0*	*0.0*	*95.9*	*0.0*
Red Palm & Canola, Carotino*	1 Tsp/5ml	41.0	5.0	812	0.0	0.0	92.0	0.0
Rice Bran, Average	1 Tbsp/14g	120.0	14.0	884	0.0	0.0	100.0	0.0
Safflower, Average	*1 Tsp/5ml*	*45.0*	*5.0*	*899*	*0.0*	*0.0*	*99.9*	*0.0*
Sesame, Average	*1 Tsp/5ml*	*45.0*	*5.0*	*892*	*0.1*	*0.0*	*99.9*	*0.0*
Soya, Average	*1 Tsp/5ml*	*45.0*	*5.0*	*899*	*0.0*	*0.0*	*99.9*	*0.0*
Stir Fry, Sharwood's*	1 fl oz/30ml	269.0	30.0	897	0.0	0.0	99.7	0.0
Sunflower, Average	*1 Tsp/5ml*	*43.0*	*5.0*	*869*	*0.0*	*0.0*	*96.6*	*0.0*
Sunflower, Spray, Fry Light*	1 Spray/0.2ml	1.0	0.0	522	0.0	0.0	55.2	0.0
Ultimate Blend, Ugo's*	1 Capsule/1ml	9.0	1.0	900	1.3	0.0	96.8	0.0
Vegetable, Average	*1 Tbsp/15ml*	*129.0*	*14.0*	*858*	*0.0*	*0.0*	*95.3*	*0.0*
Walnut, Average	*1 Tsp/5ml*	*45.0*	*5.0*	*899*	*0.0*	*0.0*	*99.9*	*0.0*
Wheatgerm, Average	*1 Tsp/5ml*	*45.0*	*5.0*	*899*	*0.0*	*0.0*	*99.9*	*0.0*
OKRA								
Boiled in Unsalted Water, Average	*1 Serving/80g*	*22.0*	*1.0*	*28*	*2.5*	*2.7*	*0.9*	*3.6*
Canned, Drained, Average	*1 Serving/80g*	*17.0*	*1.0*	*21*	*1.4*	*2.5*	*0.7*	*2.6*
Raw, Average	*1 Serving/80g*	*25.0*	*1.0*	*31*	*2.8*	*3.0*	*1.0*	*4.0*
Stir-Fried in Corn Oil, Average	*1 Serving/80g*	*215.0*	*21.0*	*269*	*4.3*	*4.4*	*26.1*	*6.3*
OLIVES								
Black & Green, with Greek Feta Cheese, Tesco*	1 Pot/100g	200.0	20.0	200	3.4	0.3	20.1	4.6
Black, Pitted, Average	*½ Jar/82g*	*135.0*	*13.0*	*164*	*1.0*	*3.5*	*16.2*	*3.1*
Green, Garlic Stuffed, Asda*	1 Olive/3g	6.0	1.0	174	1.8	3.5	17.0	0.0
Green, Lightly Flavoured with Lemon & Garlic, Attis*	1 Serving/50g	82.0	8.0	164	1.7	2.2	16.5	0.0
Green, Pimiento Stuffed, Somerfield*	1 Olive/3g	4.0	0.0	126	1.0	4.0	12.0	0.0
Green, Pitted, Average	*1 Olive/3g*	*4.0*	*0.0*	*129*	*1.1*	*0.9*	*13.3*	*2.5*
Green, Pitted, Stuffed with Anchovies, Sainsbury's*	1 Serving/50g	77.0	8.0	155	1.8	0.6	16.1	3.2
Green, Stuffed with Almonds, Pitted, Waitrose*	1 Serving/50g	90.0	8.0	180	3.8	3.2	16.9	2.5
Green, Stuffed with Anchovy, Waitrose*	½ Can/40g	38.0	3.0	94	1.5	4.7	7.7	2.3
Green, with Chilli & Garlic, Delicious, Boots*	1 Pack/60g	97.0	9.0	161	1.3	4.4	15.0	2.0
Kalamata, Kalamata	*1 Olive/3g*	*9.0*	*1.0*	*300*	*1.0*	*6.7*	*30.0*	*0.0*
Marinated, Mixed, M & S*	1 Serving/20g	33.0	3.0	165	1.6	6.5	14.9	3.0
Marinated, Selection, M & S*	4 Olives/20g	44.0	4.0	225	1.4	3.9	22.6	2.1
Mixed, Chilli & Garlic, Asda*	1 Serving/30g	43.0	5.0	144	0.9	0.0	15.6	6.1
Mixed, Marinated, Anti Pasti, Asda*	1 Serving/100g	215.0	22.0	215	1.8	0.7	22.0	3.1
Mixed, Marinated, with Feta & Red Peppers, Asda*	1 Pot/120g	233.0	22.0	194	5.8	2.2	18.0	1.7
Pimento Stuffed, in Brine, Tesco*	1 Serving/25g	38.0	4.0	153	0.8	0.1	16.4	2.1
Pitted, with Anchovy Paste, Safeway*	1/3 Can/50g	69.0	7.0	139	2.7	0.1	14.2	2.0

	Measure INFO/WEIGHT	per Measure KCAL	FAT	Nutrition Values per 100g / 100ml KCAL	PROT	CARB	FAT	FIBRE
OMELETTE								
Cheese & Mushroom, Apetito*	1 Serving/320g	486.0	25.0	152	6.2	14.4	7.8	1.9
Cheese, 2 Egg, Average	1 Omelette/180g	479.0	41.0	266	15.9	0.0	22.6	0.0
Cheese, Asda*	1 Omelette/119g	268.0	23.0	225	12.0	1.5	19.0	0.0
Cheese, Findus*	1 Serving/200g	400.0	26.0	200	9.5	14.0	13.0	0.0
Ham & Mushroom, Farmfoods*	1 Omelette/120g	200.0	17.0	167	8.7	1.8	13.9	0.1
Mushroom & Cheese, Tesco*	1 Omelette/120g	248.0	21.0	207	9.8	1.6	17.9	0.2
Plain, 2 Egg	1 Omelette/120g	229.0	20.0	191	10.9	0.0	16.4	0.0
Spanish	1oz/28g	34.0	2.0	120	5.7	6.2	8.3	1.4
ONION RINGS								
Battered, Asda*	1 Serving/100g	343.0	23.0	343	3.8	31.0	22.7	1.7
Battered, Oven Baked, Tesco*	1 Serving/50g	109.0	5.0	219	3.9	28.4	10.0	3.5
Battered, Sainsbury's*	1 Ring/12g	26.0	1.0	219	3.9	28.4	10.0	3.5
Breadcrumbs, Tesco*	1 Serving/100g	294.0	16.0	294	4.3	34.1	15.6	2.3
Breaded, Asda*	1 Serving/10g	29.0	1.0	289	4.4	34.0	15.0	2.7
Breaded, Iceland*	1 Ring/11g	33.0	2.0	293	4.4	34.2	15.4	2.7
Breaded, Sainsbury's*	1 Serving/100g	280.0	12.0	280	4.6	37.6	12.4	4.1
Oven Crisp Batter, Tesco*	1 Ring/17g	40.0	2.0	236	4.2	24.8	13.3	2.5
ONIONS								
Baked	*1oz/28g*	*29.0*	*0.0*	*103*	*3.5*	*22.3*	*0.6*	*3.9*
Boiled in Unsalted Water	*1oz/28g*	*5.0*	*0.0*	*17*	*0.6*	*3.7*	*0.1*	*0.7*
Borettane, Char-Grilled, Sacla*	1 Serving/100g	90.0	6.0	90	0.9	8.9	5.6	2.5
Dried, Raw, Average	*1oz/28g*	*88.0*	*0.0*	*313*	*10.2*	*68.6*	*1.7*	*12.1*
Fried, Average	*1oz/28g*	*46.0*	*3.0*	*164*	*2.3*	*14.1*	*11.2*	*3.1*
Pickled, Average	*1 Onion/15g*	*3.0*	*0.0*	*23*	*0.8*	*4.9*	*0.1*	*0.7*
Raw, Average	*1 Med/180g*	*55.0*	*0.0*	*31*	*1.3*	*6.0*	*0.2*	*1.4*
Red, Raw, Average	*1 Med/180g*	*66.0*	*0.0*	*37*	*1.2*	*7.9*	*0.2*	*1.5*
Spring Or Scallion, Raw, Average	*1 Med/15g*	*5.0*	*0.0*	*33*	*1.8*	*7.3*	*0.2*	*2.6*
Sweet, TTD, Sainsbury's*	1 Serving/100g	39.0	0.0	39	1.3	7.9	0.2	1.4
OPTIONS								
Choca Mocha Drink, Ovaltine*	1 Sachet/11g	39.0	1.0	359	14.1	50.1	11.4	7.0
Chocolate Au Lait, Ovaltine*	1 Sachet/10g	35.0	1.0	355	11.8	54.5	10.0	7.3
Coffee, Dreamy Cappuccion, Cafe, Ovaltine*	1 Sachet/25g	64.0	4.0	256	12.9	58.1	16.9	0.0
Cracking Hazelnut, Ovaltine*	1 Sachet/11g	40.0	1.0	361	16.0	57.0	11.0	0.0
Irish Cream, Ovaltine*	1 Sachet/11g	39.0	1.0	357	13.9	50.0	11.3	8.1
Mint Madness, Ovaltine*	1 Serving/11g	40.0	1.0	365	15.0	50.6	11.4	0.0
Outrageous Orange, Ovaltine*	1 Serving/11g	32.0	1.0	289	11.7	43.3	7.7	18.0
Tempting Toffee, Ovaltine*	1 Sachet/11g	43.0	1.0	391	13.6	66.4	9.1	0.0
Wicked White Chocolate, Ovaltine*	1 Sachet/11g	46.0	1.0	414	10.3	68.1	11.1	0.5
ORANGE DRINK								
Sparkling, Diet, Tesco*	1 Glass/250ml	7.0	0.0	3	0.1	0.5	0.1	0.0
Sparkling, Florida, M & S*	1 Serving/500ml	250.0	0.0	50	0.0	12.5	0.0	0.0
Sparkling, Shapers, Boots*	1 Bottle/500ml	15.0	0.0	3	0.1	0.4	0.1	0.0
Sparkling, Tesco*	1 Serving/100ml	35.0	0.0	35	0.0	8.5	0.0	0.0
Sugar Free, Tesco*	1 Glass/250ml	2.0	0.0	1	0.0	0.0	0.0	0.0
ORANGES								
Blood, Average	*1 Orange/140g*	*82.0*	*0.0*	*58*	*0.8*	*13.3*	*0.0*	*2.5*
Cherry, Graze*	1 Pack /120g	56.0	0.0	47	0.9	11.8	0.1	0.0
Fresh Cut, Graze*	1 Pack /120g	47.0	0.0	39	1.1	8.5	0.1	0.0
Fresh, Weighed with Peel, Average	*1 Med/185g*	*115.0*	*0.0*	*62*	*1.0*	*15.6*	*0.3*	*3.2*
Fresh, without Peel, Average	*1 Med/145g*	*90.0*	*0.0*	*62*	*1.0*	*15.6*	*0.3*	*3.2*
Peel Only, Raw, Average	*1 Tbsp/6g*	*6.0*	*0.0*	*97*	*1.5*	*25.0*	*0.2*	*10.6*
Ruby Red, Tesco*	1 Med/130g	51.0	0.0	39	1.1	8.5	0.1	1.7
TTD, Sainsbury's*	1 Serving/100g	37.0	0.0	37	1.1	8.5	0.1	1.7

O

	Measure INFO/WEIGHT	per Measure KCAL	FAT	Nutrition Values per 100g / 100ml KCAL	PROT	CARB	FAT	FIBRE
OREGANO								
Dried,	*1 Tsp/1g*	*3.0*	*0.0*	*306*	*11.0*	*49.5*	*10.3*	*0.0*
Fresh	*1 Tsp/1.25g*	*1.0*	*0.0*	*66*	*2.2*	*9.7*	*2.0*	*0.0*
OVALTINE*								
Hi Malt, Light, Instant Drink, Ovaltine*	1 Sachet/20g	72.0	1.0	358	9.1	67.1	5.9	2.8
Powder, Made Up with Semi-Skimmed Milk, Ovaltine*	1 Mug/227ml	179.0	4.0	79	3.9	13.0	1.7	0.0
Powder, Made Up with Whole Milk, Ovaltine*	1 Mug/227ml	220.0	9.0	97	3.8	12.9	3.8	0.0
OXTAIL								
Raw	*1oz/28g*	*48.0*	*3.0*	*171*	*20.0*	*0.0*	*10.1*	*0.0*
Stewed	*1oz/28g*	*68.0*	*4.0*	*243*	*30.5*	*0.0*	*13.4*	*0.0*
OYSTERS								
in Vegetable Oil, Smoked, John West*	1oz/28g	64.0	4.0	230	16.0	10.0	14.0	0.0
Raw, Shucked	*1 Oyster/14g*	*9.0*	*0.0*	*65*	*10.8*	*2.7*	*1.3*	*0.0*

O

	Measure INFO/WEIGHT	per Measure KCAL	FAT	Nutrition Values per 100g / 100ml KCAL	PROT	CARB	FAT	FIBRE
PAELLA								
Bistro, Waitrose*	1 Serving/300g	534.0	20.0	178	7.4	22.2	6.6	0.7
Chicken & Chorizo, Asda*	1 Pack/390g	484.0	9.0	124	10.0	16.0	2.2	2.6
Chicken & Chorizo, Big Dish, M & S*	1 Pack/450g	630.0	18.0	140	7.9	18.4	3.9	1.6
Chicken & King Prawn, HL, Tesco*	1 Pack/385g	346.0	6.0	90	5.3	12.7	1.6	2.0
Chicken & Prawn, Asda*	1 Pack/400g	352.0	4.0	88	5.8	13.7	1.1	1.4
Chicken & Vegetable, HL, Tesco*	1 Pack/450g	441.0	6.0	98	9.7	11.8	1.3	1.1
Chicken, Chorizo & King Prawn, Finest, Tesco*	½ Pack/400g	520.0	20.0	130	7.0	14.2	4.9	1.2
Chicken, King Prawns, British, Sainsbury's*	1 Pack/400g	380.0	5.0	95	7.6	13.3	1.2	0.9
Chicken, Tesco*	1 Serving/475g	575.0	14.0	121	7.9	15.7	3.0	1.6
Diet Chef Ltd*	1 Pack/250g	355.0	3.0	142	11.2	21.7	1.2	0.4
Enjoy, Birds Eye*	1 Pack/500g	620.0	16.0	124	7.7	16.2	3.2	0.6
King Prawn, Chicken & Chorizo, City Kitchen, Tesco*	1 Pack/400g	540.0	20.0	135	4.7	17.0	5.0	1.4
Seafood, Finest, Tesco*	1 Pack/400g	756.0	24.0	189	6.8	27.2	5.9	1.0
Seafood, M & S*	1 Pack/450g	517.0	17.0	115	6.4	13.7	3.8	3.2
Seafood, Sainsbury's*	1 Pack/400g	504.0	5.0	126	8.3	20.3	1.3	0.6
Tesco*	1 Serving/460g	584.0	17.0	127	4.6	18.9	3.7	1.0
TTD, Sainsbury's*	½ Pack/374g	475.0	21.0	127	9.4	9.9	5.6	4.8
Vegetable, Waitrose*	1 Serving/174g	202.0	3.0	116	2.2	22.7	1.8	1.5
with Prawns, Chicken, Cod & Salmon, Sainsbury's*	1 Pack/750g	772.0	1.0	103	8.3	16.9	0.2	3.1
PAIN AU CHOCOLAT								
Asda*	1 Serving/58g	244.0	14.0	420	8.0	43.0	24.0	3.3
Extra Special, Asda*	1oz/28g	113.0	6.0	405	8.0	46.0	21.0	3.3
M & S*	1 Pastry/60g	210.0	12.0	350	5.9	38.0	19.2	1.6
Mini, Asda*	1 Pastry/23g	96.0	5.0	420	8.0	43.0	24.0	3.3
Mini, Cafe Simple*	1 Pastry/27g	122.0	7.0	452	10.2	42.8	26.7	2.5
Sainsbury's*	1 Serving/58g	241.0	14.0	415	7.9	42.5	23.7	3.3
Small, Asda*	1 Serving/23g	106.0	6.0	462	8.0	49.0	26.0	0.0
Waitrose*	1 Pastry/52.9g	230.0	13.0	435	8.8	45.5	23.9	3.7
PAIN AU RAISIN								
Twist, Extra Special, Asda*	1 Pastry/110g	421.0	21.0	383	7.0	46.0	19.0	2.5
PAK CHOI								
Raw, Average	*1 Leaf/14g*	*2.0*	*0.0*	*13*	*1.5*	*2.2*	*0.2*	*1.0*
PAKORA								
Bhaji, Onion, Fried in Vegetable Oil	1oz/28g	76.0	4.0	271	9.8	26.2	14.7	5.5
Bhajia, Potato Carrot & Pea, Fried in Vegetable Oil	1oz/28g	100.0	6.0	357	10.9	28.8	22.6	6.1
Bhajia, Vegetable, Retail	1oz/28g	66.0	4.0	235	6.4	21.4	14.7	3.6
Chicken, Tikka, Asda*	1 Pack/350g	696.0	38.0	199	16.0	9.0	11.0	1.1
Potato & Spinach, Waitrose*	1 Pakora/50g	120.0	8.0	240	5.5	17.3	16.5	4.7
Prawn, Indian Appetisers, Waitrose*	1 Pakora/21g	35.0	2.0	165	16.8	5.9	8.2	1.5
Sainsbury's*	1 Pakora/55g	166.0	10.0	302	7.3	26.8	18.3	1.1
Spinach, Mini, Indian Selection, Somerfield*	1 Serving/22g	61.0	4.0	277	6.2	26.9	16.1	4.9
Spinach, Sainsbury's*	1 Pakora/17.9g	35.0	2.0	195	5.1	19.4	10.8	3.8
Vegetable, Indian Selection, Party, Co-Op*	1 Pakora/23g	47.0	2.0	205	6.0	28.0	7.0	4.0
Vegetable, Indian Starter Selection, M & S*	1 Pakora/23g	61.0	4.0	265	6.3	19.6	18.1	2.9
Vegetable, Mini, Indian Snack Collection, Tesco*	1 Pakora/21g	36.0	2.0	173	6.0	16.8	9.1	4.9
PANCAKE								
Apple & Sultana, M & S*	1 Serving/80g	160.0	6.0	200	2.2	30.2	7.9	1.2
Apple, GFY, Asda*	1 Pancake/74g	100.0	2.0	135	4.2	24.0	2.5	1.0
Asda*	1 Pancake/23g	59.0	2.0	254	4.8	43.0	7.0	4.0
Big, Crafty, Genesis*	1 Pancake/71g	171.0	4.0	241	6.2	42.3	5.2	2.1
Bramley Apple, Sainsbury's*	1 Pancake/85g	114.0	2.0	134	4.2	23.6	2.5	1.0
Cherry, GFY, Asda*	1 Serving/206g	206.0	4.0	100	1.9	18.9	1.8	1.8
Chinatown, Asda*	1 Pancake/10g	33.0	1.0	335	10.9	51.7	9.2	2.4

	Measure INFO/WEIGHT	per Measure KCAL	FAT	Nutrition Values per 100g / 100ml KCAL	PROT	CARB	FAT	FIBRE
PANCAKE								
Chinese Roll, Farmfoods*	1 Pancake/88g	125.0	4.0	142	4.3	21.6	4.3	1.0
Chinese Style, Cherry Valley*	1 Pancake/8g	25.0	0.0	310	9.2	54.7	6.0	0.0
Chocolate, M & S*	1 Pancake/80g	125.0	5.0	156	3.1	22.1	6.1	0.2
for Duck, Sainsbury's*	1 Pancake/10g	33.0	1.0	333	10.9	51.7	9.3	2.4
for Honey Chicken, Sainsbury's*	1 Pack/50g	146.0	3.0	293	8.0	51.6	6.1	5.3
HL, Tesco*	1 Pancake/25g	60.0	0.0	240	5.8	48.8	2.0	1.9
Lemon, M & S*	1 Pancake/38g	90.0	3.0	235	4.5	38.5	7.2	2.8
Light Choices, Tesco*	1 Pancake/27g	66.0	1.0	243	6.9	47.7	2.6	0.0
Maple & Raisin, M & S*	1 Pancake/33g	88.0	2.0	269	6.5	49.7	5.4	2.2
Mini, for, Kids, Tesco*	1 Pancake/16g	45.0	1.0	283	6.6	51.7	5.5	1.3
Mini, Scotch, Tesco*	1 Pancake/16g	44.0	1.0	277	6.7	50.0	5.6	1.4
Morrisons*	1 Pancake/60g	133.0	3.0	221	8.4	37.3	5.0	1.5
North Staffordshire Oatcakes Ltd*	1 Pancake/71g	166.0	4.0	234	5.0	40.9	6.1	1.0
Perfect, Kingsmill*	1 Pancake/27g	71.0	1.0	264	6.2	49.7	4.5	1.2
Plain, Sainsbury's*	1 Pancake/46g	102.0	2.0	221	6.9	36.1	5.3	1.2
Raisin & Lemon, Asda*	1 Serving/30g	92.0	2.0	304	6.0	52.0	8.0	1.4
Raisin & Lemon, Sainsbury's*	1 Pancake/35g	95.0	2.0	272	6.3	51.8	4.4	2.2
Savoury, Made with Skimmed Milk, Average	1 6"/77g	192.0	11.0	249	6.4	24.1	14.7	0.8
Savoury, Made with Whole Milk, Average	1 6"/77g	210.0	13.0	273	6.3	24.0	17.5	0.8
Scotch	1 Pancake/50g	146.0	6.0	292	5.8	43.6	11.7	1.4
Scotch, BGTY, Sainsbury's*	1 Pancake/30g	76.0	1.0	252	5.3	48.5	4.1	1.3
Scotch, Low Fat, Asda*	1 Pancake/32g	87.0	1.0	272	6.0	57.0	2.2	1.3
Scotch, M & S*	1 Pancake/34g	95.0	1.0	280	6.5	54.5	4.0	1.6
Scotch, Sainsbury's*	1 Pancake/30g	84.0	2.0	280	6.3	47.6	7.2	1.7
Sultana & Syrup Scotch, Sainsbury's*	1 Pancake/35g	113.0	3.0	322	6.7	55.2	8.3	1.7
Sultana & Syrup, Asda*	1 Pancake/34g	89.0	2.0	263	5.9	43.7	7.2	1.5
Sultana & Syrup, Iceland*	1 Pancake/35g	95.0	1.0	270	5.3	53.0	4.1	1.2
Sweet, Made with Skimmed Milk	1oz/28g	78.0	4.0	280	6.0	35.1	13.8	0.8
Sweet, Made with Whole Milk	1oz/28g	84.0	5.0	301	5.9	35.0	16.2	0.8
Sweet, Raspberry Ripple Sauce, Findus*	1 Pancake/38g	80.0	2.0	210	3.9	37.1	4.7	0.9
Syrup, Tesco*	1 Pancake/30g	79.0	2.0	265	4.7	42.1	8.2	1.5
Traditional, Aunt Bessie's*	1 Pancake/60g	90.0	2.0	150	6.1	24.6	3.1	1.1
Traditional, Tesco*	1 Pancake/62g	137.0	3.0	221	8.4	35.6	5.0	1.5
Vegetable Roll	1 Roll/85g	185.0	11.0	218	6.6	21.0	12.5	0.0
Warburton's*	1 Pancake/35g	84.0	2.0	239	7.6	37.7	6.4	2.4
with Golden Syrup, Value, Tesco*	1 Pancake/27g	72.0	2.0	265	4.7	47.4	6.3	1.5
with Maple Sauce & Fromage Frais, BGTY, Sainsbury's*	1 Serving/100g	163.0	2.0	163	5.0	30.0	2.5	0.8
with Syrup, American Style, Large, Tesco*	1 Pancake/38g	102.0	1.0	268	5.1	54.2	3.4	0.9
PANCAKE MIX								
Fresh, M & S*	1 Pancake/38g	90.0	5.0	235	7.5	22.4	13.1	0.5
Glutano*	1 Tbs/15g	57.0	0.0	378	8.9	75.6	2.2	0.0
Traditional, Asda*	1 Pack/256g	545.0	23.0	213	6.0	27.0	9.0	1.8
PANCETTA								
Average	**½ Pack/65g**	**212.0**	**19.0**	**326**	**17.0**	**0.1**	**28.7**	**0.0**
Cubes, Tesco*	1 Serving/38g	135.0	12.0	355	17.5	0.5	32.2	0.0
PANINI								
Bacon, British Midland*	1 Serving/150g	273.0	10.0	182	9.1	21.6	6.6	0.0
Chargrilled Chicken, Mozzarella & Pesto, Ugo's*	1 Panini/170g	389.0	15.0	229	16.4	21.6	8.6	2.0
Cheese, Tesco*	1 Panini/100g	249.0	9.0	249	10.5	31.3	9.1	3.1
Mozzarella & Tomato, M & S*	1 Serving/176g	484.0	29.0	275	11.3	21.3	16.2	2.1
Tuna & Sweetcorn, Tesco*	1 Serving/250g	559.0	16.0	224	12.0	29.3	6.6	1.4
PANNA COTTA								
BGTY, Sainsbury's*	1 Pot/150g	150.0	3.0	100	2.4	18.2	1.9	1.4

P

	Measure INFO/WEIGHT	per Measure KCAL	FAT	Nutrition Values per 100g / 100ml KCAL	PROT	CARB	FAT	FIBRE
PANNA COTTA								
Caramel, Sainsbury's*	1 Pot/120g	335.0	16.0	279	2.5	34.6	13.1	3.3
Sainsbury's*	1 Pot/100g	304.0	16.0	304	3.0	41.5	15.7	4.0
Strawberry, COU, M & S*	1 Pot/145g	145.0	4.0	100	2.6	15.7	2.6	0.8
PAPAYA								
Dried, Pieces, Nature's Harvest*	1 Serving/50g	177.0	0.0	355	0.2	85.4	0.0	2.6
Dried, Strips, Tropical Wholefoods*	1 Strip/10g	31.0	0.0	310	3.9	71.4	0.9	1.5
Dried, Sweetened, Tesco*	4 Pieces/25g	59.0	0.0	235	0.4	56.3	0.9	2.9
Raw, Flesh Only, Average	*1 Serving/140g*	*37.0*	*0.0*	*26*	*0.4*	*6.6*	*0.1*	*1.2*
Raw, Weighed with Seeds & Skin	*1 Cup/140g*	*55.0*	*0.0*	*39*	*0.6*	*9.8*	*0.1*	*1.8*
Unripe, Raw, Weighed with Seeds & Skin	*1oz/28g*	*8.0*	*0.0*	*27*	*0.9*	*5.5*	*0.1*	*1.5*
PAPPADS								
Green Chilli & Garlic, Sharwood's*	1 Pappad/14g	38.0	0.0	268	23.2	39.4	1.9	14.6
PAPPARDELLE								
Basil, Fresh, Sainsbury's*	1 Serving/240g	281.0	3.0	117	5.0	21.2	1.4	2.0
Buitoni*	1 Serving/65g	242.0	3.0	373	15.0	67.5	4.8	0.0
Chilli, Fresh, Sainsbury's*	1 Serving/250g	302.0	4.0	121	5.7	20.7	1.7	2.0
Egg & Spinach, Extra Special, Asda*	½ Pack/200g	328.0	4.0	164	6.5	30.5	1.8	1.4
Egg, Dry, Average	*1 Serving/100g*	*364.0*	*4.0*	*364*	*14.1*	*68.5*	*3.7*	*2.1*
Egg, Fresh, Waitrose*	¼ Pack/125g	350.0	3.0	280	12.9	51.0	2.7	1.9
Saffron, Eat Well, M & S*	1 Serving/100g	360.0	2.0	360	14.0	69.0	2.5	3.2
The Best Fresh, Morrisons*	¼ Pack/240g	353.0	4.0	147	6.3	26.9	1.6	1.9
with Salmon, COU, M & S*	1 Pack/358g	340.0	7.0	95	6.3	13.0	1.9	0.8
PAPRIKA								
Average	*1 Tsp/2g*	*6.0*	*0.0*	*289*	*14.8*	*34.9*	*13.0*	*0.0*
PARATHA								
Average	*1 Paratha/80g*	*258.0*	*11.0*	*322*	*8.0*	*43.2*	*14.3*	*4.0*
Lachha, Waitrose*	1 Paratha/75g	322.0	18.0	429	7.8	46.0	23.8	1.8
Roti, Plain, Crown Farms*	1 Slice/80g	250.0	10.0	312	5.0	46.2	12.5	1.2
PARSLEY								
Dried	*1 Tsp/1g*	*2.0*	*0.0*	*181*	*15.8*	*14.5*	*7.0*	*26.9*
Fresh, Average	*1 Tbsp/3.8g*	*1.0*	*0.0*	*34*	*3.0*	*2.7*	*1.3*	*5.0*
PARSNIP								
Boiled, Average	*1 Serving/80g*	*53.0*	*1.0*	*66*	*1.6*	*12.9*	*1.2*	*4.7*
Fragrant, Tesco*	1 Serving/50g	33.0	1.0	67	1.8	12.5	1.1	4.6
Honey Glazed, Roasting, Cooked, Betty Smith's*	1 Serving/100g	144.0	7.0	144	2.6	23.4	7.2	6.3
Honey Roasted, Tesco*	1 Serving/125g	202.0	10.0	162	1.9	20.0	8.2	2.2
Raw, Unprepared, Average	*1oz/28g*	*19.0*	*0.0*	*66*	*1.8*	*12.5*	*1.1*	*4.6*
Roast, Honey Glazed, Baked, Aunt Bessie's*	1 Serving/125g	162.0	9.0	130	1.7	14.0	7.5	4.1
PARTRIDGE								
Meat Only, Roasted	*1oz/28g*	*59.0*	*2.0*	*212*	*36.7*	*0.0*	*7.2*	*0.0*
PASANDA								
Chicken, M & S*	½ Pack/150g	240.0	16.0	160	11.3	3.8	10.9	1.3
Chicken, Sainsbury's*	1 Serving/200g	368.0	25.0	184	14.7	3.4	12.4	2.3
Chicken, Waitrose*	1oz/28g	52.0	3.0	185	14.8	3.8	12.3	1.1
Chicken, with Pilau Rice, HL, Tesco*	1 Pack/440g	466.0	11.0	106	5.7	15.2	2.5	0.9
PASSATA								
Basil, Del Monte*	1 Jar/500g	160.0	1.0	32	1.4	5.9	0.2	0.0
Classic, Italian, with Onion & Garlic, Sainsbury's*	1oz/28g	10.0	0.0	37	1.4	7.7	0.1	1.3
Napolina*	1 Bottle/690g	172.0	1.0	25	1.4	4.5	0.1	0.0
Sieved Tomato, Valfrutta*	1 Pack/500g	110.0	0.0	22	1.2	4.0	0.1	0.0
Smart Price, Asda*	1 Serving/100g	25.0	0.0	25	1.4	4.5	0.1	0.2
So Organic, Sainsbury's*	¼ Jar/175g	38.0	1.0	22	0.9	3.8	0.4	0.9
with Fresh Leaf Basil, Waitrose*	¼ Jar/170g	44.0	0.0	26	1.0	5.2	0.1	0.8

P

	Measure INFO/WEIGHT	per Measure KCAL	per Measure FAT	Nutrition Values per 100g / 100ml KCAL	PROT	CARB	FAT	FIBRE
PASSATA								
with Garlic & Herbs, Roughly Chopped, Tesco*	1 Serving/200g	56.0	0.0	28	1.4	5.5	0.0	1.0
with Garlic & Italian Herbs, Tesco*	1 Serving/165g	53.0	0.0	32	1.2	6.4	0.2	1.1
PASSION FRUIT								
Raw, Fresh	*1 Fruit/30g*	*18.0*	*0.0*	*60*	*0.7*	*14.4*	*0.2*	*0.2*
Weighed with Skin	*1oz/28g*	*6.0*	*0.0*	*22*	*1.7*	*3.5*	*0.2*	*2.0*
PASTA								
& Chargrilled Mushrooms, Finest, Tesco*	1 Pack/200g	410.0	22.0	205	6.1	19.6	11.2	1.4
& Flame Grilled Chicken, M & S*	1 Pack/180g	414.0	25.0	230	8.2	17.5	14.0	0.8
& Roasted Vegetables, Waitrose*	1oz/28g	43.0	3.0	154	2.4	14.2	9.7	1.0
Arrabbiata Nodini, Asda*	1 Serving/150g	301.0	9.0	201	7.8	29.3	5.8	2.7
Bean & Tuna, BGTY, Sainsbury's*	1 Serving/200g	176.0	2.0	88	7.3	12.6	0.9	2.8
Blue Cheese, Bacon & Spinach, M & S*	1 Pack/400g	640.0	34.0	160	6.5	13.8	8.5	0.7
Boccoletti, Dried, Sainsbury's*	1 Serving/90g	321.0	2.0	357	12.3	73.1	1.7	2.5
Bolognese, Diet Chef Ltd*	1 Pack/300g	255.0	10.0	85	7.9	5.8	3.4	4.4
Cajun Chicken, GFY, Asda*	1 Serving/297g	312.0	8.0	105	8.0	12.0	2.8	2.1
Cannelloni, Tubes, Dry, Average	*1oz/28g*	*101.0*	*1.0*	*361*	*12.5*	*69.1*	*3.6*	*1.2*
Carbonara, with Cheese & Bacon, Slim Fast*	1 Serving/70g	240.0	4.0	343	22.7	48.9	6.3	5.7
Chargrilled Chicken & Bacon, Tesco*	1 Pack/200g	420.0	24.0	210	6.7	18.8	11.8	1.3
Chargrilled Chicken, Asda*	1 Serving/250g	537.0	27.0	215	7.0	22.0	11.0	1.7
Cheddar, Country, Bowl, Haribo*	1 Serving/269g	400.0	19.0	149	5.6	15.2	7.1	1.5
Cheese & Broccoli, Light Choices, Tesco*	1 Pack/348g	435.0	8.0	125	4.4	21.2	2.3	2.4
Cheese & Broccoli, Tubes, Tesco*	1 Serving/202g	319.0	14.0	158	5.0	19.1	6.9	2.3
Cheese, Tomato, & Pesto, Boots*	1 Pack/250g	355.0	11.0	142	5.9	20.0	4.4	2.0
Cheesy Spirals, Curly Whirly, Asda*	1/3 Pack/200g	214.0	5.0	107	6.0	15.0	2.6	0.5
Chicken & Asparagus, GFY, Asda*	1 Pack/400g	388.0	9.0	97	10.9	8.5	2.2	1.5
Chicken & Green Pesto, HL, Tesco*	1 Serving/376g	440.0	5.0	117	8.3	18.5	1.2	1.4
Chicken & Ham, Easy Steam, Tesco*	1 Pack/400g	572.0	26.0	143	9.8	11.2	6.6	0.6
Chicken & Mushroom Flavour, Quick, Sainsbury's*	1 Pot/220g	235.0	6.0	107	3.3	16.1	2.8	1.9
Chicken & Mushroom, Big Eat, Heinz*	1 Pot/350g	339.0	16.0	97	4.8	9.2	4.5	0.5
Chicken & Mushroom, Pasta & Sauce, Dry, Tesco*	1 Pack/120g	427.0	4.0	356	16.0	65.0	3.6	3.9
Chicken & Pineapple, Shapers, Boots*	1 Pack/221g	210.0	3.0	95	5.4	15.0	1.5	0.9
Chicken & Roasted Tomato, HL, Tesco*	1 Serving/374g	426.0	7.0	114	7.4	16.7	1.9	1.3
Chicken & Tomato, Classic, Mini, Tesco*	1 Pack/300g	165.0	7.0	55	6.6	1.7	2.4	1.7
Chicken & Vegetable, Mediterranean, Waitrose*	1 Serving/400g	375.0	9.0	94	7.5	10.5	2.3	2.2
Chicken, Tomato & Basil, GFY, Asda*	1 Pack/400g	404.0	9.0	101	6.4	13.6	2.3	1.4
Chicken, Tomato & Basil, HL, Tesco*	1 Pack/400g	264.0	2.0	66	7.9	7.5	0.5	1.1
Chicken, Tomato & Herb, Easy Steam, Tesco*	1 Serving/400g	528.0	25.0	132	8.9	10.2	6.2	1.3
Chicken, Tomato & Mascarpone, Easy Steam, Tesco*	1 Pack/400g	468.0	16.0	117	9.7	10.3	4.1	0.9
Chicken, Tomato & Mascarpone, HL, Tesco*	1 Pack/450g	504.0	11.0	112	7.5	14.8	2.5	1.1
Chicken, Tomato, & Basil, Asda*	1 Pack/400g	474.0	10.0	118	6.5	17.5	2.5	1.2
Chicken, Tomato, & Mascarpone, Italiano, Tesco*	1 Pack/400g	572.0	25.0	143	7.4	14.3	6.2	1.3
Creamy Cheese, Big Eat, Heinz*	1 Pot/350g	437.0	32.0	125	3.7	7.0	9.2	1.8
Creamy Mushroom, Light Choices, Tesco*	1 Pack/350g	455.0	5.0	130	4.3	25.0	1.4	1.3
Creamy Mushroom, Sainsbury's*	1 Serving/63g	148.0	9.0	237	4.5	21.7	14.6	1.2
Creamy Tomato & Chicken, Great Stuff, Asda*	1 Pack/300g	351.0	12.0	117	7.0	13.5	3.9	2.3
Creamy Vegetable, Meal in 5, Ainsley Harriott*	1 Pot/386.9g	414.0	10.0	107	2.8	18.1	2.6	0.8
Dischi Volanti, Tesco*	1 Serving/50g	177.0	1.0	355	12.5	73.0	1.4	2.6
Elicoidali, Waitrose*	1 Serving/200g	682.0	3.0	341	11.5	70.7	1.3	3.7
Fagottini, Wild Mushroom, Sainsbury's*	½ Pack/125g	274.0	9.0	219	10.2	27.7	7.5	2.7
Feta & Black Olive Girasole, Extra Special, Asda*	½ Pack/150g	360.0	15.0	240	8.3	28.4	10.3	0.0
Fiorelli, Egg, M & S*	1 Serving/100g	355.0	3.0	355	13.9	68.5	2.8	3.0
Fiorelli, Mozzarella, Tomato & Basil, Waitrose*	1 Serving/125g	352.0	12.0	282	10.8	38.9	9.3	1.7
Florentina, with Broccoli & Spinach, Slim Fast*	1 Serving/71g	239.0	3.0	336	23.0	50.5	4.6	5.8

	Measure INFO/WEIGHT	per Measure KCAL	FAT	Nutrition Values per 100g / 100ml KCAL	PROT	CARB	FAT	FIBRE
PASTA								
Fusilloni, TTD, Sainsbury's*	1 Serving/90g	321.0	2.0	357	12.3	73.1	1.7	2.5
Garlic Mushroom Filled, Extra Special, Asda*	1 Serving/125g	224.0	9.0	179	8.0	21.0	7.0	2.5
Girasole, Filled with Red Pepper & Goats Cheese, Asda*	½ Pack/150g	261.0	10.0	174	7.2	21.4	6.6	1.8
Green & White, Duetto, Pasta Reale*	1oz/28g	79.0	2.0	281	10.9	49.4	6.0	3.6
High Fibre, Uncooked, Fiber Gourmet*	1 Serving/56g	130.0	1.0	232	12.5	75.0	1.8	32.1
Honey & Mustard Chicken, Light Choices, Tesco*	1 Pack/375g	881.0	48.0	235	6.7	22.0	12.9	1.2
Honey & Mustard Chicken, Tesco*	1 Pack/375g	865.0	48.0	231	6.7	21.9	12.9	0.0
Hot Smoked Salmon, Tesco*	1 Pack/275g	426.0	17.0	155	7.1	16.6	6.2	4.1
King Prawn & Pesto, Asda*	1 Pack/400g	488.0	18.0	122	7.6	12.9	4.4	1.2
Linguine, Dry Weight, De Cecco*	1 Serving/100g	350.0	1.0	350	13.0	71.0	1.5	2.9
Lumaconi, TTD, Sainsbury's*	1 Serving/90g	321.0	2.0	357	12.3	73.1	1.7	2.5
Macaroni Cheese, Meal in 5, Ainsley Harriott*	1 Pot/386.9g	467.0	16.0	121	3.7	17.3	4.1	1.0
Margherite, Basil & Pinenut, TTD, Sainsbury's*	½ Pack/150g	309.0	10.0	206	12.6	23.2	7.0	2.7
Meat Feast, Italian, Sainsbury's*	1 Pack/450g	508.0	18.0	113	7.4	11.8	4.0	0.6
Medaglioni, Bolognese, Rich Red Wine, Waitrose*	½ Pack/125g	266.0	7.0	213	12.5	28.1	5.6	2.6
Mediterranean Vegetable, Weight Watchers*	1 Pack/400g	262.0	3.0	65	2.6	12.0	0.8	1.6
Mini Spirals, in Cheese Sauce, Heinz*	1 Can/154g	120.0	4.0	78	3.9	10.4	2.3	0.3
Organic, Gluten Free, Dove's Farm*	1 Serving/100g	338.0	1.0	338	7.9	70.3	1.5	4.1
Paccheri, Finest, Tesco*	1 Serving/100g	360.0	1.0	360	13.5	72.5	1.5	1.6
Parcels, Basil & Parmesan, Fresh, Sainsbury's*	1 Serving/162g	357.0	13.0	220	10.0	26.4	8.3	3.3
Penne, Creamy Mushroom, Prepared, Tesco*	½ Pack/200g	288.0	13.0	144	4.5	17.4	6.4	3.3
Penne, Mediterranean, HL, Tesco*	1 Pack/400g	296.0	11.0	74	2.9	9.6	2.7	1.5
Pennoni, TTD, Sainsbury's*	1 Serving/90g	321.0	2.0	357	12.3	73.1	1.7	2.5
Pepper & Tomato, Asda*	1 Serving/250g	340.0	17.0	136	3.2	15.0	7.0	2.4
Pomodoro, with Tomato & Herbs, Slim Fast*	1 Serving/71g	235.0	3.0	331	21.5	51.5	4.3	6.0
Quadrotti, Pumpkin, TTD, Sainsbury's*	½ Pack/159g	287.0	8.0	180	7.6	25.8	5.1	3.0
Riccioli, Dry Weight, Buitoni*	1 Serving/75g	264.0	1.0	352	11.2	72.6	1.9	0.0
Sausage & Tomato, Italiano, Tesco*	1 Serving/450g	679.0	27.0	151	5.7	18.8	5.9	1.6
Seafood, Retail	1oz/28g	31.0	1.0	110	8.9	7.6	4.8	0.4
Spicy Tomato, Meal in 5, Ainsley Harriott*	1 Pot/386.9g	369.0	2.0	95	2.6	19.9	0.5	1.5
Spinach & Pine Nut, Finest, Tesco*	1 Pack/195g	546.0	35.0	280	6.4	23.1	17.9	1.5
Stuffed Mushroom & Emmental, Sainsbury's*	1 Pack/250g	650.0	23.0	260	11.3	33.5	9.2	3.7
Sundried Tomato, Sainsbury's*	1 Serving/50g	196.0	18.0	393	4.5	13.4	35.7	6.2
Tomato & Bacon, Value, Tesco*	1 Pack/300g	300.0	4.0	100	4.0	17.8	1.4	1.1
Tomato & Basil Chicken, Boots*	1 Serving/320g	621.0	29.0	194	9.0	19.0	9.0	1.4
Tomato & Chicken Spiralli, HL, Tesco*	1 Pack/350g	402.0	5.0	115	7.8	17.3	1.5	1.6
Tomato & Mascarpone, GFY, Asda*	½ Can/200g	128.0	4.0	64	2.1	9.0	2.2	0.0
Tomato & Mascarpone, Tesco*	1 Pack/400g	468.0	16.0	117	9.7	10.3	4.1	0.9
Tomato & Onion, Shells, Tesco*	1 Serving/193g	643.0	3.0	333	12.5	67.1	1.6	6.3
Tomato & Pepper, GFY, Asda*	1 Pack/400g	344.0	8.0	86	3.1	14.0	1.9	1.1
Tomato & Vegetable, Diet Chef Ltd*	1 Pack/300g	216.0	6.0	72	2.6	10.9	2.0	1.8
Tortelloni, Spinach & Ricotta, Emma Giordani*	1 Pack/250g	685.0	15.0	274	10.0	45.0	6.0	0.0
Twists, with Tuna, Italian, Weight Watchers*	1 Can/385g	239.0	5.0	62	4.3	8.2	1.4	0.6
Vegetable Rice, Dry Weight, Orgran*	1 Serving/66g	233.0	1.0	353	6.8	80.0	2.0	4.8
Vegetable, Creamy, BGTY, Sainsbury's*	1 Pack/400g	348.0	6.0	87	4.0	14.3	1.5	1.9
Vegetable, Mediterranean, Sainsbury's*	1 Pack/400g	504.0	12.0	126	4.0	20.9	2.9	1.8
Wheat Free, Delverde*	1 Serving/63g	229.0	1.0	366	0.5	86.9	1.9	1.2
Whole Wheat, Bella Terra*	1 Serving/100g	375.0	2.0	375	12.5	78.5	1.7	10.7
Whole Wheat, Penne, Asda*	1 Serving/100g	333.0	2.0	333	12.1	66.3	2.1	6.9
Wholewheat, Cooked, Tesco*	1 Serving/200g	284.0	2.0	142	5.7	27.9	0.9	4.5
PASTA BAKE								
Aberdeen Angus Meatball, Waitrose*	½ Pack/350g	501.0	28.0	143	5.2	12.5	8.0	0.9
Bacon & Leek, Sainsbury's*	1 Pack/400g	660.0	28.0	165	7.3	18.5	6.9	1.8

P

PASTA BAKE

INFO/WEIGHT	per Measure KCAL	FAT	Nutrition Values per 100g / 100ml KCAL	PROT	CARB	FAT	FIBRE
PASTA BAKE							
Bacon & Leek, Tesco*	1 Pack/450g	774.0	37.0	172	8.1	16.1	8.3	2.0
Bolognese, Asda*	¼ Pack/375g	514.0	24.0	137	7.3	12.7	6.3	1.8
Bolognese, GFY, Asda*	1 Pack/400g	376.0	8.0	94	5.8	13.1	2.1	0.9
Bolognese, Italiano, Tesco*	1/3 Pack/284g	409.0	14.0	144	8.7	15.7	5.1	2.3
Bolognese, Weight Watchers*	1 Pack/400g	324.0	8.0	81	6.1	9.6	2.0	1.3
Cheese & Bacon, Asda*	1 Serving/120g	168.0	14.0	140	2.9	5.2	12.0	0.3
Cheese & Bacon, Fresh Italian, Asda*	1 Serving/250g	265.0	20.0	106	6.0	2.6	8.0	0.5
Cheese & Tomato, Tesco*	1 Pack/400g	388.0	6.0	97	3.4	17.8	1.4	1.2
Chicken & Bacon, Asda*	1 Pack/400g	592.0	25.0	148	8.6	14.2	6.3	3.0
Chicken & Broccoli, Morrisons*	1 Pack/400g	452.0	16.0	113	6.1	13.3	4.0	0.6
Chicken & Broccoli, Pasta Presto, Findus*	1 Pack/321g	449.0	22.0	140	7.5	12.0	7.0	0.0
Chicken & Broccoli, Weight Watchers*	1 Bake/305g	290.0	5.0	95	6.0	14.2	1.5	0.9
Chicken & Courgette, Asda*	½ Pack/387g	519.0	23.0	134	6.0	14.0	6.0	0.6
Chicken & Leek, HL, Tesco*	1 Pack/400g	460.0	8.0	115	10.8	13.1	1.9	1.6
Chicken & Mushroom, Waitrose*	1 Pack/400g	532.0	31.0	133	6.7	9.1	7.7	0.8
Chicken & Roast Mushroom, HL, Tesco*	1 Pack/390g	413.0	0.0	106	8.6	17.6	0.1	1.3
Chicken & Spinach, GFY, Asda*	1 Pack/400g	374.0	6.0	93	5.0	15.0	1.5	1.2
Chicken & Spinach, Sainsbury's*	1 Pack/340g	286.0	9.0	84	4.9	10.0	2.7	0.6
Chicken & Sweetcorn, Eat Smart, Safeway*	1 Pack/400g	380.0	7.0	95	6.5	13.0	1.8	1.8
Chicken, BGTY, Sainsbury's*	1 Pack/400g	348.0	8.0	87	9.7	7.5	2.0	0.8
Chicken, Italiano, Tesco*	1 Serving/190g	218.0	8.0	115	8.4	11.2	4.1	3.1
Chicken, Morrisons*	1 Pack/402g	442.0	14.0	110	4.6	14.8	3.6	0.9
Chicken, Mozzarella & Tomato, Birds Eye*	1 Pack/360g	468.0	7.0	130	7.1	14.3	1.9	0.3
Chicken, Tomato, & Mascarpone, Tesco*	1 Serving/400g	448.0	8.0	112	8.0	15.2	2.1	1.7
Chilli & Cheese, American Style, Tesco*	1 Pack/425g	637.0	17.0	150	6.8	21.8	3.9	1.5
Creamy Mushroom, Dolmio*	½ Jar/245g	267.0	23.0	109	1.1	5.5	9.2	0.0
Creamy Tomato, Dolmio*	1 Serving/125g	141.0	9.0	113	2.3	8.4	7.2	0.0
Findus*	1 Pack/320g	448.0	22.0	140	7.5	12.0	7.0	0.0
Ham & Broccoli, Asda*	1 Pack/340g	309.0	14.0	91	3.4	10.0	4.1	0.5
Ham & Mushroom, Italiano, Tesco*	1 Pack/425g	646.0	20.0	152	5.8	21.3	4.8	1.7
Italian Creamy Tomato & Bacon, Asda*	1 Serving/125g	131.0	11.0	105	2.0	3.9	9.0	0.6
King Prawn & Salmon, GFY, Asda*	1 Pack/400g	420.0	12.0	105	6.9	12.7	2.9	1.2
Leek & Bacon, Morrisons*	1 Pack/401g	553.0	36.0	138	4.8	9.9	9.0	0.2
Meatball, Tesco*	1 Pack/400g	576.0	19.0	144	5.9	19.3	4.8	0.5
Meatfeast, Italian, Tesco*	1 Serving/500g	675.0	19.0	135	6.4	17.8	3.8	2.3
Mediterranean Style, Tesco*	1 Pack/450g	423.0	2.0	94	2.9	19.6	0.4	2.0
Mediterranean, Weight Watchers*	1 Pack/397g	262.0	3.0	66	2.6	12.0	0.8	1.6
Mix, Tuna, Colman's*	1 Sachet/45g	145.0	2.0	323	9.2	60.0	5.2	4.7
Mozzarella & Tomato, Asda*	1 Pack/400g	532.0	19.0	133	4.4	18.1	4.8	1.8
Mushroom, Creamy, Asda*	¼ Jar/118g	204.0	20.0	173	1.8	3.3	17.0	0.5
Penne Mozzarella, Tesco*	1 Pack/340g	408.0	8.0	120	4.7	19.7	2.5	0.6
Pepperoni & Ham, Tesco*	½ Pack/425g	501.0	3.0	118	8.9	19.3	0.6	2.5
Roast Vegetable, Eat Smart, Safeway*	1 Pack/330g	379.0	6.0	115	3.8	19.6	1.9	1.3
Roasted Mediterranean Vegetables, Dolmio*	1 Portion/125g	66.0	2.0	53	1.3	8.1	1.7	1.2
Spicy Tomato & Pepperoni, Asda*	1 Pack/440g	431.0	26.0	98	1.1	10.0	6.0	1.2
Three Bean, Asda*	¼ Jar/125g	187.0	15.0	150	2.4	8.0	12.0	1.3
Tomato & Cheese, Light Choices, Tesco*	1 Pack/350g	385.0	5.0	110	3.2	20.9	1.3	1.5
Tomato & Mozzarella, Italiano, Tesco*	1 Pack/340g	398.0	8.0	117	4.8	18.9	2.5	1.7
Tomato & Mozzarella, Light Choices, Tesco*	1 Pack/400g	368.0	8.0	92	3.7	14.8	2.0	1.5
Tomato & Red Pepper, with Crunch Topping, Homepride*	1 Jar/535g	417.0	9.0	78	1.8	14.1	1.6	0.9
Tuna & Sweetcorn, Asda*	1 Serving/250g	332.0	22.0	133	5.0	8.0	9.0	0.9
Tuna & Tomato, BGTY, Sainsbury's*	1 Pack/450g	553.0	19.0	123	8.7	12.6	4.2	0.4
Tuna Conchiglie, M & S*	1 Pack/400g	520.0	17.0	130	8.6	14.3	4.3	1.1

	Measure INFO/WEIGHT	per Measure KCAL	FAT	Nutrition Values per 100g / 100ml KCAL	PROT	CARB	FAT	FIBRE
PASTA BAKE								
Tuna, COU, M & S*	1 Pack/360g	432.0	15.0	120	8.0	11.9	4.3	0.8
Tuna, Lean Cuisine*	1 Pack/346g	380.0	9.0	110	5.0	16.0	2.5	1.5
Tuna, Light Choices, Tesco*	1 Pack/400g	380.0	5.0	95	10.8	10.0	1.3	2.2
Tuna, Tesco*	1oz/28g	36.0	2.0	129	6.9	11.7	6.1	0.9
Tuna, Weight Watchers*	1 Pack/400g	292.0	3.0	73	7.0	9.4	0.8	1.4
Vegetable, Findus*	1 Pack/331g	430.0	22.0	130	6.0	13.0	6.5	0.0
Vegetable, M & S*	1 Pack/350g	455.0	20.0	130	4.8	14.6	5.7	1.6
Vegetable, Mediterranean, Tesco*	1 Serving/450g	495.0	21.0	110	4.3	12.9	4.6	1.3
Vegetable, Ready Meals, Waitrose*	1oz/28g	44.0	2.0	157	5.9	14.4	8.6	1.0
Vegetable, Tesco*	1 Pack/380g	467.0	21.0	123	5.6	12.6	5.6	1.6
with Tomato & Mozzarella, Sainsbury's*	1 Pack/400g	480.0	13.0	120	5.0	17.9	3.2	2.1
PASTA IN								
Arrabiata Sauce, Pasta King*	1 Serving/100g	104.0	1.0	104	3.5	19.5	1.4	1.8
Basilico Sauce, Pasta King*	1 Serving/100g	123.0	3.0	123	3.8	19.5	3.3	2.1
Bolognese Sauce, Pasta King*	1 Serving/100g	121.0	3.0	121	5.1	19.3	2.6	1.9
Carbonara Sauce, Pasta King*	1 Serving/100g	122.0	3.0	122	5.1	19.3	2.9	1.2
Cheese Sauce, Pasta King*	1 Serving/100g	117.0	2.0	117	5.0	19.2	2.3	1.1
Chicken Italiano Sauce, Pasta King*	1 Serving/100g	125.0	3.0	125	5.5	18.9	3.2	1.9
Chicken, Garlic & Wine Flavour Sauce, Dry Weight, Tesco*	1 Pack/120g	438.0	5.0	365	14.2	66.8	4.3	5.0
Chilli Beef Sauce, Pasta King*	1 Serving/100g	125.0	3.0	125	5.4	20.5	2.6	2.2
Garlic & Herb, Asda*	1 Serving/120g	487.0	12.0	406	10.0	69.0	10.0	2.3
Herb Sauce, Sainsbury's*	1 Pack/420g	441.0	1.0	105	3.5	22.4	0.2	0.8
Peperonata Sauce, Pasta King*	1 Serving/100g	104.0	1.0	104	3.5	19.4	1.4	1.8
Pomodoro Sauce, Pasta King*	1 Serving/100g	109.0	2.0	109	3.6	19.6	1.8	1.8
Vegetable Chilli, Pasta King*	1 Serving/100g	121.0	2.0	121	5.2	20.9	2.1	2.3
Vegetarian Bolognese, Pasta King*	1 Serving/100g	117.0	2.0	117	4.9	19.7	2.1	1.9
Zingy Pepper Sauce, Pasta King*	1 Serving/100g	106.0	1.0	106	3.6	19.6	1.5	1.8
PASTA 'N' SAUCE								
Bolognese Flavour, Dry, Batchelors*	½ Pack/64.6g	228.0	2.0	353	15.1	67.2	2.6	3.9
Carbonara Flavour, Dry, Batchelors*	1 Pack/120g	463.0	6.0	386	14.3	71.0	5.0	3.1
Cheese, Leek & Ham, Batchelors*	1 Pack/120g	454.0	6.0	378	16.1	67.0	5.1	2.0
Chicken & Mushroom, Batchelors*	½ Pack/63g	227.0	1.0	361	14.1	72.3	1.7	2.8
Chicken & Roasted Garlic Flavour, Dry, Batchelors*	½ Pack/60g	223.0	2.0	372	12.6	73.8	2.9	3.4
Creamy Tikka Masala, Dry, Batchelors*	1 Pack/122g	426.0	3.0	349	12.7	69.5	2.2	4.4
Creamy Tomato & Mushroom, Dry, Batchelors*	1 Pack/125g	457.0	4.0	366	13.0	71.0	3.3	3.2
Macaroni Cheese, Dry, Batchelors*	1 Pack/108g	402.0	5.0	372	17.2	65.2	4.7	2.7
Mild Cheese & Broccoli, Batchelors*	½ Pack/61g	221.0	2.0	363	15.0	67.0	3.9	4.0
Mushroom & Wine, Batchelors*	½ Pack/50.1g	242.0	3.0	483	18.5	89.9	5.5	4.4
Mushroom & Wine, Dry, Batchelors*	1 Pack/132g	498.0	6.0	377	12.0	71.3	4.9	2.5
Tomato & Bacon Flavour, Dry, Batchelors*	1 Pack/134g	476.0	3.0	355	13.0	70.0	2.6	3.0
Tomato & Mascarpone, BGTY, Sainsbury's*	1 Pack/380g	555.0	7.0	146	6.6	25.6	1.9	1.3
Tomato, Onion & Herbs, Dry, Batchelors*	1 Pack/135g	455.0	2.0	337	12.8	68.5	1.3	5.8
PASTA QUILLS								
Dry, Average	*1 Serving/75g*	*256.0*	*1.0*	*342*	*12.0*	*72.3*	*1.2*	*2.0*
Gluten Free, Salute*	1 Serving/75g	269.0	1.0	359	7.5	78.0	1.9	0.0
PASTA SALAD								
& Mixed Leaf, with Basil Pesto Dressing, Tesco*	1 Pack/220g	528.0	38.0	240	4.7	16.9	17.1	0.7
Bacon, Budgens*	1 Salad/200g	570.0	48.0	285	5.1	12.6	23.9	0.7
Basil & Parmesan, Tesco*	1 Serving/50g	65.0	2.0	130	4.3	20.2	3.6	0.6
BBQ Bean, Tesco*	1 Pack/850g	1139.0	43.0	134	3.6	18.5	5.1	1.8
BBQ Chicken, Positive Eating, Scottish Slimmers*	1 Serving/240g	223.0	4.0	93	6.4	14.0	1.8	1.3
Caesar & Santa Tomatoes, M & S*	1 Serving/220g	495.0	34.0	225	5.2	15.9	15.3	0.8
Caesar, Chicken, Shapers, Boots*	1 Pack/218g	288.0	8.0	132	6.7	18.0	3.8	1.8

P

PASTA SALAD

	Measure INFO/WEIGHT	per Measure KCAL	FAT	Nutrition Values per 100g / 100ml KCAL	PROT	CARB	FAT	FIBRE
Carbonara, Waitrose*	1oz/28g	72.0	6.0	257	5.4	8.1	22.6	0.5
Chargrilled Chicken & Pesto Pasta, Sainsbury's*	1 Pack/240g	454.0	22.0	189	7.2	19.4	9.2	0.0
Chargrilled Chicken & Red Pepper, Tesco*	1 Pack/270g	553.0	24.0	205	9.8	20.3	8.9	3.1
Chargrilled Chicken, Italian Style, Fresh, Asda*	1 Pack/200g	318.0	14.0	159	7.0	17.0	7.0	0.4
Chargrilled Chicken, M & S*	1 Serving/190g	285.0	6.0	150	9.6	23.6	2.9	1.6
Chargrilled Red Pepper & Sunblush Tomato, Finest, Tesco*	1 Serving/100g	165.0	4.0	165	4.9	26.0	4.3	3.3
Chargrilled Vegetables & Tomato, Shapers, Boots*	1 Pack/175g	187.0	5.0	107	2.8	17.0	3.1	1.5
Cheddar Cheese, Tesco*	1 Pot/215g	546.0	44.0	254	5.7	12.0	20.4	0.8
Cheese Layered, Asda*	1 Pack/440g	471.0	22.0	107	5.2	10.4	4.9	2.0
Cheese, Asda*	1 Serving/40g	118.0	9.0	296	6.5	16.6	22.6	0.5
Cheese, Layered, Asda*	1 Pack/440g	647.0	41.0	147	4.5	11.4	9.3	0.0
Cheese, with Mayonnaise & Vinaigrette, Sainsbury's*	¼ Pot/50g	124.0	9.0	249	6.1	17.0	17.3	1.7
Chicken & Bacon, Tesco*	½ Pack/200g	450.0	29.0	225	6.3	16.8	14.5	3.2
Chicken & Smoked Bacon, M & S*	1 Pack/380g	817.0	47.0	215	7.5	19.0	12.3	1.9
Chicken & Sweetcorn, Eat Smart, Safeway*	1 Serving/200g	230.0	4.0	115	7.5	16.3	1.8	1.0
Chicken Caesar, Asda*	1 Pack/297g	683.0	41.0	230	9.6	16.6	13.9	2.5
Chicken Caesar, Ginsters*	1 Pack/220g	504.0	35.0	229	7.5	13.6	16.1	0.0
Chicken, Asda*	1 Pot/250g	322.0	12.0	129	5.8	15.5	4.9	1.3
Chilli & Cheese, Sainsbury's*	1 Serving/300g	384.0	17.0	128	4.3	15.5	5.6	0.3
Crayfish, Rocket & Lemon, Finest, Tesco*	1 Serving/250g	727.0	40.0	291	8.9	28.0	15.9	4.2
Crayfish, Shapers, Boots*	1 Pack/280g	269.0	6.0	96	6.0	13.0	2.3	0.7
Farfalle, Prawns Tomatoes & Cucumber, Sainsbury's*	1 Serving/260g	270.0	12.0	104	4.5	10.9	4.7	0.7
Fire Roasted Tomato, So Good, Somerfield*	½ Pack/100g	199.0	11.0	199	4.4	21.6	10.6	1.5
Garlic Mushroom, Salad Bar, Asda*	1oz/28g	59.0	5.0	212	2.5	12.5	16.9	0.8
Goats Cheese, & Mixed Pepper, Sainsbury's*	1 Pack/200g	366.0	19.0	183	6.4	18.2	9.4	1.5
Ham & Pineapple, Salad Bar, Asda*	1oz/28g	62.0	5.0	221	3.3	15.6	16.2	1.4
Ham, Sainsbury's*	1 Pot/250g	610.0	48.0	244	4.1	13.4	19.3	0.8
Honey & Mustard Chicken, M & S*	1 Serving/190g	304.0	5.0	160	8.7	26.7	2.5	1.5
Honey & Mustard Chicken, Sainsbury's*	1 Pack/190g	344.0	17.0	181	7.1	18.0	8.9	0.0
Honey & Mustard Chicken, Shapers, Boots*	1 Serving/252g	350.0	6.0	139	8.4	22.0	2.2	2.8
Hot Smoked Salmon, No Mayonnaise, Tesco*	1 Pack/275g	426.0	17.0	155	7.1	16.6	6.2	4.1
Italian Style, Sainsbury's*	1/3 Pot/84g	129.0	5.0	153	3.5	20.5	6.3	1.4
Italian Style, Snack, Asda*	1 Pack/150g	141.0	6.0	94	3.4	11.0	4.0	4.1
Italian, Bowl, Sainsbury's*	1 Serving/210g	309.0	16.0	147	3.1	16.9	7.4	1.9
Italian, Tesco*	½ Pack/225g	315.0	8.0	140	3.5	22.6	3.7	2.3
Lime & Coriander Chicken, M & S*	1 Serving/190g	370.0	23.0	195	7.6	14.4	12.2	0.6
Mediterranean Chicken, Waitrose*	1 Serving/200g	314.0	14.0	157	7.0	16.9	6.8	2.1
Mediterranean Style, Layered, Waitrose*	1 Pot/275g	190.0	4.0	69	2.6	11.8	1.3	1.0
Mediterranean Tuna, Shapers, Boots*	1 Serving/239g	232.0	3.0	97	6.2	15.0	1.3	0.9
Mediterranean Vegetable & Bean, BGTY, Sainsbury's*	1 Serving/66g	53.0	1.0	80	3.2	12.5	1.9	2.8
Mediterranean, Tesco*	1oz/28g	24.0	1.0	87	2.1	9.6	4.5	1.4
Mexican Chicken, Weight Watchers*	1 Pack/249g	284.0	4.0	114	7.8	16.9	1.7	3.6
Mozzarella & Plum Tomatoes, COU, M & S*	1 Bowl/255g	204.0	4.0	80	4.6	11.5	1.6	1.7
Mozzarella & Sun Dried Tomato, Waitrose*	1 Serving/150g	312.0	18.0	208	5.8	18.8	12.2	1.3
Pepper & Tomato, Fire Roasted, Finest, Tesco*	1 Pack/200g	260.0	8.0	130	3.7	19.4	4.1	2.5
Pepper, Side, Tesco*	1 Serving/46g	56.0	3.0	122	2.4	13.0	6.5	1.3
Poached Salmon, M & S*	1 Serving/200g	340.0	17.0	170	7.8	16.2	8.4	1.4
Poached Salmon, Sainsbury's*	1 Serving/200g	472.0	31.0	236	6.7	17.9	15.3	12.0
Prawn, Layered, Asda*	½ Pack/220g	205.0	6.0	93	4.2	12.8	2.8	2.0
Prawn, Shapers, Boots*	1 Pot/250g	250.0	8.0	100	4.1	14.0	3.1	0.4
Prawn, Tesco*	½ Pack/250g	487.0	28.0	195	4.9	18.9	11.1	2.0
Prawns, King, & Juicy Fresh Tomatoes, COU, M & S*	1 Serving/270g	256.0	4.0	95	5.1	16.4	1.5	0.9
Roasted Mushroom, Spinach & Tarragon, Tesco*	1 Pot/200g	216.0	5.0	108	4.3	17.2	2.4	0.8

P

	Measure INFO/WEIGHT	per Measure KCAL	FAT	Nutrition Values per 100g / 100ml KCAL	PROT	CARB	FAT	FIBRE
PASTA SALAD								
Roasted Vegetable, Waitrose*	1 Pack/190g	270.0	9.0	142	6.8	18.2	4.6	1.1
Sainsbury's*	½ Pack/160g	235.0	10.0	147	3.2	20.0	6.0	1.5
Salmon, M & S*	1 Serving/380g	817.0	58.0	215	6.8	12.7	15.2	0.7
Spicy Chicken, Geo Adams*	1 Pack/230g	580.0	44.0	252	5.1	14.9	19.1	2.9
Spicy Chilli Pesto, Sainsbury's*	¼ Pot/63g	170.0	12.0	272	3.8	20.1	19.6	1.6
Sun Dried Tomato Dressing, Sainsbury's*	1 Pack/320g	442.0	14.0	138	3.7	20.8	4.4	3.6
Sweetcorn, & Pepper, GFY, Asda*	1 Serving/175g	68.0	1.0	39	1.9	7.0	0.4	0.0
Sweetcorn, Waitrose*	1oz/28g	31.0	0.0	112	6.4	18.9	1.2	1.1
Tiger Prawn & Tomato, GFY, Asda*	1 Serving/200g	250.0	6.0	125	4.6	20.0	2.9	2.0
Tiger Prawn, Waitrose*	1 Serving/225g	544.0	38.0	242	5.4	16.7	17.1	0.4
Tomato & Basil Chicken, M & S*	1 Serving/279g	446.0	22.0	160	7.0	14.8	7.9	1.8
Tomato & Basil with Red & Green Pepper, Sainsbury's*	¼ Pot/63g	89.0	4.0	141	3.2	16.4	6.9	3.8
Tomato & Basil, M & S*	1 Pot/225g	484.0	36.0	215	2.9	15.0	15.9	1.2
Tomato & Basil, Perfectly Balanced, Waitrose*	1 Serving/100g	97.0	2.0	97	3.7	16.8	1.7	0.0
Tomato & Basil, Pot, HL, Tesco*	1 Pot/200g	242.0	5.0	121	2.0	22.1	2.7	2.2
Tomato & Basil, Sainsbury's*	1 Serving/62g	87.0	4.0	141	3.2	16.4	6.9	3.8
Tomato & Chargrilled Vegetable, Tesco*	1 Serving/200g	248.0	8.0	124	3.7	18.6	3.9	1.4
Tomato & Mozzarella, Leaf, Shapers, Boots*	1 Pack/185g	356.0	22.0	192	5.1	16.0	12.0	2.5
Tomato & Mozzarella, Sainsbury's*	1 Pack/200g	440.0	23.0	220	7.5	22.2	11.3	1.3
Tomato & Mozzarella, Waitrose*	1 Pack/225g	380.0	28.0	169	4.3	10.0	12.4	0.6
Tomato & Pepper, HL, Tesco*	1 Serving/200g	162.0	3.0	81	2.6	13.9	1.6	1.4
Tomato & Tuna, Snack, Sainsbury's*	1 Serving/200g	238.0	2.0	119	5.3	21.7	1.2	1.2
Tomato, Bacon & Cheese, Ginsters*	1 Pack/220g	381.0	20.0	173	7.4	15.6	9.0	0.0
Tuna & Spinach, COU, M & S*	1 Pack/270g	256.0	5.0	95	6.8	14.3	1.8	3.8
Tuna & Sweetcorn, COU, M & S*	1 Pack/200g	210.0	2.0	105	7.1	18.3	0.9	1.2
Tuna & Sweetcorn, Sainsbury's*	1 Serving/100g	111.0	1.0	111	7.1	18.3	1.2	1.2
Tuna Crunch, Shapers, Boots*	1 Pack/250g	352.0	7.0	141	9.8	19.0	2.7	2.8
Tuna Nicoise, Waitrose*	1 Pot/190g	306.0	17.0	161	5.1	14.9	9.0	1.1
Tuna, Arrabbiata, BGTY, Sainsbury's*	1 Serving/200g	196.0	3.0	98	6.8	14.7	1.3	0.0
Tuna, Mediterranean, Johnsons*	1 Serving/225g	148.0	6.0	66	2.8	7.5	2.8	0.9
Tuna, Perfectly Balanced, Waitrose*	1 Tub/190g	180.0	4.0	95	7.0	11.5	2.3	1.1
Tuna, Tesco*	1 Pot/300g	399.0	22.0	133	6.2	10.5	7.3	0.0
PASTA SAUCE								
Amatriciana, Asda*	1 Jar/320g	496.0	42.0	155	4.4	5.0	13.0	1.0
Amatriciana, Italiano, Tesco*	½ Pot/175g	124.0	7.0	71	4.1	5.3	3.8	0.9
Amatriciana, M & S*	1 Jar/340g	425.0	32.0	125	3.4	6.3	9.5	2.9
Amatriciana, Tesco*	1 Serving/175g	108.0	7.0	62	2.3	4.0	4.1	0.7
Arrabbiata, Barilla*	1 Serving/100g	47.0	3.0	47	1.5	3.5	3.0	0.0
Arrabbiata, Fresh, Morrisons*	1 Pot/350g	139.0	5.0	40	1.9	5.4	1.5	0.0
Arrabbiata, GFY, Asda*	1 Serving/350g	133.0	4.0	38	1.1	6.0	1.1	0.0
Arrabbiata, Italian, Waitrose*	1 Jar/320g	115.0	3.0	36	1.5	6.7	1.0	1.4
Arrabbiata, M & S*	1 Jar/320g	240.0	17.0	75	1.2	6.2	5.3	0.8
Arrabbiata, Red Pepper, Sainsbury's*	½ Pot/175g	79.0	5.0	45	1.4	3.3	2.9	1.6
Arrabbiata, Romano*	1 Serving/100g	69.0	3.0	69	2.5	7.0	3.4	0.6
Arrabbiata, Stir in, BGTY, Sainsbury's*	1 Serving/75g	53.0	3.0	71	1.3	7.6	3.9	0.7
Arrabiata, Morrisons*	½ Pot/175g	148.0	9.0	85	2.5	7.1	5.1	1.6
Aubergine & Pepper, Sacla*	½ Pot/95g	237.0	23.0	250	1.8	5.6	24.5	0.0
Basil & Oregano, Ragu, Knorr*	1 Jar/500g	215.0	0.0	43	1.3	9.4	0.0	1.1
Bolognese with Beef, Tesco*	½ Can/213g	179.0	10.0	84	4.9	5.5	4.7	0.0
Bolognese, Carb Check, Heinz*	1 Serving/150g	79.0	4.0	53	3.8	3.6	2.6	0.4
Bolognese, Dolmio*	1 Serving/100g	56.0	1.0	56	1.5	9.4	1.5	1.1
Bolognese, Finest, Tesco*	1 Serving/175g	170.0	11.0	97	7.0	3.8	6.1	0.5
Bolognese, Fresh, Sainsbury's*	½ Pot/150g	120.0	6.0	80	6.0	4.7	4.1	1.2

	Measure INFO/WEIGHT	per Measure		Nutrition Values per 100g / 100ml				
		KCAL	FAT	KCAL	PROT	CARB	FAT	FIBRE
PASTA SAUCE								
Bolognese, Italiano, Tesco*	1 Serving/175g	194.0	13.0	111	5.9	4.8	7.5	0.8
Bolognese, Light, Original, Ragu, Knorr*	1 Jar/515g	196.0	1.0	38	1.4	8.2	0.1	1.2
Bolognese, Mediterranean Vegetable, Chunky, Dolmio*	½ Jar/250g	137.0	4.0	55	1.3	8.8	1.6	1.1
Bolognese, Organic, Seeds of Change*	1 Jar/500g	290.0	6.0	58	1.3	10.4	1.2	0.8
Bolognese, Original, Light, Dolmio*	1 Serving/125g	44.0	0.0	35	1.5	6.7	0.3	0.9
Bolognese, Original, Sainsbury's*	¼ Jar/136g	90.0	3.0	66	1.9	9.9	2.1	1.3
Bolognese, Spicy, Ragu, Knorr*	1 Jar/500g	220.0	0.0	44	1.3	9.6	0.1	1.1
Bolognese, Tomato, Beef & Red Wine, Fresh, Waitrose*	1 Pot/350g	301.0	17.0	86	5.4	5.3	4.9	2.0
Bolognese, Traditional, Ragu, Knorr*	1 Jar/320g	157.0	5.0	49	1.3	7.1	1.7	1.2
Bolognese, VLH Kitchens	1 Serving/380g	316.0	16.0	83	6.0	4.7	4.1	1.2
Cacciatore, Fresh, Sainsbury's*	½ Pot/150g	151.0	9.0	101	5.4	8.1	5.9	1.5
Carbonara, Creamy, Stir in Sauce, Dolmio*	1 Serving/75g	136.0	12.0	181	5.5	4.3	15.8	0.0
Carbonara, Fresh, BGTY, Sainsbury's*	1 Tub/300g	255.0	11.0	85	5.4	7.8	3.6	0.5
Carbonara, Fresh, Chilled, Finest, Tesco*	½ Tub/175g	297.0	25.0	170	5.5	4.2	14.2	0.0
Carbonara, Fresh, Chilled, Italiano, Tesco*	½ Tub/175g	201.0	11.0	115	6.1	7.2	6.5	0.1
Carbonara, Italian, Asda*	½ Pack/175g	359.0	30.0	205	7.0	6.0	17.0	0.1
Carbonara, Italian, Fresh, Sainsbury's*	½ Pot/176g	209.0	16.0	119	5.4	3.4	9.3	0.9
Carbonara, Reduced Fat, BFY, Morrisons*	½ Pot/175g	135.0	6.0	77	6.6	5.1	3.3	0.5
Carbonara, with Pancetta, Loyd Grossman*	½ Pack/170g	209.0	15.0	123	2.8	7.5	9.1	0.1
Chargrilled Vegetable with Extra Virgin Olive Oil, Bertolli*	½ Jar/250g	150.0	5.0	60	2.1	8.7	1.9	2.4
Cheese, Fresh, Perfectly Balanced, Waitrose*	½ Pot/175g	143.0	5.0	82	6.1	7.9	2.9	0.5
Cherry Tomato & Basil, Sacla*	1 Serving/96g	90.0	7.0	94	1.2	5.3	7.4	0.0
Cherry Tomato & Roasted Pepper, Asda*	1 Jar/172g	91.0	5.0	53	1.5	5.0	3.0	2.4
Chilli with Jalapeno Peppers, Seeds of Change*	1 Jar/350g	322.0	5.0	92	3.6	16.0	1.5	2.2
Chunky Vegetable, Asda*	1 Serving/250g	122.0	4.0	49	1.4	7.0	1.7	1.2
Country Mushroom, for Bolognese, Ragu, Knorr*	1 Jar/510g	347.0	11.0	68	2.0	9.5	2.1	1.2
Cream & Mushroom, M & S*	1oz/28g	45.0	4.0	160	1.5	6.6	14.3	0.6
Creamy Mushroom, Dolmio*	1 Pack/150g	166.0	15.0	111	1.3	3.7	10.0	0.0
Creamy Mushroom, Express, Dolmio*	1 Serving/150g	160.0	14.0	107	1.4	3.8	9.6	0.0
Creamy Tomato & Basil, BGTY, Sainsbury's*	½ Jar/250g	172.0	9.0	69	1.7	7.6	3.6	1.0
Creamy Tomato, Carb Check, Heinz*	1 Serving/150g	91.0	6.0	61	2.0	4.2	4.0	0.5
Fiorentina, Fresh, Sainsbury's*	½ Pot/157g	165.0	13.0	105	3.2	4.3	8.4	0.9
Five Cheese, Italiano, Tesco*	½ Tub/175g	271.0	20.0	155	6.8	6.0	11.5	0.0
for Bolognese, Extra Mushrooms, Dolmio*	1 Jar/500g	240.0	6.0	48	1.6	7.6	1.3	1.1
for Bolognese, Extra Onion & Garlic, Dolmio*	1 Serving/125g	66.0	1.0	53	1.7	9.0	1.0	0.0
for Bolognese, Extra Spicy, Dolmio*	1 Jar/500g	260.0	5.0	52	1.7	8.8	1.1	0.8
for Lasagne, Tomato, Red, Ragu, Knorr*	1 Jar/500g	215.0	0.0	43	1.1	9.7	0.0	1.1
for Lasagne, White, Light, Ragu, Knorr*	¼ Jar/122g	88.0	6.0	72	0.5	6.3	5.0	0.2
for Lasagne, White, Ragu, Knorr*	1 Jar/475g	755.0	72.0	159	0.5	5.1	15.2	0.3
Four Cheese, BGTY, Sainsbury's*	1 Serving/150g	103.0	6.0	69	2.9	5.5	4.0	0.1
Four Cheese, Loyd Grossman*	1 Jar/350g	476.0	42.0	136	2.6	4.6	11.9	0.0
Four Cheese, Sainsbury's*	1 Serving/150g	295.0	25.0	197	6.6	4.5	17.0	0.8
Garlic & Chilli, Slow Roasted, Seeds of Change*	½ Jar/175g	157.0	9.0	90	1.7	8.7	5.3	2.0
Garlic & Onion, Finest, Tesco*	1 Serving/126g	43.0	1.0	34	0.8	6.9	0.4	1.3
Garlic, Perfectly Balanced, Waitrose*	1 Jar/440g	330.0	7.0	75	2.3	12.7	1.7	2.3
Grilled Vegetables, Bertolli*	1 Jar/400g	215.0	10.0	43	1.4	4.9	2.0	1.1
Ham & Mushroom, Creamy, Stir & Serve, Homepride*	1 Serving/92g	124.0	11.0	135	1.8	5.5	11.7	0.0
Hot & Spicy, Morrisons*	1 Serving/130g	81.0	3.0	62	1.4	8.5	2.4	1.1
Hot Mixed Peppers Bolognese, Sainsbury's*	1oz/28g	18.0	1.0	66	2.0	9.7	2.1	1.5
Hot Pepper & Mozzarella, Stir Through, Sacla*	½ Jar/95g	229.0	20.0	241	4.7	7.2	21.5	0.0
Hot, Heinz*	1 Serving/200g	120.0	7.0	60	1.2	5.7	3.6	0.9
Italian Cheese, Finest, Tesco*	½ Pot/175g	171.0	9.0	98	4.8	8.4	5.1	0.0
Italian Mushroom, Sainsbury's*	1 Serving/85g	56.0	2.0	66	2.0	9.8	2.1	1.7

	Measure INFO/WEIGHT	per Measure KCAL	per Measure FAT	Nutrition Values per 100g / 100ml KCAL	PROT	CARB	FAT	FIBRE
PASTA SAUCE								
Italian Tomato & Herb, for Pasta, Sainsbury's*	½ Jar/146g	102.0	3.0	70	2.0	11.1	2.0	1.4
Italian, Amatriciana, Sainsbury's*	½ Pot/175g	136.0	3.0	78	2.6	5.7	1.7	0.5
Italian, Tomato, Mushroom & Pancetta, Sainsbury's*	½ Jar/75g	125.0	11.0	167	2.2	6.1	14.9	1.3
Italian, Vongole, Waitrose*	1 Serving/175g	115.0	6.0	66	4.2	5.2	3.2	0.7
Italian, with Tomato & Herbs, Somerfield*	1 Jar/340g	153.0	4.0	45	1.2	7.7	1.1	0.9
Layered Tomato & Mozzarella, Finest, Tesco*	1 Jar/160g	232.0	16.0	145	6.6	6.9	10.1	0.7
Light Choices, Tesco*	1oz/28g	9.0	0.0	33	0.7	6.9	0.3	1.2
Mediterranean Tomato, Asda*	1 Jar/500g	285.0	6.0	57	1.5	10.0	1.2	0.0
Mediterranean Vegetable Pasta, Tesco*	1 Serving/166g	95.0	3.0	57	1.4	9.0	1.7	1.2
Mediterranean Vegetable, Organic, Pasta Reale*	1 Pack/300g	183.0	14.0	61	1.0	3.9	4.6	0.3
Mediterranean Vegetable, Organic, Seeds of Change*	1 Jar/350g	245.0	12.0	70	1.5	8.3	3.5	1.1
Mediterranean Vegetable, Rustico, Bertolli*	½ Jar/160g	141.0	12.0	88	1.7	4.1	7.2	0.7
Mediterranean, BGTY, Sainsbury's*	1oz/28g	23.0	1.0	82	1.9	9.0	4.3	1.4
Mediterranean, Fresh, Waitrose*	1 Pot/350g	213.0	14.0	61	1.4	5.0	3.9	2.4
Mushroom & Garlic, 98% Fat Free, Homepride*	1 Jar/450g	229.0	6.0	51	1.1	8.9	1.4	0.5
Mushroom & Garlic, Deliciously Good, Homepride*	1/3 Jar/147g	109.0	7.0	74	0.9	6.9	4.8	0.3
Mushroom & Marsala Wine, Sacla*	½ Pot/85g	165.0	16.0	194	2.2	3.9	18.8	0.0
Mushroom & Mascarpone, Morrisons*	½ Pot/175g	199.0	17.0	114	2.3	4.3	9.7	0.0
Mushroom & White Wine, Knorr*	1oz/28g	27.0	2.0	98	1.0	4.0	8.0	0.0
Mushroom, Fresh, Waitrose*	1 Serving/175g	142.0	10.0	81	1.6	5.7	5.7	0.5
Mushroom, Microwaveable, Dolmio*	1 Serving/150g	160.0	14.0	107	1.4	3.8	9.6	0.0
Mushroom, Perfectly Balanced, Waitrose*	1 Jar/440g	330.0	8.0	75	2.6	11.8	1.9	2.2
Mushroom, Romano*	1/3 Jar/156g	94.0	3.0	60	1.6	9.5	1.7	0.8
Mushroom, Sainsbury's*	1 Serving/100g	66.0	2.0	66	2.0	9.8	2.1	1.7
Napoletana, BGTY, Sainsbury's*	½ Pot/151g	71.0	4.0	47	1.2	5.0	2.5	1.3
Napoletana, Buitoni*	½ Jar/200g	146.0	8.0	73	1.6	7.3	4.1	2.2
Napoletana, Fresh, Sainsbury's*	1oz/28g	25.0	2.0	91	1.9	7.9	5.8	1.1
Napoletana, Fresh, Waitrose*	1 Serving/175g	82.0	3.0	47	1.3	6.6	1.7	1.0
Napoletana, GFY, Asda*	1 Serving/175g	58.0	2.0	33	1.0	5.0	1.0	0.0
Napoletana, Morrisons*	1 Serving/175g	82.0	3.0	47	2.6	6.7	1.5	0.0
Napoletana, Sainsbury's*	½ Pot/150g	126.0	8.0	84	1.9	6.6	5.6	0.9
Olive & Tomato, Sacla*	1 Serving/95g	87.0	8.0	92	1.3	3.6	8.0	0.0
Olive, Barilla*	1 Serving/100g	92.0	5.0	92	1.5	10.3	5.0	0.0
Onion & Garlic, Tesco*	1 Serving/125g	35.0	0.0	28	1.2	5.6	0.1	2.6
Onion & Roasted Garlic, Knorr*	1 Jar/500g	210.0	0.0	42	1.3	9.2	0.0	1.1
Original, BFY, Morrisons*	1/3 Jar/200g	100.0	2.0	50	1.6	10.6	0.1	1.2
Original, Tesco*	1 Jar/300g	123.0	4.0	41	1.0	6.1	1.4	2.3
Original, with Tomato & Onions, BFY, Morrisons*	1 Serving/125g	51.0	1.0	41	1.4	6.3	1.1	1.2
Original, with Tomatoes & Onions, Morrisons*	1 Serving/100g	64.0	2.0	64	1.2	9.3	2.5	1.0
Parmesan & Pesto, Weight Watchers*	½ Jar/175g	86.0	3.0	49	1.8	6.7	1.6	1.0
Pepper & Tomato, M & S*	1 Jar/320g	224.0	13.0	70	1.6	6.1	4.2	0.9
Pomodoro, Cirio*	1 Serving/200g	116.0	5.0	58	1.4	8.4	2.3	0.0
Porcini Mushroom & Pepperoni, Asda*	½ Jar/140g	158.0	8.0	113	3.8	11.0	6.0	0.0
Porcini Mushroom Stir in, BGTY, Sainsbury's*	½ Jar/75g	57.0	3.0	76	3.8	5.7	4.2	1.9
Primavera, Fresh, Morrisons*	½ Pot/175g	152.0	10.0	87	2.4	6.1	5.9	0.0
Primavera, Loyd Grossman*	1 Jar/350g	343.0	26.0	98	1.4	6.3	7.4	0.9
Puttanesca, Italian, Waitrose*	1 Jar/350g	195.0	10.0	56	1.5	6.1	2.8	1.3
Puttanesca, Loyd Grossman*	1 Jar/350g	315.0	22.0	90	1.7	6.8	6.2	0.9
Puttanesca, M & S*	1 Jar/320g	256.0	18.0	80	1.5	6.2	5.5	1.9
Puttanesca, Sainsbury's*	1 Serving/110g	132.0	10.0	120	2.0	8.1	8.8	0.0
Red Pepper & Italian Cheese, Stir Through, Asda*	½ Jar/95g	85.0	5.0	90	2.9	8.5	4.9	0.9
Red Pepper & Plum, Finest, Tesco*	1 Serving/63g	109.0	7.0	173	3.7	14.0	11.4	5.4
Red Wine & Shallots, Bertolli*	1 Jar/500g	225.0	8.0	45	1.5	6.0	1.7	1.0

P

PASTA SAUCE

	Measure INFO/WEIGHT	per Measure KCAL	per Measure FAT	KCAL	PROT	CARB	FAT	FIBRE
Rich Tomato with Basil Pesto, Express, Dolmio*	1 Pack/170g	146.0	10.0	86	2.0	6.2	5.9	0.0
Roasted Garlic, Weight Watchers*	½ Jar/176.5g	60.0	1.0	34	1.3	6.4	0.4	1.2
Roasted Red Pepper & Tomato, Finest, Tesco*	1 Serving/145g	117.0	8.0	81	1.2	6.8	5.4	2.2
Roasted Vegetable, GFY, Asda*	½ Pot/175g	84.0	3.0	48	1.3	7.0	1.6	0.5
Roasted Vegetable, Microwaveable, Dolmio*	½ Pack/190g	103.0	4.0	54	1.4	7.6	2.0	0.0
Roasted Vegetable, Sainsbury's*	½ Pot/151g	103.0	6.0	68	1.6	6.7	3.9	0.4
Roasted Vegetable, Tesco*	1 Pack/175g	114.0	5.0	65	1.5	8.0	3.0	0.8
Roasted Vegetables & Tuna, BGTY, Sainsbury's*	½ Pot/150g	73.0	3.0	49	3.5	4.5	1.9	3.1
Romano*	1 Serving/235g	141.0	5.0	60	1.7	8.8	2.0	1.1
Rustico Mushroom, Garlic & Oregano, Bertolli*	1 Serving/100g	90.0	7.0	90	1.9	3.8	7.5	0.0
Rustico Sweet Chilli & Red Onion, Bertolli*	½ Jar/160g	146.0	12.0	91	1.7	4.9	7.2	0.7
Salsina with Onions & Garlic, Valfrutta*	1 Serving/150g	36.0	0.0	24	1.6	4.5	0.0	1.4
Siciliana, Sainsbury's*	1/3 Jar/113g	168.0	15.0	149	1.8	6.2	13.0	0.0
Sliced Mushroom, Tesco*	1 Jar/460g	161.0	1.0	35	1.3	7.0	0.2	0.8
Smoky Bacon, Loyd Grossman*	1 Jar/350g	343.0	25.0	98	3.1	5.4	7.2	0.7
Spicy Italian Chilli, Express, Dolmio*	1 Serving/170g	87.0	3.0	51	1.5	7.5	1.6	0.0
Spicy Pepper & Tomato, Sacla*	½ Jar/95g	132.0	11.0	139	1.4	6.8	11.8	0.0
Spicy Pepper, Tesco*	1 Jar/500g	245.0	5.0	49	1.7	8.4	1.0	1.0
Spicy Red Pepper & Roasted Vegetable, Asda*	1 Serving/175g	140.0	8.0	80	1.2	9.0	4.4	1.0
Spicy Roasted Garlic, Seeds of Change*	1 Serving/195g	123.0	4.0	63	1.5	9.7	2.0	1.2
Spicy Tomato, Asda*	1 Serving/155g	76.0	2.0	49	1.5	8.0	1.2	1.0
Spicy with Peppers, Tesco*	1 Jar/455g	177.0	1.0	39	1.2	7.9	0.3	1.1
Spinach & Ricotta, Asda*	½ Pot/175g	175.0	12.0	100	3.2	6.0	7.0	0.5
Spinach & Ricotta, BGTY, Sainsbury's*	1 Serving/150g	73.0	4.0	49	2.7	3.4	2.7	2.2
Spinach & Ricotta, Fresh, Perfectly Balanced, Waitrose*	½ Pot/175g	96.0	4.0	55	3.3	5.7	2.1	0.9
Spinach & Ricotta, Stir Through, Sacla*	½ Jar/95g	196.0	19.0	206	3.7	3.7	19.6	0.0
Stir & Serve, Homepride*	1 Jar/480g	187.0	6.0	39	1.2	6.0	1.2	0.0
Sun Dried Tomato & Basil, Free From, Sainsbury's*	½ Jar/172g	124.0	5.0	72	2.9	8.7	2.8	1.5
Sun Dried Tomato & Garlic, Sacla*	1 Serving/95g	177.0	14.0	186	3.0	10.3	14.7	0.0
Sun Dried Tomato, Asda*	½ Jar/159g	165.0	13.0	104	1.9	6.0	8.0	1.5
Sun Dried Tomato, Garlic & Basil, Finest, Tesco*	1 Jar/340g	493.0	39.0	145	1.8	7.7	11.5	2.3
Sun Dried Tomato, Stir In, Light, Dolmio*	1 Serving/75g	62.0	4.0	83	1.7	9.8	4.7	0.0
Sun Ripened Tomato & Basil, Dolmio*	1 Serving/150g	117.0	7.0	78	1.3	7.9	4.6	0.0
Sun Ripened Tomato & Basil, Express, Dolmio*	1 Pouch/170g	88.0	3.0	52	1.5	7.9	1.6	0.0
Sun Ripened Tomato & Basil, Microwaveable, Dolmio*	½ Pack/190g	106.0	4.0	56	1.4	7.9	2.1	0.0
Sundried Tomato & Basil, Organic, Seeds of Change*	½ Jar/100g	155.0	13.0	155	1.6	7.7	13.1	0.0
Sundried Tomato & Garlic, M & S*	½ Jar/95g	147.0	13.0	155	2.9	4.4	13.7	0.8
Sundried Tomato, Heinz*	½ Jar/150g	55.0	0.0	37	1.5	7.3	0.2	1.1
Sweet Pepper, Dolmio*	1 Serving/150g	238.0	20.0	159	1.6	8.8	13.4	0.0
Sweet Red Pepper, Loyd Grossman*	1 Jar/350g	304.0	20.0	87	1.7	7.3	5.6	1.2
Tomato & Basil, Bertolli*	1 Jar/500g	215.0	5.0	43	1.2	7.3	1.0	0.4
Tomato & Basil, Carb Check, Heinz*	1 Serving/150g	84.0	5.0	56	1.5	4.4	3.6	0.6
Tomato & Basil, Classic, Sacla*	1 Serving/100g	137.0	11.0	137	2.0	7.2	11.1	2.8
Tomato & Basil, Dolmio*	1 Serving/170g	95.0	4.0	56	1.4	7.9	2.1	0.0
Tomato & Basil, Loyd Grossman*	½ Jar/175g	157.0	10.0	90	1.7	7.9	5.7	0.8
Tomato & Basil, Organic, Pasta Reale*	1 Pack/300g	216.0	16.0	72	1.0	5.1	5.3	0.4
Tomato & Basil, Organic, Simply Organic*	1 Pot/300g	183.0	13.0	61	1.5	4.2	4.3	0.6
Tomato & Black Olive, Carb Control, Tesco*	1 Serving/110g	74.0	5.0	67	1.3	6.0	4.3	2.3
Tomato & Chargrilled Vegetable, Loyd Grossman*	1 Serving/150g	133.0	8.0	89	1.8	7.9	5.6	0.9
Tomato & Chilli, Loyd Grossman*	½ Jar/175g	154.0	10.0	88	1.7	7.3	5.7	0.9
Tomato & Chilli, Pour Over, M & S*	1 Jar/330g	231.0	13.0	70	1.3	7.6	3.8	1.8
Tomato & Chunky Mushroom, Dolmio*	1 Pack/475g	323.0	18.0	68	1.2	7.6	3.7	0.0
Tomato & Creme Fraiche, Perfectly Balanced, Waitrose*	½ Pot/177g	85.0	2.0	48	1.8	7.1	1.3	2.0

	Measure INFO/WEIGHT	per Measure KCAL	FAT	Nutrition Values per 100g / 100ml KCAL	PROT	CARB	FAT	FIBRE
PASTA SAUCE								
Tomato & Herb, M & S*	1 Jar/500g	400.0	15.0	80	2.6	10.1	3.1	1.7
Tomato & Herb, Organic, M & S*	1 Jar/550g	302.0	20.0	55	1.4	4.2	3.6	2.6
Tomato & Herb, Organic, Meridian Foods*	½ Jar/220g	141.0	6.0	64	1.6	8.1	2.8	1.1
Tomato & Herb, Perfectly Balanced, Waitrose*	½ Tub/175.7g	65.0	2.0	37	1.3	5.3	1.2	2.3
Tomato & Herb, with Extra Garlic, Sainsbury's*	½ Pot/150g	61.0	2.0	41	1.4	6.3	1.1	1.6
Tomato & Mascarpone, BGTY, Sainsbury's*	1 Pot/300g	150.0	9.0	50	2.0	3.6	3.0	3.6
Tomato & Mascarpone, Fresh, Sainsbury's*	1 Serving/150g	177.0	15.0	118	2.2	4.2	10.3	1.1
Tomato & Mascarpone, Italiano, Tesco*	½ Pot/175g	168.0	12.0	96	2.8	5.5	7.0	0.7
Tomato & Mascarpone, Pasta Reale*	1 Pack/300g	318.0	24.0	106	2.9	5.9	7.9	0.5
Tomato & Mascarpone, Sacla*	½ Jar/95g	161.0	14.0	169	2.2	6.2	15.0	0.0
Tomato & Mascarpone, Waitrose*	½ Pot/175g	184.0	15.0	105	1.9	5.5	8.4	1.1
Tomato & Mushroom, Organic, Sainsbury's*	1 Serving/150g	87.0	4.0	58	1.6	7.1	2.6	1.5
Tomato & Olives, La Doria*	1 Jar/90g	76.0	6.0	84	1.2	5.0	6.6	0.0
Tomato & Parmesan, Seeds of Change*	1 Serving/150g	100.0	4.0	67	2.5	7.8	2.9	1.1
Tomato & Pesto, Planet Cook, Heinz*	1 Jar/300g	237.0	17.0	79	1.7	5.2	5.7	1.0
Tomato & Ricotta, Italian, Sainsbury's*	1 Pack/390g	238.0	12.0	61	2.5	6.1	3.0	1.2
Tomato & Roasted Garlic, Loyd Grossman*	½ Jar/175g	161.0	10.0	92	2.0	8.8	5.5	0.8
Tomato & Smokey Bacon, Dolmio*	1 Pot/150g	240.0	20.0	160	5.5	5.8	13.1	0.0
Tomato & Spicy Sausages, M & S*	1 Jar/330g	214.0	10.0	65	4.0	5.5	3.0	0.8
Tomato & Tuna, Loyd Grossman*	½ Jar/175g	154.0	8.0	88	4.4	7.5	4.4	0.8
Tomato & Wild Mushroom, Loyd Grossman*	½ Jar/175g	154.0	10.0	88	2.1	7.4	5.6	1.5
Tomato & Wild Mushroom, Waitrose*	1 Serving/175g	65.0	1.0	37	1.7	6.0	0.7	0.9
Tomato Bacon, Stir & Serve, Homepride*	1 Serving/96g	81.0	4.0	84	2.7	8.1	4.5	0.0
Tomato, Bacon & Mushroom, Asda*	½ Pot/50g	33.0	2.0	66	2.5	6.0	3.6	0.0
Tomato, Basil & Parmesan Stir in, BGTY, Sainsbury's*	1 Serving/75g	69.0	4.0	92	2.9	7.8	5.5	1.0
Tomato, Black Olive, Caper, Finest, Tesco*	1 Serving/145g	146.0	11.0	101	1.5	6.4	7.7	3.3
Tomato, Blue Parrot Cafe, Sainsbury's*	1/3 Jar/63g	91.0	6.0	144	3.6	11.5	9.3	1.9
Tomato, Chilli & Onion, Bertolli*	1 Serving/100g	49.0	2.0	49	1.8	6.7	1.7	1.8
Tomato, Garlic & Chilli, Finest, Tesco*	1 Serving/145g	199.0	16.0	137	2.0	7.1	11.2	3.4
Tomato, Ginger & Basil, Cranks*	½ Jar/175g	129.0	8.0	74	1.7	6.3	4.7	1.1
Tomato, Mushroom & Roasted Garlic, Bertolli*	1 Jar/500g	235.0	9.0	47	1.9	5.3	1.9	0.0
Tomato, Organic, Evernat*	1oz/28g	18.0	0.0	64	2.8	10.2	1.3	0.0
Tomato, Pecorino Romano Cheese & Garlic, Bertolli*	1 Serving/125g	76.0	3.0	61	2.3	6.5	2.8	0.9
Tomato, Red Pepper and Chilli, Slow Cooked, Dress Italian*	1 Jar/350g	318.0	22.0	91	1.9	6.6	6.4	1.3
Tomato, Red Wine, Shallots, Bertolli*	½ Jar/250g	112.0	4.0	45	1.7	7.2	1.7	1.5
Tomato, with Red Wine & Herbs, Ragu, Knorr*	1 Jar/500g	215.0	0.0	43	1.3	9.3	0.1	1.1
Vegetable & Garlic, Dolmio*	1 Serving/150g	108.0	6.0	72	1.3	7.4	4.1	0.0
Vegetable, Chunky, Tesco*	1 Jar/455g	223.0	6.0	49	0.7	8.6	1.3	1.1
Veneziana, M & S*	½ Jar/140g	196.0	15.0	140	5.7	5.5	10.7	1.6
Vine Ripened Tomato & Black Olive, Bertolli*	½ Jar/93g	145.0	12.0	157	2.3	7.3	13.3	0.0
Whole Cherry Tomato & Roasted Pepper, Sacla*	½ Jar/145g	93.0	6.0	64	1.5	5.2	4.1	0.0
Wild Mushroom & Herb, Seeds of Change*	1 Serving/190g	103.0	3.0	54	1.6	8.8	1.4	1.2
PASTA SHAPES								
Alphabetti, in Tomato Sauce, Heinz*	1 Can/200g	118.0	1.0	59	1.8	11.7	0.5	1.5
Bob The Builder, in Tomato Sauce, Heinz*	1 Can/205g	111.0	1.0	54	1.7	11.3	0.3	1.5
Cooked, Tesco*	1 Serving/260g	356.0	2.0	137	5.1	26.3	0.8	1.1
Disney Princess, in Tomato Sauce, Heinz*	1 Can/200g	114.0	1.0	57	1.8	11.9	0.3	1.5
Dried, Tesco*	1 Serving/100g	345.0	2.0	345	13.2	68.5	2.0	2.9
Durum Wheat, Dry, Basics, Sainsbury's*	1 Serving/75g	259.0	1.0	346	12.0	70.0	2.0	4.0
Funky Fish, in Tomato Sauce, Heinz*	1 Can/200g	108.0	1.0	54	1.4	11.6	0.3	0.4
in a Cheese & Broccoli Sauce, Tesco*	1 Serving/84g	317.0	6.0	377	13.1	66.2	6.6	4.1
Pirates of the Caribbean, with Cannon Balls, Heinz*	1 Can/200g	182.0	7.0	91	4.2	10.9	3.3	1.5
Postman Pat, HP*	1 Can/410g	279.0	2.0	68	1.8	14.3	0.4	0.7

	Measure INFO/WEIGHT	per Measure KCAL	FAT	Nutrition Values per 100g / 100ml KCAL	PROT	CARB	FAT	FIBRE
PASTA SHAPES								
Scooby Doo, HP*	1 Can/410g	279.0	2.0	68	1.8	14.3	0.4	0.7
Shrek, Multigrain, in Tomato Sauce, with Omega 3, Heinz*	1 Can/200g	120.0	1.0	60	1.9	12.0	0.5	1.5
Spiderman, in Tomato Sauce, Heinz*	½ Can/200g	114.0	1.0	57	1.7	11.4	0.5	1.5
Spiderman, with Mini Sausages, in Tomato Sauce, Heinz*	1 Can/200g	178.0	6.0	89	3.6	11.6	3.1	0.5
Teletubbies, in Tomato Sauce, Heinz*	1 Can/400g	244.0	2.0	61	2.0	12.3	0.4	0.6
Thomas Tank Engine, in Tomato Sauce, Heinz*	1 Can/205g	109.0	0.0	53	1.7	11.0	0.2	0.5
Tweenies, in Tomato Sauce, Heinz*	1 Can/205g	121.0	1.0	59	1.8	11.7	0.5	1.5
PASTA SHELLS								
Dry, Average	**1 Serving/75g**	**265.0**	**1.0**	**353**	**11.1**	**71.8**	**2.0**	**2.0**
Egg, Fresh, Average	**1 Serving/125g**	**344.0**	**4.0**	**275**	**11.5**	**49.7**	**2.8**	**3.4**
Fresh, Dry, Average	**1 Serving/125g**	**216.0**	**2.0**	**173**	**7.4**	**32.0**	**1.6**	**1.5**
PASTA SPIRALS								
Co-Op*	1 Serving/100g	350.0	1.0	350	12.0	73.0	1.0	3.0
Glutenfree, Glutano*	1oz/28g	100.0	0.0	357	4.0	83.0	1.0	0.0
PASTA TWIRLS								
Dry, Asda*	1 Serving/50g	173.0	1.0	346	12.0	71.0	1.5	3.0
Tri-Colour, Sainsbury's*	1 Serving/75g	268.0	1.0	357	12.3	73.1	1.7	2.5
PASTA TWISTS								
Dry, Average	**1oz/28g**	**99.0**	**0.0**	**354**	**12.2**	**71.8**	**1.5**	**2.2**
Wheat & Gluten Free, Glutafin*	1 Serving/75g	262.0	1.0	350	8.0	75.0	2.0	0.1
PASTA WITH								
Chargrilled Vegetables & Tomatoes, BGTY, Sainsbury's*	1 Serving/100g	96.0	2.0	96	2.9	17.4	1.6	0.0
Cheese & Tomato, Al Forno, Sainsbury's*	½ Pack/499g	749.0	29.0	150	5.5	18.9	5.8	1.8
Feta Cheese & Slow Roasted Tomatoes, M & S*	1 Pack/190g	332.0	13.0	175	6.0	22.3	7.0	2.5
Honey Mustard Chicken, COU, M & S*	1 Pack/300g	360.0	7.0	120	8.4	16.2	2.4	1.9
Meatballs, Sainsbury's*	1 Can/300g	339.0	15.0	113	6.6	10.6	4.9	1.6
Pesto, Spinach & Pine Nuts, Tesco*	1 Pack/300g	480.0	22.0	160	5.2	17.1	7.4	1.5
Salmon & Broccoli, Lemon Dressed, Sainsbury's*	1 Serving/300g	486.0	18.0	162	6.9	20.4	5.9	2.1
Spicy Chicken, Sainsbury's*	1 Pot/300g	489.0	18.0	163	7.1	20.1	6.1	2.3
Tomato & Basil Chicken, BGTY, Sainsbury's*	1 Pack/189.4g	250.0	2.0	132	9.2	21.2	1.1	2.7
Tuna & Roasted Peppers, M & S*	1 Serving/220g	308.0	9.0	140	9.1	17.7	3.9	0.9
PASTE								
Bacon & Tomato, Tesco*	1 Serving/20g	46.0	4.0	232	14.0	3.4	18.0	0.1
BBQ Bean, Princes*	1 Serving/33g	35.0	0.0	106	5.7	19.8	0.4	0.0
BBQ Chicken, Princes*	1oz/28g	69.0	5.0	246	14.3	9.5	16.8	0.0
Beef, Asda*	1 Serving/37g	72.0	5.0	194	17.0	0.1	14.0	0.0
Beef, Princes*	1 Serving/18g	40.0	3.0	220	14.4	5.2	15.8	0.0
Beef, Sainsbury's*	1 Jar/75g	142.0	10.0	189	16.0	1.5	13.2	1.4
Chicken & Ham, Asda*	½ Jar/38g	82.0	6.0	217	14.0	2.1	17.0	0.0
Chicken & Ham, Princes*	1 Jar/100g	233.0	19.0	233	13.6	2.8	18.6	0.0
Chicken & Ham, Sainsbury's*	1 Thin Spread/9g	14.0	1.0	158	16.0	1.1	10.0	1.1
Chicken & Ham, Tesco*	1 Serving/19g	44.0	4.0	231	12.5	1.4	19.5	0.0
Chicken & Mushroom, Princes*	1 Serving/50g	93.0	5.0	187	17.1	5.0	11.0	0.0
Chicken & Stuffing, Asda*	½ Jar/35g	71.0	5.0	203	16.0	3.3	14.0	0.0
Chicken & Stuffing, Princes*	1 Jar/100g	229.0	17.0	229	15.7	3.3	17.0	0.0
Chicken, Asda*	1 Thin Spread/7g	13.0	1.0	184	16.0	0.8	13.0	0.0
Chicken, Princes*	1 Thin Spread/9g	22.0	2.0	240	12.6	5.6	18.5	0.0
Chicken, Tesco*	1 Serving/12g	30.0	2.0	248	14.8	2.3	20.0	0.1
Chicken, Value, Tesco*	1 Thin Spread/9g	18.0	1.0	196	15.1	1.8	14.3	0.1
Crab, Princes*	1 Pot/35g	36.0	1.0	104	13.4	4.8	3.5	0.0
Crab, Tesco*	1 Jar/75g	116.0	6.0	155	14.4	4.6	8.4	0.1
Fruit, Golden Quince, Lowry Peaks*	1 Tsp/5g	16.0	0.0	321	0.8	83.6	0.2	0.0
Salmon & Shrimp, Tesco*	1 Jar/75g	83.0	3.0	111	15.1	5.0	3.4	0.1

	Measure INFO/WEIGHT	per Measure KCAL	FAT	Nutrition Values per 100g / 100ml KCAL	PROT	CARB	FAT	FIBRE
PASTE								
Salmon, Asda*	1 Serving/53g	76.0	4.0	143	15.0	5.0	7.0	0.0
Salmon, Princes*	1 Serving/30g	58.0	4.0	195	13.5	6.5	12.8	0.0
Salmon, Value, Tesco*	1 Serving/10g	16.0	1.0	165	14.0	4.6	10.1	0.8
Sardine & Tomato, Asda*	1 Thin Spread/9g	11.0	1.0	123	14.0	3.3	6.0	0.0
Sardine & Tomato, Princes*	1 Jar/75g	109.0	5.0	146	15.4	5.0	7.2	0.0
Sardine & Tomato, Sainsbury's*	1 Mini Pot/35g	59.0	4.0	170	16.9	1.2	10.8	1.3
Sardine & Tomato, Tesco*	1 Jar/75g	97.0	4.0	130	14.6	4.8	5.8	0.1
Smokey Bacon, Princes*	1 Serving/30g	60.0	4.0	199	17.3	5.4	12.0	0.0
Tagine, Lemon, Spicy, Al'fez*	1 Tsp/6g	13.0	1.0	216	3.1	17.6	14.8	4.6
Tuna & Mayonnaise, Princes*	1 Pot/75g	86.0	12.0	115	16.8	3.8	16.4	0.0
Tuna & Mayonnaise, Sainsbury's*	1 Tbsp/17g	41.0	3.0	242	19.2	0.6	18.1	1.6
Tuna & Mayonnaise, Tesco*	1 Serving/15g	31.0	2.0	209	14.9	2.1	15.7	0.1
Vegetable, Sainsbury's*	1 Serving/17g	26.0	2.0	154	7.4	5.9	11.2	3.4
PASTILLES								
Blackcurrant, Rowntree's*	1 Tube/53.3g	188.0	0.0	353	4.4	84.0	0.0	0.0
Fruit, Average	1 Tube/33g	108.0	0.0	327	2.8	84.2	0.0	0.0
Fruit, Rowntree's*	1 Tube/53g	186.0	0.0	351	4.4	83.7	0.0	0.0
Wine, Maynards*	1 Pack/52g	161.0	0.0	310	3.9	72.1	0.0	0.0
PASTRAMI								
Beef, Average	*1 Serving/40g*	*51.0*	*1.0*	*128*	*23.1*	*1.1*	*3.6*	*0.2*
Turkey, Average	*½ Packet/35g*	*38.0*	*1.0*	*107*	*21.8*	*1.7*	*1.5*	*0.5*
PASTRY								
Case, From Supermarket, Average	*1 Case/230g*	*1081.0*	*59.0*	*470*	*5.8*	*55.9*	*25.6*	*1.2*
Choux, Cooked, Average	*1oz/28g*	*91.0*	*6.0*	*325*	*8.5*	*29.8*	*19.8*	*1.2*
Choux, Raw, Average	*1oz/28g*	*59.0*	*4.0*	*211*	*5.5*	*19.4*	*12.9*	*0.8*
Filo, Average	*1 Sheet/45g*	*137.0*	*1.0*	*304*	*9.0*	*61.4*	*2.7*	*0.9*
Filo, Frozen, Jus-Rol*	1 Sheet/45g	105.0	1.0	234	8.1	52.1	2.7	2.1
Flaky, Chinese, Average	*1oz/28g*	*110.0*	*5.0*	*392*	*5.4*	*59.3*	*16.4*	*0.0*
Flaky, Cooked, Average	*1oz/28g*	*157.0*	*11.0*	*560*	*5.6*	*45.9*	*40.6*	*1.8*
Flaky, Raw, Average	*1oz/28g*	*119.0*	*9.0*	*424*	*4.2*	*34.8*	*30.7*	*1.4*
Flan Case, Average	*1 Case/113g*	*615.0*	*38.0*	*544*	*7.1*	*56.7*	*33.6*	*1.8*
Greek, Average	*1oz/28g*	*90.0*	*5.0*	*322*	*4.7*	*40.0*	*17.0*	*0.0*
Puff, Fresh, Sainsbury's*	½ Pack/250g	1112.0	86.0	445	5.4	28.8	34.3	1.3
Puff, Frozen, Average	*1 Serving/47g*	*188.0*	*12.0*	*400*	*5.0*	*29.2*	*25.6*	*0.0*
Shortcrust, Cooked, Average	*1oz/28g*	*146.0*	*9.0*	*521*	*6.6*	*54.2*	*32.3*	*2.2*
Shortcrust, Raw, Average	*1oz/28g*	*127.0*	*8.0*	*453*	*5.6*	*44.0*	*29.1*	*1.3*
Spring Roll Wrapper, TYJ Food Manufacturing*	1 Lge Sheet/18g	54.0	0.0	300	0.0	73.0	0.0	0.0
Wholemeal, Cooked, Average	*1oz/28g*	*140.0*	*9.0*	*499*	*8.9*	*44.6*	*32.9*	*6.3*
Wholemeal, Raw, Average	*1oz/28g*	*121.0*	*8.0*	*431*	*7.7*	*38.5*	*28.4*	*5.4*
PASTY								
Beef, Port Royal*	1 Pattie/130g	299.0	13.0	230	10.2	24.4	10.2	0.0
Bite Size Pasties, Food to Go, Sainsbury's*	1 Serving/60g	226.0	15.0	377	8.2	31.2	24.4	1.5
Cheddar & Onion, Hand Crimped, Waitrose*	1 Pasty/200g	546.0	42.0	273	8.8	22.5	21.1	2.2
Cheese & Onion, Aldi*	1oz/28g	80.0	5.0	287	7.0	22.9	18.6	1.0
Cheese & Onion, Co-Op*	1 Pasty/75g	235.0	15.0	313	9.2	24.5	19.8	1.7
Cheese & Onion, Farmfoods*	1 Pasty/191g	485.0	27.0	254	6.6	25.5	14.0	2.0
Cheese & Onion, Freshbake*	1 Pastry/135g	368.0	22.0	272	5.6	25.5	16.6	1.1
Cheese & Onion, Geo Adams*	1 Pasty/150g	420.0	23.0	280	6.9	27.9	15.6	1.1
Cheese & Onion, Sainsbury's*	1 Serving/150g	486.0	33.0	324	7.4	24.5	21.8	1.3
Cheese & Onion, Tesco*	1 Pasty/150g	415.0	26.0	277	5.9	23.7	17.6	2.2
Chicken & Vegetable, Proper Cornish Ltd*	1 Pasty/255g	671.0	35.0	263	7.4	30.2	13.6	2.4
Chicken, Port Royal*	1 Pattie/130g	289.0	11.0	222	5.5	31.2	8.4	0.0
Corned Beef, Mega, M & S*	1oz/28g	87.0	6.0	310	9.5	22.3	20.2	0.9

P

	Measure	per Measure		Nutrition Values per 100g / 100ml				
	INFO/WEIGHT	KCAL	FAT	KCAL	PROT	CARB	FAT	FIBRE

PASTY

Cornish Roaster, Ginsters*	1 Pasty/130g	417.0	24.0	321	8.5	29.9	18.6	1.3
Cornish, Asda*	1 Pasty/100g	287.0	19.0	287	7.0	22.0	19.0	1.2
Cornish, BGTY, Sainsbury's*	1 Pasty/135g	308.0	13.0	228	7.7	28.2	9.4	1.6
Cornish, Cheese & Onion, Ginsters*	1 Pasty/130g	511.0	33.0	393	10.4	30.7	25.4	2.3
Cornish, Chicken & Bacon, Ginsters*	1 Pasty/227g	574.0	35.0	253	6.9	22.2	15.2	0.8
Cornish, Co-Op*	1 Pasty/75g	200.0	12.0	267	6.4	23.4	16.4	1.6
Cornish, Crimped, TTD, Sainsbury's*	1 Pasty/200g	515.0	29.0	258	8.3	23.7	14.4	1.2
Cornish, Ginsters*	1 Pasty/227g	549.0	32.0	242	5.3	23.2	14.2	3.1
Cornish, Mega, M & S*	1oz/28g	84.0	6.0	300	6.0	18.7	22.1	1.2
Cornish, Mini, Iceland*	1 Pasty/70g	215.0	15.0	306	7.0	22.1	21.1	1.2
Cornish, Mini, M & S*	1 Pasty/75g	244.0	18.0	325	7.3	21.9	23.4	1.8
Cornish, Mini, Sainsbury's*	1 Pasty/70g	280.0	20.0	400	7.3	28.1	28.7	1.5
Cornish, Mini, Tesco*	1 Pasty/24g	66.0	4.0	274	5.6	23.2	17.7	0.5
Cornish, Morrisons*	1 Pasty/200g	626.0	37.0	313	7.5	29.1	18.5	0.0
Cornish, Pork Farms*	1 Pasty/250g	672.0	41.0	269	7.7	22.8	16.3	0.0
Cornish, Safeway*	1 Pasty/170g	490.0	32.0	288	7.5	22.6	18.6	1.5
Cornish, Sainsbury's*	1 Pasty/150g	489.0	32.0	326	6.7	26.6	21.4	2.0
Cornish, Smart Price, Asda*	1 Pasty/94g	286.0	15.0	304	8.0	32.0	16.0	1.7
Cornish, Somerfield*	1oz/28g	85.0	5.0	303	6.0	28.0	18.0	0.0
Cornish, Tesco*	1 Pasty/150g	466.0	33.0	311	6.8	21.9	21.8	1.6
Cornish, Traditional Style, Geo Adams*	1 Pasty/165g	488.0	30.0	296	7.1	25.4	18.4	1.3
Cornish, Value, Tesco*	1 Pasty/150g	425.0	27.0	283	6.7	24.2	17.7	2.2
Lamb, Port Royal*	1 Pattie/130g	352.0	17.0	271	7.2	30.5	13.4	0.0
Olive & Cheese, Tapas, Waitrose*	1 Pack/130g	455.0	25.0	350	8.1	35.8	19.4	1.3
Salt Fish, Port Royal*	1 Pattie/130g	300.0	13.0	231	6.8	27.8	10.3	0.0
Tandoori & Vegetable, Holland & Barrett*	1 Pack/110g	232.0	9.0	211	4.3	29.4	8.5	1.8
Vegetable	1oz/28g	77.0	4.0	274	4.1	33.3	14.9	1.9
Vegetable, Hand Crimped, Waitrose*	1 Pasty/200g	454.0	23.0	227	4.5	26.8	11.3	2.2
Vegetarian, Country Slice, Linda McCartney*	1 Pasty/150g	373.0	20.0	249	5.6	26.5	13.5	2.9
Vegetarian, Port Royal*	1 Pattie/130g	315.0	14.0	242	12.5	24.1	10.6	0.0

PATE

Apricot, Asda*	1 Serving/50g	156.0	14.0	312	12.0	3.0	28.0	0.0
Ardennes, Asda*	1 Serving/50g	143.0	12.0	286	13.9	3.6	24.0	1.3
Ardennes, BGTY, Sainsbury's*	¼ Pack/50g	90.0	6.0	180	16.6	2.9	11.4	0.0
Ardennes, HL, Tesco*	½ Pack/87.5g	154.0	11.0	176	12.1	3.6	12.6	1.8
Ardennes, Iceland*	1 Serving/70g	223.0	20.0	318	12.0	3.4	28.5	0.5
Ardennes, Reduced Fat, Safeway*	1 Serving/50g	97.0	6.0	194	18.5	3.1	11.9	0.1
Ardennes, Reduced Fat, Waitrose*	¼ Pack/42g	94.0	7.0	224	15.4	2.6	16.9	0.5
Ardennes, Safeway*	1 Serving/50g	165.0	14.0	331	12.8	6.0	28.4	0.8
Ardennes, Tesco*	1 Tbsp/15g	53.0	5.0	354	13.3	0.5	33.2	1.2
Ardennes, with Bacon, Tesco*	½ Pack/85g	241.0	21.0	284	11.4	5.1	24.2	1.1
Asparagus, Sainsbury's*	½ Pot/58g	88.0	8.0	153	3.4	5.4	13.1	1.0
Bean Feast, The Redwood Co*	1 Serving/60g	161.0	10.0	268	7.3	21.1	17.0	3.8
Breton, Country, with Apricots, Coarse, Sainsbury's*	1 Serving/21g	60.0	5.0	285	13.5	7.0	22.5	0.5
Brie & Cranberry, M & S*	1 Serving/55g	192.0	18.0	350	6.0	7.3	33.3	1.5
Brussels Style, Organic, The Redwood Co*	¼ Pack/30g	82.0	6.0	273	15.2	8.0	20.4	1.3
Brussels, & Garlic, Reduced Fat, Tesco*	1 Serving/65g	135.0	8.0	208	16.2	8.1	12.3	0.6
Brussels, & Garlic, Tesco*	1 Serving/40g	145.0	14.0	363	8.7	6.0	33.8	0.0
Brussels, & Mushroom, Mini, GFY, Asda*	1 Pack/40g	67.0	4.0	167	14.7	2.3	11.0	3.9
Brussels, 25% Less Fat, Morrisons*	¼ Pack/43g	106.0	9.0	249	14.2	0.7	20.6	0.0
Brussels, BGTY, 50% Less Fat, Sainsbury's*	1 Serving/100g	223.0	16.0	223	14.6	5.1	16.0	0.1
Brussels, Co-Op*	1 Serving/15g	51.0	5.0	340	11.0	4.0	31.0	2.0
Brussels, Fat Reduced, Somerfield*	1 Serving/50g	96.0	7.0	192	14.0	2.0	14.0	0.0

P

PATE

	Measure INFO/WEIGHT	per Measure KCAL	FAT	Nutrition Values per 100g / 100ml KCAL	PROT	CARB	FAT	FIBRE
Brussels, Finest, Tesco*	½ Pack/85g	306.0	29.0	360	8.6	5.2	33.8	0.8
Brussels, HL, Tesco*	1 Serving/29g	66.0	4.0	229	14.4	8.4	15.3	1.8
Brussels, M & S*	1 Pot/170g	518.0	45.0	305	13.3	2.8	26.6	1.0
Brussels, Reduced Fat, Waitrose*	1 Serving/40g	92.0	7.0	229	13.2	2.4	18.5	0.5
Brussels, Sainsbury's*	1 Pack/170g	663.0	65.0	390	10.6	1.1	38.2	0.1
Brussels, Sanpareil*	¼ Pack/37g	121.0	11.0	326	13.0	1.0	30.0	0.0
Brussels, Smooth, 50% Less Fat, Tesco*	1 Pack/175g	350.0	27.0	200	14.1	1.2	15.3	1.8
Brussels, Smooth, Reduced, Tesco*	1 Serving /40g	82.0	6.0	205	10.7	4.5	16.0	0.6
Brussels, Smooth, Safeway*	1 Pack/170g	552.0	50.0	325	11.5	3.9	29.3	1.6
Brussels, Smooth, Spreadable, Sainsbury's*	1 Serving/30g	97.0	9.0	323	10.7	4.7	29.0	0.0
Brussels, Tesco*	1 Serving/28g	92.0	9.0	330	11.0	3.0	30.5	1.1
Brussels, with Forest Mushroom, Co-Op*	1 Serving/57g	180.0	17.0	315	12.0	2.0	29.0	1.0
Brussels, with Garlic, Asda*	1 Serving/50g	170.0	16.0	340	10.7	4.0	31.3	2.5
Brussels, with Herbs, Tesco*	1 Serving/25g	87.0	8.0	347	8.4	6.4	32.6	1.5
Brussels, with Wild Mushrooms, The Best, Safeway*	1 oz/28g	89.0	8.0	319	11.6	2.9	29.0	1.0
Carrot, Ginger & Spring Onion, M & S*	1 Serving/50g	72.0	5.0	145	1.5	9.6	11.0	0.9
Celery, Stilton & Walnut, Waitrose*	1 Pot/115g	294.0	26.0	256	9.0	3.2	23.0	2.2
Chargrilled Vegetable, BGTY, Sainsbury's*	½ Pot/57g	43.0	1.0	75	4.9	10.8	1.3	2.7
Chick Pea & Black Olive, Cauldron Foods*	1 Pot/113g	193.0	12.0	171	7.6	11.4	10.5	6.6
Chicken & Brandy, Morrisons*	1 Serving/44g	133.0	12.0	303	10.8	4.3	26.9	0.8
Chicken Liver, & Brandy, Asda*	1 Serving/50g	176.0	16.0	353	9.0	5.5	32.8	3.2
Chicken Liver, & Garlic, Smooth, Asda*	1 Serving/31g	119.0	11.0	388	9.0	7.0	36.0	3.2
Chicken Liver, Asda*	1 Serving/65g	131.0	10.0	202	13.0	4.0	16.0	0.8
Chicken Liver, BGTY, Sainsbury's*	1 Serving/30g	64.0	5.0	214	11.5	6.0	16.0	0.5
Chicken Liver, M & S*	1oz/28g	79.0	7.0	281	14.0	1.9	24.1	0.1
Chicken Liver, Organic, Waitrose*	½ Tub/88g	204.0	16.0	233	12.6	1.8	18.4	1.4
Chicken Liver, with Brandy, Tesco*	1oz/28g	82.0	7.0	293	11.8	3.5	25.8	1.4
Chicken Liver, with Madeira, Sainsbury's*	1 Serving/30g	84.0	7.0	279	13.1	1.9	24.3	0.0
Chicken, with Sauternes, TTD, Sainsbury's*	1 Serving/30g	114.0	11.0	381	6.5	5.3	37.1	0.6
Chickpea, Moroccan, Organic, Cauldron Foods*	½ Pot/57.5g	119.0	8.0	207	6.8	16.3	13.7	4.9
Coarse Farmhouse, Organic, Sainsbury's*	1 Serving/56g	138.0	11.0	246	13.3	3.7	19.7	0.8
Coarse Pork Liver with Garlic, Asda*	1 Pack/40g	130.0	12.0	326	13.0	1.0	30.0	0.0
Crab, M & S*	1oz/28g	63.0	5.0	225	12.1	5.9	17.3	0.0
Crab, Terrine, Orkney, Luxury, Castle MacLellan*	1 Tub/113g	250.0	21.0	221	7.3	5.5	18.9	0.9
Crab, Waitrose*	1oz/28g	59.0	5.0	209	14.5	0.5	16.6	0.0
De Campagne, Sainsbury's*	1 Serving/55g	129.0	10.0	235	16.3	1.4	18.2	0.0
Duck & Champagne, Luxury, M & S*	1oz/28g	106.0	10.0	380	8.3	8.3	35.2	7.8
Duck & Orange, Asda*	1 Serving/40g	94.0	7.0	235	16.0	2.2	18.0	0.0
Duck & Orange, Smooth, Tesco*	1 Serving/50g	188.0	18.0	377	10.5	4.0	35.4	0.5
Duck & Truffle, Medallions, M & S*	1 Serving/25g	91.0	9.0	365	9.0	4.8	35.0	1.4
Farmhouse Mushroom, Asda*	1 Serving/50g	126.0	10.0	252	13.0	5.0	20.0	0.7
Farmhouse Style, Finest, Tesco*	1 Serving/28g	83.0	7.0	295	11.9	3.6	25.9	1.0
Farmhouse Style, M & S*	¼ Pack/42g	90.0	7.0	215	14.4	1.9	16.9	1.2
Farmhouse Style, Weight Watchers*	1 Serving/37g	49.0	2.0	133	14.8	5.5	5.7	0.5
Farmhouse with Christmas Ale, Sainsbury's*	1oz/28g	67.0	5.0	239	15.4	1.6	19.1	0.0
Farmhouse with Herbes De Provence, Tesco*	1 Serving/50g	136.0	11.0	273	13.9	5.4	21.6	1.0
Farmhouse with Mushrooms & Garlic, Tesco*	1 Serving/90g	256.0	23.0	285	13.8	0.6	25.3	1.3
Forestiere, M & S*	1 Serving/20g	61.0	5.0	305	11.5	4.2	26.6	1.4
Herb, Organic, Suma*	1 Serving/25g	58.0	4.0	234	12.0	6.0	18.0	0.0
Kipper, Waitrose*	¼ Tub/28g	105.0	9.0	370	16.8	2.0	32.7	0.6
Liver & Bacon, Tesco*	1 Serving/10g	28.0	2.0	276	12.9	4.3	23.0	0.4
Liver Spreading, Somerfield*	1oz/28g	77.0	6.0	275	14.0	3.0	23.0	0.0
Liver, Value, Tesco*	1 Serving/50g	151.0	13.0	302	13.0	4.1	26.0	0.5

P

	Measure INFO/WEIGHT	per Measure KCAL	per Measure FAT	Nutrition Values per 100g / 100ml KCAL	PROT	CARB	FAT	FIBRE

PATE

	Measure INFO/WEIGHT	KCAL	FAT	KCAL	PROT	CARB	FAT	FIBRE
Mackerel, Smoked	1oz/28g	103.0	10.0	368	13.4	1.3	34.4	0.0
Mackerel, Tesco*	1 Serving/29g	102.0	9.0	353	14.3	0.5	32.6	0.0
Mediterranean Roast Vegetable, Tesco*	1 Serving/28g	31.0	3.0	112	2.4	4.3	9.4	1.2
Mousse De Canard, French, Weight Watchers*	1 Portion/50g	122.0	9.0	245	14.0	4.4	19.0	0.0
Mushroom & Herb, Somerfield*	1oz/28g	81.0	8.0	289	4.0	8.0	27.0	0.0
Mushroom & Tarragon, Cauldron Foods*	1 Pot/113g	118.0	9.0	104	2.7	5.9	8.3	1.2
Mushroom & Tarragon, Waitrose*	1 Serving/30g	46.0	4.0	155	2.8	5.5	13.5	1.4
Mushroom, BGTY, Sainsbury's*	½ Pot/58g	29.0	0.0	50	4.6	6.7	0.5	3.0
Mushroom, COU, M & S*	1oz/28g	17.0	1.0	60	2.9	7.4	1.9	0.9
Mushroom, M & S*	1 Pot/115g	224.0	20.0	195	4.2	4.8	17.5	1.5
Mushroom, Organic, Cauldron Foods*	1 Pot/113g	169.0	15.0	150	2.9	6.2	13.3	1.5
Mushroom, Roast, Tesco*	1 Serving/25g	36.0	3.0	145	3.6	3.6	12.9	4.5
Mushroom, Tesco*	1oz/28g	39.0	3.0	138	3.3	9.8	9.5	1.0
Poached Salmon & Watercress, Tesco*	1 Serving/25g	59.0	4.0	238	19.2	0.4	17.7	0.2
Pork & Garlic, Somerfield*	1oz/28g	83.0	7.0	295	14.0	3.0	25.0	0.0
Pork & Mushroom, Somerfield*	1oz/28g	95.0	9.0	339	11.0	3.0	31.0	0.0
Pork with Port & Cranberry, Tesco*	1 Serving/28g	83.0	7.0	296	12.1	4.3	25.6	0.6
Pork, with Apple & Cider, Sainsbury's*	1 Serving/50g	151.0	13.0	303	12.5	6.3	25.3	1.1
Pork, with Peppercorns, Tesco*	1 Serving/28g	84.0	8.0	300	12.9	1.4	26.8	0.7
Red Pepper, M & S*	1oz/28g	52.0	5.0	185	3.0	6.6	16.2	0.9
Ricotta, Sundried Tomato & Basil, Princes*	1 Jar/110g	343.0	32.0	312	5.2	8.3	28.7	0.0
Roasted Carrot, Ginger & Spring Onion, M & S*	1 Serving/50g	72.0	5.0	145	1.5	9.6	11.0	0.9
Roasted Parsnip & Carrot, Organic, Cauldron Foods*	1 Pot/115g	132.0	8.0	115	3.5	10.2	6.7	4.9
Roasted Red Pepper & Houmous, Princes*	¼ Jar/27g	32.0	2.0	120	4.6	12.4	5.8	0.0
Roasted Red Pepper, Oven Roasted, Castle MacLellan*	1oz/28g	46.0	4.0	163	3.3	8.2	13.5	0.8
Roasted Red Pepper, Princes*	1 Serving/35g	47.0	2.0	135	4.8	17.6	5.0	0.0
Roasted Vegetable & Feta, Cauldron Foods*	1 Pot/115g	148.0	8.0	129	4.3	10.0	7.1	2.1
Roasted Vegetable, COU, M & S*	1 Pot/115g	86.0	2.0	75	6.2	9.1	1.5	1.4
Salmon Dill, Princes*	1 Serving/70g	124.0	8.0	177	15.4	4.0	11.1	0.5
Salmon, John West*	1 Serving/50g	136.0	12.0	272	14.9	0.0	23.5	0.2
Salmon, Organic, M & S*	1oz/28g	76.0	6.0	270	16.9	0.0	22.5	0.0
Salmon, Smoked, Isle of Skye, TTD, Sainsbury's*	½ Pot/58g	133.0	10.0	231	17.5	1.8	17.1	0.2
Salmon, Smoked, M & S*	1oz/28g	74.0	6.0	265	16.9	0.0	22.0	0.0
Salsa, Princes*	1 Serving/25g	21.0	0.0	84	3.6	16.7	0.3	0.0
Scottish Smoked Salmon, Castle MacLellan*	¼ Tub/28g	62.0	4.0	220	13.5	5.6	16.0	0.0
Scottish Smoked Salmon, M & S*	1 Serving/30g	81.0	7.0	270	17.0	0.2	22.3	0.0
Smoked Mackerel, M & S*	1oz/28g	104.0	10.0	370	13.4	0.7	34.7	0.3
Smoked Mackerel, Sainsbury's*	½ Pot/57g	215.0	20.0	378	14.2	0.8	35.3	0.0
Smoked Mackerel, Scottish, M & S*	½ Pot/58g	158.0	13.0	275	15.9	0.6	23.2	0.1
Smoked Salmon, Luxury, Morrisons*	½ Pot/57g	150.0	12.0	266	16.0	0.9	22.0	0.5
Smoked Salmon, Organic, Waitrose*	1oz/28g	83.0	7.0	296	13.9	2.4	25.6	0.0
Smoked Salmon, Tesco*	1 Pack/115g	282.0	22.0	245	15.0	3.0	19.1	1.0
Smoked Salmon, Waitrose*	½ Pot/56.5g	120.0	9.0	212	17.1	0.5	15.7	0.6
Smoked Trout, Waitrose*	½ Pot/56g	130.0	10.0	232	15.8	0.9	18.4	0.6
Soya & Mushroom, Cauldron Foods*	1 Pot/115g	199.0	11.0	173	8.8	6.4	9.4	6.5
Spiced Parsnip & Carrot, Organic, Asda*	½ Pot/58g	63.0	3.0	109	3.7	10.0	6.0	2.6
Spicy Bean, BGTY, Sainsbury's*	½ Pot/58g	56.0	1.0	97	5.0	15.1	1.9	5.4
Spicy Bean, Princes*	½ Pot/55g	46.0	0.0	84	3.6	16.7	0.3	0.0
Spicy Bean, Weight Watchers*	1 Serving/37g	33.0	1.0	89	5.7	12.9	1.6	4.2
Spicy Mexican, Organic, Waitrose*	1 Serving/50g	57.0	3.0	115	6.2	8.6	6.2	3.5
Spinach, Cheese & Almond, Organic, Cauldron Foods*	½ Pot/57.5g	103.0	8.0	179	7.7	5.1	14.2	3.2
Sun-Dried Tomato & Basil, Cauldron Foods*	1 Pot/115g	189.0	12.0	164	6.9	11.1	10.2	4.6
Tofu, Spicy Mexican, Organic, GranoVita*	1 Serving/50g	108.0	10.0	216	6.0	3.0	20.0	0.0

	Measure INFO/WEIGHT	per Measure KCAL	per Measure FAT	Nutrition Values per 100g / 100ml KCAL	PROT	CARB	FAT	FIBRE
PATE								
Tomato, Lentil & Basil, Cauldron Foods*	1 Pot/115g	161.0	8.0	140	6.8	14.0	6.8	3.2
Tomato, Organic, GranoVita*	1 Tsp/5g	11.0	1.0	215	5.0	6.0	19.0	0.0
Tuna with Butter & Lemon Juice, Sainsbury's*	½ Pot/58g	209.0	18.0	360	19.0	0.1	31.6	0.3
Tuna, M & S*	1oz/28g	99.0	9.0	355	18.0	0.0	31.3	0.0
Tuna, Tesco*	1 Pack/115g	332.0	27.0	289	19.8	0.3	23.2	0.2
Vegetable	1oz/28g	48.0	4.0	173	7.5	5.9	13.4	0.0
Vegetable, Cauldron Foods*	1 Pack/113g	220.0	13.0	195	9.2	14.1	11.3	4.4
Vegetarian, with Mushrooms, Organic, Tartex*	¼ Tube/50g	101.0	8.0	203	7.7	7.0	16.0	0.0
Yeast with Red & Green Peppers, Vessen*	1 Pot/50g	111.0	9.0	222	6.0	9.0	18.0	0.0
Yeast, Garlic & Herb, Tartex*	1 Serving/30g	69.0	5.0	230	7.0	10.0	18.0	0.0
Yeast, Pateole, GranoVita*	1 Portion/30g	66.0	5.0	219	10.2	4.5	17.8	0.0
Yeast, Wild Mushroom, GranoVita*	1oz/28g	60.0	5.0	213	10.0	5.0	17.0	0.0
PAVLOVA								
Bucks Fizz Mini Champagne, Co-Op*	1 Pavlova/19g	62.0	3.0	325	3.0	38.0	18.0	0.5
Mandarin, Mini, Iceland*	1 Pavlova/22g	59.0	3.0	268	2.1	37.9	12.0	1.7
Raspberry & Lemon, Asda*	1 Serving/43g	102.0	2.0	235	2.8	46.0	4.4	0.5
Raspberry, Co-Op*	1/6 Pavlova/49g	147.0	6.0	300	3.2	44.8	12.0	1.1
Raspberry, Individual, M & S*	1 Pavlova/65g	133.0	2.0	205	4.0	41.8	2.4	0.2
Raspberry, M & S*	1 Serving/84g	193.0	8.0	230	2.3	33.3	9.6	0.3
Raspberry, Mini, Co-Op*	1 Pavlova/19g	61.0	2.0	320	3.0	56.0	9.0	0.6
Raspberry, Mini, Iceland*	1 Pavlova/21g	58.0	3.0	273	2.3	35.1	13.7	2.6
Raspberry, Safeway*	1 Serving/53g	163.0	7.0	307	2.9	44.6	13.0	0.5
Raspberry, Sara Lee*	1/6 Pavlova/55g	168.0	8.0	303	2.7	38.5	15.3	1.1
Raspberry, Tesco*	1 Serving/65g	191.0	8.0	294	2.7	41.8	12.9	1.1
Sticky Toffee, Farmfoods*	1/6 Pavlova/49g	186.0	10.0	380	3.4	47.8	19.5	0.3
Sticky Toffee, Sainsbury's*	1/6 Pavlova/60g	249.0	10.0	415	3.7	63.1	16.4	0.9
Strawberry & Champagne, Mini, Co-Op*	1 Pavlova/19g	65.0	4.0	340	3.0	40.0	19.0	0.8
Strawberry, Co-Op*	1 Serving/52g	177.0	7.0	340	3.0	50.0	14.0	0.4
Strawberry, COU, M & S*	1 Pot/95g	147.0	2.0	155	2.4	30.5	2.4	0.8
Strawberry, Farmfoods*	1/6 Pavlova/52g	152.0	8.0	292	2.3	36.9	15.0	2.2
Toffee Pecan, M & S*	1oz/28g	118.0	7.0	420	3.9	41.5	26.6	0.4
Toffee, Co-Op*	1/6 Pavlova/53g	193.0	8.0	365	3.0	52.0	16.0	0.6
Toffee, Mini, Co-Op*	1 Pavlova/18g	69.0	2.0	385	4.0	64.0	13.0	0.0
Toffee, Mini, Iceland*	1 Pavlova/19g	68.0	3.0	353	3.0	51.5	15.0	1.9
PAW-PAW								
Raw, Fresh	*1oz/28g*	*10.0*	*0.0*	*36*	*0.5*	*8.8*	*0.1*	*2.2*
Raw, Weighed with Skin & Pips	*1oz/28g*	*8.0*	*0.0*	*27*	*0.4*	*6.6*	*0.1*	*1.7*
PEACH								
Dried, Average	*1 Pack/250g*	*472.0*	*2.0*	*189*	*2.5*	*44.9*	*0.6*	*6.9*
in Fruit Juice, Average	*1oz/28g*	*13.0*	*0.0*	*47*	*0.5*	*11.2*	*0.0*	*0.7*
in Syrup, Average	*1oz/28g*	*19.0*	*0.0*	*67*	*0.4*	*16.3*	*0.1*	*0.4*
Pieces in Strawberry Jelly, Fruitini, Del Monte*	1 Can/140g	91.0	0.0	65	0.3	15.3	0.1	0.0
Raw, Average	*1 Peach/125g*	*39.0*	*0.0*	*31*	*0.9*	*7.2*	*0.1*	*1.4*
Raw, Stoned	1oz/28g	11.0	0.0	39	0.9	9.5	0.2	1.5
Slices, in Fruit Juice, Average	1 Serving/100g	49.0	0.0	49	0.6	11.5	0.0	0.5
Slices, in Fruit Juice, Tesco*	½ Can/125g	51.0	0.0	41	0.6	9.7	0.0	0.8
PEANUT BRITTLE								
Thorntons*	2 Pieces/32g	163.0	9.0	509	12.4	54.3	26.9	2.6
PEANUT BUTTER								
Creamy, Smooth, Sun Pat*	1 Serving/15g	93.0	8.0	620	24.0	17.5	50.2	6.1
Crunchy, Asda*	1 Serving/10g	61.0	5.0	611	28.0	12.0	51.0	6.0
Crunchy, Bettabuy, Morrisons*	1 Serving/10g	61.0	5.0	606	22.5	17.3	52.2	5.7
Crunchy, Budgens*	1oz/28g	166.0	14.0	592	23.6	12.5	49.7	6.9

P

PEANUT BUTTER

	Measure INFO/WEIGHT	per Measure KCAL	FAT	Nutrition Values per 100g / 100ml KCAL	PROT	CARB	FAT	FIBRE
Crunchy, Harvest Spread*	1 Serving/25g	148.0	12.0	592	23.6	12.5	49.7	6.9
Crunchy, No Added Sugar, Organic, Whole Earth*	1 Serving/25g	148.0	13.0	592	24.9	10.1	50.2	7.3
Crunchy, Organic, Evernat*	1 Tsp/10g	64.0	5.0	641	29.0	13.0	53.0	7.0
Crunchy, Organic, No Added Sugar, Waitrose*	1 Serving/12g	71.0	6.0	595	14.6	9.9	50.8	7.1
Crunchy, Organic, Tesco*	1 Serving/25g	149.0	12.0	595	23.6	12.5	49.7	6.9
Crunchy, Original Style, No Added Sugar, Whole Earth*	1 Serving/20g	127.0	10.0	637	25.7	16.8	51.1	8.7
Crunchy, Route 66*	1 Serving/10g	65.0	6.0	648	20.0	13.0	58.0	5.4
Crunchy, Sainsbury's*	1 Serving/10g	59.0	5.0	594	23.2	12.4	50.2	6.7
Crunchy, Somerfield*	1 Tsp/10g	59.0	5.0	586	24.4	11.8	49.0	7.1
Crunchy, Sun Pat*	1 Serving/50g	300.0	24.0	601	25.3	15.1	48.9	6.8
Crunchy, Tesco*	1 Serving/20g	123.0	10.0	614	27.8	12.0	50.5	6.5
Crunchy, Value, Tesco*	1 Serving/20g	123.0	11.0	615	21.5	11.7	53.6	5.4
Crunchy, Whole Nut, Organic, Meridian Foods*	1 Serving/28g	171.0	14.0	612	31.2	12.2	48.7	6.5
Extra Crunchy, Sun Pat*	1 Serving/20g	119.0	10.0	597	21.9	12.6	51.0	7.3
GFY, Asda*	1 Serving/15g	80.0	5.0	531	28.0	31.0	35.0	0.0
Organic, Rapunzel*	1 Serving/5g	31.0	3.0	613	29.0	4.5	53.0	0.0
Smart Price, Asda*	1 Serving/15g	87.0	7.0	582	23.0	10.0	50.0	6.0
Smooth Original, No Added Sugar, Whole Earth*	1 Serving/10g	59.0	5.0	595	24.6	9.9	50.8	7.1
Smooth, 25% Less Fat, Tesco*	1 Serving/15g	85.0	6.0	555	20.5	31.0	38.7	5.5
Smooth, 33% Less Fat, BGTY, Sainsbury's*	1 Serving/10g	53.0	4.0	533	22.6	31.7	35.1	6.7
Smooth, Average	1 Serving/20g	125.0	11.0	623	22.6	13.1	53.7	5.4
Smooth, Kernel King, Duerr's*	1 Serving/15g	89.0	8.0	596	23.3	12.4	50.3	6.8
Smooth, Kraft*	1 Serving/20g	127.0	11.0	636	23.1	17.6	53.5	0.0
Smooth, Light, Kraft*	1 Serving/20g	114.0	8.0	571	16.3	40.1	38.6	0.0
Smooth, Morrisons*	1 Serving/15g	92.0	8.0	616	23.1	14.5	51.8	6.2
Smooth, No Added Sugar, Organic, Whole Earth*	1 Serving/20g	119.0	10.0	595	24.5	9.9	50.8	7.1
Smooth, Organic, Meridian Foods*	1 Serving/10g	61.0	5.0	612	31.2	12.2	48.7	6.5
Smooth, Organic, Tesco*	1 Serving/15g	90.0	8.0	600	23.3	12.4	50.3	6.5
Smooth, Organic, Waitrose*	1 Serving/12g	71.0	6.0	595	24.6	9.9	50.8	7.1
Smooth, Somerfield*	1 Tsp/10g	59.0	5.0	592	24.0	11.0	50.0	0.0
Smooth, Sun Pat*	1 Serving/20g	120.0	10.0	601	25.0	15.2	48.9	6.7
Smooth, Tesco*	1 Serving/20g	123.0	10.0	614	27.8	12.0	50.5	6.5
Stripy, Sun Pat*	1 Tsp/10g	62.0	5.0	617	13.0	35.0	47.0	3.0
Whole Nut, Crunchy, Average	1 Tsp/10g	61.0	5.0	606	24.9	7.7	53.1	6.0
Wholenut, Sainsbury's*	1 Serving/15g	90.0	8.0	598	24.2	9.8	51.3	7.0
Wholenut, Tesco*	1 Tbsp/15.3g	95.0	8.0	620	24.0	12.9	52.1	6.9

PEANUT SHOOTS

	Measure INFO/WEIGHT	per Measure KCAL	FAT	Nutrition Values per 100g / 100ml KCAL	PROT	CARB	FAT	FIBRE
Cooked with Oil, Sainsbury's*	1 Pack/80g	177.0	14.0	221	10.6	4.1	16.9	2.5
Raw, without Oil, Sainsbury's*	1 Serving/80g	48.0	0.0	60	10.6	4.1	0.0	2.5

PEANUTS

	Measure INFO/WEIGHT	per Measure KCAL	FAT	Nutrition Values per 100g / 100ml KCAL	PROT	CARB	FAT	FIBRE
Chilli, Average	½ Pack/50g	303.0	25.0	605	28.2	9.3	50.6	6.8
Dry Roasted, Average	1 Serving/20g	117.0	10.0	587	25.7	11.5	48.8	6.5
Honey Roasted, Average	1oz/28g	169.0	13.0	605	26.8	23.5	47.0	5.5
Hot Chilli, Holland & Barrett*	1 Pack/100g	523.0	31.0	523	14.0	47.0	31.0	5.5
Milk Chocolate Coated, Graze*	1 Pack/35g	187.0	13.0	533	14.6	34.9	37.3	0.0
Mixed, Average	1 Pack/40g	174.0	10.0	435	15.3	37.5	26.0	4.4
Plain, Average	*10 Whole/10g*	*59.0*	*5.0*	*592*	*24.7*	*11.0*	*50.0*	*6.3*
Roast, Salted, Average	10 Whole/12g	74.0	6.0	614	27.8	7.9	52.4	4.9
Salted, Average	10 Whole/6g	37.0	3.0	609	27.0	8.3	52.0	5.4
White Chocolate Coated, Graze*	1 Pack/30g	166.0	12.0	553	14.7	37.8	39.3	0.0
Yoghurt Coated, Graze*	1 Pack/35g	189.0	12.0	540	9.9	48.1	35.1	0.0

PEARL BARLEY

	Measure INFO/WEIGHT	per Measure KCAL	FAT	Nutrition Values per 100g / 100ml KCAL	PROT	CARB	FAT	FIBRE
Boiled	*1oz/28g*	*34.0*	*0.0*	*123*	*2.3*	*28.2*	*0.4*	*0.0*

	Measure INFO/WEIGHT	per Measure KCAL	FAT	Nutrition Values per 100g / 100ml KCAL	PROT	CARB	FAT	FIBRE
PEARL BARLEY								
Raw, Average	**1oz/28g**	**99.0**	**0.0**	**352**	**9.9**	**77.7**	**1.2**	**15.6**
PEARS								
Abate Fetel, Average	**1 Med/133g**	**48.0**	**0.0**	**36**	**0.4**	**8.3**	**0.1**	**2.2**
Asian, Nashi, Raw, Average	**1 Lge/209g**	**88.0**	**0.0**	**42**	**0.5**	**10.6**	**0.2**	**3.6**
Blush, Morrisons*	1 Sm/148g	86.0	0.0	58	0.4	15.5	0.1	3.1
Cape, Quartered, Tesco*	1 Serving/100g	35.0	0.0	35	0.3	8.5	0.0	1.4
Comice, Raw, Weighed with Core	**1 Med/170g**	**56.0**	**0.0**	**33**	**0.3**	**8.5**	**0.0**	**2.0**
Conference, Average	**1 Lge/209g**	**88.0**	**0.0**	**42**	**0.3**	**10.1**	**0.1**	**2.0**
Dessert, Green, Sainsbury's*	1 Sm/135g	53.0	0.0	39	0.3	9.2	0.1	2.0
Dried, Average	**1 Pear Half/16g**	**33.0**	**0.0**	**204**	**1.9**	**48.4**	**0.5**	**9.7**
in Fruit Juice, Average	**1 Serving/225g**	**102.0**	**0.0**	**45**	**0.3**	**10.9**	**0.0**	**1.2**
in Syrup, Average	**1oz/28g**	**16.0**	**0.0**	**58**	**0.2**	**14.4**	**0.1**	**1.4**
Prickly, Raw, Fresh	**1oz/28g**	**14.0**	**0.0**	**49**	**0.7**	**11.5**	**0.3**	**0.0**
Raw, Weighed with Core, Average	**1 Lge/209g**	**78.0**	**0.0**	**37**	**0.3**	**9.1**	**0.1**	**1.4**
Red, Tesco*	1 Med/180g	65.0	0.0	36	0.4	8.3	0.1	2.2
TTD, Sainsbury's*	1 Serving/100g	40.0	0.0	40	0.3	10.0	0.1	2.2
William, Raw, Average	**1 Med/170g**	**58.0**	**0.0**	**34**	**0.4**	**8.3**	**0.1**	**2.2**
PEAS								
Dried, Boiled in Unsalted Water, Average	**1oz/28g**	**31.0**	**0.0**	**109**	**6.9**	**19.9**	**0.8**	**5.5**
Dried, Raw, Average	**1oz/28g**	**85.0**	**1.0**	**303**	**21.6**	**52.0**	**2.4**	**13.0**
Edible Podded, Whole, Raw	**1 Cup/63g**	**26.0**	**0.0**	**42**	**2.8**	**7.6**	**0.2**	**2.6**
Frozen, Average	**1 Serving/85g**	**55.0**	**1.0**	**64**	**5.4**	**9.0**	**0.8**	**4.9**
Frozen, Boiled, Average	**1 Serving/75g**	**51.0**	**1.0**	**68**	**6.0**	**9.4**	**0.9**	**5.1**
Garden, Canned, No Sugar Or Salt, Average	**1 Can/80g**	**36.0**	**0.0**	**45**	**4.4**	**6.0**	**0.4**	**2.8**
Garden, Canned, with Sugar & Salt, Average	**1 Serving/90g**	**59.0**	**1.0**	**66**	**5.3**	**9.3**	**0.7**	**5.1**
Garden, Frozen, Average	**1 Serving/90g**	**66.0**	**1.0**	**74**	**6.3**	**9.7**	**1.1**	**3.3**
Garden, Minted, Average	**1 Serving/80g**	**59.0**	**1.0**	**74**	**6.3**	**9.7**	**1.1**	**5.9**
Garden, TTD, Sainsbury's*	1 Serving/79g	54.0	1.0	68	5.9	9.0	0.9	5.5
Hand Shelled, & Baby Leeks, Sainsbury's*	1 Serving/120g	59.0	1.0	49	4.0	5.8	1.2	3.3
Marrowfat, Average	**1 Sm Can/160g**	**140.0**	**1.0**	**88**	**6.4**	**14.3**	**0.6**	**3.9**
Mushy, Average	**1 Can/200g**	**173.0**	**1.0**	**86**	**6.2**	**14.3**	**0.5**	**2.2**
Processed, Canned, Average	**1 Sm Can/220g**	**176.0**	**2.0**	**80**	**6.1**	**12.3**	**0.8**	**3.6**
Snow	**1 Serving/80g**	**24.0**	**0.0**	**29**	**3.3**	**3.9**	**0.2**	**2.1**
Sugar Snap, Average	**1 Serving/80g**	**27.0**	**0.0**	**34**	**3.3**	**4.9**	**0.2**	**1.4**
Wasabi, Average	1 Av Serving/28g	114.0	4.0	406	15.2	54.0	13.7	8.6
PEASE PUDDING								
Canned, Re-Heated, Drained	1oz/28g	26.0	0.0	93	6.8	16.1	0.6	1.8
PECAN NUTS								
Average	**3 Nuts/18g**	**125.0**	**13.0**	**692**	**10.0**	**5.6**	**70.1**	**4.7**
Honey, Golden, Graze*	1 Pack/26g	168.0	15.0	647	7.6	23.4	59.4	0.0
PENNE								
Arrabbiata, BGTY, Sainsbury's*	1 Pack/450g	414.0	7.0	92	2.9	16.5	1.6	1.9
Chicken & Red Wine, Italiana, Weight Watchers*	1 Pack/395g	249.0	3.0	63	3.7	10.1	0.7	0.6
Chicken & Tomato, Italian, Sainsbury's*	½ Pack/350g	472.0	11.0	135	7.6	19.0	3.2	1.6
Chilli & Garlic, Asda*	1 Serving/75g	259.0	1.0	346	12.0	71.0	1.5	3.0
Chilli, Asda*	1 Serving/100g	148.0	1.0	148	5.1	30.2	0.7	2.4
Cooked, Average	**1 Serving/185g**	**244.0**	**1.0**	**132**	**4.7**	**26.7**	**0.7**	**1.1**
Corn, Free From, Dry Weight, Sainsbury's*	1 Serving/100g	348.0	2.0	348	7.6	74.2	2.3	5.2
Creamy Sun Dried Tomato & Mascarpone, Somerfield*	1 Pack/500g	775.0	30.0	155	5.0	21.0	6.0	0.0
Dry, Average	**1 Serving/100g**	**352.0**	**2.0**	**352**	**12.4**	**71.3**	**1.9**	**2.7**
Egg, Fresh, Average	**1 Serving/125g**	**352.0**	**4.0**	**282**	**11.1**	**52.2**	**3.2**	**2.0**
Free From, Tesco*	1 Serving/100g	340.0	2.0	340	8.0	72.5	2.0	2.5
Fresh, Dry, Average	**1 Serving/125g**	**222.0**	**2.0**	**178**	**7.3**	**32.2**	**1.9**	**1.6**

P

	Measure INFO/WEIGHT	KCAL	FAT	KCAL	PROT	CARB	FAT	FIBRE
PENNE								
Hickory Steak, American, Sainsbury's*	1 Pack/450g	544.0	8.0	121	6.5	19.8	1.8	1.5
Hickory Steak, COU, M & S*	1oz/28g	22.0	0.0	80	5.6	11.9	1.0	1.3
Hickory Steak, M & S*	1 Pack/400g	540.0	12.0	135	6.9	19.3	3.1	1.3
in Tomato & Basil Sauce, Sainsbury's*	½ Pack/110g	118.0	1.0	107	3.6	21.8	0.6	1.1
Leek & Bacon, Al Forno, Asda*	½ Pack/300g	531.0	39.0	177	5.0	10.0	13.0	0.5
Mozzarella, Safeway*	1 Serving/400g	480.0	15.0	120	5.2	16.3	3.8	1.5
Napoletana Chicken, BFY, Morrisons*	1 Pack/350g	252.0	6.0	72	6.4	7.2	1.6	0.2
Organic, Dry, Average	*1 Serving/100g*	*352.0*	*2.0*	*352*	*12.4*	*71.6*	*1.8*	*1.9*
Rigate, Dry Weight, Average	*1 Serving/90g*	*318.0*	*2.0*	*353*	*12.3*	*72.1*	*1.8*	*1.8*
Roasted Red Pepper, GFY, Asda*	1 Pack/400g	212.0	2.0	53	1.9	10.0	0.6	0.8
Tomato & Basil Sauce, Asda*	½ Pack/314g	185.0	11.0	59	0.8	6.0	3.5	2.0
Tomato & Roasted Vegetable, Big Eat, Heinz*	1 Pot/351.3g	281.0	11.0	80	2.5	10.7	3.0	4.6
Tuna, Tomato & Olive, Asda*	1 Pack/340g	173.0	6.0	51	4.2	4.2	1.9	0.6
with Chicken & Vegetables, Eat Positive, Birds Eye*	1 Meal/396g	325.0	5.0	82	7.7	9.8	1.3	1.2
with Chilli & Red Peppers, Asda*	1 Can/400g	224.0	5.0	56	1.3	10.0	1.2	0.6
with Roasted Vegetables, Waitrose*	1 Pack/400g	424.0	16.0	106	2.8	15.0	3.9	0.8
PENNETTE								
Tricolore, Sainsbury's*	1 Serving/100g	357.0	2.0	357	12.3	73.1	1.7	2.5
PEPERAMI*								
Firestick, Peperami*	1 Stick/25g	127.0	11.0	508	24.5	3.5	44.0	1.2
Hot, Peperami*	1 Stick/25g	126.0	11.0	504	24.5	2.5	44.0	1.2
Mini, 30% Less Fat, Peperami*	1 Stick/10g	38.0	3.0	379	25.0	1.5	30.0	3.0
Original, Peperami*	1 Stick/25g	126.0	11.0	504	24.0	2.5	44.0	0.1
PEPPER								
Black, Freshly Ground, Average	*1 Tsp/2g*	*5.0*	*0.0*	*255*	*10.9*	*64.8*	*3.3*	*26.5*
Cayenne, Ground	*1 Tsp/2g*	*6.0*	*0.0*	*318*	*12.0*	*31.7*	*17.3*	*0.0*
White	*½ Tsp/1g*	*3.0*	*0.0*	*296*	*10.4*	*68.6*	*2.1*	*26.2*
PEPPERONATA								
Salmon, BGTY, Sainsbury's*	1 Pack/380g	300.0	9.0	79	5.8	8.8	2.3	0.9
PEPPERS								
Capsicum, Green, Boiled in Salted Water	*1oz/28g*	*5.0*	*0.0*	*18*	*1.0*	*2.6*	*0.5*	*1.8*
Capsicum, Green, Raw, Unprepared, Average	*1 Med/160g*	*24.0*	*0.0*	*15*	*0.8*	*2.6*	*0.3*	*1.6*
Capsicum, Red, Boiled in Salted Water	*1oz/28g*	*10.0*	*0.0*	*34*	*1.1*	*7.0*	*0.4*	*1.7*
Capsicum, Red, Raw, Unprepared, Average	*1 Med/160g*	*51.0*	*1.0*	*32*	*1.0*	*6.4*	*0.4*	*1.6*
Capsicum, Sweet, Raw, Average	*1 Serving/100g*	*16.0*	*0.0*	*16*	*0.8*	*2.6*	*0.3*	*1.6*
Capsicum, Yellow, Raw, Unprepared, Average	*1 Med/160g*	*42.0*	*0.0*	*26*	*1.2*	*5.3*	*0.2*	*1.7*
Chilli, Chopped, Stir Fry, Schwartz*	1 Tbsp/18.8g	24.0	1.0	130	2.2	15.6	6.5	0.0
Chilli, Crushed, Schwartz*	1 Tsp/0.5g	2.0	0.0	321	12.0	29.0	17.0	27.0
Chilli, Dried, Whole, Red, Schwartz*	1 Tsp/0.5g	2.0	0.0	425	15.9	56.4	15.1	0.0
Chilli, Green, Raw, Unprepared, Average	*1 Med/13g*	*5.0*	*0.0*	*40*	*2.0*	*9.5*	*0.2*	*1.5*
Chilli, Green, Very Lazy, The English Provender Co.*	1 Serving/10g	11.0	1.0	114	4.2	15.3	4.0	0.5
Chilli, Red, Chopped, In Marinade, Chef Kuo*	1 Tbsp/15g	10.0	1.0	69	1.6	11.5	4.2	5.3
Chilli, Red, Raw, Unprepared, Average	*1 Pepper/13g*	*5.0*	*0.0*	*40*	*2.0*	*9.5*	*0.2*	*1.5*
Chilli, Red, Very Lazy, The English Provender Co.*	1 Serving/15g	17.0	1.0	114	4.2	15.3	4.0	0.5
Flame Seared, with Greek Feta, M & S*	½ Tub/85g	106.0	8.0	125	3.6	5.4	9.7	1.8
Green, Filled, Tesco*	1 Pepper/150g	117.0	5.0	78	2.6	9.0	3.5	0.7
Italian Style, Sainsbury's*	1 Serving/150g	160.0	7.0	107	3.5	14.1	5.0	2.1
Jalapeno, Crushed, Schwartz*	1 Tsp/0.5g	1.0	0.0	136	15.9	56.4	15.1	0.0
Jalapeno, Raw	*1 Cup/90g*	*27.0*	*1.0*	*30*	*1.3*	*5.9*	*0.6*	*2.8*
Mixed Bag, From Supermarket, Average	*1oz/28g*	*7.0*	*0.0*	*25*	*1.0*	*4.4*	*0.4*	*1.7*
Pickled, Hot, Turkish, Melis, Melis*	1 Serving/25g	9.0	0.0	35	1.0	7.9	0.0	1.0
Ramiro, Red, Sainsbury's*	1 Serving/100g	30.0	0.0	30	1.6	5.1	0.3	2.2
Red, Filled with Feta, COU, M & S*	1 Pepper/154g	200.0	11.0	130	4.1	12.4	7.2	0.6

	Measure INFO/WEIGHT	per Measure KCAL	FAT	Nutrition Values per 100g / 100ml KCAL	PROT	CARB	FAT	FIBRE
PEPPERS								
Red, Filled, Halves, Vegetarian, M & S*	1 Pack/250g	200.0	8.0	80	2.8	12.1	3.3	1.8
Red, Roasted, Melis*	1 Serving/100g	90.0	1.0	90	1.1	18.8	1.0	0.2
Red, Sweet, Pointed, TTD, Sainsbury's*	1 Serving/100g	32.0	0.0	32	1.0	6.4	0.4	0.0
Stuffed with Rice Based Filling, Average	1oz/28g	24.0	1.0	85	1.5	15.4	2.4	1.3
Sweet, Orange, Raw, Average	*1oz/28g*	*8.0*	*0.0*	*30*	*1.8*	*5.0*	*0.3*	*1.5*
Sweet, Tinned, Sainsbury's*	½ Can/125g	45.0	0.0	36	1.1	7.0	0.4	1.7
PERCH								
Raw, Atlantic	*1oz/28g*	*26.0*	*0.0*	*94*	*18.6*	*0.0*	*1.6*	*0.0*
PERNOD*								
*19% Volume, Pernod**	*1 Shot/35ml*	*45.0*	*0.0*	*130*	*0.0*	*0.0*	*0.0*	*0.0*
PESTO								
Green, Alla Genovese, TTD, Sainsbury's*	1 Serving/30g	192.0	20.0	640	6.2	5.4	65.9	3.1
Sauce, Green, Fresh, Sainsbury's*	1 Serving/60g	328.0	32.0	546	9.4	8.3	52.8	0.1
Sauce, Green, Fresh, Tesco*	1oz/28g	141.0	13.0	505	6.5	12.2	48.0	0.1
Sauce, Green, GFY, Asda*	1 Jar/190g	338.0	30.0	178	5.0	4.3	15.6	3.3
Sauce, Green, Italiano, Tesco*	1 Serving/50g	251.0	24.0	502	9.6	5.6	49.0	1.2
Sauce, Green, Jamie Oliver*	1 Serving/25g	107.0	11.0	430	6.9	5.2	42.4	2.4
Sauce, Green, Less Than 60% Fat, BGTY, Sainsbury's*	¼ Jar/48g	61.0	5.0	128	4.2	2.6	11.2	0.0
Sauce, Green, Morrisons*	1 Serving/50g	255.0	25.0	510	10.7	4.7	49.8	0.0
Sauce, Green, Sainsbury's*	1 Tsp/5g	23.0	2.0	451	5.9	10.1	41.0	2.0
Sauce, Green, Tesco*	¼ Jar/47.5g	192.0	20.0	405	5.6	0.6	42.2	4.4
Sauce, Green, Verde, Bertolli*	¼ Jar/46g	266.0	28.0	575	5.7	4.3	59.5	0.0
Sauce, Italian Style, Stir Thru, Asda*	1 Serving/15g	55.0	5.0	369	4.4	9.0	35.0	0.9
Sauce, M & S*	1oz/28g	115.0	12.0	411	3.2	3.5	43.3	3.9
Sauce, Red, Italian, Tesco*	1 Serving/37.5g	127.0	11.0	340	8.2	8.2	30.6	1.2
Sauce, Red, M & S*	1oz/28g	93.0	9.0	331	3.6	6.9	33.2	3.5
Sauce, Red, Morrisons*	1 Tbsp/15g	47.0	4.0	311	5.7	6.6	29.0	5.9
Sauce, Red, Rosso, Bertolli*	1 Jar/185g	703.0	65.0	380	6.8	9.5	35.0	2.0
Sauce, Red, Tesco*	¼ Jar/50g	162.0	15.0	325	5.6	6.3	30.3	6.0
Sauce, Roasted Red Pepper, Sacla*	1 Serving/30g	72.0	7.0	241	4.3	4.6	22.8	5.3
Sauce, Spinach & Parmesan, Sainsbury's*	¼ Jar/46.4g	162.0	16.0	349	4.6	5.3	34.4	2.5
Sauce, Sun Dried Tomato, Sacla*	1 Serving/30g	87.0	8.0	289	4.2	5.2	27.9	0.0
PETIT FOURS								
Milk Chocolate, Belgian, Safeway*	1 Cake/11g	55.0	3.0	525	6.2	49.9	33.2	1.8
PETIT POIS								
& Baby Carrots, Safeway*	1 Can/138g	57.0	0.0	41	2.5	7.4	0.0	1.0
Average	*1 Serving/65g*	*34.0*	*0.0*	*53*	*5.0*	*6.8*	*0.7*	*3.5*
Freshly Frozen, Boiled, Asda*	1 Serving/80g	39.0	1.0	49	5.0	5.5	0.9	4.5
Frozen, M & S*	1 Serving/80g	56.0	1.0	70	5.0	5.5	0.9	4.5
in Water, Sugar & Salt Added, Sainsbury's*	½ Tin/140g	81.0	1.0	58	4.0	9.4	0.5	2.0
PHEASANT								
Meat Only, Roasted	*1oz/28g*	*62.0*	*3.0*	*220*	*27.9*	*0.0*	*12.0*	*0.0*
Meat Only, Roasted, Weighed with Bone	*1oz/28g*	*61.0*	*3.0*	*219*	*27.9*	*0.0*	*11.9*	*0.0*
Stuffed, Easy Carve, Finest, Tesco*	1 Serving/200g	540.0	37.0	270	23.2	2.2	18.7	0.9
PHYSALIS								
Raw, without Husk, Average	*5 Fruits/30g*	*16.0*	*0.0*	*53*	*1.9*	*11.2*	*0.7*	*0.4*
PICCALILLI								
Dijon, Sainsbury's*	1 Dtsp/15g	14.0	0.0	91	1.8	19.0	0.9	0.7
Haywards*	1 Serving/28g	18.0	0.0	66	1.4	13.9	0.5	0.0
Heinz*	1 Serving/10g	10.0	0.0	99	1.0	20.5	0.6	0.6
Morrisons*	1 Serving/50g	37.0	0.0	75	1.6	15.0	0.7	0.6
Sainsbury's*	1 Dtsp/15g	9.0	0.0	60	1.8	11.9	0.6	0.7
Sandwich, Tesco*	1 Serving/20g	16.0	0.0	80	0.4	18.5	0.0	1.6

P

	Measure INFO/WEIGHT	per Measure KCAL	FAT	Nutrition Values per 100g / 100ml KCAL	PROT	CARB	FAT	FIBRE
PICCALILLI								
Sweet, Asda*	1 Tbsp/15g	17.0	0.0	112	0.5	27.0	0.2	0.6
Sweet, Somerfield*	1 Tsp/10g	11.0	0.0	107	1.0	24.0	1.0	0.0
Tesco*	1 Serving/50g	51.0	2.0	102	0.5	17.8	3.6	2.0
Three Mustard, Finest, Tesco*	1 Serving/30g	40.0	0.0	134	1.3	30.7	0.7	1.0
TTD, Sainsbury's*	1 Serving/19g	13.0	0.0	67	0.7	13.9	0.9	1.8
PICKLE								
Beetroot, Branston*	1 Teaspoon/20g	25.0	0.0	123	1.2	28.2	0.3	1.6
Branston, Crosse & Blackwell*	1 Tsp/10g	11.0	0.0	109	0.8	26.1	0.2	1.1
Brinjal, Patak's*	1 Tsp/16g	59.0	4.0	367	2.2	34.6	24.4	0.9
Chilli Tomato, Patak's*	1oz/28g	27.0	1.0	95	2.5	16.0	3.2	1.5
Chilli, Branston*	1 Tsp/16g	21.0	0.0	130	0.7	30.0	0.7	1.5
Chilli, Patak's*	1 Tsp/16g	52.0	5.0	325	4.3	1.3	33.7	0.0
Dill, Cucumbers, Safeway*	1oz/28g	5.0	0.0	19	0.9	3.5	0.2	0.0
Garlic, Patak's*	1 Tsp/16g	42.0	3.0	261	3.6	20.0	18.5	1.6
Lime, Hot, Asda*	1 Dtsp/10g	12.0	1.0	123	2.2	6.0	10.0	1.0
Lime, Hot, Patak's*	1 Tsp/16g	31.0	3.0	194	2.2	4.0	18.7	0.4
Lime, M & S*	1 Tsp/16g	34.0	1.0	215	0.8	42.5	4.8	2.4
Lime, Sharwood's*	1 Tsp/16g	24.0	1.0	152	2.2	15.0	9.3	2.9
Mango, Hot, Patak's*	1 Tsp/16g	43.0	4.0	270	2.3	7.4	25.7	1.9
Mild Mustard, Heinz*	1 Tbsp/10g	13.0	0.0	129	2.2	25.7	1.3	0.9
Mixed, Haywards*	½ Jar/120g	22.0	0.0	18	1.4	2.4	0.3	0.0
Mixed, Patak's*	1 Serving/30g	78.0	8.0	259	2.3	4.7	25.7	0.8
Sandwich, Branston*	1 Tsp/10g	14.0	0.0	140	0.7	34.2	0.3	1.3
Sandwich, Somerfield*	1 Tsp/10g	15.0	0.0	150	1.0	36.0	0.0	0.0
Sandwich, Tesco*	1 Serving/5g	7.0	0.0	138	1.0	33.1	0.2	1.0
Small Chunk, Branston*	1 Serving/20g	22.0	0.0	109	0.8	26.1	0.2	1.1
Spicy, Branston*	1 Tsp/15g	21.0	0.0	140	0.7	34.7	0.3	1.3
Sweet	***1 Tsp/10g***	***14.0***	***0.0***	***141***	***0.6***	***36.0***	***0.1***	***1.2***
Sweet Harvest, Asda*	1 Serving/25g	38.0	0.0	154	0.8	37.0	0.3	0.8
Sweet, Branston*	1 Serving/30g	33.0	0.0	109	0.8	26.1	0.2	1.1
Sweet, Budgens*	1 Tsp/10g	14.0	0.0	141	0.8	34.0	0.2	0.0
Sweet, Country, Morrisons*	1 Tbsp/15g	19.0	0.0	130	0.9	31.1	0.2	0.0
Sweet, Frank Cooper*	1 Pot/20g	21.0	0.0	104	0.5	25.3	0.1	0.8
Sweet, Hartley's*	1 Tsp/16g	22.0	0.0	140	0.5	36.2	0.0	0.0
Sweet, Low Price, Sainsbury's*	1 Serving/23g	23.0	0.0	98	0.7	23.2	0.3	0.7
Sweet, Value, Tesco*	1 Serving/10g	10.0	0.0	96	0.6	23.0	0.2	0.7
Tangy, Sandwich, Heinz*	1 Tsp/10g	13.0	0.0	134	0.7	31.4	0.2	0.9
Tomato, Tangy, Heinz*	1 Tsp/10g	10.0	0.0	102	2.0	22.0	0.3	1.5
PICKLES								
Cornichons, in Sweet & Sour Vinegar, Waitrose*	1 Serving/10g	3.0	0.0	28	0.6	6.1	0.1	0.6
Mixed, Salad Bar, Asda*	1oz/28g	11.0	0.0	40	0.5	9.2	0.1	0.0
Red Cabbage, Asda*	1 Serving/50g	16.0	0.0	32	1.6	6.0	0.1	0.0
PIE								
Admiral's, Light & Easy, Youngs*	1 Pack/360g	342.0	14.0	95	4.1	10.9	3.9	0.8
Admiral's, Ross*	1 Pie/340g	357.0	16.0	105	4.8	10.9	4.6	0.7
Apple & Blackberry, Lattice Topped, BGTY, Sainsbury's*	¼ Pie/100g	256.0	7.0	256	2.8	44.4	7.5	3.1
Apple & Blackberry, Shortcrust, M & S*	1 Serving/142g	469.0	18.0	330	4.3	50.2	12.5	1.1
Apple & Blackberry, Tesco*	1 Serving/106g	287.0	12.0	271	4.2	38.4	11.2	1.7
Apple & Blackcurrant, Mr Kipling*	1 Pie/66g	211.0	8.0	320	3.3	47.9	12.8	1.2
Apple Meringue, Frozen, Sara Lee*	1/6 Pie/74g	179.0	7.0	242	2.7	37.9	8.8	1.5
Apple, & Blackberry, Fruit, Finest, Tesco*	1 Pie/95g	265.0	11.0	279	13.7	29.3	11.9	2.8
Apple, American, Iceland*	1 Serving/92g	258.0	11.0	280	4.8	39.2	11.6	2.2
Apple, Asda*	¼ Pack/107g	287.0	12.0	269	3.6	39.0	11.0	1.7

PIE

INFO/WEIGHT	Measure	per Measure		Nutrition Values per 100g / 100ml				
		KCAL	FAT	KCAL	PROT	CARB	FAT	FIBRE
Apple, Bramley, Aunt Bessie's*	¼ Pie/138g	351.0	15.0	255	2.8	36.2	11.0	1.2
Apple, Bramley, Free From, Tesco*	1 Pie/60g	185.0	5.0	309	2.5	55.4	8.6	1.4
Apple, Bramley, Individual, Sainsbury's*	1 Pie/54g	165.0	5.0	307	3.6	52.2	9.3	1.3
Apple, Bramley, Individual, Tesco*	1 Pie/61g	210.0	8.0	344	3.4	53.1	13.0	1.5
Apple, Bramley, Large, Tesco*	1/8 Pie/87g	311.0	13.0	358	3.9	51.9	15.0	1.9
Apple, Bramley, Tesco*	1 Serving/106g	284.0	12.0	268	3.6	38.8	10.9	1.7
Apple, Cooked, Speedibake*	1 Serving/120g	340.0	15.0	283	3.4	38.5	12.8	1.5
Apple, Deep Filled, Amanda Smith*	1/5 Pie/150g	420.0	20.0	280	2.8	37.4	13.2	1.2
Apple, Deep Filled, Iceland*	1 Serving/116g	332.0	15.0	286	2.5	39.2	13.2	1.1
Apple, Deep Filled, Sainsbury's*	¼ Pie/137g	374.0	18.0	273	3.8	35.6	12.8	1.6
Apple, Family, Asda*	1/6 Pie/118.5g	314.0	13.0	265	3.6	38.0	11.0	2.9
Apple, Family, Morrisons*	1/6 Pie/116g	326.0	14.0	281	3.1	39.9	12.1	3.1
Apple, Lattice, Tesco*	1 Serving/145g	325.0	13.0	224	2.2	33.2	9.2	1.4
Apple, Low Price, Sainsbury's*	¼ Pie/103g	291.0	15.0	283	4.4	33.5	14.6	1.3
Apple, McVitie's*	1 Serving/117g	316.0	13.0	270	3.0	39.0	11.0	2.0
Apple, Pastry Top & Bottom	1oz/28g	74.0	4.0	266	2.9	35.8	13.3	1.7
Apple, Puff Pastry, M & S*	1 Pie/135g	337.0	17.0	250	2.4	31.3	12.7	1.0
Apple, Ready Baked, Sara Lee*	1/6 Pie/90g	249.0	12.0	277	2.8	35.4	13.8	1.2
Apple, Sainsbury's*	1/6 Pie/118g	314.0	14.0	266	3.4	37.1	11.5	0.6
Apple, Smart Price, Asda*	1 Serving/47g	178.0	8.0	379	3.5	53.0	17.0	1.3
Apple, Sultana & Cinnamon, Finest, Tesco*	1 Slice/83g	193.0	7.0	233	2.8	35.6	8.8	5.0
Apple, Tesco*	1 Pie/47g	191.0	8.0	406	3.3	59.4	17.2	1.5
Apple, Value, Tesco*	1 Pie/47g	133.0	7.0	284	4.0	34.3	14.5	0.9
Apple, VLH Kitchens	1 Serving/50g	136.0	6.0	272	3.7	40.0	11.2	1.7
Apricot Fruit, GFY, Asda*	1 Serving/52g	162.0	5.0	311	3.3	52.0	10.0	0.0
Apricot, Weight Watchers*	1 Serving 40g	123.0	0.0	308	4.6	56.4	0.9	14.6
Banoffee Cream, American Dream, Heinz*	1/6 Pie/70g	239.0	15.0	342	3.7	33.7	21.4	3.9
Banoffee Cream, American Dream, McVitie's*	1 Serving/70g	277.0	18.0	396	4.3	36.7	25.5	0.8
Banoffee, Individual, Sainsbury's*	1 Pie/104g	365.0	21.0	351	3.2	39.2	20.2	2.2
Banoffee, Tesco*	1/6 Pie/94g	365.0	20.0	390	3.9	45.8	21.1	1.5
Beef & Kidney, Farmfoods*	1oz/28g	68.0	4.0	242	5.6	23.9	13.8	1.1
Beef & Vegetable, Macdougalls, McDougalls*	¼ Pie/114g	292.0	19.0	256	5.3	20.6	16.9	0.3
Beef Steak, Aberdeen Angus, Top Crust, Waitrose*	½ Pie/280g	476.0	24.0	170	10.0	13.4	8.6	4.1
Beef, Lean, BGTY, Sainsbury's*	1 Serving/212g	280.0	13.0	132	7.3	12.2	6.0	1.5
Beef, Minced, Aberdeen Angus, Shortcrust, M & S*	1 Pie/170.6g	435.0	27.0	255	9.3	19.3	15.6	3.0
Beef, Sainsbury's*	1 Pie/210g	535.0	30.0	255	10.3	21.2	14.3	2.0
Blackberry & Apple, Sara Lee*	1 Serving/100g	272.0	14.0	272	2.9	34.0	13.9	0.0
Blackcurrant, Deep Filled, Sainsbury's*	1 Slice/137g	440.0	19.0	321	5.8	42.6	14.1	2.2
Blackcurrant, Shortcrust, M & S*	1 Pie/142g	412.0	14.0	290	3.9	45.6	10.1	1.3
Bramley Apple & Blackberry, Aunt Bessie's*	¼ Pie/137.5g	344.0	13.0	250	2.1	40.1	9.1	2.6
Bramley Apple & Blackberry, M & S*	¼ Pie/146g	380.0	14.0	260	3.4	39.8	9.9	1.3
Bramley Apple & Custard, Lattice Topped, Mr Kipling*	1 Pie/64g	236.0	10.0	369	3.8	53.7	15.4	1.1
Bramley Apple & Damson, M & S*	¼ Pie/142g	370.0	14.0	260	3.3	39.7	9.8	2.1
Bramley Apple, Deep Filled, Sainsbury's*	1/6 Pie/120g	329.0	14.0	274	3.7	38.0	11.9	1.9
Bramley Apple, Individual, Mr Kipling*	1 Pie/66g	228.0	9.0	346	3.4	53.8	13.0	1.4
Bramley Apple, Less Than 10% Fat, Sainsbury's*	1 Pie/54g	165.0	5.0	307	3.6	52.2	9.3	1.3
Bramley Apple, M & S*	1 Pie/55g	184.0	6.0	335	2.9	57.6	11.7	1.6
Bramley Apple, Reduced Fat, Asda*	1 Pie/56g	176.0	5.0	314	3.3	55.1	9.4	1.3
Bramley Apple, Rowan Hill Bakery*	1 Pie/64g	216.0	8.0	337	3.6	51.5	13.0	1.4
Butternut Squash, Skinny, & Red Pepper, Little, Higgidy*	1 Pie/180g	367.0	24.0	204	4.2	17.2	13.1	1.6
Cheese & Onion, Hollands*	1 Pie/200g	516.0	24.0	258	6.3	30.9	12.2	0.0
Cheese & Onion, Oven Baked, Average	1 Serving/200g	654.0	40.0	327	8.2	30.4	20.0	1.2
Cheese & Potato	1oz/28g	39.0	2.0	139	4.8	12.6	8.1	0.7

	Measure INFO/WEIGHT	per Measure KCAL	per Measure FAT	Nutrition Values per 100g / 100ml KCAL	PROT	CARB	FAT	FIBRE

PIE

	Measure INFO/WEIGHT	KCAL	FAT	KCAL	PROT	CARB	FAT	FIBRE
Cheese & Potato, Aunt Bessie's*	¼ Serving/200g	288.0	19.0	144	4.6	11.7	9.4	1.5
Cherry Bakewell Meringue, Sara Lee*	1 Slice/70g	228.0	8.0	326	4.1	51.9	11.3	1.4
Cherry, Asda*	1/6 Pie/116.7g	337.0	14.0	289	3.1	41.2	12.4	1.8
Cherry, Sainsbury's*	1 Serving/117g	325.0	14.0	278	3.9	39.6	11.6	1.7
Cherry, Tesco*	1 Serving/106g	294.0	13.0	277	4.0	38.3	12.0	1.8
Chicken & Asparagus, Lattice, Waitrose*	1 Serving/100g	295.0	20.0	295	7.4	22.3	19.6	1.8
Chicken & Asparagus, McDougalls*	1 Serving/170g	394.0	22.0	232	7.4	21.6	12.9	1.5
Chicken & Asparagus, Tesco*	1 Serving/170g	467.0	29.0	275	8.3	22.4	16.9	0.8
Chicken & Bacon, Filo Pastry, Finest, Tesco*	1 Serving/160g	362.0	19.0	226	11.3	18.9	11.7	1.7
Chicken & Bacon, Puff Pastry, Deep Fill, Sainsbury's*	1/3 Pie/200g	532.0	34.0	266	9.1	19.1	17.0	1.3
Chicken & Bacon, with Cheese Sauce, Tesco*	1 Serving/200g	540.0	34.0	270	12.0	17.6	16.8	0.8
Chicken & Basil, M & S*	1oz/28g	59.0	3.0	210	8.9	17.0	11.9	1.1
Chicken & Broccoli Lattice, Sainsbury's*	½ Pie/192g	520.0	31.0	271	9.3	22.4	16.0	0.9
Chicken & Broccoli Potato, Top, Asda*	1 Pack/400g	319.0	7.0	80	5.2	10.7	1.7	0.6
Chicken & Broccoli, BGTY, Sainsbury's*	1 Pack/450g	297.0	4.0	66	5.9	8.9	0.8	1.8
Chicken & Broccoli, COU, M & S*	1 Serving/320g	272.0	6.0	85	8.1	8.8	1.9	1.3
Chicken & Broccoli, Lattice, Tesco*	½ Pie/200g	496.0	31.0	248	8.5	18.9	15.4	2.1
Chicken & Broccoli, Light Choices, Tesco*	1 Pack/450g	337.0	9.0	75	6.6	6.8	1.9	1.7
Chicken & Gravy, Deep Fill, Asda*	1 Serving/130g	370.0	22.0	285	10.0	23.0	17.0	0.8
Chicken & Gravy, Light Choices, Tesco*	1 Pack/450g	337.0	7.0	75	5.4	9.4	1.6	1.2
Chicken & Gravy, Shortcrust Pastry, Large, Tesco*	1 Pie/600g	1578.0	91.0	263	8.2	23.4	15.2	1.0
Chicken & Gravy, Shortcrust Pastry, Sainsbury's*	1 Serving/250g	637.0	35.0	255	8.0	24.1	14.1	1.0
Chicken & Gravy, Shortcrust Pastry, Tesco*	1 Pie/250g	617.0	34.0	247	6.8	23.9	13.8	1.0
Chicken & Ham, Deep Filled, Sainsbury's*	1 Pie/210g	594.0	37.0	283	8.0	23.0	17.7	1.0
Chicken & Ham, Morrisons*	¼ Pie/115g	267.0	14.0	232	8.7	22.5	11.9	0.8
Chicken & Ham, Sainsbury's*	1 Pie/128g	461.0	29.0	360	11.0	28.5	22.4	2.0
Chicken & Ham, Tesco*	1 Serving/113g	293.0	18.0	259	9.4	20.2	15.6	1.2
Chicken & Leek, Deep Filled, Puff Pastry, Sainsbury's*	1/3 Pie/451g	1109.0	65.0	246	10.1	18.7	14.5	1.5
Chicken & Leek, Light Choices, Tesco*	1 Pie/350g	297.0	6.0	85	6.6	10.3	1.6	1.3
Chicken & Leek, M & S*	1oz/28g	70.0	4.0	250	10.1	18.8	15.1	1.1
Chicken & Leek, Shortcrust, TTD, Sainsbury's*	½ Pie/300g	824.0	49.0	275	12.2	19.8	16.3	1.1
Chicken & Mushroom, Asda*	1 Pie/ 150g	384.0	24.0	256	9.0	19.0	16.0	1.0
Chicken & Mushroom, Deep Filled, Frozen, Tesco*	¼ Pie/197.9g	465.0	22.0	235	9.0	23.8	11.2	1.2
Chicken & Mushroom, Dietary Specials*	1 Pie/140g	300.0	14.0	214	6.3	24.7	10.0	0.9
Chicken & Mushroom, Favourites, Morrisons*	¼ Pie/352g	989.0	61.0	281	7.2	23.8	17.4	0.9
Chicken & Mushroom, Finest, Tesco*	1 Pie/250g	742.0	47.0	297	9.3	21.1	18.7	0.9
Chicken & Mushroom, Fray Bentos*	1 Pie/425g	684.0	40.0	161	6.7	11.5	9.5	0.0
Chicken & Mushroom, Individual, Co-Op*	1 Pie/149g	465.0	30.0	312	8.6	24.5	19.9	1.2
Chicken & Mushroom, Individual, Frozen, Tesco*	1 Pie/141.75	347.0	18.0	245	8.9	23.5	12.6	1.2
Chicken & Mushroom, Luxury, M & S*	½ Pie/275g	880.0	62.0	320	9.9	20.0	22.5	1.0
Chicken & Mushroom, Morrisons*	1 Serving/100g	261.0	15.0	261	7.6	22.9	15.4	0.9
Chicken & Mushroom, Puff Pastry, Birds Eye*	1 Pie/152.0g	415.0	21.0	273	11.9	24.9	14.0	1.6
Chicken & Mushroom, Puff Pastry, Sainsbury's*	1 Pie/150g	450.0	25.0	300	7.8	29.6	16.7	0.9
Chicken & Mushroom, Weight Watchers*	1 Pie/136g	317.0	15.0	233	8.0	25.1	11.1	1.5
Chicken & Vegetable, Farmfoods*	1 Pie/128g	384.0	24.0	300	7.2	25.4	18.8	1.4
Chicken & Vegetable, Freshbake*	1 Pie/125g	319.0	20.0	255	6.5	21.8	15.7	2.7
Chicken & Vegetable, Kids, Tesco*	1 Serving/235g	235.0	11.0	100	5.9	9.1	4.5	0.7
Chicken & Vegetable, Microbake, Freshbake*	1 Pie/100g	348.0	16.0	348	10.2	40.8	16.1	1.8
Chicken & Vegetable, Perfectly Balanced, Waitrose*	1 Serving/375g	285.0	5.0	76	5.1	10.8	1.4	1.3
Chicken & Vegetable, Value, Tesco*	1 Pie/150g	378.0	22.0	252	8.0	21.9	14.7	1.3
Chicken & Wiltshire Ham, Finest, Tesco*	1 Pie/250g	687.0	37.0	275	11.6	22.7	14.9	1.1
Chicken Curry, Iceland*	1 Pie/156g	440.0	24.0	282	10.2	26.2	15.2	2.0
Chicken, Aunt Bessie's*	¼ Pie/200g	474.0	24.0	237	10.6	21.4	12.1	2.1

P

PIE

	Measure INFO/WEIGHT	per Measure KCAL	FAT	Nutrition Values per 100g / 100ml KCAL	PROT	CARB	FAT	FIBRE
Chicken, Bacon & Cheddar Cheese, Lattice, Birds Eye*	1 Pie/155g	454.0	27.0	293	13.4	21.0	17.3	1.5
Chicken, Broccoli & White Wine, Waitrose*	1 Serving/200g	605.0	40.0	302	12.5	17.7	20.2	2.3
Chicken, Cheese & Broccoli Lattice, Birds Eye*	1 Pie/155g	446.0	25.0	288	12.6	22.7	16.3	1.1
Chicken, Cheese & Leek Lattice, Sun Valley*	1 Lattice/125g	315.0	22.0	252	15.2	8.6	17.5	1.0
Chicken, Cottage, Frozen, Tesco*	1 Pack/450g	292.0	2.0	65	2.8	11.7	0.5	1.0
Chicken, Deep Filled, Puff Pastry, Sainsbury's*	1 Pie/210g	538.0	32.0	256	10.0	19.9	15.2	3.1
Chicken, Eat Smart, Safeway*	1 Pack/400g	340.0	7.0	85	8.2	9.0	1.7	1.2
Chicken, Finest, Tesco*	1 Pie/250g	615.0	32.0	246	10.7	21.9	12.9	1.2
Chicken, Individual Shortcrust, Asda*	1 Pie/175g	534.0	30.0	305	10.0	28.0	17.0	1.0
Chicken, Individual, Made with 100% Breast, Birds Eye*	1 Pie/153.7g	455.0	28.0	296	7.9	25.0	18.3	1.0
Chicken, Leek & Bacon Filo, Willow Farm, Finest, Tesco*	½ Pie/225g	574.0	33.0	255	11.1	18.5	14.7	1.4
Chicken, Leek & Ham, Morrisons*	1 Serving/113g	305.0	17.0	270	8.8	25.7	14.7	1.1
Chicken, Newgate*	1 Pie/142g	358.0	24.0	252	6.1	23.1	16.6	1.0
Chicken, Puff Pastry, Tesco*	¼ Pie/114g	250.0	13.0	220	8.6	21.3	11.2	1.4
Chicken, Roast, In Gravy, Deep Fill, Tesco*	1 Pie/800g	1640.0	78.0	205	9.3	20.2	9.7	3.0
Chicken, Roast, Puff Pastry, Deep Fill, Asda*	½ Pie/259g	739.0	44.0	285	10.0	23.0	17.0	0.8
Chicken, Roast, Sainsbury's*	1/3 Pie/173g	538.0	31.0	311	10.5	27.2	17.8	0.9
Chicken, Roast, Shortcrust, Sainsbury's*	1 Pie/200g	1012.0	56.0	506	19.2	44.4	28.0	2.4
Chicken, Short Crust, M & S*	1 Pie/170g	510.0	30.0	300	9.7	26.2	17.4	1.7
Chicken, Tomato & Basil Lattice, Birds Eye*	1 Serving/155g	340.0	20.0	220	10.8	15.7	12.7	1.4
Chocolate, Mini, Waitrose*	1 Pie/24.0g	109.0	6.0	455	5.3	51.4	25.3	1.7
Cod & Prawn, M & S*	1oz/28g	43.0	2.0	155	10.6	8.7	8.9	0.7
Cod & Smoked Haddock, COU, M & S*	1 Pack/400g	320.0	10.0	80	6.1	9.0	2.4	1.2
Cottage, Aberdeen Angus, Large, Chilled, Finest, Tesco*	½ Pack/400g	420.0	18.0	105	8.2	7.7	4.6	3.0
Cottage, Aberdeen Angus, Waitrose*	1 Pie/350g	339.0	12.0	97	5.3	11.0	3.5	0.9
Cottage, Asda*	1 Pack/400g	360.0	10.0	90	6.5	10.6	2.4	1.0
Cottage, Aunt Bessie's*	1 Pack/350g	413.0	18.0	118	4.8	12.1	5.2	1.0
Cottage, British Pies, Chilled, Tesco*	1 Pack/500g	450.0	14.0	90	4.6	10.3	2.8	1.5
Cottage, Chicken, Tesco*	1 Pack/400g	340.0	3.0	85	6.0	12.8	0.7	1.7
Cottage, Classic British, Sainsbury's*	1 Pack/450g	499.0	21.0	111	6.3	11.1	4.6	0.6
Cottage, Family, Iceland*	¼ Pack/259g	262.0	11.0	101	4.2	11.8	4.1	0.8
Cottage, Fresh, M & S*	1 Pie/400g	460.0	22.0	115	6.8	9.9	5.6	0.6
Cottage, Healthy Options, Birds Eye*	1oz/28g	23.0	1.0	83	4.9	11.9	1.8	1.0
Cottage, Individual, Smart Price, Asda*	1 Pie/159g	149.0	6.0	94	3.1	12.0	3.7	0.7
Cottage, Light Choices, Tesco*	1 Pack/500g	400.0	8.0	80	4.5	11.4	1.7	1.7
Cottage, Luxury, M & S*	½ Pack/310g	403.0	22.0	130	7.9	8.3	7.0	1.8
Cottage, Meal for One, M & S*	1 Pack/445g	356.0	16.0	80	5.4	6.2	3.6	1.7
Cottage, Meatfree, Sainsbury's*	1 Pack/400g	364.0	12.0	91	4.4	11.7	3.0	0.7
Cottage, Mini, Waitrose*	1 Pack/250g	267.0	10.0	107	6.4	11.1	4.2	1.4
Cottage, Ross*	1 Pack/320g	240.0	7.0	75	3.0	10.9	2.2	0.3
Cottage, Sainsbury's*	1 Pack/300g	297.0	10.0	99	6.4	10.7	3.4	1.1
Cottage, Salmon, Sainsbury's*	1 Serving/299g	218.0	4.0	73	4.6	10.4	1.4	1.3
Cottage, Vegetarian, Sainsbury's*	1 Pack/450g	328.0	10.0	73	3.0	10.2	2.2	1.8
Cottage, Vegetarian, Tesco*	1 Pie/448g	345.0	13.0	77	3.6	8.9	3.0	1.9
Cottage, Waitrose*	1 Pack/400g	424.0	20.0	106	3.4	12.1	4.9	1.2
Cottage, Weight Watchers*	1 Pack/300g	186.0	4.0	62	3.6	9.0	1.3	0.3
Country, Vegetarian, Tesco*	1 Pie/142g	381.0	22.0	268	5.6	27.3	15.2	1.2
Cumberland, Asda*	1 Pack/400g	504.0	22.0	126	6.3	12.7	5.6	1.5
Cumberland, Beef, HL, Tesco*	1 Pack/500g	460.0	13.0	92	5.0	11.8	2.7	0.9
Cumberland, BGTY, Sainsbury's*	1 Pack/450g	360.0	9.0	80	5.3	10.1	2.0	1.6
Cumberland, Cod & Prawn, Tesco*	1 Pack/450g	427.0	11.0	95	7.9	9.5	2.5	1.3
Cumberland, GFY, Asda*	1 Pack/451g	469.0	10.0	104	11.4	11.4	2.2	2.1
Cumberland, HL, Tesco*	1 Pie/500g	430.0	13.0	86	4.5	10.8	2.7	1.2

PIE

INFO/WEIGHT	Measure	per Measure KCAL	FAT	Nutrition Values per 100g / 100ml KCAL	PROT	CARB	FAT	FIBRE
Cumberland, M & S*	1 Pie/195g	312.0	20.0	160	6.9	10.1	10.4	1.1
Festive, BGTY, Sainsbury's*	1 Pie/58g	222.0	5.0	383	6.2	69.9	8.7	2.6
Fish	1 Serving/250g	262.0	7.0	105	8.0	12.3	3.0	0.7
Fish & Prawn, Perfectly Balanced, Waitrose*	1 Serving/375g	379.0	13.0	101	6.8	10.4	3.6	0.7
Fish with Cheese, Ross*	1 Pack/300g	321.0	13.0	107	4.7	12.0	4.5	0.8
Fish with Vegetables, Ross*	1 Pack/300g	255.0	9.0	85	4.4	10.2	2.9	1.3
Fish, BFY, Morrisons*	1 Pack/350g	301.0	10.0	86	5.0	10.0	2.9	0.9
Fish, Chilled, GFY, Asda*	1 Pie/450g	405.0	13.0	90	6.8	9.3	2.8	1.4
Fish, Creamy, Classics, Tesco*	½ Pack/350g	472.0	28.0	135	7.5	7.7	8.0	0.7
Fish, Cumberland, BGTY, Sainsbury's*	1 Serving/450g	342.0	9.0	76	7.3	7.3	1.9	1.8
Fish, Extra Special, Asda*	1 Pack/400g	540.0	31.0	135	9.8	6.5	7.7	1.1
Fish, Frozen, GFY, Asda*	1 Pack/360g	342.0	9.0	95	5.8	12.5	2.4	0.9
Fish, Healthy Options, Birds Eye*	1 Pack/350g	238.0	3.0	68	3.7	11.6	0.8	0.7
Fish, HL, Tesco*	1 Pack/400g	316.0	9.0	79	4.0	10.8	2.2	1.7
Fish, Kids, Great Stuff, Asda*	1 Pack/300g	276.0	9.0	92	7.8	8.4	3.0	1.4
Fish, Luxury, M & S*	1 Pack/300g	330.0	17.0	110	7.3	7.6	5.6	1.5
Fish, Mariner's, Frozen, Youngs*	1 Pack/360g	382.0	16.0	106	5.3	11.0	4.5	1.0
Fish, Mix, Tesco*	1 Pack/320g	480.0	26.0	150	19.3	0.0	8.0	0.0
Fish, Ocean Crumble, Low Fat, Light & Easy, Youngs*	1 Pack/300g	261.0	6.0	87	4.6	12.9	1.9	1.4
Fish, Seasonal, Mix, Sainsbury's*	1 Pack/320g	480.0	28.0	150	17.7	0.0	8.8	0.0
Fish, with Cheddar & Parsley Sauce, Go Cook, Asda*	½ Pack/450g	427.0	16.0	95	7.8	7.9	3.6	0.8
Fish, with Grated Cheddar, Asda*	¼ Pie/250g	262.0	12.0	105	7.0	8.0	5.0	1.0
Fisherman's, Asda*	1 Serving/300g	429.0	21.0	143	7.0	13.0	7.0	0.0
Fishermans, British Recipe, Waitrose*	1 Pack/400g	408.0	16.0	102	7.7	8.5	4.1	1.2
Fisherman's, Chilled, Co-Op*	1 Pie/300g	345.0	18.0	115	4.0	11.0	6.0	0.7
Fisherman's, Famous, Chilled, Youngs*	1 Pack/400g	448.0	23.0	112	7.6	7.6	5.7	0.9
Fisherman's, Healthy Options, Asda*	1 Pie/406g	337.0	10.0	83	5.0	10.0	2.5	0.9
Fisherman's, M & S*	1 Pie/248g	335.0	16.0	135	9.3	9.8	6.4	0.3
Fisherman's, Nisa Heritage*	1 Serving/550g	588.0	31.0	107	5.2	9.0	5.6	0.2
Fisherman's, Perfectly Balanced, Waitrose*	1 Pack/376g	380.0	14.0	101	6.8	10.4	3.6	0.7
Fisherman's, Sainsbury's*	1 Pack/300g	195.0	4.0	65	3.9	9.7	1.2	1.2
Fruit, Pastry Top & Bottom	1oz/28g	73.0	4.0	260	3.0	34.0	13.3	1.8
Fruit, Selection, Mr Kipling*	1 Pie/66g	232.0	9.0	350	3.5	53.5	13.6	1.3
Gala, Tesco*	1 Serving/70g	241.0	18.0	344	10.6	24.5	25.2	0.0
Haddock & Broccoli, M & S*	1 Serving/250g	262.0	10.0	105	8.1	9.3	4.0	0.5
Key Lime, Sainsbury's*	¼ Pie/80g	280.0	11.0	350	4.2	51.8	14.0	0.7
Lamb & Mint, Shortcrust Pasty, Tesco*	¼ Pack/150g	412.0	26.0	275	5.9	23.6	17.4	1.6
Lemon Meringue	1oz/28g	89.0	4.0	319	4.5	45.9	14.4	0.7
Lemon Meringue, 90% Fat Free, Sara Lee*	1/6 Pie/75g	204.0	7.0	272	2.4	46.1	8.9	0.9
Lemon Meringue, Lyons*	1 Serving/100g	310.0	14.0	310	0.0	45.9	14.4	0.0
Lemon Meringue, Mr Kipling*	1 Pie/51g	184.0	6.0	360	2.9	59.9	12.1	3.0
Lemon Meringue, Ready to Bake, Aunt Bessie's*	¼ Pie/106g	305.0	9.0	288	3.8	49.8	8.2	2.0
Lemon Meringue, Sara Lee*	1oz/28g	77.0	3.0	276	2.6	46.6	9.2	0.9
Lemon Meringue, Weight Watchers*	1 Serving/85g	161.0	0.0	189	2.4	43.1	0.5	0.6
Macaroni Cheese, Countryside*	1 Serving/144g	282.0	10.0	196	4.9	28.3	7.0	1.2
Mariner's, Light & Easy, Youngs*	1 Pack/350g	367.0	14.0	105	5.0	12.0	4.1	1.1
Mariner's, Ross*	1 Pie/340g	435.0	20.0	128	5.0	13.9	5.9	1.0
Mashed Potato Topped Cumberland, M & S*	1/3 Pack/300g	360.0	18.0	120	5.8	9.6	5.9	1.0
Meat & Potato, Hollands*	1 Pie/175g	409.0	19.0	234	6.1	27.5	11.0	0.0
Meat & Potato, Tesco*	1 Serving/150g	414.0	27.0	276	5.1	23.6	17.9	1.6
Meat, Freshbake*	1 Pie/49g	152.0	10.0	313	6.6	23.2	21.6	1.0
Mediterranean Vegetable, Cheesy, COU, M & S*	1 Pack/400g	280.0	8.0	70	2.1	10.6	2.1	2.1
Mince Puff, Tesco*	1 Pie/25g	105.0	4.0	420	3.3	62.0	17.6	2.0

PIE

Measure INFO/WEIGHT		per Measure		Nutrition Values per 100g / 100ml				
		KCAL	FAT	KCAL	PROT	CARB	FAT	FIBRE
Mince, Christmas, Sainsbury's*	1 Pie/37g	147.0	6.0	397	4.5	58.0	16.3	2.6
Mince, Deep, Morrisons*	1 Pie/65g	243.0	9.0	371	3.7	57.8	13.9	1.5
Mince, Dusted, Mini, Finest, Tesco*	1 Pie/20g	76.0	2.0	379	7.3	62.9	12.2	5.0
Mince, Extra Special, Asda*	1 Pie/60g	225.0	8.0	378	3.9	59.0	14.0	2.2
Mince, Finest, Tesco*	1 Pie/61g	234.0	9.0	384	4.3	59.9	14.1	2.7
Mince, Iced Top, Asda*	1 Pie/57g	214.0	7.0	375	2.8	61.0	12.0	1.1
Mince, Iced Top, Oakdale Bakeries*	1 Pie/49g	190.0	5.0	388	2.4	71.0	10.5	0.0
Mince, Iceland*	1 Pie/39g	156.0	6.0	405	4.4	59.6	16.6	3.8
Mince, Individual, Average	1 Pie/48g	203.0	10.0	423	4.3	59.0	20.4	2.1
Mince, Lattice, Classics, M & S*	1 Pie/52.5g	210.0	8.0	400	4.0	61.7	15.2	2.4
Mince, Rowan Hill Bakery*	1 Pie/55g	202.0	8.0	370	3.8	54.8	15.1	0.0
Mince, Shortcrust, Waitrose*	1 Pie/55g	210.0	8.0	385	3.6	60.0	14.6	20.9
Mince, Star Motif, Mini, Finest, Tesco*	1 Pie/20g	75.0	2.0	377	4.2	62.8	12.1	3.6
Mince, Topped with Nibbed Almonds, Mini, Finest, Tesco*	1 Pie/20g	77.0	3.0	383	4.9	59.0	14.1	3.4
Minced Beef & Onion, Birds Eye*	1 Pie/145g	419.0	25.0	289	7.1	26.3	17.3	0.7
Minced Beef & Onion, Denny*	1 Sm Pie/140g	288.0	20.0	206	6.1	17.3	14.1	0.0
Minced Beef & Onion, Tesco*	1 Pie/150g	454.0	28.0	303	5.7	27.4	19.0	1.7
Minced Beef & Vegetable, Pot, M & S*	1/3 Pie/183g	366.0	27.0	200	7.8	9.1	14.5	7.1
Minced Beef, Plate, M & S*	1oz/28g	71.0	4.0	253	7.6	20.7	16.0	2.0
Mississippi Mud, Tesco*	1 Serving/104g	399.0	27.0	384	5.3	33.1	25.6	1.8
Moroccan Vegetable & Feta, Little, Higgidy*	1 Pie/180g	418.0	22.0	232	5.1	24.7	12.5	0.6
Mushroom & Leaf Spinach, Little, Higgidy*	1 Pie/180g	441.0	26.0	245	6.6	22.3	14.4	0.7
Mushroom & Parsley Potato, Waitrose*	1 Pack/350g	346.0	17.0	99	2.5	10.9	5.0	1.2
Ocean, Basics, Sainsbury's*	1 Serving/302g	196.0	4.0	65	3.9	9.7	1.2	1.2
Ocean, BGTY, Sainsbury's*	1 Pack/350g	285.0	5.0	81	6.3	11.1	1.3	0.8
Ocean, Frozen, BGTY, Sainsbury's*	1 Pack/350g	318.0	5.0	91	7.0	12.4	1.5	0.9
Ocean, M & S*	1 Pie/650g	617.0	23.0	95	8.2	7.6	3.5	0.9
Ocean, Original, Frozen, Youngs*	1 Pack/375g	420.0	21.0	112	7.6	7.6	5.7	0.9
Ocean, The Original, Light & Easy, Youngs*	1 Pack/415g	432.0	19.0	104	6.4	9.5	4.5	1.0
Ocean, Weight Watchers*	1 Pack/300g	207.0	4.0	69	4.5	9.5	1.4	0.2
Pork, & Egg, M & S*	¼ Pie/108g	379.0	28.0	351	9.7	19.8	25.9	0.8
Pork, & Pickle, Bowyers*	1 Pie/150g	576.0	41.0	384	10.0	26.3	27.3	0.0
Pork, Buffet, Bowyers*	1 Pie/60g	217.0	15.0	362	10.4	24.9	24.5	0.0
Pork, Buffet, Farmfoods*	1 Pie/65g	252.0	17.0	388	8.8	28.2	26.7	1.0
Pork, Cheese & Pickle, Mini, Tesco*	1 Pie/49g	191.0	13.0	389	9.2	29.3	26.1	1.2
Pork, Crusty Bake, Sainsbury's*	1 Pie/75g	292.0	20.0	390	10.5	27.0	26.7	1.0
Pork, Geo Adams*	1 Pie/125g	487.0	35.0	390	11.8	23.1	27.8	0.9
Pork, Medium, Pork Farms*	1 Pie/200g	744.0	53.0	372	9.5	23.6	26.5	1.7
Pork, Melton Mowbray, Cured, M & S*	1 Pie/290g	1044.0	71.0	360	10.1	25.9	24.5	1.0
Pork, Melton Mowbray, Cured, Mini, M & S*	1 Pie/50g	192.0	12.0	385	9.8	32.6	24.4	1.0
Pork, Melton Mowbray, Ginsters*	1 Pie/75g	317.0	23.0	423	12.3	25.2	30.3	0.9
Pork, Melton Mowbray, Individual, Sainsbury's*	1 Pie/75g	296.0	21.0	395	10.2	26.1	27.7	2.4
Pork, Melton Mowbray, Lattice, Sainsbury's*	1 Serving/100g	342.0	24.0	342	10.8	21.7	23.6	1.2
Pork, Melton Mowbray, Mini, Tesco*	1 Pie/50g	196.0	14.0	392	12.6	20.8	28.7	2.9
Pork, Melton Mowbray, Tesco*	1 Sm Pie/148g	679.0	50.0	459	10.0	29.0	33.7	1.3
Pork, Melton, Mini, Pork Farms*	1 Pie/50g	199.0	15.0	399	8.9	26.2	29.2	0.0
Pork, Mini, Christmas, Tesco*	1 Pie/50g	194.0	13.0	389	10.7	26.3	26.8	2.3
Pork, Mini, Tesco*	1 Pie/45g	162.0	11.0	359	10.2	25.9	23.8	1.0
Pork, VLH Kitchens	1 Serving/36g	168.0	13.0	466	11.0	26.0	36.0	0.0
Pork, with Cheese & Pickle, Waitrose*	1 Pack/150g	568.0	37.0	379	10.3	29.1	24.6	2.7
Potato & Meat, Farmfoods*	1 Pie/158g	416.0	27.0	263	5.4	22.0	17.0	1.0
Rhubarb, Sara Lee*	1 Serving/90g	224.0	12.0	250	2.9	28.7	13.8	1.3
Roast Chicken & Vegetable, Pot, M & S*	1/3 Pie/183g	366.0	23.0	200	7.7	13.5	12.5	4.5

P

PIE

INFO/WEIGHT	Measure	per Measure KCAL	FAT	KCAL	PROT	CARB	FAT	FIBRE
Roast Chicken, COU, M & S*	1 Pack/320g	272.0	3.0	85	9.4	9.7	1.0	0.8
Salmon & Broccoli Lattice Bar, Asda*	1/3 Bar/133g	360.0	20.0	271	6.0	28.0	15.0	0.8
Salmon & Broccoli, Birds Eye*	1 Pie/351g	449.0	22.0	128	6.6	11.4	6.2	0.7
Salmon & Broccoli, Light Choices, Tesco*	1 Pack/400g	365.0	11.0	90	6.9	9.5	2.7	1.1
Salmon & Broccoli, Premium, Tesco*	1 Serving/170g	425.0	29.0	250	6.1	17.7	17.2	0.7
Salmon, Crumble, Light & Easy, Youngs*	1 Pack/320g	282.0	6.0	88	5.7	11.8	2.0	1.0
Salmon, Value, Tesco*	1 Pack/300g	312.0	13.0	104	4.5	11.3	4.5	1.0
Sausage & Onion, Lattice, Puff Pastry, Tesco*	1/3 Pie/133g	480.0	22.0	361	9.1	20.6	16.9	4.6
Sausage & Onion, Tesco*	1 Pack/300g	333.0	18.0	111	2.3	11.7	6.1	0.5
Scotch, Co-Op*	1 Pie/132g	408.0	25.0	309	7.3	27.3	18.9	1.5
Shepherd's, Average	1oz/28g	31.0	2.0	112	6.0	9.3	5.9	0.7
Shepherd's, Baked Bean Cuisine, Heinz*	**1 Pie/340g**	**299.0**	**10.0**	**88**	**4.1**	**11.6**	**2.8**	**1.5**
Shepherd's, BGTY, Sainsbury's*	1 Pack/300g	225.0	7.0	75	3.6	10.2	2.2	1.7
Shepherd's, COU, M & S*	1 Pack/300g	210.0	4.0	70	5.2	8.6	1.3	1.6
Shepherd's, Frozen, Tesco*	1 Pack/400g	508.0	28.0	127	4.2	11.7	7.1	1.0
Shepherd's, GFY, Asda*	1 Pack/399g	339.0	11.0	85	4.0	11.1	2.7	1.4
Shepherd's, Great Value, Asda*	1 Pack/400g	376.0	12.0	94	4.7	12.0	3.0	0.6
Shepherd's, Weight Watchers*	1 Pack/320g	221.0	7.0	69	3.2	8.8	2.3	0.3
Shepherd's, Welsh Hill Lamb, Gastropub, M & S*	½ Pack/330g	313.0	12.0	95	5.4	10.2	3.5	1.5
Steak & Ale, Deep Fill, Puff Pastry, Tesco*	¼ Pie/150g	324.0	20.0	216	8.0	16.6	13.1	2.3
Steak & Ale, Fray Bentos*	1 Pie/425g	697.0	39.0	164	7.6	13.0	9.1	0.0
Steak & Ale, Puff Pastry, Asda*	1/3 Pie/200g	520.0	30.0	260	10.6	20.4	15.1	1.6
Steak & Ale, Sainsbury's*	1 Serving/190g	445.0	23.0	234	8.3	22.6	12.3	0.9
Steak & Ale, TTD, Sainsbury's*	1 Pie/250g	681.0	36.0	272	11.6	24.4	14.2	1.4
Steak & Guinness, Sainsbury's*	¼ Pie/137g	399.0	25.0	291	8.7	22.2	18.6	1.0
Steak & Kidney, Birds Eye*	1 Pie/146g	447.0	28.0	306	9.0	23.7	19.5	2.3
Steak & Kidney, Deep Fill, Sainsbury's*	½ Pie/125g	314.0	19.0	251	8.4	21.0	14.9	2.0
Steak & Kidney, Family, Co-Op*	1/6 Pie/87g	278.0	17.0	320	9.0	26.0	20.0	0.9
Steak & Kidney, Family, Iceland*	1/3 Pie/225g	502.0	29.0	223	10.2	16.3	13.0	2.1
Steak & Kidney, Individual	1 Pie/200g	646.0	42.0	323	9.1	25.6	21.2	0.9
Steak & Kidney, Princes*	½ Pack/212g	379.0	20.0	179	8.8	14.8	9.4	0.0
Steak & Kidney, Puff Pastry, Sainsbury's*	1 Pie/150g	423.0	24.0	282	8.2	26.9	15.7	0.9
Steak & Kidney, Tinned, Fray Bentos*	½ Pie/212g	346.0	19.0	163	8.2	12.9	8.8	0.0
Steak & Mushroom, Asda*	1 Pie/130g	350.0	18.0	270	9.0	27.0	14.0	1.4
Steak & Mushroom, Deep Fill, Asda*	1/3 Pie/175g	476.0	28.0	272	11.0	21.0	16.0	1.1
Steak & Mushroom, Deep Fill, Puff Pastry, Tesco*	1 Slice/150g	339.0	21.0	226	9.1	16.3	13.8	1.9
Steak & Mushroom, Home Comforts, Weight Watchers*	1 Pie/136g	322.0	16.0	237	5.8	26.9	11.7	1.4
Steak & Mushroom, Individual, Birds Eye*	1 Pie/142g	389.0	24.0	274	7.5	22.7	17.0	2.0
Steak & Mushroom, McDougalls*	1 Pack/340g	779.0	58.0	229	9.0	10.0	17.0	0.9
Steak & Mushroom, Sainsbury's*	¼ Pie/130g	372.0	21.0	286	8.6	26.0	16.4	1.0
Steak & Mushroom, Tesco*	1 Pie/138g	345.0	19.0	250	8.3	22.2	14.1	1.8
Steak & Onion, Minced, Aberdeen Angus, Tesco*	½ Pie/300g	897.0	58.0	299	9.4	22.1	19.2	0.7
Steak & Potato, Asda*	1/3 Pie/173g	442.0	26.0	255	6.9	23.1	15.0	0.9
Steak & Red Wine, Puff Pastry, Pub, Sainsbury's*	1 Pie/240g	497.0	30.0	207	7.2	16.8	12.3	2.1
Steak, Au Gratin, Tesco*	1 Pack/450g	594.0	27.0	132	8.7	10.7	6.0	1.1
Steak, Braised, Shortcrust Pastry, Asda*	½ Pack/260g	785.0	47.0	302	9.0	26.0	18.0	0.9
Steak, Deep Fill, Tesco*	¼ Pie/195g	468.0	26.0	240	9.7	20.0	13.1	1.5
Steak, Dietary Specials*	1 Pie/140g	328.0	14.0	234	9.8	25.7	10.3	0.4
Steak, in Rich Gravy, Aunt Bessie's*	¼ Pie/200g	440.0	21.0	220	9.6	22.0	10.3	1.5
Steak, Individual, British Classics, Tesco*	1 Pie/150g	450.0	28.0	300	9.1	23.3	18.4	2.5
Steak, Large, Glenfell*	¼ Pie/170g	445.0	28.0	262	6.8	21.8	16.4	1.0
Steak, M & S*	1oz/28g	64.0	4.0	230	10.0	19.0	12.7	1.2
Steak, Mini, Asda*	1 Serving/67g	117.0	5.0	176	9.0	17.0	8.0	0.9

	Measure INFO/WEIGHT	per Measure KCAL	FAT	Nutrition Values per 100g / 100ml KCAL	PROT	CARB	FAT	FIBRE
PIE								
Steak, Mushroom & Ale, Topcrust, Waitrose*	1 Pie/250g	500.0	29.0	200	11.1	12.2	11.8	1.1
Steak, Puff Pastry, Deep Filled, Sainsbury's*	1 Pie/210g	535.0	30.0	255	10.3	21.2	14.3	2.0
Steak, Safeway*	¼ Pie/130g	381.0	21.0	293	9.4	27.4	16.2	1.1
Steak, Scotch, Bell's Bakery*	1 Serving/150g	378.0	20.0	252	13.6	18.6	13.5	0.7
Steak, Short Crust, Sainsbury's*	½ Pie/117.5g	314.0	24.0	267	10.9	22.2	20.5	1.7
Steak, Shortcrust Pastry, Finest, Tesco*	1 Pie/250g	660.0	38.0	264	10.9	21.2	15.1	0.8
Steak, Tesco*	1 Serving/205g	556.0	34.0	271	7.2	23.3	16.5	1.4
Steak, Top Crust, TTD, Sainsbury's*	½ Pie/299g	530.0	23.0	177	15.4	11.4	7.7	0.5
Steak, TTD, Sainsbury's*	½ Pie/300g	713.0	35.0	238	12.6	20.3	11.8	1.0
Summer Fruits, Orchard Tree*	1/8 Pie/75g	242.0	10.0	323	3.0	46.6	13.8	1.2
Teviot, Minced Beef, Morrisons*	½ Pie/250g	382.0	17.0	153	8.0	14.5	6.9	1.6
Tuna & Sweetcorn, HL, Tesco*	1 Pack/450g	391.0	12.0	87	7.1	8.6	2.7	2.0
Turkey & Ham, Farmfoods*	1 Pie/147g	404.0	22.0	275	8.6	26.5	14.9	1.4
Turkey & Ham, Shortcrust, M & S*	1/3 Pie/183g	494.0	29.0	270	11.9	19.5	15.9	1.0
Vegetable	1oz/28g	42.0	2.0	151	3.0	18.9	7.6	1.5
Vegetable & Cheddar Cheese, Waitrose*	1 Pie/210g	475.0	31.0	226	4.9	17.8	15.0	1.2
Vegetable & Cheese, Asda*	1 Pie/141g	330.0	16.0	234	5.8	26.9	11.5	1.0
Vegetarian, Deep Country, Linda McCartney*	1 Pie/166.1g	412.0	23.0	248	5.1	26.1	13.7	1.4
Vegetarian, Shepherd's, Linda McCartney*	1 Pack/340g	286.0	7.0	84	3.7	12.3	2.2	2.3
Vegetarian, Vegetable Cumberland, M & S*	½ Pack/211g	190.0	5.0	90	2.8	13.4	2.6	1.6
Welsh Lamb, Sainsbury's*	¼ Pie/120g	290.0	17.0	242	9.1	19.2	14.3	0.8
West Country Chicken, Sainsbury's*	1 Serving/240g	614.0	37.0	256	11.9	17.1	15.6	2.1
PIE FILLING								
Apple, Sainsbury's*	1 Serving/75g	67.0	0.0	89	0.1	22.1	0.1	1.0
Black Cherry, Fruit, Sainsbury's*	1 Serving/100g	73.0	0.0	73	0.3	17.7	0.1	0.3
Blackcurrant, Fruit, Sainsbury's*	1 Serving/100g	82.0	0.0	82	0.4	20.0	0.1	1.6
Cherry	1oz/28g	23.0	0.0	82	0.4	21.5	0.0	0.4
Fruit	1oz/28g	22.0	0.0	77	0.4	20.1	0.0	1.0
Lemon, Sainsbury's*	1 Sachet/280g	218.0	1.0	78	0.1	18.6	0.4	0.0
Summer Fruits, Fruit, Tesco*	1 Can/385g	377.0	0.0	98	0.4	24.1	0.0	0.9
PIGEON								
Meat Only, Roasted, Average	**1 Pigeon/115g**	**215.0**	**9.0**	**187**	**29.0**	**0.0**	**7.9**	**0.0**
Meat Only, Roasted, Weighed with Bone, Average	**1oz/28g**	**25.0**	**1.0**	**88**	**13.6**	**0.0**	**3.7**	**0.0**
PIKELETS								
Classics, M & S*	1 Pikelet/35g	70.0	0.0	200	7.3	39.1	1.3	1.6
Free From, Tesco*	1 Pikelet/30g	58.0	1.0	194	2.8	36.2	4.3	1.4
Tesco*	1 Pikelet/35g	68.0	0.0	193	5.8	40.9	0.7	1.7
PILAF								
Bulgar Wheat, Sainsbury's*	1 Pack/381.3g	347.0	11.0	91	3.9	12.3	2.9	6.3
Forest Mushroom & Pine Nut, Bistro, Waitrose*	1 Serving/225g	337.0	15.0	150	7.0	15.8	6.5	1.5
with Tomato, Average	1oz/28g	40.0	1.0	144	2.5	28.0	3.3	0.4
PILCHARDS								
Fillets, in Tomato Sauce, Average	1 Can/120g	158.0	8.0	132	16.2	2.2	6.5	0.1
Fillets, in Virgin Olive Oil, Glenryck*	1 Serving/92g	223.0	14.0	242	23.3	2.0	15.7	0.0
in Brine, Average	**½ Can/77g**	**114.0**	**6.0**	**148**	**20.8**	**0.0**	**7.3**	**0.0**
PIMMS*								
& Lemonade, Premixed, Canned, Pimms*	1 Can/250ml	85.0	0.0	34	0.0	8.0	0.0	0.0
*25% Volume, Pimms**	**1 Serving/25ml**	**40.0**	**0.0**	**160**	**0.0**	**5.0**	**0.0**	**0.0**
PINE NUTS								
Average	**1oz/28g**	**195.0**	**19.0**	**695**	**15.7**	**3.9**	**68.6**	**1.9**
PINEAPPLE								
& Papaya, Dried, Garden Gang, Asda*	1 Pack/50g	141.0	1.0	283	2.8	64.0	1.7	8.0
Dried, Sweetened, Ready to Eat, Tesco*	1/5 Pack/50g	117.0	1.0	235	0.4	52.9	1.9	1.7

	Measure INFO/WEIGHT	per Measure KCAL	FAT	Nutrition Values per 100g / 100ml KCAL	PROT	CARB	FAT	FIBRE
PINEAPPLE								
Dried, Tropical Wholefoods*	1 Slice/10g	35.0	0.0	355	1.8	84.2	1.2	8.6
Dried, Unsweetened, Sainsbury's*	1 Bag/75g	255.0	1.0	340	1.7	84.7	2.0	6.0
in Juice, Average	*1 Can/106g*	*57.0*	*0.0*	*53*	*0.3*	*12.9*	*0.0*	*0.6*
in Syrup, Average	*1 Can/240g*	*158.0*	*0.0*	*66*	*0.3*	*16.1*	*0.0*	*0.8*
Pieces, Yoghurt Coated, Holland & Barrett*	1 Pack/100g	344.0	19.0	344	2.1	46.8	19.3	0.6
Raw, Average	*1 Fruit/472g*	*233.0*	*1.0*	*49*	*0.4*	*11.6*	*0.1*	*0.9*
Sliced, Snack, Shapers, Boots*	1 Pack/80g	35.0	0.0	44	0.4	10.0	0.2	1.2
Tidbits, Dried, Graze*	1 Pack/30g	79.0	0.0	263	0.6	72.0	0.6	1.0
PISTACHIO NUTS								
Roasted & Salted, Average	*1 Serving/25g*	*152.0*	*14.0*	*608*	*19.6*	*9.9*	*54.5*	*6.1*
Roasted, Graze*	1 Pack/50g	166.0	15.0	333	9.9	4.6	31.0	0.0
Salted, Lemon, Graze*	1 Box/26g	148.0	12.0	568	21.4	26.8	46.0	0.0
PIZZA								
American Hot, 8 Inch, Supermarket, Pizza Express*	1 Pizza/295g	652.0	22.0	221	11.0	27.3	7.6	3.5
American Hot, Chicago Town*	1 Pizza/170g	445.0	20.0	262	8.2	30.8	11.8	0.9
Bacon & Mushroom Pizzeria, Sainsbury's*	1 Pizza/355g	880.0	25.0	248	11.7	34.5	7.0	3.7
Bacon & Mushroom, Stone Bake, M & S*	1 Pizza/375g	750.0	24.0	200	9.9	27.2	6.4	1.6
Bacon & Mushroom, Stonebaked, Tesco*	1 Serving/157g	352.0	15.0	224	10.5	24.3	9.4	3.3
Bacon & Mushroom, Thin & Crispy, Sainsbury's*	½ Pizza/150g	396.0	16.0	264	12.9	29.2	10.6	1.7
Bacon, Mushroom & Tomato, Deep Pan, Loaded, Tesco*	½ Pizza/219g	464.0	13.0	212	9.3	30.6	5.8	1.5
Bacon, Mushroom & Tomato, HL, Tesco*	1 Pizza/231g	395.0	6.0	171	10.6	25.9	2.7	1.5
Bacon, Mushroom & Tomato, Stonebaked, Tesco*	1 Serving/173g	351.0	13.0	203	9.9	24.1	7.4	2.0
Baguette, Cheese & Tomato, Tesco*	1 Baguette/125g	275.0	8.0	220	11.0	28.0	6.8	2.8
Balsamic Roast Vegetable & Mozzarella, Sainsbury's*	½ Pizza/200g	444.0	16.0	222	8.5	29.4	7.8	2.4
BBQ Chicken Stuffed Crust, Asda*	½ Pizza/245g	612.0	24.0	250	13.0	27.0	10.0	2.7
BBQ Chicken, M & S*	½ Pizza/210g	430.0	12.0	205	11.6	27.5	5.6	1.8
BBQ Chicken, Stonebaked, Tesco*	½ Pizza/158g	285.0	9.0	180	10.5	20.9	6.0	3.9
BBQ Chicken, Thin & Crispy, Sainsbury's*	½ Pizza/147g	384.0	12.0	261	13.8	33.1	8.2	1.6
BBQ Chicken, Thin & Crispy, Tesco*	1 Serving/165g	355.0	7.0	215	11.9	31.6	4.5	1.2
BBQ Chicken, Weight Watchers*	1 Pizza/224g	412.0	8.0	184	11.5	26.5	3.5	2.7
Bianca, Bistro, Waitrose*	½ Pizza/207g	618.0	33.0	298	12.9	26.2	15.7	2.3
Big American, Dr Oetker*	1 Serving/225g	571.0	25.0	254	9.7	28.9	11.0	0.0
Bistro Caramelised Onion, Feta & Rosemary, Waitrose*	½ Pizza/230g	607.0	32.0	264	8.6	26.1	13.9	2.4
Bistro Salami & Pepperoni, Waitrose*	½ Pizza/190g	492.0	19.0	259	12.9	28.8	10.2	1.5
Cajun Chicken, BGTY, Sainsbury's*	½ Pizza/165g	363.0	6.0	220	11.0	36.0	3.6	1.7
Cajun Chicken, Pizzatilla, M & S*	½ Pizza/240g	636.0	36.0	265	10.5	21.8	15.1	1.3
Cajun Chicken, Sainsbury's*	½ Pizza/146g	285.0	3.0	195	12.9	31.8	1.8	2.6
Cajun Style Chicken, Stonebaked, Tesco*	1 Pizza/561g	1318.0	55.0	235	11.9	24.8	9.8	1.4
Calzone Speciale, Ristorante, Dr Oetker*	½ Pizza/145g	378.0	23.0	261	11.5	22.1	16.0	0.0
Charged Up Chilli Beef, Goodfella's*	½ Pizza/357g	857.0	33.0	240	12.8	26.4	9.2	1.6
Chargrilled Chicken & Vegetable, GFY, Asda*	½ Pizza/166g	355.0	3.0	214	13.0	36.0	2.0	2.0
Chargrilled Chicken & Vegetable, Low Fat, Bertorelli*	1 Pizza/180g	439.0	8.0	244	14.2	39.3	4.4	2.3
Chargrilled Chicken, Iceland*	1 Pizza/381g	804.0	26.0	211	12.3	25.4	6.7	2.0
Chargrilled Chicken, Thin & Crispy, Asda*	1 Pizza/373g	780.0	19.0	209	9.0	32.0	5.0	1.6
Chargrilled Vegetable, Frozen, BGTY, Sainsbury's*	1 Pizza/290g	548.0	13.0	189	10.2	26.7	4.6	3.0
Chargrilled Vegetable, Thin & Crispy, GFY, Asda*	1 Serving/188g	290.0	4.0	154	6.0	28.0	2.0	3.1
Cheese & Onion, Tesco*	1 Serving/22g	56.0	2.0	255	10.5	32.7	9.1	2.7
Cheese & Tomato French Bread, Findus*	1 Serving/143g	322.0	12.0	225	9.4	29.0	8.1	0.0
Cheese & Tomato Range, Italiano, Tesco*	1 Pizza/380g	969.0	35.0	255	11.4	31.7	9.2	3.3
Cheese & Tomato Slice, Ross*	1 Slice/77g	148.0	7.0	192	6.5	22.2	8.6	2.0
Cheese & Tomato Thin & Crispy, Stonebaked, Tesco*	1 Pizza/155g	355.0	12.0	229	11.6	28.1	7.8	1.3
Cheese & Tomato, Average	1 Serving/300g	711.0	35.0	237	9.1	25.2	11.8	1.4
Cheese & Tomato, Big Value, Ross*	1 Pizza/716g	1446.0	34.0	202	7.8	32.2	4.7	2.7

PIZZA

	Measure INFO/WEIGHT	per Measure KCAL	FAT	Nutrition Values per 100g / 100ml KCAL	PROT	CARB	FAT	FIBRE
Cheese & Tomato, Bistro, Waitrose*	½ Pizza/205g	488.0	20.0	238	10.0	27.6	9.7	1.2
Cheese & Tomato, Blue Parrot Cafe, Sainsbury's*	¼ Pizza/88g	217.0	8.0	248	12.7	29.5	8.8	1.2
Cheese & Tomato, Deep & Crispy, Tesco*	1 Serving/197g	455.0	13.0	231	10.8	31.7	6.8	1.2
Cheese & Tomato, Deep Pan, Goodfella's*	¼ Pizza/102g	259.0	11.0	253	11.5	29.6	10.5	3.7
Cheese & Tomato, Economy, Sainsbury's*	1 Pizza/60g	142.0	4.0	237	11.2	34.1	6.2	1.8
Cheese & Tomato, French Bread, Co-Op*	1 Pizza/135g	270.0	8.0	200	9.0	27.0	6.0	2.0
Cheese & Tomato, Frozen, Sainsbury's*	1 Serving/122g	300.0	11.0	246	13.7	28.0	8.8	3.0
Cheese & Tomato, Micro, McCain*	1 Pizza/121.8g	319.0	12.0	262	13.4	29.7	10.0	2.4
Cheese & Tomato, Mini, Bruschetta, Iceland*	1 Pizza/34g	63.0	2.0	188	8.0	23.0	7.0	2.1
Cheese & Tomato, Piccadella, Tesco*	1 Pizza/295g	684.0	31.0	232	9.1	24.8	10.6	1.5
Cheese & Tomato, Retail, Frozen	1oz/28g	70.0	3.0	250	7.5	32.9	10.7	1.4
Cheese & Tomato, Square, Sainsbury's*	1 Square/160g	435.0	12.0	272	14.0	37.6	7.3	2.1
Cheese & Tomato, Stonebaked, Co-Op*	1 Pizza/325g	699.0	26.0	215	10.0	26.0	8.0	3.0
Cheese & Tomato, Stonebaked, Thin & Crispy, Tesco*	½ Pizza/161g	388.0	14.0	241	11.6	29.4	8.6	2.1
Cheese & Tomato, Thin & Crispy, Asda*	1 Pizza/366g	827.0	37.0	226	11.0	23.0	10.0	2.0
Cheese & Tomato, Thin & Crispy, Carlos*	1 Pizza/155g	405.0	13.0	261	11.4	35.0	8.4	1.2
Cheese & Tomato, Thin & Crispy, Morrisons*	1 Pizza/335g	734.0	24.0	219	11.2	27.7	7.1	3.1
Cheese & Tomato, Thin & Crispy, Organic, Tesco*	½ Pizza/147g	369.0	14.0	251	10.6	30.1	9.8	1.3
Cheese & Tomato, Thin & Crispy, Sainsbury's*	1 Serving/135g	344.0	10.0	255	14.9	32.2	7.4	5.0
Cheese & Tomato, Thin & Crispy, Stonebaked, Tesco*	1/3 Pizza/212g	509.0	20.0	240	10.1	29.2	9.2	1.4
Cheese & Tomato, Thin & Crispy, Waitrose*	1 Pizza/280g	658.0	28.0	235	12.3	23.6	10.1	2.3
Cheese Feast, Deep Pan, Asda*	½ Pizza/210g	422.0	19.0	201	13.0	17.0	9.0	2.3
Cheese Feast, Thin Crust, Chilled, Tesco*	½ Pizza/175g	467.0	22.0	267	14.7	23.4	12.8	2.5
Cheese Suprema, Freschetta, Schwan's*	½ Pizza/150g	391.0	14.0	261	12.4	32.4	9.3	1.8
Cheese Supreme, New Recipe, Goodfella's*	¼ Pizza/102g	269.0	10.0	264	12.3	31.2	10.0	2.2
Cheese, Deep Pan, Tesco*	½ Pizza/455g	990.0	26.0	218	11.4	29.8	5.8	3.1
Cheese, Onion & Garlic, Pizzeria, Waitrose*	½ Pizza/245g	684.0	29.0	279	10.8	29.8	11.8	2.5
Cheese, Stuffed, Crust, Sainsbury's*	1 Pizza/525g	1428.0	52.0	272	14.0	31.5	10.0	2.0
Cheese, Thin & Crispy, Goodfella's*	1 Serving/275g	729.0	28.0	265	15.7	27.6	10.1	1.8
Cheese, Three, Slice, Microwaveable, Tesco*	1 Slice/160g	486.0	19.0	304	13.3	36.7	11.7	1.6
Cheesefeast, Deep & Crispy 12", Takeaway, Iceland*	1 Slice/132g	342.0	11.0	259	13.1	32.8	8.4	1.5
Chesse & Tomato, Kids Crew, Iceland*	1 Pizza/90g	204.0	6.0	227	9.6	32.4	6.5	1.2
Chicken & Bacon Carbonara, Thin Crust, Italian, Asda*	1 Pizza/492g	1156.0	34.0	235	12.0	31.0	7.0	3.4
Chicken & Bacon, Loaded, Tesco*	1 Serving/258g	622.0	25.0	241	12.8	25.4	9.8	1.9
Chicken & Bacon, Pizzeria, Italian, Sainsbury's*	½ Pizza/169.5g	508.0	24.0	300	13.6	29.4	14.2	2.7
Chicken & Chorizo, 12", TTD, Sainsbury's*	½ Pizza/290g	702.0	21.0	242	12.2	32.1	7.2	2.6
Chicken & Maple Bacon Carbonara, Asda*	½ Pizza/195g	484.0	16.0	248	11.0	33.0	8.0	2.2
Chicken & Pesto, Californian Style, Asda*	½ Pizza/235g	533.0	16.0	227	10.0	31.0	7.0	2.0
Chicken & Pesto, with Red Peppers, Italian, Sainsbury's*	½ Pizza/192.2g	471.0	19.0	245	12.0	27.3	9.7	2.7
Chicken & Sweetcorn, Stonebaked, Tesco*	1 Serving/177g	354.0	10.0	200	11.9	26.0	5.4	2.0
Chicken & Vegetable, Chargrill, Italiano, Tesco*	½ Pizza/184g	383.0	15.0	208	10.6	23.3	8.0	2.4
Chicken & Vegetable, Stone Baked, GFY, Asda*	½ Pizza/161g	349.0	4.0	217	13.0	36.0	2.3	1.7
Chicken Alfredo, Chicago Town*	1 Pizza/265g	583.0	25.0	220	11.9	21.9	9.4	1.8
Chicken Arrabbiata, Italian Style, M & S*	½ Pizza/225g	495.0	16.0	220	12.3	26.3	7.0	2.0
Chicken Arrabiata, Sainsbury's*	½ Pizza/191g	444.0	12.0	232	12.1	31.4	6.4	1.7
Chicken Provencal, Goodfella's*	½ Pizza/143g	388.0	18.0	272	13.7	25.9	12.6	2.1
Chicken Salsa, HL, Tesco*	½ Pizza/169g	269.0	4.0	159	11.1	24.0	2.1	2.2
Chicken Tikka, Stonebaked, Tesco*	1 Serving/153g	326.0	10.0	213	10.7	27.3	6.8	1.3
Chicken, Thin & Crispy, Iceland*	½ Pizza/157g	469.0	20.0	299	13.0	33.2	12.7	3.1
Chilli Beef, Stone Bake, M & S*	1 Pizza/395g	790.0	23.0	200	9.6	26.7	5.8	1.9
Cream Cheese & Pepperonata, Calzone, Waitrose*	½ Pizza/165g	383.0	16.0	232	7.0	29.4	9.6	1.5
Deep South, Chicago Town*	1 Pizza/171g	363.0	12.0	212	6.9	30.0	7.1	0.0
Double Cheese, Chicago Town*	1 Pizza/405g	931.0	27.0	230	11.7	30.6	6.7	0.0

P

PIZZA

	Measure INFO/WEIGHT	per Measure KCAL	FAT	Nutrition Values per 100g / 100ml KCAL	PROT	CARB	FAT	FIBRE
Double Cheese, Square Snacks, Food Explorer, Waitrose*	1 Pizza/146g	416.0	11.0	286	12.4	40.2	7.5	1.9
Easy Cheesy, Deep Pan, Chicago Town*	½ Pizza/547g	1455.0	59.0	266	11.4	30.9	10.8	1.7
Etruscan Pepperoni, TTD, Sainsbury's*	½ Pizza/252g	676.0	21.0	268	13.2	35.1	8.3	2.4
Fajita Chicken, COU, M & S*	1 Pizza/255g	433.0	6.0	170	9.9	25.5	2.4	1.2
Fajita Vegetable, BGTY, Sainsbury's*	1 Pizza/214g	366.0	3.0	171	8.9	30.8	1.4	2.9
Farmhouse, Tesco*	½ Pizza/190g	353.0	14.0	186	9.7	20.3	7.4	2.7
Fingers & Curly Fries, M & S*	1 Pack/212g	360.0	10.0	170	7.9	22.9	4.9	1.6
Fingers, Oven Baked, McCain*	1 Finger/30g	78.0	2.0	261	12.6	34.8	7.9	2.4
Fire Roasted Pepper, Sainsbury's*	1 Pizza/344g	605.0	5.0	176	5.3	35.3	1.5	1.6
Fire Roasted Peppers & Vegetables, Waitrose*	½ Pizza/235g	442.0	17.0	188	9.8	21.3	7.1	2.7
Five Cheese & Pepperoni, Deep & Crispy, Waitrose*	1/3 Pizza/200g	560.0	23.0	280	11.7	32.3	11.6	1.3
Flamed Chicken & Vegetables, BGTY, Sainsbury's*	1 Pizza/260g	660.0	11.0	254	14.2	39.3	4.4	2.3
Flamin' Hot, Deep Dish, Chicago Town*	1 Pizza/170g	454.0	20.0	267	8.6	31.1	12.0	0.0
Four Cheese & Tomato, Pizzatilla, M & S*	1 Serving/69g	225.0	14.0	324	10.5	26.0	19.9	1.5
Four Cheese, Freschetta, Schwan's*	¼ Slice/75g	205.0	7.0	273	11.3	34.8	9.8	1.4
Four Cheese, M & S*	1oz/28g	67.0	2.0	240	13.2	30.3	7.5	1.2
Four Cheese, Stuffed Crust, Takeaway, Chicago Town*	¼ Pizza/149g	410.0	16.0	275	12.6	31.4	11.0	2.2
Four Cheese, Thin & Crispy, Sainsbury's*	1 Pizza/265g	729.0	33.0	275	11.8	29.3	12.3	3.5
Four Cheese, Thin Crust, Tesco*	½ Pizza/142g	386.0	14.0	272	14.5	31.8	9.6	1.8
Four Cheese, Weight Watchers*	1 Pizza/186g	400.0	7.0	215	10.7	34.9	3.8	1.6
French Bread, Blue Parrot Cafe, Sainsbury's*	1 Pizza/132g	271.0	6.0	205	10.7	30.8	4.3	1.3
Funghi, Ristorante, Dr Oetker*	1 Pizza/365g	865.0	43.0	237	7.9	22.5	11.9	0.0
Garlic & Mushroom, Thin & Crispy, Sainsbury's*	1 Pizza/260g	829.0	43.0	319	11.1	31.2	16.6	1.7
Garlic Bread, Stonebaked, Italiono, Tesco*	1 Serving/117g	403.0	18.0	346	7.8	43.6	15.6	1.5
Garlic Chicken & Spinach, Perfectly Balanced, Waitrose*	½ Pizza/172g	351.0	5.0	204	13.3	30.8	3.1	2.3
Garlic Chicken, Deep Pan, Sainsbury's*	½ Pizza/214g	464.0	14.0	217	11.2	28.3	6.5	3.3
Garlic Chicken, Thin & Crispy, Stonebake, Sainsbury's*	½ Pizza/160g	386.0	17.0	241	10.7	25.2	10.8	3.5
Garlic Mushroom, BGTY, Sainsbury's*	½ Pizza/123g	262.0	2.0	213	11.6	37.2	2.0	2.7
Garlic Mushroom, Classico, Tesco*	½ Pizza/207.5g	415.0	14.0	200	10.0	24.9	6.7	2.6
Garlic Mushroom, Thin & Crispy, Chicago Town*	Pizza/115g	283.0	13.0	246	9.0	26.4	11.6	1.9
Garlic Mushroom, Thin & Crispy, Weight Watchers*	1 Pizza/240g	410.0	3.0	171	11.2	28.8	1.3	3.0
Garlic Mushroom, Thin Crust, Tesco*	½ Pizza/163g	340.0	15.0	209	11.0	21.1	9.0	3.6
Giardiniera, From Supermarket, Pizza Express*	½ Pizza/144g	291.0	11.0	202	8.6	25.5	7.3	2.1
Grilled Pepper, Weight Watchers*	1 Pizza/220g	392.0	5.0	178	10.0	29.3	2.3	1.8
Ham & Cheese, Chunky, Asda*	1 Serving/90g	211.0	3.0	234	12.0	39.0	3.3	4.7
Ham & Mushroom Calzone, Waitrose*	½ Pizza/145g	362.0	13.0	250	10.0	31.6	9.3	1.6
Ham & Mushroom Slices, Farmfoods*	1 Slice/89g	170.0	2.0	191	8.0	34.0	2.6	0.9
Ham & Mushroom, BGTY, Sainsbury's*	1 Pizza/248g	526.0	3.0	212	12.1	37.8	1.4	2.9
Ham & Mushroom, Deep & Crispy, Tesco*	1 Serving/210g	420.0	10.0	200	9.7	29.2	4.9	1.1
Ham & Mushroom, Deep Pan, Waitrose*	½ Pizza/220g	453.0	14.0	206	10.9	26.6	6.2	1.0
Ham & Mushroom, Finest, Tesco*	½ Pizza/240g	576.0	26.0	240	9.5	25.9	11.0	2.2
Ham & Mushroom, New, BGTY, Sainsbury's*	1 Pizza/248g	526.0	3.0	212	12.1	37.8	1.4	2.9
Ham & Mushroom, Stone Baked, Goodfella's*	½ Pizza/175g	439.0	20.0	251	9.6	27.6	11.4	1.2
Ham & Mushroom, Thin & Crispy, Tesco*	1 Serving/166g	349.0	11.0	210	13.0	23.9	6.9	2.4
Ham & Onion, Tesco*	1 Serving/181g	452.0	17.0	250	11.8	29.0	9.6	2.2
Ham & Pineapple, American Deep Pan, Sainsbury's*	1 Pizza/412g	1001.0	32.0	243	10.5	32.6	7.8	1.7
Ham & Pineapple, Chicago Town*	1 Pizza/435g	866.0	20.0	199	10.0	29.7	4.5	0.0
Ham & Pineapple, Deep Dish, Individual, Chicago Town*	1 Pizza/170g	410.0	15.0	241	9.9	30.4	8.9	1.6
Ham & Pineapple, Deep Pan, Ciabatta, Iceland*	½ Pizza/185g	440.0	14.0	238	11.6	30.3	7.8	0.8
Ham & Pineapple, Deep Pan, Tesco*	1 Pizza/237g	437.0	7.0	184	9.8	29.8	2.9	1.9
Ham & Pineapple, HL, Tesco*	¼ Pizza/105g	170.0	2.0	162	10.0	25.9	2.1	2.4
Ham & Pineapple, Loaded, Tesco*	½ Pizza/265g	556.0	15.0	210	11.3	28.7	5.5	1.4
Ham & Pineapple, Pizzerai, Simply Italian, Sainsbury's*	½ Pizza/178g	434.0	15.0	244	11.5	30.4	8.5	2.4

PIZZA	Measure INFO/WEIGHT	per Measure KCAL	FAT	KCAL	PROT	CARB	FAT	FIBRE
Ham & Pineapple, Stone Bake, M & S*	1 Pizza/345g	690.0	20.0	200	10.1	28.3	5.7	1.6
Ham & Pineapple, Stonebaked, Tesco*	1 Pizza/161g	293.0	9.0	182	9.2	23.5	5.7	3.5
Ham & Pineapple, Thin & Crispy Italian, Morrisons*	1 Pizza/375g	746.0	23.0	199	10.2	24.9	6.1	0.0
Ham & Pineapple, Thin & Crispy, 2 Pack, Sainsbury's*	1 Pizza/163g	417.0	13.0	256	13.8	32.0	8.1	1.7
Ham & Pineapple, Thin & Crispy, Goodfella's*	1 Serving/163g	333.0	13.0	204	10.6	22.8	7.8	2.4
Ham & Pineapple, Thin & Crispy, Iceland*	1 Serving/110g	301.0	13.0	274	9.9	31.9	11.9	3.0
Ham & Pineapple, Thin & Crispy, Waitrose*	1 Pizza/220g	616.0	21.0	280	12.8	33.3	9.6	2.2
Ham & Roast Onion, Classico, Italiano, Tesco*	1 Serving/182g	470.0	19.0	259	12.1	29.1	10.5	1.6
Ham, Mushroom & Gruyere, Sainsbury's*	¼ Pizza/169.0g	404.0	14.0	239	10.2	31.3	8.1	3.7
Ham, Mushroom & Mascarpone, Italian Style, M & S*	1 Pizza/224g	515.0	22.0	230	10.0	25.5	9.7	2.9
Ham, Mushroom & Tomato, BGTY, Sainsbury's*	½ Pizza/150g	309.0	6.0	206	11.8	30.4	4.1	1.2
Ham, Pepperoni & Milano, M & S*	1 Pizza/290g	696.0	28.0	240	14.0	23.3	9.8	1.1
Hawaiian, San Marco*	¼ Pizza/90g	208.0	8.0	231	8.9	29.7	9.2	1.5
Hawaiian, Thin Crust, Tesco*	½ Pizza/192g	365.0	9.0	190	10.3	25.6	4.9	1.8
Hickory Steak, M & S*	1 Pizza/400g	820.0	27.0	205	9.9	25.7	6.7	1.4
Honey Roast Salmon & Broccoli, BGTY, Sainsbury's*	1 Serving/280g	613.0	13.0	219	10.2	34.4	4.5	3.5
Hot & Spicy Chicken, Deep Pan, Tesco*	½ Pizza/222g	423.0	7.0	191	10.5	30.0	3.3	2.1
Hot & Spicy, Deep Dish, Chicago Town*	1 Pizza/177g	434.0	18.0	245	8.6	30.4	9.9	0.9
Hot & Spicy, Deep Dish, Schwan's*	1 Pizza/170g	423.0	19.0	249	9.1	27.6	11.4	0.0
Hot & Spicy, Pizzeria Style, Sainsbury's*	1 Pizza/376g	986.0	46.0	262	12.5	25.5	12.3	2.4
Hot & Spicy, Thin & Crispy, Morrisons*	½ Pizza/170g	393.0	16.0	231	10.5	26.5	9.3	3.2
Hot Chicken, Stone Bake, M & S*	1 Pizza/380g	798.0	26.0	210	11.5	25.1	6.8	1.3
Hot Dog, Kids, Tesco*	1 Pizza/95g	233.0	6.0	245	9.8	36.6	6.6	2.0
Italian Cheese & Ham, The Little Big Food Company*	1 Pizza/95g	236.0	6.0	248	10.9	36.2	6.5	1.0
Italian Meat Feast, Thin & Crispy, Waitrose*	1 Pizza/182g	477.0	23.0	262	10.7	26.5	12.6	1.8
Italian Meats, Finest, Tesco*	½ Pizza/217g	449.0	8.0	207	13.6	29.4	3.9	1.3
Italian Mozzarella & Black Forest Ham, Asda*	¼ Pizza/110g	227.0	7.0	206	10.0	28.0	6.0	2.7
Italian Sausage & Roasted Peppers, Finest, Tesco*	1 Pizza/325g	650.0	14.0	200	7.8	31.7	4.2	1.9
Le Reine, 8 Inch, Supermarket, Pizza Express*	1 Pizza/283g	546.0	16.0	193	10.2	25.0	5.8	2.7
Leggera, Dr Oetker*	½ Pizza/175g	317.0	10.0	181	8.8	23.1	5.8	2.7
Loaded Cheese, Goodfella's*	1 Pizza/410g	1115.0	50.0	272	11.4	29.4	12.1	1.7
Margherita Classico, Italiano, Tesco*	½ Pizza/191g	414.0	12.0	217	11.2	29.1	6.2	2.5
Margherita, 12 Inch, Supermarket, Pizza Express*	½ Pizza/246.5g	542.0	17.0	220	9.8	29.9	6.8	2.6
Margherita, 12", Finest, Tesco*	½ Pizza/255g	433.0	9.0	170	8.1	26.4	3.6	2.7
Margherita, Cheese & Tomato, San Marco*	½ Pizza/200g	454.0	14.0	227	10.7	29.8	7.2	1.2
Margherita, Classico, Tesco*	1 Serving/150g	342.0	11.0	228	11.3	28.5	7.6	1.8
Margherita, Finest, Tesco*	1 Serving/207g	441.0	11.0	213	11.0	30.5	5.2	1.2
Margherita, HL, Tesco*	½ Pizza/125g	222.0	2.0	178	10.8	29.3	2.0	2.5
Margherita, Italian Stonebaked, Asda*	¼ Pizza/134.6g	323.0	11.0	240	11.0	31.0	8.0	1.8
Margherita, Italiano, Tesco*	½ Pizza/168g	395.0	12.0	235	11.7	29.9	7.2	1.2
Margherita, Light Choices, Tesco*	1 Pizza/200g	410.0	5.0	205	11.0	33.8	2.5	1.7
Margherita, Pizzeria, Italian, Sainsbury's*	½ Pizza/168.5g	426.0	17.0	253	12.2	27.9	10.3	2.5
Margherita, Primafresco, Tesco*	½ Pizza/204.1g	500.0	20.0	245	10.7	27.4	10.0	2.4
Margherita, Stone Baked, GFY, Asda*	¼ Pizza/73g	158.0	1.0	217	11.0	39.0	1.9	1.8
Margherita, Stone Baked, Goodfella's*	1 Slice/36g	95.0	4.0	263	10.9	31.9	11.4	7.6
Margherita, Stonebaked Ciabatta, Goodfella's*	½ Pizza/150g	404.0	17.0	270	11.3	32.8	11.5	2.6
Margherita, Stonebaked, Co-Op*	1 Pizza/350g	840.0	29.0	240	13.2	27.6	8.3	3.0
Margherita, Thin & Crispy, Iceland*	½ Pizza/170g	391.0	14.0	230	12.7	25.9	8.5	2.8
Margherita, Thin Crust, Tesco*	1 Serving/170g	354.0	13.0	208	10.1	24.1	7.9	3.6
Margherita, Tuscan, Finest, Tesco*	½ Pack/247.5g	557.0	22.0	225	8.2	27.7	8.9	1.3
Marinated Tomato & Mascarpone, Piccadella, Tesco*	1 Pizza/260g	634.0	27.0	244	6.4	31.6	10.2	2.2
Massive on Meat, Deep Pan, Goodfella's*	1 Serving/106g	259.0	9.0	244	10.4	30.6	8.9	3.0
Meat Feast, American Style, Sainsbury's*	½ Pizza/263g	642.0	26.0	244	12.6	26.2	9.9	2.9

P

PIZZA

INFO/WEIGHT	Measure		Nutrition Values per 100g / 100ml				
	KCAL	FAT	KCAL	PROT	CARB	FAT	FIBRE
Meat Feast, Deep & Crispy, Iceland* — 1/6 Pizza/136g	345.0	11.0	254	11.2	33.7	8.3	2.0
Meat Feast, Deep & Loaded, Sainsbury's* — ½ Pizza/298g	818.0	30.0	275	13.2	32.7	10.1	2.6
Meat Feast, Hot & Spicy, Thin & Crispy, Sainsbury's* — ½ Pizza/170g	462.0	22.0	272	13.0	26.5	12.7	3.2
Meat Feast, Large, Tesco* — 1 Pizza/735g	1904.0	69.0	259	10.9	32.6	9.4	2.0
Meat Feast, Loaded, Deep Pan, Large, Tesco* — ½ Pizza/282g	775.0	38.0	275	12.0	26.1	13.6	1.9
Meat Feast, Mega, Asda* — ½ Pizza/428g	1044.0	34.0	244	9.5	33.6	7.9	3.2
Meat Feast, Stuffed Crust, Asda* — ½ Pizza/238g	597.0	24.0	251	14.6	25.5	10.1	3.1
Meat Feast, Thin & Crispy, Asda* — ½ Pizza/183g	410.0	15.0	224	11.0	27.0	8.0	1.4
Meat Feast, Thin Crust, Tesco* — ½ Pizza/178g	430.0	20.0	242	13.6	21.3	11.4	2.3
Meat Mayhem, Goodfella's* — 1 Pizza/436.5g	1100.0	42.0	252	10.6	30.9	9.6	2.5
Meat, Mediterranean Style, Pizzeria, Waitrose* — ¼ Pizza/174g	395.0	15.0	227	11.1	25.8	8.8	2.0
Mediterranean Madness, Goodfella's* — ¼ Pizza/109g	235.0	9.0	216	9.1	27.0	8.0	3.9
Mediterranean Vegetable, Pizzeria, Sainsbury's* — 1 Serving/211g	397.0	14.0	188	8.0	24.7	6.4	3.2
Mediterranean Vegetable, Stonebaked, Sainsbury's* — ½ Pizza/260g	622.0	16.0	239	9.8	35.7	6.3	3.1
Mediterranean, Delicia, Goodfella's* — ½ Pizza/150g	371.0	18.0	247	9.1	25.3	12.2	2.1
Mexican Style, Morrisons* — ½ Pizza/180g	437.0	17.0	243	13.7	26.0	9.4	2.0
Mini, Party, Tesco* — 1 Pizza/11g	26.0	1.0	248	11.4	28.6	10.5	1.9
Mozzarella & Sunblush Tomato, 12", TTD, Sainsbury's* — ½ Pizza/251g	638.0	18.0	254	12.4	35.0	7.1	2.6
Mozzarella & Tomato, Asda* — 1 Pizza/360g	824.0	32.0	229	12.0	25.0	9.0	2.4
Mozzarella E Provolone, La Bottega, Goodfella's* — ½ Pizza/156g	372.0	15.0	238	10.1	27.9	9.6	2.4
Mushroom & Ham, COU, M & S* — 1 Pizza/245g	355.0	4.0	145	8.8	24.0	1.8	2.2
Mushroom & Mascarpone, 12", TTD, Sainsbury's* — ½ Pizza/255g	638.0	19.0	250	12.1	34.0	7.3	2.4
Mushroom & Roasted Onion, Waitrose* — ½ Pizza/187g	403.0	13.0	215	9.8	28.9	6.7	1.3
Napoletana, Sainsbury's* — ½ Pizza/186g	424.0	14.0	228	9.7	29.9	7.7	3.1
Napoli Ham & Mushroom, San Marco* — ½ Pizza/219g	449.0	13.0	205	10.0	27.5	6.1	2.8
Napoli, Tesco* — ½ Pizza/184g	431.0	12.0	235	11.9	32.6	6.3	1.4
Oval, Ham & Pineapple, Weight Watchers* — 1 Pizza/130g	220.0	2.0	169	11.6	26.7	1.8	3.0
Pasta, Ristorante, Dr Oetker* — ½ Pizza/205g	449.0	18.0	219	8.0	26.6	8.9	0.0
Pepper Steak, Deep Dish, Chicago Town* — 1 Pack/365g	372.0	10.0	102	6.1	13.4	2.7	0.0
Pepperonata, Delicata, Sainsbury's* — 1 Pizza/330g	917.0	48.0	278	12.9	24.3	14.4	2.6
Pepperoni & Cheese, Asda* — ½ Pizza/150g	385.0	13.0	257	10.0	34.0	9.0	2.7
Pepperoni & Jalapeno Chill, Asda* — 1 Pizza/277g	742.0	22.0	268	10.0	39.0	8.0	1.8
Pepperoni & Onion, 9", Sainsbury's* — ½ Pizza/207g	615.0	27.0	297	13.4	31.7	13.0	1.9
Pepperoni Bacon, Primo* — ½ Pizza/111g	360.0	15.0	324	10.5	42.5	13.1	0.0
Pepperoni, American Style Deep Pan, Co-Op* — 1 Pizza/395g	987.0	39.0	250	12.0	28.0	10.0	1.0
Pepperoni, Chicago Town* — 1 Pizza/170g	471.0	22.0	277	11.5	28.8	12.9	0.0
Pepperoni, Deep & Crispy, Iceland* — 1 Serving/175g	490.0	21.0	280	11.9	31.1	12.0	1.8
Pepperoni, Deep Filled, Chicago Town* — 1 Serving/202g	621.0	34.0	307	11.5	28.0	16.6	1.3
Pepperoni, Deep Pan, Frozen, Tesco* — ½ Pizza/215g	527.0	17.0	245	11.9	31.1	8.1	2.6
Pepperoni, Deep Pan, Goodfella's* — ¼ Pizza/109g	294.0	13.0	270	12.7	28.9	11.6	1.6
Pepperoni, Deep Pan, Sainsbury's* — ½ Pizza/191g	477.0	21.0	250	9.9	28.3	10.8	3.2
Pepperoni, Deluxe, American Deep Pan, Sainsbury's* — 1 Pizza/424g	1077.0	40.0	254	13.3	28.7	9.5	2.7
Pepperoni, Double, Italian, Chilled, Tesco* — ½ Pizza/159.6g	455.0	23.0	285	12.4	25.6	14.6	2.4
Pepperoni, Extra, Chicago Town* — 1 Pizza/460g	994.0	34.0	216	9.6	27.7	7.4	0.0
Pepperoni, Feast, Deep Dish, Schwan's* — 1 Pizza/435g	1188.0	62.0	273	9.9	26.3	14.2	0.0
Pepperoni, Freschetta, Schwan's* — 1 Pizza/310g	846.0	36.0	273	10.8	31.6	11.5	0.0
Pepperoni, Goodfella's* — 1 Pizza/337g	900.0	43.0	267	13.2	26.3	12.9	1.7
Pepperoni, Hot & Spicy, Stuffed Crust, Asda* — 1 Pizza/245g	666.0	30.0	272	13.9	26.5	12.2	2.4
Pepperoni, Hot & Spicy, Thin Crust, Chilled, Tesco* — ½ Pizza/173.5g	486.0	26.0	280	12.4	24.0	14.7	2.2
Pepperoni, Italian Stonebaked, Asda* — ¼ Pizza/131.6g	329.0	13.0	250	12.0	28.0	10.0	2.8
Pepperoni, Italian Style, Stonebaked, Stateside Foods* — ½ Pizza/168g	436.0	18.0	260	11.8	29.0	10.7	2.1
Pepperoni, Italian, Tesco* — ½ Pizza/186g	484.0	21.0	260	11.4	28.0	11.1	1.1
Pepperoni, Mini, Tesco* — 1 Serving/22g	71.0	4.0	323	11.8	30.5	16.8	2.7

PIZZA

INFO/WEIGHT	Measure	per Measure		Nutrition Values per 100g / 100ml				
		KCAL	FAT	KCAL	PROT	CARB	FAT	FIBRE
Pepperoni, Pizzeria Style, Sainsbury's*	½ Pizza/183g	515.0	23.0	281	13.5	28.0	12.7	2.2
Pepperoni, Pizzeria, Sainsbury's*	½ Pizza/197g	559.0	26.0	284	13.4	28.3	13.1	2.4
Pepperoni, Speciale, Sainsbury's*	½ Pizza/179g	447.0	20.0	250	11.9	26.6	10.9	2.3
Pepperoni, Stone Baked, Carlos*	1 Pizza/330g	832.0	40.0	252	13.0	23.0	12.0	0.0
Pepperoni, Stone Baked, Pizzaroma, Safeway*	½ Pizza/178g	480.0	19.0	269	12.9	30.6	10.6	2.2
Pepperoni, Stonebake, 10", Asda*	½ Pizza/170g	435.0	19.0	256	12.9	25.9	11.2	2.5
Pepperoni, Stonebaked Ciabatta, Goodfella's*	½ Pizza/181g	503.0	26.0	278	11.9	27.4	14.4	2.4
Pepperoni, Stonebaked, American Hot, Sainsbury's*	½ Pizza/276g	674.0	31.0	244	11.6	24.1	11.2	2.9
Pepperoni, Thin & Crispy, Essential, Waitrose*	½ Pizza/133g	380.0	18.0	286	12.3	28.8	13.5	1.0
Pepperoni, Thin & Crispy, Goodfella's*	1 Pizza/593g	1595.0	70.0	269	13.8	26.9	11.8	2.3
Pepperoni, Thin & Crispy, Sainsbury's*	½ Pizza/132g	405.0	19.0	307	13.9	30.7	14.3	2.6
Pepperoni, Thin Crust, Chilled, Tesco*	½ Pizza/163g	479.0	24.0	295	13.5	25.4	15.0	1.8
Pepperoni, Xxx Hot, Deep & Crispy, Chilled, Tesco*	½ Pizza/262.5	656.0	27.0	250	9.1	30.1	10.3	2.0
Pepperoni, Zingy, Asda*	1 Serving/90g	255.0	6.0	283	12.0	43.0	7.0	4.0
Pleasure with Fire Roasted Vegetables, Heinz*	½ Pizza/200g	418.0	16.0	209	9.5	24.8	8.0	2.4
Pollo, Ristorante, Dr Oetker*	½ Pizza/178g	383.0	17.0	216	8.9	23.4	9.5	0.0
Prosciutto & Mascarpone, Safeway*	½ Pizza/200g	522.0	21.0	261	12.3	29.8	10.3	2.2
Prosciutto, Classico, Tesco*	½ Pizza/205g	461.0	10.0	225	11.7	33.6	4.9	2.5
Prosciutto, Italian Style, Co-Op*	½ Pizza/183g	421.0	13.0	230	13.0	29.0	7.0	3.0
Prosciutto, Pizzaria, Sainsbury's*	1 Pizza/325g	806.0	23.0	248	11.4	34.7	7.1	3.2
Prosciutto, Ristorante, Dr Oetker*	1 Pizza/330g	752.0	32.0	228	10.3	24.6	9.8	0.0
Quattro Formaggi Pizzeria, Sainsbury's*	½ Pizza/175g	490.0	21.0	280	12.8	30.8	12.1	2.5
Quattro Formaggi, 8 Inch, Supermarket, Pizza Express*	1 Pizza/266g	646.0	26.0	243	12.1	26.5	9.8	2.3
Quattro Formaggi, Ristorante, Dr Oetker*	½ Pizza/175g	472.0	25.0	270	11.4	23.9	14.3	0.0
Quattro Formaggio, Tesco*	½ Pizza/219g	583.0	27.0	266	13.3	25.1	12.5	1.8
Roasted Tomato & Mozzarella, BGTY, Sainsbury's*	1 Pizza/204g	526.0	16.0	258	17.8	28.6	8.0	6.0
Roasted Vegetable, for One, GFY, Asda*	1 Pizza/96.0g	190.0	4.0	198	9.0	32.0	3.8	1.5
Salame, Ristorante, Dr Oetker*	½ Pizza/160g	455.0	24.0	285	10.4	26.3	15.3	0.0
Salami & Ham, Pizzeria, Waitrose*	½ Pizza/205g	443.0	14.0	216	10.1	28.7	6.7	1.8
Salami & Pepperoni, Waitrose*	½ Pizza/190g	578.0	31.0	304	13.4	23.9	16.2	2.1
Salami, Ultra Thin Italian, Tesco*	1 Serving/263g	692.0	26.0	263	12.0	31.9	9.7	1.0
Sicilian, Premium, Co-Op*	1 Pizza/600g	1320.0	48.0	220	9.0	27.0	8.0	2.0
Siciliana, Frozen, Finest, Tesco*	1 Serving/248g	431.0	14.0	174	8.5	21.9	5.8	3.2
Simply Cheese, Goodfella's*	¼ Pizza/82g	226.0	11.0	276	16.3	22.5	13.4	1.9
Slice Selection, M & S*	1 Serving/52g	120.0	4.0	230	9.4	30.3	7.8	1.9
Smoked Ham & Mushroom, Thin & Crispy, Co-Op*	1 Pizza/400g	792.0	18.0	198	9.0	30.3	4.5	1.7
Smoked Ham & Peppers, HL, Tesco*	1 Serving/282g	386.0	6.0	137	8.7	21.1	2.0	1.8
Smoked Ham & Pineapple, Deep Pan, Co-Op*	1 Pizza/395g	1142.0	42.0	289	11.6	36.7	10.6	1.7
Smoked Ham & Pineapple, Weight Watchers*	1 Pizza/241g	429.0	7.0	178	10.3	27.6	2.9	1.5
Spicy Beef, Goodfella's*	½ Pizza/148g	391.0	18.0	265	12.4	26.5	12.1	2.2
Spicy Chicken, Foccacia, Sainsbury's*	½ Pizza/245g	581.0	19.0	237	12.0	30.3	7.6	2.5
Spicy Chicken, HL, Tesco*	1 Serving/252g	418.0	4.0	166	10.9	27.1	1.6	2.7
Spicy Chicken, Iceland*	1 Pizza/345g	797.0	23.0	231	13.4	29.9	6.6	1.5
Spicy Chicken, Micro, McCain*	1 Pizza/133g	388.0	20.0	292	12.4	26.9	15.0	0.0
Spicy Chicken, Somerfield*	1 Serving/133g	304.0	8.0	229	13.4	29.7	6.3	0.0
Spicy Chorizo, Red Pepper & Chilli, Classico, Tesco*	1 Serving/218g	474.0	17.0	218	10.3	26.4	8.0	2.5
Spicy Vegetable Nacho, GFY, Asda*	1 Pizza/283g	636.0	13.0	225	10.0	36.0	4.5	3.3
Spicy Vegetable, Low Fat, Bertorelli*	1 Pizza/180g	243.0	4.0	135	6.0	23.4	2.4	1.9
Spinach & Bacon, Thin & Crispy, M & S*	1 Pizza/290g	739.0	35.0	255	10.6	26.8	12.1	1.0
Spinach & Ricotta, BGTY, Sainsbury's*	1 Pizza/265g	535.0	7.0	202	10.4	34.4	2.5	2.6
Spinach & Ricotta, Extra Special, Asda*	1 Pizza/400g	940.0	28.0	235	9.0	34.0	7.0	1.9
Spinach & Ricotta, Italian, Chilled, Sainsbury's*	1 Pizza/361g	859.0	35.0	238	9.3	28.7	9.6	2.3
Spinach & Ricotta, Italian, Somerfield*	1 Pizza/370g	918.0	37.0	248	10.3	29.2	10.0	2.2

P

PIZZA

INFO/WEIGHT	Measure	per Measure		Nutrition Values per 100g / 100ml				
		KCAL	FAT	KCAL	PROT	CARB	FAT	FIBRE
Spinach & Ricotta, Perfectly Balanced, Waitrose*	½ Pizza/165g	272.0	3.0	165	9.7	27.7	1.7	2.6
Spinach & Ricotta, Pizzaria, Waitrose*	½ Pizza/238g	501.0	21.0	211	10.7	21.9	8.9	2.6
Spinach & Ricotta, Thin Crust, Italian, Tesco*	½ Pizza/190g	365.0	17.0	192	9.6	18.7	8.8	1.9
Spinach with Bacon & Mushroom, GFY, Asda*	1 Serving/270g	618.0	12.0	229	13.0	34.0	4.5	2.6
Sunblushed Tomato & Mascarpone, Pizzadella, Tesco*	1 Serving/275g	894.0	44.0	325	8.5	36.7	16.0	1.5
Super Supreme, Family, Chicago Town*	¼ Pizza/225g	526.0	24.0	234	9.6	24.5	10.8	0.0
Supreme, Deep Dish, Individual, Chicago Town*	1 Pizza/170g	456.0	20.0	268	9.2	30.8	12.0	1.0
Supreme, Deep Pan, Safeway*	1 Serving/189g	450.0	18.0	238	10.8	27.0	9.6	4.7
Supreme, McCain*	1 Serving/125g	267.0	9.0	214	10.9	27.0	6.9	0.0
Supreme, Square to Share, Farmfoods*	1 Serving/93g	196.0	8.0	211	10.7	22.9	8.6	1.1
Sweet & Sour Chicken, Thin Crust, Tesco*	½ Pizza/186g	366.0	13.0	197	11.9	21.9	6.9	2.3
Sweet Chilli Chicken, BGTY, Sainsbury's*	½ Pizza/138g	276.0	2.0	200	13.0	33.2	1.7	2.1
The Big Cheese, Deep Pan, Goodfella's*	1/6 Pizza/118g	295.0	13.0	250	12.2	25.9	10.8	1.1
The Big Eat Meat X-Treme, Deep Pan, Goodfella's*	½ Pizza/352g	806.0	29.0	229	11.6	27.1	8.2	3.6
Three Cheese & Cherry Tomato, Weight Watchers*	1 Pizza/256g	399.0	4.0	156	9.8	25.6	1.6	2.3
Three Cheese Calzone, Waitrose*	1 Pizza/265g	747.0	32.0	282	10.4	33.0	12.0	1.4
Three Cheese, Ultra Thin, Sodebo*	1 Pizza/180g	450.0	18.0	250	10.9	28.5	10.2	1.8
Three Cheeses & Tomato, Stonebaked, Co-Op*	1 Pizza/415g	888.0	34.0	214	10.0	25.2	8.1	1.5
Three Meat, Thin & Crispy, Sainsbury's*	½ Pizza/147g	344.0	16.0	234	12.5	23.4	10.7	1.3
Tomato	1oz/28g	54.0	3.0	193	3.3	22.6	10.6	1.4
Tomato & Cheese, Ross*	1 Pizza/81g	181.0	6.0	224	7.4	31.5	7.6	2.5
Tomato & Cheese, Savers, Safeway*	1 Pizza/140g	371.0	11.0	265	9.5	38.4	8.1	3.0
Tomato & Cheese, Stone Bake, M & S*	1 Pizza/340g	782.0	29.0	230	10.8	30.1	8.4	1.6
Tomato & Cheese, Thin & Crispy, M & S*	1 Pizza/300g	705.0	28.0	235	11.0	27.7	9.4	1.2
Tomato & Mascarpone Piccadella, Slow Roasted, Tesco*	½ Pizza/128g	280.0	10.0	220	8.4	29.8	7.6	1.5
Tomato & Pesto, Tesco*	1 Serving/176g	449.0	23.0	256	8.4	25.9	13.2	1.1
Tomato & Red Pepper, Perfectly Balanced, Waitrose*	½ Pizza/163g	313.0	2.0	192	6.6	38.1	1.5	1.9
Tomato & Ricotta, Waitrose*	½ Pizza/208g	444.0	18.0	214	7.8	25.7	8.9	2.2
Tomato, Aubergine & Spinach, Pizzeria, Waitrose*	½ Pizza/193g	403.0	8.0	209	7.8	35.4	4.0	3.6
Tomato, Basil & Garlic, Weight Watchers*	1 Serving/85g	169.0	3.0	199	12.3	29.8	3.4	1.6
Tomato, Mushroom & Bacon, Deep Pan, Co-Op*	1 Pizza/420g	882.0	34.0	210	9.0	25.0	8.0	2.0
Triple Cheese, Deep Dish, Chicago Town*	1 Serving/170g	418.0	18.0	246	9.9	27.6	10.7	0.0
Triple Cheese, Deep Pan, Morrisons*	1/6 Pizza/75g	198.0	9.0	265	10.4	28.2	12.3	1.9
Tuna & Caramelised Red Onion, COU, M & S*	1 Pizza/245g	429.0	6.0	175	9.6	26.7	2.3	1.2
Tuna Sweetcorn, BGTY, Sainsbury's*	1 Pizza/304g	602.0	6.0	198	13.5	31.7	1.9	2.7
Tuscana, Finest, Tesco*	1 Serving/255g	643.0	36.0	252	13.2	18.4	14.0	5.9
Ultimate Meat Feast, Sainsbury's*	1 Pizza/465g	1302.0	48.0	280	13.5	35.1	10.3	1.7
Vegetable Feast, Thin & Crispy, Iceland*	1 Slice/63g	148.0	7.0	237	7.8	26.5	11.1	1.8
Vegetable Supreme, Safeway*	¼ Pizza/170g	352.0	12.0	207	10.4	25.9	6.9	2.9
Vegetable, COU, M & S*	1 Pizza/294g	397.0	7.0	135	6.4	23.2	2.4	1.9
Vegetable, Deep Pan, Co-Op*	1 Pizza/425g	829.0	30.0	195	8.0	25.0	7.0	2.0
Vegetable, Frozen, HL, Tesco*	1 Pizza/400g	604.0	11.0	151	8.1	23.5	2.7	4.4
Vegetable, GFY, Asda*	¼ Pizza/94g	141.0	3.0	150	7.0	24.0	2.9	3.7
Vegetable, HL, Tesco*	1 Serving/200g	302.0	5.0	151	8.1	23.5	2.7	4.4
Vegetable, Stone Bake, M & S*	1 Serving/465g	837.0	26.0	180	7.8	25.0	5.6	1.5
Vegetable, Stonebake, Thin & Crispy, Sainsbury's*	½ Pizza/156g	329.0	13.0	211	8.3	25.5	8.6	3.5
Vegetale, Ristorante, Dr Oetker*	½ Pizza/185g	386.0	17.0	209	8.1	23.9	9.0	0.0
Verona, Frozen, Finest, Tesco*	1 Serving/238g	541.0	23.0	228	11.6	23.2	9.8	2.7

PIZZA BASE

INFO/WEIGHT	Measure	per Measure		Nutrition Values per 100g / 100ml				
Deep Pan, Italian, Sainsbury's*	1 Base/220g	684.0	11.0	311	7.0	59.5	5.0	1.4
Deep Pan, Napolina*	1 Base/260g	757.0	8.0	291	7.9	58.0	3.0	0.2
Garlic Bread, Sainsbury's*	¼ Base/58.7g	109.0	4.0	186	5.1	25.4	7.1	1.8
Gluten & Wheat Free, Glutafin*	1 Base/110g	309.0	5.0	281	3.0	56.0	5.0	6.0

	Measure INFO/WEIGHT	per Measure		Nutrition Values per 100g / 100ml				
		KCAL	FAT	KCAL	PROT	CARB	FAT	FIBRE
PIZZA BASE								
Gluten Free, Glutafin*	1 Base/110g	278.0	5.0	253	3.0	49.0	5.0	4.5
Italian, Classic, Sainsbury's*	1 Base/150g	451.0	7.0	301	7.6	57.0	4.8	1.5
Italian, The Pizza Company*	1 Base/260g	624.0	7.0	240	7.6	46.5	2.6	0.0
Italiana, Parmalat*	1 Base/150g	450.0	7.0	300	9.0	55.0	4.9	0.0
Light & Crispy, Napolina*	1 Base/150g	436.0	4.0	291	7.9	58.0	3.0	0.2
Mini, Napolina*	1 Base/75g	218.0	2.0	291	7.9	58.0	3.0	0.2
Thin & Crispy, Sainsbury's*	1 Base/135g	338.0	4.0	251	8.4	47.3	3.1	4.4
Thin & Crispy, Tesco*	1 Serving/110g	348.0	8.0	316	9.2	52.9	7.5	1.5
Trufree*	1 Base/110g	345.0	7.0	314	3.0	63.0	6.0	4.0
Value, Tesco*	1 Base/150g	432.0	5.0	288	8.1	56.2	3.4	3.2
PIZZA BASE MIX								
Morrisons*	1 Serving/77g	313.0	4.0	407	12.7	77.9	5.0	3.6
Sainsbury's*	1 Pack/145g	486.0	6.0	335	12.8	62.3	3.8	2.9
Tesco*	1 Serving/36g	99.0	2.0	272	10.2	43.0	6.6	3.8
PLAICE								
Fillets, in Breadcrumbs, Average	1 Serving/150g	331.0	18.0	221	12.8	15.5	11.9	0.8
Fillets, Lightly Dusted, Average	1 Fillet/113g	188.0	9.0	166	12.9	10.4	8.1	0.6
Fillets, Raw, Average	*1oz/28g*	*24.0*	*0.0*	*87*	*18.2*	*0.0*	*1.5*	*0.0*
Goujons, Baked	1oz/28g	85.0	5.0	304	8.8	27.7	18.3	0.0
Goujons, Fried in Blended Oil	1oz/28g	119.0	9.0	426	8.5	27.0	32.3	0.0
Grilled	*1oz/28g*	*27.0*	*0.0*	*96*	*20.1*	*0.0*	*1.7*	*0.0*
in Batter, Fried in Blended Oil	1oz/28g	72.0	5.0	257	15.2	12.0	16.8	0.5
Steamed	*1oz/28g*	*26.0*	*1.0*	*93*	*18.9*	*0.0*	*1.9*	*0.0*
PLAICE WITH								
Mushrooms & Prawns, Sainsbury's*	1 Serving/170g	354.0	18.0	208	12.0	15.9	10.7	1.7
Mushrooms, Filled, Somerfield*	1 Serving/170g	338.0	18.0	199	10.2	15.7	10.6	1.2
Prawns, Fillets, Asda*	1oz/28g	24.0	1.0	86	11.0	0.4	4.5	0.7
Spinach & Cheddar Cheese, Fillets, Sainsbury's*	1 Serving/154g	222.0	13.0	144	13.6	3.1	8.6	0.8
Spinach & Ricotta Cheese, Whole, Sainsbury's*	1 Serving/159g	334.0	17.0	210	11.6	17.2	10.5	0.8
PLANTAIN								
Boiled in Unsalted Water	*1oz/28g*	*31.0*	*0.0*	*112*	*0.8*	*28.5*	*0.2*	*1.2*
Raw, Average	*1 Med/179g*	*218.0*	*1.0*	*122*	*1.3*	*31.9*	*0.4*	*2.3*
Ripe, Fried in Vegetable Oil	*1oz/28g*	*75.0*	*3.0*	*267*	*1.5*	*47.5*	*9.2*	*2.3*
PLUMS								
Average, Stewed without Sugar	*1oz/28g*	*8.0*	*0.0*	*30*	*0.5*	*7.3*	*0.1*	*1.3*
Soft Dried, Blue Parrot Cafe, Sainsbury's*	1 Pack/50g	118.0	0.0	237	2.6	55.6	0.5	7.1
Weighed with Stone, Average	*1 Plum/90g*	*32.0*	*0.0*	*36*	*0.6*	*8.6*	*0.1*	*1.6*
Whole, Dried, Graze*	1 Pack/60g	143.0	0.0	239	2.6	56.0	0.5	0.0
Yellow, Waitrose*	1 Plum/50g	19.0	0.0	39	0.6	8.8	0.1	1.5
POLENTA								
Merchant Gourmet*	1 Serving/65g	232.0	1.0	357	7.4	78.8	1.4	1.3
Organic, Kallo*	1 Serving/150g	543.0	3.0	362	8.5	78.0	1.8	0.0
POLLOCK								
Breaded, Asda*	1 Serving/97g	200.0	10.0	206	12.0	17.0	10.0	1.0
POLO								
Citrus Sharp, Nestle*	1 Tube/34g	134.0	0.0	393	0.0	96.6	1.0	0.0
Fruits, Nestle*	1 Tube/37g	142.0	0.0	383	0.0	96.0	0.0	0.0
Mints, Clear Ice, Nestle*	1 Sweet/4g	16.0	0.0	390	0.0	97.5	0.0	0.0
Mints, Original, Nestle*	1 Sweet/2g	8.0	0.0	404	0.0	98.9	1.1	0.0
Smoothies, Nestle*	1 Sweet/4g	16.0	0.0	408	0.1	86.9	6.8	0.0
Spearmint, Nestle*	1 Tube/35g	141.0	0.0	402	0.0	98.2	1.1	0.0
POMEGRANATE								
Raw, Fresh, Flesh Only, Average	*1 Sm Fruit/86g*	*59.0*	*0.0*	*68*	*0.9*	*17.2*	*0.3*	*0.6*

P

	Measure INFO/WEIGHT	per Measure KCAL	FAT	Nutrition Values per 100g / 100ml KCAL	PROT	CARB	FAT	FIBRE
POMEGRANATE								
Raw, Weighed with Rind & Skin, Average	*1 Sm Fruit/154g*	*105.0*	*0.0*	*68*	*0.9*	*17.2*	*0.3*	*0.1*
POMELO								
Fresh, Raw, Weighed with Skin & Seeds	*100 Grams/100g*	*18.0*	*0.0*	*18*	*0.4*	*4.1*	*0.1*	*0.0*
Raw, Flesh Only, Average	1 Av Fruit/340g	129.0	0.0	38	0.8	9.6	0.0	1.0
POP TARTS								
Bustin' Berry, Kellogg's*	1 Tart/50g	200.0	6.0	400	4.0	69.0	12.0	2.0
Chocomallow, Kellogg's*	1 Tart/50g	198.0	6.0	396	6.0	66.0	12.0	2.5
Cookies 'n' Creme, Kellogg's*	1 Tart/50g	197.0	5.0	394	4.0	72.0	10.0	1.5
Cream Cheese & Cherry Swirl, Kellogg's*	1 Tart/62g	250.0	11.0	403	3.2	59.7	17.7	1.0
Frosted Brown Sugar Cinnamon, Kellogg's*	1 Tart/50g	210.0	7.0	420	6.0	68.0	14.0	2.0
Strawberry Sensation, Kellogg's*	1 Tart/50g	197.0	5.0	395	4.0	70.0	11.0	2.0
POPCORN								
94% Fat Free, Orville Redenbacher's*	1 Bag/76g	220.0	0.0	289	13.2	65.8	0.0	0.0
Air Popped, Plain, Average	1oz/28g	110.0	1.0	387	12.9	77.9	4.5	14.5
Butter Flavour, Microwave, Popz*	1 Serving/100g	480.0	27.0	480	7.5	51.1	27.5	9.2
Butter Toffee, Asda*	1 Serving/100g	364.0	8.0	364	2.1	71.0	8.0	4.1
Butter Toffee, Belgian Milk Chocolate Coated, M & S*	1 Pack/100g	495.0	26.0	495	5.7	59.0	26.3	2.3
Butter Toffee, Snack-A-Jacks, Quaker Oats*	1 Bag/35g	149.0	3.0	425	3.5	86.0	9.0	4.5
Butter Toffee, Tesco*	1 Pack/350g	1417.0	27.0	405	2.2	81.7	7.7	4.3
Butter Toffee, Yummies*	1 Serving/50g	227.0	6.0	455	2.5	82.4	12.8	3.1
Butter, 6% Fat, Orville Redenbacher's*	1 Portion/21g	86.0	1.0	410	11.9	77.6	5.7	14.3
Butter, Microwave, 94% Fat Free, Act II*	½ Bag/41g	130.0	3.0	317	9.8	68.3	6.1	12.2
Butter, Microwave, Act II*	1 Bag/90g	425.0	16.0	472	9.0	69.0	18.0	9.0
Chocolate Flavour, Toffee, Snack-A-Jacks, Quaker Oats*	1 Bag/35g	126.0	3.0	359	2.2	65.0	9.8	3.0
Lightly Salted, Snack-A-Jack, Quaker Oats*	1 Bag/13g	48.0	1.0	370	12.1	58.0	9.9	14.6
Plain, Oil Popped, Average	1 Bag/74g	439.0	32.0	593	6.2	48.7	42.8	0.0
Ready Salted, Microwave, Popz*	1 Serving/20g	101.0	6.0	504	7.0	51.5	30.0	9.2
Salt & Vinegar, Snack-A-Jacks, Quaker Oats*	1 Sm Pack/13g	47.0	1.0	360	12.0	55.0	9.9	14.0
Salted, Blockbuster*	1 Bowl/25g	99.0	3.0	397	10.6	62.2	11.7	8.6
Salted, Bop, Microwave, Zanuy*	1 Serving/25g	119.0	6.0	477	10.7	56.9	23.0	0.0
Salted, Light, Microwave, Act II*	1 Pack/85g	336.0	6.0	395	10.6	71.0	7.6	15.8
Salted, Microwave, 93% Fat Free, Act II*	1 Pack/85g	345.0	6.0	406	10.0	76.0	7.0	13.0
Salted, Sold At Cinema, Playtime Popcorn*	1 Av Sm/74g	384.0	25.0	519	8.3	45.9	33.6	0.0
Super, Perri*	1 Packet/30g	139.0	7.0	464	8.4	55.5	23.2	8.5
Sweet, Best-In*	1 Serving/34g	161.0	6.0	473	7.3	72.6	17.0	0.0
Sweet, Butterkist, Butterkist*	1 Pack/120g	612.0	30.0	510	2.8	68.5	24.8	5.6
Sweet, Cinema Style, Butterkist*	1 Serving/100g	391.0	7.0	391	4.9	76.2	7.4	0.0
Sweet, Microwave, Cinema, Popz*	1 Bag/85g	420.0	22.0	494	6.0	60.0	25.5	8.2
Sweet, Vanilla & Sugar, Microwave, Act II*	1 Pack75g	369.0	18.0	492	7.9	60.8	24.1	10.4
Toffee, 90% Fat Free, Butterkist*	1 Pack/35g	142.0	3.0	406	2.8	77.7	9.3	0.0
Toffee, Best-In*	1 Bag/90g	356.0	3.0	396	5.0	85.9	3.6	0.0
Toffee, Butterkist*	1 Serving/35g	135.0	3.0	385	1.8	76.4	8.0	3.5
Toffee, Chicago Joes*	1 Serving/10g	31.0	0.0	314	3.1	84.6	4.8	0.0
Toffee, Milk Chocolate Coated, Sainsbury's*	¼ Bag/25g	130.0	7.0	520	6.5	64.1	26.4	1.3
Toffee, Sainsbury's*	1 Serving/50g	207.0	6.0	415	1.8	73.8	12.7	3.3
Vanilla, Cinema Sweet Microwave, Act II*	½ Pack/50g	234.0	8.0	468	9.0	71.0	16.0	12.0
Yellow, Kernel, (Unpopped), Jolly Time*	2 Tbsp/33g	110.0	1.0	333	12.1	78.8	3.0	21.2
POPCORN CAKES								
Caramel, Orville Redenbacher's*	1 Cake/12g	47.0	0.0	392	7.2	89.0	0.9	6.0
POPPADOM BITES								
Lime & Coriander Chutney, Sensations, Walkers*	1 Serving/18g	83.0	4.0	460	7.0	59.0	22.0	4.5
Spicy Tandoori Masala, Sensations, Walkers*	1 Sm Bag/18g	88.0	4.0	490	7.5	59.0	25.0	4.0

P

	Measure INFO/WEIGHT	per Measure KCAL	FAT	Nutrition Values per 100g / 100ml KCAL	PROT	CARB	FAT	FIBRE
POPPADOMS								
Fried in Vegetable Oil, Takeaway, Average	1 Poppadom/13g	65.0	5.0	501	11.5	28.3	38.8	5.8
Indian, Asda*	1 Pack/45g	232.0	16.0	516	14.5	36.2	34.8	7.8
Mercifully Mild, Phileas Fogg*	1 Serving/30g	150.0	10.0	499	14.8	36.8	32.6	6.0
Mini, Sainsbury's*	½ Pack/50g	249.0	16.0	498	14.9	36.9	32.3	7.6
Plain, Asda*	1 Poppadom/9g	44.0	3.0	484	18.0	40.0	28.0	0.0
Plain, Indian to Go, Sainsbury's*	1 Poppadom/8g	34.0	1.0	405	18.4	43.4	17.5	9.0
Plain, Tesco*	1 Serving/9.4	41.0	2.0	439	17.8	44.4	21.1	4.6
Plain, Waitrose*	1 Serving/9g	37.0	2.0	408	21.0	39.3	18.6	9.1
Spicy, COU, M & S*	1 Pack/26g	84.0	1.0	325	23.5	51.9	2.4	8.1
POPPETS*								
Chocolate Raisins, Poppets*	1 Pack/35g	140.0	5.0	401	4.9	65.4	13.3	0.0
Mint Cream, Poppets*	1oz/28g	119.0	4.0	424	2.0	75.0	13.0	0.0
Peanut, Poppets*	1 Box/100g	544.0	37.0	544	16.4	37.0	37.0	0.0
Toffee, Milk Chocolate, Poppets*	1 Box/100g	491.0	23.0	491	5.3	68.0	23.0	0.0
POPPING CORN								
Average	1 Serving/30g	112.0	1.0	375	10.9	73.1	4.3	12.7
Organic, Evernat*	1oz/28g	165.0	12.0	588	6.2	44.4	42.8	6.6
PORK								
Belly, Fresh, Raw, Weighed with Skin, Average	1 Serving/100g	518.0	53.0	518	9.3	0.0	53.0	0.0
Belly, Roasted, Lean & Fat	1oz/28g	82.0	6.0	293	25.1	0.0	21.4	0.0
Chop, Lean & Fat, Boneless, Raw, Average	*1oz/28g*	*67.0*	*4.0*	*240*	*29.2*	*0.0*	*13.7*	*0.0*
Cooked, with Herbs, Italian, Finest, Tesco*	2 Slices/50g	117.0	9.0	234	18.0	1.0	17.5	0.0
Diced, Lean, Average	*1oz/28g*	*31.0*	*0.0*	*109*	*22.0*	*0.0*	*1.7*	*0.0*
Escalope, Average	*1 Escalope/75g*	*108.0*	*2.0*	*144*	*31.0*	*0.0*	*2.2*	*0.0*
Haslet, Somerfield*	1oz/28g	57.0	3.0	205	15.0	10.0	12.0	0.0
Joint, Ready to Roast, Average	*½ Joint/254g*	*375.0*	*18.0*	*147*	*19.2*	*2.3*	*7.1*	*0.1*
Joint, with Crackling, Ready to Roast, Average	*1 Joint/567g*	*1283.0*	*80.0*	*226*	*24.2*	*0.8*	*14.1*	*0.0*
Loin, Applewood Smoked, Asda*	1 Slice/15g	18.0	1.0	122	21.8	0.5	3.6	0.0
Loin, Chops, Boneless, Grilled, Average	*1oz/28g*	*90.0*	*4.0*	*320*	*29.0*	*0.0*	*15.7*	*0.0*
Loin, Chops, Grilled, Lean	*1oz/28g*	*52.0*	*2.0*	*184*	*31.6*	*0.0*	*6.4*	*0.0*
Loin, Joint, Roast, Lean	*1oz/28g*	*51.0*	*2.0*	*182*	*30.1*	*0.0*	*6.8*	*0.0*
Loin, Joint, Roasted, Lean & Fat	*1oz/28g*	*71.0*	*4.0*	*253*	*26.3*	*0.0*	*15.3*	*0.0*
Loin, Roasted, with Rosemary, Arista, Sainsbury's*	1 Slice/17g	24.0	1.0	144	20.8	0.1	6.8	0.7
Loin, Steak, Fried, Lean	*1oz/28g*	*53.0*	*2.0*	*191*	*31.5*	*0.0*	*7.2*	*0.0*
Loin, Steak, Fried, Lean & Fat	*1oz/28g*	*77.0*	*5.0*	*276*	*27.5*	*0.0*	*18.4*	*0.0*
Loin, Steak, Lean, Raw, Average	*1 Serving/175g*	*345.0*	*20.0*	*197*	*22.7*	*1.8*	*11.2*	*0.4*
Loin, Stuffed, Roast, M & S*	1 Slice/12g	22.0	1.0	180	24.4	2.4	7.9	0.0
Medallions, Average	*1 Pack/220g*	*359.0*	*5.0*	*163*	*35.1*	*0.0*	*2.5*	*0.4*
Mince, Lean, Healthy Range, Average	*1 Pack/400g*	*504.0*	*20.0*	*126*	*19.7*	*0.4*	*5.0*	*0.3*
Mince, Raw	*1oz/28g*	*46.0*	*3.0*	*164*	*19.2*	*0.0*	*9.7*	*0.0*
Mince, Stewed	*1oz/28g*	*53.0*	*3.0*	*191*	*24.4*	*0.0*	*10.4*	*0.0*
Rashers, Streaky, British, Sainsbury's*	1 Serving/100g	320.0	23.0	320	27.4	0.0	23.4	0.0
Raw, Lean, Average	*1oz/28g*	*42.0*	*1.0*	*151*	*28.6*	*0.0*	*4.1*	*0.0*
Roast, Lean Only, Average	*1oz/28g*	*34.0*	*1.0*	*121*	*22.7*	*0.3*	*3.3*	*0.0*
Roast, Slices, Average	*1 Slice/30g*	*40.0*	*1.0*	*133*	*22.7*	*0.4*	*4.5*	*0.0*
Shoulder, Slices, Cured	*1oz/28g*	*29.0*	*1.0*	*103*	*16.9*	*0.9*	*3.6*	*0.0*
Shoulder, Whole, Lean & Fat, Raw, Average	*100g*	*236.0*	*18.0*	*236*	*17.2*	*0.0*	*18.0*	*0.0*
Slow Cooked, With Smoked Chilli Beans, HL, Tesco*	1 Pack/365g	255.0	5.0	70	6.6	8.0	1.3	2.5
Steak, Lean & Fat, Average	*1oz/28g*	*61.0*	*4.0*	*219*	*23.8*	*0.0*	*13.7*	*0.1*
Steak, Lean, Stewed	*1oz/28g*	*49.0*	*1.0*	*176*	*33.6*	*0.0*	*4.6*	*0.0*
Tenderloin, Lean, Boneless, Raw, Average	1 Serving/100g	109.0	2.0	109	20.9	0.0	2.2	0.0
Tenderloin, Roulade, Waitrose*	1 Pack/171g	282.0	13.0	165	18.4	5.9	7.5	1.8
Tenderloin, Separable Lean & Fat, Raw, Average	1 Av Loin/265g	318.0	9.0	120	20.6	0.0	3.5	0.0

P

	Measure INFO/WEIGHT	per Measure KCAL	per Measure FAT	Nutrition Values per 100g / 100ml KCAL	PROT	CARB	FAT	FIBRE
PORK &								
Apricots, Aromatic, Cafe Culture, M & S*	½ Pack/420g	672.0	31.0	160	10.3	12.5	7.4	2.1
Chestnut Stuffing, M & S*	1oz/28g	64.0	5.0	230	5.3	12.6	17.1	3.7
PORK CHAR SUI								
Chinese, Tesco*	1 Pack/400g	520.0	17.0	130	7.2	15.7	4.3	0.6
in Cantonese Sauce, Asda*	1 Pack/360g	623.0	8.0	173	9.8	28.4	2.2	0.5
Oriental, Finest, Tesco*	1 Pack/350g	245.0	5.0	70	6.8	6.2	1.5	2.1
Takeaway, Iceland*	1 Pack/400g	412.0	10.0	103	7.9	12.5	2.4	1.2
with Chicken, & Egg Fried Rice, Tesco*	1 Serving/450g	602.0	16.0	134	7.1	18.3	3.6	0.9
PORK CHINESE								
Sliced, M & S*	1 Serving/140g	224.0	4.0	160	26.4	6.1	3.1	0.0
Style, GFY, Asda*	1 Serving/170g	286.0	6.0	168	18.8	15.3	3.5	0.4
with Noodles, Tesco*	1 Serving/450g	612.0	26.0	136	7.0	14.2	5.7	1.1
PORK DINNER								
Roast, Birds Eye*	1 Pack/340g	410.0	12.0	121	7.6	14.7	3.5	1.6
PORK IN								
Kentish Cider, With Bramley Apple Mash, Tesco*	1 Pack/450g	495.0	22.0	110	5.6	10.6	4.8	1.1
Light Mustard Sauce, Fillet, COU, M & S*	1 Pack/390g	312.0	9.0	80	10.9	3.5	2.4	0.7
Mustard & Cream, Chops	1oz/28g	73.0	6.0	261	14.5	2.4	21.6	0.3
Rich Sage & Onion Gravy, Steaks, Tesco*	1 Serving/160g	218.0	10.0	136	16.0	3.2	6.5	1.5
PORK SCRATCHINGS								
Crunch, Mr Porky*	1 Pack/30g	159.0	10.0	531	60.4	0.5	31.9	4.6
KP Snacks*	1 Pack/20g	125.0	10.0	624	47.3	0.5	48.1	0.5
Tavern Snacks*	1 Pack/30g	187.0	14.0	624	47.3	0.5	48.1	0.5
PORK WITH								
Apricot & Orange Stuffing, Joint, Sainsbury's*	¼ Joint/200g	566.0	36.0	283	29.0	0.9	18.1	1.4
Cheese & Pineapple, Loin Steaks, M & S*	1 Steak/141g	240.0	14.0	170	14.0	6.3	9.9	0.0
Herbes De Provence, Joint, Sainsbury's*	¼ Joint/200g	302.0	16.0	151	19.2	0.1	8.2	0.6
Honey & Mustard Sauce, Steaks, Tesco*	½ Pack/160g	258.0	12.0	161	16.3	8.7	7.4	1.4
Honey & Soy, Sainsbury's*	1 Serving/260g	260.0	7.0	100	12.3	6.2	2.9	0.3
Leek & Bacon Stuffing, Roast, Shoulder, Sainsbury's*	1 Serving/150g	237.0	12.0	158	18.8	2.4	8.3	0.5
Leek & Cheese Stuffing, Joint, Sainsbury's*	1 Serving/100g	231.0	10.0	231	31.0	3.0	10.5	1.1
Maple & BBQ Sauce, Loin Steaks, Somerfield*	½ Pack/160g	336.0	16.0	210	20.4	9.2	10.0	0.0
Medallions, with Bramley Apple, M & S*	1 Serving/380g	418.0	13.0	110	17.7	2.5	3.4	0.5
Noodles, Chinese, Tesco*	1 Serving/450g	463.0	13.0	103	5.3	13.7	3.0	1.4
Peppers, Marinated, Tapas, Waitrose*	1 Serving/105g	181.0	7.0	172	26.3	2.2	6.4	0.3
Roasted Rosemary Potatoes, Porchetta, Finest, Tesco*	½ Pack/370g	455.0	32.0	123	6.9	4.6	8.6	0.5
Sage & Onion Stuffing, Joint, BGTY, Sainsbury's*	1 Serving/150g	246.0	5.0	164	29.5	3.3	3.6	1.3
Sage & Onion Stuffing, Joint, Tesco*	1 Serving/200g	208.0	6.0	104	17.1	2.7	2.8	0.0
Sage, Onion & Lemon Stuffing, Joint, Sainsbury's*	1 Serving/260g	699.0	43.0	269	27.4	2.2	16.7	1.4
Spiced Apple Stuffing, Steaks, Easy Cook, Waitrose*	1 Serving/190g	236.0	8.0	124	19.3	2.4	4.1	0.5
Stuffing, Belly, Norfolk Outdoor Reared, Finest, Tesco*	1 Serving/180g	524.0	45.0	291	14.9	1.7	24.9	0.0
Thai Style Butter, Steaks, Asda*	4 Steaks/300g	810.0	54.0	270	26.0	1.0	18.0	0.0
Tomato & Apricot Sauce, Loin Steaks, Sainsbury's*	½ Pack/110g	216.0	11.0	196	24.4	3.1	9.6	0.6
PORRIDGE								
Apple & Cinnamon, Diet Chef Ltd*	1 Pack/40g	143.0	2.0	357	8.9	65.5	4.6	9.0
Chocolate, Instant, Grasshopper*	1 Pot/60g	221.0	3.0	368	15.0	68.3	5.0	0.0
Cinnamon & Raisin, Instant, Grasshopper*	1 Pot/60g	208.0	2.0	346	13.3	68.3	3.3	0.0
Strawberry, Diet Chef Ltd*	1 Pack/40g	153.0	3.0	382	11.2	65.5	7.8	10.3
Vanilla & Banana, Diet Chef Ltd*	1 Pack/40g	151.0	2.0	377	10.7	70.6	5.6	9.8
with Cocoa Nib, Diet Chef Ltd*	1 Pack/40g	159.0	3.0	397	10.9	67.3	8.7	9.2
PORT								
Average	*1 Serving/50ml*	*78.0*	*0.0*	*157*	*0.1*	*12.0*	*0.0*	*0.0*

	Measure INFO/WEIGHT	KCAL	FAT	Nutrition Values per 100g / 100ml KCAL	PROT	CARB	FAT	FIBRE
POT NOODLE*								
Balti Curry, Made Up, Pot Noodle*	1 Pot/301g	268.0	2.0	89	3.1	17.8	0.5	0.5
Beef & Tomato, Made Up, Pot Noodle*	1 Pot/300g	378.0	14.0	126	3.1	18.1	4.7	1.1
Beef & Tomato, Mini, Pot Noodle*	1 Pot/190g	254.0	9.0	134	3.5	18.7	5.0	1.7
Beef & Tomato, Pot Noodle*	1 Pot/319g	424.0	15.0	133	3.4	19.4	4.6	1.3
Bombay Bad Boy, Made Up, Pot Noodle*	1 Pot/305g	384.0	14.0	126	3.1	17.9	4.6	1.1
Chicken & Mushroom, King, Pot Noodle*	1 Pack/401g	513.0	19.0	128	3.2	18.1	4.8	1.1
Chicken & Mushroom, Made Up, Pot Noodle*	1 Pot/300g	384.0	14.0	128	3.2	18.0	4.7	1.1
Chicken & Mushroom, Mini, Made Up, Pot Noodle*	1 Pot/190g	243.0	9.0	128	3.8	18.2	4.5	1.4
Chicken Curry, Hot, Made Up, Pot Noodle*	1 Pot/300g	384.0	14.0	128	2.8	18.7	4.7	1.1
Hot Dog & Ketchup, Fun Pots, Made Up, Pot Noodle*	1 Pot/190g	243.0	9.0	128	3.6	18.3	4.5	1.5
Hot, Made Up, Pot Noodle*	1 Pot/300g	378.0	16.0	126	3.0	16.9	5.2	1.1
Korma Curry, Made Up, Pot Noodle*	1 Pot/300g	273.0	3.0	91	2.9	17.4	1.1	0.4
Nice & Spicy, Made Up, Pot Noodle*	1 Pot/300g	381.0	14.0	127	2.8	18.3	4.7	1.1
Seedy Sanchez, Made Up, Pot Noodle*	1 Pot/300g	396.0	14.0	132	3.1	19.1	4.8	1.1
Spicy Chilli, Posh, Made Up, Pot Noodle*	1 Pot/301g	328.0	18.0	109	2.5	11.7	5.9	1.0
Spicy Curry, Made Up, Pot Noodle*	1 Pot/300g	393.0	14.0	131	2.9	19.1	4.8	1.1
Sweet & Sour, Dry, Pot Noodle*	1 Pot/86g	376.0	14.0	437	12.1	60.9	16.1	3.1
Sweet & Sour, King, Dry, Pot Noodle*	1 Pot/105g	473.0	20.0	450	8.8	60.0	19.1	4.8
Sweet & Sour, Oriental, Posh, Pot Noodle*	1 Pot/300g	375.0	14.0	125	1.7	19.2	4.6	0.5
POT RICE								
Chicken & Sweetcorn, Dry, Pot Rice*	1 Pot/68g	243.0	3.0	357	13.1	65.8	4.6	4.0
Chicken Curry, Dry, Pot Rice*	1 Pot/74g	253.0	2.0	342	11.0	67.2	2.3	3.3
POTATO BITES								
Barbecue, Baked, COU, M & S*	1 Pack/26g	92.0	1.0	355	7.1	76.7	2.4	4.2
Butter & Chive, Baked, COU, M & S*	1 Serving/26g	92.0	1.0	355	7.6	77.2	2.0	4.7
Crispy, Morrisons*	1 Serving/115g	240.0	8.0	209	3.5	32.6	7.2	2.2
POTATO BOMBAY								
Average	1oz/28g	33.0	2.0	117	2.0	13.7	6.8	1.2
Flavours of India, Canned, Sainsbury's*	½ Can/200g	160.0	4.0	80	2.4	13.3	1.9	1.8
Indian Meal for Two, Sainsbury's*	½ Pack/151g	154.0	8.0	102	1.6	11.4	5.6	3.1
Indian Takeaway for 1, Sainsbury's*	1 Serving/200g	202.0	10.0	101	1.8	11.8	5.2	1.7
POTATO CAKES								
Average	1 Cake/70g	127.0	1.0	180	3.8	37.5	1.7	2.4
Fried, Average	1oz/28g	66.0	3.0	237	4.9	35.0	9.0	0.8
POTATO CHIPS								
Beef & Horseradish, Tyrells*	¼ Pack/37.4g	177.0	9.0	473	9.0	58.6	24.8	2.4
Hand Fried Mature Cheddar, Burts*	1 Serving/40g	202.0	11.0	504	6.4	57.4	27.7	0.0
Lightly Sea Salted, Tyrells*	1 Pack/150g	739.0	38.0	493	7.7	58.9	25.4	2.6
Mature Cheese & Chives, Tyrells*	1 Bag/50g	261.0	14.0	522	6.1	56.5	27.9	0.0
Ready Salted, Sainsbury's*	¼ Pack/33g	174.0	11.0	526	5.6	51.7	33.0	3.8
Reduced Fat, Cape Cod*	1 Bag/140g	664.0	36.0	474	7.9	53.5	25.4	6.4
Sweet Chilli & Red Pepper, Tyrells*	¼ Pack/37.4g	180.0	9.0	481	7.9	59.7	24.5	2.4
Worcester Sauce, with Sun Dried Tomato, Tyrells*	1 Bag/50g	241.0	12.0	482	7.6	60.1	24.8	2.5
POTATO MASH								
Bacon & Cheese, Tesco*	1 Serving/200g	252.0	13.0	126	3.1	13.9	6.4	1.3
Bacon & Spring Onion, Finest, Tesco*	½ Pack/200g	214.0	10.0	107	4.3	10.8	5.2	1.6
Carrot And Swede, Sainsbury's*	½ Pack/225g	101.0	4.0	45	0.7	6.8	1.7	2.8
Cheddar, Irish, Finest, Tesco*	½ Pack/250g	350.0	20.0	140	6.3	10.2	7.9	1.4
Cheese & Chive, Snack in a Pot, Tesco*	1 Pot/230g	304.0	22.0	132	2.2	9.6	9.4	0.9
Cheese & Onion, Eat Smart, Morrisons*	1 Pack/400g	340.0	6.0	85	4.4	13.2	1.6	1.3
Cheese & Onion, Tesco*	1 Serving/200g	210.0	9.0	105	3.2	12.6	4.7	1.0
Leek & Bacon, Tesco*	1 Serving/400g	356.0	14.0	89	3.0	11.1	3.6	1.9
Leek & Cheese, COU, M & S*	½ Pack/225g	180.0	5.0	80	3.0	12.0	2.1	1.3

P

	Measure INFO/WEIGHT	per Measure KCAL	per Measure FAT	Nutrition Values per 100g / 100ml KCAL	PROT	CARB	FAT	FIBRE
POTATO MASH								
Mustard, with Caramelised Onions, Finest, Tesco*	1 Serving/200g	232.0	9.0	116	2.6	16.0	4.6	1.8
Roast Onion, Snack in a Pot, Tesco*	1 Pot/218g	257.0	13.0	118	1.6	14.7	5.9	0.6
Savoy Cabbage & Spring Onion, M & S*	1 Serving/225g	250.0	16.0	111	2.0	10.2	6.9	1.3
Sun Dried Tomato & Basil, COU, M & S*	1 Serving/170g	127.0	3.0	75	1.0	14.4	1.5	1.2
with Cracked Pepper & Sea Salt, Luxury, Sainsbury's*	½ Pack/225g	389.0	28.0	173	1.6	13.2	12.6	1.0
with Sweetcorn & Flaked Tuna, Quick, Sainsbury's*	1 Pot/224g	240.0	9.0	107	2.4	15.0	4.1	2.1
with Vegetables, GFY, Asda*	1 Pack/290g	186.0	3.0	64	1.6	12.0	1.1	2.3
with Vegetables, Sainsbury's*	½ Pack/229.0g	142.0	2.0	62	1.8	11.4	1.0	3.1
POTATO RINGS								
Mature Cheddar & Red Onion, GFY, Asda*	1 Pack/10g	36.0	0.0	360	5.2	81.6	1.5	2.9
Ready Salted, M & S*	1 Serving/75g	375.0	21.0	500	3.5	58.9	28.1	2.6
Ready Salted, Sainsbury's*	1 Serving/50g	257.0	14.0	514	3.2	61.5	28.4	1.8
Salt Vinegar, Sainsbury's*	1 Pack/25g	114.0	5.0	456	3.6	65.6	19.6	2.8
POTATO SKINS								
¼ Cut, Deep Fried, McCain*	1oz/28g	52.0	2.0	186	3.0	30.1	6.0	0.0
American Style, Loaded, Asda*	1 Serving/78g	294.0	18.0	375	15.0	27.0	23.0	2.4
American Style, Loaded, Tesco*	1 Serving/340g	388.0	8.0	114	6.8	16.3	2.4	3.3
Cheese & Bacon, Loaded, Asda*	½ Pack/125g	275.0	15.0	220	13.0	15.0	12.0	3.3
Cheese & Bacon, Sainsbury's*	1 Serving/140g	349.0	22.0	249	10.3	17.3	15.4	2.5
Cheese & Bacon, Waitrose*	1 Serving/75g	146.0	9.0	195	7.3	13.1	12.6	3.5
Cheese & Chive, Sainsbury's*	2 Skins/150g	286.0	18.0	191	7.7	13.3	11.9	2.8
Cheese & Ham, Iceland*	2 Skins/108.4g	155.0	5.0	143	6.3	19.3	4.5	2.0
Soured Cream, Loaded, M & S*	½ Pack/150g	307.0	18.0	205	9.1	15.8	11.9	0.9
POTATO SMILES								
Weighed Baked, McCain*	1 Serving/100g	237.0	10.0	237	3.4	33.4	10.1	3.1
Weighed Frozen, McCain*	1 Serving/100g	191.0	8.0	191	2.6	27.0	8.0	2.7
POTATO SUMTHINGS								
Weighed Baked, McCain*	1 Serving/100g	220.0	9.0	220	3.4	31.3	9.0	2.8
Weighed Frozen, McCain*	1 Serving/100g	187.0	8.0	187	2.9	26.2	7.9	2.4
POTATO TWIRLS								
Sainsbury's*	1 Serving/50g	217.0	7.0	435	3.0	72.8	14.6	3.1
POTATO WAFFLES								
Birds Eye*	1 Waffle/60g	105.0	5.0	175	2.5	21.6	8.7	1.5
Frozen, Cooked	1oz/28g	56.0	2.0	200	3.2	30.3	8.2	2.3
Frozen, Grilled, Asda*	1 Waffle/57g	104.0	6.0	183	2.0	21.0	10.1	1.7
Mini, Farmfoods*	1oz/28g	41.0	2.0	145	1.9	21.6	5.7	1.7
Mini, Sainsbury's*	1 Waffle/11g	27.0	2.0	242	2.8	20.1	16.7	1.0
Oven Baked, Mini, McCain*	1oz/28g	62.0	2.0	221	3.9	32.0	8.6	0.0
Sainsbury's*	1 Waffle/56g	108.0	6.0	194	2.9	22.8	10.1	1.1
Southern Fried, Asda*	1 Waffle/51g	107.0	5.0	209	2.8	27.0	10.0	2.1
POTATO WEDGES								
& Dip, M & S*	1 Pack/450g	697.0	33.0	155	2.5	20.4	7.4	1.8
Aldi*	1 Serving/100g	150.0	7.0	150	2.1	20.2	6.8	0.0
Asda*	1 Wedge/40g	57.0	2.0	142	3.4	21.0	4.9	1.7
Baked, GFY, Asda*	1 Pack/450g	616.0	12.0	137	3.4	25.0	2.6	3.4
BBQ Chicken Spicy, Good Intentions, Somerfield*	1 Pack/400g	380.0	5.0	95	7.4	13.6	1.2	1.4
BBQ Flavour, Asda*	1 Serving/100g	185.0	9.0	185	2.9	23.0	9.0	1.7
BGTY, Sainsbury's*	½ Pack/190g	179.0	3.0	94	3.0	16.4	1.8	3.4
Bombay, with Yoghurt & Mint Dip, HL, Tesco*	1 Serving/170g	139.0	4.0	82	1.3	14.5	2.1	0.9
Co-Op*	1oz/28g	38.0	2.0	135	2.0	20.0	6.0	2.0
Crispy, M & S*	1 Serving/200g	340.0	14.0	170	1.3	25.3	7.1	1.7
Four Cheese & Red Onion, Chicago Town*	1 Serving/150g	210.0	8.0	140	2.1	21.0	5.3	2.4
Garlic & Herb Crusted, Chicago Town*	1 Serving/150g	216.0	6.0	144	1.9	24.4	4.3	2.2

	Measure INFO/WEIGHT	per Measure KCAL	FAT	Nutrition Values per 100g / 100ml KCAL	PROT	CARB	FAT	FIBRE
POTATO WEDGES								
Garlic & Herb, COU, M & S*	1 Pack/300g	300.0	8.0	100	2.3	16.4	2.6	3.2
Garlic & Herb, Kitchen Range Foods*	1oz/28g	42.0	2.0	151	1.6	18.5	7.8	0.0
Jacket, Spicy, American Style, Frozen, Sainsbury's*	1 Serving/125g	156.0	5.0	125	1.9	20.3	4.0	1.1
Jumbo, Finest, Tesco*	1 Serving/126g	145.0	3.0	115	1.4	22.7	2.1	1.7
Mexican, Inspire, Asda*	1 Pack/500g	525.0	17.0	105	2.2	16.5	3.4	1.8
Micro, Tesco*	1 Pack/100g	170.0	7.0	170	2.6	24.5	6.8	2.3
New York Style, HL, Tesco*	1 Serving/125g	129.0	3.0	103	2.0	18.3	2.4	2.3
Only 5% Fat, Weighed Baked, McCain*	1 Serving/100g	173.0	4.0	173	3.3	30.2	4.3	2.8
Only 5% Fat, Weighed Frozen, McCain*	1 Serving/100g	123.0	3.0	123	2.2	21.8	3.0	1.9
Oven Baked, Waitrose*	1oz/28g	46.0	1.0	165	2.4	29.2	4.3	2.1
Perfectly Balanced, Waitrose*	1 Serving/275g	278.0	5.0	101	2.5	19.0	1.7	3.5
Savoury, Waitrose*	1/3 Bag/250g	350.0	11.0	140	2.3	22.9	4.3	1.9
Sour Cream & Chives, McCain*	1 Serving/100g	132.0	4.0	132	2.4	24.0	4.1	0.0
Southern Fried Flavour, Champion*	1oz/28g	41.0	2.0	147	2.1	20.8	6.2	2.8
Southern Fried Style, Tesco*	1 Serving/155g	232.0	14.0	150	3.0	14.1	9.1	2.0
Southern Fried, Asda*	1 Serving/100g	157.0	4.0	157	3.0	26.0	4.5	3.5
Spicy, & Garlic Dip, Linda McCartney*	1 Pack/300g	366.0	17.0	122	2.6	15.3	5.6	3.1
Spicy, Asda*	1 Serving/100g	145.0	6.0	145	1.8	21.8	5.7	2.1
Spicy, Deep Fried, McCain*	1oz/28g	52.0	2.0	187	3.6	27.3	8.1	0.0
Spicy, M & S*	½ Pack/225g	349.0	15.0	155	2.4	21.8	6.5	1.3
Spicy, Occasions, Sainsbury's*	1 Serving/100g	144.0	4.0	144	2.5	23.7	4.3	0.4
Spicy, Simple Solutions, Tesco*	1 Serving/150g	141.0	4.0	94	4.6	12.2	3.0	1.4
With A Parsley & Oil Dressing, Tesco*	½ Pack/280g	168.0	3.0	60	1.0	11.5	1.0	1.8
with Broccoli & Mozzarella Cheese, Weight Watchers*	1 Pack/320g	294.0	10.0	92	3.1	13.3	3.0	1.0
with Chilli, COU, M & S*	1 Pack/400g	380.0	11.0	95	5.2	13.7	2.7	2.3
with Olive Oil & Parsley Dressing, Inspire, Asda*	½ Pack/300g	219.0	7.0	73	0.1	12.7	2.4	2.1
POTATOES								
Alphabites, Captain Birds Eye, Birds Eye*	9 Bites/56g	75.0	3.0	134	2.0	19.5	5.3	1.4
Anya, Raw, TTD, Sainsbury's*	1 Serving/100g	75.0	0.0	75	1.5	17.8	0.3	1.1
Baby, Dressed with Garlic & Rosemary, M & S*	1 Serving/185g	129.0	5.0	70	2.0	9.0	2.8	2.4
Baby, Garlic & Sea Salt Roasted, Finest, Tesco*	1 Serving/200g	192.0	7.0	96	3.1	13.5	3.3	1.0
Baby, New, with Butter, Mint & Parsley, Organic, Asda*	1 Pack/360g	414.0	10.0	115	1.7	20.4	2.9	2.5
Baby, Oven Bake, Aunt Bessie's*	1 Serving/120g	103.0	2.0	86	2.2	16.3	1.4	3.0
Baby, with Butter & Herbs, Sainsbury's*	¼ Pack/142.7g	107.0	2.0	75	1.3	14.7	1.2	2.1
Baby, with Herb Butter, Safeway*	1 Serving/200g	158.0	2.0	79	1.4	15.6	1.2	1.4
Baked, Flesh & Skin, Average	*1 Med/200g*	*218.0*	*0.0*	*109*	*2.3*	*25.2*	*0.1*	*2.4*
Baked, Flesh Only, Weighed with Skin, Average	*1oz/28g*	*26.0*	*0.0*	*93*	*2.0*	*21.6*	*0.1*	*1.5*
Baked, in Microwave, Flesh & Skin, Average	*1oz/28g*	*29.0*	*0.0*	*105*	*2.4*	*24.1*	*0.1*	*2.3*
Baked, in Microwave, Flesh Only, Average	*1oz/28g*	*28.0*	*0.0*	*100*	*2.1*	*23.3*	*0.1*	*1.6*
Baked, in Microwave, Skin Only, Average	*1oz/28g*	*37.0*	*0.0*	*132*	*4.4*	*29.6*	*0.1*	*5.5*
Baked, Jacket, Baby, Veg, COOK!, M & S*	1 Pack/675g	776.0	38.0	115	2.1	14.3	5.6	2.3
Baked, Jacket, Beef Chilli Filled, GFY, Asda*	1 Serving/300g	261.0	1.0	87	4.6	16.0	0.5	3.2
Baked, Jacket, Beef Chilli Filled, Mini, Classic, Asda*	1 Pack/300g	233.0	2.0	78	3.9	13.7	0.8	1.5
Baked, Jacket, Cheddar Cheese, COU, M & S*	1 Potato/164g	164.0	3.0	100	2.9	17.3	1.9	2.0
Baked, Jacket, Cheese & Beans, Somerfield*	1 Pack/340g	306.0	7.0	90	4.1	13.8	2.0	2.2
Baked, Jacket, Cheese Filled, Farmfoods*	2 Halves/255g	349.0	10.0	137	4.7	21.0	3.8	1.9
Baked, Jacket, Cheese, M & S*	1oz/28g	24.0	1.0	85	4.5	11.1	2.5	1.6
Baked, Jacket, Cheesy, GFY, Asda*	1 Serving/155g	129.0	2.0	83	2.6	16.0	1.0	2.1
Baked, Jacket, Chicken Tikka, COU, M & S*	1 Serving/300g	240.0	5.0	80	5.4	10.9	1.6	1.3
Baked, Jacket, Chicken Tikka, Spar*	1 Serving/300g	309.0	3.0	103	5.5	19.2	1.0	5.0
Baked, Jacket, Chilli Con Carne, COU, M & S*	1 Pack/300g	270.0	6.0	90	6.0	11.1	2.1	1.2
Baked, Jacket, Chilli Con Carne, Pro Cuisine*	1 Pack/340g	347.0	3.0	102	4.6	18.7	1.0	0.0
Baked, Jacket, Chilli Con Carne, Somerfield*	1 Pack/340g	319.0	12.0	94	5.5	10.3	3.4	1.2

POTATOES

INFO/WEIGHT	Measure	per Measure KCAL	FAT	Nutrition Values per 100g / 100ml KCAL	PROT	CARB	FAT	FIBRE
Baked, Jacket, Chilli, BGTY, Sainsbury's*	1 Pack/350g	318.0	5.0	91	5.3	14.3	1.4	1.2
Baked, Jacket, Creamy Mushroom, Asda*	1 Serving/100g	124.0	2.0	124	3.5	22.0	2.4	1.7
Baked, Jacket, Garlic Butter Filling, Morrisons*	1 Potato/210g	239.0	12.0	114	1.7	13.6	5.9	0.9
Baked, Jacket, Garlic Butter, Mini, Safeway*	1 Pack/450g	495.0	21.0	110	1.8	14.6	4.6	2.4
Baked, Jacket, Garlic Mushrooms, BGTY, Sainsbury's*	1 Pack/350g	262.0	3.0	75	2.3	14.4	0.9	1.2
Baked, Jacket, Garlic Mushrooms, Eat Smart, Safeway*	1 Pack/300g	210.0	8.0	70	2.7	8.1	2.7	1.6
Baked, Jacket, Garlic, Mini, Asda*	1 Serving/65g	59.0	2.0	91	2.2	13.0	3.3	0.0
Baked, Jacket, Halves, M & S*	1 Serving/250g	187.0	3.0	75	2.0	14.2	1.1	1.7
Baked, Jacket, Ham & Cheddar Cheese, Asda*	1 Pack/300g	435.0	11.0	145	7.0	21.0	3.7	1.6
Baked, Jacket, Herb & Rock Salt Seasoning, M & S*	1 Pack/500g	375.0	5.0	75	2.0	14.2	1.1	1.7
Baked, Jacket, Leek & Cheese, M & S*	1 Serving/206g	206.0	6.0	100	3.8	13.4	3.1	3.2
Baked, Jacket, Mature Cheddar Cheese, Finest, Tesco*	1 Potato/245g	360.0	18.0	147	5.4	14.6	7.5	2.3
Baked, Jacket, Mature Cheddar Cheese, M & S*	½ Pack/206g	225.0	7.0	109	3.6	16.9	3.2	1.0
Baked, Jacket, Mature Cheddar Cheese, Morrisons*	1 Serving/400g	520.0	20.0	130	4.4	16.6	5.1	1.5
Baked, Jacket, Spicy Chilli Con Carne, Spar*	1 Pack/340g	265.0	5.0	78	3.4	12.4	1.6	1.5
Baked, Jacket, Stuffed, Garlic & Herb Butter, Tesco*	1 Pack/435g	570.0	33.0	131	1.3	14.6	7.5	1.0
Baked, Jacket, Tuna & Sweetcorn, Average	1 Serving/300g	273.0	7.0	91	5.0	12.5	2.2	0.9
Baked, Jacket, Tuna & Sweetcorn, BGTY, Sainsbury's*	1 Pack/350g	360.0	9.0	103	6.5	13.2	2.7	1.3
Baked, Jacket, Tuna & Sweetcorn, COU, M & S*	1 Pack/300g	270.0	5.0	90	5.1	12.8	1.8	1.4
Baked, Jacket, Tuna & Sweetcorn, Morrisons*	1 Serving/300g	243.0	2.0	81	5.1	13.5	0.7	0.0
Baked, Jacket, Tuna & Sweetcorn, Somerfield*	1 Pack/340g	333.0	13.0	98	3.2	12.5	3.9	1.0
Baked, Jacket, with Baked Bean & Sausage, Asda*	1 Pack/300g	447.0	10.0	149	5.0	25.0	3.2	2.7
Baked, Jacket, with Baked Bean Toppers, Safeway*	1 Serving/92g	165.0	7.0	180	5.0	22.1	7.8	4.5
Baked, Jacket, with Baked Beans, Pro Cuisine*	1 Pack/340g	374.0	1.0	110	4.3	22.3	0.4	0.0
Baked, Jacket, with Beef Chilli, Asda*	1 Pack/300g	381.0	8.0	127	5.0	21.0	2.6	2.0
Baked, Jacket, with Beef Chilli, M & S*	1 Pack/360g	288.0	7.0	80	5.9	9.6	2.0	0.9
Baked, Jacket, with Cheese & Bacon, Finest, Tesco*	1 Potato/245g	360.0	20.0	147	6.0	12.6	8.0	2.5
Baked, Jacket, with Cheese & Butter, Tesco*	1 Potato/224.8g	263.0	11.0	117	3.1	14.9	5.0	2.3
Baked, Jacket, with Cheese & Vegetarian Bacon, Tesco*	½ Pack/225g	279.0	11.0	124	4.7	15.5	4.8	1.3
Baked, Jacket, with Cheese Mash, GFY, Asda*	1 Potato/200g	192.0	6.0	96	4.8	13.0	2.8	2.2
Baked, Jacket, with Cheese, Freshly Prepared, Tesco*	½ Pack/215g	150.0	3.0	70	3.9	9.7	1.4	2.8
Baked, Jacket, with Cheese, HL, Tesco*	1 Potato/225g	202.0	5.0	90	4.5	13.0	2.2	1.8
Baked, Jacket, with Cheese, Safeway*	1 Potato/200g	165.0	2.0	82	2.1	16.3	0.8	2.0
Baked, Jacket, with Smoked Bacon, Finest, Tesco*	½ Pack/200g	165.0	6.0	85	3.0	9.9	3.3	1.3
Baked, Jackets, Stuffed, Mini, Tesco*	1 Serving/108g	130.0	6.0	120	2.3	14.6	5.8	2.3
Baked, Skin Only, Average	**1oz/28g**	**55.0**	**0.0**	**198**	**4.3**	**46.1**	**0.1**	**7.9**
Baked, with Cheddar Cheese, Farmfoods*	1 Potato/143g	196.0	5.0	137	4.7	21.0	3.8	1.9
Baked, with Chicken & Mushroom, Homepride*	1 Serving/105g	128.0	12.0	122	2.3	1.9	11.7	0.0
Baking, Raw, Average	**1 Med/250g**	**197.0**	**0.0**	**79**	**2.1**	**18.0**	**0.1**	**1.6**
Boiled, Average	**1 Serving/120g**	**86.0**	**0.0**	**72**	**1.8**	**17.0**	**0.1**	**1.2**
Boiled, with Skin	**1 Potato/125g**	**97.0**	**0.0**	**78**	**2.9**	**17.2**	**0.1**	**3.3**
Bombay, TTD, Sainsbury's*	½ Pack/113g	79.0	3.0	70	1.9	9.3	2.8	3.9
Boulangere, M & S*	½ Pack/225g	180.0	2.0	80	2.8	15.9	0.9	0.9
Charlotte, Average	**1 Serving/184g**	**139.0**	**0.0**	**76**	**1.6**	**17.4**	**0.2**	**3.3**
Crispy Bites, Weighed Frozen, McCain*	1 Serving/100g	141.0	4.0	141	2.5	20.4	4.4	1.5
Crispy Slices, Weighed Baked, McCain*	1 Serving/100g	240.0	11.0	240	3.2	32.1	11.0	2.1
Crispy Slices, Weighed Frozen, McCain*	1 Portion/100g	163.0	7.0	163	2.1	21.9	7.4	1.4
Dauphinoise, Average	**1 Serving/200g**	**335.0**	**24.0**	**167**	**2.2**	**12.7**	**11.9**	**1.5**
Dauphinoise, TTD, Sainsbury's*	½ Pack/174g	240.0	16.0	138	2.9	10.8	9.3	2.7
Desiree, Average	**1 Serving/200g**	**152.0**	**0.0**	**76**	**2.1**	**16.3**	**0.2**	**0.6**
Exquisa, Finest, Tesco*	¼ Pack/247g	185.0	1.0	75	1.7	16.1	0.3	1.0
Frites, Fries, Golden, Crunchy, M & S*	½ Pack/100g	158.0	6.0	158	2.2	23.4	6.2	1.0
Garlic, Tapas Selection, Sainsbury's*	1 Serving/22g	49.0	4.0	224	2.6	10.4	19.1	0.7

	Measure INFO/WEIGHT	per Measure KCAL	FAT	Nutrition Values per 100g / 100ml KCAL	PROT	CARB	FAT	FIBRE
Hasselback, Average	*1 Serving/175g*	*182.0*	*2.0*	*104*	*1.9*	*22.0*	*0.9*	*2.9*
Italian Style, & Vegetables, Waitrose*	1 Serving/126g	138.0	4.0	110	2.0	19.2	2.8	3.4
Jacket, Filled with Cheese & Chives, GFY, Asda*	1 Pack/340g	289.0	4.0	85	4.1	14.2	1.3	2.3
Jersey Royal with Mint Butter, Extra Special, Asda*	½ Pack/172.1g	148.0	5.0	86	1.6	13.0	3.1	1.5
Jersey Royal, Canned, Average	*1 Can/186g*	*116.0*	*0.0*	*62*	*1.4*	*14.0*	*0.1*	*1.2*
Jersey Royal, New, Raw, Average	*1oz/28g*	*21.0*	*0.0*	*75*	*1.6*	*17.2*	*0.2*	*1.5*
Juliette, Sainsbury's*	1 Serving/250g	200.0	0.0	80	1.4	19.7	0.1	1.0
King Edward, Tesco*	1 Serving/100g	77.0	0.0	77	2.1	16.8	0.2	1.3
Lemon & Rosemary, Finest, Tesco*	½ Pack/200g	200.0	7.0	100	2.1	14.7	3.7	2.0
Maris Piper, Raw, Average	*1 Serving/200g*	*151.0*	*0.0*	*75*	*2.0*	*16.5*	*0.2*	*1.4*
Mashed, Buttery, Sainsbury's*	1 Pack /450g	454.0	26.0	101	1.3	11.1	5.7	3.0
Mashed, Colcannon, Co-Op*	1 Pack/500g	325.0	10.0	65	2.0	10.0	2.0	2.0
Mashed, Colcannon, Sainsbury's*	½ Pack/300g	192.0	12.0	64	0.4	6.7	4.0	1.4
Mashed, Colcannon, Tesco*	1 Serving/250g	225.0	13.0	90	1.6	8.4	5.4	1.8
Mashed, Colcannon, Waitrose*	½ Pack/150g	138.0	6.0	92	1.7	12.8	3.8	1.4
Mashed, Fresh Mash, Light Choices, Tesco*	1 Pack/450g	292.0	10.0	65	2.0	9.3	2.2	1.6
Mashed, From Supermarket, Average	½ Pack/200g	197.0	8.0	98	1.8	13.3	4.1	1.5
Mashed, From Supermarket, Premium, Average	1 Serving/225g	305.0	18.0	136	1.7	14.4	7.9	1.1
Mashed, Maris Piper, Tesco*	½ Pack/228g	182.0	4.0	80	1.5	14.0	1.7	0.9
Mashed, Maris Piper, with Cream & Butter, M & S*	½ Pack/200g	180.0	7.0	90	1.1	12.9	3.6	0.4
Mashed, Vintage Cheddar Cheese, M & S*	½ Pack/225g	247.0	12.0	110	4.6	12.6	5.3	1.0
Mashed, with Carrot & Swede, COU, M & S*	1oz/28g	20.0	1.0	70	1.1	12.1	2.1	2.9
Mashed, with Carrot & Swede, M & S*	1 Serving/225g	214.0	14.0	95	1.6	8.3	6.4	1.4
Mashed, with Carrot & Swede, Morrisons*	1 Serving/100g	71.0	2.0	71	1.5	12.6	1.6	2.2
Mashed, with Carrot & Swede, Sainsbury's*	½ Pack/225.5g	230.0	12.0	102	1.9	11.7	5.3	1.5
Mashed, with Creme Fraiche & Seasoning, Waitrose*	½ Pack/225g	189.0	6.0	84	2.0	12.7	2.8	1.4
Mashed, with Leeks, Creamy, Birds Eye*	1 Pack/300g	300.0	21.0	100	2.0	7.3	7.0	0.8
Mashed, with Spring Onion, Weight Watchers*	1 Serving/100g	79.0	2.0	79	2.0	11.2	2.4	1.1
New, Average	*1 Serving/100g*	*75.0*	*0.0*	*75*	*1.5*	*17.8*	*0.3*	*1.1*
New, Baby, Average	*1 Serving/180g*	*135.0*	*0.0*	*75*	*1.7*	*17.1*	*0.3*	*1.6*
New, Baby, Canned, Average	*1 Can/120g*	*70.0*	*0.0*	*59*	*1.4*	*13.2*	*0.2*	*1.4*
New, Baby, with Mint Butter, The Best, Safeway*	½ Pack/190g	161.0	3.0	85	1.2	15.4	1.8	2.2
New, Crushed, The Best, Safeway*	1 Pack/400g	440.0	21.0	110	2.2	12.6	5.2	1.3
New, Easy Steam, With Herbs & Butter, Tesco*	1 Serving/125g	94.0	3.0	75	1.8	9.6	2.8	1.7
New, Garlic, Herb & Parsley Butter, Co-Op*	1 Serving/100g	115.0	5.0	115	1.0	15.0	5.0	2.0
New, in a Herb Marinade, Tesco*	¼ Pack/150g	151.0	7.0	101	1.3	13.0	4.9	1.5
New, with Butter, Chives & Mint, M & S*	¼ Pack/145g	116.0	2.0	80	1.1	16.2	1.4	2.3
New, with English Churned Butter, M & S*	1 Pack/180g	261.0	4.0	145	1.3	29.5	2.2	2.1
New, with Herbs & Butter, Asda*	½ Pack/169.8g	146.0	3.0	86	1.7	16.0	1.7	1.5
New, with Herbs & Butter, Waitrose*	1 Serving/385g	443.0	23.0	115	1.7	13.8	5.9	1.2
New, with Sunblush Tomato, M & S*	1 Pack/385g	346.0	7.0	90	1.6	17.2	1.8	1.3
Pan Fried, Aldi*	1 Serving/250g	182.0	2.0	73	2.7	13.7	0.8	0.0
Red, Flesh Only, Average	*1 Serving/300g*	*217.0*	*0.0*	*72*	*1.9*	*16.3*	*0.1*	*1.2*
Roast, Basted in Beef Dripping, Waitrose*	1 Serving/165g	213.0	9.0	129	2.2	18.0	5.4	1.9
Roast, Extra Crispy, Oven Baked, Aunt Bessie's*	1 Serving/100g	223.0	12.0	223	2.9	26.1	11.8	3.6
Roast, Frozen, Average	1 Potato/70g	105.0	3.0	149	2.6	23.5	5.0	1.4
Roast, Frozen, Healthy Range, Average	1 Potato/70g	70.0	2.0	100	2.5	18.1	2.4	2.1
Roast, Garlic, Sainsbury's*	½ Pack/225g	358.0	22.0	159	3.2	14.6	9.7	1.4
Roast, in Lard, Average	*1oz/28g*	*42.0*	*1.0*	*149*	*2.9*	*25.9*	*4.5*	*1.8*
Roast, in Oil, Average	*1oz/28g*	*42.0*	*1.0*	*149*	*2.9*	*25.9*	*4.5*	*1.8*
Roast, New, Rosemary, Ainsley Harriott*	1 Serving/150g	133.0	4.0	89	2.0	16.0	2.7	1.3
Roast, Oven Baked, Aunt Bessie's*	1 Serving/165g	305.0	15.0	185	2.3	22.9	9.3	1.8
Roast, Pepper & Basil Layer, Safeway*	1 Pack/260g	195.0	9.0	75	1.7	8.8	3.4	1.9

P

	Measure INFO/WEIGHT	per Measure KCAL	FAT	Nutrition Values per 100g / 100ml KCAL	PROT	CARB	FAT	FIBRE
POTATOES								
Roast, Seasoned, Butter Basted, Tesco*	½ Pack/225g	337.0	13.0	150	2.3	21.9	5.7	2.4
Roast, with Caramelised Onions, Finest, Tesco*	½ Pack/200g	500.0	16.0	250	5.5	38.6	8.2	2.9
Roasted with Goose Fat, TTD, Sainsbury's*	½ Pack/185g	216.0	4.0	117	2.7	21.1	2.4	3.0
Roasting, Average	***1 Serving/150g***	***202.0***	***5.0***	***135***	***2.5***	***23.3***	***3.5***	***1.6***
Salad, Value, Tesco*	1 Serving/150g	111.0	0.0	74	1.7	16.1	0.3	1.0
Saute, Deep Fried, McCain*	1oz/28g	47.0	2.0	167	2.6	23.3	7.0	0.0
Saute, Oven Baked, McCain*	1oz/28g	56.0	1.0	199	4.4	36.9	3.8	0.0
Saute, with Onion, & Bacon, Country Supper, Waitrose*	¼ Pack/100g	112.0	4.0	112	1.9	16.4	4.3	1.3
Slices, Garlic & Herb, Heinz*	1oz/28g	23.0	1.0	82	1.7	10.2	3.9	0.7
Slices, in Batter, Crispy, Ready To Bake, Waitrose*	1 Pack/475g	860.0	45.0	181	2.5	21.4	9.5	3.1
Slices, in Rich Crispy Batter, Crispy, Chilled, Sainsbury's*	½ Pack/237.5g	591.0	37.0	249	2.4	24.8	15.6	2.8
Slices, Spicy Coated, Safeway*	½ Pack/150g	305.0	19.0	203	2.5	19.7	12.4	2.5
Spicy, with Chorizo, Tapas, Waitrose*	1 Serving/260g	512.0	36.0	197	6.7	11.8	13.7	1.1
Vivaldi, Boiled in Unsalted Water, Sainsbury's*	1 Serving/200g	144.0	0.0	72	1.8	17.0	0.1	1.2
Wedges, Jumbo, TTD, Sainsbury's*	1 Serving/165g	279.0	7.0	169	2.4	30.7	4.1	3.1
White, Raw, Weighed with Skin, Flesh Only, Average	***1 Med/213g***	***160.0***	***0.0***	***75***	***2.0***	***16.8***	***0.2***	***1.3***
White, Vivaldi, TTD, Sainsbury's*	1 Serving/100g	76.0	0.0	76	1.8	17.0	0.1	1.2
with Garlic & Parsley Butter, Herb Oil Dressed, Co-Op*	1 Serving/178g	205.0	9.0	115	1.0	15.0	5.0	2.0
with Seafood & Seasoned Butter, Tapas, Waitrose*	Pack/170g	330.0	19.0	194	6.2	16.7	11.4	2.1
With Smoked Bacon, Oven Roasted, Extra Special, Asda*	½ Pack/200g	242.0	10.0	121	3.9	15.5	4.8	2.6
POTATOES INSTANT								
Mashed, Dry, Tesco*	1 Serving/70g	225.0	0.0	321	7.7	72.0	0.2	7.1
Mashed, Dry, Value, Tesco*	1/6 Pack/42g	157.0	0.0	373	7.0	84.0	1.0	6.9
Mashed, Made Up with Water, Average	1 Serving/180g	118.0	0.0	66	1.7	14.5	0.2	1.3
Mashed, Original, Dry Weight, Smash*	1 Serving/30g	107.0	1.0	358	10.7	68.1	4.8	3.4
Mashed, with Fried Onion, Smash*	½ Pack/269g	191.0	3.0	71	1.6	13.4	1.3	0.7
Mashed, with Smoked Bacon, Smash*	1 Serving/169g	137.0	4.0	81	1.7	13.6	2.2	0.6
POUSSIN								
Meat & Skin, Raw, Average	***1oz/28g***	***57.0***	***4.0***	***202***	***19.1***	***0.0***	***13.9***	***0.0***
Spatchcock, British, Waitrose*	½ Poussin/225g	364.0	20.0	162	19.0	1.2	9.0	0.0
Spatchcock, with Garlic & Herbs, Finest, Tesco*	½ Poussin/235g	348.0	17.0	148	19.7	1.0	7.3	0.5
POWERADE								
Berry & Tropical Fruit, Coca-Cola*	1 Bottle/500ml	120.0	0.0	24	0.0	5.6	0.0	0.0
Citrus Charge, Coca-Cola*	1 Bottle/500ml	120.0	0.0	24	0.0	6.0	0.0	0.0
Gold Rush, Coca-Cola*	1 Bottle/500ml	120.0	0.0	24	0.0	6.0	0.0	0.0
Ice Storm, Coca-Cola*	1 Bottle/500ml	120.0	0.0	24	0.0	6.0	0.0	0.0
Isotonic, Sports Drink, Coca-Cola*	1 Bottle/500ml	120.0	0.0	24	0.0	5.6	0.0	0.0
PRAWN COCKTAIL								
20% More Prawns, M & S*	½ Pack/100g	330.0	32.0	330	8.9	2.2	31.6	0.2
Asda*	1oz/28g	124.0	12.0	443	8.6	3.3	43.6	0.0
BFY, Morrisons*	1 Serving/100g	149.0	10.0	149	4.7	9.7	10.3	0.1
BGTY, Sainsbury's*	1 Pack/200g	330.0	23.0	165	10.1	4.8	11.7	0.9
Delicious, Boots*	1 Pack/250g	285.0	6.0	114	5.5	17.0	2.6	1.2
Half Fat, Safeway*	1 Serving/200g	362.0	28.0	181	8.0	6.4	13.8	0.6
HL, Tesco*	1 Serving/200g	276.0	23.0	138	6.8	2.3	11.3	0.6
King, Sainsbury's*	1 Pack/260g	328.0	15.0	126	5.8	12.7	5.8	2.3
Light Choices, Tesco*	1 Pot/140g	210.0	16.0	150	7.5	4.3	11.4	1.3
Light, Asda*	1oz/28g	45.0	3.0	160	9.9	4.8	11.2	0.0
Reduced Fat, M & S*	1 Pack/200g	260.0	15.0	130	11.9	3.2	7.5	0.7
Reduced Fat, Tesco*	1 Serving/200g	304.0	21.0	152	7.6	6.5	10.6	0.4
Safeway*	½ Pot/100g	373.0	36.0	373	7.6	3.4	36.5	0.2
Sainsbury's*	1 Serving/200g	706.0	69.0	353	7.9	2.7	34.5	0.5
Tesco*	1 Tub/200g	834.0	83.0	417	7.3	3.5	41.5	0.1

	Measure INFO/WEIGHT	KCAL	FAT	Nutrition Values per 100g / 100ml KCAL	PROT	CARB	FAT	FIBRE
PRAWN COCKTAIL								
TTD, Sainsbury's*	1 Serving/100g	333.0	31.0	333	11.5	2.9	30.6	0.5
PRAWN CRACKERS								
Asda*	1 Serving/25g	134.0	9.0	535	2.0	53.0	35.0	0.0
Cooked in Sunflower Oil, Sharwood's*	1 Cracker/2g	10.0	0.0	479	0.7	68.3	22.6	0.8
Food to Go, Sainsbury's*	1 Bag/40g	214.0	13.0	534	2.9	60.2	31.3	0.4
Green Thai Curry, M & S*	1 Pack/50g	250.0	13.0	500	3.2	62.2	25.8	1.6
M & S*	1 Bag/50g	262.0	16.0	525	2.8	57.4	31.3	0.8
Ready to Eat, Sharwood's*	1 Bag/60g	316.0	18.0	527	0.5	62.0	30.8	1.2
Red Mill*	1 Bag/50g	281.0	19.0	563	2.8	53.1	37.7	0.7
Sainsbury's*	1 Cracker/3g	16.0	1.0	537	2.4	60.4	31.7	0.8
Tesco*	1/3 Pack/20g	114.0	7.0	570	2.5	56.5	37.1	0.9
Uncooked, Sharwood's*	1oz/28g	136.0	8.0	487	0.7	52.7	29.7	1.7
Waitrose*	1 Pack/50g	266.0	16.0	533	2.4	58.6	32.1	1.6
PRAWN CREOLE								
with Rice, Perfectly Balanced, Waitrose*	1 Serving/404g	275.0	4.0	68	4.2	10.3	1.1	2.9
PRAWN PINWHEEL								
Oriental Style, BGTY, Sainsbury's*	1 Pack/189.0g	274.0	2.0	145	6.0	26.7	1.1	0.0
PRAWN TOAST								
Chinese Selection, Tesco*	1 Toast/9.9g	36.0	3.0	362	8.2	20.7	27.5	1.7
Chinese Snack Selection, Morrisons*	1 Toast/12.5g	41.0	3.0	328	11.3	23.1	21.2	6.6
Dim Sum Selection, Sainsbury's*	1 Toast/8g	23.0	1.0	283	9.9	19.2	18.5	2.0
Mini, Oriental Selection, Party, Iceland*	1 Toast/15.1g	52.0	4.0	345	10.5	22.0	23.9	2.1
Oriental Selection, Waitrose*	1 Toast/14g	38.0	2.0	272	11.1	18.3	17.2	2.1
Sesame Prawn, Toasted Triangles, M & S*	1 Pack/220g	616.0	40.0	280	12.4	17.3	18.0	2.0
Sesame, Occasions, Sainsbury's*	1 Toast/12g	34.0	2.0	283	9.9	19.2	18.5	2.0
Sesame, Oriental Snack Selection, Sainsbury's*	1 Toast/12g	40.0	3.0	335	9.3	23.0	22.9	5.1
Waitrose*	1 Toast/21g	47.0	4.0	223	9.7	7.4	17.2	5.8
PRAWNS								
Atlantic, Extra Large, TTD, Sainsbury's*	¼ Pack/100g	79.0	1.0	79	17.4	0.1	1.0	0.5
Batter Crisp, Lyons*	1 Pack/160g	350.0	20.0	219	8.0	18.2	12.7	1.1
Boiled	*1 Prawn/3g*	*3.0*	*0.0*	*99*	*22.6*	*0.0*	*0.9*	*0.0*
Brine, John West*	½ Can/60g	58.0	1.0	97	21.0	1.0	1.0	0.0
Cooked & Peeled, Average	*1oz/28g*	*21.0*	*0.0*	*77*	*17.6*	*0.2*	*0.6*	*0.0*
Crevettes, Asda*	1oz/28g	11.0	0.0	41	8.6	0.0	0.7	0.0
Dried, Average	*1 Prawn/3g*	*8.0*	*0.0*	*281*	*62.4*	*0.0*	*3.5*	*0.0*
Filo Wrapped & Breaded, M & S*	1 Serving/19g	45.0	2.0	235	9.5	20.4	13.0	1.4
Honduran, & Cocktail Sauce Dipper, M & S*	1 Pack/120g	258.0	22.0	215	13.6	0.0	18.0	1.1
Hot & Spicy, Average	1 Serving/170g	461.0	27.0	271	9.4	22.8	15.8	2.1
Icelandic, Raw, Average	*1oz/28g*	*30.0*	*0.0*	*105*	*22.7*	*0.0*	*1.5*	*0.0*
King, Crevettes, Sainsbury's*	1 Pack/225g	205.0	1.0	91	21.8	0.1	0.5	0.3
King, in Filo, Finest, Tesco*	1 Prawn/20g	38.0	1.0	189	13.0	27.8	2.9	1.6
King, in Sweet Chilli Sauce, with Noodles, COU, M & S*	1 Pack/400g	260.0	2.0	65	4.8	10.3	0.4	1.5
King, Jumbo, TTD, Sainsbury's*	½ Pack/90g	63.0	1.0	70	15.7	0.1	0.7	0.5
King, Raw, Average	*1 Bag/200g*	*145.0*	*2.0*	*72*	*15.8*	*0.2*	*0.9*	*0.1*
King, Shell On, TTD, Sainsbury's*	1 Serving/100g	67.0	1.0	67	14.3	0.8	0.7	0.5
King, Sizzler, with Rice Noodles, BGTY, Sainsbury's*	1 Pack/400g	276.0	5.0	69	3.8	10.6	1.3	1.6
King, Tandoori, Average	1 Prawn/59g	33.0	1.0	55	5.7	5.9	1.1	0.7
King, with Garlic Butter, M & S*	1 Serving/100g	165.0	9.0	165	12.5	9.1	9.0	0.5
King, with Ginger & Spring Onion, Waitrose*	1 Pack/300g	207.0	5.0	69	6.4	7.1	1.7	1.9
North Atlantic, Peeled, Cooked, Average	*1oz/28g*	*22.0*	*0.0*	*80*	*17.5*	*0.0*	*1.1*	*0.0*
North Atlantic, Raw, Average	*1oz/28g*	*17.0*	*0.0*	*61*	*14.4*	*0.0*	*0.4*	*0.0*
Peeled, TTD, Sainsbury's*	1 Serving/100g	65.0	1.0	65	14.1	0.1	0.9	0.5
Raw, Average	*1oz/28g*	*22.0*	*0.0*	*79*	*17.8*	*0.2*	*0.7*	*0.0*

	Measure INFO/WEIGHT	per Measure KCAL	per Measure FAT	Nutrition Values per 100g / 100ml KCAL	PROT	CARB	FAT	FIBRE
PRAWNS								
Raw, Jumbo, TTD, Sainsbury's*	½ Pack/85g	115.0	2.0	135	25.5	2.0	2.8	0.5
Spirals, Shapers, Boots*	1 Pack/100g	468.0	22.0	468	3.1	64.0	22.0	2.8
Succulent King, With A Sweet Chilli Sauce, Birds Eye*	1 Serving/140g	251.0	17.0	179	10.5	6.5	12.3	0.1
Sweet Chilli, Skewers, Tesco*	1 Skewer/22g	26.0	0.0	120	20.4	6.9	0.9	0.5
Thai, M & S*	1oz/28g	29.0	1.0	103	5.2	13.6	3.1	1.3
Tiger, Cooked & Peeled, Average	*1 Pack/180g*	*151.0*	*2.0*	*84*	*18.4*	*0.1*	*1.1*	*0.0*
Tiger, Jumbo, Average	*1 Serving/50g*	*39.0*	*0.0*	*78*	*18.2*	*0.3*	*0.5*	*0.0*
Tiger, Raw, Average	*1 Av Prawn/30g*	*19.0*	*0.0*	*64*	*14.2*	*0.0*	*0.7*	*0.0*
Tiger, Vegetarian, Crispy, Tkc*	½ Pack/150g	225.0	6.0	150	12.0	17.0	4.0	5.0
Tiger, Wrapped, M & S*	1 Pack/190g	477.0	26.0	251	11.3	20.7	13.6	1.3
PRAWNS CHILLI								
& Coriander, King, Honduran, M & S*	½ Pack/70g	70.0	2.0	100	17.2	0.1	3.2	0.4
& Coriander, King, Sainsbury's*	1 Pack/140g	133.0	6.0	95	13.8	0.5	4.2	0.5
Battered, Cantonese, King, Sainsbury's*	1 Pack/300g	570.0	23.0	190	10.0	20.2	7.7	0.8
Battered, M & S*	1oz/28g	63.0	3.0	225	7.2	23.8	11.5	0.5
Sweet, Crispy, Dipping Sauce, M & S*	1 Pack/240g	515.0	28.0	215	7.5	19.9	11.6	2.3
Sweet, Thai, King, Sainsbury's*	1 Serving/150g	177.0	6.0	118	6.4	13.9	4.1	1.9
with Spicy Chilli Dip, King, Sainsbury's*	½ Pack/150g	282.0	11.0	188	8.6	22.2	7.2	1.0
PRAWNS CREOLE								
GFY, Asda*	1 Serving/300g	222.0	3.0	74	3.2	13.0	1.0	1.4
Spicy, BGTY, Sainsbury's*	1 Pack/350g	357.0	8.0	102	4.8	15.6	2.4	0.4
with Vegetable Rice, King, COU, M & S*	1 Pack/400g	300.0	2.0	75	4.5	13.3	0.6	0.7
PRAWNS GULNARI								
with Rice, COU, M & S*	1 Pack/400g	400.0	3.0	100	4.0	18.7	0.8	1.6
PRAWNS IN								
Creamy Garlic Sauce, Youngs*	1 Serving/158g	261.0	23.0	165	8.5	0.3	14.5	0.0
Sweet Chilli Sauce, Asda*	1 Pack/360g	500.0	25.0	139	4.1	15.0	6.9	0.3
PRAWNS ORIENTAL								
M & S*	1 Pack/200g	440.0	23.0	220	11.9	16.9	11.7	0.9
PRAWNS SZECHUAN								
Spicy, COU, M & S*	1 Pack/400g	380.0	4.0	95	4.5	16.9	0.9	1.5
PRAWNS WITH								
a Spicy Cajun Dip, King, Sainsbury's*	1 Pack/240g	254.0	4.0	106	14.8	9.1	1.8	1.4
Caribbean Style Sauce, GFY, Asda*	1 Serving/400g	408.0	7.0	102	4.7	17.0	1.7	2.1
Chilli, Coriander & Lime, King, Waitrose*	1 Pack/140g	143.0	3.0	102	19.9	0.5	2.3	0.6
Garlic & Herb Butter, King, Fresh, M & S*	1 Serving/200g	330.0	18.0	165	12.5	9.1	9.0	0.5
Ginger & Spring Onion, Sainsbury's*	1 Pack/300g	198.0	9.0	66	4.7	4.7	3.1	0.3
Green Thai Sauce, Tiger, Waitrose*	½ Pack/117g	108.0	3.0	92	16.1	0.8	2.3	0.1
Lemon & Pepper, Honduran, King, M & S*	1 Pack/140g	133.0	4.0	95	17.4	0.4	2.6	0.7
Rice, Sweet Chilli, Tesco*	1 Pack/460g	488.0	10.0	106	2.4	19.2	2.2	0.5
with Creamy Lime Dip, King, Waitrose*	1 Pot/230g	517.0	41.0	225	15.8	0.8	17.7	0.2
PRETZELS								
American Style, Salted, Sainsbury's*	1 Serving/50g	201.0	2.0	403	10.8	79.7	4.5	1.8
Cheddar Cheese, Penn State Pretzels*	1 Sm Bag/30g	124.0	3.0	412	10.0	71.6	9.3	3.8
Giant, Penn State Pretzels*	1 Pretzel/17.6g	66.0	1.0	374	10.5	74.7	3.7	4.1
Jumbo, Tesco*	1 Serving/50g	194.0	3.0	388	9.7	71.9	6.8	5.4
Lightly Salted, Tesco*	1 Serving/25g	99.0	2.0	395	9.3	73.4	7.1	5.5
Mini, 99% Fat Free, Free Natural*	1 Serving/50g	188.0	0.0	376	10.1	81.7	1.0	0.0
Mini, M & S*	1 Pack/45g	193.0	6.0	430	10.4	66.6	13.4	4.9
New York Style, Salted, Mini, Shapers, Boots*	1 Bag/25g	94.0	1.0	375	10.0	79.0	2.1	4.2
Salt & Cracked Black Pepper, COU, M & S*	1 Pack/25g	95.0	1.0	380	9.7	83.3	2.4	2.7
Salted, Average	1 Serving/30g	114.0	1.0	380	10.3	79.8	2.6	3.0
Salted, Mini, M & S*	1 Pack/25g	94.0	1.0	375	10.0	79.0	2.1	4.2

	Measure INFO/WEIGHT	per Measure KCAL	per Measure FAT	Nutrition Values per 100g / 100ml KCAL	PROT	CARB	FAT	FIBRE
PRETZELS								
Salted, Sainsbury's*	1 Serving/50g	200.0	2.0	401	9.8	82.4	3.6	3.4
Salted, Stars, Tesco*	1oz/28g	104.0	1.0	371	8.2	73.7	4.8	3.1
Sea Salt & Black Pepper, Penn State Pretzels*	1 Serving/25g	94.0	1.0	375	10.4	73.7	4.2	4.7
Sea Salt & Black Pepper, Tesco*	1 Serving/50g	189.0	1.0	379	10.0	79.0	2.6	4.1
Selection Tray, M & S*	1oz/28g	112.0	2.0	401	9.7	75.5	6.7	3.4
Snacks, Fabulous Bakin' Boys*	1 Pack/24g	96.0	1.0	401	9.0	79.5	4.9	2.5
Soft, Almond, Auntie Anne's*	1 Pretzel/112g	350.0	2.0	312	7.1	66.1	1.8	1.8
Soft, Almond, with Butter, Auntie Anne's*	1 Pretzel/112g	390.0	6.0	348	7.1	66.1	5.4	1.8
Soft, Cinnamon Sugar, Auntie Anne's*	1 Pretzel/112g	380.0	1.0	339	7.1	75.0	0.9	1.8
Soft, Cinnamon Sugar, with Butter, Auntie Anne's*	1 Pretzel/112g	470.0	12.0	420	7.1	75.0	10.7	1.8
Soft, Garlic, Auntie Anne's*	1 Pretzel/112g	310.0	1.0	277	7.1	58.0	0.9	1.8
Soft, Garlic, with Butter, Auntie Anne's*	1 Pretzel/112g	350.0	5.0	312	7.1	58.0	4.5	1.8
Soft, Jalapeno, Auntie Anne's*	1 Pretzel/126g	300.0	1.0	238	6.3	50.0	0.8	1.6
Soft, Jalapeno, with Butter, Auntie Anne's*	1 Pretzel/126g	330.0	5.0	262	6.3	50.0	4.0	1.6
Soft, Raisin, Auntie Anne's*	1 Pretzel/112g	330.0	1.0	295	7.1	61.6	0.9	1.8
Soft, Raisin, with Butter, Auntie Anne's*	1 Pretzel/112g	360.0	5.0	321	7.1	61.6	4.5	1.8
Soft, Salted, Original, Auntie Anne's*	1 Pretzel/112g	310.0	1.0	277	7.1	58.0	0.9	1.8
Soft, Salted, with Butter, Original, Auntie Anne's*	1 Pretzel/112g	340.0	5.0	304	7.1	26.2	4.5	1.8
Soft, Sesame, Auntie Anne's*	1 Pretzel/112g	360.0	6.0	321	8.9	59.8	5.4	2.7
Soft, Sesame, with Butter, Auntie Anne's*	1 Pretzel/112g	400.0	10.0	357	8.9	59.8	8.9	2.7
Soft, Sour Cream & Onion, Auntie Anne's*	1 Pretzel/112g	330.0	2.0	295	8.0	60.7	1.3	1.8
Soft, Sour Cream & Onion, with Butter, Auntie Anne's*	1 Pretzel/112g	360.0	5.0	321	8.0	60.7	4.5	1.8
Soft, Whole Wheat, Auntie Anne's*	1 Pretzel/112g	355.0	2.0	317	10.0	65.2	1.4	6.3
Soft, Whole Wheat, with Butter, Auntie Anne's*	1 Pretzel/112g	375.0	5.0	335	10.0	65.2	4.1	6.3
Sour Cream & Chive Flavour, Mini, Shapers, Boots*	1 Packet/25g	93.0	1.0	371	11.0	74.0	2.7	7.3
Sour Cream & Chive, Hoops, BGTY, Sainsbury's*	1 Bag/25g	98.0	1.0	391	10.4	80.9	2.3	1.6
Sour Cream & Chive, Mini, HL, Tesco*	1 Pack/25g	92.0	1.0	369	10.9	76.3	2.2	4.6
Sour Cream & Chive, Penn State Pretzels*	1 Serving/25g	102.0	2.0	410	9.8	72.8	8.8	3.9
Sour Cream & Onion, M & S*	1 Serving/30g	136.0	4.0	455	11.0	70.9	14.5	0.7
Sour Cream & Onion, Tesco*	1 Serving/25g	114.0	4.0	457	8.4	67.7	17.0	2.3
Spicy Salsa, Penn State Pretzels*	1 Serving/25g	105.0	3.0	420	9.5	72.4	10.4	1.3
Sweet Thai Chilli Twists, Penn State Pretzels*	1 Serving/25g	98.0	2.0	393	9.8	70.1	8.2	6.8
Wheat, Gluten Free, Trufree*	1 Bag/60g	282.0	12.0	470	2.4	70.0	20.0	1.0
with Sea Salt, Giant, M & S*	1 Pretzel/8g	31.0	1.0	390	9.7	77.3	6.8	5.4
PRINGLES*								
Barbecue, Pringles*	1 Serving/50g	266.0	18.0	533	4.9	48.0	36.0	5.1
BBQ Spare Rib, Rice Infusions, Pringles*	1 Pack/23g	108.0	5.0	469	5.1	60.0	23.0	2.6
Cheese & Onion, Pringles*	1 Serving/25g	132.0	8.0	528	4.1	50.0	34.0	3.4
Hot & Spicy, Pringles*	1 Serving/25g	132.0	8.0	530	4.6	49.0	34.0	3.7
Light, Aromas, Greek Cheese & Avocado Oil, Pringles*	1 Serving/25g	122.0	6.0	488	4.6	57.0	25.0	3.6
Light, Original, Pringles*	1 Serving/25g	121.0	6.0	484	4.3	59.0	25.0	3.6
Light, Sour Cream & Onion, Pringles*	1 Serving/25g	122.0	6.0	487	4.7	57.0	25.0	3.6
Minis, Original, Pringles*	1 Pack/23g	118.0	7.0	514	5.1	55.0	30.0	3.7
Minis, Salt & Vinegar, Pringles*	1 Pack/23g	115.0	6.0	502	4.5	55.0	28.0	3.6
Minis, Sour Cream & Onion, Pringles*	1 Pack/23g	118.0	7.0	511	5.2	56.0	29.0	3.5
Minis, Texas BBQ Sauce, Pringles*	1 Pack/23g	116.0	6.0	504	5.0	56.0	28.0	3.8
Original, Pringles*	1 Serving/25g	131.0	8.0	526	3.9	52.0	34.0	2.6
Paprika, Pringles*	1 Serving/25g	132.0	8.0	529	4.9	49.0	34.0	6.5
Salt & Vinegar, Pringles*	1 Serving/25g	132.0	8.0	527	3.9	50.0	34.0	3.4
Sour Cream & Onion, Pringles*	1 Serving/25g	133.0	9.0	531	4.5	49.0	35.0	3.6
Texas BBQ Sauce, Pringles*	1 Serving/25g	132.0	8.0	527	4.2	50.0	34.0	3.5
PROBIOTIC DRINK								
Cranberry & Raspberry, Dairy, Asda*	1 Bottle/100ml	64.0	1.0	64	2.3	12.0	0.8	2.4

	Measure INFO/WEIGHT	per Measure KCAL	FAT	Nutrition Values per 100g / 100ml KCAL	PROT	CARB	FAT	FIBRE
PROBIOTIC DRINK								
Peach, Dairy, Asda*	1 Bottle/100ml	68.0	1.0	68	2.3	13.0	0.8	2.3
Strawberry, Dairy, Asda*	1 Bottle/100ml	64.0	1.0	64	2.3	12.0	0.8	2.3
Yoghurt, Original, Tesco*	1 Bottle/100g	68.0	1.0	68	1.7	13.1	1.0	1.4
PROFITEROLES								
Asda*	1 Serving/64g	218.0	17.0	343	5.0	20.0	27.0	0.0
Chocolate Covered, Tesco*	1 Serving/72g	295.0	21.0	410	5.7	29.3	29.5	2.0
Chocolate, 8 Pack, Co-Op*	¼ Pack/112g	330.0	18.0	295	6.0	31.0	16.0	2.0
Chocolate, Co-Op*	1Pot/91g	260.0	14.0	285	6.0	33.0	15.0	3.0
Chocolate, Sainsbury's*	1/6 Pot/95.0g	192.0	8.0	202	5.4	25.1	8.9	0.8
Chocolate, Stack, Sainsbury's*	¼ Pack/76g	311.0	19.0	409	5.3	39.3	25.6	2.0
Chocolate, Tesco*	1 Serving/76g	293.0	22.0	386	5.1	26.9	28.7	0.5
Choux & Chocolate Sauce, Tesco*	1 Serving/77g	295.0	22.0	386	5.1	26.9	28.7	0.5
Classic French, Sainsbury's*	1 Serving/90g	284.0	15.0	316	6.6	33.7	17.2	0.1
Dairy Cream, Co-Op*	¼ Pack/70g	241.0	17.0	345	6.0	24.0	25.0	0.5
Dairy Cream, Safeway*	¼ Pack/67g	275.0	18.0	410	5.5	35.3	26.9	2.2
Filled with Cream, Stack, Fresh, M & S*	1 Serving/75g	281.0	21.0	375	5.3	23.6	28.5	1.9
in a Pot, Waitrose*	1 Pot/80g	207.0	11.0	259	6.3	25.6	14.1	2.9
Somerfield*	1 Serving/100g	273.0	14.0	273	5.0	31.0	14.0	0.0
Waitrose*	4 Roles/75g	269.0	18.0	359	4.8	31.1	23.9	0.7
PROTEIN POWDER								
Soya, Holland & Barrett*	1oz/28g	109.0	1.0	390	88.0	0.5	4.0	0.0
PROVENCALE								
Cabillaud à la, Weight Watchers*	1 Pack/380g	327.0	10.0	86	5.1	10.3	2.7	0.0
Chicken, M & S*	1 Pack/430g	365.0	12.0	85	13.2	2.3	2.7	0.6
Chicken, Steam Cuisine, M & S*	1oz/28g	34.0	1.0	120	9.6	12.7	3.8	1.4
King Prawn & Mushroom, M & S*	½ Pack/185g	120.0	5.0	65	7.2	3.9	2.5	0.9
Mushroom, Fresh, COU, M & S*	½ Pack/150g	60.0	2.0	40	2.6	4.1	1.5	1.8
Prawn & Mushroom with Pasta, COU, M & S*	1 Pack/400g	360.0	2.0	90	5.9	15.7	0.5	0.0
Ratatouille, Asda*	½ Can/195g	97.0	4.0	50	1.0	7.0	2.0	1.0
PRUNES								
Dried, Average	*1 Serving/50g*	*79.0*	*0.0*	*157*	*2.5*	*36.4*	*0.4*	*5.8*
in Apple Juice, Average	*1 Serving/90g*	*76.0*	*0.0*	*84*	*0.8*	*19.8*	*0.1*	*1.4*
in Fruit Juice, Average	*1oz/28g*	*25.0*	*0.0*	*88*	*0.9*	*21.4*	*0.2*	*3.0*
in Syrup, Average	*1oz/28g*	*26.0*	*0.0*	*92*	*1.0*	*22.1*	*0.2*	*2.6*
Stewed with Sugar	*1oz/28g*	*29.0*	*0.0*	*103*	*1.3*	*25.5*	*0.2*	*3.1*
Stewed without Sugar	*1oz/28g*	*23.0*	*0.0*	*81*	*1.4*	*19.5*	*0.3*	*3.3*
PUDDING								
Apple & Custard, Sainsbury's*	1 Serving/115g	132.0	2.0	115	5.4	19.0	1.9	0.1
Banana Fudge Crunch, Bird's*	1oz/28g	125.0	4.0	445	5.4	75.0	14.0	0.8
Black, VLH Kitchens	1 Serving/40g	105.0	6.0	262	11.0	20.3	15.6	0.4
Blackberry & Bramley Apple, M & S*	¼ Pudding/152g	365.0	12.0	240	3.3	38.2	8.2	2.0
Butterscotch, Instant, Fat Free, Jell-O*	1 Serving/8g	25.0	0.0	333	1.3	78.7	1.3	0.0
Cherry Cobbler, GFY, Asda*	1 Pudding/100g	158.0	2.0	158	2.1	33.0	2.0	0.9
Chocolate with Cream, Delice, Campina*	1 Pot/100g	136.0	5.0	136	2.5	18.9	5.4	0.0
Chocolate, Gu*	1 Pack/240g	780.0	27.0	325	3.9	51.8	11.4	1.6
Chocolate, Low Fat, Good Intentions, Somerfield*	1 Pudding/110g	200.0	2.0	182	3.0	37.6	2.2	2.4
Chocolate, M & S*	¼ Pudding/76g	265.0	12.0	350	4.1	48.0	15.8	2.1
Chocolate, Melting Middle, M & S*	1 Pudding/154g	510.0	28.0	330	5.8	36.2	18.0	3.1
Chocolate, Perfectly Balanced, Waitrose*	1 Pot/105g	196.0	3.0	187	3.8	36.0	3.1	0.8
Chocolate, Tesco*	1 Serving/110g	348.0	21.0	316	3.1	32.9	19.1	1.9
Christmas, VLH Kitchens	1 Serving/114g	310.0	3.0	272	3.1	59.3	2.5	4.6
Creamed Sago, Ambrosia*	1 Serving/200g	158.0	3.0	79	2.5	13.6	1.6	0.2
Creme Aux Oeufs a la Vanille, Weight Watchers*	1 Pot/100g	116.0	3.0	116	4.8	17.0	3.2	0.0

	Measure INFO/WEIGHT	per Measure KCAL	FAT	Nutrition Values per 100g / 100ml KCAL	PROT	CARB	FAT	FIBRE

PUDDING

	Measure INFO/WEIGHT	KCAL	FAT	KCAL	PROT	CARB	FAT	FIBRE
Creme Aux Oeufs Au Chocolat, Weight Watchers*	1 Pot/100g	136.0	4.0	136	4.7	19.7	4.3	0.0
Diat, in Schoko-Creme, Onken*	1oz/28g	24.0	1.0	85	3.8	10.8	2.9	0.0
Eve's, Average	1oz/28g	67.0	4.0	241	3.5	28.9	13.1	1.4
Eve's, BGTY, Sainsbury's*	1 Pudding/145g	164.0	2.0	113	2.2	23.4	1.2	0.7
Eve's, with Custard, Less Than 5% Fat, M & S*	1 Pudding/205g	318.0	9.0	155	3.4	24.7	4.6	0.7
Jam Roly Poly & Custard, Co-Op*	1 Serving/105g	262.0	7.0	250	3.0	44.0	7.0	0.8
Lemon Crunch, Bird's*	1oz/28g	125.0	4.0	445	5.5	74.0	14.0	0.7
Lemon, BGTY, Sainsbury's*	1 Serving/100g	151.0	2.0	151	2.9	31.0	1.9	0.5
Lemon, M & S*	1 Pudding/105g	328.0	16.0	312	4.3	39.4	15.2	2.3
Lemon, Perfectly Balanced, Waitrose*	1 Serving/105g	212.0	3.0	202	3.4	41.7	2.4	0.6
Plum, Spiced, Safeway*	1 Pudding/125g	275.0	3.0	220	2.7	45.7	2.5	0.9
Protein, Cnp*	1 Serving/39g	129.0	2.0	330	61.0	10.0	5.0	1.0
Queen of Puddings	1oz/28g	60.0	2.0	213	4.8	33.1	7.8	0.2
Rhubarb & Custard, BGTY, Sainsbury's*	1 Pudding/140g	137.0	3.0	98	2.0	18.4	2.0	1.4
Rhubarb Crumble, Custard Style, Somerfield*	1oz/28g	33.0	1.0	119	3.0	16.0	5.0	0.0
Rich Chocolate, Tryton Foods*	1oz/28g	76.0	3.0	273	4.7	41.7	9.5	1.8
Sticky Toffee, Co-Op*	¼ Pudding/100g	355.0	20.0	355	3.0	40.0	20.0	0.7
Sticky Toffee, Extra Special, Asda*	¼ Pudding/100g	378.0	18.0	378	1.9	52.0	18.0	1.8
Sticky Toffee, Farmfoods*	¼ Pudding/186g	627.0	12.0	337	4.1	65.7	6.4	0.3
Sticky Toffee, HL, Tesco*	1 Pack/125g	245.0	6.0	196	4.0	34.9	4.5	0.6
Sticky Toffee, Tesco*	1 Serving/110g	287.0	15.0	261	3.3	31.8	13.4	0.7
Sticky Toffee, Tryton Foods*	1oz/28g	88.0	2.0	314	3.7	62.7	5.4	1.0
Sticky Toffee, with Custard, Somerfield*	1 Pack/245g	576.0	20.0	235	3.0	38.0	8.0	0.0
Strawberry Jam with Custard, Farmfoods*	1 Serving/145g	525.0	35.0	362	3.2	35.5	23.9	0.9
Summer Fruits, Co-Op*	1 Pack/260g	273.0	1.0	105	1.0	25.0	0.2	1.0
Summer Fruits, Eat Well, M & S*	1 Pudding/135g	128.0	1.0	95	1.7	20.8	0.5	3.0
Summer Pudding, BGTY, Sainsbury's*	1 Pot/110g	223.0	5.0	203	3.2	40.9	4.6	2.4
Summer Pudding, Safeway*	1 Pudding/135g	196.0	1.0	145	2.5	32.9	0.4	3.1
Summer Pudding, Waitrose*	1 Pot/120g	125.0	0.0	104	2.0	23.1	0.4	1.4
Syrup, Individual, Co-Op*	1 Pudding/170g	603.0	36.0	355	3.0	38.0	21.0	1.0
Syrup, M & S*	1 Serving/105g	370.0	10.0	352	3.9	61.7	10.0	0.8
Truffle, Chocolate Amaretto, Gu*	1 Pot/80g	272.0	15.0	340	3.2	34.9	19.4	1.6
Truffle, Chocolate, with Raspberry Compote, Gu*	1 Pot/80g	250.0	15.0	312	2.7	28.7	18.2	1.7
Truffle, Double Chocolate, Cheeky Chocolate, Gu*	1 Pot/50g	216.0	18.0	433	3.2	24.1	35.9	2.1

PULSES

Mixed, in Water, Sainsbury's*	½ Can/120g	131.0	3.0	109	8.7	13.6	2.2	4.6

PUMPKIN

Boiled in Salted Water	*1oz/28g*	*4.0*	*0.0*	*13*	*0.6*	*2.1*	*0.3*	*1.1*
Kabocha, Tesco*	1 Serving 50g	19.0	0.0	39	1.1	8.3	0.1	1.6
Solid Pack, 100% Pure, Canned, Libby's*	1 Can/425g	139.0	2.0	33	1.6	7.4	0.4	4.1

PUPPODUMS

Cracked Black Pepper, Ready to Eat, Sharwood's*	1 Puppodum/9g	41.0	2.0	461	16.7	37.2	27.3	7.3
Extra Large, Cook to Eat, Sharwood's*	1oz/28g	78.0	0.0	279	21.3	44.7	1.7	10.3
Garlic & Coriander, Ready to Eat, Sharwood's*	1 Puppodum/9g	39.0	2.0	438	18.4	43.0	21.4	6.5
Plain, Cook to Eat, Sharwood's*	1 Puppodum/12g	32.0	0.0	273	21.9	45.7	1.0	10.1
Plain, Mini, Cook to Eat, Sharwood's*	1 Puppodum/4g	11.0	0.0	273	21.9	45.7	0.3	10.1
Plain, Ready to Eat, Sharwood's*	1 Puppodum/9g	41.0	2.0	461	17.0	40.6	25.6	0.0
Spicy, Cook to Eat, Sharwood's*	1 Puppodum/12g	30.0	0.0	257	20.2	43.0	0.5	13.0

P

	Measure INFO/WEIGHT	per Measure KCAL	FAT	Nutrition Values per 100g / 100ml KCAL	PROT	CARB	FAT	FIBRE
QUADRELLI								
Organic, M & S*	1 Serving/75g	262.0	1.0	350	13.4	71.1	1.4	3.0
QUAVERS								
Cheese, Walkers*	1 Std Bag/16.4g	87.0	5.0	530	2.5	62.0	30.0	1.1
Prawn Cocktail, Walkers*	1 Bag/16.4g	90.0	5.0	550	1.9	63.7	31.9	1.2
Salt & Vinegar, Walkers*	1 Bag/16.4g	86.0	5.0	525	1.9	62.0	30.0	1.2
QUICHE								
Asparagus & Mushroom, Tesco*	½ Quiche/200g	474.0	33.0	237	5.1	17.2	16.4	1.2
Baby Spinach & Gruyere, Sainsbury's*	¼ Quiche/93g	228.0	16.0	245	7.4	15.1	17.2	1.0
Bacon & Cheese, Pork Farms*	1 Pack/120g	378.0	24.0	315	11.1	20.8	20.0	0.0
Bacon & Cheese, Sainsbury's*	¼ Quiche/100g	237.0	15.0	237	7.0	18.6	15.0	0.7
Bacon & Leek, Asda*	¼ Quiche/100g	252.0	16.0	252	8.4	18.9	15.9	1.5
Bacon & Leek, Individual, Tesco*	1 Quiche/175g	485.0	32.0	277	8.3	19.4	18.5	0.9
Bacon & Leek, Tesco*	¼ Quiche/100g	260.0	18.0	260	6.9	17.5	18.0	1.2
Bacon & Tomato, Asda*	1 Serving/107g	201.0	9.0	188	8.0	21.0	8.0	1.1
Bacon, Leek & Mushroom, M & S*	¼ Quiche/100g	245.0	16.0	245	6.9	17.2	16.4	1.3
Bacon, Leek, & Cheese, Weight Watchers*	1 Quiche/165g	307.0	13.0	186	7.4	21.0	8.1	1.8
Brie & Smoked Bacon, Asda*	¼ Quiche/90g	249.0	17.0	277	8.9	17.8	18.9	1.0
Broccoli & Cheddar Cheese, Safeway*	1 Pack/300g	813.0	54.0	271	7.7	19.8	17.9	1.9
Broccoli & Gruyere Cheese, Waitrose*	1 Serving/100g	241.0	18.0	241	7.3	13.0	17.8	2.9
Broccoli & Stilton, Mini, Sainsbury's*	1 Quiche/14g	52.0	3.0	369	8.8	35.2	21.4	3.3
Broccoli, Budgens*	1 Serving/88g	213.0	16.0	243	6.3	14.8	17.7	1.0
Broccoli, Extra, Value, Tesco*	1 Serving/125g	341.0	24.0	273	10.0	15.1	19.2	0.8
Broccoli, Tesco*	1 Serving/100g	249.0	17.0	249	6.0	17.6	17.2	1.4
Broccoli, Tomato & Cheese, BGTY, Sainsbury's*	1 Quiche/390g	632.0	32.0	162	6.4	15.7	8.2	1.3
Broccoli, Tomato & Cheese, Deep Filled, Sainsbury's*	¼ Quiche/100g	203.0	13.0	203	5.2	16.9	12.9	2.3
Cheese & Bacon, Crustless, Tesco*	1 Serving/85g	170.0	12.0	200	8.8	9.6	13.8	3.3
Cheese & Bacon, Smart Price, Asda*	¼ Quiche/82g	211.0	14.0	257	6.0	20.0	17.0	0.7
Cheese & Broccoli, Morrisons*	1/3 Quiche/134g	338.0	22.0	253	7.1	18.4	16.8	1.7
Cheese & Egg	1oz/28g	88.0	6.0	314	12.5	17.3	22.2	0.6
Cheese & Ham, Basics, Somerfield*	¼ Quiche/81g	187.0	11.0	231	7.0	20.1	13.6	0.7
Cheese & Ham, Sainsbury's*	1 Serving/100g	266.0	19.0	266	9.3	14.4	19.0	1.2
Cheese & Ham, Somerfield*	1 Quiche/325g	835.0	58.0	257	7.0	18.0	18.0	0.0
Cheese & Mushroom, Budgens*	½ Quiche/170g	474.0	33.0	279	7.8	18.4	19.3	1.4
Cheese & Onion, 25% Reduced Fat, Asda*	½ Quiche/78g	163.0	7.0	209	11.0	21.0	9.0	2.4
Cheese & Onion, Asda*	½ Quiche/200g	578.0	40.0	289	9.0	18.6	19.8	1.5
Cheese & Onion, Crustless, Asda*	1 Quiche/160g	277.0	15.0	173	7.6	14.3	9.5	1.3
Cheese & Onion, Deep Filled, Sainsbury's*	¼ Quiche/100g	254.0	17.0	254	7.3	17.2	17.2	2.2
Cheese & Onion, Finest, Tesco*	1 Serving/130g	346.0	24.0	266	9.1	15.3	18.7	2.5
Cheese & Onion, HL, Tesco*	1 Quarter/100g	180.0	8.0	180	9.4	17.6	7.8	1.8
Cheese & Onion, Individual, Sainsbury's*	1 Quiche/180g	542.0	35.0	301	9.9	21.6	19.4	1.5
Cheese & Onion, M & S*	1 Slice/100g	250.0	17.0	250	8.2	16.1	17.2	1.5
Cheese & Onion, Mini, Somerfield*	1oz/28g	110.0	8.0	394	9.0	27.0	28.0	0.0
Cheese & Onion, Reduced Fat, Eat Smart, Morrisons*	1 Quiche/400g	824.0	37.0	206	7.7	16.9	9.2	0.7
Cheese & Onion, Sainsbury's*	1oz/28g	67.0	4.0	241	6.8	18.3	15.6	2.6
Cheese & Onion, Shell*	1 Slice/150g	361.0	23.0	241	7.9	16.1	15.4	0.0
Cheese & Onion, Snack, Tasty Pastry*	1 Quiche/50g	137.0	9.0	274	4.9	24.9	17.2	1.2
Cheese & Onion, VLH Kitchens	1 Serving/80g	134.0	5.0	167	9.6	18.1	6.0	1.8
Cheese & Onion, Weight Watchers*	1 Quiche/165g	325.0	15.0	197	7.0	21.2	9.3	1.6
Cheese & Tomato, Asda*	¼ Quiche/105g	274.0	18.0	261	8.0	19.0	17.0	0.9
Cheese & Tomato, M & S*	1 Serving/100g	230.0	16.0	230	7.7	15.1	15.6	1.6
Cheese & Tomato, Morrisons*	½ Quiche/64g	195.0	13.0	304	7.3	22.8	20.5	1.0
Cheese & Tomato, Somerfield*	1 Quiche/135g	416.0	26.0	308	10.0	23.0	19.0	0.0
Cheese Potato & Onion, Safeway*	1/3 Quiche/115g	361.0	23.0	314	8.8	24.1	20.3	1.5

P

QUICHE

	INFO/WEIGHT	KCAL	FAT	KCAL	PROT	CARB	FAT	FIBRE
Cheese, Onion & Chive, Smart Price, Asda*	¼ Quiche/83g	213.0	14.0	257	6.0	20.0	17.0	0.7
Cheese, Onion & Chive, Somerfield*	1oz/28g	87.0	6.0	310	9.0	16.0	23.0	0.0
Cheese, Onion & Chive, Tesco*	1oz/28g	90.0	7.0	320	10.6	15.5	24.0	0.6
Chicken & Basil, Finest, Tesco*	1 Serving/134g	381.0	25.0	284	9.3	19.8	18.6	1.3
Chicken & Mushroom, Somerfield*	1oz/28g	90.0	6.0	320	12.0	22.0	21.0	0.0
Chicken, Garlic & Herb, Asda*	1/8 Quiche/52g	137.0	8.0	264	10.0	20.0	16.0	1.2
Crustless, Green Vegetable, Light Choices, Tesco*	1 Quiche/160g	200.0	9.0	125	6.0	11.9	5.8	4.7
Cumberland Sausage & Onion, Sainsbury's*	1 Serving/180g	486.0	33.0	270	7.0	18.8	18.5	1.3
Farmhouse Cheddar & Onion, Waitrose*	¼ Quiche/100g	257.0	18.0	257	8.1	15.4	18.1	1.3
Gammon, Leek & Cheddar Cheese, Somerfield*	¼ Quiche/95g	251.0	16.0	264	7.6	19.9	17.1	0.9
Gammon, Leek & Mustard, Weight Watchers*	1 Quiche/165g	305.0	15.0	185	5.7	20.7	8.8	3.4
Garlic Mushroom, Asda*	¼ Quiche/105g	273.0	17.0	260	7.0	22.0	16.0	0.7
Goats Cheese & Red Pepper, Finest, Tesco*	1 Serving/200g	600.0	45.0	300	5.9	18.5	22.5	1.5
Ham & Mustard, GFY, Asda*	1 Quiche/155g	327.0	17.0	211	9.0	19.0	11.0	3.9
Ham & Soft Cheese, Tesco*	¼ Quiche/100g	280.0	20.0	280	7.4	17.5	20.1	1.9
Ham & Tomato, M & S*	½ Pack/200g	440.0	31.0	220	8.1	12.4	15.5	2.9
Ham, Cheese & Chive, GFY, Asda*	1 Serving/78g	173.0	8.0	222	9.0	24.0	10.0	1.5
Leek & Sweet Potato, Waitrose*	½ Quiche/200g	440.0	29.0	220	5.3	17.0	14.5	2.3
Lorraine, Asda*	¼ Quiche/100g	246.0	16.0	246	6.6	18.5	16.2	4.2
Lorraine, Average	1oz/28g	109.0	8.0	391	16.1	19.8	28.1	0.7
Lorraine, BGTY, Sainsbury's*	1 Serving/128g	273.0	14.0	213	10.9	17.7	10.9	0.7
Lorraine, Budgens*	1 Pack/180g	520.0	31.0	289	8.2	25.6	17.1	0.8
Lorraine, Co-Op*	1/3 Quiche/108g	313.0	23.0	290	11.0	20.0	21.0	3.0
Lorraine, Crustless, Asda*	1 Quiche/160g	259.0	13.0	162	9.3	13.5	7.9	1.1
Lorraine, Crustless, Light Choices, Tesco*	1 Pack/160g	280.0	13.0	175	12.6	11.8	8.4	2.5
Lorraine, Extra Special, Asda*	¼ Quiche/100g	270.0	18.0	270	8.0	19.0	18.0	2.3
Lorraine, Finest, Tesco*	1 Serving/100g	330.0	25.0	330	8.4	17.5	25.1	1.5
Lorraine, Half Fat, Waitrose*	¼ Quiche/100g	189.0	9.0	189	8.1	19.0	8.9	1.4
Lorraine, Light Choices, Tesco*	¼ Pack/100g	170.0	6.0	170	12.3	15.5	6.4	3.2
Lorraine, Meat Free, Tesco*	1 Quiche/139.6g	335.0	19.0	240	9.4	19.1	13.8	2.8
Lorraine, Mini, M & S*	1oz/28g	95.0	7.0	340	11.6	21.0	23.6	1.6
Lorraine, Quiche Selection, M & S*	1 Slice/56g	160.0	12.0	285	12.8	12.3	20.6	2.1
Lorraine, Reduced Fat, Eat Smart, Morrisons*	¼ Quiche/100g	209.0	10.0	209	9.4	17.8	9.8	0.5
Lorraine, Reduced Fat, Safeway*	¼ Quiche/100g	231.0	12.0	231	11.0	18.9	12.4	1.4
Lorraine, Sainsbury's*	½ Quiche/200g	598.0	42.0	299	10.6	16.3	21.2	0.9
Lorraine, Small, Waitrose*	1 Pack/170g	507.0	35.0	298	9.8	18.4	20.6	2.3
Lorraine, Smoked Bacon & Cheese, M & S*	¼ Quiche/100g	270.0	18.0	270	9.7	16.4	18.4	1.6
Lorraine, Snack, Morrisons*	1 Serving/50g	142.0	9.0	285	10.2	19.0	18.7	2.0
Lorraine, Somerfield*	¼ Quiche/87g	260.0	18.0	299	10.1	17.1	21.1	0.7
Lorraine, Spar*	1 Quiche/340g	979.0	66.0	288	10.6	17.9	19.3	0.8
Lorraine, Tesco*	1 Serving/81g	215.0	13.0	265	8.9	20.0	16.6	0.8
Lorraine, Weight Watchers*	1 Quiche/165g	292.0	13.0	177	8.7	17.5	8.0	3.2
Lorraine, with a Creamy Filling, Safeway*	1 Quiche/485g	1576.0	110.0	325	9.8	19.4	22.7	1.2
Mature Cheddar & Onion, Deep Fill, Somerfield*	¼ Quiche/100g	280.0	18.0	280	8.4	22.1	17.6	1.1
Meat Feast, Tesco*	1 ¼ /100g	265.0	19.0	265	6.2	17.2	19.0	2.5
Mediterranean Vegetable, BGTY, Sainsbury's*	½ Quiche/90g	160.0	7.0	178	7.3	19.2	8.0	1.7
Mediterranean Vegetable, Mini, M & S*	1oz/28g	78.0	5.0	280	6.8	23.9	17.5	1.6
Mediterranean Vegetable, Weight Watchers*	1 Quiche/165g	285.0	14.0	173	3.8	21.1	8.2	4.0
Mediterranean, GFY, Asda*	1 Serving/25g	54.0	2.0	217	9.0	25.0	9.0	2.4
Mediterranean, M & S*	1oz/28g	64.0	4.0	230	6.6	16.6	15.3	0.9
Mushroom	1oz/28g	80.0	5.0	284	10.0	18.3	19.5	0.9
Mushroom Medley, Waitrose*	¼ Quiche/100g	222.0	15.0	222	6.4	15.0	15.2	2.9
Mushroom, M & S*	¼ Quiche/100g	235.0	17.0	235	6.1	14.6	16.7	2.8

Q

	Measure INFO/WEIGHT	per Measure KCAL	per Measure FAT	Nutrition Values per 100g / 100ml KCAL	PROT	CARB	FAT	FIBRE
QUICHE								
Mushroom, Somerfield*	¼ Quiche/82g	212.0	13.0	258	9.0	20.0	16.0	0.0
Mushroom, Tesco*	¼ Quiche/100g	250.0	17.0	250	5.6	17.4	17.5	1.0
Red Pepper, Goats Cheese & Spinach, Waitrose*	1 Serving/100g	218.0	14.0	218	6.5	15.8	14.3	2.6
Red Pepper, Rocket & Parmesan, Waitrose*	1 Serving/100g	236.0	17.0	236	6.1	14.8	16.9	1.9
Roast Sweet Potato, Carrot & Coriander, Asda*	½ Quiche/208g	523.0	33.0	252	7.0	20.0	16.0	1.0
Salmon & Broccoli, Asda*	¼ Quiche/106g	289.0	18.0	273	10.0	20.0	17.0	2.6
Salmon & Broccoli, Budgens*	½ Quiche/187g	539.0	36.0	288	11.2	17.7	19.1	0.6
Salmon & Broccoli, Sainsbury's*	1 Serving	346.0	23.0	260	7.9	18.5	17.1	0.8
Salmon & Broccoli, Tesco*	1 Serving/133g	311.0	20.0	234	7.9	16.6	15.1	0.9
Salmon & Spinach, Sainsbury's*	1/3 Quiche/125g	318.0	22.0	254	8.2	15.9	17.5	1.0
Sausage & Onion, Sainsbury's*	1 Serving/100g	287.0	20.0	287	7.1	19.7	20.0	1.2
Smoked Bacon & Cheddar, Little, Higgidy*	1 Quiche/155g	485.0	34.0	313	11.5	17.6	21.8	1.0
Spinach & Gruyere, Sainsbury's*	¼ Quiche/100g	258.0	19.0	258	7.7	13.9	19.1	1.0
Spinach & Ricotta, M & S*	1oz/28g	73.0	5.0	260	8.0	14.9	18.8	1.7
Spinach & Ricotta, Tesco*	¼ Quiche/100g	237.0	15.0	237	5.8	19.9	14.9	1.0
Spinach & Roast Red Pepper, Little, Higgidy*	1 Quiche/155g	397.0	27.0	256	9.1	15.2	17.6	1.2
Spinach Ricotta Cheese & Red Pepper, Safeway*	1 Serving/120g	304.0	20.0	253	6.2	20.2	16.4	1.2
Spinach, Feta & Roasted Red Pepper, Higgidy*	1 Quiche/400g	888.0	53.0	222	5.8	19.9	13.3	2.2
Sunblush Tomato, Basil & Mozzarella, Somerfield*	¼ Quiche/88g	221.0	15.0	251	7.7	17.9	16.5	1.0
Sweet Cherry Pepper & Fontal Cheese, Finest, Tesco*	¼ Quiche/100g	293.0	22.0	293	6.7	16.9	22.1	0.9
Sweetfire Pepper, Feta & Olive, Waitrose*	¼ Quiche/100g	238.0	17.0	238	5.7	15.7	16.9	1.4
Three Cheese & Onion, GFY, Asda*	1 Serving/73g	188.0	10.0	258	10.0	23.0	14.0	3.1
Tomato & Cheese, Sainsbury's*	1/3 Quiche/133g	374.0	24.0	281	7.9	20.9	18.4	1.5
Tomato Cheese & Courgette, GFY, Asda*	1 Serving/155g	333.0	17.0	215	7.0	22.0	11.0	3.3
Tomato, Cheese & Courgette, Asda*	1 Quiche/100g	333.0	17.0	333	11.0	34.0	17.0	5.0
Tomato, GFY, Asda*	¼ Quiche/50g	94.0	4.0	188	8.0	21.0	8.0	0.8
Tomato, Mozzarella, & Basil, Weight Watchers*	1 Quiche/165g	300.0	12.0	182	6.1	22.8	7.4	1.3
Tomato, Mushroom & Bacon, Sainsbury's*	1 Serving/187g	447.0	31.0	239	7.5	15.2	16.5	1.1
Tomato, Pesto & Mozzarella, TTD, Sainsbury's*	1/3 Quiche/158g	370.0	26.0	234	5.5	16.5	16.2	2.1
Tuna, Tomato & Basil, Asda*	1 Serving/125g	305.0	20.0	244	9.0	16.0	16.0	1.5
Vegetable, Tesco*	1 Serving/100g	257.0	18.0	257	6.9	17.5	17.7	1.5
QUICK SNACK								
Mash, Roasted Onion, Sainsbury's*	1 Pot/58g	75.0	4.0	130	1.8	14.8	7.1	0.0
Rice, Chilli, Sainsbury's*	1 Pack/280g	241.0	1.0	86	2.5	18.6	0.2	0.0
Rice, Sweet & Sour, Sainsbury's*	1 Serving/237g	230.0	1.0	97	2.5	20.5	0.5	0.0
QUINCE								
Average	*1oz/28g*	*7.0*	*0.0*	*26*	*0.3*	*6.3*	*0.1*	*0.0*
QUINOA								
Dry Weight, Average	*1 Serving/70g*	*262.0*	*4.0*	*374*	*13.1*	*68.9*	*5.8*	*5.9*
QUORN*								
Bacon Style, Slices, Smoky, Frozen, Quorn*	¼ Pack/37.5g	75.0	6.0	199	11.8	3.0	15.5	5.0
Balls, Al Forno, Quorn*	1 Serving/400g	348.0	7.0	87	4.7	13.1	1.8	1.8
Balls, Swedish Style, Quorn*	1 Pack/300g	354.0	6.0	118	17.0	8.0	2.0	2.0
Beef Style Pieces, in Red Wine Sauce, Quorn*	1 Pack/275g	165.0	4.0	60	5.0	6.5	1.5	1.7
Beef Style Pieces, Quorn*	½ Pack/75g	69.0	2.0	92	13.5	4.5	2.2	5.0
Bites, BBQ, Quorn*	1 Pack/140g	147.0	3.0	105	13.5	7.0	2.5	5.5
Bites, Indian, Quorn*	1 Bite/15.3g	34.0	2.0	222	6.0	27.0	10.0	3.0
Bites, Quorn*	½ Pack/70g	77.0	2.0	110	13.8	8.0	2.5	5.0
Burgers, Chicken Style, Quorn*	1 Burger/70g	136.0	7.0	194	11.0	16.0	9.6	4.6
Burgers, Minted Lamb Style, Quorn*	1 Burger/80g	86.0	3.0	108	12.0	6.0	4.0	4.0
Burgers, Original, Quorn*	1 Burger/50g	73.0	2.0	146	18.9	6.7	4.8	3.0
Burgers, Premium, Quorn*	1 Burger/82g	88.0	3.0	107	11.3	6.5	4.0	3.5
Burgers, Quarter Pounder, Mexican Style, Quorn*	1 Burger/113g	180.0	6.0	159	18.3	8.9	5.6	3.8

Q

	Measure INFO/WEIGHT	per Measure KCAL	FAT	Nutrition Values per 100g / 100ml KCAL	PROT	CARB	FAT	FIBRE
Burgers, Quarter Pounder, Quorn*	1 Burger/113.5g	158.0	5.0	139	18.0	6.5	4.5	4.5
Burgers, Sizzling, Quorn*	1 Burger/80g	123.0	5.0	154	18.0	7.0	6.0	3.0
Burgers, Southern Style, Quorn*	1 Burger/63g	119.0	6.0	189	10.7	14.5	9.8	3.1
Chicken Style Dippers, Quorn*	1 Dipper/19.2g	32.0	2.0	167	11.0	7.2	10.5	4.0
Chicken Style Pieces, Frozen Or Chilled, Quorn*	1 Serving/87g	90.0	2.0	103	14.0	5.8	2.6	5.5
Chilli, Quorn*	1oz/28g	23.0	1.0	81	4.7	6.9	4.2	2.5
Cottage Pie, Quorn*	1 Lg Pack/500g	345.0	6.0	69	2.4	12.1	1.2	2.3
Curry & Rice, Quorn*	1 Pack/400g	412.0	8.0	103	3.8	17.5	2.0	1.5
Curry, Red Thai, Quorn*	1 Pack/400g	464.0	16.0	116	4.6	15.5	3.9	4.0
Eggs, Picnic, Quorn*	1 Egg/20g	50.0	2.0	248	15.0	21.0	11.5	4.6
En Croute, Cheddar Cheese & Ham Style, Quorn*	1 Pastry/200g	486.0	28.0	243	7.2	22.0	14.0	3.0
En Croute, Creamy Mushroom & Garlic, Quorn*	1 Pastry/200g	460.0	29.0	230	5.9	19.0	14.5	3.2
Enchiladas, Quorn*	1 Pack/401g	405.0	15.0	101	5.3	11.7	3.7	1.9
Escalope, Mozzarella & Pesto, Quorn*	1 Piece/120g	260.0	16.0	217	10.0	15.0	13.0	4.5
Escalope, Turkey Style, Sage & Onion, Quorn*	1 Piece/100g	195.0	9.0	195	9.1	19.2	9.1	3.3
Escalopes, Creamy Garlic & Mushroom, Quorn*	1 Piece/120g	266.0	15.0	222	7.9	19.4	12.5	3.1
Escalopes, Creamy Peppercorn, Quorn*	1 Piece/120g	252.0	15.0	210	7.8	16.0	12.7	4.0
Escalopes, Feta & Tomato, Quorn*	1 Piece/120g	257.0	15.0	214	8.0	18.0	12.2	4.0
Escalopes, Garlic & Herb, Quorn*	1 Piece/140g	293.0	17.0	209	8.9	16.9	11.8	3.8
Escalopes, Goats Cheese & Cranberry, Quorn*	1 Piece/120g	281.0	17.0	234	10.0	17.0	14.0	4.0
Escalopes, Gruyere Cheese And Leek, Quorn*	1 Piece/120g	244.0	13.0	203	9.0	17.0	11.0	5.0
Escalopes, Gruyere Cheese, Quorn*	1 Piece/110g	262.0	15.0	238	10.0	18.0	14.0	2.6
Escalopes, Korma, Quorn*	1 Piece/120g	270.0	16.0	225	7.0	20.0	13.0	3.0
Escalopes, Lemon & Black Pepper, Quorn*	1 Piece/110g	249.0	13.0	226	9.6	20.5	11.7	2.1
Escalopes, Mature Cheddar & Broccoli, Quorn*	1 Piece/120g	244.0	14.0	203	8.7	16.5	11.4	2.9
Escalopes, Spinach & Soft Cheese, Quorn*	1 Piece/120g	236.0	13.0	197	8.5	16.1	11.0	2.9
Escalopes, Sweet Pepper & Mozzarella, Quorn*	1 Piece/120g	231.0	12.0	193	8.7	16.1	10.4	3.8
Escalopes, Wensleydale & Blueberry, Quorn*	1 Piece/120g	281.0	17.0	234	10.0	17.0	14.0	4.0
Fajita Meal Kit, Quorn*	½ Pack/214g	268.0	5.0	125	7.0	18.5	2.5	3.5
Fillets, Cajun Spice, Quorn*	1 Serving/100g	176.0	8.0	176	10.9	14.7	8.2	3.4
Fillets, Chargrilled Tikka Style, Mini, Quorn*	½ Pack/85g	110.0	2.0	129	12.5	14.4	2.4	5.0
Fillets, Chinese Style Chargrilled, Mini, Quorn*	1 Serving/85g	115.0	2.0	135	12.1	15.6	2.7	4.7
Fillets, Crispy, Quorn*	1 Fillet/100g	197.0	10.0	197	13.0	14.2	9.8	4.0
Fillets, Garlic & Herb, Quorn*	1 Fillet/100g	208.0	10.0	208	13.9	16.1	9.8	4.1
Fillets, Hot & Spicy, Quorn*	1 Fillet/100g	176.0	8.0	176	10.9	14.7	8.2	6.4
Fillets, in a Mediterranean Marinade, Quorn*	1 Fillet/80g	90.0	2.0	112	12.5	8.8	3.0	4.0
Fillets, Lemon & Pepper, Quorn*	1 Fillet/100g	195.0	8.0	195	13.3	16.2	8.5	3.5
Fillets, Mushroom & White Wine Sauce, Quorn*	1oz/28g	18.0	1.0	65	6.3	6.0	1.8	2.1
Fillets, Plain, Quorn*	1 Fillet/52g	47.0	1.0	90	12.6	5.9	1.8	4.7
Fillets, Thai, Quorn*	1 Serving/79g	96.0	4.0	121	11.0	9.0	4.5	4.0
Florentine, Deli, Quorn*	1 Slice/15g	21.0	1.0	140	15.0	5.8	6.3	3.0
Goujons, Quorn*	1 Goujon/31g	57.0	3.0	187	10.2	15.0	9.6	4.5
Goujons, with Chunky Salsa Dip, Quorn*	1oz/28g	57.0	3.0	204	10.4	17.0	10.5	3.0
Grills, Lamb Style, Quorn*	1 Grill/89.0g	97.0	3.0	109	11.2	7.6	3.7	4.3
Kievs, Mini, Quorn*	1 Kiev/20g	41.0	2.0	207	14.0	13.0	11.0	6.5
Lasagne, Quorn*	1 Pack/400g	332.0	12.0	83	3.7	10.6	2.9	1.8
Mince, Frozen Or Chilled, Quorn*	1 Serving/87g	82.0	2.0	94	14.5	4.5	2.0	5.5
Mini Savoury Eggs, Quorn*	1 Egg/20g	50.0	2.0	248	15.0	21.0	11.5	4.6
Moussaka, Quorn*	1 Pack/400g	364.0	16.0	91	3.6	9.8	4.1	1.2
Noodles, Sweet Chilli, Quorn*	1 Pack/400g	352.0	9.0	88	4.2	12.7	2.3	1.5
Nuggets, Chicken Style, Quorn*	1 Nugget/20g	41.0	2.0	207	10.3	16.7	11.0	3.8
Nuggets, Crispy, Chicken Style, Quorn*	1 Nugget/15.9g	29.0	2.0	182	12.0	9.9	10.5	4.0
Pasty, Cornish Style, Quorn*	1 Pasty/150g	399.0	24.0	266	5.5	25.0	16.0	3.0

	Measure INFO/WEIGHT	per Measure		Nutrition Values per 100g / 100ml				
		KCAL	FAT	KCAL	PROT	CARB	FAT	FIBRE
QUORN*								
Pate, Brussels Style, Deli, Quorn*	1/3 Pack/43.3g	55.0	2.0	128	11.3	8.5	5.4	4.0
Pate, Country Style Coarse, Quorn*	½ Pot/65g	68.0	3.0	104	9.2	7.3	4.2	2.7
Pie, & Vegetable, Quorn*	1oz/28g	52.0	3.0	186	6.9	14.7	11.5	2.0
Pie, Creamy Mushroom, Quorn*	1 Pie/141.9g	359.0	21.0	253	4.5	26.0	14.5	2.0
Pie, Mince & Onion, Quorn*	1 Pie/141.75	360.0	20.0	254	5.0	27.0	14.0	1.5
Pieces, Bacon Style, Quorn*	1 Pack/100g	103.0	2.0	103	15.0	5.0	2.5	5.0
Pizza, Bolognese, Quorn*	1 Pizza/240g	485.0	16.0	202	9.2	26.5	6.6	3.0
Pork Style Ribsters, Quorn*	2 Ribsters/85g	105.0	3.0	124	15.9	6.3	3.9	2.1
Roast, Chicken Style, Quorn*	1/5 Roast/91g	87.0	2.0	96	15.0	4.5	2.0	4.9
Satay Skewers, Quorn*	1 Skewer/10g	19.0	1.0	183	16.7	14.0	6.7	4.5
Satay Sticks, Quorn*	½ Pack/90.2g	149.0	8.0	165	13.0	7.1	9.4	3.2
Sausage Roll, Chilled, Quorn*	1 Roll/75.2g	194.0	10.0	258	12.0	24.0	12.7	4.0
Sausage, Seasoned with Chopped Onion, Quorn*	1 Sausage/42g	51.0	2.0	120	14.9	6.7	3.7	3.3
Sausages, Bangers, Bramley Apple, Quorn*	1 Sausage/50g	59.0	2.0	117	11.5	7.5	4.6	3.0
Sausages, Bangers, Quorn*	1 Sausage/50g	58.0	2.0	116	11.7	6.6	4.8	3.0
Sausages, Bangers, Sizzling, Quorn*	1 Sausage/50g	86.0	6.0	171	13.0	5.0	11.0	5.0
Sausages, Cocktail, Quorn*	1 Sausage/10g	15.0	1.0	155	13.0	11.0	6.5	4.5
Sausages, Cumberland, Quorn*	1 Sausage/50g	60.0	2.0	120	13.1	7.0	4.4	2.4
Sausages, Frankfurter, Quorn*	1 sausage/45g	82.0	6.0	183	12.5	4.0	13.0	3.0
Sausages, Frozen, Quorn*	1 Sausage/50g	56.0	2.0	113	14.9	4.9	3.7	3.3
Sausages, Leek & Pork Style, Quorn*	1 Sausage/44g	56.0	2.0	127	15.1	5.5	4.9	4.3
Sausages, Pork & Apple Style, Quorn*	1 Sausage/50g	58.0	2.0	117	11.5	7.5	4.6	3.0
Sausages, Quorn*	1 Sausage/43g	48.0	2.0	113	14.9	4.9	3.7	3.3
Sausages, Red Leicester & Onion, Quorn*	1 Sausage/50g	72.0	3.0	144	13.0	10.0	5.8	3.0
Sausages, Sizzlers, BBQ, Quorn*	1 Sausage/50g	83.0	5.0	165	13.0	4.0	10.8	4.0
Sausages, Smoky Red Pepper Sizzlers, Quorn*	1 Sausage/50g	83.0	5.0	165	13.0	4.0	10.8	4.0
Sausages, Spinach & Cheese, Quorn*	1 Sausage/50g	60.0	2.0	120	15.1	6.0	4.0	2.8
Sausages, Sweet Chilli, Quorn*	1 Sausage/50g	63.0	2.0	125	14.0	7.0	4.5	3.0
Sausages, Tomato & Basil, Quorn*	1 Sausage/50g	51.0	1.0	102	14.3	6.0	2.3	2.8
Seasoned Steak, Strips, Quorn*	½ Pack/70g	76.0	1.0	109	14.0	7.5	1.3	5.5
Slices, Chicken Style, Wafer Thin, Deli, Quorn*	1/3 Pack/60g	64.0	2.0	107	16.3	4.5	2.6	5.9
Slices, Ham Style, Deli, Quorn*	½ Pack/50g	55.0	1.0	110	16.0	6.5	2.2	5.8
Slices, Ham Style, Smoky, Quorn*	½ Pack/50g	55.0	1.0	110	16.5	5.7	2.4	5.0
Slices, Ham Style, Wafer Thin, Deli, Quorn*	1/3 Pack/60g	66.0	1.0	110	16.0	6.5	2.2	5.8
Slices, Peppered Beef Style, Quorn*	½ Pack/50g	53.0	1.0	107	14.5	7.6	2.1	4.0
Slices, Roast Chicken Style, Quorn*	½ Pack/50g	54.0	1.0	109	16.0	6.4	2.2	5.6
Slices, Turkey Style & Cranberry, Quorn*	½ Pack/50g	56.0	1.0	113	14.5	8.0	2.5	4.0
Slices, Turkey Style, with Stuffing, Deli, Quorn*	½ Pack/50g	53.0	1.0	107	14.9	6.6	2.3	4.7
Southern Style, Strips, Quorn*	Per Strip/31g	62.0	3.0	200	9.5	19.0	9.5	3.5
Spaghetti Bolognese, Quorn*	1 Pack/400g	240.0	4.0	60	3.7	9.2	0.9	1.6
Spaghetti Carbonara, Quorn*	1 Pack/400g	460.0	26.0	115	5.0	9.1	6.5	1.1
Spring Rolls, Mini, Quorn*	1 Roll/20g	41.0	2.0	205	4.5	23.0	10.5	2.4
Steaks, Peppered, Quorn*	1 Steak/98g	107.0	4.0	109	11.4	7.4	3.8	4.0
Stir Fry, Spicy Chilli with Vegetables & Rice, Quorn*	½ Pack/170g	161.0	2.0	95	5.9	15.6	1.0	1.8
Sweet & Sour, with Long Grain Rice, Quorn*	1 Pack/400g	380.0	4.0	95	4.0	17.5	1.0	2.0
Tandoori Pieces, Quorn*	½ Pack/70g	93.0	3.0	133	12.0	11.0	4.5	5.0
Tikka Masala, with Rice, Quorn*	1 Pack/400g	333.0	12.0	83	3.7	10.6	2.9	1.8

	Measure INFO/WEIGHT	per Measure KCAL	FAT	Nutrition Values per 100g / 100ml KCAL	PROT	CARB	FAT	FIBRE
RABBIT								
Meat Only, Raw	*1oz/28g*	*38.0*	*2.0*	*137*	*21.9*	*0.0*	*5.5*	*0.0*
Meat Only, Stewed	*1oz/28g*	*32.0*	*1.0*	*114*	*21.2*	*0.0*	*3.2*	*0.0*
Meat Only, Stewed, Weighed with Bone	*1oz/28g*	*19.0*	*1.0*	*68*	*12.7*	*0.0*	*1.9*	*0.0*
RADDICCIO								
Raw	*1oz/28g*	*4.0*	*0.0*	*14*	*1.4*	*1.7*	*0.2*	*1.8*
RADISH								
Red, Unprepared, Average	*1 Radish/8g*	*1.0*	*0.0*	*12*	*0.7*	*1.9*	*0.2*	*0.9*
White, Mooli, Raw	1oz/28g	4.0	0.0	15	0.8	2.9	0.1	0.0
RAISINS								
& Apricot, The Fruit Factory*	1 Box/14g	41.0	0.0	290	3.5	67.9	0.5	6.3
& Cranberries, Waitrose*	1 Serving/30g	94.0	0.0	312	1.5	75.7	0.3	3.4
& Sultanas, Jumbo, M & S*	1 Serving/80g	212.0	0.0	265	2.4	62.4	0.5	2.6
& Sultanas, Little Herberts, Nature's Harvest*	1 Pack/40g	128.0	0.0	319	3.1	75.5	0.5	3.7
& Sultanas, The Fruit Factory*	1 Box/14g	43.0	0.0	305	3.0	72.3	0.5	4.0
RAITA								
Cucumber & Mint, Patak's*	1oz/28g	18.0	1.0	64	3.4	8.4	1.8	0.0
Plain, Average	1oz/28g	16.0	1.0	57	4.2	5.8	2.2	0.0
RASPBERRIES								
Dried, Graze*	1 Pack/30g	85.0	1.0	284	3.2	62.0	2.6	0.0
Fresh, Raw, Average	*1 Serving/80g*	*20.0*	*0.0*	*25*	*1.3*	*4.7*	*0.3*	*6.5*
in Fruit Juice, Average	*1oz/28g*	*9.0*	*0.0*	*31*	*0.8*	*6.7*	*0.1*	*1.7*
In Fruit Juice, Canned, John West*	1 Can/290g	93.0	1.0	32	0.9	6.7	0.2	1.5
in Syrup, Canned	*1oz/28g*	*25.0*	*0.0*	*88*	*0.6*	*22.5*	*0.1*	*1.5*
RATATOUILLE								
Average	1oz/28g	23.0	2.0	82	1.3	3.8	7.0	1.8
Chicken, Finest, Tesco*	1 Pack/550g	407.0	12.0	74	7.8	5.9	2.1	0.0
Provencale, French Style Mixed Vegetables, Tesco*	½ Can/195g	76.0	4.0	39	1.1	4.2	2.0	1.9
Roasted Vegetable, Sainsbury's*	1 Pack/300g	134.0	3.0	45	1.4	7.5	1.0	2.3
RAVIOLI								
Asparagus, Waitrose*	1 Serving/150g	303.0	9.0	202	10.5	26.4	6.0	2.0
Basil & Parmesan, Organic, Sainsbury's*	½ Pack/192g	290.0	10.0	151	7.4	21.1	5.2	2.1
Beef & Red Wine, Italiano, Tesco*	½ Pack/150g	315.0	10.0	210	7.3	30.0	6.5	2.3
Beef & Shiraz, Finest, Tesco*	½ Pack/200g	358.0	9.0	179	8.4	26.1	4.5	1.8
Beef in Tomato Sauce, Canned, Asda*	1 Can/400g	352.0	8.0	88	3.6	14.0	2.0	3.0
Beef, GFY, Asda*	½ Pack/150g	288.0	5.0	192	7.0	33.9	3.2	1.9
Beef, Tesco*	1 Serving/194g	175.0	5.0	90	4.3	12.3	2.6	1.5
Cheese & Asparagus, Waitrose*	1 Serving/100g	242.0	7.0	242	12.6	31.7	7.2	2.4
Cheese & Tomato, Fresh, Organic, Tesco*	1 Serving/125g	342.0	14.0	274	12.5	30.8	11.2	1.1
Cheese & Tomato, Heinz*	1 Can/400g	340.0	8.0	85	2.4	13.9	2.1	0.9
Cheese, Garlic, & Herb, Fresh, Organic, Tesco*	1 Serving/125g	382.0	19.0	306	11.3	30.1	15.6	0.9
Cheese, Garlic, & Herb, Safeway*	½ Pack/125g	262.0	9.0	210	9.1	26.5	7.6	2.0
Cheese, in Tomato Sauce, Canned, Tesco*	1 Can/410g	328.0	8.0	80	2.5	13.0	2.0	0.5
Cheese, Tomato & Basil, Italiano, Tesco*	½ Pack/125g	309.0	11.0	247	13.1	28.5	8.8	2.1
Chicken & Bacon, Sainsbury's*	½ Pack/150g	238.0	8.0	159	5.5	22.2	5.4	2.0
Chicken & Mushroom, Finest, Tesco*	½ Pack/125g	267.0	9.0	214	11.6	25.8	7.1	1.1
Chicken & Rosemary, Perfectly Balanced, Waitrose*	½ Pack/125g	266.0	4.0	213	14.9	30.4	3.5	2.1
Chicken & Tomato, Perfectly Balanced, Waitrose*	1 Serving/125g	265.0	3.0	212	13.5	33.4	2.7	2.8
Chicken, Tomato & Basil, Finest, Tesco*	1 Serving/200g	358.0	12.0	179	9.6	21.7	6.0	1.0
Feta Cheese, M & S*	1 Serving/100g	195.0	8.0	195	9.1	20.5	8.5	1.3
Five Cheese, Weight Watchers*	1 Pack/330g	271.0	9.0	82	3.2	11.1	2.8	0.8
Florentine, Weight Watchers*	1 Serving/241g	220.0	5.0	91	3.7	14.1	2.1	1.2
Four Cheese, Italian Choice, Asda*	1 Pack/449g	467.0	27.0	104	3.4	9.0	6.0	2.1
Fresh, Bolognese, Safeway*	1 Serving/120g	200.0	6.0	167	8.8	22.6	4.6	2.0

R

	Measure INFO/WEIGHT	per Measure KCAL	per Measure FAT	Nutrition Values per 100g / 100ml KCAL	PROT	CARB	FAT	FIBRE
RAVIOLI								
Fresh, Pasta Reale*	1 Serving/150g	459.0	9.0	306	13.1	53.3	5.9	0.0
Garlic & Herb, Italiano, Tesco*	1 Serving/100g	318.0	13.0	318	11.1	39.1	13.0	2.6
Garlic Mushroom, Finest, Tesco*	1 Serving/250g	552.0	18.0	221	8.9	30.0	7.3	2.0
Goat's Cheese & Pesto, Asda*	½ Pack/150g	204.0	5.0	136	6.0	20.0	3.6	0.0
Goats Cheese & Roasted Red Pepper, Finest, Tesco*	½ Pack/125g	307.0	10.0	246	11.4	32.8	7.7	1.8
Grana Padano & Rocket, Finest, Tesco*	½ Pack/150g	270.0	7.0	180	7.5	26.0	5.0	1.8
in Tomato Sauce, Canned, Carlini*	1 Can/400g	324.0	4.0	81	3.1	15.0	1.0	0.5
in Tomato Sauce, Canned, Sainsbury's*	½ Can/200g	166.0	2.0	83	3.1	15.5	1.0	0.5
in Tomato Sauce, Heinz*	1 Can/400g	308.0	7.0	77	2.4	13.2	1.7	0.9
in Tomato Sauce, Meat Free, Heinz*	1 Can/410g	307.0	3.0	75	2.4	14.4	0.8	0.5
Meat, Italian, Fresh, Asda*	½ Pack/150g	261.0	6.0	174	8.0	26.0	4.2	0.0
Mozzarella Tomato & Basil, Tesco*	1 Serving/125g	304.0	13.0	243	13.6	24.1	10.2	0.5
Mushroom & Mascarpone, The Best, Safeway*	1 Pack/175g	465.0	19.0	266	9.9	31.8	11.0	1.0
Mushroom, Fresh, Sainsbury's*	½ Pack/125g	196.0	5.0	157	7.4	22.6	4.1	1.9
Mushroom, Italiano, Tesco*	1 Serving/125g	332.0	16.0	266	10.4	27.0	12.9	3.0
Mushroom, Safeway*	½ Pack/125g	242.0	9.0	194	7.5	25.5	6.9	1.8
Mushroom, Wild, Finest, Tesco*	1 Serving/200g	472.0	12.0	236	10.8	34.4	6.1	1.9
Pancetta & Mozzarella, Finest, Tesco*	1 Serving/125g	344.0	13.0	275	12.2	32.8	10.6	1.8
Red Pepper, Basil & Chilli, Waitrose*	½ Pack/125g	312.0	10.0	250	11.6	32.0	8.4	1.7
Rich Beef & Red Wine, Morrisons*	1 Pack/300g	813.0	21.0	271	12.0	42.8	6.9	2.6
Roast Garlic & Herb, Tesco*	½ Pack/125g	342.0	14.0	274	12.8	31.1	10.9	1.1
Roasted Pepper, M & S*	1 Pack/400g	540.0	31.0	135	5.4	11.0	7.7	1.1
Roasted Vegetable, Asda*	½ Pack/150g	217.0	1.0	145	6.0	29.0	0.5	0.0
Salmon & Dill, Sainsbury's*	1 Pack/300g	615.0	21.0	205	8.7	26.5	7.1	3.0
Smart Price, Asda*	1 Can/400g	272.0	0.0	68	2.7	14.0	0.1	1.3
Smoked Ham, Bacon & Tomato, Italiano, Tesco*	1 Can/125g	302.0	10.0	242	10.8	32.3	7.7	2.9
Smoked Salmon & Dill, Sainsbury's*	1 Serving/125g	256.0	9.0	205	8.7	26.5	7.1	0.7
Spinach & Ricotta, Waitrose*	1 Serving/125g	309.0	9.0	247	10.5	35.0	7.2	1.9
Sweet Pepper & Chilli, Tesco*	½ Pack/125g	324.0	14.0	259	12.5	27.1	11.2	2.7
Tomato, Cheese & Meat, Sainsbury's*	1 Serving/125g	314.0	16.0	251	12.4	21.4	12.9	2.2
Vegetable in Tomato Sauce, Italiana, Weight Watchers*	1 Can/385g	266.0	8.0	69	1.7	11.0	2.1	0.5
Vegetable, Canned, Sainsbury's*	1 Can/400g	328.0	3.0	82	2.6	16.3	0.7	0.7
Vegetable, Morrisons*	1 Can/400g	276.0	2.0	69	2.4	13.9	0.4	0.0
Vegetable, Tesco*	½ Can/200g	164.0	1.0	82	2.6	16.3	0.7	0.7
Vegetable, with Omega 3, Heinz*	1 Can/200g	144.0	3.0	72	2.2	12.2	1.6	0.6
RED BULL*								
Energy Shot, Red Bull*	1 Can/60ml	27.0	0.0	45	0.0	10.7	0.0	0.0
Regular, Red Bull*	1 Can/250ml	112.0	0.0	45	0.0	11.3	0.0	0.0
REDCURRANTS								
Raw, Average	*1oz/28g*	*6.0*	*0.0*	*21*	*1.1*	*4.4*	*0.0*	*3.4*
REEF*								
Orange & Passionfruit, Reef*	1 Bottle/275ml	179.0	0.0	65	0.0	9.5	0.0	0.0
REFRESHERS								
Bassett's*	1oz/28g	106.0	0.0	377	4.3	78.1	0.0	0.0
RELISH								
Barbeque, Sainsbury's*	1 Serving/50g	50.0	1.0	100	1.0	19.3	2.1	1.1
Burger, Juicy, Asda*	1 Tbsp/15g	17.0	0.0	113	1.2	25.4	0.7	0.7
Caramelised Onion & Chilli, M & S*	1 Serving/20g	47.0	0.0	235	1.4	55.1	1.1	1.0
Caramelised Red Onion, Tesco*	1 Serving/10g	28.0	0.0	280	0.6	69.1	0.1	0.7
Onion & Garlic, Spicy, Waitrose*	1 Tbsp/15g	35.0	0.0	232	0.8	54.2	1.1	1.7
Onion, M & S*	1oz/28g	46.0	1.0	165	1.0	32.1	3.0	1.1
Onion, Sainsbury's*	1 Serving/15g	23.0	0.0	151	0.9	36.0	0.4	0.7
Onion, Sweet, Heinz*	1 Tbsp/37.5g	38.0	0.0	102	1.0	23.5	0.4	0.6

R

	Measure INFO/WEIGHT	per Measure KCAL	FAT	Nutrition Values per 100g / 100ml KCAL	PROT	CARB	FAT	FIBRE
RELISH								
Sweet Onion, Branston*	1 Serving/10g	14.0	0.0	145	1.0	34.2	0.4	0.6
Sweetcorn, American Style, Maryland, Tesco*	1 Serving/15g	15.0	0.0	101	1.1	23.9	0.1	0.9
Sweetcorn, Bick's*	1 Tbsp/22g	23.0	0.0	103	1.3	24.3	0.2	0.0
Tomato & Chilli Texan Style, Tesco*	1 Tbsp/14g	20.0	0.0	140	1.7	32.0	0.1	1.1
Tomato Spicy, Bick's*	1 Serving/28g	28.0	0.0	99	1.3	23.2	0.2	0.0
Tomato, M & S*	1oz/28g	36.0	0.0	130	1.8	30.2	0.3	1.5
Tomato, Sweet, Heinz*	1 Serving/25g	34.0	0.0	136	0.9	32.6	0.2	0.9
REVELS								
Mars*	1 Packet/35g	168.0	7.0	480	5.1	68.0	20.9	0.0
RHUBARB								
Raw, Average	*1 Stalk/51g*	*11.0*	*0.0*	*21*	*0.9*	*4.5*	*0.2*	*1.8*
Stewed with Sugar, Average	*1oz/28g*	*32.0*	*0.0*	*116*	*0.4*	*31.2*	*0.0*	*2.0*
RIBENA*								
Apple Juice Drink, Ribena*	1 Carton/287ml	132.0	0.0	46	0.0	11.1	0.0	0.0
Blackcurrant & Cranberry, Ribena*	1 Bottle/500ml	205.0	0.0	41	0.0	9.9	0.0	0.0
Blackcurrant Juice Drink, Ribena*	1 Carton/288ml	147.0	0.0	51	0.0	12.6	0.0	0.0
Blackcurrant, Diluted with Water, Ribena*	1 Serving/100ml	46.0	0.0	46	0.0	11.4	0.0	0.0
Blackcurrant, Original, Undiluted, Ribena*	1 Serving/20ml	46.0	0.0	230	0.0	57.0	0.0	0.0
Blackcurrant, Really Light, No Added Sugar, Ribena*	1 Carton/250ml	7.0	0.0	3	0.0	0.7	0.0	0.0
Light, Ribena*	1 Carton/288ml	26.0	0.0	9	0.1	2.1	0.0	0.0
Orange, Juice Drink, Ribena*	1 Serving/288ml	98.0	0.0	34	0.1	8.1	0.0	0.0
Really Light, Undiluted, Ribena*	1 Serving/25ml	20.0	0.0	80	0.0	2.5	0.0	0.0
Strawberry Juice Drink, Ribena*	1 Carton/288ml	138.0	0.0	48	0.0	11.8	0.0	0.0
RIBS								
in a Chinese Style Coating, Tesco*	1 Serving/250g	420.0	22.0	168	19.5	5.3	8.7	2.5
Loin, BBQ, Sainsbury's*	1 Rib/42g	104.0	6.0	247	24.7	7.3	13.2	0.9
Loin, Chinese, Sainsbury's*	1 Rib/42g	103.0	5.0	246	27.2	7.2	12.0	0.9
Loin, Chinese, Taste Summer, Sainsbury's*	1 Serving/30g	38.0	2.0	128	11.7	2.8	7.8	0.1
Pork, Barbecue, Average	1 Serving/100g	275.0	18.0	275	21.4	7.2	17.9	0.3
Pork, Chinese Style, Average	1 Serving/300g	736.0	45.0	245	17.9	10.0	14.9	0.7
Pork, Full Rack, Sainsbury's*	1 Serving/225g	567.0	39.0	252	18.0	6.5	17.2	0.9
Pork, Raw, Average	1oz/28g	47.0	3.0	169	18.6	1.8	9.9	0.2
Spare, Barbecue, Chinese Style, Farmfoods*	1 Pack/400g	464.0	25.0	116	9.3	5.6	6.3	0.1
Spare, Cantonese, Mini, Sainsbury's*	1 Rib/38g	97.0	5.0	259	17.2	17.3	13.4	1.0
Spare, Sweet, Sticky, Mini, M & S*	1 Pack/300g	615.0	34.0	205	16.6	8.6	11.5	0.2
RIBSTEAKS								
Smokey Barbecue Style, Dalepak*	1 Serving/75g	164.0	10.0	219	16.1	8.8	13.1	0.8
RICCOLI								
Egg, Fresh, Waitrose*	1oz/28g	81.0	1.0	289	11.4	53.1	3.4	2.1
RICE								
Arborio, Dry, Average	*1 Serving/80g*	*279.0*	*1.0*	*348*	*7.1*	*78.3*	*0.8*	*0.8*
Basmati, & Wild, Cooked, Sainsbury's*	½ Pack/125g	150.0	1.0	120	3.1	25.7	0.6	1.3
Basmati, & Wild, Dry Weight, Tilda*	1 Serving/70g	244.0	0.0	349	9.4	77.0	0.5	1.0
Basmati, Boil in the Bag, Dry, Average	1 Serving/50g	176.0	0.0	352	8.4	77.8	0.8	0.4
Basmati, Brown, Dry, Average	*1 Serving/50g*	*177.0*	*2.0*	*353*	*9.5*	*71.8*	*3.0*	*2.2*
Basmati, Cooked, Average	*1 Serving/140g*	*189.0*	*2.0*	*135*	*3.6*	*26.0*	*1.8*	*0.7*
Basmati, Dry Weight, Average	*1 Serving/60g*	*212.0*	*1.0*	*353*	*8.1*	*77.9*	*1.0*	*0.6*
Basmati, Indian, Dry, Average	*1 Serving/75g*	*260.0*	*1.0*	*346*	*8.4*	*76.1*	*0.9*	*0.1*
Basmati, Microwave, Cooked, Average	1 Serving/125g	182.0	2.0	145	2.7	30.0	1.8	0.0
Basmati, White, Dry, Average	*1 Serving/75g*	*262.0*	*0.0*	*349*	*8.1*	*77.1*	*0.6*	*2.2*
Basmati, Wholegrain, Cooked, Tilda*	1 Serving/60g	68.0	1.0	113	3.3	23.0	0.9	3.2
BBQ & Spicy, M & S*	1 Pack/250g	462.0	18.0	185	6.1	23.7	7.2	1.2
Beef, Savoury, Batchelors*	1 Pack/120g	431.0	3.0	359	8.9	75.7	2.3	2.5

R

RICE

	Measure INFO/WEIGHT	per Measure KCAL	FAT	Nutrition Values per 100g / 100ml KCAL	PROT	CARB	FAT	FIBRE
Black, Artemide, Eat Well, M & S*	1 Serving/75g	251.0	2.0	335	8.5	73.3	2.6	4.0
Brown Basmati, Butternut Squash, Tilda*	½ Pack/125g	164.0	5.0	131	3.3	20.3	4.1	1.2
Brown, Cooked, Average	**1 Serving/140g**	**173.0**	**1.0**	**123**	**2.6**	**26.6**	**1.1**	**0.9**
Brown, Dry, Average	**1 Serving/75g**	**266.0**	**2.0**	**355**	**7.5**	**76.2**	**3.0**	**1.4**
Brown, Long Grain, Dry, Average	**1 Serving/50g**	**182.0**	**1.0**	**363**	**7.6**	**76.8**	**2.8**	**2.0**
Brown, Short Grain, Dry, Average	**1 Serving/50g**	**175.0**	**1.0**	**351**	**6.8**	**77.6**	**2.8**	**0.9**
Brown, Whole Grain, Cooked, Average	**1 Serving/170g**	**223.0**	**2.0**	**131**	**2.6**	**27.8**	**1.1**	**1.2**
Brown, Whole Grain, Dry, Average	**1 Serving/40g**	**138.0**	**1.0**	**344**	**7.4**	**71.6**	**2.9**	**3.0**
Chicken & Sweetcorn, Savoury, Asda*	½ Pack/60g	195.0	2.0	325	10.0	65.0	2.8	10.0
Chicken, Savoury, Batchelors*	1 Pack/124g	455.0	2.0	367	8.9	79.4	1.5	2.6
Chicken, Savoury, Smart Price, Asda*	½ Pack/168g	210.0	2.0	125	3.2	26.0	0.9	2.4
Chilli & Coriander, TTD, Sainsbury's*	1 Pack/446g	522.0	12.0	117	6.5	16.5	2.8	2.2
Chinese Five Spice, Special Recipe, Sainsbury's*	1oz/28g	37.0	0.0	133	2.9	29.9	0.3	0.9
Chinese Savoury, Batchelors*	1 Serving/50g	177.0	1.0	354	9.9	73.1	2.4	2.8
Chinese Style Savoury Five Spice, Made Up, Tesco*	1 Serving/141g	217.0	4.0	154	3.2	28.2	3.1	2.2
Chinese Style, Express, Uncle Ben's*	1 Pack/250g	392.0	5.0	157	3.4	30.9	2.2	0.4
Coconut & Lime, Asda*	1 Pack/360g	695.0	18.0	193	4.5	32.7	4.9	0.9
Coconut, M & S*	½ Pack/124g	217.0	5.0	175	3.1	31.8	4.0	0.3
Coconut, Thai, Sainsbury's*	½ Pack/100g	178.0	9.0	178	2.6	21.3	9.1	1.9
Coriander & Herb, Packet, Cooked, Sainsbury's*	¼ Pack/150g	204.0	1.0	136	2.5	30.4	0.5	1.5
Coriander & Herbs, Batchelors*	1/3 Pack/76g	280.0	3.0	369	7.9	79.6	3.5	5.0
Curry Style Savoury, Safeway*	1 Serving/100g	112.0	1.0	112	2.2	23.4	1.1	1.6
Curry, Savoury, Somerfield*	½ Pack/160g	194.0	1.0	121	2.2	26.0	0.9	1.3
Egg Fried, Average	1 Serving/300g	624.0	32.0	208	4.2	25.7	10.6	0.4
Egg Fried, Chinese Style, Tesco*	1 Portion/250g	417.0	10.0	167	4.4	27.9	4.2	0.7
Egg Fried, Chinese Takeaway, Tesco*	1 Serving/200g	250.0	3.0	125	4.7	23.3	1.5	1.8
Egg Fried, Express, Uncle Ben's*	½ Pack/124.9g	216.0	5.0	173	4.0	29.9	4.2	0.3
Egg Fried, Micro, Tesco*	1 Pack/250g	312.0	9.0	125	4.6	18.3	3.7	6.4
Egg, Chinese Style, Morrisons*	1 Serving/250g	285.0	12.0	114	2.1	16.8	4.8	0.7
Egg, Fried, 2 Minute Meals, Sainsbury's*	1 Pack/250g	342.0	1.0	137	3.8	29.2	0.6	0.8
Express Microwave, Uncle Ben's*	1 Serving/250g	370.0	4.0	148	3.2	30.0	1.7	0.0
Fried, Chicken, Chinese Takeaway, Iceland*	1 Pack/340g	510.0	16.0	150	6.5	20.7	4.6	0.6
Fried, Duck, Chicken & Pork Celebration, Sainsbury's*	1 Pack/450g	544.0	16.0	121	7.9	14.2	3.6	1.5
Garlic & Coriander Flavoured, Patak's*	1 Serving/125g	186.0	3.0	149	2.6	28.9	2.2	0.0
Golden Savoury, Dry Weight, Batchelors*	1 Pack/120g	437.0	3.0	364	10.1	74.7	2.8	2.4
Golden Savoury, Nirvana*	1 Pack/120g	142.0	1.0	118	2.5	25.4	0.7	2.9
Golden Vegetable, Freshly Frozen, Asda*	1 Sachet/200g	238.0	3.0	119	3.2	23.6	1.3	1.3
Golden Vegetable, Savoury, Morrisons*	1 Serving/50g	70.0	0.0	141	3.4	30.1	0.8	1.1
Golden Vegetable, Savoury, Sainsbury's*	¼ Pack/100g	122.0	1.0	122	2.9	25.4	1.0	0.3
Ground, Whitworths*	1 Serving/28g	98.0	0.0	349	7.7	77.7	0.8	0.7
Lemon Pepper Speciality, Asda*	1 Serving/52g	67.0	1.0	129	2.0	27.0	1.4	0.1
Lemon Pepper, in 5, Crosse & Blackwell*	½ Pack/163g	201.0	2.0	123	2.7	25.2	1.3	4.0
Long Grain, & Wild, Dry, Average	**1 Serving/75g**	**254.0**	**1.0**	**338**	**7.6**	**72.6**	**2.0**	**1.7**
Long Grain, American, Cooked, Average	**1 Serving/160g**	**229.0**	**3.0**	**143**	**3.0**	**28.7**	**1.7**	**0.2**
Long Grain, American, Dry, Average	**1 Serving/50g**	**175.0**	**1.0**	**350**	**7.1**	**77.8**	**1.1**	**0.6**
Long Grain, Dry, Average	**1 Serving/50g**	**169.0**	**0.0**	**337**	**7.4**	**75.5**	**1.0**	**1.7**
Long Grain, Microwavable, Cooked, Average	1 Serving/150g	180.0	1.0	120	2.7	25.8	0.6	0.7
Mexican Style, Cooked, Express, Uncle Ben's*	1 Pack/250g	385.0	5.0	154	3.2	31.1	1.9	0.7
Mexican Style, Old El Paso*	1 Serving/75g	268.0	1.0	357	9.0	78.0	1.0	0.0
Mexican, Ready Meals, Waitrose*	1 Pack/300g	432.0	7.0	144	2.6	27.8	2.5	0.5
Mild Curry, Cooked, Tesco*	1 Serving/154g	217.0	2.0	141	3.1	29.7	1.1	2.1
Mild Curry, Savoury, Batchelors*	1 Pack/120g	426.0	3.0	355	8.0	76.1	2.1	1.6
Mixed Vegetable, Savoury, Dry Weight, Tesco*	1 Pack/120g	450.0	3.0	375	7.8	79.1	2.7	2.9

R

RICE

Measure INFO/WEIGHT	per Measure KCAL	per Measure FAT	KCAL	PROT	CARB	FAT	FIBRE
RICE							
Mushroom & Coconut, Organic, Waitrose* — 1 Pack/300g	474.0	15.0	158	3.7	24.5	5.0	1.4
Mushroom & Pepper, Savoury, Cooked, Morrisons* — 1 Serving/200g	204.0	2.0	102	2.3	21.5	0.8	0.0
Mushroom & Pepper, Savoury, Safeway* — ½ Pack/194g	227.0	1.0	117	2.7	25.4	0.5	0.7
Mushroom Pilau, Bombay Brasserie, Sainsbury's* — 1 Pack/400g	672.0	17.0	168	3.7	28.6	4.3	0.7
Mushroom Savoury, Batchelors* — ½ Pack/61g	217.0	1.0	356	10.7	73.6	2.1	2.8
Mushroom Savoury, Bettabuy, Morrisons* — 1 Serving/128g	131.0	1.0	102	2.3	21.5	0.8	0.0
Nine Jewel, Chef's Special, Waitrose* — ½ A Pot/175g	257.0	5.0	147	4.4	26.3	2.7	4.2
Paella, Savoury, Tesco* — 1 Serving/60g	220.0	3.0	367	8.4	72.7	4.7	4.5
Pilau, Cooked, Average — **1 Serving/140g**	**244.0**	**6.0**	**174**	**3.5**	**30.3**	**4.4**	**0.8**
Pilau, Dry, Average — **1oz/28g**	**101.0**	**1.0**	**361**	**8.4**	**78.2**	**2.3**	**3.4**
Pilau, Indian Mushroom, Sainsbury's* — 1 Serving/100g	119.0	2.0	119	3.0	21.3	2.4	1.9
Pilau, Mushroom, Sainsbury's* — 1 Pack/250g	400.0	14.0	160	3.4	24.1	5.5	2.4
Pilau, Spinach & Carrot, Waitrose* — 1 Pack/350g	465.0	8.0	133	3.1	24.8	2.4	1.2
Pilau, Spinach, Bombay Brasserie, Sainsbury's* — 1 Pack/401g	642.0	17.0	160	3.5	26.9	4.3	0.8
Pudding, Dry Weight, Average — 1 Serving/100g	355.0	1.0	355	6.9	82.0	1.1	0.3
Risotto, Dry, Average — **1 Serving/50g**	**174.0**	**1.0**	**348**	**7.8**	**76.2**	**1.3**	**2.4**
Saffron, Cooked, Average — **1 Serving/150g**	**208.0**	**5.0**	**139**	**2.5**	**25.3**	**3.1**	**0.5**
Special Fried, Cantonese, Sainsbury's* — ½ Pack/250g	442.0	10.0	177	4.9	30.4	4.0	1.2
Special Fried, Chinese Takeaway, Iceland* — 1 Pack/350g	630.0	17.0	180	5.5	28.2	5.0	1.2
Special Fried, Chinese, Tesco* — 1 Serving/300g	618.0	33.0	206	6.5	19.9	11.1	0.8
Special Fried, M & S* — 1 Pack/450g	922.0	35.0	205	6.2	27.2	7.8	0.5
Special Fried, Sainsbury's* — 1 Serving/166g	272.0	8.0	164	5.1	25.5	4.6	0.7
Special Fried, Waitrose* — 1 Serving/350g	532.0	22.0	152	6.1	17.6	6.4	3.2
Spicy Mexican Style, Savoury, Made Up, Tesco* — 1 Serving/164g	213.0	3.0	130	2.9	26.3	1.5	2.4
Stir Fry, Oriental Style, Oriental Express* — 1 Serving/150g	216.0	5.0	144	4.2	24.1	3.4	1.9
Sweet & Sour, Rice Bowl, Uncle Ben's* — 1 Pack/350g	364.0	2.0	104	5.2	19.5	0.6	0.0
Sweet & Sour, Savoury, Batchelors* — 1 Serving/135g	418.0	3.0	310	9.4	75.6	2.1	3.1
Sweet & Sour, Savoury, Sainsbury's* — 1 Serving/145g	198.0	1.0	137	2.4	30.8	0.5	1.0
Sweet & Spicy, Express, Uncle Ben's* — 1 Pack/250g	417.0	10.0	167	2.7	30.1	4.0	0.0
Tandoori, Savoury, Batchelors* — 1 Serving/120g	430.0	3.0	358	10.3	73.5	2.5	3.0
Thai Sticky, Tesco* — 1 Serving/250g	357.0	6.0	143	2.5	27.6	2.5	0.4
Thai Style Lemon Chicken, Made Up, Tesco* — ½ Pack/138g	192.0	2.0	139	3.4	27.5	1.7	2.1
Thai, Cooked, Average — **1 Serving/100g**	**135.0**	**2.0**	**135**	**2.5**	**27.4**	**1.7**	**0.3**
Thai, Dry, Average — **1 Serving/50g**	**174.0**	**0.0**	**348**	**7.1**	**78.9**	**0.4**	**0.9**
Thai, Fragrant, Dry, Average — **1 Serving/75g**	**272.0**	**1.0**	**363**	**7.2**	**82.0**	**0.7**	**0.3**
Three Grain Mix, Wholefoods, Tesco* — 1 Portion/75g	266.0	2.0	355	9.6	73.3	2.2	2.3
Valencia for Paella, Asda* — 1 Serving/125g	435.0	1.0	348	6.0	79.0	0.8	0.0
Vegetable, Golden, Safeway* — 1 Serving/125g	111.0	1.0	89	2.9	18.2	0.5	1.9
Vegetable, Savoury, Co-Op* — ½ Pack/60g	210.0	1.0	350	9.0	76.0	1.0	3.0
White, Cooked, Average — **1 Serving/140g**	**182.0**	**1.0**	**130**	**2.6**	**28.7**	**0.8**	**0.1**
White, Cooked, Frozen, Average — **1 Serving/150g**	**168.0**	**1.0**	**112**	**2.9**	**23.8**	**0.5**	**1.1**
White, Flaked, Dry Weight, Average — **1oz/28g**	**97.0**	**1.0**	**346**	**6.6**	**77.5**	**1.2**	**0.0**
White, Fried — 1oz/28g	37.0	1.0	131	2.2	25.0	3.2	0.6
White, Long Grain, Dry Weight, Average — **1 Serving/50g**	**181.0**	**1.0**	**362**	**7.1**	**79.1**	**1.9**	**0.4**
White, Microwave, Cooked, Average — 1 Serving/150g	157.0	1.0	105	2.7	22.4	0.5	1.1
Whole Grain, Dry, Average — **1 Serving/50g**	**171.0**	**1.0**	**341**	**8.2**	**72.0**	**2.3**	**4.0**
Wild, Coronation, Sainsbury's* — ¼ Pot/75g	139.0	5.0	186	3.1	29.1	6.4	0.9
Wild, Giant Canadian, Dry Weight, Tilda* — 1 Serving/75g	262.0	1.0	350	11.5	74.2	0.8	1.9
Yellow, Ready Cooked, Tesco* — 1oz/28g	32.0	0.0	113	2.7	27.1	1.3	0.1
RICE BOWL							
Beef with Black Bean Sauce, Uncle Ben's* — 1 Pack/350g	367.0	5.0	105	5.6	17.4	1.4	0.0
Chicken Tikka Masala, Uncle Ben's* — 1 Pack/350g	381.0	8.0	109	5.9	15.9	2.4	0.0
Free From, Sainsbury's* — 1 Serving/182g	146.0	1.0	80	1.6	17.1	0.6	1.4

R

	Measure INFO/WEIGHT	per Measure KCAL	per Measure FAT	Nutrition Values per 100g / 100ml KCAL	PROT	CARB	FAT	FIBRE
RICE BOWL								
Honey BBQ Chicken, Uncle Ben's*	1 Pack/350g	420.0	2.0	120	5.4	23.1	0.6	0.0
Sweet 'n' Sour, Sharwood's*	1 Serving/350g	437.0	12.0	125	4.8	18.6	3.5	0.8
Thai Green, Sharwood's*	1 Bowl/350g	549.0	27.0	157	4.8	17.3	7.6	0.9
Thai Red, Sharwood's*	1 Bowl/350g	486.0	19.0	139	4.7	18.1	5.3	1.0
RICE CAKES								
Apple & Cinnamon Flavour, Kallo*	1 Cake/11g	41.0	0.0	376	6.2	83.1	2.2	3.9
Asda*	1 Cake/8g	31.0	0.0	386	8.7	81.1	3.0	2.8
Bacon, Asda*	1 Cake/9g	42.0	2.0	462	8.0	67.0	18.0	0.0
Barbecue, Sainsbury's*	1 Pack/30g	121.0	3.0	403	7.9	73.5	8.6	2.7
Caramel Flavour, Kallo*	1 Cake/10g	38.0	0.0	383	6.2	78.9	4.8	3.9
Caramel, Large, Tesco*	1 Cake/10g	34.0	0.0	344	6.5	73.9	2.5	5.1
Caramel, Less Than 3% Fat, Sainsbury's*	1 Pack/35g	134.0	1.0	382	5.6	86.4	1.6	1.8
Caramel, Snack Size, Tesco*	1 Pack/35g	133.0	1.0	379	5.5	82.7	2.9	0.9
Caramel, Tesco*	1 Serving/2g	9.0	0.0	379	5.5	98.2	2.9	0.9
Chocolate Flavour, Happy Shopper*	2 Portions/33g	156.0	6.0	469	5.1	69.9	18.8	2.4
Chocolate, Fabulous Bakin' Boys*	1 Biscuit/17g	83.0	4.0	490	6.4	66.7	22.0	1.6
Co-Op*	1 Cake/20g	80.0	1.0	402	8.0	84.0	3.1	0.0
Dark Chocolate, Organic, Kallo*	1 Cake/12g	57.0	3.0	471	6.8	57.2	24.1	7.4
Five Grain, Finn Crisp*	1 Cake/10g	36.0	0.0	356	9.8	73.9	1.7	9.7
Honey, Kallo*	1 Cake/10g	40.0	0.0	388	5.4	86.6	2.2	1.6
Japanese, Black Sesame, Clearspring*	1 Cake/7.5g	29.0	0.0	385	7.4	82.2	2.9	0.0
Japanese, Miso, Clearspring*	1 Cake/7.4g	27.0	0.0	365	9.2	77.0	3.0	2.0
Lightly Salted, Perfectly Balanced, Waitrose*	1 Cake/8g	31.0	0.0	387	8.3	82.4	2.7	2.1
Lightly Salted, Thick Slice, Low Fat, Kallo*	1 Cake/7.5g	28.0	0.0	372	8.0	78.7	2.8	5.1
Low Fat, Kallo*	1 Cake/10g	37.0	0.0	375	6.2	83.1	2.2	3.9
Milk Chocolate, Organic, Kallo*	1 Cake/11g	57.0	3.0	509	6.5	56.2	28.7	3.5
Multigrain, Ryvita*	3 Cakes/11g	43.0	1.0	384	9.1	76.2	4.7	5.3
Organic, Tesco*	1 Cake/7.6g	29.0	0.0	380	7.2	80.7	2.9	3.4
Plain, Finger Foods, Organic, Organix*	3 Cakes/6g	22.0	0.0	370	6.5	82.9	1.4	3.2
Salt & Vinegar, Jumbo, Tesco*	1 Cake/8.9g	31.0	0.0	347	8.4	72.7	2.5	6.0
Salt & Vinegar, Sainsbury's*	1 Pack/30g	121.0	2.0	403	8.3	73.3	8.3	2.7
Savoury, Jumbo, HL, Tesco*	1 Cake/8.4g	31.0	0.0	369	11.9	75.0	2.4	3.6
Sea Salt & Balsamic Vinegar, Kallo*	1 Cake/9g	32.0	0.0	361	6.5	78.1	2.5	3.0
Sesame Garlic, Clearspring*	1 Serving/8g	29.0	0.0	382	7.8	82.3	2.4	0.0
Sesame Teriyaki, Clearspring*	1 Cake/7.4g	28.0	0.0	377	6.5	82.8	2.2	0.0
Sesame, No Added Salt, Thick Sliced, Organic, Kallo*	1 Cake/10g	37.0	0.0	373	8.0	78.0	3.2	5.4
Sesame, Slightly Salted, Thin Slice, Organic, Kallo*	1 Cake/4.6g	17.0	0.0	373	8.0	78.0	3.2	5.4
Slightly Salted, Mrs Crimble's*	1 Slice/5.5g	21.0	0.0	380	7.6	80.4	3.1	3.2
Slightly Salted, Organic, Thin Slice, Kallo*	1 Cake/4.6g	17.0	0.0	372	8.0	78.7	2.8	5.1
Sour Cream & Chive Flavour, Sainsbury's*	1 Pack/30g	119.0	3.0	396	7.9	72.0	8.5	2.9
Thin Slice, No Added Salt, Organic, Kallo*	1 Cake/5g	19.0	0.0	372	8.0	78.7	2.8	5.1
Thin Slice, Organic, Hawkwood*	1 Cake/5.5g	21.0	0.0	378	7.6	79.1	3.5	3.4
Thin Slice, Organic, Waitrose*	1 Serving/5g	17.0	0.0	340	8.0	70.0	2.0	4.0
Toasted Sesame, Ryvita*	1 Pack/11g	43.0	1.0	391	8.4	78.4	4.9	3.5
Whole Grain, No Added Salt, Thick Slice, Organic, Kallo*	1 Cake/9g	33.0	0.0	365	7.6	80.0	3.1	3.4
Wholegrain, No Added Salt, BGTY, Sainsbury's*	1 Cake/8g	30.0	0.0	372	8.0	78.7	2.8	5.1
Wholegrain, Salt & Vinegar, Tesco*	1 Cake/9g	28.0	0.0	314	8.4	61.9	2.6	6.0
with Sesame, Organic, Evernat*	1 Cake/4g	15.0	0.0	368	8.5	74.5	4.0	0.0
with Yeast Extract, Snack Size, Kallo*	1 Cake/2g	7.0	0.0	364	12.6	71.1	2.8	4.7
RICE CRACKERS								
Authentic Thai Chilli, Tyrells*	½ Pack/75g	389.0	20.0	519	5.0	64.0	27.0	1.0
Barbecue Flavour, Tesco*	1 Pack/25g	102.0	2.0	409	6.7	78.8	7.4	1.7
Barbecue, Sakata*	½ Pack/50g	203.0	1.0	407	7.3	85.2	2.6	1.6

R

	Measure INFO/WEIGHT	per Measure KCAL	FAT	Nutrition Values per 100g / 100ml KCAL	PROT	CARB	FAT	FIBRE
RICE CRACKERS								
Brown, Wakama*	1 Cracker/5g	19.0	0.0	375	8.0	84.8	0.4	0.0
Cheese, Tesco*	1 Serving/25g	104.0	2.0	416	7.9	78.1	8.0	1.8
Chilli, Temptations, Tesco*	1 Serving/25g	128.0	7.0	512	4.4	58.0	28.8	0.0
Choco Noir, Bonvita*	1 Cracker/18g	79.0	3.0	440	6.8	64.0	18.5	0.0
Cracked Pepper, Sakata*	½ Pack/50g	200.0	1.0	400	7.3	84.4	3.0	2.0
Crispy, Chilli & Lime, Go Ahead, McVitie's*	1 Serving/25g	101.0	1.0	405	7.1	83.6	3.6	2.1
Crispy, Sea Salt & Vinegar, Go Ahead, McVitie's*	1 Serving/25g	102.0	1.0	408	6.6	80.6	5.4	1.8
Crispy, Sour Cream & Herbs, Go Ahead, McVitie's*	1 Serving/25g	105.0	2.0	422	7.1	78.2	8.0	1.8
Japanese Style, Tesco*	1 Serving/25g	101.0	2.0	405	11.7	75.2	6.1	3.3
Japanese, Apollo*	1 Pack/75g	297.0	4.0	396	9.6	78.8	4.7	0.9
Japanese, Graze*	1 Pack/40g	159.0	2.0	397	9.0	79.7	4.7	0.0
Japanese, Hider*	1 Pack/70g	303.0	12.0	433	11.3	61.7	17.3	0.0
Japanese, Julian Graves*	1 Serving/25g	92.0	0.0	369	8.8	79.5	1.7	3.8
Japanese, Mini, Sunrise*	1 Serving/50g	180.0	0.0	360	7.0	83.0	0.0	7.0
Korean Chilli, Graze*	1 Pack/20g	117.0	8.0	585	3.5	54.4	39.3	0.0
Mix, M & S*	½ Pack/63g	225.0	0.0	360	6.5	82.9	0.1	1.6
Paprika Flavour, Namchow*	1 Serving/38g	141.0	1.0	375	7.5	78.9	3.3	0.0
Sainsbury's*	1 Serving/20g	87.0	2.0	433	11.2	74.3	9.4	1.0
Salt & Pepper, Asda*	1 Cracker/5g	19.0	0.0	385	7.0	87.0	1.0	2.2
Salt & Vinegar, Namchow*	1 Serving/38g	139.0	1.0	370	6.7	77.5	3.7	0.0
Sour Cream & Chive, Sakata*	1 Serving/25g	107.0	2.0	430	7.8	80.6	7.9	0.0
Spicy Mix, Asda*	1 Serving/25g	115.0	4.0	461	6.4	71.2	16.7	0.2
Thai, M & S*	1 Serving/55g	209.0	2.0	380	7.0	80.2	3.3	1.2
Thai, Sesame & Soy Sauce, M & S*	1 Pack/55g	210.0	3.0	385	7.6	77.8	4.8	1.4
Thai, Wakama*	1 Cracker/2g	8.0	0.0	400	6.9	86.9	2.7	0.5
Thin, Blue Dragon*	3 Crackers/5g	20.0	0.0	395	6.1	84.4	3.7	0.0
with Tamari, Clearspring*	1 Bag/50g	190.0	1.0	380	8.2	83.4	1.5	0.3
RICE MILK								
Organic, Provamel*	1 Serving/250ml	122.0	4.0	49	0.1	9.5	1.5	0.0
Original, Rice Dream*	1 Serving/150ml	70.0	1.0	47	0.1	9.4	1.0	0.1
RICE PUDDING								
& Conserve, M & S*	1oz/28g	53.0	3.0	190	2.3	17.4	12.5	0.3
50% Less Fat, Asda*	½ Can/212g	180.0	2.0	85	3.3	16.2	0.8	0.2
Apple, Mullerrice, Muller*	1 Pot/200g	224.0	4.0	112	3.2	19.8	2.2	0.4
Banana, Ambrosia*	1 Pot/150g	153.0	4.0	102	3.2	16.6	2.5	0.0
Canned, Average	1oz/28g	25.0	1.0	89	3.4	14.0	2.5	0.2
Caramel, Ambrosia*	1 Pot/150g	149.0	4.0	99	3.1	16.1	2.5	0.0
Clotted Cream, Cornish, Waitrose*	1 Serving/150g	304.0	20.0	203	3.0	17.6	13.4	0.5
Clotted Cream, M & S*	1 Pudding/185g	431.0	31.0	233	3.0	19.2	16.6	0.2
COU, M & S*	1 Pot/170.6g	145.0	3.0	85	2.4	15.5	1.7	0.5
Creamed, Canned, Ambrosia*	1 Can/425g	382.0	8.0	90	3.1	15.2	1.9	0.0
Creamed, Canned, Sainsbury's*	½ Can/212g	195.0	3.0	92	3.1	16.2	1.6	0.1
Creamed, HL, Tesco*	1 Can/425g	340.0	3.0	80	3.0	15.1	0.6	0.2
Creamed, Pot, Ambrosia*	1 Pot/150g	156.0	4.0	104	3.3	17.0	2.5	0.1
Creamed, Weight Watchers*	1 Pot/130g	108.0	1.0	83	3.2	16.0	0.7	0.3
Creamy Rice, Shape, Danone*	1 Serving/175g	149.0	2.0	85	3.5	15.4	1.0	0.4
Creamy, Ambrosia*	½ Can/212g	197.0	4.0	93	3.2	15.7	1.9	0.0
Creamy, Delicious, Taste of Home, Heinz*	½ Can/212g	225.0	4.0	106	3.4	18.6	1.9	0.2
Libby's*	1 Serving/200g	180.0	3.0	90	3.3	16.2	1.6	0.2
Light, Creamy, Delicious, Taste of Home, Heinz*	½ Can/213g	194.0	1.0	91	3.4	18.0	0.6	0.2
Low Fat, Ambrosia*	½ Can/212g	176.0	2.0	83	3.2	15.7	0.8	0.0
Low Fat, No Added Sugar, Canned, Weight Watchers*	½ Can/212g	155.0	3.0	73	3.7	11.4	1.5	0.0
Organic, Ambrosia*	1 Can/425g	455.0	16.0	107	3.4	15.1	3.7	0.0

R

	Measure			Nutrition Values per 100g / 100ml				
	INFO/WEIGHT	per Measure KCAL	FAT	KCAL	PROT	CARB	FAT	FIBRE

RICE PUDDING

Organic, Evernat*	1oz/28g	39.0	1.0	141	5.5	22.9	3.0	0.0
Original, Mullerrice, Muller*	1 Pot/200g	212.0	5.0	106	3.7	16.9	2.6	0.3
Raspberry, BGTY, Sainsbury's*	1 Pot/135g	126.0	2.0	93	3.2	17.2	1.2	1.3
Raspberry, Mullerice, Muller*	1 Std Pot/200g	218.0	4.0	109	3.2	19.1	2.2	0.6
Rhubarb, Muller*	1 Pot/200g	226.0	4.0	113	3.2	20.0	2.2	0.0
Strawberry, Mullerrice, Muller*	1 Pot/200g	220.0	4.0	110	3.2	19.3	2.2	0.4
Thick & Creamy, Nestle*	1 Can/425g	527.0	24.0	124	3.1	15.4	5.6	0.2
Vanilla Custard, Mullerrice, Muller*	1 Pot/200g	230.0	5.0	115	3.4	19.8	2.5	0.3
with Peach, Apricot & Passion Fruit, Onken*	1oz/28g	33.0	1.0	118	2.5	18.7	3.7	0.5
with Strawberry Compote, Onken*	1 Pot/160g	184.0	5.0	115	2.6	18.6	3.4	0.5
with Strawberry Sauce, Ambrosia*	1 Pot/160g	174.0	3.0	109	2.7	19.8	2.0	0.1
with Sultanas & Nutmeg, Ambrosia*	1 Pack/425g	446.0	12.0	105	3.2	16.6	2.9	0.1
with Summer Fruit Compote, Onken*	1 Pot/160g	195.0	5.0	122	2.5	20.3	3.4	0.5

RICE SALAD

Chicken Tikka, COU, M & S*	1 Pack/390g	409.0	4.0	105	5.1	18.7	1.0	0.6
Hot Smoked Salmon, Deli Meal, M & S*	1 Pack/380g	570.0	26.0	150	6.5	15.1	6.9	0.2
Indian Style, with Chickpeas & Yoghurt Dressing, M & S*	1 Pack/220g	264.0	7.0	120	3.7	19.3	3.2	3.4
Mexican, with Beans, COU, M & S*	1 Serving/250g	250.0	3.0	100	6.0	15.6	1.4	1.2
Rainbow, M & S*	1 Serving/262g	340.0	8.0	130	2.5	23.3	3.2	1.5
Red, with Feta, M & S*	1 Pack/244g	440.0	21.0	180	4.8	21.0	8.5	1.3
Spanish Style, with Chicken, M & S*	1 Serving/220g	319.0	13.0	145	5.8	17.4	5.8	0.5

RICE WINE

Sake, Average	*1oz/28g*	*38.0*	*0.0*	*134*	*0.5*	*5.0*	*0.0*	*0.0*

RIGATONI

Carbonara, Tesco*	1 Serving/205g	236.0	12.0	115	5.2	10.6	5.8	1.2
Dry, Average	*1 Serving/80g*	*272.0*	*1.0*	*339*	*11.4*	*68.4*	*1.5*	*2.7*
Tomato & Cheese, Perfectly Balanced, Waitrose*	1 Pack/400g	664.0	9.0	166	7.6	28.6	2.3	2.3
Tuna, Diet Chef Ltd*	1 Pack/300g	336.0	13.0	112	5.9	12.2	4.4	1.0

RISOTTO

Balls, Mushroom, Occasions, Sainsbury's*	1 Ball/25g	76.0	3.0	304	3.8	41.2	13.8	1.7
Balls, Sun Dried Tomato, Occasions, Sainsbury's*	1 Ball/25g	71.0	4.0	285	6.8	30.8	15.0	2.9
Beef, Vesta*	1 Serving/100g	346.0	6.0	346	15.3	57.8	5.9	5.6
Caramelised Onion & Gruyere Cheese, M & S*	1 Pack/200g	350.0	21.0	175	3.0	17.8	10.3	1.7
Chargrilled Chicken, Ready Meal, M & S*	1 Pack/365g	493.0	25.0	135	6.4	11.6	6.9	0.7
Cheese Flavour, Made Up, Ainsley Harriott*	1 Sachet/140g	565.0	15.0	404	7.8	69.6	10.4	9.1
Cheese, Onion & Wine, Rice & Simple, Ainsley Harriott*	1 Pack/140g	253.0	7.0	181	3.1	31.0	5.0	1.6
Cherry Tomato, COU, M & S*	1 Pack/360g	324.0	8.0	90	2.0	15.4	2.3	1.8
Chicken & Asparagus, Eat Smart, Safeway*	1 Pack/380g	418.0	6.0	110	6.2	16.8	1.5	0.6
Chicken & Bacon, Italiano, Tesco*	1 Pack/450g	652.0	20.0	145	5.9	20.2	4.5	1.5
Chicken & Lemon, Weight Watchers*	1 Pack/330g	330.0	9.0	100	5.9	13.0	2.7	0.4
Chicken & Mushroom, Finest, Tesco*	1 Pack/400g	496.0	11.0	124	7.4	17.2	2.8	0.5
Chicken & Mushroom, Waitrose*	1 Pack/350g	364.0	16.0	104	6.0	9.7	4.6	0.8
Chicken & Mushroom, Weight Watchers*	1 Pack/320g	323.0	8.0	101	5.7	13.8	2.5	0.3
Chicken & Sun Dried Tomato, Waitrose*	1 Pack/350g	385.0	22.0	110	6.0	7.2	6.3	0.3
Chicken, BGTY, Sainsbury's*	1 Pack/327g	356.0	6.0	109	7.5	15.5	1.9	1.0
Chicken, Enjoy, Birds Eye*	1 Pack/500g	735.0	31.0	147	8.5	14.0	6.3	0.5
Chicken, Lemon & Wild Rocket, Sainsbury's*	1 Pack/360g	683.0	41.0	190	16.2	5.6	11.4	0.1
Chicken, Ready Meal, M & S*	1 Pack/360g	450.0	16.0	125	6.7	14.4	4.4	0.9
Chicken, Tomato & Mozzarella, GFY, Asda*	1 Pack/400g	356.0	4.0	89	8.1	11.9	1.0	1.2
Green Bean, Asparagus & Pecorino, Finest, Tesco*	1 Pack/400g	460.0	16.0	115	4.4	15.0	3.9	1.5
Haddock & Mushroom, COU, M & S*	1 Pack/400g	320.0	3.0	80	6.4	12.1	0.8	2.0
Hot Smoked Salmon & Spinach, M & S*	½ Pack/300g	420.0	24.0	140	6.4	11.0	8.0	0.6
Italian Red Wine with Creamed Spinach, Sainsbury's*	1 Pack/400g	596.0	28.0	149	2.4	19.3	6.9	0.4

R

	Measure INFO/WEIGHT	per Measure KCAL	FAT	Nutrition Values per 100g / 100ml KCAL	PROT	CARB	FAT	FIBRE
RISOTTO								
King Prawn & Snow Crab, M & S*	1 Pack/365g	401.0	16.0	110	4.1	12.7	4.5	0.5
King Prawn, Pea & Mint, M & S*	½ Pack/300g	405.0	19.0	135	3.8	15.9	6.2	0.9
Lemon & Mint, Perfectly Balanced, Waitrose*	1 Pack/350g	462.0	13.0	132	3.9	20.7	3.7	1.0
Mushroom, Asda*	1 Pack/340g	340.0	12.0	100	2.3	15.0	3.4	0.6
Mushroom, BGTY, Sainsbury's*	1 Pack/400g	387.0	9.0	102	2.7	17.6	2.3	1.0
Mushroom, COU, M & S*	1 Pack/373g	317.0	6.0	85	2.9	14.2	1.7	1.5
Mushroom, Italiano, Tesco*	1 Pack/340g	367.0	7.0	108	2.4	20.0	2.0	4.6
Mushroom, Perfectly Balanced, Waitrose*	1 Pack/400g	384.0	6.0	96	4.3	16.1	1.6	2.1
Roasted Red Pepper & Italian Cheese, M & S*	1 Pack/400g	500.0	13.0	125	2.9	20.4	3.3	1.0
Roasted Vegetable & Sunblush Tomato, Finest, Tesco*	½ Pack/200g	306.0	18.0	153	3.7	14.5	9.0	1.4
Roasted Vegetables, Stir-In, Uncle Ben's*	½ Pack/75g	86.0	7.0	115	1.7	5.0	9.7	0.0
Salmon & Prawn, Eat Smart, Morrisons*	1 Pack/380.9g	339.0	5.0	89	4.9	14.1	1.4	0.8
Seafood, HL, Tesco*	1 Pack/365g	328.0	4.0	90	5.3	14.1	1.0	0.9
Seafood, Youngs*	1 Pack/350g	423.0	13.0	121	4.5	17.4	3.7	0.1
Spring Vegetable, M & S*	1 Serving/330g	330.0	13.0	100	2.0	14.2	4.0	0.9
Tomato & Cheese, GFY, Asda*	1 Pack/400g	428.0	12.0	107	3.1	17.0	3.0	0.7
Tomato & Mascarpone, M & S*	1 Pack/360g	468.0	19.0	130	2.7	17.5	5.3	0.9
Vegetable, Average	1oz/28g	41.0	2.0	147	4.2	19.2	6.5	2.2
Vegetable, Brown Rice, Average	1oz/28g	40.0	2.0	143	4.1	18.6	6.4	2.4
ROCKET								
Fresh, Raw, Average	*1 Serving/80g*	*20.0*	*1.0*	*25*	*2.6*	*3.6*	*0.7*	*1.6*
ROE								
Cod, Average	*1 Can/100g*	*96.0*	*3.0*	*96*	*17.1*	*0.5*	*2.8*	*0.0*
Cod, Hard, Coated in Batter, Fried	1oz/28g	53.0	3.0	189	12.4	8.9	11.8	0.2
Cod, Hard, Fried in Blended Oil	1oz/28g	57.0	3.0	202	20.9	3.0	11.9	0.1
Herring, Soft, Fried in Blended Oil	1oz/28g	74.0	4.0	265	26.3	4.7	15.8	0.2
Herring, Soft, Raw	*1oz/28g*	*25.0*	*1.0*	*91*	*16.8*	*0.0*	*2.6*	*0.0*
ROGAN JOSH								
Chicken & Rice, Sainsbury's*	1 Pack/500g	675.0	27.0	135	6.7	14.1	5.4	2.4
Chicken, with Pilau Rice, Farmfoods*	1 Pack/325g	354.0	7.0	109	5.3	17.1	2.1	0.4
King Prawn, with Rice, HL, Tesco*	1 Pack/400g	365.0	6.0	91	4.8	14.6	1.5	1.6
Lamb, & Pilau Rice, Tesco*	1 Pack/550g	770.0	29.0	140	6.0	16.9	5.3	1.0
Lamb, Sainsbury's*	1 Pack/400g	660.0	44.0	165	11.3	4.9	11.1	1.9
Lamb, Tesco*	1 Pack/350g	402.0	20.0	115	10.2	5.0	5.8	1.3
Lamb, Waitrose*	1 Serving/60g	79.0	5.0	131	12.3	3.0	7.8	1.3
Prawn & Pilau Rice, BGTY, Sainsbury's*	1 Pack/401g	353.0	3.0	88	4.8	15.3	0.8	1.9
Prawn, COU, M & S*	1 Pack/400g	360.0	2.0	90	4.9	16.2	0.6	0.8
ROLL								
All Day Breakfast, Asda*	1 Roll/220g	581.0	26.0	264	10.0	29.0	12.0	0.0
Beef, Weight Watchers*	1 Roll/174g	276.0	4.0	159	10.8	23.1	2.5	1.0
Brie & Grapes, M & S*	1 Roll/57g	174.0	10.0	306	11.1	24.5	18.2	1.4
Cheese & Chutney, M & S*	1 Roll/165g	256.0	1.0	155	13.9	23.1	0.7	1.2
Cheese & Onion, Asda*	1 Serving/67g	199.0	12.0	298	7.0	27.0	18.0	2.0
Cheese & Onion, M & S*	1 Roll/25g	80.0	5.0	320	9.6	24.7	20.5	1.3
Cheese & Onion, Sainsbury's*	1 Roll/67g	205.0	14.0	306	8.0	22.9	20.3	1.9
Cheese & Onion, Tesco*	1 Roll/67g	203.0	12.0	305	7.3	28.0	18.1	1.9
Cheese & Pickle, Sainsbury's*	1 Roll/136g	359.0	14.0	264	10.6	35.1	10.0	0.0
Chicken & Beef Duo, M & S*	1 Serving/147g	235.0	4.0	160	12.0	22.1	2.6	2.7
Chicken & Herb, Shapers, Boots*	1 Roll/168g	290.0	5.0	173	12.0	25.0	2.8	1.7
Chicken & Stuffing, Tesco*	1 Roll/323g	1043.0	59.0	323	10.4	29.4	18.2	1.0
Chicken & Sun Dried Tomato, Weight Watchers*	1 Pack/170g	272.0	3.0	160	12.9	22.7	1.9	1.2
Chicken & Sweetcorn, Sainsbury's*	1 Serving/170g	462.0	24.0	272	12.5	24.2	13.9	0.0
Chicken Salsa, BGTY, Sainsbury's*	1 Pack/197g	323.0	5.0	164	11.1	24.8	2.3	0.0

R

	Measure INFO/WEIGHT	per Measure KCAL	FAT	Nutrition Values per 100g / 100ml KCAL	PROT	CARB	FAT	FIBRE
ROLL								
Chicken, Salad, Mini, Selection Pack, British, M & S*	1 Roll/61g	134.0	4.0	220	11.9	28.1	6.8	2.1
Chunky Cheese & Mustard, Finest, Tesco*	1 Roll/88g	260.0	9.0	295	10.9	40.0	10.2	2.4
Chunky Herbes De Provence, Finest, Tesco*	1 Roll/82g	196.0	3.0	239	7.4	45.2	3.2	2.6
Cornish, in Pastry, Pork Farms*	1 Roll/75g	226.0	15.0	301	6.6	24.5	20.1	0.0
Egg & Bacon, Sub, Shapers, Boots*	1 Serving/169g	320.0	7.0	189	11.0	27.0	4.3	1.3
Egg & Cress, HL, Tesco*	1 Pack/175g	322.0	7.0	184	9.6	27.7	3.9	1.2
Egg & Tomato, Shapers, Boots*	1 Roll/166g	301.0	5.0	181	8.0	30.0	3.2	2.6
Egg Mayonnaise & Cress, Sub, Delicious, Boots*	1 Pack/204.6g	399.0	14.0	195	10.0	23.0	6.9	2.4
Ham & Cheese, in Pastry, Pork Farms*	1 Roll/70g	216.0	13.0	308	8.0	28.8	17.9	0.0
Ham & Tomato, Taste!*	1 Serving/112g	211.0	5.0	188	10.4	27.0	4.3	0.0
Ham Salad, BGTY, Sainsbury's*	1 Roll/178g	292.0	3.0	164	10.8	25.9	1.9	0.0
Ham Salad, HL, Tesco*	1 Roll/203g	284.0	5.0	140	9.8	19.3	2.6	0.0
Ham, Darwins Deli*	1 Serving/125g	298.0	7.0	238	11.0	37.4	6.0	0.0
Lincolnshire Sausage, COU, M & S*	1 Roll/175g	280.0	5.0	160	10.0	23.2	2.7	2.6
Mushroom & Bacon, Crusty, M & S*	1 Roll/160g	424.0	20.0	265	8.7	29.0	12.6	2.3
Oak Smoked Salmon, M & S*	1 Roll/55g	139.0	6.0	252	14.6	23.1	11.3	1.2
Roast Chicken & Mayonnaise, Big, Sainsbury's*	1 Pack/185g	479.0	27.0	259	9.6	21.8	14.8	0.0
Roast Chicken & Sweetcure Bacon, Boots*	1 Pack/245g	690.0	34.0	282	13.0	26.0	14.0	1.6
Roast Chicken Salad, Improved, Shapers, Boots*	1 Pack/188g	302.0	4.0	161	11.0	25.0	1.9	1.6
Roast Pork, Stuffing & Apple Sauce, Boots*	1 Roll/218g	602.0	26.0	276	10.0	32.0	12.0	1.8
Sausage & Egg, Burger King*	1 Roll/162g	386.0	18.0	238	12.3	21.0	11.1	1.8
Spicy Chicken, Crusty, M & S*	1 Roll/150g	382.0	17.0	255	12.8	25.8	11.1	2.0
Steak & Onion, M & S*	1 Serving/150g	307.0	10.0	205	11.0	24.5	7.0	3.8
Tomato & Basil, Sub, COU, M & S*	1 Roll/35g	93.0	1.0	265	11.0	48.7	2.7	2.4
Tuna & Sweetcorn with Mayonnaise, Shell*	1 Pack/180g	536.0	26.0	298	13.1	28.6	14.6	0.0
Tuna Cheese Melt, Boots*	1 Roll/199g	612.0	36.0	308	13.0	23.0	18.0	1.2
Tuna Mayo & Cucumber, Taste!*	1 Serving/111g	274.0	13.0	247	9.0	27.3	11.3	0.0
Tuna Mayonnaise, with Cucumber, Yummies*	1 Serving/132g	340.0	19.0	257	10.4	22.5	14.0	0.0
Turkey Salad, Northern Bites*	1 Roll/231g	323.0	8.0	140	8.6	19.6	3.6	3.0
Turkey, Stuffed, GFY, Asda*	½ Pack/225g	319.0	9.0	142	14.0	12.0	4.2	0.8
White, Cheese & Onion, Shell*	1 Roll/178g	554.0	26.0	311	14.5	30.2	14.8	0.0
ROLO								
Giant, Nestle*	1 Sweet/9g	42.0	2.0	470	3.1	70.1	19.7	0.3
Little, Nestle*	1 Pack/40g	196.0	9.0	491	4.0	65.5	23.5	0.5
Nestle*	1 Sweet/5g	24.0	1.0	471	3.2	68.5	20.5	0.3
ROLY POLY								
Frozen, Tesco*	1 Serving/81g	287.0	11.0	354	4.4	52.7	14.0	0.5
Jam & Custard, Safeway*	1 Serving/112g	299.0	10.0	267	3.8	43.0	8.9	0.8
Jam, & Custard, Co-Op*	¼ Pack/100g	235.0	8.0	235	4.0	36.0	8.0	0.7
Jam, Aunt Bessie's*	1 Serving/100g	384.0	16.0	384	5.4	53.9	16.3	1.7
Jam, Sainsbury's*	¼ Pack/81g	291.0	12.0	359	4.4	53.3	14.2	0.5
Jam, Tesco*	1 Serving/90g	320.0	11.0	356	4.3	59.0	12.1	13.9
ROOT BAKES								
Herby, Red Sky*	1 Bag/30g	120.0	4.0	400	6.9	63.2	13.3	10.4
Spiced, Red Sky*	1 Bag/30g	122.0	4.0	408	8.0	62.9	13.8	9.2
ROOT BEER								
Average	1 Can/330ml	135.0	0.0	41	0.0	10.6	0.0	0.0
ROSE WATER								
English Provender*	1 Tsp/5g	0.0	0.0	2	0.1	0.6	0.1	0.1
ROSEMARY								
Dried	*1 Tsp/1g*	*3.0*	*0.0*	*331*	*4.9*	*46.4*	*15.2*	*0.0*
Fresh	*1 Tsp/0.7g*	*1.0*	*0.0*	*99*	*1.4*	*13.5*	*4.4*	*0.0*

R

	Measure INFO/WEIGHT	per Measure KCAL	per Measure FAT	Nutrition Values per 100g / 100ml KCAL	PROT	CARB	FAT	FIBRE
ROSTI								
Garlic & Mushroom, Finest, Tesco*	1 Serving/200g	346.0	20.0	173	5.7	15.4	9.8	1.7
Honey & Parsnip, Tesco*	1 Rosti/75g	79.0	2.0	105	1.8	17.0	3.2	3.9
Oven Baked, McCain*	1 Rosti/100g	194.0	9.0	194	2.6	25.0	9.3	2.3
Peppered Steak, British Classics, Tesco*	1 Pack/450g	598.0	28.0	133	9.0	10.7	6.2	1.7
Potato & Leek, Sainsbury's*	½ Pack/190g	296.0	21.0	156	4.5	9.8	11.0	0.3
Potato & Root Vegetable, COU, M & S*	1 Rosti/100g	85.0	3.0	85	1.6	13.3	2.7	1.5
Potato Cakes, Baby, M & S*	1 Rosti/23g	40.0	2.0	175	3.5	25.1	6.7	1.6
Potato, Chicken & Sweetcorn Bake, Asda*	1 Serving/400g	440.0	19.0	110	7.0	10.0	4.7	0.6
Potato, Fresh, Safeway*	1 Rosti/100g	138.0	5.0	138	2.8	19.2	5.5	2.8
Potato, McCain*	1 Rosti/95g	161.0	9.0	169	2.2	19.6	9.1	0.0
Potato, Mini, Party Bites, Sainsbury's*	1 Serving/100g	218.0	11.0	218	2.5	26.2	11.5	3.0
Potato, Mini, Party Range, Tesco*	1 Rosti/17g	32.0	2.0	193	2.1	20.6	11.4	3.3
Potato, Onion & Gruyere, Finest, Tesco*	½ Pack/200g	206.0	11.0	103	3.2	10.5	5.3	2.0
Potato, Spinach & Mozzarella, Tesco*	1 Serving/140g	228.0	8.0	163	3.8	24.5	5.5	2.0
Spinach & Mozzarella, Vegetarian, Tesco*	1 Rosti/140g	245.0	14.0	175	4.8	17.0	9.7	2.3
Waitrose*	1 Rosti/45g	112.0	7.0	248	3.8	22.5	15.9	2.7
ROULADE								
Chocolate, Finest, Tesco*	1 Serving/80g	222.0	4.0	277	3.4	53.2	5.6	2.3
Chocolate, Sainsbury's*	1 Serving/72g	264.0	16.0	367	5.7	36.9	21.8	1.8
Lemon, Asda*	1 Serving/100g	343.0	12.0	343	2.7	56.0	12.0	0.0
Mini, M & S*	1 Serving/63g	201.0	19.0	321	8.5	3.0	30.5	0.0
Orange & Lemon Meringue, Co-Op*	1 Serving/82g	287.0	10.0	350	3.0	57.0	12.0	0.3
Raspberry, Finest, Tesco*	1 Serving/67g	203.0	12.0	303	3.3	33.2	17.4	1.7
Raspberry, M & S*	1oz/28g	88.0	3.0	315	3.3	50.3	11.0	0.1
Smoked Salmon & Asparagus, Sainsbury's*	1 Serving/60g	122.0	10.0	204	13.0	2.2	16.0	0.3
Smoked Salmon & Spinach, Finest, Tesco*	1 Serving/60g	91.0	6.0	152	11.5	3.6	10.2	0.6
Toffee Pecan, Finest, Tesco*	1 Serving/60g	218.0	9.0	363	3.6	53.8	14.8	0.5
Toffee, M & S*	1oz/28g	104.0	4.0	371	4.1	56.0	14.5	0.3
RUM								
*21% Volume, Malibu**	*1 Shot/35ml*	*70.0*	*0.0*	*200*	*0.0*	*29.0*	*0.0*	*0.0*
37.5% Volume	*1 Shot/35ml*	*72.0*	*0.0*	*207*	*0.0*	*0.0*	*0.0*	*0.0*
40% Volume	*1 Shot/35ml*	*78.0*	*0.0*	*222*	*0.0*	*0.0*	*0.0*	*0.0*
White	*1 Shot/35ml*	*72.0*	*0.0*	*207*	*0.0*	*0.0*	*0.0*	*0.0*
RUSKS								
Banana, Farleys*	1 Serving/17g	70.0	2.0	409	7.3	75.1	8.8	2.9
Mini, Farleys*	1 Serving/30g	121.0	2.0	405	7.0	77.7	7.3	2.1
Original, Farleys*	1 Rusk/17g	69.0	1.0	406	7.1	77.6	7.1	2.3

R

	Measure INFO/WEIGHT	per Measure KCAL	FAT	Nutrition Values per 100g / 100ml KCAL	PROT	CARB	FAT	FIBRE
SAAG								
Aloo Gobi, Waitrose*	1 Pack/300g	240.0	14.0	80	2.6	7.1	4.6	2.9
Aloo, Canned, Tesco*	½ Can/200g	124.0	4.0	62	1.8	9.3	1.9	2.0
Aloo, Fresh, Sainsbury's*	1 Pack/400g	388.0	13.0	97	2.0	14.7	3.3	4.8
Aloo, Jar, Sainsbury's*	½ Jar/135g	121.0	6.0	90	1.6	11.0	4.3	1.7
Aloo, North Indian, Sainsbury's*	1 Pack/300g	354.0	24.0	118	2.4	9.0	8.0	1.6
Aloo, Packet, Sainsbury's*	½ Pack/150g	184.0	12.0	123	2.1	9.9	8.3	2.7
Aloo, Sainsbury's*	1 Pack/300g	441.0	32.0	147	2.1	10.7	10.6	3.5
Chicken, Masala, M & S*	½ Pack/175g	227.0	12.0	130	13.3	3.1	7.1	5.2
Chicken, Masala, Sainsbury's*	1oz/28g	36.0	2.0	127	13.2	2.4	7.2	2.3
Chicken, Masala, Waitrose*	1 Pack/400g	520.0	30.0	130	13.8	1.8	7.5	2.5
Gobi Aloo, Indian, Tesco*	1 Pack/225g	225.0	16.0	100	2.1	6.5	7.3	1.8
Gobi Aloo, M & S*	1 Pack/225g	270.0	19.0	120	1.9	9.3	8.5	2.4
Gobi Aloo, Tesco*	1 Serving/175g	166.0	9.0	95	2.1	9.5	5.1	1.9
Paneer, Sainsbury's*	1 Pack/300g	387.0	29.0	129	6.0	4.3	9.7	2.3
SAFFRON								
Average	*1 Tsp/1g*	*2.0*	*0.0*	*310*	*11.4*	*61.5*	*5.9*	*0.0*
SAGE								
Dried, Ground	*1 Tsp/1g*	*3.0*	*0.0*	*315*	*10.6*	*42.7*	*12.7*	*0.0*
Fresh	*1oz/28g*	*33.0*	*1.0*	*119*	*3.9*	*15.6*	*4.6*	*0.0*
SAGO								
Raw	*1oz/28g*	*99.0*	*0.0*	*355*	*0.2*	*94.0*	*0.2*	*0.5*
SALAD								
3 Bean, Sainsbury's*	1 Tub/270g	281.0	6.0	104	7.1	13.6	2.3	5.9
Alfresco Style, Tesco*	1 Serving/200g	40.0	1.0	20	0.9	3.3	0.3	2.1
American Ranch, Asda*	1 Serving/220g	253.0	20.0	115	2.5	6.0	9.0	2.0
American Style, Morrisons*	1 Serving/25g	5.0	0.0	22	1.1	3.9	0.3	2.3
Aromatic Herb, Waitrose*	¼ Pack/27g	4.0	0.0	15	0.9	1.7	0.5	1.0
Assorted, Asda*	1 Serving/100g	22.0	1.0	22	2.4	1.7	0.6	0.0
Avocado & Feta, Gourmet To Go, M & S*	1 Pack/320g	512.0	32.0	160	5.4	12.1	10.0	3.1
Baby Leaf & Herb, Asda*	1 Serving/50g	7.0	0.0	14	2.3	0.7	0.2	2.4
Baby Leaf, Florette*	1 Serving/40g	5.0	0.0	12	2.0	0.4	0.3	1.0
Baby Leaf, Italian Style, M & S*	1 Serving/55g	11.0	0.0	20	1.3	2.3	0.5	1.3
Baby Leaf, M & S*	1 Pack/100g	20.0	0.0	20	3.0	1.7	0.2	0.5
Baby Leaf, Sainsbury's*	1 Serving/60g	12.0	1.0	20	2.8	1.1	1.9	1.9
Baby Leaf, Seasonal, Organic, Sainsbury's*	1 Serving/30g	3.0	0.0	10	1.6	0.4	0.3	1.2
Baby Leaf, Seasonal, Tesco*	½ Pack/45g	9.0	0.0	20	1.8	1.6	0.7	2.1
Baby Leaf, Sweet, Seasonal, M & S*	½ Bag/60g	9.0	0.0	15	2.4	0.6	0.4	1.8
Baby Leaf, with Purple Basil, Finest, Tesco*	½ Pack/42.5g	7.0	0.0	17	2.9	0.9	0.2	1.8
Baby Leaf, with Watercress, Tesco*	1 Serving/30g	6.0	0.0	19	1.8	1.3	0.7	1.8
Baby Tomato, Tesco*	1 Pack/205g	35.0	1.0	17	0.8	2.8	0.3	0.9
Bacon Caesar, M & S*	1oz/28g	48.0	4.0	170	5.5	5.7	14.0	1.2
Bacon Caesar, Sainsbury's*	1 Pack/256g	415.0	33.0	162	4.7	12.0	12.7	1.4
Bag, Tesco*	1 Serving/200g	38.0	1.0	19	0.9	3.0	0.4	1.4
Basil, Pesto & Pine Nuts, Italian Style, Finest, Tesco*	½ Pack/90g	144.0	13.0	160	5.1	3.6	13.9	1.2
Bean & Chorizo, Tapas Selection, Sainsbury's*	1 Serving/22g	29.0	1.0	132	8.1	10.7	6.3	1.9
Bean & Sweetcorn, Side, M & S*	1 Serving/125g	131.0	9.0	105	2.5	7.0	7.2	1.3
Bean, Mint & Coriander, Somerfield*	1 Pack/250g	287.0	3.0	115	7.0	19.4	1.1	4.7
Bean, Mixed, Vinaigrette, Tesco*	1 Can/400g	280.0	2.0	70	3.2	13.1	0.5	1.9
Bean, Retail	1oz/28g	41.0	3.0	147	4.2	12.8	9.3	3.0
Bean, Three, M & S*	1 Pack/225g	225.0	3.0	100	5.8	16.7	1.3	3.9
Beetroot	1oz/28g	28.0	2.0	100	2.0	8.4	6.8	1.7
Beetroot & Carrot, Continental, Iceland*	1 Serving/100g	24.0	0.0	24	1.2	4.3	0.2	2.1
Beetroot & Cherry Tomato, & Lemon Dressing, M & S*	1 Pack/215g	129.0	8.0	60	1.3	5.2	3.8	1.5

S

SALAD

	Measure INFO/WEIGHT	per Measure KCAL	per Measure FAT	Nutrition Values per 100g / 100ml KCAL	PROT	CARB	FAT	FIBRE
Beetroot & Lettuce, Asda*	1 Serving/30g	5.0	0.0	16	1.4	2.7	0.0	2.5
Beetroot, 1% Fat, M & S*	1 Serving/225g	130.0	6.0	58	1.1	7.7	2.7	1.7
Beetroot, Cous Cous & Quinoa, Tesco*	1 Serving/100g	70.0	1.0	70	2.3	12.9	0.6	2.3
Beetroot, Freshly Prepared, Tesco*	1 Pack/240g	58.0	1.0	24	1.9	3.3	0.3	2.7
Beetroot, GFY, Asda*	1 Pack/250g	130.0	1.0	52	1.1	11.0	0.4	2.3
Beetroot, Organic, M & S*	1oz/28g	20.0	1.0	73	1.5	9.1	3.4	1.9
Beetroot, Roast, with Quinoa & Feta, Tesco*	1 Pack/400g	452.0	20.0	113	4.8	12.4	4.9	2.3
Beetroot, With Balsamic Dressing, Finest, Tesco*	1 Portion/75g	49.0	1.0	65	1.1	11.9	1.5	2.4
Bistro Style, Morrisons*	¼ Pack/45g	11.0	0.0	24	1.2	4.1	0.3	2.0
Bistro, Morrisons*	1 Serving/20g	5.0	0.0	23	1.2	4.2	0.2	2.0
Bistro, Sainsbury's*	1 Pack/150g	25.0	0.0	17	1.9	2.0	0.2	2.0
Bistro, Washed Ready to Eat, Tesco*	1 Pack/140g	22.0	1.0	16	1.1	1.7	0.5	1.0
Bocconcini Mozzarella, with Sun Ripened Tomato, M & S*	½ Pack/100g	250.0	21.0	250	9.8	4.9	21.4	2.0
British Ham & Free Range Egg, M & S*	1 Pack/280g	182.0	6.0	65	6.1	5.3	2.3	1.0
Brown Rice, Tossed UK*	1 Pack/200g	335.0	2.0	167	13.3	19.9	0.9	0.0
Cabbage & Leek, Crunchy Mix, Sainsbury's*	½ Pack/126g	24.0	1.0	19	1.2	2.1	0.6	1.9
Caesar, & New Potatoes with Asparagus, M & S*	1 Pack/200g	270.0	15.0	135	3.1	13.8	7.6	1.7
Caesar, Bacon, M & S*	1 Serving/250g	400.0	31.0	160	7.1	4.1	12.5	1.3
Caesar, Chicken & Bacon, Gourmet, M & S*	1 Salad/250g	550.0	43.0	220	9.0	7.3	17.4	0.7
Caesar, Chicken & Bacon, Tesco*	1 Pack/200g	506.0	40.0	253	6.6	11.4	20.1	1.0
Caesar, Finest, Tesco*	1 Bowl/220g	374.0	31.0	170	4.9	5.1	13.9	1.6
Caesar, Florette*	1 Serving/100g	163.0	12.0	163	2.7	10.2	12.4	1.8
Caesar, GFY, Asda*	½ Pack/87g	76.0	3.0	87	8.0	7.0	3.0	1.5
Caesar, M & S*	1 Pack/268.4g	510.0	41.0	190	5.7	8.3	15.1	1.3
Caesar, Sainsbury's*	½ Bag/128g	227.0	19.0	177	3.6	6.7	15.1	1.0
Caesar, with Dressing, Croutons & Parmesan, M & S*	1 Serving/115g	190.0	16.0	165	4.3	6.4	13.5	1.4
Caesar, with Parmigiano Reggiano, Tesco*	1 Bag/275g	552.0	49.0	201	4.1	5.8	17.8	1.3
Caesar, with Romaine Lettuce, Kit, BGTY, Sainsbury's*	½ Pack/130g	139.0	8.0	107	3.7	9.2	6.1	1.4
Cannelini Bean & Chorizo, Sainsbury's*	1 Pack/250g	227.0	8.0	91	5.3	10.2	3.2	1.6
Cannellini Bean & Chicken, M & S*	1 Serving/225g	250.0	15.0	111	5.9	7.4	6.5	3.1
Cannellini Bean & Tuna, M & S*	1 Serving/255g	215.0	12.0	84	5.3	5.4	4.5	2.1
Caponata, Organic, Florentin*	1 Serving/100g	111.0	12.0	111	1.5	3.7	12.3	0.0
Carrot & Beetroot, Classic, Tesco*	½ Pack/83g	17.0	0.0	20	0.9	3.7	0.2	1.6
Carrot & Nut, with French Dressing, Average	1oz/28g	61.0	5.0	218	2.1	13.7	17.6	2.4
Carrot & Sultana, BGTY, Sainsbury's*	½ Pack/100g	55.0	0.0	55	0.6	12.4	0.3	0.0
Carrot, M & S*	1 Pack/215g	280.0	7.0	130	3.1	22.4	3.4	2.7
Carrot, Orange & Ginger, Good Intentions, Somerfield*	1 Serving/250g	275.0	3.0	110	2.0	22.4	1.4	1.4
Carrot, Peanut & Sultana, Asda*	1 Serving/20g	54.0	4.0	272	8.0	15.0	20.0	4.5
Carrot, with Fresh Coriander Vinaigrette, M & S*	½ Pack/105g	136.0	4.0	130	2.8	21.9	3.4	3.5
Celery, Nut & Sultana, Waitrose*	1oz/28g	54.0	5.0	192	2.8	8.4	16.4	1.0
Chargrilled Chicken & Bacon, Tesco*	1 Pack/300g	657.0	38.0	219	7.8	18.7	12.6	0.9
Chargrilled Chicken & Pesto, Sainsbury's*	1 Pack/250g	375.0	15.0	150	7.9	15.8	6.1	1.3
Chargrilled Chicken & Quinoa, Shapers, Boots*	1 Pack/185g	139.0	2.0	75	6.2	10.0	1.0	1.8
Chargrilled Chicken Wholefood, M & S*	1 Pot/219g	230.0	4.0	105	10.1	11.6	1.9	4.8
Chargrilled Chicken, Tesco*	1 Serving/300g	384.0	14.0	128	6.1	15.0	4.8	2.4
Chargrilled Chicken, Weight Watchers*	1 Pack/181.5g	265.0	4.0	146	11.7	20.0	2.1	2.2
Chargrilled Pepper with Cous Cous, Asda*	1 Pack/325g	426.0	11.0	131	4.3	21.0	3.3	0.0
Chargrilled Vegetable, M & S*	1 Tub/165g	91.0	5.0	55	1.4	5.3	3.3	2.6
Cheese & Coleslaw, Tesco*	1 Serving/125g	135.0	11.0	108	3.4	3.4	8.7	1.1
Cheese, HL, Tesco*	1 Serving/30g	32.0	1.0	107	18.0	2.0	3.0	0.0
Cheese, Layered, Tesco*	1 Serving/225g	437.0	32.0	194	5.8	10.8	14.2	0.8
Cheese, Ploughmans, Asda*	1 Bowl/300g	246.0	11.0	82	3.6	8.9	3.6	1.0
Cherry Tomato, All Good Things*	1 Pack/185g	31.0	1.0	17	0.8	2.8	0.3	1.4

SALAD

	Measure INFO/WEIGHT	per Measure KCAL	FAT	Nutrition Values per 100g / 100ml KCAL	PROT	CARB	FAT	FIBRE
Cherry Tomato, Tesco*	1 Pack/210g	136.0	9.0	65	0.9	4.2	4.5	1.1
Chick Pea & Cous Cous, Tesco*	1 Serving/250g	245.0	6.0	98	3.2	15.5	2.6	0.0
Chick Pea & Spinach, M & S*	1 Serving/260g	299.0	11.0	115	7.3	12.5	4.1	2.7
Chicken & Bacon Ranch, Sainsbury's*	1 Pack/210g	315.0	16.0	150	8.4	12.1	7.5	0.9
Chicken & Bacon, Asda*	1 Pack/381.0g	480.0	23.0	126	7.0	11.0	6.0	0.0
Chicken & Bacon, Carb Control, Tesco*	1 Serving/188g	244.0	15.0	130	13.2	1.7	7.8	0.5
Chicken & Bacon, Layered, Asda*	1 Serving/375g	472.0	22.0	126	7.0	11.0	6.0	1.6
Chicken & Bacon, Layered, Tesco*	1 Bowl/380g	475.0	28.0	125	4.8	9.1	7.5	2.7
Chicken & Rice, Safeway*	1 Serving/200g	220.0	3.0	110	6.4	17.6	1.3	1.4
Chicken Caesar, Eat Well, M & S*	1 Pack/397g	595.0	25.0	150	9.9	18.7	6.2	2.1
Chicken Caesar, Fresh, Sainsbury's*	1 Serving/200g	278.0	20.0	139	6.0	6.2	10.0	1.2
Chicken Caesar, M & S*	½ Pack/140g	266.0	20.0	190	6.7	8.7	14.3	0.8
Chicken Fajita, Shapers, Boots*	1 Pack/258g	181.0	3.0	70	7.0	7.4	1.3	2.7
Chicken Noodle & Sweet Chilli, Shapers, Boots*	1 Pack/197g	266.0	5.0	135	12.0	16.0	2.6	0.9
Chicken Noodle, Thai Style, Sainsbury's*	1 Pack/260g	283.0	8.0	109	6.6	14.2	2.9	1.3
Chicken with Mayonnaise, Waitrose*	1 Pack/208g	406.0	20.0	195	10.3	17.1	9.5	2.5
Chicken, Avocado & Bacon, M & S*	1 Serving/235g	235.0	14.0	100	8.5	2.8	5.8	2.8
Chicken, Italian Style, Snack Pot, Carb Check, Heinz*	1 Pot/218g	131.0	4.0	60	5.9	4.3	2.0	1.0
Chicken, Roast, & Coleslaw, Boots*	1 Serving/245g	392.0	34.0	160	4.5	3.9	14.0	1.3
Chicken, Roast, 93 Cals, Shapers, Boots*	1 Pack/232.5g	93.0	1.0	40	8.6	0.6	0.4	1.8
Chicken, Sweet Chilli, BGTY, Sainsbury's*	1 Serving/200g	206.0	1.0	103	6.0	18.7	0.4	0.0
Chicken, Sweetcorn & Pasta, Safeway*	1 Serving/200g	230.0	4.0	115	7.5	16.3	1.8	1.0
Chicken, Tesco*	1 Serving/300g	348.0	22.0	116	5.3	7.0	7.4	1.0
Chicken, Tomato Chilli, & Rice, COU, M & S*	1 Pack/340g	357.0	5.0	105	6.8	16.0	1.5	0.9
Chicken, Tomato, & Basil, Safeway*	1 Serving/200g	330.0	18.0	165	6.9	14.2	8.9	0.6
Chilli, Tomato, Chick Pea & Butterbean, Tesco*	1 Pack/130g	146.0	6.0	112	3.4	14.3	4.6	0.5
Classic Caesar, M & S*	½ Pack/112g	174.0	14.0	155	2.9	6.8	12.7	0.5
Classic Caesar, Reduced Fat, M & S*	1 Serving/115g	132.0	6.0	115	4.8	12.7	4.9	0.5
Classic with Green Herb Dressing, Co-Op*	1 Serving/90g	85.0	8.0	95	1.0	2.0	9.0	1.0
Classic, Complete Salad, Sainsbury's*	1 Pack/220g	112.0	8.0	51	1.0	3.3	3.8	1.4
Classic, with Chive Dressing, M & S*	½ Pack/137.5g	76.0	6.0	55	0.9	3.3	4.2	1.6
Classics, M & S*	1 Pack/255g	140.0	12.0	55	1.1	2.4	4.7	1.3
Club, Safeway*	1 Serving/215g	226.0	18.0	105	1.3	6.0	8.4	1.3
Coleslaw Layered, Fresh, Asda*	1 Tub/197g	209.0	18.0	106	1.2	5.0	9.0	1.5
Coleslaw, Classics, M & S*	1 Pot/190g	123.0	4.0	65	1.9	8.8	2.3	1.3
Coleslaw, Layered, Fresh Tastes, Asda*	1oz/28g	17.0	1.0	59	1.1	3.4	4.5	1.6
Complete Hot Greek, Sainsbury's*	1 Pack/299g	287.0	22.0	96	4.3	2.9	7.5	1.7
Continental Four Leaf, Sainsbury's*	½ Pack/100g	13.0	0.0	13	1.2	1.7	0.2	1.9
Continental, Budgens*	1 Serving/55g	8.0	0.0	14	1.2	1.4	0.4	2.1
Continental, Co-Op*	1 Serving/80g	12.0	0.0	15	1.0	2.0	0.4	1.0
Cosmopolitan, Fresh, Sainsbury's*	1 Bag/135g	20.0	1.0	15	1.2	1.6	0.4	1.9
Country Style, Co-Op*	½ Pack/100g	20.0	0.0	20	1.0	3.0	0.4	2.0
Cous Cous & Roast Vegetable, GFY, Asda*	1 Serving/100g	120.0	2.0	120	3.5	23.0	1.6	2.7
Cous Cous, & Roasted Vegetable, Waitrose*	1 Pack/220g	396.0	13.0	180	5.1	26.1	6.1	1.2
Cous Cous, BGTY, Sainsbury's*	1 Pot/200g	236.0	4.0	118	4.7	19.7	2.2	2.8
Crisp & Crunchy with French Dressing, GFY, Asda*	1/3 Pack/116g	26.0	1.0	22	0.8	3.3	0.6	1.4
Crisp & Crunchy, Asda*	1 Pack/250g	55.0	1.0	22	0.8	3.3	0.6	1.4
Crisp & Light, M & S*	1 Serving/170g	51.0	1.0	30	0.5	5.4	0.8	1.0
Crisp & Sweet Lettuce Leaves, Florette*	¼ Pack/70g	10.0	0.0	14	0.8	1.7	0.5	0.9
Crisp Mixed, Tesco*	1 Pack/200g	40.0	1.0	20	1.1	3.2	0.3	2.0
Crisp, Mixed, Morrisons*	1 Pack/230g	39.0	1.0	17	1.0	2.8	0.3	0.0
Crispy Duck & Herb, M & S*	½ Pack/140g	378.0	26.0	270	20.7	3.7	18.3	1.4
Crispy Green, Sainsbury's*	1 Serving/70g	8.0	0.0	12	0.9	1.6	0.2	0.8

SALAD

INFO/WEIGHT	Measure	per Measure		Nutrition Values per 100g / 100ml				
		KCAL	FAT	KCAL	PROT	CARB	FAT	FIBRE
Crispy Leaf, Sainsbury's*	½ Pack/67.5g	9.0	0.0	14	1.0	1.7	0.4	1.7
Crispy Medley, Waitrose*	1 Serving/50g	7.0	0.0	15	0.8	1.7	0.5	0.9
Crispy, Florette*	1 Portion/100g	22.0	0.0	22	1.5	3.4	0.3	3.0
Crispy, Tesco*	1oz/28g	6.0	0.0	20	1.2	3.0	0.3	1.6
Crunchy Layered, Tesco*	1 Serving/54g	15.0	0.0	27	1.1	4.9	0.3	1.7
Crunchy Shredded, Safeway*	1 Serving/50g	9.0	0.0	19	1.2	2.9	0.3	1.5
Crunchy Spring, Side, M & S*	1 Serving/160g	32.0	0.0	20	0.9	4.1	0.2	1.3
Crunchy, Basics, Sainsbury's*	1 Pack/200g	40.0	0.0	20	1.3	3.4	0.2	2.2
Crunchy, Waitrose*	½ Pack100g	18.0	0.0	18	1.0	2.6	0.4	1.5
Edamame & Butterbean, TTD, Sainsbury's*	1/3 Pack/62g	70.0	3.0	113	6.6	9.9	4.1	4.9
Edamame Bean, Oriental Style, Asda*	1 Pack/220g	183.0	8.0	83	4.8	7.3	3.8	4.0
Egg & Baby Spinach, Waitrose*	1 Pack/215g	167.0	13.0	78	3.5	1.8	6.3	1.0
Egg & Coleslaw, Boots*	1 Pot/233g	405.0	37.0	174	3.0	4.6	16.0	1.0
Egg & Ham, with Salad Cream Dressing, M & S*	1 Pack/240g	168.0	8.0	70	5.2	4.0	3.5	0.6
Egg & Potato, Fresh, M & S*	1 Serving/250g	150.0	7.0	60	3.0	4.6	2.9	0.9
Endive & Radicchio, Somerfield*	1 Pack/150g	19.0	0.0	13	2.0	1.0	0.0	0.0
English Garden, Tesco*	1 Serving/180g	22.0	0.0	12	0.7	1.8	0.2	0.7
Family, Florette*	1 Serving/50g	14.0	0.0	29	1.1	5.5	0.2	3.0
Feta Cheese & Sunblushed Tomato, M & S*	1 Serving/190g	361.0	21.0	190	5.5	17.2	11.1	2.1
Fine Cut, Asda*	1oz/28g	7.0	0.0	24	1.2	4.1	0.3	2.1
Fine Noodle with Duck Breast, COU, M & S*	1 Pack/280g	294.0	3.0	105	5.5	18.9	1.1	1.1
Florida, Retail, Average	1oz/28g	63.0	6.0	224	0.9	9.7	20.5	1.0
Four Bean, Finest, Tesco*	1 Pack/225g	259.0	9.0	115	5.0	14.2	4.2	4.6
Four Leaf, M & S*	1 Serving/130g	19.0	0.0	15	0.9	2.0	0.3	1.4
French Goat's Cheese, Extra Fine, Asda*	1 Pack/185g	462.0	35.0	250	8.4	11.4	19.0	0.8
French Style, M & S*	1 Pack/140g	140.0	14.0	100	1.0	2.5	9.7	0.9
French Style, Waitrose*	½ Pack/82g	149.0	12.0	182	5.1	7.2	14.8	1.8
Garden with Watercress, M & S*	1 Salad/80g	10.0	0.0	12	1.5	1.4	0.1	1.4
Garden with Yoghurt & Mint Dressing, GFY, Asda*	1 Serving/195g	51.0	2.0	26	1.1	3.2	1.0	0.0
Garden, Tesco*	1 Serving/225g	34.0	1.0	15	1.0	2.0	0.3	0.9
Garden, Tray, Asda*	½ Pack/87.5g	16.0	0.0	18	0.7	3.1	0.3	1.6
Garden, Value, Tesco*	¼ Pack/50g	9.0	0.0	18	1.0	2.9	0.3	2.1
Gourmet Chargrilled Chicken & Bacon, Atkins*	1 Pack/245g	311.0	20.0	127	12.0	2.5	8.2	1.0
Gourmet Continental, Waitrose*	1 Serving/150g	22.0	1.0	15	0.8	1.7	0.5	0.9
Greek	1oz/28g	36.0	3.0	130	2.7	1.9	12.5	0.8
Greek Feta & Pepper, with Cous Cous, Asda*	1 Pack /316g	262.0	10.0	83	3.2	10.2	3.3	0.0
Greek Style Feta, Tip & Mix, M & S*	1 Pack/195g	214.0	18.0	110	4.0	2.5	9.4	1.6
Greek Style Layered, Perfectly Balanced, Waitrose*	1 Pack/280g	134.0	8.0	48	2.4	3.2	2.8	0.7
Greek Style, Delphi*	1 Serving/220g	306.0	27.0	139	3.7	3.5	12.3	0.9
Greek Style, Fresh, Food Counter, Sainsbury's*	1 Serving/166g	247.0	23.0	149	1.9	2.7	14.0	0.0
Greek Style, Waitrose*	½ Pack/125g	54.0	3.0	43	1.9	4.0	2.2	1.2
Greek Style, with Herb Dressing, Tesco*	1 Pack/240g	305.0	28.0	127	3.2	2.0	11.8	1.0
Greek Style, with White Wine Vinaigrette, Tesco*	1 Pack/235g	256.0	22.0	109	3.5	2.3	9.5	1.5
Greek, with Basil and Mint Oil Dressing, M & S*	1 Pack/200g	220.0	20.0	110	3.6	2.2	9.8	1.5
Green Lentil, Red Pepper & Spinach, Waitrose*	1 Pack/250g	485.0	20.0	194	8.6	22.0	8.0	2.9
Green Side, M & S*	1 Serving/200g	30.0	0.0	15	0.9	2.5	0.2	0.0
Green Side, Sainsbury's*	1 Pack/200g	28.0	0.0	14	1.2	2.1	0.1	1.4
Green with Chives, Tesco*	½ Pack/90g	13.0	0.0	14	1.0	1.6	0.4	1.7
Green with Honey & Mustard Dressing, M & S*	1 Pack/200g	120.0	10.0	60	0.9	2.7	4.8	0.8
Green with Sweetcorn & Radish, Fresh, Safeway*	1 Pack/210g	55.0	1.0	26	1.1	4.8	0.3	1.1
Green, Average	1oz/28g	4.0	0.0	13	0.8	1.8	0.3	0.9
Green, Complete, Sainsbury's*	1/3 Pack/55g	92.0	7.0	168	4.2	10.3	12.2	1.4
Ham & Free Range Egg, Fresh Tastes, Asda*	1 Bowl/265g	167.0	9.0	63	5.7	2.2	3.5	0.8

	Measure INFO/WEIGHT	KCAL	FAT	Nutrition Values per 100g / 100ml				
		per Measure		KCAL	PROT	CARB	FAT	FIBRE

SALAD

	Measure INFO/WEIGHT	KCAL	FAT	KCAL	PROT	CARB	FAT	FIBRE
Ham Hock, Waitrose*	1 Pack/350g	245.0	9.0	70	6.6	4.8	2.7	2.0
Ham, Antony Worrall Thompson's*	1 Pack/202.4g	257.0	3.0	127	9.8	19.1	1.3	2.7
Herb, Asda*	1 Serving/20g	2.0	0.0	12	1.8	0.6	0.3	2.0
Herb, M & S*	1 Pack/100g	20.0	0.0	20	2.9	1.4	0.4	1.9
Herb, Organic, Sainsbury's*	1 Serving/100g	17.0	0.0	17	1.8	1.3	0.5	1.8
Herb, Sainsbury's*	1 Pack/120g	22.0	1.0	18	2.7	0.8	0.5	2.2
Honey Smoked Salmon & New Potato, M & S*	1 Pack/270g	270.0	14.0	100	5.5	7.5	5.3	1.5
Houmous, Delicious, Boots*	1 Pack/230g	154.0	4.0	67	5.3	7.4	1.9	3.1
Iceberg & Cabbage, Asda*	½ Pack/125g	24.0	0.0	19	1.0	3.1	0.3	1.5
Italian Style, Organic, Waitrose*	½ Pack/45g	7.0	0.0	15	0.8	1.7	0.5	0.9
Italian Style, Tesco*	1/3 Pack/40g	6.0	0.0	16	1.0	1.9	0.5	1.2
Italian Style, With Rocket & Lambs Lettuce, M & S*	½ Bag/60g	12.0	0.0	20	1.3	2.3	0.5	1.3
Italian Wild Rocket & Parmesan, Sainsbury's*	1 Serving/50g	88.0	7.0	177	7.5	3.4	14.8	0.5
Italian, Complete, Sainsbury's*	1 Pack/160g	237.0	14.0	148	5.4	11.4	9.0	1.6
Jardin, Tesco*	1 Serving/50g	7.0	0.0	14	0.8	1.8	0.6	1.4
King Prawn & New Potato, COU, M & S*	1 Pack/300g	180.0	7.0	60	3.0	6.9	2.3	0.8
King Prawn, GFY, Asda*	1 Serving/175g	112.0	3.0	64	4.7	8.0	1.5	1.3
King Prawn, Thai Style, M & S*	1 Pack/295g	265.0	7.0	90	4.4	12.6	2.5	1.3
Leafy, Organic, Sainsbury's*	½ Pack/50g	7.0	0.0	15	1.7	1.3	0.3	1.8
Leafy, with Tatsoi, Sainsbury's*	1 Bag/115g	17.0	0.0	15	1.0	1.6	0.3	1.7
Leaves, Oriental Mix, Waitrose*	1 Bag/100g	18.0	1.0	18	1.5	1.7	0.6	1.9
Lemon Cous Cous & Roasted Pepper, COU, M & S*	1 Pack/340g	306.0	8.0	90	3.2	14.6	2.3	1.8
Mediterranean, Side, Sainsbury's*	1 Pack/170g	44.0	2.0	26	0.9	2.7	1.3	1.3
Mexican Style Bean & Cheese, M & S*	½ Pot/150g	150.0	5.0	100	6.1	11.2	3.5	4.8
Mix, Crisp & Sweet Lettuce Leaves, Florette*	1 Portion/67g	15.0	0.0	23	1.5	3.7	0.3	2.5
Mixed Leaf & Baby Basil, A Taste of Italy, Florette*	1 Pack/155g	143.0	8.0	92	2.7	8.5	5.3	1.0
Mixed Leaf Medley, Waitrose*	1 Serving/25g	4.0	0.0	15	0.8	1.7	0.5	1.4
Mixed Leaf Tomato & Olive, Tesco*	1 Serving/170g	150.0	13.0	88	1.0	3.4	7.8	2.0
Mixed Leaf, Tomato & Olive, Tesco*	1 Serving/170g	150.0	13.0	88	1.0	3.4	7.8	0.0
Mixed Leaf, Tomato, Feta, Boots*	1 Pack/179g	218.0	17.0	122	3.7	5.4	9.5	1.0
Mixed Leaves, with Beetroot, Earthy, Waitrose*	1 Bag/140g	34.0	1.0	24	1.5	3.6	0.4	2.1
Mixed Pepper, Asda*	½ Pack/100g	24.0	0.0	24	1.0	4.3	0.3	1.7
Mixed, Florette*	1 Serving/100g	20.0	0.0	20	1.3	3.4	0.2	3.0
Mixed, Sainsbury's*	1 Serving/100g	21.0	0.0	21	1.4	3.4	0.2	2.1
Mixed, Tesco*	1 Serving/100g	24.0	0.0	24	1.0	4.2	0.3	2.0
Moroccan Styles, COU, M & S*	½ Pack/100g	160.0	1.0	160	5.0	32.8	1.2	4.8
Mozarella & Cherry Tomato, Shapers, Boots*	1 Bowl/194g	184.0	14.0	95	4.1	3.3	7.3	0.9
Mozzarella & Rocket, Asda*	1 Serving/265g	435.0	32.0	164	7.0	7.0	12.0	1.5
Mozzarella & Sunkissed Tomato, Tesco*	1 Bag/160g	270.0	23.0	169	4.6	4.3	14.3	2.1
Mozzarella & Tomato, M & S*	1 Serving/310g	400.0	15.0	129	5.5	15.5	4.8	0.9
Nicoise Style, Layered, Waitrose*	1 Bowl/275g	129.0	4.0	47	2.7	5.8	1.4	1.0
Nicoise, Tesco*	1 Pack/260g	286.0	22.0	110	3.2	5.3	8.4	1.4
Noodle & King Prawn, Perfectly Balanced, Waitrose*	1 Pack/225g	223.0	2.0	99	5.0	17.4	1.0	1.0
Noodle with Thai Style Chicken, M & S*	½ Pot/145g	159.0	7.0	110	5.2	11.6	4.9	1.4
Noodle, Sweet Chilli Chicken, Shapers, Boots*	1 Serving/197g	256.0	4.0	130	11.0	17.0	2.1	1.1
Noodle, Thai Style, BGTY, Sainsbury's*	1 Pack/185g	150.0	4.0	81	2.7	13.5	1.9	0.0
Orzo & Sunbaked Tomato, BGTY, Sainsbury's*	1 Tub/275.5g	292.0	6.0	106	3.1	18.5	2.2	2.5
Potato & Cheese, Pasta & Mixed Leaf, Waitrose*	1 Serving/205g	266.0	17.0	130	3.2	10.1	8.5	1.1
Potato & Cheese, Sainsbury's*	1 Serving/125g	200.0	16.0	160	2.7	7.9	13.1	3.4
Potato & Egg, Fresh, Safeway*	1 Serving/105g	84.0	4.0	80	8.4	3.0	3.6	1.6
Potato & Egg, with Mayonnaise, Tesco*	½ Tub/150g	115.0	9.0	77	2.9	3.1	5.7	1.2
Potato Layered, Tesco*	1 Pack/350g	283.0	17.0	81	1.3	7.8	4.9	1.3
Potato, 30% Less Fat, BGTY, Sainsbury's*	1 Serving/60g	64.0	4.0	106	1.7	11.1	6.1	1.1

S

SALAD	Measure INFO/WEIGHT	per Measure KCAL FAT	Nutrition Values per 100g / 100ml KCAL PROT CARB FAT FIBRE

SALAD

	Measure INFO/WEIGHT	per Measure KCAL	FAT	KCAL	PROT	CARB	FAT	FIBRE
Potato, Creamy, Waitrose*	1 Serving/100g	163.0	12.0	163	1.3	12.7	11.9	1.1
Potato, Finest, Tesco*	1 Tub/250g	587.0	51.0	235	2.4	9.7	20.6	1.2
Potato, From Salad Selection, Sainsbury's*	1 Serving/50g	102.0	9.0	204	1.0	10.5	17.5	1.3
Potato, GFY, Asda*	½ Pack/125g	145.0	9.0	116	1.3	12.0	7.0	0.0
Potato, Heinz*	½ Can/97g	137.0	8.0	141	1.4	14.8	8.5	0.8
Potato, Light Choices, Tesco*	1 Pack/100g	110.0	6.0	110	1.3	12.5	5.9	0.9
Potato, Luxury, Asda*	1 Serving/50g	118.0	10.0	237	1.0	11.0	21.0	0.0
Potato, Side, Waitrose*	1 Pack/250g	181.0	11.0	72	3.0	5.2	4.4	1.0
Potato, with Onions & Chives, Co-Op*	1 Serving/50g	80.0	6.0	160	1.0	12.0	12.0	1.0
Prawn & Avocado, M & S*	1 Serving/220g	176.0	15.0	80	3.0	2.0	6.8	3.1
Prawn & Egg, Leaf, Shapers, Boots*	1 Pack/182g	193.0	14.0	106	6.7	2.1	7.9	1.0
Prawn Cocktail, HL, Tesco*	1 Serving/300g	279.0	3.0	93	5.7	15.3	1.0	2.0
Prawn Cocktail, Shapers, Boots*	1 Pack/245g	120.0	6.0	49	4.7	2.2	2.4	0.7
Prawn Cocktail, Tesco*	1 Pack/300g	360.0	18.0	120	5.7	10.9	6.0	0.8
Prawn Layer, Eat Well, M & S*	1 Pack/220g	143.0	5.0	65	4.3	6.9	2.1	1.4
Prawn Satay & Noodle, Tesco*	1 Serving/250g	320.0	17.0	128	7.1	9.5	6.8	1.2
Prawn, King & Rice Noodle, M & S*	1 Pack/320g	208.0	3.0	65	2.9	11.6	0.8	0.9
Prawn, King, with Noodles, Delicious, Boots*	1 Pack/228g	251.0	4.0	110	6.3	18.0	1.6	1.8
Prawn, Layered, Sainsbury's*	1 Pack/275g	355.0	21.0	129	3.6	11.2	7.7	1.1
Prawn, Layered, Single Size, Asda*	1 Serving/197g	217.0	10.0	110	4.3	12.0	5.0	1.0
Prawn, Layered, Tesco*	1 Pack/180g	243.0	13.0	135	4.2	13.1	7.2	2.0
Red Cabbage & Sweetcorn, Crunchy, M & S*	1 Serving/80g	28.0	0.0	35	1.3	6.6	0.5	1.2
Red Hot, Very Special, Asda*	1 Serving/85g	9.0	0.0	11	1.9	0.9	0.0	1.4
Red Thai Chicken with Noodles, Tesco*	1 Pack/300g	342.0	1.0	114	7.2	20.2	0.5	1.4
Rice, Courgette & Pine Nut, BGTY, Sainsbury's*	1/3 Pot/65g	68.0	1.0	105	2.7	20.0	1.6	1.5
Roast Chicken, Layered, HL, Tesco*	1 Salad/400g	268.0	4.0	67	5.8	8.4	1.1	2.1
Roast Chicken, Tesco*	1 Salad/300g	348.0	22.0	116	5.3	7.0	7.4	1.0
Roast Pepper Cous Cous, HL, Tesco*	1 Pot/220g	308.0	5.0	140	5.6	24.3	2.1	1.7
Roasted Artichoke & Pepper, M & S*	1 Serving/220g	638.0	54.0	290	4.1	12.8	24.5	5.1
Rocket, Leafy, Asda*	1 Serving/75g	10.0	0.0	13	1.5	1.4	0.1	1.8
Rocket, Morrisons*	1 Serving/100g	14.0	0.0	14	0.8	1.7	0.5	0.0
Ruby, Tesco*	1 Serving/48g	12.0	0.0	25	1.4	4.1	0.4	2.2
Salmon & Roquette, M & S*	1 Serving/255g	306.0	20.0	120	3.9	8.5	8.0	1.0
Salmon, Hot Smoked with Potato Salad, M & S*	1 Pack/338g	270.0	7.0	80	4.5	10.3	2.2	1.3
Santa Plum Tomato & Avocado, M & S*	1 Pack/240g	348.0	32.0	145	1.7	4.1	13.4	0.2
Santa Plum Tomato with Dressing, M & S*	1 Pack/225g	135.0	11.0	60	0.9	3.1	4.8	0.9
Seafood, Marinated, M & S*	1 Serving/90g	108.0	6.0	120	13.4	2.3	6.4	0.8
Selection, Fresh, M & S*	1 Pack/230g	32.0	1.0	14	0.7	2.1	0.3	0.9
Selection, Side, M & S*	1 Serving/255g	153.0	13.0	60	1.1	2.5	5.0	1.3
Side, Fresh & Crispy, Tesco*	1 Salad/230g	30.0	1.0	13	0.7	1.9	0.3	1.3
Side, Garden, with Cherry Tomatoes, Waitrose*	1 Pack/170g	25.0	1.0	15	0.8	2.0	0.4	1.3
Simply Chicken, Ginsters*	1 Pack/187g	317.0	7.0	170	11.4	22.7	3.7	0.0
Skipjack Tuna, John West*	1 Can/192g	190.0	12.0	99	7.3	3.7	6.1	0.0
Smoked Ham, Weight Watchers*	1 Pack/181g	233.0	4.0	129	11.0	16.6	2.0	3.0
Spicy Bean, Tesco*	1 Serving/125g	111.0	3.0	89	4.9	12.1	2.3	2.5
Spicy Chickpea, BGTY, Sainsbury's*	½ Pack/125g	119.0	2.0	95	4.7	15.3	1.7	5.5
Spicy Rice, Waitrose*	1 Serving/200g	318.0	13.0	159	3.2	21.7	6.6	0.9
Spinach, Waitrose*	1 Pack/100g	25.0	1.0	25	2.8	1.6	0.8	2.1
Sprouted Pea & Bean, Mint Dressing, Eat Well, M & S*	1 Pot/165g	181.0	9.0	110	7.3	8.7	5.3	7.4
Sugar Plum Tomato, Fresh, Safeway*	1 Serving/160g	46.0	2.0	29	1.1	3.2	1.3	1.2
Sweet & Crispy, Fresh, Safeway*	1 Serving/90g	19.0	0.0	21	0.9	3.7	0.3	1.5
Sweet & Crispy, M & S*	1 Serving/140g	49.0	1.0	35	1.7	4.7	1.0	1.6
Sweet & Crunchy, Sainsbury's*	1 Pack/150g	22.0	0.0	15	0.9	2.6	0.1	1.8

S

	Measure INFO/WEIGHT	per Measure KCAL	FAT	Nutrition Values per 100g / 100ml KCAL	PROT	CARB	FAT	FIBRE
SALAD								
Sweet, Layered, Tesco*	1 Serving/285g	80.0	1.0	28	1.1	5.0	0.4	1.6
Sweet, Shredded, Tesco*	1 Serving/100g	20.0	0.0	20	1.1	2.9	0.4	1.9
Tabbouleh & Feta, Tesco*	1 Pack/225g	301.0	11.0	134	5.4	16.7	5.0	0.6
Tabbouleh Feta, Finest, Tesco*	1 Pack/225g	265.0	12.0	118	4.2	13.7	5.2	0.6
Tabbouleh Style, Perfectly Balanced, Waitrose*	1 Pack/225g	234.0	9.0	104	2.8	14.3	3.9	2.6
Tabbouleh, HL, Tesco*	1 Serving/200g	194.0	4.0	97	3.5	16.8	1.8	1.3
Tenderleaf, with Mizuna, Sainsbury's*	1 Serving/50g	10.0	0.0	20	3.6	0.2	0.6	2.2
Thai Style Chicken, M & S*	1 Serving/195g	205.0	4.0	105	6.7	15.1	1.9	1.9
Three Bean & Pesto, Italian Style, Boots*	1 Serving/290g	374.0	12.0	129	8.3	14.0	4.3	1.8
Three Bean, Sainsbury's*	1 Serving/125g	108.0	6.0	86	4.2	6.0	5.0	0.0
Three Bean, Tinned, Tesco*	1 Tin/160g	176.0	2.0	110	7.7	17.6	1.0	5.3
Three Bean, with Mint Vinaigrette, M & S*	1 Pack/250g	175.0	6.0	70	5.9	6.4	2.4	13.0
Tomato & Mozzarella, M & S*	1 Pack/220g	264.0	16.0	120	9.8	2.8	7.5	1.1
Tomato & Onion	1oz/28g	20.0	2.0	72	0.8	4.0	6.1	1.0
Tomato, Avocado & Rocket, M & S*	1 Pack/350g	507.0	47.0	145	1.7	4.1	13.4	0.2
Tomato, Lettuce & Cucumber, Classics, M & S*	1 Serving/275g	151.0	12.0	55	0.9	3.3	4.2	1.6
Tuna & Three Bean, Healthily Balanced, M & S*	1 Serving/350g	332.0	10.0	95	8.7	8.8	2.9	4.6
Tuna & Tomato, Boots*	1 Pack/171g	150.0	10.0	88	6.5	2.0	6.0	1.0
Tuna Layered, Waitrose*	1 Bowl/300g	636.0	59.0	212	4.0	4.8	19.6	1.0
Tuna Nicoise, BGTY, Sainsbury's*	1 Pack/300g	315.0	6.0	105	6.3	15.5	2.0	2.5
Tuna Nicoise, No Mayonnaise, Shapers, Boots*	1 Pack/276g	133.0	4.0	48	4.0	5.0	1.3	0.8
Tuna, Breton Style, Snack Pot, Carb Check, Heinz*	1 Pot/219g	239.0	14.0	109	8.4	4.6	6.3	1.5
Tuna, Layered, Tesco*	1 Serving/370g	466.0	29.0	126	4.4	9.4	7.9	1.0
Tuna, with Lemon Dressing, Tesco*	1 Serving/300g	282.0	24.0	94	4.2	1.4	8.0	1.0
Tuscan Style Bean & Sunblush Tomato, Waitrose*	1 Pot/225g	308.0	11.0	137	5.6	17.9	4.8	1.0
Vegetable, Canned	1oz/28g	40.0	3.0	143	1.6	13.0	9.8	1.2
Vegetable, Heinz*	1 Can/195g	259.0	17.0	133	1.5	12.6	8.5	1.3
Waldorf, Average	1 Serving/100g	193.0	18.0	193	1.4	7.5	17.7	1.3
Watercress & Spinach, Asda*	1 Serving/50g	10.0	0.0	21	2.8	1.2	0.6	1.9
Watercress, Morrisons*	1 Bag/100g	17.0	1.0	17	1.7	1.2	0.7	0.0
Watercress, Mustard Leaf & Mizuna, M & S*	½ Pack/60g	9.0	0.0	15	2.4	0.4	0.3	3.0
Watercress, Spinach & Rocket, Waitrose*	1 Bag/145g	30.0	1.0	21	2.2	1.2	0.8	1.5
Wheat with Roasted Vegetables, Sainsbury's*	1 Pack/220g	339.0	18.0	154	3.3	17.0	8.3	4.5
Wild Rocket & Chard, Waitrose*	½ Bag/53.3g	8.0	0.0	15	0.8	1.7	0.5	1.4
Wild Rocket, Safeway*	1 Serving/75g	13.0	0.0	18	1.3	2.1	0.5	1.1
SALAD BOWL								
Chicken & Bacon, Layered, Tesco*	1 Serving/350g	437.0	23.0	125	5.3	10.2	6.7	1.8
Coleslaw, Budgens*	1 Pack/163g	220.0	18.0	135	1.5	7.1	11.2	1.4
Coleslaw, M & S*	1 Pack/325g	292.0	24.0	90	1.3	4.9	7.4	1.3
Coleslaw, Tesco*	1 Bowl/300g	327.0	30.0	109	1.0	3.4	10.1	1.3
Crispy, M & S*	1 Serving/250g	87.0	1.0	35	1.3	6.6	0.5	1.2
Egg Layered, Tesco*	1 Pack/410g	726.0	58.0	177	4.2	8.4	14.1	1.3
French Style, Sainsbury's*	1oz/28g	15.0	1.0	55	1.0	4.8	3.5	1.5
French Style, Way to Five, Sainsbury's*	1 Pack/264g	103.0	6.0	39	0.7	4.2	2.2	2.2
Goats Cheese, Sainsbury's*	1 Serving/100g	161.0	12.0	161	5.8	7.6	11.9	1.3
Greek Style, M & S*	1 Bowl/255g	242.0	21.0	95	2.5	2.4	8.2	0.7
Honey & Mustard Chicken, Fresh, Sainsbury's*	1 Serving/300g	408.0	24.0	136	5.9	10.3	7.9	1.7
Italian Avocado & Tomato, Sainsbury's*	1 Bowl/180g	97.0	5.0	54	1.0	6.7	2.6	1.3
Large, Sainsbury's*	1/6 Pack/52g	12.0	0.0	23	0.9	4.3	0.3	1.1
Mixed, Medley, Waitrose*	¼ Pack/60g	9.0	0.0	15	0.9	1.7	0.5	1.0
Mushrooms in Tomato Sauce, Sainsbury's*	1 Serving/100g	72.0	5.0	72	2.5	3.3	4.8	0.5
Pasta, Somerfield*	1 Pack/320g	541.0	26.0	169	3.3	20.8	8.1	1.5
Prawn, Sainsbury's*	1 Bowl/400g	632.0	47.0	158	3.7	9.4	11.7	1.2

S

	Measure INFO/WEIGHT	per Measure KCAL	FAT	Nutrition Values per 100g / 100ml KCAL	PROT	CARB	FAT	FIBRE
SALAD BOWL								
Red Cheddar & Edam, Way to Five, Sainsbury's*	½ Pack/224g	240.0	9.0	107	4.4	12.8	4.2	1.1
Tomato & Basil, M & S*	1 Serving/225g	225.0	23.0	100	0.8	3.7	10.1	1.1
Tomato, Sainsbury's*	½ Bowl/150g	93.0	7.0	62	0.9	4.4	4.5	1.6
Tomato, Way to Five, Sainsbury's*	1 Bowl/300g	174.0	12.0	58	0.8	4.5	4.1	2.8
Tuna, BGTY, Sainsbury's*	½ Pack/175g	180.0	3.0	103	7.0	15.4	1.5	1.7
Tuna, Fresh, Asda*	1 Serving/160g	184.0	11.0	115	8.0	5.0	7.0	0.0
Tuna, Sainsbury's*	1 Serving/200g	336.0	21.0	168	6.1	11.7	10.7	1.5
with Crunchy Coleslaw, M & S*	1 Pack/325g	455.0	45.0	140	1.0	2.5	13.8	2.0
SALAD CREAM								
Average	*1 Tsp/5g*	*17.0*	*1.0*	*335*	*1.7*	*18.6*	*27.8*	*0.1*
Reduced Calorie, Average	*1 Tsp/5g*	*6.0*	*0.0*	*130*	*1.0*	*12.9*	*7.9*	*0.1*
SALAD KIT								
Caesar, HL, Tesco*	½ Pack/133g	148.0	11.0	112	3.3	5.9	8.3	1.4
Caesar, New Improved, Tesco*	½ Pack/138g	279.0	25.0	202	4.7	4.5	18.3	1.3
Caesar, Tesco*	½ Pack/150g	237.0	20.0	158	3.2	6.7	13.2	0.7
Caesar, Waitrose*	1 Bag/250g	445.0	39.0	178	5.0	4.2	15.7	1.1
Ranch, HL, Tesco*	1 Serving/115g	69.0	3.0	60	4.4	5.0	2.5	1.8
SALAD SNACK								
Chargrilled Chicken, Tesco*	1 Pot/300g	384.0	14.0	128	6.1	15.0	4.8	2.4
Cheese & Tomato, Tesco*	1 Pot/300g	519.0	20.0	173	6.3	21.7	6.8	2.2
Cheese Layered, Sainsbury's*	1 Pack/190g	397.0	29.0	209	5.4	12.4	15.3	0.0
Chicken & Bacon, Tesco*	1 Pack/300g	501.0	31.0	167	7.2	10.9	10.5	3.2
Chicken Caesar, Sainsbury's*	1 Pack/182g	164.0	9.0	90	5.9	5.3	5.0	1.0
Chicken Caesar, Tesco*	1 Serving/300g	420.0	20.0	140	8.2	11.4	6.8	1.7
Chicken Noodle, Sainsbury's*	1 Snack/240g	278.0	12.0	116	5.2	12.4	5.1	1.4
Greek Style, BGTY, Sainsbury's*	1 Pack/199g	133.0	5.0	67	2.0	9.0	2.5	0.8
Ham & Mushroom, Tesco*	1 Pot/300g	600.0	32.0	200	4.7	21.2	10.7	1.4
Pasta & Tuna, BGTY, Sainsbury's*	1 Pack/260g	218.0	4.0	84	6.0	11.5	1.6	2.3
Pasta & Tuna, Healthy Selection, Somerfield*	1 Pot/190g	194.0	5.0	102	6.5	13.0	2.7	1.1
Pasta, Egg Mayo, Asda*	1 Serving/180g	364.0	27.0	202	4.0	12.8	15.0	0.3
Pasta, Tuna, Asda*	1 Serving/180g	196.0	7.0	109	5.5	13.2	3.8	0.9
Roast Chicken, Tesco*	1 Pack/300g	324.0	22.0	108	6.0	4.8	7.2	1.9
Salmon & Dill, Tesco*	1 Pack/300g	600.0	38.0	200	7.7	13.4	12.8	0.8
Sausage & Tomato, Tesco*	1 Serving/300g	529.0	27.0	176	4.5	19.1	9.1	4.0
Tuna & Pasta, BGTY, Sainsbury's*	1 Pack/260g	255.0	6.0	98	5.7	13.9	2.2	1.3
Tuna & Sweetcorn, Tesco*	1 Pack/300g	540.0	18.0	180	7.3	23.9	6.1	0.7
Tuna, HL, Tesco*	1 Serving/300g	237.0	3.0	79	7.2	10.1	1.1	1.7
SALAMI								
Ardennes Pepper, Waitrose*	1 Serving/7g	30.0	3.0	429	18.6	1.9	38.5	1.1
Average	*1 Slice/5g*	*18.0*	*1.0*	*360*	*28.4*	*1.8*	*26.1*	*0.0*
Danish, Average	*1 Serving/17g*	*89.0*	*9.0*	*524*	*13.2*	*1.3*	*51.7*	*0.0*
Emiliano, Sainsbury's*	1 Serving/70g	209.0	14.0	298	28.8	0.1	20.3	0.0
German, Average	*1 Serving/60g*	*200.0*	*16.0*	*333*	*20.3*	*1.6*	*27.3*	*0.1*
German, Peppered, Average	*3 Slices/25g*	*86.0*	*7.0*	*342*	*22.2*	*2.5*	*27.1*	*0.2*
Healthy Range, Average	*4 Slices/25g*	*55.0*	*4.0*	*220*	*22.3*	*0.6*	*14.3*	*0.0*
Milano, Average	*1 Serving/70g*	*278.0*	*23.0*	*397*	*25.9*	*0.9*	*32.2*	*0.0*
Napoli, Average	*1 Slice/5g*	*17.0*	*1.0*	*341*	*27.1*	*0.7*	*25.5*	*0.0*
Pepperoni, Italian, Morrisons*	1 Slice/5.7g	23.0	2.0	406	24.0	0.9	34.0	0.0
Spanish, Wafer Thin, Tesco*	1 Pack/80g	273.0	19.0	341	25.5	6.8	23.5	0.0
Ungherese, Tesco*	1 Serving/35g	136.0	11.0	388	24.5	0.5	32.0	0.0
SALMON								
Alaskan, Wild, TTD, Sainsbury's*	1 Fillet/115g	173.0	8.0	150	21.2	0.1	7.2	0.1
Fillet, Dinner, Light & Easy, Youngs*	1 Pack/375g	315.0	10.0	84	6.7	7.9	2.8	1.6

S

	Measure INFO/WEIGHT	per Measure KCAL	FAT	Nutrition Values per 100g / 100ml KCAL	PROT	CARB	FAT	FIBRE
SALMON								
Fillet, Skin On, TTD, Sainsbury's*	1 Fillet/126g	249.0	14.0	197	23.5	0.2	11.3	0.0
Fillets, Cajun, Waitrose*	1 Serving/150g	214.0	10.0	143	20.6	0.4	6.5	0.0
Fillets, Chargrilled, Sainsbury's*	1 Serving/270g	270.0	20.0	243	20.9	0.2	17.6	0.0
Fillets, Honey Roast, Co-Op*	1 Fillet/100g	250.0	14.0	250	26.7	4.7	13.8	0.1
Fillets, Lightly Smoked, TTD, Sainsbury's*	1 Serving/100g	201.0	13.0	201	20.2	0.3	13.2	0.6
Fillets, Raw, Average	*1 Fillet/79g*	*149.0*	*9.0*	*189*	*20.9*	*0.1*	*11.7*	*0.1*
Fillets, with Lemon & Herb Butter, Asda*	1 Fillet/125g	305.0	22.0	244	20.0	0.4	18.0	0.0
Fillets, with Orange & Dill Dressing, Tesco*	1 Serving/300g	540.0	31.0	180	17.7	4.1	10.3	0.7
Fillets, with Sicilian Citrus Glaze, Sainsbury's*	1 Fillet/145g	371.0	26.0	256	21.9	2.3	17.8	0.0
Flakes, Honey Roast, Average	*1oz/28g*	*56.0*	*3.0*	*198*	*24.0*	*1.9*	*10.7*	*0.2*
Goujons, Average	1 Pack/150g	321.0	16.0	214	16.4	12.4	10.9	1.1
Gravadlax, Finest, Tesco*	1 Serving/70g	125.0	7.0	178	22.1	0.2	9.9	0.0
Gravadlax, M & S*	1 Serving/140g	294.0	16.0	210	18.4	5.3	11.4	0.5
Gravadlax, with Mustard Sauce, Waitrose*	1 Serving/100g	191.0	11.0	191	21.8	1.0	11.1	0.4
Grilled	*1oz/28g*	*60.0*	*4.0*	*215*	*24.2*	*0.0*	*13.1*	*0.0*
Hot Smoked, Average	*1 Serving/62g*	*103.0*	*4.0*	*166*	*24.0*	*0.9*	*7.2*	*0.1*
Lemon & Rosemary, Easy Steam, BGTY, Sainsbury's*	1 Pack/350g	329.0	13.0	94	6.4	9.0	3.6	1.3
Lime & Coriander, Tesco*	1 Serving/120g	176.0	4.0	147	21.4	7.0	3.7	0.7
Mild Oak Smoked, Average	*1 Slice/25g*	*45.0*	*3.0*	*182*	*22.6*	*0.1*	*10.2*	*0.0*
Moroccan Style, Light Lunch, John West*	1 Pack/240g	199.0	1.0	83	5.5	14.0	0.6	3.1
Mousse, Tesco*	1 Mousse/57g	100.0	7.0	177	13.5	2.9	12.4	0.2
Pink, Average	*1 Serving/125g*	*162.0*	*7.0*	*130*	*19.5*	*0.1*	*5.8*	*0.1*
Pink, in Brine, Average	*1oz/28g*	*43.0*	*2.0*	*153*	*23.5*	*0.0*	*6.6*	*0.0*
Poached, Average	*1 Serving/90g*	*176.0*	*10.0*	*195*	*22.5*	*0.2*	*11.7*	*0.3*
Potted, M & S*	1 Serving/75g	184.0	15.0	245	17.1	0.5	19.4	1.2
Red, Average	*½ Can/90g*	*141.0*	*7.0*	*156*	*20.4*	*0.1*	*8.2*	*0.1*
Red, in Brine, Average	*1oz/28g*	*47.0*	*2.0*	*169*	*22.4*	*0.0*	*8.9*	*0.0*
Rillettes, John West*	½ Can/62g	169.0	15.0	272	14.9	0.1	23.5	0.0
Scottish Lochmuir Sashimi Smoked, M & S*	1 Pack/130g	214.0	11.0	165	18.6	3.3	8.5	0.5
Smoked, Appetisers, Tesco*	1/3 Pack/33g	80.0	6.0	240	16.3	1.1	18.5	0.0
Smoked, Average	*1 Serving/70g*	*126.0*	*7.0*	*179*	*21.9*	*0.5*	*10.0*	*0.1*
Smoked, Trimmings, Average	*1 Serving/55g*	*101.0*	*6.0*	*184*	*22.8*	*0.2*	*10.3*	*0.0*
Steaks	*1 Serving/100g*	*180.0*	*11.0*	*180*	*20.2*	*0.0*	*11.0*	*0.0*
Steamed	*1oz/28g*	*55.0*	*4.0*	*197*	*20.1*	*0.0*	*13.0*	*0.0*
Whole, Raw, Average	1 Serving/100g	228.0	14.0	228	25.6	0.0	13.9	0.0
SALMON EN CROUTE								
Retail, Average	1oz/28g	81.0	5.0	288	11.8	18.0	19.1	0.0
SALMON IN								
a Creamy Horseradish Sauce, Fillets, Wonnemeyer*	1 Serving/300g	459.0	31.0	153	9.4	5.3	10.5	0.0
Creamy Watercress Sauce, Fillets, Scottish, Seafresh*	1 Pack 300g	528.0	39.0	176	13.7	1.2	12.9	0.1
Dill Sauce, Youngs*	1 Pack/435g	265.0	10.0	61	6.1	4.2	2.3	0.1
Lemon Mayonnaise, From Heinz, Weight Watchers*	1 Can/80g	130.0	8.0	163	10.2	6.4	10.6	0.1
Pancetta, Wrapped, Finest, Tesco*	1 Serving/150g	328.0	26.0	219	14.9	1.0	17.2	0.1
Tomato & Mascarpone Sauce, Fillets, Asda*	½ Pack/181.0g	279.0	20.0	154	13.0	0.8	11.0	0.6
Watercress Sauce, Pink, Wild Alaskan, Sainsbury's*	½ Pack/180g	194.0	10.0	108	13.9	0.9	5.4	0.8
Watercress Sauce, Waitrose*	½ Pack/150g	264.0	19.0	176	13.7	1.2	12.9	0.1
White Wine & Cream Sauce, Tesco*	1 Serving/170g	279.0	19.0	164	13.5	2.0	11.3	1.2
White Wine & Parsley Dressing, Fillets, Tesco*	1 Fillet/150g	291.0	20.0	194	17.5	0.3	13.6	0.6
SALMON WITH								
a Cream Sauce, Scottish Fillets, M & S*	1 Serving/200g	360.0	26.0	180	13.8	1.0	13.0	0.1
Asparagus & Rice, Fillets, Perfectly Balanced, Waitrose*	1 Serving/400g	348.0	4.0	87	8.2	11.4	1.0	0.9
Coriander & Lime, Pacific, Asda*	1 Serving/113g	154.0	3.0	137	27.0	0.5	3.0	0.0
Garlic & Herb Butter, Tesco*	1 Fillet/112g	291.0	23.0	260	17.6	0.0	20.6	0.0

	Measure INFO/WEIGHT	per Measure KCAL	per Measure FAT	Nutrition Values per 100g / 100ml KCAL	PROT	CARB	FAT	FIBRE
SALMON WITH								
Mozzarella & Tomato Crust, Just Cook, Sainsbury's*	½ Pack/171g	220.0	9.0	129	15.0	5.2	5.4	0.4
Pasta, Frozen, Youngs*	½ Bag/175g	234.0	8.0	134	7.4	16.3	4.4	1.2
Penne Pasta & Dill Sauce, SteamFresh, Birds Eye*	1 Pack/424g	335.0	6.0	79	6.4	9.9	1.5	1.1
Potatoes, Honey Roast, Light Choices, Tesco*	1 Pack/350g	332.0	12.0	95	6.6	8.5	3.5	2.4
Prawns, & Fusilli Pasta, Frozen, Youngs*	1 Pack/375g	439.0	28.0	117	5.6	7.0	7.4	1.1
Rice, Oriental Style, M & S*	1 Pot/210g	252.0	7.0	120	5.9	16.5	3.3	3.3
Sweet Chilli Lime & Ginger, Simply Fish, Tesco*	½ Pack/98g	235.0	17.0	240	17.4	3.2	17.5	0.0
Sweet Chilli, Fillets, Roasted, Tesco*	1 Fillet/100g	210.0	11.0	210	26.1	1.7	10.6	0.6
Sweet Chilli, Hot Smoked, Scottish, Tesco*	1 Fillet/120g	252.0	13.0	210	26.1	1.7	10.6	0.6
Sweet Soy Sauce, Fillets, Inspired To Cook, Sainsbury's*	1 Fillet/142g	278.0	16.0	196	17.5	5.3	11.6	0.4
SALSA								
Bottled, M & S*	½ Jar/136g	95.0	3.0	70	1.2	12.0	2.4	1.5
Chunky, Sainsbury's*	½ Pot/84g	43.0	1.0	51	1.1	7.8	1.7	1.2
Cool, Sainsbury's*	1 Serving/100g	31.0	0.0	31	1.0	6.1	0.3	1.2
GFY, Asda*	½ Pot/236g	85.0	1.0	36	1.1	7.0	0.4	0.7
Hot, Fresh, Chilled, Tesco*	1 Tub/200g	120.0	5.0	60	1.4	7.5	2.4	1.2
Medium Hot, Discovery*	1 Serving/30g	17.0	0.0	56	1.4	11.7	0.4	0.8
Mild, Heinz*	1 Serving/20g	16.0	0.0	79	1.2	17.9	0.1	0.8
Mild, Original, Old El Paso*	1 Sachet/144g	60.0	1.0	42	1.6	9.0	0.5	0.0
Original, From Dinner Kit, Old El Paso*	1 Jar/226g	71.0	1.0	32	1.2	6.0	0.3	0.0
Prawn & Tomato, Fresh, Anti Pasti, Asda*	1 Pot/150g	100.0	4.0	67	8.0	3.1	2.5	1.3
Red Onion & Tomato, Tapas Selection, Sainsbury's*	1 Serving/22g	17.0	1.0	77	3.0	6.0	4.5	0.9
Red Pepper, Sainsbury's*	1 Serving/85g	31.0	1.0	37	1.7	3.8	1.7	1.5
Smokey BBQ, Weight Watchers*	1 Serving/56g	20.0	0.0	36	1.1	7.6	0.1	2.3
Spiced Mango, Ginger & Chilli, Weight Watchers*	½ Pot/50g	42.0	0.0	85	1.0	19.9	0.2	2.6
Spicy Mango & Lime, Morrisons*	½ Pot/85g	62.0	0.0	73	1.0	15.9	0.4	1.3
Spicy Red Pepper, Fresh, Waitrose*	½ Pot/85g	27.0	1.0	32	1.9	4.1	0.9	1.6
Spicy Red Pepper, Sainsbury's*	1 Pot/170g	54.0	2.0	32	1.4	3.2	1.4	1.3
Spicy, Less Than 3% Fat, M & S*	½ Pot/85g	30.0	1.0	35	1.3	5.6	0.8	0.8
Sweetcorn, Fresh, Sainsbury's*	¼ Pot/51g	32.0	1.0	63	1.1	10.5	1.8	1.3
Tomato & Avocado, Chunky, COU, M & S*	½ Pack/86g	30.0	1.0	35	0.8	5.4	1.4	1.4
Tomato, Chunky, Tesco*	1 Pot/170g	68.0	2.0	40	1.1	5.9	1.3	1.1
Tomato, Chunky, Tex Mex, Tesco*	1 Serving/50g	26.0	1.0	52	1.0	6.4	2.5	1.0
Tomato, Onion, Coriander & Chilli, Fresh, Waitrose*	1 Tub/170g	110.0	5.0	65	1.3	8.0	3.1	1.2
Tomato, Reduced Fat, Waitrose*	1 Serving/1g	0.0	0.0	27	1.5	4.7	0.2	1.4
Tomato, Spicy, Worldwide Sauces*	1 Serving/25g	7.0	0.0	30	1.2	5.9	0.2	1.2
Tomato, Sun Ripened, Tesco*	1 Serving/40g	46.0	2.0	115	5.0	14.2	4.2	4.6
Vine Ripened Tomato & Jalapeno, Sainsbury's*	¼ Tub/50g	34.0	2.0	68	1.1	8.0	3.5	1.2
SALT								
Alternative, Reduced Sodium, Losalt*	1 Serving/10g	0.0	0.0	0	0.0	0.0	0.0	0.0
Table, Average	*1 Tsp/5g*	*0.0*	*0.0*	*0*	*0.0*	*0.0*	*0.0*	*0.0*
SAMBUCA								
Average	*1 Shot/35ml*	*122.0*	*0.0*	*348*	*0.0*	*37.2*	*0.0*	*0.0*
SAMOSAS								
Chicken Tikka, Sainsbury's*	1 Samosa/50g	119.0	6.0	239	8.3	22.5	12.9	3.1
Chicken, Mumtaz*	1 Serving/105g	177.0	8.0	169	19.6	4.9	7.9	0.0
Dim Sum Selection, Sainsbury's*	1 Samosa/12g	24.0	1.0	196	3.4	28.6	7.6	2.8
Indian Style Selection, Co-Op*	1 Samosa/21g	50.0	3.0	240	5.0	27.0	13.0	3.0
Lamb, Waitrose*	1oz/28g	87.0	6.0	310	8.5	18.1	22.6	0.8
Vegetable Lightly Spiced, Sainsbury's*	1 Samosa/50g	112.0	6.0	223	4.0	23.5	12.5	1.2
Vegetable, Mini, Indian, Party Selection, Tesco*	1 Samosa/30g	58.0	1.0	195	3.6	33.9	5.0	2.2
Vegetable, Mini, Waitrose*	1 Samosa/29g	70.0	4.0	242	3.6	27.1	13.2	3.1
Vegetable, Retail, Average	1 Samosa/110g	239.0	10.0	217	5.1	30.0	9.3	2.5

S

	Measure INFO/WEIGHT	per Measure KCAL	per Measure FAT	Nutrition Values per 100g / 100ml KCAL	PROT	CARB	FAT	FIBRE
SAMPHIRE								
Raw, Fresh	1 Serving/80g	24.0	0.0	30	12.0	0.0	0.0	3.0
SANDWICH								
All Day Breakfast, BGTY, Sainsbury's*	1 Pack/188g	294.0	5.0	156	9.6	22.7	2.4	0.0
All Day Breakfast, Finest, Tesco*	1 Pack/275g	660.0	42.0	240	9.7	16.4	15.1	1.6
All Day Breakfast, Ginsters*	1 Pack/241g	538.0	27.0	223	10.8	20.3	11.0	0.0
All Day Breakfast, HL, Tesco*	1 Pack/223g	328.0	8.0	147	11.9	16.8	3.6	2.7
All Day Breakfast, Shapers, Boots*	1 Pack/207g	323.0	5.0	156	11.0	23.0	2.5	2.2
All Day Breakfast, Weight Watchers*	1 Pack/158g	298.0	4.0	189	11.0	30.2	2.7	1.9
Avocado, & Spinach, M & S*	1 Pack/242g	580.0	27.0	240	4.0	21.0	11.3	4.8
Avocado, Mozzarella & Tomato, M & S*	1 Pack/273g	655.0	36.0	240	8.8	21.7	13.2	2.3
Bacon, & Brie, Asda*	1 Pack/181g	603.0	38.0	333	13.3	22.9	21.1	1.3
Bacon, & Brie, Finest, Tesco*	1 Pack/201g	571.0	34.0	284	14.1	19.4	16.7	2.1
Bacon, & Egg, Boots*	1 Pack/179g	480.0	29.0	268	12.0	19.0	16.0	1.4
Bacon, & Egg, Deep Fill, Ginsters*	1 Pack/210g	590.0	38.0	281	11.5	18.8	18.2	0.0
Bacon, & Egg, Free Range, Daily Bread*	1 Serving/175g	425.0	23.0	243	10.1	21.5	13.1	0.0
Bacon, & Egg, Ginsters*	1 Pack/210g	523.0	24.0	249	13.2	22.0	11.6	0.0
Bacon, & Egg, HL, Tesco*	1 Serving/178g	328.0	9.0	184	11.5	22.7	5.2	1.7
Bacon, & Egg, Sainsbury's*	1 Pack/215g	535.0	26.0	249	12.3	23.2	11.9	0.0
Bacon, & Egg, Scottish Slimmers, Tesco*	1 Pack/139g	279.0	6.0	201	13.6	26.3	4.6	1.2
Bacon, & Egg, Shell*	1 Pack/191g	579.0	38.0	303	12.2	18.7	19.9	0.0
Bacon, & Tomato, COU, M & S*	1 Pack/169g	270.0	5.0	160	9.5	25.6	2.7	2.5
Bacon, Brie, & Mango Chutney, Daily Bread*	1 Serving/213g	555.0	23.0	261	12.7	28.6	10.7	0.0
Bacon, Cheese & Chicken, Triple, BGTY, Sainsbury's*	1 Serving/266g	506.0	17.0	190	12.7	20.7	6.3	2.6
Bacon, Lettuce & Tomato, Shapers, Boots*	1 Pack/175.2g	272.0	8.0	155	11.0	18.0	4.3	5.9
Bacon, Lettuce & Tomato, Weight Watchers*	1 Pack/153g	237.0	2.0	155	9.4	25.8	1.6	2.4
Bap, Chicken, & Sweetcorn, Sainsbury's*	1 Serving/170g	462.0	24.0	272	12.5	24.2	13.9	0.0
Beef, & Horseradish Mayonnaise, Roast, Rare, Waitrose*	1 Pack/197g	415.0	15.0	211	12.2	23.1	7.8	2.0
Beef, & Horseradish Mayonnaise, Shapers, Boots*	1 Pack/159g	266.0	3.0	167	12.0	25.0	2.1	2.6
Beef, & Horseradish, Deep Filled, BGTY, Sainsbury's*	1 Pack/202g	313.0	5.0	155	11.4	22.0	2.4	2.4
Beef, & Horseradish, Sainsbury's*	1 Pack/187g	389.0	13.0	208	12.0	24.1	7.1	0.0
Beef, & Horseradish, Shapers, Boots*	1 Pack/156g	276.0	3.0	177	12.0	28.0	1.7	1.8
Beef, & Onion, Roast, Deep Filled, Asda*	1 Pack/258g	550.0	28.0	213	11.3	22.6	10.8	1.1
Beef, & Onion, Roast, HL, Tesco*	1 Pack/185g	278.0	4.0	150	13.3	20.0	1.9	2.7
Beef, & Pate, M & S*	1 Pack/188g	310.0	7.0	165	11.2	21.6	3.9	2.4
Beef, Roast, Feel Good, Shell*	1 Pack/153g	390.0	15.0	255	17.6	24.2	9.7	0.0
Beef, Roast, Handmade, Tesco*	1 Pack/223g	439.0	16.0	197	12.5	20.7	7.1	1.6
Beef, Roast, Sainsbury's*	1 Pack/174g	426.0	17.0	245	9.4	29.3	10.0	0.0
Beef, Salt, with Gherkins, & Mustard Mayo, Sainsbury's*	1 Pack/242g	486.0	18.0	201	9.3	24.1	7.5	3.1
Beef, Tomato & Horseradish, Asda*	1 Pack/169g	255.0	4.0	151	10.0	22.0	2.6	2.7
BLT, BGTY, Sainsbury's*	1 Pack/196g	331.0	4.0	169	10.4	27.0	2.2	0.0
BLT, Classic, Somerfield*	1 Pack/160g	338.0	6.0	211	11.2	33.6	3.5	3.9
BLT, COU, M & S*	1 Pack/174g	278.0	5.0	160	9.5	25.6	2.7	2.5
BLT, Deep Fill, Tesco*	1 Pack/231g	635.0	38.0	275	11.8	19.8	16.5	1.2
BLT, Ginsters*	1 Pack/192g	516.0	30.0	269	15.6	21.2	15.6	0.0
BLT, M & S*	1 Serving/181g	381.0	15.0	210	10.7	23.8	8.1	1.8
BLT, Max, Shell*	1 Pack/249g	665.0	35.0	267	10.8	24.1	14.1	0.0
BLT, Shapers, Boots*	1 Pack/169g	254.0	6.0	150	10.7	18.9	3.7	5.9
BLT, Tesco*	1 Pack/203g	520.0	29.0	256	11.9	19.5	14.4	1.5
BLT, Waitrose*	1 Pack/184g	398.0	16.0	216	9.5	24.5	8.9	2.3
BLT, With Mayo, Seeded Malted Bread, Deep Fill, Heinz*	1 Pack/182g	444.0	20.0	244	10.3	26.2	10.9	3.0
Brie, & Grape, Finest, Tesco*	1 Pack/209g	527.0	32.0	252	8.5	20.6	15.1	1.5
Brie, with Apple & Grapes, Sainsbury's*	1 Pack/220g	473.0	24.0	215	8.2	20.8	11.0	0.0
British Chicken & Sweetcorn, Eat Well, M & S*	1 Pack/194g	340.0	10.0	175	11.4	19.6	5.4	3.1

S

SANDWICH

Chargrilled Vegetable & Houmous, HL, Tesco*	1 Pack/167g	250.0	4.0	150	5.9	25.3	2.4	2.0
Cheddar, & Celery, M & S*	1 Pack/200g	540.0	32.0	270	9.7	22.4	15.9	1.5
Cheddar, & Coleslaw, Simply, Boots*	1 Pack/185g	538.0	33.0	291	9.2	23.0	18.0	1.8
Cheddar, & Ham, British, M & S*	1 Serving/165g	395.0	19.0	240	15.1	20.0	11.3	1.7
Cheddar, & Ham, M & S*	1 Pack/165g	396.0	19.0	240	15.1	20.0	11.3	1.7
Cheddar, & Ham, Smoked, Deep Filled, Tesco*	1 Serving/203g	573.0	33.0	282	14.3	19.5	16.3	1.2
Cheddar, & Ham, with Pickle, Smoked, Finest, Tesco*	1 Pack/217g	532.0	25.0	245	11.9	23.7	11.4	3.9
Cheddar, & Pickle, Mature, Sainsbury's*	1 Pack/171g	588.0	27.0	344	14.3	38.7	15.8	7.0
Cheddar, & Tomato, Mature, Big, Sainsbury's*	1 Pack/233g	596.0	26.0	256	12.9	26.3	11.0	0.0
Cheddar, & Tomato, Red, Tesco*	1 Pack/182g	526.0	32.0	289	9.2	24.0	17.4	1.1
Cheddar, Red Leicester, & Onion, Tesco*	1 Pack/182g	604.0	39.0	332	11.0	23.8	21.4	2.5
Cheese, & Apple & Grape, COU, M & S*	1 Pack/186g	270.0	2.0	145	8.5	24.9	1.2	2.0
Cheese, & Apple, & Celery, Asda*	1 Pack/173g	244.0	5.0	141	8.0	21.0	2.8	2.7
Cheese, & Celery, Shapers, Boots*	1 Pack/181g	288.0	4.0	159	11.0	24.0	2.3	3.0
Cheese, & Coleslaw, Asda*	1 Pack/262g	799.0	51.0	305	10.1	22.1	19.6	3.3
Cheese, & Coleslaw, M & S*	1 Pack/186g	498.0	32.0	268	10.2	17.6	17.4	3.2
Cheese, & Ham, & Pickle, HL, Tesco*	1 Pack/201g	312.0	4.0	155	13.1	21.0	2.1	1.7
Cheese, & Ham, & Pickle, Shapers, Boots*	1 Pack/184g	318.0	8.0	173	13.0	20.0	4.6	2.5
Cheese, & Ham, & Pickle, Tesco*	1 Serving/215g	497.0	25.0	231	11.7	20.3	11.5	1.8
Cheese, & Onion, Deep Fill, Tesco*	1 Pack/212g	742.0	52.0	350	12.3	20.2	24.5	1.3
Cheese, & Onion, HL, Tesco*	1 Pack/168g	314.0	10.0	187	10.3	23.2	5.9	1.7
Cheese, & Onion, M & S*	1 Serving/188g	460.0	24.0	245	11.2	21.3	12.9	2.9
Cheese, & Onion, Tesco*	1 Pack/178g	573.0	38.0	322	11.6	21.0	21.3	3.5
Cheese, & Onion, Waitrose*	1 Pack/176g	579.0	39.0	329	12.5	20.2	22.0	2.8
Cheese, & Pickle, Heinz*	1 Pack/178g	543.0	27.0	305	13.8	28.4	15.1	3.8
Cheese, & Pickle, Shapers, Boots*	1 Pack/165g	342.0	8.0	207	9.8	31.0	4.9	2.3
Cheese, & Pickle, Tesco*	1 Pack/140g	400.0	19.0	286	12.7	27.8	13.8	1.4
Cheese, & Pickle, Virgin Trains*	1 Pack/158g	444.0	20.0	281	11.5	31.1	12.4	0.0
Cheese, & Salad, COU, M & S*	1 Pack/188g	244.0	3.0	130	12.1	17.0	1.6	2.4
Cheese, & Salad, Shapers, Boots*	1 Pack/205g	307.0	5.0	150	9.7	22.0	2.5	2.2
Cheese, & Salad, Tesco*	1 Serving/188g	429.0	22.0	228	10.1	20.2	11.9	2.1
Cheese, & Spring Onion, Asda*	1 Pack/160g	576.0	40.0	361	13.0	21.0	25.0	1.9
Cheese, & Spring Onion, Sainsbury's*	1 Serving/177g	605.0	39.0	342	11.4	24.0	22.3	1.1
Cheese, & Tomato, Asda*	1 Pack/154g	388.0	20.0	252	11.0	23.2	12.8	3.7
Cheese, & Tomato, Organic, M & S*	1 Pack/165g	559.0	35.0	339	11.8	24.8	21.4	1.9
Cheese, & Tomato, Sainsbury's*	1 Pack/216g	542.0	26.0	251	12.9	22.8	12.2	0.0
Cheese, & Tomato, Tesco*	1 Pack/182g	582.0	39.0	320	9.2	22.6	21.4	1.1
Cheese, Asda*	1 Pack/262g	618.0	31.0	236	12.2	20.3	12.0	3.0
Cheese, Three, & Onion, Boots*	1 Pack/169g	566.0	34.0	335	11.0	28.0	20.0	1.9
Cheese, Three, & Spring Onion, Shell*	1 Pack/168g	672.0	51.0	400	11.1	20.8	30.3	0.0
Chicken Salad, HL, Tesco*	1 Serving/190g	247.0	3.0	130	12.3	15.8	1.8	4.5
Chicken Salad, Light Choices, Tesco*	1 Pack/207g	290.0	4.0	140	13.9	16.8	1.9	2.7
Chicken, & Avocado, Tesco*	1 Serving/219g	559.0	32.0	255	11.9	19.5	14.4	2.4
Chicken, & Bacon & Tomato, Paprika, Shapers, Boots*	1 Pack/184g	296.0	8.0	161	11.0	19.0	4.6	2.3
Chicken, & Bacon, & Salad, Big, Sainsbury's*	1 Pack/249g	610.0	32.0	245	11.1	21.7	12.7	0.0
Chicken, & Bacon, Baton, Tesco*	1 Pack/201g	511.0	26.0	254	9.4	24.7	13.1	1.7
Chicken, & Bacon, BGTY, Sainsbury's*	1 Pack/211g	315.0	5.0	149	11.7	20.8	2.3	0.0
Chicken, & Bacon, COU, M & S*	1 Pack/178.6g	250.0	4.0	140	13.5	15.8	2.0	3.8
Chicken, & Bacon, Deep Filled, Ginsters*	1 Pack/200g	540.0	32.0	270	13.1	18.3	16.1	0.0
Chicken, & Bacon, HL, Tesco*	1 Pack/193g	318.0	6.0	165	13.5	19.5	3.2	2.7
Chicken, & Bacon, M & S*	1 Pack/185g	509.0	27.0	275	15.9	20.2	14.7	2.1
Chicken, & Bacon, on Pepper Bread, M & S*	1 Serving/177g	265.0	2.0	150	13.2	22.7	0.9	2.1
Chicken, & Bacon, Roast, Boots*	1 Pack/175g	413.0	14.0	236	15.4	26.3	8.0	2.2

	Measure INFO/WEIGHT	per Measure KCAL	FAT	Nutrition Values per 100g / 100ml KCAL	PROT	CARB	FAT	FIBRE

SANDWICH

	Measure INFO/WEIGHT	KCAL	FAT	KCAL	PROT	CARB	FAT	FIBRE
Chicken, & Bacon, Tesco*	1 Pack/195g	486.0	24.0	249	14.3	20.0	12.4	2.7
Chicken, & Bacon, Waitrose*	1 Serving/191g	495.0	24.0	259	11.8	25.3	12.3	2.2
Chicken, & Balsamic Roasted Tomatoes, COU, M & S*	1 Pack/200g	280.0	5.0	140	11.6	18.1	2.3	2.6
Chicken, & Coleslaw, Tesco*	1 Pack/160g	305.0	7.0	191	12.0	25.7	4.4	2.4
Chicken, & Coriander, with Lime, BGTY, Sainsbury's*	1 Pack/168g	282.0	6.0	168	10.6	23.5	3.5	0.0
Chicken, & Ham, Roast, Tesco*	1 Pack/228g	561.0	32.0	246	13.3	16.6	14.0	1.2
Chicken, & Mayonnaise, Country Harvest*	1 Pack/120g	268.0	9.0	223	13.1	27.6	7.5	0.0
Chicken, & Pepperonata, COU, M & S*	1 Pack/171g	240.0	3.0	140	10.4	20.9	1.7	1.3
Chicken, & Pesto Salad, Bells*	1 Pack/196g	430.0	23.0	220	12.0	16.6	11.7	0.0
Chicken, & Pesto, Shapers, Boots*	1 Pack/181g	311.0	4.0	172	12.0	26.0	2.3	1.7
Chicken, & Roasted Peppers, Chargrilled, BHS*	1 Pack/183g	295.0	6.0	161	11.5	22.0	3.1	3.1
Chicken, & Salad with Mayo, Roast, Big, Sainsbury's*	1 Pack/269g	559.0	24.0	208	11.0	20.9	8.9	9.0
Chicken, & Salad, COU, M & S*	1 Pack/194g	262.0	4.0	135	9.8	19.0	1.9	1.6
Chicken, & Salad, Deep Filled, Asda*	1 Pack/247g	551.0	18.0	223	18.1	22.2	7.4	1.3
Chicken, & Salad, Deep Filled, Tesco*	1 Pack/238g	440.0	19.0	185	13.1	14.6	8.2	2.8
Chicken, & Salad, GFY, Asda*	1 Pack/194g	252.0	3.0	130	12.0	17.0	1.5	2.6
Chicken, & Salad, Heinz*	1 Pack/166g	331.0	16.0	200	8.6	19.9	9.6	2.0
Chicken, & Salad, HL, Tesco*	1 Pack/207g	290.0	4.0	140	13.9	16.8	1.9	2.7
Chicken, & Salad, Low Fat, Heinz*	1 Pack/166g	246.0	2.0	148	11.8	22.3	1.3	5.3
Chicken, & Salad, Low Fat, Waitrose*	1 Pack/188g	291.0	8.0	155	10.4	18.6	4.3	2.1
Chicken, & Salad, Roast, COU, M & S*	1 Pack/196g	265.0	5.0	135	8.9	19.6	2.3	2.2
Chicken, & Salad, Roast, Feel Good, Shell*	1 Pack/191g	326.0	9.0	171	9.8	22.4	4.7	0.0
Chicken, & Salad, Roast, Waitrose*	1 Pack/217g	482.0	24.0	222	9.4	21.1	11.1	2.0
Chicken, & Salad, Roast, Weight Watchers*	1 Pack/186g	266.0	8.0	143	10.3	15.8	4.3	2.8
Chicken, & Salad, Sainsbury's*	1 Pack/240g	425.0	14.0	177	12.1	18.8	5.9	0.0
Chicken, & Salad, Shell*	1 Pack/201g	404.0	20.0	201	8.7	19.4	9.8	0.0
Chicken, & Salad, Tesco*	1 Pack/193g	386.0	18.0	200	11.9	17.6	9.1	1.5
Chicken, & Salad, Waitrose*	1 Pack/208g	406.0	20.0	195	10.3	17.1	9.5	2.5
Chicken, & Stuffing, Light Choices, Tesco*	1 Pack/172g	275.0	5.0	160	14.4	18.7	2.8	6.9
Chicken, & Stuffing, M & S*	1 Pack/166g	398.0	17.0	240	13.9	23.1	10.3	5.6
Chicken, & Stuffing, Roast, Weight Watchers*	1 Pack/159g	283.0	4.0	178	14.1	24.2	2.8	3.1
Chicken, & Stuffing, Waitrose*	1 Pack/183g	450.0	19.0	246	12.8	25.6	10.3	1.5
Chicken, & Sweet Chilli, Flora Light, Flora*	1 Pack/154g	296.0	6.0	192	13.1	27.0	3.7	1.9
Chicken, & Sweetcorn, Scottish Slimmers*	1 Pack/147g	289.0	7.0	197	11.1	27.4	4.9	2.2
Chicken, & Sweetcorn, Shapers, Boots*	1 Pack/180g	324.0	6.0	180	12.0	25.0	3.5	2.0
Chicken, & Tomato Relish, Chargrilled, Shapers, Boots*	1 Pack/190g	294.0	6.0	155	12.0	20.0	3.0	3.1
Chicken, & Watercress, Chargrilled, M & S*	1 Pack/173g	285.0	3.0	165	12.8	23.9	1.7	2.1
Chicken, & Watercress, COU, M & S*	1 Pack/164g	266.0	3.0	162	12.8	23.9	1.7	2.1
Chicken, Bacon & Sweet Chilli, Feel Good, Shell*	1 Pack/174g	366.0	9.0	211	14.1	29.2	5.0	0.0
Chicken, Bacon & Tomato, BGTY, Sainsbury's*	1 Pack/190g	270.0	4.0	142	11.4	19.0	2.3	0.0
Chicken, Bacon, & Avocado, M & S*	1 Pack/242g	508.0	28.0	210	10.7	15.8	11.7	3.2
Chicken, Bacon, & Cheese, Club, M & S*	1 Pack/383g	805.0	37.0	210	11.9	18.5	9.7	1.9
Chicken, Basil & Sunblush Tomato, Harry Mason*	1 Pack/164g	272.0	5.0	166	13.0	21.8	3.2	0.6
Chicken, Breast, BGTY, Sainsbury's*	1 Pack/165g	251.0	1.0	152	12.2	24.7	0.5	0.0
Chicken, Caesar, & Salad, GFY, Asda*	1 Pack/163g	289.0	5.0	177	11.0	27.0	2.8	2.1
Chicken, Caesar, & Salad, Sainsbury's*	1 Pack/186g	299.0	7.0	161	11.2	20.4	3.8	0.0
Chicken, Caesar, Boots*	1 Pack/226g	531.0	27.0	235	9.8	22.0	12.0	1.7
Chicken, Caesar, Chargrilled, Big, Sainsbury's*	1 Pack/216g	657.0	37.0	304	12.2	25.3	17.1	0.0
Chicken, Caesar, COU, M & S*	1 Pack/181g	244.0	4.0	135	12.2	19.9	2.4	4.3
Chicken, Chargrilled, Ginsters*	1 Pack/209g	431.0	17.0	206	11.3	21.6	8.3	0.0
Chicken, Chargrilled, Pitta Pocket, M & S*	1 Pack/208g	279.0	7.0	134	11.2	14.5	3.5	1.6
Chicken, Chargrilled, with Salad, Weight Watchers*	1 Pack/181g	264.0	4.0	146	11.7	20.0	2.1	2.2
Chicken, Cheese, Bacon, Big, Sainsbury's*	1 Pack/254g	734.0	45.0	289	11.7	18.0	17.9	0.0

SANDWICH

	Measure INFO/WEIGHT	per Measure KCAL	FAT	KCAL	PROT	CARB	FAT	FIBRE
Chicken, Chinese, Low Calorie, Tesco*	1 Pack/169g	270.0	4.0	160	11.8	22.6	2.5	2.0
Chicken, Chinese, Malted Brown Bread, Waitrose*	1 Pack/164g	333.0	11.0	203	13.5	21.9	6.8	3.3
Chicken, Chinese, Snack & Shop, Esso*	1 Pack/178g	409.0	16.0	230	13.0	22.8	9.0	4.0
Chicken, Coronation, M & S*	1 Pack/210g	420.0	20.0	200	11.2	20.2	9.7	3.1
Chicken, Flame Grilled, Rustlers*	1 Pack/150g	346.0	14.0	231	16.3	20.1	9.5	0.0
Chicken, Healthier Choice, Ginsters*	1 Pack/183g	247.0	3.0	135	10.2	20.5	1.4	0.0
Chicken, Honey & Mustard, BGTY, Sainsbury's*	1 Pack/171g	296.0	5.0	173	13.1	24.0	2.7	0.0
Chicken, Lemon, & Relish, Perfectly Balanced, Waitrose*	1 Pack/151g	243.0	4.0	161	12.3	21.4	2.9	3.5
Chicken, Lime & Coriander, BP*	1 Pack/155g	292.0	6.0	189	12.5	25.2	4.2	0.0
Chicken, Mexican, Healthy Choices, Shell*	1 Serving/168g	376.0	12.0	224	12.2	28.1	7.0	0.0
Chicken, Moroccan, Sainsbury's*	½ Pack/100g	185.0	4.0	186	10.6	27.9	3.6	0.0
Chicken, No Mayo, M & S*	1 Pack/142g	220.0	4.0	155	15.0	17.5	3.0	3.1
Chicken, No Mayonnaise, Waitrose*	1 Pack/173g	332.0	10.0	192	11.6	24.0	5.5	2.1
Chicken, Red Thai, BGTY, Sainsbury's*	1 Pack/195g	326.0	4.0	167	11.3	26.4	1.9	0.0
Chicken, Roast, Breast, BGTY, Sainsbury's*	1 Pack/174g	275.0	4.0	158	14.8	20.9	2.5	1.8
Chicken, Roast, HL, Tesco*	1 Pack/155g	288.0	5.0	186	13.5	25.4	3.4	1.4
Chicken, Roast, Salad, BGTY, Sainsbury's*	1 Pack/182g	268.0	4.0	147	11.9	19.9	2.2	2.7
Chicken, Roast, Shapers, Boots*	1 Pack/163g	259.0	2.0	159	16.0	21.0	1.3	2.5
Chicken, Roast, Tesco*	1 Pack/158g	412.0	20.0	261	13.1	23.9	12.5	1.5
Chicken, Salad, M & S*	1 Pack/226g	350.0	9.0	155	10.6	18.8	4.1	3.0
Chicken, Salad, On Malted Bread, BGTY, Sainsbury's*	1 Pack/216g	346.0	7.0	160	12.7	19.7	3.4	2.7
Chicken, Shell*	1 Pack/121g	334.0	16.0	276	13.9	25.9	13.0	0.0
Chicken, Smokey, BGTY, Sainsbury's*	1 Pack/178g	276.0	2.0	155	11.1	25.6	1.0	0.0
Chicken, Southern Fried Breast, Microwave, Tesco*	1 Burger/135g	381.0	17.0	282	13.0	28.9	12.7	1.6
Chicken, Southern Fried, Rustlers*	1 Serving/145g	436.0	21.0	301	11.7	30.6	14.7	0.0
Chicken, Southern Spiced, M & S*	1 Pack/179g	421.0	23.0	235	11.2	21.7	13.0	3.1
Chicken, Tangy Lime & Ginger, Shapers, Boots*	1 Pack/168g	319.0	11.0	190	12.0	21.0	6.4	5.1
Chicken, Thai, BGTY, Sainsbury's*	1 Pack/196g	280.0	5.0	143	10.2	19.6	2.6	0.6
Chicken, Thai, Tesco*	1 Pack/244g	634.0	38.0	260	8.5	21.1	15.7	1.5
Chicken, Tikka, COU, M & S*	1 Pack/185g	268.0	3.0	145	12.1	20.5	1.8	3.2
Chicken, Tikka, M & S*	1 Pack/180g	391.0	20.0	217	10.4	19.5	10.9	2.0
Chicken, Tikka, Naan, Ready to Go, M & S*	1 Pack/298g	641.0	23.0	215	9.9	26.5	7.8	4.0
Chicken, Tikka, on Pepper Chilli Bread, Shapers, Boots*	1 Pack/172g	296.0	4.0	172	13.0	25.0	2.6	2.5
Chicken, Tikka, Thai Style, Korma, Big, Sainsbury's*	1 Pack/268g	581.0	26.0	217	11.9	20.5	9.7	0.0
Chicken, Tikka, Weight Watchers*	1 Pack/158g	250.0	2.0	158	13.1	23.2	1.4	2.9
Chicken, Tomato & Rocket, Light Choices, Tesco*	1 Pack/184g	285.0	4.0	155	10.3	23.4	2.1	2.6
Chicken, Tzatziki, Perfectly Balanced, Waitrose*	1 Pack/189g	270.0	3.0	143	12.4	19.4	1.7	1.7
Chicken, with Fresh Herb Salad, Roast, British, Asda*	1 Pack/214g	447.0	19.0	209	11.0	21.0	9.0	2.0
Chicken, with Pork Sage & Onion Stuffing, Tesco*	1 Pack/136g	376.0	17.0	276	12.1	28.1	12.5	1.4
Classic Feast, M & S*	1 Serving/295g	841.0	52.0	285	10.6	21.3	17.5	4.7
Club, New York Style, Sainsbury's*	1 Serving/212g	608.0	33.0	287	13.3	22.8	15.8	2.7
Coronation Chicken, in Pitta Bread, COU, M & S*	1 Serving/207g	269.0	2.0	130	9.2	20.4	1.2	2.0
Crab, Marie Rose, Brown Bread, Royal London Hospital*	1 Pack/158g	293.0	11.0	185	9.7	22.0	7.1	0.0
Crayfish & Rocket, Finest, Tesco*	1 Pack/178g	365.0	11.0	205	9.8	27.5	5.9	2.1
Cream Cheese, & Ham, Tesco*	1 Pack/212g	655.0	37.0	309	11.0	27.2	17.3	1.2
Cream Cheese, & Peppers, Taste!*	1 Pack/154g	296.0	10.0	192	7.3	25.5	6.8	0.0
Cream Cheese, & Salad, Sandwich Box*	1 Pack/138g	250.0	8.0	181	5.6	26.3	5.8	0.0
Duck, Peking, No Mayo, Boots*	1 Pack/222g	399.0	10.0	180	7.7	27.0	4.6	1.7
Edam, & Tomato, & Spring Onion, BHS*	1 Serving/184g	313.0	9.0	170	8.6	22.5	5.1	3.2
Egg & Cress, BGTY, Sainsbury's*	1 Pack/145g	268.0	8.0	185	9.1	25.4	5.2	2.7
Egg & Cress, No Mayo, Light Choices, Tesco*	1 Pack/160g	280.0	7.0	175	9.5	24.2	4.3	2.7
Egg & Cress, on Wheat Germ Bread, Tesco*	1 Pack/174g	365.0	16.0	210	11.0	20.5	9.1	2.1
Egg & Cress, Reduced Fat, Asda*	1 Pack/164g	290.0	9.0	177	9.8	22.4	5.3	0.0

SANDWICH

	Measure INFO/WEIGHT	per Measure KCAL	FAT	Nutrition Values per 100g / 100ml KCAL	PROT	CARB	FAT	FIBRE
Egg Mayonnaise, & Bacon, Boots*	1 Serving/200g	426.0	14.0	213	13.5	23.5	7.0	2.8
Egg Mayonnaise, & Cress, Go Simple, Asda*	1 Pack/169g	370.0	19.0	219	10.0	20.0	11.0	1.7
Egg Mayonnaise, & Cress, Reduced Fat, Waitrose*	1 Pack/162g	300.0	13.0	185	10.4	18.1	7.9	3.4
Egg Mayonnaise, & Cress, Shapers, Boots*	1 Pack/156g	292.0	8.0	187	11.0	25.0	4.9	2.6
Egg Mayonnaise, & Cress, Weight Watchers*	1 Pack/126g	238.0	4.0	189	8.8	31.1	3.3	3.3
Egg Mayonnaise, & Cress, Wheatgerm Bread, Asda*	1 Pack/158g	371.0	20.0	235	9.7	21.3	12.4	1.9
Egg Mayonnaise, & Cress, Wholemeal Bread, Oldfields*	1 Pack/128g	301.0	14.0	235	9.7	24.0	11.2	3.6
Egg Mayonnaise, HL, Tesco*	1 Pack/162g	253.0	6.0	156	9.3	21.4	3.7	2.8
Egg Mayonnaise, Shell*	1 Pack/189g	522.0	29.0	276	9.8	24.7	15.4	0.0
Egg Mayonnaise, Waitrose*	1 Pack/180g	396.0	21.0	220	10.1	19.1	11.4	3.4
Egg, & Bacon, & Lincolnshire Sausage, Waitrose*	1 Pack/249g	655.0	33.0	263	11.3	24.7	13.2	0.9
Egg, & Bacon, Weight Watchers*	1 Pack/139g	246.0	5.0	177	10.1	26.1	3.6	1.9
Egg, & Cress, COU, M & S*	1 Pack/192g	240.0	5.0	125	9.8	15.5	2.7	2.8
Egg, & Cress, Free Range, M & S*	1 Pack/192g	307.0	9.0	160	10.7	17.8	4.7	3.0
Egg, & Cress, Free Range, Sainsbury's*	1 Pack/204g	404.0	17.0	198	10.5	20.3	8.3	3.3
Egg, & Cress, Heinz*	1 Pack/200g	610.0	22.0	305	14.4	37.5	10.8	4.0
Egg, & Cress, M & S*	1 Pack/182g	331.0	18.0	182	10.1	13.6	9.7	3.2
Egg, & Gammon, Safeway*	1 Pack/233g	490.0	19.0	210	12.9	20.4	8.0	0.0
Egg, & Ham, Asda*	1 Pack/262g	589.0	34.0	225	10.4	16.8	12.8	2.1
Egg, & Salad, Deep Filled, Asda*	1 Pack/231g	395.0	16.0	171	8.0	19.0	7.0	1.0
Egg, & Salad, Free Range, Sainsbury's*	1 Pack/225g	449.0	17.0	200	8.5	24.5	7.5	0.0
Egg, & Salad, Free Range, Waitrose*	1 Pack/180g	281.0	12.0	156	7.6	16.9	6.4	3.3
Egg, & Salad, GFY, Asda*	1 Pack/157g	229.0	5.0	146	8.0	22.0	2.9	2.9
Egg, & Salad, Weight Watchers*	1 Pack/172g	237.0	5.0	138	7.1	21.3	2.7	2.2
Egg, & Salad, with Mayonnaise, Wholemeal, Waitrose*	1 Pack/180g	257.0	9.0	143	8.3	16.5	4.9	3.6
Egg, & Tomato, on Softgrain Bread, Daily Bread*	1 Pack/160g	279.0	7.0	174	8.6	23.8	4.4	0.0
Egg, & Tomato, Organic, Waitrose*	1 Pack/192g	359.0	19.0	187	9.7	15.3	9.7	4.0
Egg, & Tomato, Tesco*	1 Pack/172g	311.0	11.0	181	8.5	22.6	6.3	2.3
Egg, & Tomato, with Salad Cream, Big, Sainsbury's*	1 Pack/266g	463.0	15.0	174	9.1	21.3	5.8	0.0
Goats Cheese, & Chargrilled Vegetables, Finest, Tesco*	1 Pack/214g	481.0	20.0	225	7.7	27.8	9.2	1.4
Goat's Cheese, & Cranberry, Shapers, Boots*	1 Pack/150g	323.0	6.0	216	8.4	36.0	4.2	2.6
Goat's Cheese, Sunblush Tomato, Deli Continental*	1 Pack/179g	480.0	29.0	268	9.5	20.5	16.4	0.0
Greek Salad, Classic, Cafe, Primo*	1 Serving/216g	513.0	27.0	238	8.6	23.1	12.5	1.8
Ham Salad, Light Choices, HL, Tesco*	1 Pack/190g	266.0	5.0	140	11.0	19.8	2.8	2.1
Ham, & Cheese, Light Choices, Tesco*	1 Pack/158g	284.0	5.0	180	14.5	22.8	3.2	5.0
Ham, & Cheese, Morrisons*	1 Serving/183g	273.0	5.0	149	12.5	19.2	2.5	4.1
Ham, & Mustard, Heinz*	1 Pack/180g	460.0	21.0	255	11.8	25.6	11.5	5.0
Ham, & Mustard, Salad, BGTY, Sainsbury's*	1 Pack/182g	261.0	4.0	143	8.7	22.4	2.1	2.6
Ham, & Mustard, Tesco*	1 Pack/147g	437.0	28.0	297	10.6	20.8	19.0	1.2
Ham, & Philadelphia Light, Dry Cured, Boots*	1 Pack/172g	339.0	9.0	197	12.8	24.4	5.4	2.5
Ham, & Pineapple Salsa, Maple Flavoured, Waitrose*	1 Pack/194g	329.0	9.0	170	8.4	23.8	4.6	3.1
Ham, & Salad, British, COU, M & S*	1 Pack/204g	255.0	4.0	125	6.7	19.9	2.1	2.9
Ham, & Salad, Leicester, Waitrose*	1 Serving/187g	325.0	9.0	174	8.6	24.0	4.8	1.6
Ham, & Salad, Shapers, Boots*	1 Pack/195g	269.0	3.0	138	9.4	22.0	1.4	1.8
Ham, & Salad, Snack & Shop, Esso*	1 Pack/191g	304.0	7.0	159	9.2	22.9	3.4	5.0
Ham, & Tomato, GFY, Asda*	1 Pack/173g	254.0	3.0	147	10.0	23.0	1.7	1.4
Ham, & Tomato, Honey Roast, Feel Good, Shell*	1 Pack/171g	388.0	19.0	227	9.8	22.1	11.0	0.0
Ham, & Turkey, Asda*	1 Pack/190g	393.0	19.0	207	12.9	15.8	10.2	2.3
Ham, Cheese & Pickle, Deep Fill, Tesco*	1 Pack/225g	495.0	21.0	220	14.6	19.4	9.2	2.4
Ham, Cheese & Pickle, in a Soft Wrap, Sainsbury's*	1 Pack/195g	503.0	23.0	258	10.9	26.8	11.9	0.9
Ham, Cheese, & Pickle, Heinz*	1 Pack/188g	466.0	24.0	248	11.3	21.7	12.9	4.8
Ham, Cheese, & Pickle, Leicester, Waitrose*	1 Pack/205g	512.0	24.0	250	11.9	23.7	11.9	2.1
Ham, Cheese, Pickle & Lettuce, No Mayo, Tesco*	1 Pack/207g	435.0	16.0	210	12.2	23.0	7.8	2.7

S

SANDWICH

INFO/WEIGHT	Measure	per Measure KCAL	per Measure FAT	Nutrition Values per 100g / 100ml KCAL	PROT	CARB	FAT	FIBRE
Ham, M & S*	1 Pack/200g	220.0	5.0	110	17.2	3.2	2.6	0.0
King Prawn, Sainsbury's*	1 Pack/204g	424.0	16.0	208	11.6	22.3	8.0	0.0
Mozzarella, & Pepperoni, Sainsbury's*	1 Pack/171g	380.0	12.0	222	10.5	29.0	7.1	0.0
Mozzarella, & Tomato, Waitrose*	1 Pack/193g	359.0	18.0	186	9.7	15.7	9.4	2.3
Mozzarella, Pesto & Pine Nuts, Sainsbury's*	1 Pack/180g	423.0	17.0	235	10.2	26.8	9.7	2.8
Ploughman's, Cheddar Cheese, Deep Fill, Asda*	1 Pack/229g	471.0	23.0	206	9.0	20.0	10.0	4.3
Ploughman's, Cheddar, Heinz*	1 Pack/208g	552.0	28.0	265	9.3	27.1	13.3	2.4
Ploughman's, Cheddar, Mature Vintage, Sainsbury's*	1 Pack/204g	439.0	20.0	215	9.3	22.3	9.9	0.0
Ploughman's, Cheese, BGTY, Sainsbury's*	1 Pack/193g	326.0	8.0	169	9.8	22.8	4.2	3.6
Ploughmans, Light Choices, Tesco*	1 Pack/178g	320.0	7.0	180	12.2	22.9	4.2	3.3
Ploughman's, Shell*	1 Pack/226g	540.0	31.0	239	9.0	19.4	13.9	1.0
Prawn Cocktail, Waitrose*	1 Pack/196g	300.0	8.0	153	8.3	20.7	4.1	2.5
Prawn Cocktail, Weight Watchers*	1 Pack/168g	252.0	8.0	150	8.9	18.1	4.6	2.8
Prawn Mayonnaise, COU, M & S*	1 Pack/155g	240.0	4.0	155	10.2	22.9	2.3	2.8
Prawn Mayonnaise, GFY, Asda*	1 Pack/160g	251.0	4.0	157	10.0	23.0	2.8	2.8
Prawn Mayonnaise, Heinz*	1 Pack/180g	493.0	28.0	274	8.9	24.0	15.8	2.5
Prawn Mayonnaise, Light Choices, HL, Tesco*	1 Pack/153g	260.0	4.0	170	11.7	23.2	2.9	1.6
Prawn Mayonnaise, M & S*	1 Pack/156g	328.0	12.0	210	10.0	24.7	7.7	2.2
Prawn Mayonnaise, Morrisons*	1 Pack/157g	234.0	4.0	149	9.0	22.7	2.5	3.0
Prawn Mayonnaise, Nutritionally Balanced, M & S*	1 Pack/162g	300.0	11.0	185	10.2	21.2	6.6	1.9
Prawn Mayonnaise, Sainsbury's*	1 Pack/151g	323.0	14.0	214	11.6	20.9	9.3	0.0
Prawn Mayonnaise, Tesco*	1 Pack/143g	300.0	10.0	210	11.6	25.3	6.8	1.8
Prawn Mayonnaise, Triple, Asda*	1 Pack/248g	635.0	40.0	256	9.0	19.0	16.0	3.4
Prawn Mayonnaise, Triple, Tesco*	1 Pack/231g	603.0	33.0	261	9.5	23.5	14.3	1.6
Prawn, & Coriander, M & S*	1 Serving/213g	575.0	35.0	270	9.5	20.6	16.6	3.7
Prawn, & Salmon, Waitrose*	1 Pack/154g	345.0	15.0	224	12.5	22.0	9.5	2.8
Prawn, & Smoked Salmon, M & S*	1 Pack/445g	1135.0	64.0	255	11.7	19.3	14.3	1.4
Prawn, & Thai Dressing, Tiger, Waitrose*	1 Pack/200g	342.0	9.0	171	9.6	23.6	4.3	2.2
Prawn, Bells, Lighter Eating, Ready to Go, Bells*	1 Serving/155g	258.0	4.0	167	12.5	24.0	2.3	0.0
Prawn, Crayfish & Rocket, Tesco*	1 Pack/193g	425.0	17.0	220	11.4	22.3	9.0	2.0
Prawn, Creme Fraiche, on Oatmeal Bread, Choice*	1 Pack/153g	265.0	5.0	173	11.7	23.8	3.4	1.9
Prawn, Egg & Chicken, Triple, Weight Watchers*	1 Pack/224g	367.0	6.0	164	10.2	24.8	2.7	2.9
Prawn, Marie Rose, Waitrose*	1 Pack/164g	226.0	6.0	138	8.8	18.0	3.4	1.9
Prawn, Salad, COU, M & S*	1 Pack/200g	230.0	4.0	115	8.0	16.6	1.8	3.8
Salmon, & Cucumber, Brown Bread, Waitrose*	1 Pack/150g	295.0	11.0	197	10.5	22.7	7.1	1.4
Salmon, & Cucumber, Light Choices, Tesco*	1 Pack/155g	262.0	4.0	169	12.3	24.1	2.5	2.1
Salmon, & Cucumber, M & S*	1 Pack/168g	329.0	14.0	196	11.0	19.5	8.3	2.6
Salmon, & Cucumber, Red, BGTY, Sainsbury's*	1 Pack/192g	278.0	4.0	145	9.4	21.7	2.3	2.4
Salmon, & Cucumber, Red, Healthy Choice, Asda*	1 Pack/149g	285.0	11.0	191	10.6	19.9	7.7	2.1
Salmon, & Cucumber, Red, Tesco*	1 Pack/144g	284.0	9.0	197	11.1	20.8	6.4	1.9
Salmon, & Soft Cheese, Smoked, Waitrose*	1 Pack/154g	300.0	10.0	195	14.8	19.2	6.5	4.2
Salmon, & Spinach, Poached, Shapers, Boots*	1 Pack/168g	284.0	8.0	169	9.2	23.0	4.5	3.1
Salmon, Poached, Prawn & Rocket, Waitrose*	1 Pack/166g	308.0	9.0	186	11.2	23.5	5.2	2.1
Salmon, Red, Wild & Cucumber, Eat Well, M & S*	1 Pack/182g	337.0	13.0	185	11.2	18.6	7.2	8.0
Salmon, Smoked & Cream Cheese, M & S*	1 Pack/184g	450.0	22.0	245	12.7	20.8	12.2	1.8
Salsa Chicken, HL, Tesco*	1 Pack/182g	300.0	3.0	165	13.4	23.6	1.8	1.9
Sausage, Egg & Bacon, Boots*	1 Pack/325g	887.0	52.0	273	9.3	23.0	16.0	2.2
Sausage, Triple Pack, GFY, Asda*	1 Pack/215g	424.0	10.0	197	9.0	30.0	4.5	2.3
Seafood Cocktail, Asda*	1 Pack/190g	486.0	30.0	256	6.7	21.3	15.8	1.6
Seafood Cocktail, Waitrose*	1 Pack/210g	267.0	6.0	127	7.3	17.6	3.0	8.1
Seafood Medley, M & S*	1 Pack/227g	468.0	28.0	206	7.2	16.3	12.4	3.5
Seafood, Mixed, Tesco*	1 Pack/184g	502.0	31.0	273	7.3	23.2	16.8	0.8
Soft Cheese, & Roasted Pepper, Weight Watchers*	1 Pack/158g	289.0	6.0	183	9.4	27.7	3.8	1.5

S

SANDWICH

	Measure INFO/WEIGHT	per Measure KCAL	FAT	Nutrition Values per 100g / 100ml KCAL	PROT	CARB	FAT	FIBRE
Sub, Beef, & Onion, M & S*	1 Pack/207g	611.0	32.0	295	13.3	25.6	15.3	1.5
Sub, Beef, & Onion, Roast, Sainsbury's*	1 Serving/174g	426.0	17.0	245	9.4	29.3	10.0	0.0
Sub, Chicken & Bacon, Sainsbury's*	1 Pack/190g	554.0	27.0	291	13.4	27.4	14.2	0.8
Sub, Chicken, & Stuffing, Shell*	1 Serving/183g	437.0	12.0	239	13.3	32.0	6.4	0.0
Sub, Chicken, Caesar, Chargrilled, Sainsbury's*	1 Pack/216g	611.0	30.0	283	13.4	25.6	14.1	0.0
Sub, Ham, & Tomato Salad, Shapers, Boots*	1 Pack/170g	286.0	4.0	168	9.2	28.0	2.3	1.4
Sweet Chilli Chicken, in Pitta Bread, Shapers, Boots*	1 Pack/178g	245.0	5.0	138	9.2	19.0	2.8	2.2
Three Cheese & Celery on Malted Brown, COU, M & S*	1 Pack/161g	250.0	4.0	155	8.0	24.7	2.6	2.1
Three Cheese & Onion, on White Bread, Weight Watchers*	1 Pack/158g	283.0	3.0	179	12.4	28.4	1.8	1.5
Three Cheese Salad, Shapers, Boots*	1 Pack/169g	248.0	2.0	147	11.0	23.0	1.3	2.7
Tuna Mayonnaise, & Cucumber, Classic*	1 Serving/185g	429.0	23.0	232	10.6	19.8	12.3	0.0
Tuna Mayonnaise, & Cucumber, Simply, Boots*	1 Pack/200g	498.0	26.0	249	12.0	21.0	13.0	2.4
Tuna Mayonnaise, & Salad, Serious About Sandwiches*	1 Pack/192g	305.0	9.0	159	8.6	20.5	4.7	2.9
Tuna Mayonnaise, & Sweetcorn, Whistlestop*	1 Pack/140g	378.0	18.0	271	13.6	25.5	12.7	0.0
Tuna Mayonnaise, Menu, Boots*	1 Pack/182g	451.0	20.0	248	13.0	23.0	11.0	1.1
Tuna, & Celery, Perfectly Balanced, Waitrose*	1 Pack/172g	272.0	6.0	158	11.7	20.5	3.2	3.9
Tuna, & Celery, Waitrose*	1 Pack/168g	254.0	6.0	151	10.2	19.5	3.6	3.0
Tuna, & Chargrilled Vegetables, BGTY, Sainsbury's*	1 Pack/196g	329.0	9.0	168	10.7	21.5	4.4	3.0
Tuna, & Cucumber, BGTY, Sainsbury's*	1 Pack/178g	268.0	3.0	151	11.3	22.3	1.8	3.1
Tuna, & Cucumber, Feel Good, Shell*	1 Pack/214g	518.0	16.0	242	12.6	31.2	7.5	0.0
Tuna, & Cucumber, Perfectly Balanced, Waitrose*	1 Pack/178g	240.0	4.0	135	11.0	18.3	2.0	3.6
Tuna, & Cucumber, Shapers, Boots*	1 Pack/167g	267.0	5.0	160	11.0	22.0	3.2	2.4
Tuna, & Cucumber, Shell*	1 Pack/188g	431.0	19.0	229	12.3	21.9	10.2	0.0
Tuna, & Cucumber, Weight Watchers*	1 Pack/173g	279.0	3.0	161	11.4	25.1	1.7	1.4
Tuna, & Green Pesto, BGTY, Sainsbury's*	1 Pack/211g	279.0	5.0	132	11.0	17.0	2.2	0.0
Tuna, & Salad, Classic*	1 Pack/230g	449.0	16.0	195	8.7	27.3	6.9	2.1
Tuna, & Salad, M & S*	1 Pack/250g	575.0	31.0	230	12.5	16.8	12.6	2.1
Tuna, & Salad, Tesco*	1 Pack/197g	339.0	15.0	172	9.9	16.5	7.4	2.8
Tuna, & Sweetcorn, BGTY, Sainsbury's*	1 Pack/187g	309.0	5.0	165	10.8	24.7	2.7	2.8
Tuna, & Sweetcorn, COU, M & S*	1 Pack/180g	270.0	4.0	150	12.6	19.0	2.4	3.8
Tuna, & Sweetcorn, Light Choices, HL, Tesco*	1 Pack/168g	285.0	3.0	170	11.2	25.9	1.9	2.8
Tuna, & Sweetcorn, on Malt Bread, Tesco*	1 Pack/175g	350.0	8.0	200	11.6	27.5	4.7	2.2
Tuna, & Sweetcorn, Safeway*	1 Pack/155g	255.0	3.0	165	12.8	23.2	1.8	1.7
Tuna, & Sweetcorn, Sainsbury's*	1 Pack/183g	392.0	16.0	214	12.1	22.3	8.5	0.0
Tuna, & Sweetcorn, Shapers, Boots*	1 Pack/170g	295.0	4.0	174	12.4	25.3	2.6	2.0
Tuna, & Tomato, & Onion, COU, M & S*	1 Pack/177g	250.0	4.0	141	11.1	18.8	2.4	2.2
Tuna, Mediterranean, COU, M & S*	1 Pack/260g	364.0	6.0	140	10.3	19.6	2.2	1.6
Turkey, & Bacon, COU, M & S*	1 Pack/165g	256.0	4.0	155	12.0	21.0	2.4	1.7
Turkey, & Cheese, & Bacon, Bernard Matthews*	1 Serving/192g	482.0	22.0	251	9.2	28.3	11.2	0.0
Turkey, & Cranberry, COU, M & S*	1 Pack/180g	279.0	3.0	155	12.1	22.8	1.7	2.9
Turkey, & Stuffing, M & S*	1 Pack/190g	351.0	9.0	185	12.3	23.1	4.9	1.9
Turkey, & Sun Dried Tomato, Festive Feast, Taste!*	1 Pack/159g	401.0	22.0	252	8.8	23.0	13.9	0.0
Turkey, Gibsons*	1 Pack/138g	260.0	5.0	188	12.5	26.0	3.8	0.0
Turkey, Just Turkey, White Bread, Sandwich King*	1 Serving/135g	317.0	7.0	235	17.3	29.7	5.2	0.0
Turkey, Northern Bites*	1 Pack/200g	354.0	9.0	177	11.9	22.8	4.3	0.0
Turkey, Pork Sausage, & Stuffing, Somerfield*	1 Pack/209g	475.0	19.0	227	11.6	24.3	9.3	2.1
Turkey, Stuffing & Cranberry, Boots*	1 Pack/192g	328.0	2.0	171	12.0	28.0	1.1	2.5
Vegetable, & Chilli Bean, Roasted, M & S*	1 Pack/200g	340.0	11.0	170	5.2	24.5	5.7	2.1
Vegetable, M & S*	1 Serving/180g	252.0	4.0	140	6.1	23.5	2.3	2.1
Vegetable, Roasted, Open, COU, M & S*	1 Pack/150g	260.0	2.0	173	8.4	31.3	1.5	4.4
Wedge, Chicken, & Salad, Tesco*	1 Serving/257g	599.0	24.0	233	11.3	25.3	9.5	1.2
Wedge, Sausage, & Egg, Tesco*	1 Pack/269g	699.0	39.0	260	9.1	23.6	14.4	1.1
Wedge, Tuna, & Salad, Tesco*	1 Pack/205g	291.0	3.0	142	8.1	23.9	1.5	0.8

	Measure INFO/WEIGHT	per Measure KCAL	FAT	Nutrition Values per 100g / 100ml KCAL	PROT	CARB	FAT	FIBRE
SANDWICH								
Wensleydale, & Carrot, M & S*	1 Pack/183g	430.0	23.0	235	9.9	21.4	12.3	2.8
SANDWICH FILLER								
Beef & Onion, Deli, Asda*	1 Serving/50g	78.0	6.0	157	10.0	0.1	13.0	1.1
Big Breakfast, Asda*	1 Serving/125g	314.0	26.0	251	12.0	3.5	21.0	0.5
Cajun Chicken, Sainsbury's*	1 Serving/60g	109.0	8.0	182	13.4	1.8	13.5	1.8
Chargrilled Vegetable, Sainsbury's*	½ Pot/85g	192.0	19.0	226	3.4	2.2	22.7	0.6
Cheese & Bacon, Tesco*	1 Serving/50g	199.0	19.0	398	12.2	2.6	37.6	1.2
Cheese & Celery, Sainsbury's*	1 Tub/250g	397.0	35.0	159	5.7	2.1	14.2	3.0
Cheese & Ham, Sainsbury's*	1 Serving/25g	124.0	12.0	497	12.4	0.8	49.3	0.3
Cheese & Onion, Deli, Asda*	1 Serving/57g	217.0	21.0	381	10.0	2.0	37.0	2.0
Cheese & Onion, Sainsbury's*	1 Tub/200g	632.0	60.0	316	8.7	3.2	29.8	2.2
Cheese & Onion, Tesco*	1 Pack/170g	721.0	72.0	424	10.0	0.2	42.6	1.5
Cheese & Spring Onion, M & S*	1 Serving/56g	199.0	19.0	355	8.5	5.0	33.6	0.2
Chicken & Bacon with Sweetcorn, Sainsbury's*	1 Serving/60g	123.0	9.0	205	12.0	4.0	15.7	0.9
Chicken & Stuffing, Sainsbury's*	½ Tub/120g	397.0	38.0	331	6.5	5.3	31.5	1.7
Chicken & Sweetcorn, Sainsbury's*	1 Tub/170g	396.0	34.0	233	11.0	2.7	19.8	1.9
Chicken Caesar, BGTY, Sainsbury's*	½ Jar/85g	117.0	6.0	137	15.6	2.5	7.2	2.2
Chicken Fajita, Tesco*	1 Serving/50g	77.0	4.0	155	13.8	5.9	8.5	1.4
Chicken Tikka & Citrus Raita, COU, M & S*	½ Pot/85g	76.0	2.0	90	12.6	4.9	2.0	0.9
Chicken Tikka, BGTY, Sainsbury's*	½ Pot/85g	99.0	3.0	117	16.5	6.0	3.0	1.0
Chicken Tikka, Mild, Heinz*	1 Serving/52g	102.0	7.0	196	5.2	12.3	14.0	0.7
Chicken with Salad Vegetables, Heinz*	1 Serving/56g	114.0	8.0	203	5.1	11.7	15.1	0.5
Chicken, Bacon & Sweetcorn, BGTY, Sainsbury's*	1 Tub/300g	399.0	18.0	133	14.0	5.5	6.1	0.5
Chicken, Stuffing & Bacon, COU, M & S*	1 Pack/170g	170.0	4.0	100	13.1	6.2	2.2	1.3
Chicken, Sweetcorn & Bacon, Tesco*	1 Serving/50g	167.0	15.0	334	12.3	4.3	29.7	1.6
Chicken, Tomato & Sweetcure Bacon, M & S*	1 Pot/170g	501.0	45.0	295	11.4	2.8	26.4	0.7
Chickpea, Moroccan Style, Sainsbury's*	½ Tub/120g	160.0	9.0	133	4.1	11.7	7.8	4.2
Chunky Egg & Smoked Ham, Tesco*	1 Serving/100g	234.0	21.0	234	11.8	0.2	20.7	0.3
Chunky Seafood Cocktail, Tesco*	1 Serving/100g	308.0	28.0	308	6.0	8.3	27.8	2.0
Corned Beef & Onion, Deli, Asda*	1 Serving/50g	170.0	15.0	340	12.0	3.3	31.0	0.7
Coronation Chicken, BGTY, Sainsbury's*	1 Portion/50g	73.0	3.0	146	11.9	8.9	7.0	1.4
Coronation Chicken, Sainsbury's*	¼ Tub/60g	183.0	15.0	305	12.1	8.9	24.6	1.2
Coronation Chicken, Tesco*	1 Tbsp/30g	84.0	7.0	279	14.7	6.1	21.8	0.7
Coronation Chicken, Waitrose*	1 Pack/170g	554.0	43.0	326	11.1	13.2	25.4	2.0
Coronation Tuna, BGTY, Sainsbury's*	1 Can/80g	90.0	2.0	112	16.5	5.7	2.6	1.0
Egg & Bacon, Fresh, Tesco*	1 Serving/45g	112.0	9.0	248	12.7	4.2	20.1	0.6
Egg & Smoked Bacon, BGTY, Sainsbury's*	½ Pot/120g	187.0	14.0	156	9.7	3.8	11.3	0.5
Egg Mayonnaise, BGTY, Sainsbury's*	1 Serving/63g	75.0	4.0	119	10.9	3.1	7.0	0.5
Egg Mayonnaise, Deli, Asda*	1 Serving/50g	113.0	10.0	227	11.0	0.8	20.0	0.3
Egg Mayonnaise, M & S*	1oz/28g	62.0	6.0	220	10.1	0.8	19.7	1.1
Egg Mayonnaise, Sainsbury's*	1 Serving/60g	129.0	11.0	215	10.4	2.0	18.4	0.5
Egg Mayonnaise, Tesco*	1 Serving/50g	114.0	10.0	228	10.2	1.9	20.0	0.5
Ham & Salad Vegetables, Heinz*	1oz/28g	57.0	4.0	204	5.3	10.0	15.9	0.4
Peppered Mackerel, Creamy, Shippam*	1 Serving/15g	27.0	3.0	177	7.8	6.5	18.6	0.0
Poached Salmon & Cucumber, Deli, M & S*	1 Pot/170g	348.0	28.0	205	14.0	1.0	16.3	0.5
Prawn Marie Rose, Sainsbury's*	1 Serving/60g	121.0	11.0	201	8.1	2.5	17.6	0.9
Prawn Mayonnaise, GFY, Asda*	1 Serving/57g	101.0	7.0	177	12.0	3.0	13.0	0.1
Prawn Mayonnaise, M & S*	½ Pack/170g	501.0	48.0	295	10.6	0.6	28.0	0.3
Prawn Mayonnaise, Waitrose*	1 Pot/170g	537.0	53.0	316	8.9	0.2	31.1	0.0
Roast Beef, Onion & Horseradish, Sainsbury's*	1 Serving/100g	372.0	37.0	372	6.4	3.7	36.8	1.2
Roast Chicken & Stuffing, Sainsbury's*	1 Serving/100g	424.0	41.0	424	10.8	1.9	41.5	1.2
Seafood Cocktail, M & S*	1oz/28g	76.0	7.0	272	6.4	8.2	23.8	0.2
Seafood Cocktail, Sainsbury's*	½ Tub/120g	314.0	28.0	262	5.7	8.1	23.0	1.0

S

	Measure INFO/WEIGHT	per Measure KCAL	FAT	Nutrition Values per 100g / 100ml KCAL	PROT	CARB	FAT	FIBRE
SANDWICH FILLER								
Seafood, BGTY, Sainsbury's*	1oz/28g	36.0	2.0	128	8.7	7.6	7.0	0.5
Smoked Ham, Roasted Onion & Mustard, Sainsbury's*	1 Serving/100g	343.0	33.0	343	7.3	3.4	33.4	0.0
Smoked Salmon & Soft Cheese, M & S*	1 Pack/170g	450.0	41.0	265	11.1	4.9	23.9	0.0
Tex-Mex Chicken, Tesco*	1 Pack/250g	255.0	2.0	102	12.3	11.2	0.9	1.2
Three Cheese & Onion, Premier Deli*	1 Serving/100g	540.0	55.0	540	10.8	1.0	54.8	2.0
Tuna & Sweetcorn with Salad Vegetables, Heinz*	1oz/28g	53.0	4.0	191	5.8	12.1	13.2	0.7
Tuna & Sweetcorn, COU, M & S*	½ Pot/85g	76.0	2.0	90	11.6	5.7	2.0	1.3
Tuna & Sweetcorn, Deli, Asda*	1 Serving/50g	148.0	13.0	296	12.0	3.4	26.0	1.4
Tuna & Sweetcorn, GFY, Asda*	1/3 Pot/57g	71.0	2.0	125	12.0	10.0	4.1	0.8
Tuna & Sweetcorn, HL, Tesco*	1 Serving/60g	69.0	3.0	115	11.2	5.0	5.3	1.4
Tuna & Sweetcorn, M & S*	1oz/28g	70.0	6.0	250	14.2	2.3	20.7	1.3
Tuna Mayonnaise, & Cucumber, Choice, Tesco*	1 Serving/200g	463.0	23.0	231	12.8	23.2	11.4	1.5
Tuna Mayonnaise, BGTY, Sainsbury's*	1 Serving/100g	114.0	3.0	114	17.6	3.5	3.4	0.1
Tuna, Carb Check, Heinz*	1 Serving/52g	84.0	6.0	161	6.6	6.3	12.0	0.7
Tuna, Tomato & Black Olive, BGTY, Sainsbury's*	1 Pack/100g	88.0	2.0	88	12.6	5.9	1.6	1.2
SANDWICH FILLING								
Cheese & Onion, Asda*	1 Serving/56g	288.0	29.0	515	9.8	4.4	50.9	0.3
Cheese & Onion, GFY, Asda*	1 Serving/80g	206.0	17.0	257	11.0	6.0	21.0	0.8
Chicken & Bacon, Asda*	1 Serving/100g	341.0	29.0	341	17.0	3.0	29.0	0.5
Chicken & Sweetcorn, Asda*	1 Serving/60g	187.0	17.0	312	11.0	4.0	28.0	2.0
Chicken Tikka, Asda*	1 Serving/28g	80.0	6.0	284	13.0	13.0	20.0	0.7
Chicken Tikka, Less Than 5% Fat, Asda*	1 Serving/56g	65.0	3.0	116	11.0	7.3	4.7	1.2
Crab, BGTY, Sainsbury's*	1oz/28g	36.0	2.0	128	8.7	7.6	7.0	0.5
Egg Mayonnaise with Chives, Asda*	1oz/28g	92.0	9.0	327	9.1	1.1	31.8	0.0
Egg Mayonnaise, Asda*	1oz/28g	72.0	7.0	258	10.3	1.9	23.3	0.7
Houmous & Vegetable, Asda*	1/3 Tub/57g	133.0	10.0	233	8.0	12.0	17.0	3.5
Prawns with Seafood Sauce, Asda*	1oz/28g	107.0	10.0	382	11.7	1.4	36.8	0.0
Tuna & Sweetcorn, Asda*	1oz/28g	83.0	7.0	295	8.2	6.0	26.5	0.6
Tuna & Sweetcorn, Reduced Fat, Morrisons*	1oz/28g	48.0	3.0	172	13.2	6.9	10.2	0.0
SANDWICH SPREAD								
Beef, Classic, Shippam*	1 Pot/75g	133.0	9.0	177	15.5	2.2	11.8	0.0
Chicken & Bacon, Asda*	¼ Jar/43g	153.0	13.0	359	18.0	2.0	31.0	1.0
Chicken Tikka, Asda*	1 Serving/50g	77.0	5.0	154	7.0	9.0	10.0	0.2
Chicken, Classic, Shippam*	1 Serving/35g	64.0	4.0	182	15.5	1.8	12.5	0.0
Crab, Classic, Shippam*	1 Jar/35g	59.0	4.0	170	13.1	4.6	10.9	0.0
Cucumber, Heinz*	1oz/28g	46.0	3.0	164	1.7	12.7	11.6	0.6
Salmon, Classic, Shippam*	1 Serving/35g	70.0	5.0	200	14.7	4.2	14.1	0.0
Tuna & Mayonnaise, Shippam*	1 Pot/75g	189.0	14.0	252	18.3	3.1	18.5	0.0
SARDINES								
Boneless, in Tomato Sauce, John West*	1 Can/120g	197.0	12.0	164	17.0	1.5	10.0	0.0
Grilled	*1oz/28g*	*55.0*	*3.0*	*195*	*25.3*	*0.0*	*10.4*	*0.0*
in Brine, Canned, Drained	*1oz/28g*	*48.0*	*3.0*	*172*	*21.5*	*0.0*	*9.6*	*0.0*
in Oil, Canned, Drained	*1oz/28g*	*62.0*	*4.0*	*220*	*23.3*	*0.0*	*14.1*	*0.0*
in Tomato Sauce, Canned	1oz/28g	45.0	3.0	162	17.0	1.4	9.9	0.0
Raw	*1oz/28g*	*46.0*	*3.0*	*165*	*20.6*	*0.0*	*9.2*	*0.0*
SATAY								
Chicken & Turkey, Sainsbury's*	1 Stick/20g	44.0	3.0	222	20.0	4.0	14.0	1.9
Chicken, Breast, Iceland*	1 Satay/9.7g	15.0	0.0	155	34.1	2.7	0.9	0.1
Chicken, Breast, Party Bites, Sainsbury's*	1 Stick/10g	16.0	0.0	157	34.1	2.7	0.9	0.1
Chicken, GFY, Asda*	1 Serving/168g	242.0	6.0	144	22.0	6.0	3.6	0.8
Chicken, Indonesian, Bighams*	1 Serving/240g	314.0	15.0	131	12.2	6.2	6.4	0.6
Chicken, Indonesian, Mini, Sainsbury's*	1 Stick/10g	17.0	1.0	171	23.0	4.0	7.0	0.7
Chicken, Kebab, Waitrose*	½ Pack/125g	246.0	13.0	197	18.9	6.0	10.8	0.5

	Measure INFO/WEIGHT	per Measure KCAL	FAT	Nutrition Values per 100g / 100ml KCAL	PROT	CARB	FAT	FIBRE
SATAY								
Chicken, M & S*	1 Satay/43g	90.0	5.0	210	19.1	4.4	12.7	0.7
Chicken, Mini, Iceland*	1 Satay/8g	19.0	1.0	236	23.0	4.5	14.0	0.7
Chicken, Morrisons*	1 Satay/10g	17.0	1.0	171	23.5	3.5	7.0	0.7
Chicken, Occasions, Sainsbury's*	1 Satay/10g	15.0	1.0	150	22.0	2.0	6.0	0.7
Chicken, Oriental, Tesco*	1 Serving/100g	160.0	5.0	160	23.6	5.1	5.0	0.4
Chicken, Party, Mini, Tesco*	1 Satay/10g	13.0	0.0	133	23.7	3.4	2.8	1.0
Chicken, Sticks, Asda*	1 Stick/20g	43.0	3.0	216	18.0	4.5	14.0	0.0
Chicken, Stuffed, Asda*	½ Pack/168g	242.0	6.0	144	22.0	6.0	3.6	0.8
Chicken, Taste Original*	1 Stick/20g	33.0	1.0	164	23.0	2.5	6.5	0.7
Chicken, with Peanut Sauce, Waitrose*	1 Pack/250g	492.0	27.0	197	18.9	6.0	10.8	0.5
Szechuan Style, Occasions, Sainsbury's*	1 Satay/10g	20.0	1.0	196	22.8	6.4	8.8	0.5
SATSUMAS								
Fresh, Raw, Flesh Only, Average	*1 Sm/56g*	*20.0*	*0.0*	*36*	*0.8*	*13.3*	*0.3*	*1.8*
Weighed with Peel, Average	*1 Med/80g*	*21.0*	*0.0*	*26*	*0.6*	*6.0*	*0.1*	*0.9*
SAUCE								
Amatrician, Sainsbury's*	1 Serving/100g	52.0	2.0	52	3.8	4.3	2.2	1.4
Apple & Brandy, Asda*	1 Serving/125g	56.0	0.0	45	0.2	11.0	0.0	0.0
Apple, Baxters*	1 Tsp/15g	7.0	0.0	49	0.1	11.1	0.4	0.7
Apple, Bramley, M & S*	1 Tbsp/15g	21.0	0.0	140	0.2	32.6	0.3	0.4
Apple, Bramley, Sainsbury's*	1 Tsp/15g	17.0	0.0	111	0.2	27.2	0.1	1.8
Apple, Heinz*	1 Tsp/15g	8.0	0.0	56	0.3	13.4	0.2	1.5
Apricot & Almond Tagine, Sainsbury's*	1/3 Jar/120g	98.0	2.0	82	2.0	17.9	1.6	2.5
Aromatic Cantonese, Express, Uncle Ben's*	1 Serving/170g	172.0	0.0	101	0.6	24.6	0.1	0.0
Arrabbiata, Don Pomodoro*	½ Pot/185g	231.0	20.0	125	0.5	6.0	11.0	0.0
Arrabbiata, Fresh, Waitrose*	1 Serving/100g	52.0	2.0	52	1.4	5.9	2.5	2.0
Arrabbiata, Italian, Tesco*	½ Pot/175g	72.0	1.0	41	1.3	8.3	0.3	1.1
Arrabbiata, Lazio, Sainsbury's*	1/3 Jar/113g	154.0	12.0	136	2.2	7.2	10.9	0.0
Arrabbiata, Weight Watchers*	½ Pot/150g	43.0	1.0	29	1.1	5.0	0.5	1.7
Balti Curry, Tesco*	1 Serving/200g	126.0	9.0	63	1.7	4.3	4.6	1.7
Balti Indian, M & S*	1oz/28g	25.0	2.0	90	1.6	5.6	6.7	1.8
Balti, 97% Fat Free, Homepride*	1 Serving/230g	133.0	4.0	58	1.1	9.1	1.9	1.8
Balti, Cooking, BGTY, Sainsbury's*	¼ Jar/129g	98.0	4.0	76	1.1	10.9	3.1	0.6
Balti, Cooking, Indian Inspired, Asda*	1 Jar/320g	243.0	11.0	76	0.9	10.5	3.4	1.8
Balti, Cooking, Organic, Perfectly Balanced, Waitrose*	1 Jar/450g	301.0	6.0	67	1.6	12.1	1.3	3.1
Balti, Cooking, Organic, Sainsbury's*	1 Serving/225g	157.0	5.0	70	2.2	10.0	2.3	0.5
Balti, Cooking, Sharwood's*	1/3 Jar/140g	105.0	5.0	75	1.6	9.4	3.5	3.0
Balti, Deliciously Good, Homepride*	1/3 Jar/153g	89.0	3.0	58	1.1	9.1	1.9	0.6
Balti, Sizzle & Stir, Chicken Tonight, Knorr*	1/3 Jar/168g	195.0	16.0	116	1.3	6.3	9.5	2.9
Balti, Tomato & Coriander, Canned, Patak's*	1 Can/283g	235.0	17.0	83	0.8	6.5	6.0	1.2
Balti, TTD, Sainsbury's*	½ Pack/175g	159.0	12.0	91	1.4	6.0	6.8	2.0
Barbecue, Chicken Tonight, Knorr*	¼ Jar/125g	76.0	0.0	61	2.0	12.4	0.4	0.9
Barbecue, Cooking, BGTY, Sainsbury's*	¼ Jar/124g	46.0	0.0	37	0.4	8.4	0.2	0.7
Barbecue, Original, Sainsbury's*	1 Tbsp/15g	19.0	0.0	127	0.9	29.6	0.1	0.3
Barbecue, Smoky, Ainsley Harriott*	1 Serving/10g	15.0	0.0	153	0.8	36.4	0.1	0.0
Barbeque, Asda*	1 Tbsp/15g	20.0	0.0	136	0.9	33.0	0.2	0.0
Barbeque, Cook in, Homepride*	1 Can/500g	375.0	7.0	75	0.7	14.6	1.5	0.6
Barbeque, Simply Sausages Ranch, Colman's*	1 Serving/130g	96.0	0.0	74	1.8	16.6	0.1	1.1
BBQ, Bick's*	1 Serving/100g	119.0	0.0	119	1.6	27.5	0.3	0.0
BBQ, Heinz*	1 Serving/20g	29.0	0.0	143	1.1	32.9	0.3	0.5
BBQ, Hellmann's*	1 Serving/10g	12.0	0.0	125	0.8	27.7	0.7	0.0
BBQ, HP*	1 Serving/20ml	29.0	0.0	143	0.8	33.1	0.2	0.0
BBQ, Smokey Tomato, HP*	1oz/28g	40.0	0.0	143	0.8	33.1	0.2	0.0
BBQ, Spicy Mayhem, HP*	1 Serving/2g	3.0	0.0	156	0.9	36.7	0.1	0.0

S

SAUCE

INFO/WEIGHT	Measure	per Measure		Nutrition Values per 100g / 100ml				
		KCAL	FAT	KCAL	PROT	CARB	FAT	FIBRE
Bearnaise, Sainsbury's*	1 Tbsp/15.0g	59.0	6.0	393	0.6	5.0	41.0	0.0
Bechamel, for Lasagne, Loyd Grossman*	1 Jar/400g	396.0	33.0	99	0.6	5.4	8.3	0.1
Beef in Ale, Cooking, Asda*	1 Jar/500g	160.0	1.0	32	1.6	6.0	0.2	0.0
Bhuna, Cooking, Sharwood's*	1/3 Jar/140g	116.0	8.0	83	1.2	7.6	5.4	1.6
Black Bean & Chilli, Stir Fry, Asda*	½ Jar/97g	158.0	12.0	163	3.7	10.0	12.0	0.8
Black Bean & Green Pepper, Stir Fry, Sharwood's*	1 Serving/150g	82.0	0.0	55	2.0	11.0	0.3	0.5
Black Bean & Red Pepper, Sharwood's*	½ Jar/213g	132.0	3.0	62	1.9	10.5	1.4	1.2
Black Bean Sauce Cantonese, Sharwood's*	1 Serving/140g	87.0	2.0	62	1.9	10.5	1.4	1.2
Black Bean, Asda*	1 Serving/55g	55.0	1.0	100	2.9	19.0	1.4	0.0
Black Bean, Canton, Stir Fry, Blue Dragon*	½ Pack/60g	53.0	1.0	88	2.8	14.8	2.0	1.5
Black Bean, Cooking, Tesco*	1 Tbsp/15g	13.0	0.0	90	2.5	14.9	2.0	0.6
Black Bean, Crushed, Stir Fry Sensations, Amoy*	1 Pouch/150g	150.0	4.0	100	2.4	16.9	2.9	1.0
Black Bean, Finest, Tesco*	1 Jar/350g	252.0	2.0	72	0.8	16.1	0.5	0.8
Black Bean, Fresh, Sainsbury's*	1 Sachet/50ml	78.0	1.0	156	6.7	27.5	2.6	1.7
Black Bean, Loyd Grossman*	1 Serving/175g	177.0	8.0	101	2.4	12.6	4.5	0.7
Black Bean, Ready to Stir Fry, M & S*	1 Sachet/120g	78.0	1.0	65	2.5	11.5	0.9	1.4
Black Bean, Sharwood's*	1 Serving/98g	96.0	1.0	98	2.2	18.8	1.5	0.6
Black Bean, Stir Fry Additions, Tesco*	1 Sachet/50g	69.0	1.0	138	4.1	23.6	3.0	0.0
Black Bean, Stir Fry, Fresh Ideas, Tesco*	½ Sachet/25g	33.0	1.0	132	4.2	22.6	2.8	0.8
Black Bean, Stir Fry, Fresh Tastea, Asda*	1 Pack/180ml	149.0	5.0	83	3.7	10.4	2.9	1.4
Black Bean, Stir Fry, Fresh, M & S*	1 Pot/120g	120.0	1.0	100	2.6	20.3	0.6	1.4
Black Bean, Stir Fry, Morrisons*	1 Serving/50g	92.0	5.0	185	4.1	17.3	10.8	1.5
Black Bean, Stir Fry, Sainsbury's*	½ Pack/75ml	91.0	3.0	121	3.3	17.6	4.3	1.7
Black Bean, Stir Fry, Sharwood's*	1 Jar/195g	191.0	3.0	98	2.2	18.8	1.5	0.6
Black Bean, Stir Fry, Tesco*	½ Jar/220g	297.0	11.0	135	3.4	18.1	4.9	2.5
Black Bean, Uncle Ben's*	1 Serving/125g	89.0	2.0	71	2.0	12.8	1.3	0.0
Black Pepper, Stir Fry, Blue Dragon*	½ Sachet/60g	47.0	3.0	79	1.6	8.4	4.4	0.1
Bolognese, Emilia Romagna, Fresh, Sainsbury's*	½ Pot/150g	99.0	5.0	66	5.9	3.4	3.2	1.7
Bolognese, for Beef, Tesco*	½ Pack/175g	177.0	10.0	101	5.4	6.9	5.8	0.8
Bolognese, Italiano, Tesco*	1 Serving/175g	194.0	13.0	111	5.9	4.8	7.5	0.8
Bolognese, Loyd Grossman*	¼ Jar/106g	79.0	3.0	75	2.0	10.2	2.9	1.4
Bolognese, Original, Deliciously Good, Homepride*	¼ Jar/112g	39.0	0.0	35	1.3	7.1	0.2	0.8
Bolognese, Tinned, Sainsbury's*	1/3 Can/141g	86.0	3.0	61	4.5	5.7	2.2	1.0
Bolognese, Waitrose*	1 Serving/175g	150.0	9.0	86	5.4	5.3	4.9	2.0
Bourguignon, Beef Tonight, Knorr*	¼ Jar/125g	71.0	3.0	57	0.6	7.6	2.6	0.4
Bramley Apple, Colman's*	1 Tbsp/15ml	16.0	0.0	107	0.2	26.5	0.0	1.3
Branston Smooth, Crosse & Blackwell*	1 Serving/25g	35.0	0.0	139	0.6	34.0	0.1	1.4
Brazilian Chicken, Chicken Tonight, Knorr*	¼ Jar/125g	49.0	1.0	39	1.2	7.0	0.7	1.3
Bread, Christmas, Tesco*	1 Serving/60g	64.0	3.0	107	3.3	11.8	5.3	0.5
Bread, Luxury, M & S*	1 Serving/115g	195.0	16.0	170	3.2	8.1	14.1	2.2
Bread, M & S*	1 Serving/85g	153.0	12.0	180	3.1	8.7	14.6	0.2
Bread, Made with Semi-Skimmed Milk	1 Serving/45g	42.0	1.0	93	4.3	12.8	3.1	0.3
Brown, Asda*	1 Serving/10g	10.0	0.0	97	0.7	23.0	0.2	0.4
Brown, Bottled	1 Tsp/6g	6.0	0.0	99	1.1	25.2	0.0	0.7
Brown, Tesco*	1 Tsp/10g	10.0	0.0	104	0.7	25.1	0.1	0.6
Burger, Hellmann's*	1 Tbsp/15g	36.0	3.0	240	1.1	12.0	21.0	0.0
Butter & Tarragon, Chicken Tonight, Knorr*	¼ Jar/125g	132.0	13.0	106	1.0	2.1	10.4	0.7
Butter Chicken, TTD, Sainsbury's*	½ Pack/174g	272.0	24.0	156	1.8	6.7	13.5	0.9
Cantonese Chow Mein Stir Fry, Sainsbury's*	½ Jar/100g	67.0	2.0	67	0.4	12.1	1.9	0.8
Cantonese, Sizzling, Uncle Ben's*	½ Jar/270g	416.0	16.0	154	0.7	24.0	6.1	0.0
Caramelised Onion & Red Wine, M & S*	1 Serving/52g	31.0	2.0	60	1.9	6.7	3.1	0.6
Carbonara, Less Than 5% Fat, GFY, Asda*	½ Tub/150g	121.0	7.0	81	5.0	5.0	4.5	0.5
Carbonara, TTD, Sainsbury's*	½ pot/175g	347.0	31.0	198	5.2	4.5	17.7	0.5

SAUCE

INFO/WEIGHT	Measure	per Measure		Nutrition Values per 100g / 100ml				
		KCAL	FAT	KCAL	PROT	CARB	FAT	FIBRE
Caribbean Curry, Levi Roots*	½ Jar/175g	182.0	14.0	104	0.4	7.2	8.1	0.3
Chasseur, Classic, Chicken Tonight, Knorr*	¼ Jar/125g	61.0	4.0	49	0.6	5.3	2.9	0.7
Chasseur, Cook in, Homepride*	1 Can/390g	160.0	0.0	41	0.7	9.2	0.1	0.4
Cheddar Cheese, Colman's*	1 Serving/85ml	348.0	13.0	410	19.2	48.5	15.4	1.9
Cheddar Cheese, Dry, Knorr*	1 Serving/10g	47.0	3.0	469	7.8	38.0	31.8	0.3
Cheese, Dry, Asda*	1 Serving/27g	101.0	3.0	373	4.4	64.0	11.0	7.0
Cheese, Fresh, Italiano, Tesco*	½ Tub/175g	236.0	16.0	135	6.8	6.2	9.2	0.0
Cheese, Fresh, Waitrose*	1 Pot/350g	458.0	34.0	131	5.1	5.7	9.8	0.0
Cheese, Italian Style, Finest, Tesco*	½ Pot/175g	355.0	21.0	203	10.1	14.0	11.9	0.0
Cheese, Italian, Tesco*	½ Carton/175g	238.0	16.0	136	5.8	8.3	8.9	0.0
Cheese, Italiano, Tesco*	1 Pot/350g	367.0	20.0	105	5.3	8.0	5.7	0.0
Cheese, Made with Semi-Skimmed Milk	1 Serving/60g	107.0	8.0	179	8.1	9.1	12.6	0.2
Cheese, Made with Whole Milk	1 Serving/60g	118.0	9.0	197	8.0	9.0	14.6	0.2
Cheese, Sainsbury's*	1 Serving/125g	140.0	9.0	112	5.0	6.1	7.5	1.2
Cherry Tomato & Fresh Basil, M & S*	1 Serving/175g	131.0	9.0	75	1.2	5.5	5.3	1.1
Cherry Tomato, Finest, Tesco*	½ Pot/171g	120.0	4.0	70	1.5	9.4	2.6	1.1
Chicken, Sizzling, Dolmio*	1 Serving/100g	102.0	7.0	102	1.2	7.5	7.5	0.0
Chickpea & Spinach, Asda*	1 Jar/500g	365.0	14.0	73	3.5	8.4	2.8	2.0
Chilli & Garlic, Blue Dragon*	1 Serving/30ml	25.0	0.0	85	1.1	19.7	0.2	0.0
Chilli & Garlic, Lea & Perrins*	1 Tsp/6g	4.0	0.0	60	1.0	14.9	0.0	0.0
Chilli & Garlic, Stir Fry, M & S*	1 Serving/83g	120.0	1.0	145	0.7	32.4	1.2	1.1
Chilli Con Carne, Asda*	1 Lge Jar/570g	370.0	4.0	65	2.6	12.0	0.7	0.0
Chilli Con Carne, Cook in, BGTY, Sainsbury's*	¼ Jar/125g	69.0	1.0	55	1.7	11.0	0.5	2.5
Chilli Con Carne, Cook in, Homepride*	1 Can/390g	234.0	2.0	60	2.5	11.2	0.6	0.0
Chilli Con Carne, Hot, Sainsbury's*	1 Serving/116g	66.0	0.0	57	2.4	11.3	0.2	1.6
Chilli Con Carne, Hot, Uncle Ben's*	1 Jar/500g	295.0	3.0	59	2.3	10.9	0.6	1.7
Chilli Con Carne, Sizzle & Stir, Knorr*	1 Jar/455g	505.0	32.0	111	2.7	9.1	7.1	2.7
Chilli Con Carne, Weight Watchers*	½ Jar/175g	84.0	0.0	48	1.8	9.7	0.2	2.0
Chilli Soy, Amoy*	1 Tbsp/15g	8.0	0.0	55	4.6	9.1	0.0	0.0
Chilli, Hot, Asda*	1 Jar/570g	445.0	3.0	78	3.7	14.4	0.6	3.2
Chilli, Hot, Blue Dragon*	1 Tbsp/15ml	14.0	0.0	96	0.5	23.0	0.2	0.0
Chilli, Hot, Heinz*	1 Portion/10g	8.0	0.0	80	1.4	18.0	0.0	0.0
Chilli, HP*	1 Tsp/6g	8.0	0.0	134	1.2	32.3	0.0	0.0
Chilli, Sweet, Thai, Dipping, Original, Blue Dragon*	1 Serving/30ml	69.0	0.0	229	0.6	55.1	0.7	1.6
Chilli, Tesco*	1 Tsp/5ml	4.0	0.0	90	1.3	14.0	3.2	1.1
Chilli, Tomato Based, Bottled, Average	*1 Tbsp/15g*	*16.0*	*0.0*	*104*	*2.5*	*19.8*	*0.3*	*5.9*
Chilli, with Kidney Beans, Old El Paso*	1 Serving/115g	92.0	1.0	80	4.3	14.8	0.4	0.0
Chinese 5 Spice, Stir It Up, Chicken Tonight, Knorr*	1 Jar/80g	478.0	40.0	597	2.4	34.1	50.1	6.6
Chinese Orange, Honey & Ginger, Cooking, Sainsbury's*	1 Serving/125g	91.0	0.0	73	0.3	17.2	0.3	0.3
Chinese Stir Fry, Sainsbury's*	½ Sachet/75g	61.0	2.0	81	0.4	14.1	2.5	1.0
Chinese Style, Stir Fry, Fresh, Asda*	½ Sachet/50ml	93.0	6.0	186	1.5	18.0	12.0	0.0
Chinese, Stir Fry, Sachet, Fresh, Sainsbury's*	½ Sachet/51ml	83.0	6.0	163	1.7	14.1	11.1	1.8
Chip Shop Curry, Knorr*	1 Sachet/150ml	145.0	7.0	97	1.7	12.4	4.6	0.7
Chocolate, Dry, Sainsbury's*	1 Serving/30g	108.0	3.0	360	1.3	62.8	11.6	0.9
Chocolate, Sainsbury's*	1 Serving/25g	81.0	2.0	323	1.8	64.7	6.3	2.7
Chop Suey, Blue Dragon*	½ Sachet/60g	34.0	1.0	57	0.5	8.3	2.4	0.5
Chop Suey, Cantonese, Sharwood's*	1 Serving/200g	146.0	3.0	73	0.6	14.4	1.4	0.4
Chop Suey, Stir Fry, Sharwood's*	1 Jar/160g	120.0	2.0	75	0.7	14.6	1.5	0.2
Chow Mein, Sainsbury's*	1 Serving/50g	35.0	1.0	71	1.8	10.5	2.4	0.0
Chow Mein, Stir Fry, Asda*	½ Jar/98g	97.0	1.0	99	1.6	21.0	1.0	0.1
Chow Mein, Stir Fry, Blue Dragon*	1 Sachet/120g	110.0	3.0	92	1.1	15.4	2.9	0.4
Coconut & Green Chilli, Noodle, Tesco*	1 Jar/320g	288.0	22.0	90	0.6	6.2	6.9	0.5
Coconut & Red Chilli, Noodle Sauce, Tesco*	1/3 Jar/110g	88.0	7.0	80	1.7	3.8	6.4	0.7

S

SAUCE

INFO/WEIGHT	Measure KCAL	FAT	KCAL	PROT	CARB	FAT	FIBRE
Coconut RunDown, Levi Roots*	½ Jar/175g	178.0	9.0	102	0.7	13.3	5.0	0.1
Coconut, Chilli & Lime, Cook-In, Homepride*	1 Serving/115g	110.0	9.0	96	1.1	5.9	7.5	0.0
Coconut, Lime & Coriander, Cooking, Nando's*	1 Serving/65g	88.0	6.0	135	1.5	12.1	10.0	1.2
Coconut, Thai Style, Stir Fry, Waitrose*	½ Pack/50ml	52.0	4.0	105	1.5	5.5	8.6	1.8
Cooking, Balti, Extra Special, Asda*	1 Jar/120g	180.0	10.0	150	2.0	17.0	8.0	1.0
Cooking, Honey & Mustard, Light Choices, Tesco*	1 Serving/124g	93.0	2.0	75	1.4	13.0	1.6	1.2
Cooking, Korma, Light Choices, Tesco*	¼ Jar/125g	100.0	4.0	80	1.6	10.2	3.2	1.6
Coronation Chicken, Cook in, Homepride*	1 Serving/250g	232.0	10.0	93	0.8	13.2	4.2	0.0
Coronation, Heinz*	1 Tbsp/10g	33.0	3.0	334	0.8	13.1	31.0	0.9
Country French, Chicken Tonight, Knorr*	¼ Jar/125g	112.0	10.0	90	0.5	4.1	8.0	0.7
Country French, Low Fat, Chicken Tonight, Knorr*	¼ Jar/125g	56.0	4.0	45	0.4	4.4	2.9	0.7
Cranberry & Port, M & S*	1 Serving/75g	71.0	0.0	95	2.3	20.2	0.4	2.1
Cranberry & Red Onion, Sizzling, Homepride*	1 Serving/100g	83.0	1.0	83	0.5	17.7	1.0	0.0
Cranberry, Sainsbury's*	1 Tsp/15g	23.0	0.0	154	0.8	37.1	0.3	1.3
Cranberry, Tesco*	1 Tsp/15g	23.0	0.0	156	0.1	38.8	0.0	0.9
Cranberry, Waitrose*	1 Tbsp/20g	31.0	0.0	156	0.2	38.5	0.2	14.0
Cranberry, with Brandy & Orange Zest, Finest, Tesco*	1 Serving/10g	23.0	0.0	235	0.3	57.2	0.6	1.3
Creamy Ham, Knorr*	1 Pouch/100ml	163.0	16.0	163	0.3	4.0	16.0	0.3
Creamy Horseradish with Garlic, So Good, Somerfield*	1 Tsp/6g	19.0	1.0	317	4.1	25.0	22.3	0.0
Creamy Mushroom, Cooking, M & S*	1 Jar/510g	663.0	58.0	130	1.3	5.4	11.3	0.5
Creamy Mushroom, Knorr*	1 Serving/125g	111.0	10.0	89	0.4	4.5	7.7	0.4
Creamy Peppercorn & Whisky, Baxters*	1 Pack/320g	422.0	35.0	132	1.9	6.7	10.8	0.2
Creamy, Curry, BGTY, Sainsbury's*	¼ Jar/125g	84.0	5.0	67	1.4	6.8	3.8	0.5
Creole, Soulful, Sauce & Spice Mix, Two Step, Discovery*	1 Jar/370g	314.0	7.0	85	1.7	18.0	1.8	3.3
Cumberland Sausage, Colman's*	¼ Jar/126g	43.0	0.0	34	0.7	7.4	0.2	0.8
Curry, 98% Fat Free, Homepride*	1oz/28g	16.0	1.0	56	1.1	8.6	1.9	0.5
Curry, Cook in, Homepride*	½ Can/250g	140.0	5.0	56	1.1	8.6	1.9	0.5
Curry, Creamy, Chicken Tonight, Knorr*	½ Jar/250g	207.0	18.0	83	0.6	3.6	7.4	0.8
Curry, Creamy, Cooking, BGTY, Sainsbury's*	¼ Jar/125g	94.0	4.0	75	1.8	10.1	3.0	1.0
Curry, Deliciously Good, Homepride*	1/3 Jar/149g	91.0	3.0	61	1.1	10.0	1.8	0.5
Curry, Green Thai, BGTY, Sainsbury's*	¼ Jar/125g	61.0	3.0	49	0.6	5.7	2.6	1.4
Curry, Green Thai, Cooking, TTD, Sainsbury's*	½ Pack/175g	152.0	12.0	87	0.9	5.5	6.8	1.0
Curry, Green Thai, Finest, Tesco*	1 Serving/350g	420.0	37.0	120	1.4	4.8	10.6	0.7
Curry, Green Thai, Sharwood's*	1 Serving/403g	431.0	31.0	107	1.1	8.4	7.6	0.1
Curry, Mild, Tesco*	1 Jar/500g	420.0	14.0	84	1.1	13.4	2.8	0.8
Curry, Red Thai, BGTY, Sainsbury's*	1 Serving/124g	77.0	5.0	62	0.6	6.0	3.9	1.4
Curry, Red Thai, Cooking, TTD, Sainsbury's*	½ Pack/175g	159.0	12.0	91	1.1	5.9	7.0	1.3
Curry, Red Thai, Finest, Tesco*	1 Jar/350g	388.0	31.0	111	1.3	6.2	9.0	0.9
Curry, Red Thai, Sainsbury's*	½ Pouch/250g	390.0	36.0	156	1.7	5.0	14.3	1.5
Curry, Red Thai, Sharwood's*	1 Serving/138g	150.0	11.0	109	1.2	7.9	8.0	0.2
Curry, Red Thai, Worldwide Sauces*	1 Jar/450g	630.0	45.0	140	1.5	10.9	10.0	0.0
Curry, Sweet	1 Serving/115g	105.0	6.0	91	1.2	9.6	5.6	1.4
Curry, Thai Coconut, Uncle Ben's*	1 Serving/125g	127.0	6.0	102	1.4	13.2	4.8	0.0
Curry, Value, Tesco*	1 Can/390g	355.0	18.0	91	1.6	11.0	4.5	1.3
Curry, Yellow Thai, Cooking, Sainsbury's*	1 Jar/500g	785.0	70.0	157	2.3	5.4	14.0	2.3
Dark Soy, Sesame & Ginger, for Fish, Schwartz*	1 Pack/300g	279.0	4.0	93	1.3	18.8	1.4	0.5
Dhansak, Medium, Sharwood's*	1 Jar/420g	370.0	13.0	88	3.6	11.1	3.2	1.0
Dhansak, Sharwood's*	1 Jar/445g	667.0	35.0	150	4.7	15.2	7.8	1.4
Dill & Lemon, Delicate, for Fish, Schwartz*	1 Pack/300g	387.0	34.0	129	1.1	5.6	11.4	0.5
Dill & Mustard, for Gravdlax, Dry, Waitrose*	1 Sachet/35g	123.0	9.0	352	2.5	27.8	25.7	0.6
Dipping for Dim Sum, Amoy*	1 Tbsp/15ml	28.0	0.0	190	0.0	48.0	0.0	0.0
Dopiaza, Cooking, Tesco*	1 Serving/166g	176.0	11.0	106	2.2	9.4	6.6	1.9
Dopiaza, Tomato & Onion, Original, in Glass Jar, Patak's*	1 Jar/540g	605.0	39.0	112	1.6	9.8	7.3	1.2

SAUCE

INFO/WEIGHT	Measure	per Measure KCAL	FAT	Nutrition Values per 100g / 100ml KCAL	PROT	CARB	FAT	FIBRE
Dopiaza,medium, Cook in, Sharwood's*	½ Bottle/210g	193.0	11.0	92	1.4	10.2	5.1	0.6
Enchilada, Medium, Old El Paso*	1 Can/270g	92.0	5.0	34	0.0	5.0	1.7	0.0
Exotic Curry, Heinz*	1 Serving/15ml	41.0	3.0	271	0.7	15.3	22.8	0.6
Fajita, Asda*	¼ Jar/125g	79.0	5.0	63	1.0	5.0	4.3	1.0
Fennel & Apricot, Tagine, Moroccan, Seasoned Pioneers*	½ Pouch/200g	136.0	10.0	68	0.9	4.6	5.0	1.2
Firery Guava, Dipping, Levi Roots*	1 Serving/20g	26.0	0.0	128	0.4	31.5	0.0	0.1
Fish Pie, Fresh, The Saucy Fish Co.*	1 Pack/230g	179.0	13.0	78	2.4	4.6	5.6	0.0
Fish, Nuoc Mam, Thai, Blue Dragon*	1 Tsp/5ml	7.0	0.0	145	5.9	30.9	0.1	0.0
Florentina, Italiano, Tesco*	½ Tub/175g	128.0	10.0	73	2.1	3.8	5.5	0.6
for Fajitas, Original Smoky BBQ, Cooking, Old El Paso*	1 Jar/395g	222.0	5.0	56	1.5	9.6	1.3	0.0
for Lasagne, White, Tesco*	1 Jar/460g	506.0	41.0	110	1.9	5.3	9.0	0.6
Four Cheese for Pasta, Asda*	½ Jar/155g	242.0	22.0	156	3.5	3.9	14.0	0.1
Four Cheese, Reduced Fat, Morrisons*	½ Tub/175g	161.0	9.0	92	6.1	4.8	5.4	0.5
Fruity, HP*	1 Tsp/6g	8.0	0.0	141	1.2	35.1	0.1	0.0
Garlic & Chive, Heinz*	1 Serving/10ml	35.0	3.0	350	1.0	11.3	33.2	0.1
Garlic & Chive, Table & Dip, Heinz*	1 Serving/10ml	32.0	3.0	323	1.0	12.1	29.9	0.2
Garlic, Heinz*	1 Serving/10ml	32.0	3.0	323	1.0	12.1	29.9	1.2
Garlic, Lea & Perrins*	1 Tsp/6g	20.0	2.0	337	1.8	17.8	29.0	0.0
Green Peppercorn, Dry, Sainsbury's*	1 Tbsp/15ml	68.0	7.0	455	0.4	3.8	48.5	0.1
Green Tandoori, M & S*	1 Jar/385g	500.0	38.0	130	3.6	6.8	9.9	1.5
Green Thai, Cooking, Perfectly Balanced, Waitrose*	½ Jar/215g	112.0	7.0	52	0.8	4.9	3.2	1.5
Green Thai, Loyd Grossman*	½ Jar/175g	182.0	11.0	104	1.6	10.0	6.4	0.8
Green Thai, Stir Fry, Additions, Tesco*	1 Pack/100g	173.0	16.0	173	2.1	6.1	15.6	0.5
Green Thai, Stir Fry, Asda*	1 Pack/180ml	344.0	27.0	191	2.4	11.1	15.2	1.0
Green Thai, Stir Fry, Fresh Ideas, Tesco*	1 Pack/50g	91.0	8.0	182	2.1	6.2	16.6	0.1
Green Thai, Stir Fry, Sainsbury's*	½ Pack/75g	112.0	8.0	149	1.2	11.9	10.7	1.0
Ham & Mushroom for Pasta, Stir & Serve, Homepride*	1 Serving/100g	95.0	9.0	95	1.5	1.3	9.3	0.0
Hoi Sin & Garlic, Blue Dragon*	1 Serving/60g	80.0	2.0	133	1.2	26.1	2.6	0.0
Hoi Sin & Plum, Chinatown, Knorr*	¼ Jar/131g	96.0	1.0	73	0.8	15.8	0.7	1.2
Hoi Sin & Plum, Sweet & Fruity, Stir Fry, Sharwood's*	1 Serving/136g	128.0	2.0	94	0.7	19.9	1.3	0.9
Hoi Sin & Spring Onion, Stir Fry, Sharwood's*	1 Jar/165g	196.0	2.0	119	1.3	26.5	0.9	0.8
Hoi Sin, M & S*	½ Pot/50ml	80.0	1.0	160	3.2	31.8	2.0	2.2
Hoi Sin, Sharwood's*	1 Tbsp/15g	32.0	0.0	211	2.7	49.5	0.3	0.1
Hoi Sin, Stir Fry, Asda*	1 Serving/100g	165.0	1.0	165	2.6	36.9	0.8	1.0
Hoisin & Plum, Dipping, Finest, Tesco*	1 Serving/50g	78.0	0.0	156	2.3	35.3	0.6	1.4
Hoisin & Plum, Stir Fry, HL, Tesco*	1 Serving/250g	147.0	3.0	59	2.1	9.7	1.3	1.3
Hollandaise, Classic, for Fish, Schwartz*	1 Sachet/300g	456.0	49.0	152	0.7	0.4	16.4	2.0
Hollandaise, Classic, Knorr*	1 Serving/100ml	202.0	20.0	202	0.6	3.9	20.5	0.4
Hollandaise, Dry, Maille*	1 Serving/30g	148.0	15.0	495	1.0	10.8	50.6	0.0
Hollandaise, Finest, Tesco*	1 Serving/98g	473.0	44.0	485	1.4	17.2	45.6	0.3
Hollandaise, Fresh, Average	1 Pack/150g	342.0	32.0	228	2.4	6.1	21.6	0.0
Hollandaise, Full Fat, Dry, M & S*	1 Tbsp/20g	67.0	7.0	336	1.1	4.5	34.9	0.1
Hollandaise, Homemade, Average	1oz/28g	198.0	21.0	707	4.8	0.0	76.2	0.0
Hollandaise, M & S*	1 Serving/10g	41.0	4.0	410	0.9	3.6	43.6	0.5
Hollandaise, Mary Berry*	1 Serving/100g	472.0	44.0	472	1.4	17.8	43.8	0.3
Hollandaise, Sainsbury's*	1 Tbsp/15g	72.0	8.0	478	0.2	5.9	50.4	0.4
Honey & Coriander, Stir Fry, Blue Dragon*	1 Pack/120g	115.0	1.0	96	0.5	22.1	0.6	0.3
Honey & Mustard, Chicken Tonight, Knorr*	¼ Jar/131.25g	139.0	6.0	106	0.8	15.1	4.7	0.6
Honey & Mustard, COU, M & S*	½ Jar/160g	112.0	5.0	70	2.3	9.2	2.9	0.7
Honey & Mustard, for Cooking, Asda*	1 Serving/200g	234.0	14.0	117	0.6	13.0	7.0	0.0
Honey & Mustard, Low Fat, Chicken Tonight, Knorr*	¼ Jar/131g	105.0	3.0	80	1.0	13.8	2.3	0.8
Horseradish, Colman's*	1 Tbsp/15ml	17.0	1.0	112	1.9	9.8	6.2	2.6
Horseradish, Creamed, Colman's*	1 Tsp/16g	37.0	2.0	229	4.3	21.4	13.3	0.0

S

SAUCE

INFO/WEIGHT	Measure		per Measure		Nutrition Values per 100g / 100ml				
			KCAL	FAT	KCAL	PROT	CARB	FAT	FIBRE
Horseradish, Creamed, M & S*	1 Tsp/5g		16.0	1.0	325	2.4	12.1	29.3	2.5
Horseradish, Creamed, Waitrose*	1 Tbsp/16g		30.0	2.0	185	2.4	19.6	9.9	2.3
Horseradish, Creamy, Sainsbury's*	1 Tsp/5g		11.0	1.0	223	2.8	28.9	11.8	1.6
Horseradish, Hot, Tesco*	1 Tsp/5g		9.0	1.0	185	2.3	19.7	10.6	2.3
Horseradish, Mustard, Sainsbury's*	1 Tsp/5g		8.0	0.0	163	7.9	18.2	6.6	3.5
Horseradish, Sainsbury's*	1 Dtsp/10g		14.0	1.0	145	1.5	17.8	6.6	2.4
Hot Bean, Har Har Pickle Food Factory*	1 Tbsp/10g		4.0	0.0	40	0.0	10.0	0.0	10.0
Hot Chilli, Deliciously Good, Homepride*	1 Serving/120g		62.0	1.0	52	1.3	10.6	0.5	1.1
Hot Chilli, Sharwood's*	1 fl oz/30ml		36.0	0.0	120	0.5	29.4	0.6	1.3
Hot Onion, Sainsbury's*	1 Serving/10g		17.0	0.0	167	0.2	41.0	0.1	0.1
Hot Pepper	1oz/28g		7.0	0.0	26	1.6	1.7	1.5	0.0
Hot Pepper, Encona*	1 Tsp/5ml		3.0	0.0	52	0.5	10.5	1.2	0.0
Hot, Cholula Hot Sauce*	1 Tbsp/12g		3.0	0.0	22	1.0	2.5	1.0	0.0
HP*	1 Tbsp/15g		18.0	0.0	119	1.1	27.1	0.2	1.3
Indian Tikka, Chicken Tonight, Knorr*	1 Serving/250g		320.0	23.0	128	1.3	10.0	9.2	1.2
Italian Hot Chilli, Dolmio*	½ Pack/150g		103.0	6.0	69	1.3	7.1	3.9	0.0
Italian Onion & Garlic, Sainsbury's*	1 Jar/500g		375.0	10.0	75	2.2	12.1	2.0	1.7
Italian Tomato & Mascarpone, Sainsbury's*	½ Tub/175g		157.0	10.0	90	2.6	6.8	5.8	1.2
Italian Tomato & Sweet Basil, Go Organic*	1 Serving/80g		51.0	4.0	64	1.2	4.3	4.7	0.9
Italian, Basil & Onion, Slow Cooked, Dolmio*	1 Jar/350g		322.0	24.0	92	1.8	5.6	7.0	1.3
Italian, Tomato & Mascarpone, Tesco*	½ Tub/175g		159.0	11.0	91	2.7	5.9	6.3	0.7
Jalfrezi, Cooking, Asda*	1 Jar/570g		519.0	36.0	91	1.2	7.4	6.3	1.7
Jalfrezi, Cooking, Sainsbury's*	1 Serving/250g		160.0	6.0	64	1.0	9.6	2.4	1.7
Jalfrezi, Stir Fry, Patak's*	1 Jar/250g		260.0	19.0	104	1.4	7.6	7.5	1.4
Jalfrezi, Sweet Pepper & Coconut, in Glass Jar, Patak's*	1 Jar/540g		626.0	38.0	116	1.7	11.3	7.0	1.4
Jalfrezi, TTD, Sainsbury's*	½ Jar/175g		205.0	17.0	117	1.3	6.4	9.6	1.5
Jamaican Jerk, Stir It Up, Chicken Tonight, Knorr*	1 Jar/80g		506.0	43.0	633	3.9	20.9	53.9	5.4
Jerk/Bbq, Levi Roots*	¼ Bottle/78g		94.0	0.0	121	1.1	28.8	0.1	0.5
Kaffir Lime Chilli & Basil, Stir Fry, Sainsbury's*	1 Serving/150g		157.0	10.0	105	1.2	10.6	6.4	1.0
Kashmiri, Chilli & Peppers, Patak's*	½ Jar/212g		159.0	9.0	75	1.3	7.7	4.4	1.1
Kashmiri, Sharwood's*	½ Bottle/210g		231.0	11.0	110	3.0	13.0	5.1	1.5
Korma With Flaked Almonds, Weight Watchers*	1 Serving/175g		107.0	4.0	61	2.0	8.5	2.1	1.6
Korma, Asda*	1 Serving/225g		434.0	34.0	193	2.5	12.0	15.0	2.2
Korma, Authentic, VLH Kitchens	1 Serving/118g		180.0	15.0	153	1.9	6.7	13.0	0.8
Korma, Cooking, BGTY, Sainsbury's*	¼ Jar/125g		100.0	3.0	80	1.1	12.9	2.7	1.2
Korma, Deliciously Good, Homepride*	1 Jar/450g		396.0	20.0	88	1.4	10.6	4.4	1.4
Korma, Free From, Sainsbury's*	½ Jar/175g		191.0	14.0	109	1.9	7.6	7.9	1.2
Korma, Royal, TTD, Sainsbury's*	½ Pack/175g		207.0	12.0	118	2.4	11.4	7.0	3.9
Korma, Sharwood's*	1 Serving/105g		150.0	10.0	143	1.4	12.2	9.8	1.8
Korma, Sizzle & Stir, Knorr*	1 Jar/455g		1092.0	96.0	240	1.2	11.2	21.2	2.7
Korma, Tesco*	¼ Jar/125g		192.0	15.0	154	2.4	9.9	11.7	1.3
Laksa, Finest, Tesco*	1/3 Jar/111g		105.0	8.0	95	1.3	5.5	7.4	1.8
Lamb Hot Pot, for Cooking, Dry, Asda*	1 Pack/42g		147.0	3.0	351	7.0	65.0	7.0	3.3
Lemon & Ginger, Stir Fry, Finest, Tesco*	¼ Jar/85g		144.0	0.0	169	0.2	41.7	0.2	0.2
Lemon & Sesame, Stir Fry, Sharwood's*	1 Serving/100g		125.0	0.0	125	0.1	30.9	0.1	0.1
Lemon, Amoy*	1 Tsp/5ml		5.0	0.0	104	0.0	26.0	0.0	0.0
Lemon, Stir Fry, Straight to Wok, Amoy*	½ Sachet/50g		81.0	0.0	162	0.3	40.0	0.2	0.0
Lemon, Stir Fry, Tesco*	1 Jar/450g		369.0	1.0	82	0.1	19.3	0.2	0.1
Madras, Cooking, HL, Tesco*	1 Serving/128g		55.0	3.0	43	1.6	4.8	2.0	2.3
Mango, Kashmiri Style, Finest, Tesco*	½ Jar/175g		285.0	24.0	163	2.4	7.7	13.6	0.9
Marie Rose, Fresh, The Saucy Fish Co.*	1 Pack/150g		589.0	60.0	393	1.6	7.0	39.8	0.0
Mediterranean Tomato, Spread & Bake, Heinz*	¼ Jar/70g		56.0	2.0	80	1.3	13.8	2.5	1.9
Mediterranean Vegetable, Chargrilled, Italiano, Tesco*	1 Pot/350g		175.0	4.0	50	1.6	8.4	1.1	1.3

SAUCE

Measure INFO/WEIGHT	per Measure KCAL	FAT	Nutrition Values per 100g / 100ml KCAL	PROT	CARB	FAT	FIBRE

	Measure INFO/WEIGHT	per Measure KCAL	per Measure FAT	KCAL	PROT	CARB	FAT	FIBRE
Mediterranean Vegetable, M & S*	1 Pot/350g	227.0	12.0	65	1.7	6.8	3.3	2.0
Mediterranean Vegetables, Stir in, BGTY, Sainsbury's*	1 Jar/150g	123.0	6.0	82	1.9	9.0	4.3	1.4
Mexican, Cooking, BGTY, Sainsbury's*	¼ Jar/124g	51.0	0.0	41	0.7	9.2	0.2	0.8
Mint Garden, Fresh, Tesco*	1 Tsp/5g	2.0	0.0	40	2.6	3.6	0.4	1.5
Mint, Sainsbury's*	1 Dtsp/10g	13.0	0.0	126	2.5	28.7	0.1	4.0
Mornay, Cheese, Asda*	¼ Pot/71g	114.0	9.0	161	6.8	6.6	12.7	0.4
Moroccan Chicken, Chicken Tonight, Knorr*	¼ Jar/125g	91.0	2.0	73	0.4	14.7	1.3	1.4
Moroccan Tagine, Loyd Grossman*	1oz/28g	16.0	1.0	58	1.1	5.9	3.3	0.4
Moroccan, Spread & Bake, Heinz*	¼ Jar/70g	64.0	2.0	91	1.7	15.8	2.3	2.1
Mushroom & Garlic, 95% Fat Free, Homepride*	1 Serving/220g	154.0	9.0	70	0.9	7.0	4.2	0.3
Mushroom & Herb, Cooking, BGTY, Sainsbury's*	¼ Jar/125g	67.0	3.0	54	1.8	6.6	2.3	0.5
Mushroom, Creamy, Asda*	1 Serving/125g	76.0	5.0	61	0.8	6.0	3.7	0.5
Mushroom, Creamy, Chicken Tonight, Knorr*	¼ Jar/125g	101.0	8.0	81	0.8	5.4	6.3	0.3
Mushroom, Creamy, Low Fat, Chicken Tonight, Knorr*	¼ Jar/125g	59.0	4.0	47	0.8	7.3	2.9	0.4
Mushroom, Creamy, Tesco*	½ Pot/175g	142.0	10.0	81	1.5	5.6	5.8	0.4
Mushroom, Not Just for Pasta, Sainsbury's*	½ Pot/150g	91.0	7.0	61	1.7	3.6	4.4	0.9
Mushroom, Schwartz*	1 Pack/170g	207.0	19.0	122	1.2	3.9	11.3	0.5
Napoletana, Fresh, Sainsbury's*	½ Pot/150g	94.0	4.0	63	1.7	7.3	3.0	2.3
Napoletana, Italian, Tesco*	1 Pot/350g	178.0	4.0	51	1.5	8.5	1.2	1.0
Napoletana, Organic, Tesco*	½ Pot/175g	70.0	1.0	40	1.3	7.3	0.6	1.0
Napoletana, Waitrose*	1 Pot/600g	252.0	8.0	42	1.8	5.5	1.4	1.7
Onion, Made with Semi-Skimmed Milk	1 Serving/60g	52.0	3.0	86	2.9	8.4	5.0	0.4
Onion, Made with Skimmed Milk	1 Serving/60g	46.0	2.0	77	2.9	8.4	4.0	0.4
Orange & Dill Sauce, for Fish, Zesty, Schwartz*	1 Pack/300g	180.0	1.0	60	0.4	13.5	0.5	0.5
Orange & Green Ginger, Blue Dragon*	1 Pack/120g	118.0	2.0	98	0.5	20.4	1.6	0.5
Oriental Orange & Ginger, Homepride*	1 Serving/100g	68.0	0.0	68	0.7	15.9	0.1	0.0
Oriental Sweet & Sour, Express, Uncle Ben's*	1 Serving/170g	221.0	3.0	130	0.8	27.5	1.9	0.0
Oriental, Cantonese, Uncle Ben's*	¼ Jar/125g	107.0	0.0	86	0.8	20.3	0.2	1.2
Oriental, Mary Berry*	1 Serving/100g	316.0	18.0	316	2.0	36.4	17.8	0.8
Oyster & Garlic, Stir Fry, Straight to Wok, Amoy*	½ Pack/50g	97.0	1.0	195	4.9	37.0	3.0	0.0
Oyster & Spring Onion, Stir Fry, Blue Dragon*	1 Sachet/120g	110.0	1.0	92	1.6	19.9	0.7	1.1
Oyster, Blue Dragon*	1 Tsp/5ml	6.0	0.0	121	3.4	26.9	0.0	0.0
Oyster, Stir Fry, Sainsbury's*	1 Tbsp/15g	9.0	0.0	61	1.6	13.3	0.1	0.2
Paprika Chicken, Chicken Tonight, Knorr*	½ Jar/250g	240.0	22.0	96	0.9	3.5	8.7	1.4
Parsley Lemon Caper, New Covent Garden Food Co*	¼ Carton/65ml	137.0	12.0	211	2.5	8.7	18.6	0.8
Parsley, Fresh, Sainsbury's*	½ Pot/150g	117.0	8.0	78	2.0	5.9	5.1	0.5
Parsley, Instant, Dry, Asda*	1 Serving/23g	82.0	2.0	355	7.0	66.0	7.0	4.4
Parsley, Instant, Made Up, Semi Skim Milk, Sainsbury's*	¼ Sachet/51ml	34.0	1.0	67	3.5	8.6	2.1	0.1
Parsley, Tesco*	½ Pack/89g	85.0	5.0	95	2.8	8.1	5.7	1.1
Peanut, Sainsbury's*	1 Sachet/70g	185.0	9.0	264	1.9	34.7	13.1	1.6
Peking Lemon, Stir Fry, Blue Dragon*	1 Serving/35g	58.0	1.0	166	0.3	36.8	1.9	0.1
Pepper & Tomato, Spicy, Stir Through, M & S*	½ Jar/95g	166.0	15.0	175	1.6	7.5	15.4	0.0
Pepper, Creamy, Schwartz*	1 Pack/170g	116.0	9.0	68	1.5	3.4	5.4	1.0
Pepper, Creamy, Tesco*	1 Serving/85ml	128.0	11.0	151	1.2	6.4	13.4	0.5
Peppercorn, Creamy, Asda*	¼ Jar/137g	137.0	11.0	100	1.1	6.0	8.0	0.2
Peppercorn, Creamy, Chicken Tonight, Knorr*	¼ Jar/125g	110.0	10.0	88	0.3	3.8	7.8	0.4
Peri-Peri, Extra Hot, Nando's*	1 Serving/5g	3.0	0.0	58	0.0	5.6	3.8	0.2
Peri-Peri, Hot, Nando's*	1 Serving/5g	3.0	0.0	65	0.0	5.2	4.8	0.6
Peri-Peri, Sweet, Nando's*	1 Tbsp/25g	35.0	1.0	142	0.5	30.7	2.1	0.0
Pesto, Green, Alla Genovese, Finest, Tesco*	1 Serving/65g	188.0	26.0	290	5.7	1.5	39.6	2.8
Pesto, Green, Classic, Sacla*	1 Serving/40g	185.0	19.0	462	5.2	7.6	46.5	0.0
Pineapple & Red Pepper, Kwazulu, New World, Knorr*	1 Pack/500g	260.0	0.0	52	0.2	12.4	0.1	0.5
Pineapple Juice & Sweet Chilli, Stir Fry, M & S*	1 Pot/120g	192.0	1.0	160	1.6	36.8	0.5	0.5

S

SAUCE

Piquant Pepper Coriander & Lime, Sainsbury's*	1/3 Pot/100g	43.0	0.0	43	1.2	8.4	0.5	0.8
Plum & Ginger, Stir Fry, Asda*	½ Jar/97g	94.0	1.0	97	0.7	22.0	0.7	0.3
Plum & Mandarin, Sichuan, Chinese, Seasoned Pioneers*	1 Pouch/400g	328.0	17.0	82	0.7	12.4	4.3	2.3
Plum & Sesame, Stir Fry, M & S*	½ Jar/115g	138.0	0.0	120	0.9	29.0	0.1	1.8
Plum, Spiced, Heinz*	1 Serving/25g	32.0	0.0	128	0.5	31.1	0.1	1.0
Prawn Cocktail, Frank Cooper*	1 Tbsp/15g	47.0	4.0	316	0.8	18.3	26.7	0.1
Puttanesca, Fresh, Waitrose*	½ Pot/176g	118.0	8.0	67	1.8	6.2	4.4	1.2
Red & Yellow Pepper, Roasted, Sacla*	1 Serving/290g	232.0	17.0	80	1.1	5.5	5.9	0.0
Red Pepper, Fresh, Asda*	¼ Pot/82g	35.0	1.0	43	1.4	6.8	1.2	1.1
Red Pepper, GFY, Asda*	1 Serving/100g	43.0	1.0	43	1.2	7.0	1.1	0.0
Red Pepper, Sainsbury's*	1 Serving/37g	118.0	12.0	320	4.3	5.0	31.4	0.0
Red Thai, Cooking, Perfectly Balanced, Waitrose*	1 Jar/430g	267.0	15.0	62	1.1	6.2	3.6	1.6
Red Wine & Onion, Rich, Simply Sausages, Colman's*	¼ Jar/125g	49.0	0.0	39	0.9	8.5	0.2	1.3
Red Wine, Cook in, Homepride*	¼ Can/98g	47.0	1.0	48	0.5	10.1	0.6	0.0
Red Wine, Cooking, BGTY, Sainsbury's*	1 Serving/125g	52.0	1.0	42	0.5	8.8	0.5	0.8
Red Wine, Cooking, Homepride*	1 Serving/250ml	115.0	1.0	46	0.4	9.8	0.6	0.0
Redcurrant, Colman's*	1 Tsp/12g	44.0	0.0	368	0.7	90.0	0.0	0.0
Reggae Reggae, Cooking, Levi Roots*	½ Jar/175g	215.0	1.0	123	1.3	28.5	0.5	0.7
Reggae Reggae, Jerk Bbq, Levi Roots*	1 Jar/310g	375.0	0.0	121	1.1	28.8	0.1	0.5
Risotto, Mushroom & White Wine, Sacla*	1 Serving/95g	151.0	12.0	159	3.7	6.9	13.0	0.0
Roast Vegetable with Basil & Tomato, M & S*	1 Serving/100g	85.0	4.0	85	2.0	9.5	4.1	1.2
Roasted Peanut Satay, Stir Fry Sensations, Amoy*	1 Pouch/160g	354.0	20.0	221	4.7	21.9	12.4	1.0
Roasted Vegetable, Finest, Tesco*	1 Serving/175g	101.0	4.0	58	1.4	7.8	2.4	1.0
Rogan Josh, 99% Fat Free, Homepride*	1/3 Jar/153g	92.0	1.0	60	1.8	11.6	0.7	2.0
Rogan Josh, Asda*	¼ Jar/125g	135.0	10.0	108	0.9	8.0	8.0	0.6
Rogan Josh, Cooking, Light Choices, Tesco*	¼ Jar/125g	57.0	3.0	46	1.4	4.8	2.4	2.5
Rogan Josh, Medium, Sharwood's*	½ Jar/210g	151.0	8.0	72	1.4	8.6	3.6	0.5
Rogan Josh, Sharwood's*	½ Jar/210g	220.0	17.0	105	1.2	7.0	8.0	1.5
Rogan Josh, Tesco*	½ Can/220g	156.0	10.0	71	1.3	5.9	4.7	1.4
Rogan Josh, VLH Kitchens	1 Serving/460g	374.0	24.0	81	1.4	6.1	5.3	1.4
Royal Korma, Tilda*	1 Pack/400ml	824.0	73.0	206	1.9	8.4	18.3	0.7
Satay, Stir Fry & Dipping, Finest, Tesco*	1 Tsp/5g	22.0	2.0	432	9.0	20.7	34.8	2.7
Sausage Casserole, Cook in, Homepride*	½ Jar/250g	92.0	0.0	37	0.7	8.0	0.2	0.6
Seafood, 25% Less Fat, Tesco*	1 Tsp/5g	17.0	1.0	344	2.7	18.2	28.5	0.3
Seafood, Colman's*	1 Tbsp/15g	44.0	3.0	296	0.9	21.5	22.9	0.4
Seafood, Sainsbury's*	1 Tbsp/15g	49.0	4.0	330	0.7	17.6	28.2	0.1
Seafood, Tesco*	1 Serving/10g	46.0	4.0	465	1.8	15.6	43.5	0.3
Sizzling Szechuan, Uncle Ben's*	1 Serving/260g	289.0	18.0	111	0.9	10.8	7.1	0.0
Smoked Bacon & Tomato, Stir in, Dolmio*	½ Tub/75g	73.0	4.0	98	4.6	7.2	5.6	1.3
Smoked Ham & Cheese, for Pasta, Eat Smart, Safeway*	1 Serving/125g	94.0	3.0	75	5.8	6.1	2.5	0.9
Smoked Paprika & Tomato, M & S*	1 Serving/300g	135.0	5.0	45	1.3	6.1	1.7	0.9
Soy & Garlic, Stir Fry, Fresh Tastes, Asda*	1 Pack/180g	175.0	7.0	97	1.7	14.1	3.7	0.5
Soy, Average	1 Tsp/5ml	3.0	0.0	64	8.7	8.3	0.0	0.0
Soy, Dark, Amoy*	1 Tsp/5ml	5.0	0.0	106	0.9	25.6	0.0	0.0
Soy, Light, Amoy*	1 Tsp/5ml	3.0	0.0	52	2.5	10.5	0.0	0.0
Soy, Light, Asda*	1 Tbsp/15ml	7.0	0.0	47	0.8	11.0	0.0	0.0
Soy, Light, Sharwood's*	1 Tsp/5ml	2.0	0.0	37	2.7	6.4	0.2	0.0
Soy, Naturally Brewed, Kikkoman*	1 Tbsp/15g	11.0	0.0	74	10.3	8.1	0.0	0.0
Soy, Premium, Light, Heinz*	1 Serving/15g	11.0	0.0	71	7.4	9.1	0.5	0.0
Soy, Reduced Salt, Amoy*	1 Tsp/5ml	3.0	0.0	56	4.0	10.0	0.0	0.0
Soy, Rich, Sharwood's*	1 Tsp/5ml	4.0	0.0	79	3.1	16.6	0.4	0.0
Soy, Wasabi & Lemon Grass, Stir Fry, Finest, Tesco*	1 Pack/125g	119.0	3.0	95	1.5	16.3	2.2	0.9
Soya, Japanese, Waitrose*	1 Tbsp/15ml	11.0	0.0	74	7.7	9.4	0.6	0.8

SAUCE

	Measure INFO/WEIGHT	per Measure KCAL	FAT	Nutrition Values per 100g / 100ml KCAL	PROT	CARB	FAT	FIBRE
Spanish Chicken, Chicken Tonight, Knorr*	½ Jar/250g	115.0	3.0	46	1.5	7.0	1.4	0.6
Spanish Style, Cooking, Light Choices, Tesco*	1 Jar/485g	131.0	1.0	27	1.0	5.0	0.3	1.4
Spiced Tomato Tagine, Sainsbury's*	1 Jar/355g	227.0	6.0	64	1.7	10.6	1.6	4.3
Spicy Durban, New World, Knorr*	1 Pack/500g	305.0	13.0	61	0.6	8.7	2.7	0.4
Spicy Pepper, Eat Smart, Safeway*	1 Serving/84g	42.0	1.0	50	1.4	7.0	1.7	1.3
Spicy Pepperoni & Tomato, Stir in, Dolmio*	½ Pack/75g	115.0	9.0	154	3.3	9.3	11.6	0.8
Spicy Red Pepper & Roasted Vegetable, Sainsbury's*	1 Pot/302g	220.0	10.0	73	1.5	8.9	3.4	1.0
Spicy Sweet & Sour, Sharwood's*	1 Serving/138g	142.0	1.0	103	0.7	23.8	0.5	0.4
Spicy Tomato & Pesto, COU, M & S*	1 Serving/100g	60.0	2.0	60	2.2	6.8	2.5	1.3
Sticky BBQ, Spread & Bake, Heinz*	¼ Jar/78g	131.0	0.0	168	1.0	39.6	0.6	1.2
Sticky Plum, Stir Fry, Blue Dragon*	1 Serving/60g	145.0	0.0	242	0.1	35.6	0.3	0.0
Sticky Ribz, Ainsley Harriott*	1 Serving/50g	107.0	0.0	214	0.4	52.2	0.1	0.0
Stir Fry, Chinese, Tesco*	1 Serving/46g	55.0	3.0	120	2.1	14.2	5.6	0.8
Stir Fry, Chinese, With Soy, Ginger & Garlic, Tesco*	1 Pack/150g	180.0	8.0	120	2.1	14.2	5.6	0.8
Stir Fry, Chow Mein, Safeway*	1 Serving/105g	79.0	1.0	75	1.1	16.2	0.6	1.3
Stir Fry, Laksa, Cook Asian, M & S*	½ Pack/75g	82.0	6.0	110	0.9	8.9	8.0	1.0
Stir Fry, Pad Thai, Tesco*	1 Pack/125g	112.0	3.0	90	1.3	15.8	2.3	0.8
Stroganoff, Asda*	1 Serving/285g	305.0	26.0	107	1.5	5.0	9.0	0.3
Stroganoff, Mushroom, Creamy, M & S*	1 Serving/75g	86.0	7.0	115	3.3	4.8	9.2	0.6
Stroganoff, Tesco*	1 Serving/100g	89.0	7.0	89	0.7	5.3	7.3	0.4
Sun Dried Tomato & Basil, Free From, Sainsbury's*	1 Serving/175g	126.0	5.0	72	2.9	8.7	2.8	1.5
Sun Dried Tomato & Basil, Seeds of Change*	1 Serving/100g	169.0	13.0	169	1.8	9.3	13.2	0.0
Sun Dried Tomato for Pasta, Stir & Serve, Homepride*	1 Serving/100g	62.0	3.0	62	1.0	7.6	3.0	0.0
Sun Dried Tomato, Heinz*	1 Serving/10ml	7.0	0.0	73	1.5	14.9	0.6	0.9
Sun Dried Tomato, Mozzarella & Basil, Safeway*	½ Pot/159g	175.0	11.0	110	3.5	8.7	6.7	1.4
Sweet & Sour, Cantonese, Loyd Grossman*	1 Serving/225g	306.0	5.0	136	1.2	28.0	2.1	0.5
Sweet & Sour, Chinese, Sainsbury's*	½ Jar/150g	222.0	0.0	148	0.2	36.6	0.1	0.1
Sweet & Sour, Classic, Canned, Homepride*	1 Can/500g	440.0	0.0	88	0.3	21.5	0.1	0.5
Sweet & Sour, Extra Pineapple, Asda*	¼ Jar/148g	138.0	0.0	93	0.5	22.0	0.3	0.3
Sweet & Sour, Fresh, Sainsbury's*	1 Sachet/50ml	102.0	4.0	205	0.8	31.2	8.6	0.3
Sweet & Sour, GFY, Asda*	½ Jar/164g	77.0	0.0	47	0.4	11.0	0.2	0.3
Sweet & Sour, Organic, Seeds of Change*	1 Jar/350g	350.0	0.0	100	0.4	24.4	0.1	0.6
Sweet & Sour, Peking Style, Finest, Tesco*	1 Serving/175g	147.0	0.0	84	0.6	20.1	0.1	0.5
Sweet & Sour, Spicy, Uncle Ben's*	1 Jar/400g	364.0	0.0	91	0.6	22.1	0.1	0.0
Sweet & Sour, Stir Fry, Blue Dragon*	1 Sachet/120g	137.0	1.0	114	0.6	25.6	1.1	0.6
Sweet & Sour, Stir Fry, M & S*	1 Pack/120g	150.0	0.0	125	0.7	29.8	0.4	1.3
Sweet & Sour, Stir Fry, Waitrose*	1 Serving/50ml	93.0	2.0	187	1.2	35.6	4.4	1.8
Sweet & Sour, Take-Away	1oz/28g	44.0	1.0	157	0.2	32.8	3.4	0.0
Sweet & Sour, Weight Watchers*	½ Jar/125g	61.0	0.0	49	0.6	11.5	0.1	0.2
Sweet Barbecue, 97% Fat Free, Homepride*	1 Serving/230g	166.0	6.0	72	1.4	11.7	2.7	2.3
Sweet Barbecue, Deliciously Good, Homepride*	1/3 Jar/149g	110.0	3.0	74	1.4	12.0	2.2	1.2
Sweet Chilli & Coriander, Sharwood's*	1 Pack/370g	407.0	4.0	110	0.3	24.4	1.2	0.1
Sweet Chilli & Coriander, Sizzling, Homepride*	1 Serving/100g	51.0	0.0	51	0.7	11.5	0.2	0.0
Sweet Chilli & Garlic Noodle, Sharwood's*	1oz/28g	30.0	1.0	107	0.9	18.9	3.1	0.4
Sweet Chilli & Garlic, Stir Fry & Dipping, Tesco*	½ Jar/95ml	78.0	0.0	82	0.3	20.1	0.0	0.1
Sweet Chilli & Lemon Grass, Stir Fry, Sharwood's*	1 Serving/155g	127.0	0.0	82	0.3	19.7	0.1	0.3
Sweet Chilli & Lime, Chinatown, Knorr*	1 Jar/525g	635.0	17.0	121	0.6	22.0	3.3	0.5
Sweet Chilli, Garlic, Stir Fry, Blue Dragon*	1 Pack/120g	192.0	0.0	160	0.1	22.8	0.3	0.2
Sweet Chilli, Heinz*	1 Serving/25g	37.0	0.0	150	0.3	36.5	0.4	6.4
Sweet Chilli, Sharwood's*	1 Bottle/150ml	325.0	1.0	217	0.7	52.8	0.4	1.7
Sweet Chilli, Stir Fry, Additions, Tesco*	1 Serving/50g	105.0	4.0	211	0.3	35.2	7.6	0.6
Sweet Chilli, Stir Fry, BGTY, Sainsbury's*	1 Pack/150ml	178.0	3.0	119	0.6	25.0	1.9	1.1
Sweet Pepper, Stir in, Dolmio*	½ Pot/75g	103.0	8.0	137	1.5	9.7	10.3	0.0

SAUCE

INFO/WEIGHT	Measure	per Measure		Nutrition Values per 100g / 100ml				
		KCAL	FAT	KCAL	PROT	CARB	FAT	FIBRE
Sweet Soy & Sesame, Uncle Ben's*	1 Serving/100g	110.0	2.0	110	0.7	23.0	1.7	0.0
Sweet Soy & Spring Onion, Stir Fry Sensations, Amoy*	1 Pouch/160g	312.0	10.0	195	2.0	31.5	6.5	0.6
Szechuan Style, Stir Fry, Fresh Ideas, Tesco*	1 Sachet/50g	114.0	5.0	228	1.9	33.4	9.7	0.1
Szechuan, Spicy Tomato, Stir Fry, Blue Dragon*	1 Sachet/120g	151.0	7.0	126	1.3	17.6	5.6	2.0
Szechuan, Stir Fry, Sharwood's*	1 Jar/150g	126.0	2.0	84	3.0	15.5	1.1	0.4
Tabasco, Tabasco*	1 Tsp/5ml	1.0	0.0	12	1.3	0.8	0.8	0.6
Tamarind & Lime, Stir Fry, Sainsbury's*	1 Serving/75g	88.0	6.0	117	1.1	11.4	7.4	0.8
Tartare	1oz/28g	84.0	7.0	299	1.3	17.9	24.6	0.0
Tartare, with Olives, The English Provender Co.*	1 Tbsp/15g	64.0	7.0	425	2.2	5.7	43.7	0.7
Teriyaki, Fresh, The Saucy Fish Co.*	1 Pack/150g	318.0	3.0	212	2.8	45.8	1.9	0.0
Teriyaki, Stir Fry, Blue Dragon*	1 Sachet/120g	208.0	0.0	173	2.0	28.6	0.0	0.0
Teriyaki, Stir Fry, Fresh Ideas, Tesco*	1 Serving/25g	33.0	1.0	133	1.1	26.9	2.3	0.0
Teriyaki, Stir Fry, Sharwood's*	1 Jar/150g	144.0	0.0	96	0.9	22.5	0.3	0.3
Thai Curry, Yellow, Loyd Grossman*	1 Serving/100g	111.0	7.0	111	1.7	9.1	7.5	1.0
Thai Green, Barts*	½ Pack/150ml	210.0	18.0	140	2.0	6.0	12.0	0.0
Thai Kaffir Lime, Chilli & Basil, Stir Fry, Sainsbury's*	½ Jar/175g	166.0	10.0	95	1.3	9.2	5.9	1.1
Thai, Lemongrass, Lime, & Chilli, Stir Fry, Sainsbury's*	1 Serving/50ml	145.0	13.0	290	4.0	10.2	26.5	3.5
Tikka Masala for One, Express, Uncle Ben's*	1 Sachet/170g	168.0	11.0	99	1.5	9.0	6.3	0.0
Tikka Masala, 98% Fat Free, Homepride*	1oz/28g	14.0	0.0	49	1.4	7.9	1.7	0.8
Tikka Masala, Cooking, Sharwood's*	1 Tsp/2g	2.0	0.0	122	1.2	11.9	7.8	0.9
Tikka Masala, GFY, Asda*	½ Jar/250g	190.0	8.0	76	2.9	9.0	3.2	0.5
Tikka Masala, Perfectly Balanced, Waitrose*	½ Jar/175g	107.0	1.0	61	2.7	10.7	0.8	1.5
Tikka Masala, Weight Watchers*	1 Jar/350g	259.0	7.0	74	2.6	11.2	2.1	0.7
Tikka, BFY, Morrisons*	½ Jar/238g	259.0	8.0	109	2.3	17.2	3.4	1.3
Tikka, Cooking, BGTY, Sainsbury's*	1 Jar/500g	370.0	9.0	74	1.2	12.9	1.9	0.3
Tikka, Indian Style, Iceland*	1 Serving/225g	283.0	17.0	126	1.7	12.9	7.5	2.2
Toffee, GFY, Asda*	1 Serving/5g	15.0	0.0	306	2.2	68.0	2.8	0.0
Toffee, Luxury, Rowse*	1 Serving/20g	67.0	1.0	336	1.9	73.9	3.7	0.4
Tomato & Basil for Pasta Stir & Serve, Homepride*	1 Jar/480g	278.0	14.0	58	1.2	6.7	2.9	0.0
Tomato & Basil, Cooking, BGTY, Sainsbury's*	1 Jar/500g	335.0	6.0	67	2.6	11.3	1.3	0.7
Tomato & Basil, Cooking, M & S*	1 Serving/130g	78.0	4.0	60	1.4	5.7	3.4	1.2
Tomato & Chilli, Table & Dip, Heinz*	1 Tsp/10ml	8.0	0.0	76	1.4	16.6	0.2	0.8
Tomato & Chilli, Waitrose*	1 Pot/350g	182.0	9.0	52	10.0	6.2	2.6	3.2
Tomato & Mascarpone, Fresh, Sainsbury's*	1/3 Pot/100g	91.0	7.0	91	2.1	5.9	6.6	1.2
Tomato & Mascarpone, Light Choices, Tesco*	½ Pot/175g	77.0	3.0	44	1.6	4.9	2.0	0.8
Tomato & Mozzarella, Finest, Tesco*	1 Serving/175g	89.0	6.0	51	1.6	4.1	3.2	0.6
Tomato & Roasted Garlic, Stir in, Dolmio*	½ Pack/75g	94.0	8.0	125	1.2	7.7	10.2	0.0
Tomato & Roasted Vegetable, M & S*	1oz/28g	17.0	1.0	60	1.8	6.9	2.5	2.1
Tomato & Smoked Bacon, Italiano, Tesco*	½ Pot/175g	96.0	4.0	55	3.0	4.7	2.5	1.0
Tomato & Wild Mushroom, Organic, Fresh, Sainsbury's*	1 Serving/152g	102.0	7.0	67	1.9	3.9	4.9	1.7
Tomato & Worcester, Table, Lea & Perrins*	1 Serving/10g	10.0	0.0	102	0.8	23.0	0.5	0.7
Vegetable, Chunky, Tesco*	1 Can/455g	155.0	1.0	34	1.2	7.0	0.2	1.0
Vegetables, Hoi Sin & Plum, Stir Fry, Sharwood's*	1 Pack/360g	367.0	5.0	102	1.1	21.4	1.3	0.2
Watercress & Creme Fraiche, COU, M & S*	½ Pack/154g	100.0	3.0	65	3.2	9.2	1.8	0.5
Watercress, & Stilton, Creamy, for Fish, Schwartz*	1 Pack/300g	141.0	12.0	47	0.6	2.0	4.1	0.7
Watercress, Fresh, The Saucy Fish Co.*	1 Pack/150g	169.0	15.0	113	2.2	5.8	9.7	0.0
White Granules, Sauce in Seconds, Dry, Asda*	1 Pack/57g	237.0	7.0	415	3.7	73.0	12.0	0.9
White Wine & Mushroom, BGTY, Sainsbury's*	¼ Jar/125g	81.0	2.0	65	2.8	9.0	2.0	0.3
White Wine & Tarragon, French, for Fish, Schwartz*	1 Pack/300g	372.0	33.0	124	1.1	5.0	11.1	0.8
White Wine and Cream, Cook in, Classic, Homepride*	¼ Can/125g	101.0	5.0	81	1.0	8.0	4.1	0.4
White Wine, Chardonnay, M & S*	1 Serving/160ml	184.0	16.0	115	1.4	4.6	10.0	0.9
White, for Lasagne, Dolmio*	1 Jar/470g	451.0	34.0	96	0.6	7.0	7.3	0.0
White, Savoury, Made with Semi-Skimmed Milk	1oz/28g	36.0	2.0	128	4.2	11.1	7.8	0.2

S

	Measure INFO/WEIGHT	per Measure KCAL	per Measure FAT	Nutrition Values per 100g / 100ml KCAL	PROT	CARB	FAT	FIBRE
SAUCE								
White, Savoury, Made with Whole Milk	1oz/28g	42.0	3.0	150	4.1	10.9	10.3	0.2
Whole Cherry Tomato & Chilli, Finest, Tesco*	1 Jar/340g	255.0	16.0	75	1.7	6.8	4.6	2.3
Wild Mushroom, Finest, Tesco*	½ Pack/175g	157.0	12.0	90	1.9	5.2	6.8	0.4
Worcestershire, Average	***1 Tsp/5g***	***3.0***	***0.0***	***65***	***1.4***	***15.5***	***0.1***	***0.0***
Worcestershire, Lea & Perrins*	1 Tsp/5ml	4.0	0.0	88	1.1	22.0	0.0	0.0
Worcestershire, Special Edition, Lea & Perrins*	1 Serving/10ml	13.0	0.0	130	1.3	28.8	0.2	0.1
Yellow Bean & Cashew, Tesco*	½ Jar/210g	170.0	6.0	81	1.6	11.9	2.9	0.3
Yellow Bean & Ginger, Stir Fry, Finest, Tesco*	1 Jar/350g	318.0	3.0	91	2.1	18.3	1.0	1.1
Yellow Bean, Stir Fry, Sainsbury's*	½ Jar/100g	126.0	1.0	126	1.8	26.7	1.3	0.8
Yellow Bean, Stir Fry, Straight to Wok, Amoy*	1oz/28g	44.0	0.0	158	1.6	36.9	0.5	0.0
Yellowbean & Cashew Nut, Asda*	1 Serving/50g	59.0	1.0	119	2.7	21.0	2.7	0.9
SAUCE MIX								
Bacon & Mushroom Tagliatelle, Schwartz*	1 Pack/33g	110.0	1.0	333	7.5	69.2	2.9	8.3
Beef Bourguignon, Colman's*	1 Pack/40g	123.0	1.0	308	4.9	68.6	1.6	2.2
Beef Stroganoff, Colman's*	1 Pack/40g	140.0	4.0	350	11.6	56.1	8.9	2.7
Bombay Potatoes, Schwartz*	1 Pack/33g	84.0	4.0	254	16.1	20.1	12.1	31.1
Bread, Colman's*	1 Pack/40g	131.0	0.0	327	11.4	67.9	1.1	3.2
Bread, Knorr*	½ Pint/40g	177.0	9.0	442	7.9	49.9	23.3	2.1
Bread, Luxury, Schwartz*	1 Pack/40g	142.0	3.0	355	12.9	61.5	6.4	6.5
Cheddar Cheese, Colman's*	1 Pack/40g	163.0	6.0	407	18.3	48.8	15.4	1.2
Cheddar Cheese, Schwartz*	1 Pack/40g	144.0	3.0	361	18.4	55.1	7.4	2.3
Cheese, Knorr*	1 Pack/58g	132.0	3.0	227	7.8	38.0	4.9	1.8
Cheese, Made Up with Skimmed Milk	1 Serving/60g	47.0	1.0	78	5.4	9.5	2.3	0.0
Cheese, Made Up, Crosse & Blackwell*	1 Pack/30g	26.0	1.0	86	5.1	9.2	3.2	0.7
Chicken Chasseur, Colman's*	1 Pack/45g	128.0	1.0	284	8.0	59.2	1.6	3.8
Chicken Chasseur, Schwartz*	1 Pack/40g	126.0	2.0	316	9.6	59.1	4.6	6.8
Chicken Korma, Colman's*	½ Pack/50g	229.0	15.0	459	6.6	38.8	30.8	13.2
Chicken Korma, Schwartz*	1 Pack/40g	154.0	4.0	385	3.5	70.5	9.9	4.3
Chicken Supreme, Colman's*	1 Pack/40g	143.0	4.0	358	12.1	56.7	9.2	2.4
Chilli Con Carne, Hot, Colman's*	1 Pack/40g	127.0	1.0	317	10.4	62.4	2.9	7.0
Chilli Con Carne, Schwartz*	1 Pack/41g	120.0	1.0	293	7.9	57.2	3.6	9.5
Chip Shop Curry, Dry Weight, Bisto*	1 Dtsp/9g	38.0	2.0	427	3.4	63.5	17.7	1.3
Coq Au Vin, Colman's*	1 Pack/50g	150.0	1.0	301	5.6	65.6	1.8	3.3
Creamy Cheese & Bacon, for Pasta, Colman's*	1 Pack/50g	182.0	4.0	364	16.7	56.1	8.1	1.9
Creamy Chicken Curry, Colman's*	1 Sachet/50g	192.0	9.0	385	11.0	46.4	17.3	7.9
Creamy Pepper & Mushroom, Colman's*	1 Pack/25g	83.0	1.0	332	9.6	64.6	3.8	3.0
Curry, Batchelors*	1 Serving/100g	359.0	8.0	359	7.1	63.9	8.3	3.9
Dauphinoise Potato Bake, Schwartz*	1 Pack/40g	161.0	11.0	402	6.8	34.7	26.3	15.8
for Garlic Mushrooms, Creamy, Schwartz*	1 Pack/35g	109.0	2.0	311	7.6	59.7	4.7	4.2
Four Cheese, Colman's*	1 Pack/35g	127.0	4.0	362	17.1	48.4	11.1	1.8
Hollandaise, Colman's*	1 Pack/28g	104.0	3.0	372	6.4	61.6	11.1	1.8
Hollandaise, Schwartz*	1 Pack/25g	98.0	3.0	394	10.6	59.2	12.8	3.7
Lamb Hotpot, Colman's*	1 Pack/40g	119.0	1.0	297	6.9	63.3	1.7	2.1
Lasagne, Schwartz*	1 Pack/36g	106.0	1.0	294	7.0	63.4	1.4	7.0
Lemon Butter, for Fish, Schwartz*	1 Pack/38g	136.0	3.0	357	6.1	65.3	8.0	5.8
Mexican Chilli Chicken, Schwartz*	1 Pack/35g	105.0	2.0	299	7.0	55.1	5.6	12.0
Moussaka, Schwartz*	1 Pack/35g	101.0	1.0	288	8.8	58.6	2.0	9.0
Onion, Colman's*	½ Pack/17g	55.0	0.0	325	9.1	69.4	1.3	4.8
Onion, Creamy, Schwartz*	1 Pack/25g	90.0	2.0	362	10.1	59.6	9.2	5.3
Paprika Chicken, Creamy, Schwartz*	1 Pack/34g	116.0	3.0	342	9.7	53.9	9.8	9.5
Parsley & Chive, for Fish, Schwartz*	1 Pack/38g	132.0	3.0	348	9.0	58.9	8.5	7.7
Parsley, Colman's*	1 Pack/20g	63.0	0.0	314	7.2	67.9	1.5	3.7
Parsley, Creamy, Schwartz*	1 Pack/26g	96.0	3.0	371	11.5	57.2	10.7	3.8

S

SAUCE MIX	Measure INFO/WEIGHT	per Measure KCAL	per Measure FAT	Nutrition Values per 100g / 100ml KCAL	PROT	CARB	FAT	FIBRE
Parsley, Knorr*	1 Sachet/48g	210.0	12.0	437	4.2	50.6	24.2	0.8
Pepper, Creamy, Colman's*	1 Pack/25g	88.0	3.0	352	13.0	50.0	11.0	0.0
Peppercorn, Mild, Creamy, Schwartz*	1 Pack/25g	88.0	2.0	352	13.8	55.0	8.6	5.0
Pork & Mushroom, Creamy, Schwartz*	1 Pack/40g	116.0	2.0	289	8.6	54.7	4.0	12.1
Rum Flavour, Kraft*	1oz/28g	116.0	3.0	415	6.1	76.5	9.5	0.0
Savoury Mince, Schwartz*	1 Pack/35g	108.0	1.0	310	14.6	58.3	2.0	1.8
Shepherd's Pie, Schwartz*	1 Pack/38g	104.0	1.0	273	7.9	54.4	2.6	11.1
Spaghetti Bolognese, Schwartz*	1 Pack/40g	114.0	1.0	285	9.2	59.0	1.6	7.0
Spaghetti Carbonara, Schwartz*	1 Pack/32g	135.0	6.0	421	10.4	49.4	20.1	7.2
Stroganoff, Beef, Schwartz*	1 Pack/35g	125.0	4.0	358	15.6	50.8	10.3	4.4
Stroganoff, Mushroom, Schwartz*	1 Pack/35g	113.0	2.0	324	10.0	59.2	5.3	9.6
Sweet & Sour, Colman's*	1 Pack/40g	133.0	0.0	333	2.6	79.9	0.4	2.2
Thai Green Curry, Schwartz*	1 Pack/41g	137.0	3.0	333	7.6	57.6	8.1	13.0
Thai Red Curry, Schwartz*	1 Pack/35g	120.0	2.0	342	5.9	63.5	7.1	7.6
Three Cheese, for Vegetables, Schwartz*	1 Pack/40g	168.0	8.0	421	17.4	41.7	20.5	4.8
Tikka Masala, Creamy, Schwartz*	1 Pack/31g	100.0	4.0	324	11.9	43.5	11.4	18.1
Tuna & Mushroom Pasta Melt, Schwartz*	1 Pack/40g	122.0	3.0	304	10.2	49.7	7.1	7.7
Tuna & Pasta Bake, Colman's*	1 Pack/45g	144.0	2.0	319	10.4	57.1	5.4	5.2
Tuna Napolitana, Schwartz*	1 Pack/30g	107.0	4.0	357	10.3	49.6	13.1	0.3
White Wine, with Herbs, Creamy, Schwartz*	1 Pack/26g	86.0	2.0	330	8.0	60.0	6.5	9.1
White, Dry Weight, Bisto*	1 Dtsp/9g	45.0	3.0	496	3.2	57.4	28.2	0.4
White, Made Up with Semi-Skimmed Milk	1oz/28g	20.0	1.0	73	4.0	9.6	2.4	0.0
White, Made Up with Skimmed Milk	1oz/28g	17.0	0.0	59	4.0	9.6	0.9	0.0
White, Savoury, Colman's*	1 Pack/25g	84.0	1.0	335	10.7	66.5	2.9	2.6
White, Savoury, Knorr*	½ Pack/16g	46.0	1.0	290	7.8	52.2	5.6	5.2
White, Savoury, Schwartz*	1 Pack/25g	108.0	6.0	434	11.5	45.6	22.9	5.9
Wholegrain Mustard, Creamy, Schwartz*	1 Pack/25g	92.0	3.0	370	12.9	54.4	11.2	7.5
SAUERKRAUT								
Average	*1oz/28g*	*4.0*	*0.0*	*13*	*1.3*	*1.9*	*0.0*	*1.1*
SAUSAGE								
BBQ Hotdog, M & S*	1 Sausage/100g	300.0	25.0	300	12.1	5.4	25.3	2.0
Beef, Average	*1 Sausage/60g*	*151.0*	*11.0*	*252*	*14.5*	*7.0*	*18.5*	*0.6*
Beef, with Onion & Red Wine, Finest, Tesco*	1 Sausage/63g	117.0	7.0	185	13.2	8.5	10.9	1.2
Billy Bear, Kids, Tesco*	1 Slice/20g	37.0	2.0	185	13.7	7.5	11.2	0.4
Bockwurst, Average	*1 Sausage/45g*	*114.0*	*10.0*	*253*	*10.7*	*0.7*	*23.0*	*0.0*
Cambridge Gluten Free, Waitrose*	1 Sausage/57g	121.0	9.0	213	14.6	1.9	16.3	1.3
Chicken & Tarragon, Butchers Choice, Sainsbury's*	1 Sausage/47g	106.0	7.0	225	18.1	5.8	14.4	0.2
Chicken & Turkey, Morrisons*	1 Sausage/57g	86.0	4.0	152	16.0	5.8	7.2	1.1
Chicken, Manor Farm*	1 Sausage/65g	126.0	8.0	194	13.7	6.6	12.5	1.2
Chilli & Coriander, TTD, Sainsbury's*	1 Sausage/44g	136.0	11.0	310	18.5	4.2	24.4	1.2
Chilli Beef, Boston Style, Waitrose*	1 Sausage/67g	135.0	10.0	203	14.7	3.4	14.6	0.9
Chipolata, Average	*1 Sausage/28g*	*81.0*	*6.0*	*291*	*12.1*	*8.7*	*23.1*	*0.7*
Chipolata, Lamb & Rosemary, Tesco*	1 Sausage/32g	69.0	5.0	218	11.3	8.3	15.5	0.0
Chipolata, Pork & Tomato, Organic, Tesco*	1 Sausage/28g	79.0	7.0	283	12.2	4.3	24.1	0.9
Chipolata, Pork, Extra Lean, BGTY, Sainsbury's*	1 Sausage/24g	46.0	2.0	189	16.9	10.9	8.6	0.5
Chipolata, Premium, Average	*1 Serving/80g*	*187.0*	*14.0*	*233*	*14.8*	*4.7*	*17.3*	*1.2*
Chorizo, & Jalapeño, Pizzadella, Tesco*	1 Pizza/600g	1272.0	41.0	212	9.9	27.9	6.8	1.7
Chorizo, Average	*1 Serving/80g*	*250.0*	*19.0*	*313*	*21.1*	*2.6*	*24.2*	*0.2*
Chorizo, Lean, Average	*1 Sausage/67g*	*131.0*	*9.0*	*195*	*15.7*	*2.3*	*13.7*	*0.8*
Cocktail, Average	*1oz/28g*	*90.0*	*7.0*	*323*	*12.1*	*8.6*	*26.7*	*0.9*
Cumberland, Average	*1 Sausage/57g*	*167.0*	*13.0*	*293*	*13.8*	*8.5*	*22.7*	*0.8*
Cumberland, Quorn*	1 Sausage/50g	60.0	2.0	120	12.3	7.0	4.8	4.0
Cumberland, with Cracked Black Pepper & Herbs, Asda*	1 Sausage/56g	127.0	8.0	225	13.6	10.8	14.2	2.2

SAUSAGE

INFO/WEIGHT	Measure	per Measure		Nutrition Values per 100g / 100ml				
		KCAL	FAT	KCAL	PROT	CARB	FAT	FIBRE
Debrecziner, Spicy Smoked, Gebirgsjager*	1 Sausage/37g	118.0	10.0	320	16.0	1.0	28.0	0.0
Extrawurst, German, Waitrose*	1 Slice/28.3g	80.0	7.0	281	13.0	1.0	25.0	0.0
Free From Wheat & Gulten, Sainsbury's*	1 Serving/23g	61.0	5.0	268	15.2	4.5	21.0	1.8
French Saucisson, Tesco*	1 Slice/5g	19.0	1.0	379	26.7	4.1	28.4	0.0
Garlic, Average	*1 Slice/11g*	*25.0*	*2.0*	*227*	*15.7*	*0.8*	*18.2*	*0.0*
German, Bierwurst, Selection, Sainsbury's*	1 Slice/4g	8.0	1.0	224	15.0	1.0	17.8	0.1
German, Extrawurst, Selection, Sainsbury's*	1 Slice/3g	9.0	1.0	279	13.1	0.5	25.0	0.1
German, Schinkenwurst, Selection, Sainsbury's*	1 Slice/3g	8.0	1.0	251	13.1	0.3	21.9	0.1
Hot & Spicy Pork Cocktail, Cooked, Asda*	1 Sausage/10g	31.0	2.0	312	13.0	11.0	24.0	1.3
Hot Mustard Porker, Tesco*	1 Sausage/52g	143.0	10.0	275	16.1	8.1	19.8	3.1
Irish Recipe, Asda*	1 Sausage/57g	120.0	7.0	212	12.1	14.0	12.0	2.7
Irish, Average	*1 Sausage/40g*	*119.0*	*8.0*	*297*	*10.7*	*17.2*	*20.7*	*0.7*
Lincolnshire, Average	*1 Sausage/42g*	*122.0*	*9.0*	*291*	*14.6*	*9.2*	*21.8*	*0.6*
Lincolnshire, Healthy Range, Average	*1 Sausage/50g*	*89.0*	*4.0*	*177*	*15.8*	*9.0*	*8.6*	*0.8*
Lorne, Average	*1 Sausage/25g*	*78.0*	*6.0*	*312*	*10.8*	*16.0*	*23.1*	*0.6*
Mediterranean Style Paprika, Waitrose*	1 Sausage/67g	190.0	16.0	283	12.1	4.6	24.0	1.9
Mediterranean Style, 95% Fat Free, Bowyers*	1 Sausage/50g	60.0	2.0	120	13.9	8.9	3.2	0.0
Mortadella, Sainsbury's*	1 Slice/13g	34.0	3.0	261	17.3	0.1	21.2	0.1
Polish Kabanos, Sainsbury's*	1 Sausage/25g	92.0	8.0	366	23.0	0.1	30.4	0.1
Polony, Slicing, Value, Tesco*	1 Serving/40g	92.0	7.0	229	10.0	10.0	16.5	1.0
Pork & Apple, Average	*1 Sausage/57g*	*146.0*	*11.0*	*255*	*14.5*	*7.5*	*18.8*	*1.9*
Pork & Beef, Average	*1 Sausage/45g*	*133.0*	*10.0*	*295*	*8.7*	*13.6*	*22.7*	*0.5*
Pork & Chilli, Tesco*	1 Sausage/67g	124.0	8.0	186	16.4	3.2	12.0	1.1
Pork & Herb, Average	*1 Sausage/75g*	*231.0*	*19.0*	*308*	*13.1*	*5.4*	*25.9*	*0.3*
Pork & Herb, Healthy Range, Average	*1 Sausage/59g*	*75.0*	*1.0*	*126*	*16.0*	*10.7*	*2.4*	*1.1*
Pork & Leek, Average	*1oz/28g*	*73.0*	*6.0*	*262*	*14.6*	*6.0*	*19.9*	*1.1*
Pork & Red Onion, TTD, Sainsbury's*	1 Sausage/48g	138.0	9.0	288	18.5	12.4	18.3	1.4
Pork & Smoked Bacon, Finest, Tesco*	1oz/28g	76.0	6.0	271	13.9	4.8	21.8	0.2
Pork & Stilton, Average	*1 Sausage/57g*	*180.0*	*15.0*	*316*	*13.2*	*5.8*	*26.7*	*0.3*
Pork & Tomato, Grilled, Average	*1 Sausage/47g*	*127.0*	*10.0*	*273*	*13.9*	*7.5*	*20.8*	*0.4*
Pork, & Sweet Chilli, Waitrose*	1 Sausage/67g	146.0	10.0	219	15.6	4.6	15.3	0.8
Pork, Apricot & Herb, Waitrose*	1 Sausage/67g	165.0	11.0	246	11.2	12.9	16.6	1.3
Pork, Average	*1 Sausage/50g*	*152.0*	*12.0*	*305*	*12.8*	*9.8*	*23.8*	*0.7*
Pork, Bacon & Cheese, Asda*	¼ Pack/114g	329.0	24.0	289	18.0	7.0	21.0	0.4
Pork, Battered, Thick, Average	1oz/28g	126.0	10.0	448	17.3	21.7	36.3	2.0
Pork, Cumberland, TTD, Sainsbury's*	1 Sausage/46g	132.0	10.0	288	21.4	3.1	21.1	0.6
Pork, Extra Lean, Average	*1 Sausage/54g*	*84.0*	*4.0*	*155*	*17.3*	*6.1*	*6.8*	*0.8*
Pork, Frozen, Fried	*1oz/28g*	*88.0*	*7.0*	*316*	*13.8*	*10.0*	*24.8*	*0.0*
Pork, Frozen, Grilled	*1oz/28g*	*81.0*	*6.0*	*289*	*14.8*	*10.5*	*21.2*	*0.0*
Pork, Garlic & Herb, Average	*1 Sausage/76g*	*203.0*	*17.0*	*268*	*12.0*	*5.9*	*21.8*	*1.1*
Pork, Ham & Asparagus, Tesco*	1 Sausage/76g	173.0	13.0	228	14.9	3.8	17.0	1.1
Pork, Lincolnshire, Traditionally Made, TTD, Sainsbury's*	1 Sausage/47g	149.0	11.0	318	20.2	4.5	24.3	0.7
Pork, Pancetta & Parmesan, TTD, Sainsbury's*	1 Sausage/47g	167.0	13.0	354	19.8	4.9	28.4	0.9
Pork, Plum Tomato & Herb, Uncooked, Finest, Tesco*	1 Sausage/55g	121.0	9.0	220	12.5	5.5	16.5	0.7
Pork, Premium, Average	*1 Sausage/74g*	*191.0*	*14.0*	*258*	*14.9*	*8.3*	*18.4*	*1.0*
Pork, Reduced Fat, Asda*	1 Sausage/54g	76.0	2.0	140	15.3	11.8	3.5	1.9
Pork, Reduced Fat, Chilled, Grilled	*1oz/28g*	*64.0*	*4.0*	*230*	*16.2*	*10.8*	*13.8*	*1.5*
Pork, Reduced Fat, Chilled, Raw	*1oz/28g*	*50.0*	*3.0*	*180*	*13.0*	*8.7*	*10.6*	*1.2*
Pork, Reduced Fat, Healthy Range, Average	*1 Sausage/57g*	*86.0*	*3.0*	*151*	*15.6*	*9.0*	*6.0*	*0.9*
Pork, Roasted Pepper & Chilli, COU, M & S*	1 Sausage/57g	57.0	1.0	100	15.2	7.1	2.0	2.1
Pork, Skinless, Average	*1oz/28g*	*81.0*	*7.0*	*291*	*11.7*	*8.2*	*23.6*	*0.6*
Pork, Smoked Bacon, & Garlic, Finest, Tesco*	1 Sausage/67g	115.0	8.0	173	14.7	0.2	12.6	0.4
Pork, Smoked, Reduced Fat, Mattessons*	½ Pack/113g	288.0	21.0	255	14.0	7.0	19.0	0.9

	Measure INFO/WEIGHT	KCAL	FAT	Nutrition Values per 100g / 100ml KCAL	PROT	CARB	FAT	FIBRE
SAUSAGE								
Pork, Thick, Average	*1 Sausage/39g*	*115.0*	*9.0*	*296*	*13.3*	*10.0*	*22.4*	*1.0*
Premium, Chilled, Fried	*1oz/28g*	*77.0*	*6.0*	*275*	*15.8*	*6.7*	*20.7*	*0.0*
Premium, Chilled, Grilled	*1oz/28g*	*82.0*	*6.0*	*292*	*16.8*	*6.3*	*22.4*	*0.0*
Schinkenwurst, German, Waitrose*	1 Slice/13g	28.0	2.0	224	16.0	0.8	17.6	0.0
Spanish, Wafer Thin, Asda*	1 Slice/4g	12.0	1.0	298	25.4	4.1	20.0	0.0
Toulouse, M & S*	1 Sausage/57g	123.0	9.0	215	12.4	5.8	15.6	1.3
Toulouse, TTD, Sainsbury's*	1 Sausage/45g	146.0	11.0	324	21.4	2.3	25.5	0.8
Turkey & Chicken, Average	*1 Sausage/57g*	*126.0*	*8.0*	*221*	*14.4*	*8.2*	*14.5*	*1.7*
Turkey & Ham, Tesco*	1 Sausage/57g	101.0	6.0	178	13.8	8.3	10.0	1.0
Turkey, Average	*1 Sausage/57g*	*90.0*	*5.0*	*157*	*15.7*	*6.3*	*8.0*	*0.0*
Tuscan, M & S*	1 Sausage/66g	145.0	11.0	220	14.9	4.6	16.0	0.6
Venison & Pork, Waitrose*	1 Sausage/63g	101.0	5.0	160	16.7	4.8	8.2	0.9
Venison & Red Wine, TTD, Sainsbury's*	1 Sausage/58g	130.0	8.0	226	19.7	6.8	13.3	1.7
Venison, Grilled, Finest, Tesco*	1 Sausage/40g	56.0	2.0	140	18.6	5.3	4.5	1.1
Wiejska, Polish, Sainsbury's*	1/8 Pack/50g	78.0	4.0	157	18.7	0.4	9.0	0.5
SAUSAGE & MASH								
British Classic, Tesco*	1 Pack/450g	675.0	43.0	150	5.1	11.1	9.5	0.9
GFY, Asda*	1 Pack/400g	330.0	10.0	82	4.2	10.7	2.5	1.7
Onion, M & S*	1 Pack/300g	315.0	17.0	105	4.1	9.0	5.7	1.5
Vegetarian, GFY, Asda*	1 Pack/400g	292.0	9.0	73	4.2	9.0	2.2	2.1
Vegetarian, Tesco*	1 Pack/410g	398.0	16.0	97	4.6	11.1	3.8	2.0
Waitrose*	1 Pack/420g	517.0	31.0	123	4.2	9.9	7.4	0.1
with Onion Gravy, Tesco*	1 Pack/500g	525.0	27.0	105	3.0	11.1	5.4	1.6
with Red Wine & Onion Gravy, BGTY, Sainsbury's*	1 Pack/379.5g	315.0	7.0	83	5.0	11.4	1.9	2.0
SAUSAGE MEAT								
Pork, Average	*1oz/28g*	*96.0*	*8.0*	*344*	*9.9*	*10.1*	*29.4*	*0.6*
SAUSAGE ROLL								
Asda*	1 Roll/64g	216.0	16.0	337	7.0	21.0	25.0	0.8
Basics, Party Size, Somerfield*	1 Roll/13g	45.0	3.0	343	7.0	29.0	22.0	0.0
BGTY, Sainsbury's*	1 Roll/65g	200.0	11.0	308	9.6	27.9	17.6	1.4
Cocktail, M & S*	1 Roll/14.3g	50.0	3.0	350	10.4	26.4	22.3	2.2
Cocktail, Mini, Sainsbury's*	1 Roll/15g	54.0	4.0	361	9.0	27.6	23.8	2.6
Farmfoods*	1 Roll/34g	101.0	7.0	297	6.7	22.9	19.8	0.4
Go Large, Asda*	1 Roll/170g	660.0	48.0	388	9.0	25.0	28.0	0.9
Jumbo, Sainsbury's*	1 Roll/145g	492.0	34.0	339	8.2	23.2	23.7	1.5
Kingsize, Pork Farms*	½ Roll/50g	241.0	16.0	483	10.5	39.9	31.8	0.0
Large, Freshbake*	1 Roll/52g	153.0	10.0	294	6.6	25.9	18.3	4.6
Large, Frozen, Tesco*	1 Roll/50g	182.0	12.0	365	6.0	31.0	23.8	0.9
Lincolnshire, Geo Adams*	1 Roll/130g	474.0	32.0	365	8.3	28.2	24.3	1.1
M & S*	1 Roll/32g	122.0	9.0	380	10.5	21.0	28.4	0.9
Mini, M & S*	1oz/28g	122.0	9.0	435	9.8	29.6	30.9	1.8
Mini, Tesco*	1 Roll/15g	53.0	4.0	356	9.0	23.9	24.9	1.5
Mini, Waitrose*	1 Roll/35g	124.0	9.0	353	13.0	16.1	26.3	1.0
Party, Sainsbury's*	1 Roll/13g	54.0	4.0	422	8.7	26.7	31.1	1.2
Party, Value, Tesco*	1 Roll/12g	33.0	1.0	274	6.8	35.9	11.5	0.6
Pork Farms*	1 Roll/54g	196.0	13.0	363	7.9	30.0	23.9	0.0
Pork, Morrisons*	1 Roll/70g	195.0	9.0	278	9.6	31.2	12.8	1.5
Puff Pastry, Sainsbury's*	1 Roll/65g	250.0	18.0	384	8.3	25.0	27.9	0.9
Reduced Fat, Sainsbury's*	1 Roll/66g	191.0	9.0	289	10.5	29.8	14.2	1.8
Sainsbury's*	1 Roll/67g	244.0	16.0	367	9.5	27.8	24.2	2.7
Snack Size, Tesco*	1 Roll/32g	118.0	9.0	369	9.1	21.7	27.4	2.3
Snack, GFY, Asda*	1 Roll/34g	112.0	7.0	329	9.4	26.5	20.6	0.9
Snack, Sainsbury's*	1 Roll/34g	130.0	8.0	383	9.7	29.9	25.0	2.1

S

	Measure INFO/WEIGHT	per Measure KCAL	FAT	Nutrition Values per 100g / 100ml KCAL	PROT	CARB	FAT	FIBRE
SAUSAGE ROLL								
Tesco*	1 Roll/67g	241.0	18.0	360	8.1	21.3	26.4	2.3
TTD, Sainsbury's*	1 Roll/115g	440.0	32.0	383	11.9	21.3	27.8	2.0
Waitrose*	1 Roll/75g	287.0	20.0	383	10.1	27.0	26.1	1.3
SAUSAGE ROLL VEGETARIAN								
Linda McCartney*	1 Roll/52g	142.0	7.0	273	9.7	28.2	13.5	2.5
SAUSAGE VEGETARIAN								
Asda*	1 Sausage/43g	81.0	4.0	189	20.0	7.0	9.0	2.9
Braai Flavour, Fry's Special Vegetarian*	1 Sausage/62g	141.0	8.0	226	20.3	9.4	12.2	0.6
Cumberland, Cauldron Foods*	1 Sausage/50g	93.0	5.0	186	9.0	16.0	9.5	4.0
Cumberland, Waitrose*	1 Sausage/50g	80.0	3.0	160	12.6	12.3	6.7	2.4
Glamorgan, Asda*	1 Sausage/50g	100.0	5.0	199	4.6	22.4	10.1	2.0
Glamorgan, Leek & Cheese, Goodlife*	1 Sausage/50g	108.0	6.0	217	5.7	20.5	12.5	2.6
Glamorgan, Organic, Cauldron Foods*	1 Sausage/41g	67.0	4.0	162	12.5	7.3	9.2	1.7
Glamorgan, Organic, Waitrose*	1 Sausage/42g	81.0	4.0	194	14.5	11.2	10.1	1.7
Granose*	1oz/28g	63.0	4.0	226	8.5	17.5	13.5	0.0
Leek & Cheese, Organic, Cauldron Foods*	1 Sausage/41g	80.0	4.0	194	14.4	11.3	10.1	1.7
Lincolnshire, Chilled, Cauldron Foods*	1 Sausage/50g	83.0	5.0	166	10.0	9.5	9.8	7.0
Linda McCartney*	1 Sausage/50g	101.0	4.0	202	22.6	8.2	8.8	1.6
Meat Free Pepperami, GranoVita*	1 Pack/50g	116.0	6.0	233	23.5	5.7	12.9	6.0
Mushroom & Herb, Waitrose*	1 Sausage/50g	61.0	3.0	123	10.2	8.1	5.4	0.5
Mushroom & Tarragon, Wicken Fen*	1 Sausage/47g	82.0	3.0	175	10.1	17.0	7.4	2.4
Roasted Garlic & Oregano, Cauldron Foods*	1 Sausage/50g	89.0	5.0	179	13.1	9.0	10.1	2.1
Smoked Paprika & Chilli, Cauldron Foods*	1 Sausage/50g	76.0	4.0	152	7.8	11.8	8.2	2.6
Sun Dried Tomato & Black Olive, Cauldron Foods*	1 Sausage/50g	71.0	4.0	142	8.7	9.4	7.7	2.6
Sun Dried Tomato & Herb, Linda McCartney*	1 Sausage/35g	93.0	5.0	266	21.8	10.1	15.4	1.7
SAVOURY EGGS								
Bites, Sainsbury's*	1 Egg/20g	55.0	4.0	277	9.6	18.8	18.2	2.1
Mini, Iceland*	1 Egg/20g	66.0	5.0	327	11.0	17.5	23.7	1.1
Mini, Tesco*	1 Egg/20g	55.0	3.0	274	9.2	20.2	17.4	2.3
Snack, Tesco*	1 Egg/45g	133.0	9.0	295	9.0	19.6	19.7	1.8
SCALLOPS								
Asda*	1oz/28g	33.0	0.0	118	23.2	1.4	1.4	0.0
Breaded, Thai Style with Plum Sauce, Finest, Tesco*	1 Serving/210g	401.0	15.0	191	11.5	20.6	7.0	0.8
Breaded, with Plum & Chilli Dipping Sauce, Tesco*	1 Pack/210g	441.0	15.0	210	10.6	25.6	7.2	0.8
Canadian, Finest, Tesco*	½ Pack/100g	80.0	0.0	80	16.4	2.6	0.2	0.1
Hotbake Shells, Sainsbury's*	1 Serving/140g	241.0	16.0	172	9.5	8.4	11.2	0.8
Lemon Grass & Ginger, Tesco*	½ Pack/112g	90.0	1.0	80	15.2	2.5	1.0	0.6
Steamed, Average	1oz/28g	33.0	0.0	118	23.2	3.4	1.4	0.0
TTD, Sainsbury's*	½ Pack/100g	68.0	0.0	68	15.5	1.2	0.1	1.2
with Roasted Garlic Butter, Finest, Tesco*	1 Serving/100g	201.0	14.0	201	16.2	1.8	14.3	0.4
SCAMPI								
Breaded, Average	½ Pack/255g	565.0	27.0	222	10.7	20.5	10.7	1.0
Wholetail, Premium, Youngs*	1 Serving/125g	256.0	11.0	205	29.5	21.6	9.1	2.1
Wholetails, in Crunchy Crumb, Morrisons*	1 Pack/250g	507.0	22.0	203	9.6	19.9	8.7	1.7
SCAMPI & CHIPS								
Chunky, Finest, Tesco*	1 Pack/280g	420.0	15.0	150	5.9	18.3	5.5	1.4
Youngs*	1oz/28g	42.0	2.0	150	5.0	20.3	5.4	1.7
SCHNITZEL VEGETARIAN								
Breaded, Tivall*	1 Piece/100g	172.0	8.0	172	16.0	9.0	8.0	5.0
SCONE								
3% Fat, M & S*	1 Scone/65g	179.0	2.0	275	7.2	55.1	2.5	2.3
All Butter, Tesco*	1 Scone/41g	126.0	3.0	308	7.2	52.3	7.8	1.6
Cheese & Black Pepper, Mini, M & S*	1 Scone/18g	67.0	3.0	370	10.2	41.1	18.3	1.7

S

	Measure INFO/WEIGHT	per Measure KCAL	per Measure FAT	Nutrition Values per 100g / 100ml KCAL	PROT	CARB	FAT	FIBRE
SCONE								
Cheese, Average	1 Scone/40g	145.0	7.0	363	10.1	43.2	17.8	1.6
Cherry, M & S*	1 Scone/60g	202.0	7.0	337	6.9	49.7	12.2	1.9
Clotted Cream, Cornish, TTD, Sainsbury's*	1 Scone/70g	269.0	13.0	384	8.4	46.6	18.2	2.1
Cream, Sainsbury's*	1 Scone/50g	172.0	9.0	345	4.6	42.5	17.4	3.1
Derby, Asda*	1 Scone/59g	202.0	6.0	342	7.0	56.0	10.0	0.0
Derby, Mother's Pride*	1 Scone/60g	208.0	8.0	347	5.2	49.8	14.0	1.5
Derby, Tesco*	1 Scone/60g	201.0	6.0	335	7.2	53.7	10.2	2.0
Devon, M & S*	1 Scone/59g	225.0	10.0	380	7.1	50.8	16.2	1.5
Devon, Sainsbury's*	1 Scone/54g	201.0	8.0	372	7.1	51.1	15.5	1.6
Devon, Waitrose*	1 Scone/72g	268.0	9.0	373	7.5	56.0	13.2	2.3
Fresh Cream with Strawberry Jam, Tesco*	1 Scone/83g	290.0	16.0	352	4.7	40.7	18.9	1.1
Fresh Cream, Finest, Tesco*	1 Serving/133g	469.0	23.0	354	4.6	44.5	17.5	1.7
Fresh Cream, Tesco*	1 Scone/80g	242.0	10.0	304	15.8	32.3	12.5	0.9
Fruit, Average	1 Scone/40g	126.0	4.0	316	7.3	52.9	9.8	0.0
Luxury, Hovis*	1 Scone/85g	267.0	8.0	314	5.6	51.8	9.3	2.2
Plain, Average	1 Scone/40g	145.0	6.0	362	7.2	53.8	14.6	1.9
Potato, Average	1 Scone/40g	118.0	6.0	296	5.1	39.1	14.3	1.6
Strawberry, Fresh Cream, BGTY, Sainsbury's*	1 Scone/50g	154.0	6.0	309	5.1	47.0	11.2	1.1
Strawberry, Fresh Cream, Sainsbury's*	1 Scone/60g	218.0	11.0	363	6.5	42.5	18.6	1.4
Sultana, BGTY, Sainsbury's*	1 Scone/63g	178.0	2.0	283	7.7	56.7	2.8	2.4
Sultana, Finest, Tesco*	1 Scone/70g	238.0	8.0	340	8.9	50.9	10.9	2.1
Sultana, GFY, Asda*	1 Scone/59g	192.0	3.0	324	7.0	64.0	4.4	2.0
Sultana, Less Than 5% Fat, Asda*	1 Scone/60g	198.0	4.0	330	7.0	62.0	6.0	1.8
Sultana, M & S*	1 Scone/66g	231.0	8.0	350	6.5	53.0	12.5	2.0
Sultana, Reduced Fat, Waitrose*	1 Scone/65g	187.0	3.0	287	6.6	53.2	5.3	2.6
Sultana, Sainsbury's*	1 Scone/54g	176.0	6.0	327	6.9	50.2	11.0	6.5
Sultana, Tesco*	1 Scone/60g	189.0	5.0	315	7.1	52.5	8.4	2.6
Wholemeal	1 Scone/40g	130.0	6.0	326	8.7	43.1	14.4	5.2
Wholemeal, Fruit	1 Scone/40g	130.0	5.0	324	8.1	47.2	12.8	4.9
SCONE MIX								
Fruit, Asda*	1 Scone/48g	143.0	2.0	301	7.0	57.0	5.0	3.7
SCOTCH EGGS								
Asda*	1 Egg/114g	286.0	19.0	251	11.2	13.7	16.8	1.4
Bar, Ginsters*	1 Bar/90g	256.0	16.0	284	11.8	20.1	17.4	1.7
Budgens*	1 Egg/113g	294.0	20.0	260	11.4	13.8	17.6	0.0
Finest, Tesco*	1 Egg/114g	280.0	20.0	247	11.6	10.4	17.7	1.1
Free Range, Sainsbury's*	1 Egg/112.7g	284.0	19.0	252	12.4	12.5	16.9	2.5
Morrisons*	1 Egg/114g	286.0	19.0	251	11.2	13.7	16.8	1.4
Retail	1 Egg/120g	301.0	21.0	251	12.0	13.1	17.1	0.0
Sainsbury's*	1 Egg/113g	311.0	22.0	275	11.1	14.2	19.3	0.9
Savoury, M & S*	1 Egg/21g	63.0	5.0	305	11.0	15.7	21.8	1.3
Super Mini, Asda*	1 Egg/13g	38.0	3.0	305	10.0	19.0	21.0	2.1
SEA BASS								
Cooked, Dry Heat, Average	*1 Fillet/101g*	*125.0*	*3.0*	*124*	*23.6*	*0.0*	*2.6*	*0.0*
Fillet, in Beurre Blanc & Dill Sauce, The Saucy Fish Co.*	2 Fillets/230g	354.0	21.0	154	17.8	0.0	9.2	0.0
Fillets, Greek, TTD, Sainsbury's*	1 Fillet/110g	131.0	3.0	119	23.9	0.0	2.6	0.0
Fillets, Skinless, Boneless, TTD, Sainsbury's*	1 Serving/100g	162.0	9.0	162	19.4	0.5	9.2	0.5
Fillets, with Lemon & Parsley Butter, Iceland*	½ Pack/110g	197.0	13.0	179	17.6	0.1	12.0	0.1
Raw, Average	*1oz/28g*	*32.0*	*1.0*	*113*	*20.3*	*0.0*	*3.5*	*0.1*
SEA BREAM								
Fillets, Raw, Average	*1oz/28g*	*27.0*	*1.0*	*96*	*17.5*	*0.0*	*2.9*	*0.0*
SEAFOOD COCKTAIL								
Average	1oz/28g	24.0	0.0	87	15.6	2.9	1.5	0.0

	Measure INFO/WEIGHT	KCAL	FAT	Nutrition Values per 100g / 100ml				
				KCAL	PROT	CARB	FAT	FIBRE
SEAFOOD COCKTAIL								
Premium Quality, Lyons Seafoods*	1 Serving/100g	76.0	1.0	76	13.2	3.7	0.9	1.1
SEAFOOD MEDLEY								
Sainsbury's*	½ Pack/175g	157.0	3.0	90	14.3	4.0	1.9	0.5
Steam Cuisine, M & S*	1 Pack/400g	320.0	12.0	80	8.5	4.5	3.1	1.3
SEAFOOD SELECTION								
Fresh, Tesco*	1 Pack/234g	187.0	2.0	80	17.7	0.1	1.0	0.0
Luxury, Safeway*	1 Pack/250g	215.0	5.0	86	13.8	3.1	2.0	0.0
M & S*	1 Serving/200g	170.0	2.0	85	17.4	1.6	1.0	0.5
Mussels, King Prawns & Squid, Frozen, Tesco*	½ Pack/200g	140.0	3.0	70	13.7	0.1	1.5	0.0
Sainsbury's*	½ Pack/125g	85.0	1.0	68	14.6	0.8	1.0	2.5
SEAFOOD STICKS								
Average	1 Stick/15g	16.0	0.0	106	8.0	18.4	0.2	0.2
with Cocktail Dip, Asda*	1 Pot/95g	126.0	5.0	133	6.0	16.0	5.0	0.1
with Garlic & Lemon Dip, Asda*	1 Pot/98g	184.0	12.0	188	7.0	13.0	12.0	0.0
SEASONING								
Aromat, Knorr*	1oz/28g	45.0	1.0	161	11.7	15.1	3.7	0.9
Sushi, Mitsukan*	2 Tbsp/30ml	50.0	1.0	167	0.0	36.7	3.3	0.0
SEASONING CUBES								
for Potato, Mint, Perfect Potato, Knorr*	1 Cube/10g	56.0	5.0	560	5.1	21.2	50.5	1.8
for Rice, Pilau, Knorr*	1 Cube/10g	30.0	2.0	305	11.4	13.9	22.6	1.4
for Rice, Saffron, Knorr*	1 Cube/10g	29.0	2.0	291	13.8	17.5	18.4	2.2
for Stir Fry, Oriental Spices, Knorr*	1 Cube/10g	41.0	3.0	414	9.7	25.0	30.6	1.1
Oriental Spice, Knorr*	1 Cube/10g	41.0	3.0	409	9.5	23.7	30.7	0.0
Perfect Pasta, Knorr*	1 Cube/10g	28.0	2.0	278	10.3	5.2	24.0	0.0
Wild Mushroom, Knorr*	1 Cube/10g	36.0	3.0	365	10.3	21.3	26.5	0.2
SEASONING MIX								
Balti, Aromatic, Schwartz*	1 Serving/10g	34.0	1.0	340	13.7	56.6	6.8	0.0
Beef Taco, Colman's*	1 Pack/30g	76.0	4.0	252	9.1	26.9	12.0	14.0
Cajun, Sizzle & Grill, Schwartz*	1 Tsp/4g	7.0	0.0	182	9.8	23.0	5.6	24.4
Chicken Fajitas, Schwartz*	1 Pack/35g	99.0	1.0	283	10.9	54.1	2.5	10.8
Chicken, Chargrilled, Grill & Sizzle, Schwartz*	1 Tsp/5g	12.0	0.0	232	8.2	40.8	4.0	13.1
Chilli, Old El Paso*	Pack/39g	117.0	2.0	301	7.0	57.0	5.0	0.0
Chinese Curry, Youngs*	1 Serving/22g	109.0	7.0	495	8.3	46.4	30.7	0.0
Fajita, Asda*	1 Serving/8g	20.0	1.0	251	6.0	41.0	7.0	0.9
Fajita, Chicken, Colman's*	1 Pack/40g	138.0	3.0	344	9.4	62.5	6.3	4.8
Fish, Schwartz*	1 Tsp/4g	9.0	0.0	222	6.5	55.5	2.3	11.6
Italian Herb, Schwartz*	1 Tsp/1g	3.0	0.0	338	11.0	64.5	4.0	0.0
Lemon & Herb, Cous Cous, Asda*	1 Tbsp/15g	46.0	1.0	305	10.6	52.0	6.5	10.2
Mediterranean Roasted Vegetable, Schwartz*	1 Pack/30g	86.0	1.0	288	6.9	56.1	4.0	10.3
Moroccan Spiced Vegetables, Schwartz*	1 Pack/40g	99.0	2.0	247	12.2	38.4	4.9	22.0
Potato Roasties, Rosemary & Garlic, Crispy, Schwartz*	1 Pack/33g	88.0	3.0	267	13.0	36.1	7.8	21.1
Potato Roasties, Southern Fried, Crispy, Schwartz*	1 Pack/35g	78.0	2.0	222	9.2	36.2	4.4	25.1
Potato Wedges, Cajun, Schwartz*	1 Pack/38g	112.0	3.0	295	9.1	47.6	7.6	14.3
Potato Wedges, Garlic & Herb, Schwartz*	1 Pack/38g	106.0	2.0	278	11.4	47.1	4.9	11.7
Potato Wedges, Nacho Cheese, Schwartz*	1 Pack/38g	114.0	4.0	299	13.6	39.3	9.7	7.7
Potato Wedges, Onion & Chive, Schwartz*	1 Pack/38g	113.0	1.0	297	10.9	59.4	1.8	6.5
Shepherd's Pie, Colman's*	1 Pack/50g	141.0	1.0	282	12.5	54.7	1.4	4.3
Shotz, Cajun Chicken Seasoning, Schwartz*	1 Pack/3g	8.0	0.0	268	9.9	45.6	5.2	0.0
Shotz, Chargrilled Chicken Seasoning, Schwartz*	1 Pack/3g	8.0	0.0	283	7.5	52.0	4.9	0.0
Shotz, Garlic Pepper Steak Seasoning, Schwartz*	1 Pack/3g	11.0	0.0	370	14.0	67.0	5.0	0.0
Shotz, Moroccan Chicken Seasoning, Schwartz*	1 Pack/3g	9.0	0.0	312	9.7	56.7	5.2	0.0
Shotz, Seven Pepper Steak Seasoning, Schwartz*	1 Pack/3g	7.0	0.0	246	8.2	47.8	2.4	0.0
Spanish Roasted Vegetables, Schwartz*	1 Pack/15g	22.0	1.0	147	9.1	14.1	6.0	22.6

S

	Measure INFO/WEIGHT	per Measure KCAL	per Measure FAT	Nutrition Values per 100g / 100ml KCAL	PROT	CARB	FAT	FIBRE
SEASONING MIX								
Taco, Old El Paso*	¼ Pack/9g	30.0	0.0	334	5.5	69.0	4.0	0.0
Thai Seven Spice, Schwartz*	1 Serving/10g	24.0	0.0	243	7.5	44.1	4.1	0.0
Whole Grain Mustard & Herb Potato Mash, Colman's*	1 Pack/30g	153.0	13.0	510	9.7	19.1	44.1	0.0
SEAWEED								
Crispy, Average	*1oz/28g*	*182.0*	*17.0*	*651*	*7.5*	*15.6*	*61.9*	*7.0*
Irish Moss, Raw	*1oz/28g*	*2.0*	*0.0*	*8*	*1.5*	*0.0*	*0.2*	*12.3*
Kombu, Dried, Raw	*1oz/28g*	*12.0*	*0.0*	*43*	*7.1*	*0.0*	*1.6*	*58.7*
Nori, Dried, Raw	*1oz/28g*	*38.0*	*0.0*	*136*	*30.7*	*0.0*	*1.5*	*44.4*
Wakame, Dried, Raw	*1oz/28g*	*20.0*	*1.0*	*71*	*12.4*	*0.0*	*2.4*	*47.1*
SEED MIX								
Boost for Breakfast, Julian Graves*	1 Serving/50g	195.0	8.0	390	10.6	60.3	16.0	7.7
Cajun, Graze*	1 Sm Pack/43g	246.0	21.0	573	26.5	18.1	49.0	11.5
Chilli, Graze*	1 Pack/25g	151.0	12.0	606	30.4	6.1	47.2	5.2
Granola, Graze*	1 Pack/25g	122.0	7.0	490	12.0	43.7	29.7	0.0
Naked, Graze*	1 Pack/25g	151.0	13.0	604	11.9	26.3	50.1	0.0
Omega, Graze*	1 Pack/25g	153.0	12.0	613	28.4	13.1	49.7	0.0
Omega, Morrisons*	¼ Pack/25g	138.0	11.0	554	20.9	15.0	45.6	6.4
Omega, Munchy Seeds*	1 Bag/30g	184.0	15.0	613	28.4	13.1	49.7	2.2
Original, The Food Doctor*	1 Serving/30g	157.0	13.0	522	28.2	3.7	44.4	17.7
Roasted, Graze*	1 Pack/25g	160.0	13.0	640	27.1	4.8	51.5	0.0
Salad Sprinkle, Nature's Harvest*	1 Serving/8g	48.0	4.0	598	20.0	14.6	51.1	4.9
Toasted, Asda*	1 Serving/28g	132.0	9.0	470	34.4	10.6	32.2	11.6
SEEDS								
Fenugreek, Average	*1 Tsp/3.7g*	*12.0*	*0.0*	*323*	*23.0*	*58.3*	*6.4*	*24.6*
Melon, Average	*1 Tbsp/15g*	*87.0*	*7.0*	*583*	*28.5*	*9.9*	*47.7*	*0.0*
Mustard, Average	*1 Tsp/3.3g*	*15.0*	*1.0*	*469*	*34.9*	*34.9*	*28.8*	*14.7*
Nigella, Average	*1 Tsp/5g*	*20.0*	*2.0*	*392*	*21.3*	*1.9*	*33.3*	*8.4*
Poppy, Average	*1 Tbsp/8.8g*	*47.0*	*4.0*	*533*	*18.0*	*23.7*	*44.7*	*10.0*
Pumpkin, Average	*1 Tbsp/10g*	*57.0*	*5.0*	*568*	*27.9*	*13.0*	*45.9*	*3.8*
Pumpkin, Whole, Roasted, Salted, Average	*1 Serving/50g*	*261.0*	*21.0*	*522*	*33.0*	*13.4*	*42.1*	*3.9*
Sesame, Average	*1oz/28g*	*171.0*	*16.0*	*610*	*22.3*	*3.6*	*56.4*	*7.7*
Sunflower, Average	*1 Tbsp/10g*	*59.0*	*5.0*	*585*	*23.4*	*15.0*	*48.7*	*5.7*
SEMOLINA								
Average	*1oz/28g*	*98.0*	*1.0*	*348*	*11.0*	*75.2*	*1.8*	*2.1*
Pudding, Creamed, Ambrosia*	1 Can/425g	344.0	7.0	81	3.3	13.1	1.7	0.2
Pudding, Creamed, Co-Op*	1 Can/425g	382.0	8.0	90	4.0	15.0	2.0	0.0
SHALLOTS								
Pickled, in Hot & Spicy Vinegar, Tesco*	1 Onion/18g	14.0	0.0	77	1.0	18.0	0.1	1.9
Raw, Average	*1 Serving/80g*	*16.0*	*0.0*	*20*	*1.5*	*3.3*	*0.2*	*1.4*
SHALLOTS IN								
Hot & Spicy Vinegar, Drained, Sainsbury's*	1 Serving/100g	76.0	0.0	76	1.0	16.0	0.2	0.8
SHANDY								
Bitter, Original, Ben Shaws*	1 Can/330ml	89.0	0.0	27	0.0	6.0	0.0	0.0
Homemade, Average	1 Pint/568ml	148.0	0.0	26	0.2	2.9	0.0	0.0
Lemonade, Schweppes*	1 Can/330ml	76.0	0.0	23	0.0	5.1	0.0	0.0
Lemonade, Traditional Style, Tesco*	1 Can/330ml	63.0	0.0	19	0.0	4.7	0.0	0.0
SHARK								
Raw	*1oz/28g*	*29.0*	*0.0*	*102*	*23.0*	*0.0*	*1.1*	*0.0*
SHARON FRUIT								
Average	*1oz/28g*	*20.0*	*0.0*	*73*	*0.8*	*18.6*	*0.0*	*1.6*
SHERBET LEMONS								
M & S*	1oz/28g	107.0	0.0	382	0.0	93.9	0.0	0.0

S

	Measure INFO/WEIGHT	per Measure KCAL FAT		Nutrition Values per 100g / 100ml				
		KCAL	FAT	KCAL	PROT	CARB	FAT	FIBRE
SHERRY								
Dry, Average	*1 Glass/120ml*	*139.0*	*0.0*	*116*	*0.2*	*1.4*	*0.0*	*0.0*
Medium	*1 Serving/50ml*	*58.0*	*0.0*	*116*	*0.1*	*5.9*	*0.0*	*0.0*
Sweet	*1 Serving/50ml*	*68.0*	*0.0*	*136*	*0.3*	*6.9*	*0.0*	*0.0*
SHORTBREAD								
All Butter, Deans*	1 Biscuit/15g	77.0	4.0	511	4.9	65.7	25.4	1.2
All Butter, Petticoat Tails, Co-Op*	1 Biscuit/13g	68.0	4.0	520	5.0	60.0	29.0	2.0
All Butter, Petticoat Tails, Gardiners of Scotland*	1 Biscuit/12g	64.0	3.0	514	5.2	62.1	27.2	0.0
All Butter, Round, Luxury, M & S*	1 Biscuit/20g	105.0	6.0	525	6.2	60.0	29.0	2.0
All Butter, Royal Edinburgh, Asda*	1 Biscuit/18g	93.0	5.0	519	5.8	60.3	28.3	1.8
All Butter, Scottish, M & S*	1 Biscuit/34g	173.0	9.0	510	5.7	58.9	27.8	2.3
All Butter, Thins, M & S*	1 Biscuit/10g	50.0	2.0	485	5.8	68.4	21.1	3.5
All Butter, Trufree*	1 Biscuit/11g	58.0	3.0	524	2.0	66.0	28.0	0.9
Assortment, Parkside*	1 Serving/30g	155.0	9.0	517	5.4	59.8	28.5	2.0
Average	1oz/28g	139.0	7.0	498	5.9	63.9	26.1	1.9
Belgian Chocolate Chunk, Asda*	1 Biscuit/20g	106.0	6.0	531	7.0	56.0	31.0	1.8
Butter, Extra Special, Asda*	1 Serving/19g	101.0	6.0	531	7.0	56.0	31.0	1.8
Caramel, Millionaires, Fox's*	1 Serving/16g	75.0	4.0	483	6.1	57.9	25.3	0.1
Choc Chip, Fair Trade, Co-Op*	1 Biscuit/19g	100.0	6.0	526	5.3	57.9	31.6	2.6
Chocolate Chip, Jacob's*	1 Biscuit/17g	87.0	5.0	513	5.2	61.2	27.5	1.8
Chocolate Chip, Tesco*	1 Serving/20g	105.0	6.0	525	7.5	55.0	30.6	3.0
Chocolate Chunk, Belgian, TTD, Sainsbury's*	1 Biscuit/19g	101.0	6.0	521	5.1	59.1	29.4	2.0
Clotted Cream, Finest, Tesco*	1 Biscuit/20g	109.0	6.0	543	5.2	58.0	32.2	1.7
Cookie, Choc Chip, Low Carb, Carbolite*	1 Biscuit/30g	120.0	9.0	400	13.3	19.0	30.0	13.3
Cookies, Organic, Evernat*	1oz/28g	149.0	9.0	532	5.9	56.7	31.3	0.0
Demerara, Rounds, TTD, Sainsbury's*	1 Biscuit/22g	113.0	6.0	508	5.1	62.2	26.5	1.8
Double Choc Chip, Petit Four, Scottish, Tesco*	1 Serving/50g	265.0	15.0	531	5.1	60.4	30.0	1.7
Dutch, M & S*	1 Biscuit/17g	90.0	5.0	530	5.7	58.2	30.6	0.9
Fingers, All Butter, Co-Op*	1 Finger/16g	85.0	5.0	520	6.0	58.0	30.0	2.0
Fingers, All Butter, Highland, Sainsbury's*	2 Biscuits/28g	146.0	8.0	520	6.3	56.7	29.8	2.2
Fingers, All Butter, Londis*	1 Finger/13g	66.0	4.0	525	5.9	59.2	29.2	1.9
Fingers, All Butter, McVitie's*	1 Finger/20g	106.0	5.0	530	6.5	64.7	27.2	0.0
Fingers, All Butter, Royal Edinburgh Bakery*	1 Biscuit/17g	88.0	5.0	519	5.8	60.3	28.3	1.8
Fingers, All Butter, Scottish, M & S*	1 Finger/18g	90.0	5.0	510	5.7	58.9	27.8	4.7
Fingers, All Butter, Tesco*	1 Finger/13g	67.0	4.0	519	5.8	60.3	28.3	1.8
Fingers, All Butter, Traditional, Scottish, Tesco*	1 Finger/18g	93.0	5.0	520	6.0	58.5	29.1	1.8
Fingers, Asda*	1 Finger/18g	93.0	5.0	519	5.8	60.3	28.3	18.0
Fingers, Cornish Cookie*	1 Finger/25g	124.0	6.0	498	6.4	61.0	25.5	0.0
Fingers, Deans*	1 Finger/24g	115.0	6.0	488	5.1	60.1	24.8	1.4
Fingers, Highland, Organic, Sainsbury's*	1 Serving/16g	84.0	5.0	527	5.8	58.7	29.9	1.9
Fingers, Safeway*	1 Finger/21g	109.0	6.0	520	5.8	58.5	29.2	18.9
Fingers, Scottish, Finest, Tesco*	1 Pack/165g	822.0	39.0	498	5.1	65.5	23.9	2.0
Free From, Sainsbury's*	1 Biscuit/20g	98.0	5.0	490	6.0	58.0	26.0	6.0
Hearts, with Milk Chocolate, M & S*	1 Biscuit/25g	125.0	6.0	500	7.2	59.5	25.8	3.0
Highland Demerara Rounds, Sainsbury's*	1 Biscuit/20g	113.0	6.0	565	5.5	70.5	29.0	2.0
Highland, Organic, Duchy Originals*	1 Biscuit/16g	80.0	4.0	515	5.2	61.8	27.4	1.7
Honey & Oatmeal, Walkers*	1 Biscuit/34g	158.0	8.0	465	6.7	64.1	22.4	3.8
Light & Buttery, Fingers, TTD, Sainsbury's*	1 Biscuit/20g	106.0	6.0	528	5.1	61.6	29.0	1.7
Mini Bites, Co-Op*	1 Biscuit/10g	53.0	3.0	530	7.0	59.0	30.0	2.0
Mini Bites, Country Table*	1 Biscuit/10g	52.0	3.0	525	7.1	59.3	29.5	1.5
Orange Marmalade & Oatflake, Deans*	1 Biscuit/20g	105.0	6.0	524	6.7	59.3	29.6	3.2
Organic, Waitrose*	1 Biscuit/13g	62.0	3.0	495	5.8	63.0	24.4	1.8
Pecan All Butter, Sainsbury's*	1 Biscuit/18g	99.0	7.0	548	5.3	49.9	36.3	2.5
Petticoat Tails, All Butter, Highland, Sainsbury's*	1 Biscuit/13g	64.0	4.0	516	6.3	58.0	28.8	2.2

S

	Measure INFO/WEIGHT	per Measure KCAL	FAT	Nutrition Values per 100g / 100ml KCAL	PROT	CARB	FAT	FIBRE
SHORTBREAD								
Pure Butter, Jacob's*	1 Biscuit/20g	105.0	6.0	525	5.7	58.6	29.7	1.8
Raspberry & Oatmeal, Deans*	1 Biscuit/20g	103.0	6.0	514	4.7	63.1	28.6	1.4
Reduced Sugar, Tesco*	1 Biscuit/17g	86.0	5.0	519	6.7	57.1	29.4	2.1
Stem Ginger, Waitrose*	1 Biscuit/15g	71.0	3.0	487	4.7	66.0	22.7	1.6
Wheat & Gluten Free, Free From Range, Tesco*	1 Biscuit/20g	98.0	5.0	490	6.0	58.0	26.0	6.0
SHRIMP								
Boiled, Average	*1 Serving/60g*	*70.0*	*1.0*	*117*	*23.8*	*0.0*	*2.4*	*0.0*
Dried, Average	*1oz/28g*	*69.0*	*1.0*	*245*	*55.8*	*0.0*	*2.4*	*0.0*
Frozen, Average	*1oz/28g*	*20.0*	*0.0*	*73*	*16.5*	*0.0*	*0.8*	*0.0*
in Brine, Canned, Drained, Average	*1oz/28g*	*26.0*	*0.0*	*94*	*20.8*	*0.0*	*1.2*	*0.0*
SKATE								
Grilled	*1oz/28g*	*22.0*	*0.0*	*79*	*18.9*	*0.0*	*0.5*	*0.0*
in Batter, Fried in Blended Oil	1oz/28g	47.0	3.0	168	14.7	4.9	10.1	0.2
Raw	*1oz/28g*	*18.0*	*0.0*	*64*	*15.1*	*0.0*	*0.4*	*0.0*
SKIPS								
Bacon, KP Snacks*	1 Bag/17g	81.0	4.0	474	6.5	62.1	22.2	2.3
Cheesy, KP Snacks*	1 Bag/17g	89.0	5.0	524	6.2	58.5	29.5	1.0
Pickled Onion, KP Snacks*	1 Bag/13g	67.0	4.0	512	3.4	56.4	30.3	1.4
Prawn Cocktail, KP Snacks*	1 Bag/17g	89.0	5.0	523	3.1	60.6	29.9	1.4
Tangy Tomato, KP Snacks*	1 Bag/17g	88.0	5.0	517	3.2	59.6	29.5	1.2
SKITTLES								
Mars*	1 Pack/55g	223.0	2.0	406	0.0	90.6	4.4	0.0
SLICES								
Bacon & Cheese, Pastry, Tesco*	1 Slice/165g	480.0	32.0	291	7.4	21.7	19.4	1.0
Bacon & Cheese, Savoury, Pastry, Somerfield*	1 Slice/165.0g	490.0	33.0	297	7.4	21.2	20.3	1.5
Beef, Minced Steak & Onion, Tesco*	1 Slice/150g	424.0	27.0	283	8.7	21.3	18.1	1.6
Beef, Minced with Onion, Sainsbury's*	1 Slice/120g	328.0	20.0	273	6.8	24.5	16.4	1.1
Beef, Minced, Morrisons*	1 Slice/143g	457.0	30.0	320	8.8	24.6	20.7	1.0
Belgian Chocolate, Weight Watchers*	1 Slice/30g	99.0	2.0	329	5.9	61.3	6.7	2.3
Cheddar Cheese & Onion, Ginsters*	1 Slice/180g	583.0	41.0	324	7.1	22.8	22.7	1.0
Cheese & Ham, Pastry, Sainsbury's*	1 Slice/118g	352.0	23.0	298	7.8	22.5	19.7	1.8
Cheese & Ham, Savoury, Pastry, Somerfield*	1 Slice/150g	399.0	24.0	266	7.0	23.0	16.0	0.0
Cheese & Onion, Pastry, Tesco*	1 Slice/150g	502.0	37.0	335	8.0	20.1	24.7	1.4
Cheese & Onion, Savoury, Pastry, Somerfield*	1 Slice/165g	518.0	34.0	314	7.4	24.0	20.9	0.6
Cheese, Potato & Onion, Pastry, Taste!*	1 Slice/155g	501.0	30.0	323	8.6	28.1	19.6	0.0
Chicken & Ham, Taste!*	1 Slice/155g	356.0	15.0	230	10.8	24.2	9.9	0.0
Chicken & Leek, Taste!*	1 Slice/155g	406.0	19.0	262	10.1	27.6	12.3	0.0
Chicken & Mushroom, Asda*	1 Slice/128g	354.0	22.0	277	7.0	24.0	17.0	2.1
Chicken & Mushroom, Ginsters*	1 Slice/180g	439.0	27.0	244	8.3	19.1	14.9	1.8
Chicken & Mushroom, Morrisons*	1 Slice/158g	446.0	28.0	282	7.3	23.3	17.8	1.0
Chicken & Mushroom, Sainsbury's*	1 Slice/164g	427.0	27.0	259	7.3	21.3	16.1	1.0
Chicken & Mushroom, Tesco*	1 Slice/165g	457.0	29.0	277	9.2	20.6	17.5	0.9
Chicken, Spicy, Deep Fill, Ginsters*	1 Slice/180g	499.0	31.0	277	9.2	21.8	17.0	1.4
Ham & Cheese, Pastry, Ginsters*	1 Slice/155g	625.0	44.0	403	9.8	31.9	28.2	4.2
Minced Steak & Onion, Sainsbury's*	1 Slice/165g	475.0	30.0	288	15.2	16.0	18.1	2.5
Mushroom, Creamy, Quorn*	1 Slice/164g	653.0	30.0	398	9.8	49.2	18.0	1.6
Peppered Steak, Asda*	1 Slice/164g	483.0	31.0	295	9.0	22.0	19.0	1.2
Pork & Egg, Gala, Tesco*	1 Slice/105g	333.0	24.0	317	10.3	17.2	23.0	3.4
Prawn & Avocado, Plait, Extra Special, Asda*	1 Serving/198g	331.0	7.0	167	11.0	23.0	3.4	1.3
Salmon, & Watercress, Honey Roast, Plait, Asda*	1 Plait/166g	421.0	17.0	254	13.0	28.0	10.0	0.4
Sausage Meat, with Onion Gravy, Lattice, Asda*	1 Serving/278g	595.0	39.0	214	10.0	12.0	14.0	1.7
Spinach & Ricotta, Safeway*	1 Slice/165g	487.0	34.0	295	6.0	21.2	20.4	2.9
Spinach & Ricotta, Sainsbury's*	1 Slice/165g	500.0	35.0	303	6.5	21.1	21.4	2.9

	Measure			Nutrition Values per 100g / 100ml				
	INFO/WEIGHT	KCAL	FAT	KCAL	PROT	CARB	FAT	FIBRE
SLICES								
Steak & Onion, Aberdeen Angus, Tesco*	1 Slice/165g	444.0	28.0	269	8.7	20.7	16.8	1.3
Steak, Peppered, Deep Fill, Ginsters*	1 Slice/180g	513.0	36.0	285	9.4	16.1	20.1	3.1
Steak, Peppered, Ginsters*	1 Slice/155g	415.0	24.0	268	9.9	21.5	15.8	1.9
SLIMFAST*								
Meal Bar, Chocolate Crunch, Slim Fast*	1 Bar/60g	206.0	6.0	343	23.9	42.8	9.9	7.7
Meal Bar, Fruits of the Forest, Slim Fast*	1 Bar/60g	211.0	6.0	351	23.7	42.1	10.1	7.3
Meal Bar, Yoghurt & Muesli, Slim Fast*	1 Bar/60g	208.0	6.0	347	23.9	42.2	10.8	7.4
Milk Shake, Banana, Canned, Slim Fast*	1 Can/325ml	214.0	8.0	66	4.2	10.6	2.6	4.9
Milk Shake, Chocolate, Powder, Dry, Slim Fast*	2 Scoops/37g	136.0	3.0	363	13.9	59.0	7.5	10.9
Milk Shake, Chocolate, Ready to Drink, Slim Fast*	1 Bottle/325ml	211.0	5.0	65	4.6	8.0	1.6	1.5
Milk Shake, Peach, Canned, Slim Fast*	1 Can/325ml	214.0	3.0	66	4.2	10.6	0.8	1.5
Milk Shake, Vanilla, Powder, Dry, Slim Fast*	2 Scoops/36g	131.0	2.0	360	13.4	60.9	6.5	11.0
Snacks, Chocolate Caramel Bar, Slim Fast*	1 Bar/26g	99.0	3.0	382	3.4	69.6	12.4	1.2
Snacks, Sour Cream & Chive Pretzels, Slim Fast*	1 Pack/23g	96.0	2.0	416	9.5	75.2	8.6	3.4
Soup, Chicken & Vegetable Pasta, Hearty's*	1 Pack/295ml	212.0	6.0	72	6.6	7.0	1.9	0.7
SMARTIES								
Biscuits, Nestle*	1 Biscuit/5g	26.0	1.0	519	7.7	57.6	28.6	0.0
Giants, Nestle*	1 Pack/186g	882.0	36.0	474	4.6	70.4	19.3	0.7
Mini Cones, Nestle*	1 Serving/44g	145.0	6.0	330	4.5	45.0	13.1	0.0
Mini Eggs, Nestle*	1 Lge Bag/112g	535.0	22.0	478	4.8	69.6	20.0	0.7
Nestle*	1 Tube/40g	184.0	7.0	461	4.0	73.6	16.6	0.6
Tree Decoration, Nestle*	1 Chocolate/18g	95.0	5.0	529	5.6	58.9	30.1	0.8
SMIRNOFF*								
Ice, Smirnoff*	1 Bottle/275ml	188.0	0.0	68	1.8	12.0	0.0	0.0
SMOOTHIE								
Apple, Grapes & Blackcurrant, PJ Smoothies*	1 Bottle/250ml	125.0	1.0	50	0.8	11.1	0.3	0.7
Apple, Kiwi & Lime, SunJuice*	1 Bottle/250ml	132.0	0.0	53	0.5	13.4	0.1	0.8
Apple, Strawberry, Cherry & Banana, M & S*	1 Bottle/250ml	125.0	1.0	50	0.5	11.2	0.3	0.6
Apricot & Peach, COU, M & S*	1 Bottle/250ml	100.0	1.0	40	0.9	8.3	0.4	0.4
Banana & Mango, Juice, Calypso*	1 Carton/200ml	106.0	0.0	53	0.0	12.8	0.0	1.0
Banana Fruit, with Yoghurt, Tesco*	1 Bottle/1000ml	610.0	7.0	61	2.1	11.3	0.7	0.4
Banana, Dairy, Probiotic, Boots*	1 Bottle/250ml	147.0	1.0	59	1.6	12.0	0.5	1.0
Blackberries & Blueberries, Innocent*	1 Bottle/250ml	120.0	0.0	48	0.5	12.0	0.1	2.1
Blackberries, Strawberries & Boysenberries, Innocent*	1 Serving/250ml	142.0	0.0	57	0.5	14.8	0.0	1.6
Blackberry & Blueberry, Wild Orchard*	1 Bottle/250ml	110.0	0.0	44	0.6	10.8	0.0	1.9
Blackcurrant & Apple, for Kids, Innocent*	1 Carton/180ml	112.0	0.0	62	0.4	14.5	0.2	0.8
Blackcurrants & Gooseberries, for Autumn, Innocent*	1 Bottle/250ml	117.0	0.0	47	0.5	12.5	0.1	1.0
Blueberry & Pear, COU, M & S*	1 Bottle/250ml	112.0	1.0	45	0.3	10.4	0.3	0.3
Blueberry Hill, King Parrot Food Company*	1 Drink/450g	252.0	1.0	56	1.2	12.0	0.3	0.6
Blueberry, Blackberry & Strawberry, COU, M & S*	1 Bottle/250ml	150.0	1.0	60	0.8	13.1	0.3	0.3
Blueberry, Blue Machine, Naked, Superfood, Nak'd*	1 Bottle/450ml	319.0	0.0	71	0.4	16.6	0.0	2.9
Cappuccino, with Yoghurt, Island Oasis*	1 Carton/473ml	300.0	4.0	63	1.7	12.5	0.7	0.0
Cherries & Strawberries, Innocent*	1 Bottle/250ml	122.0	0.0	49	0.6	12.6	0.1	0.0
Cranberries & Raspberries, Innocent*	1 Bottle/250ml	112.0	0.0	45	0.5	12.0	0.0	2.3
Cranberries & Strawberries, Innocent*	1 Bottle/250ml	102.0	0.0	41	0.5	9.5	0.2	0.0
Cranberries, Blueberries, Cherries, Innocent*	1 Serving/250ml	137.0	0.0	55	0.3	12.8	0.0	1.3
Cranberries, Yumberries & Blackcurrants, Innocent*	1 Bottle/250ml	130.0	0.0	52	0.5	14.2	0.1	1.5
Daily Detox, Mandarins & Dragonfruits, PJ Smoothies*	1 Bottle/250ml	130.0	0.0	52	0.3	12.4	0.1	0.0
Fruit Kick, Orange, Mango & Pineapple, PJ Smoothies*	1 Carton/100ml	54.0	0.0	54	0.6	12.2	0.0	0.0
Ginseng & Ace Vitamins, M & S*	1 Bottle/250ml	137.0	0.0	55	0.7	13.0	0.2	0.9
Guavas, Mangoes & Goji Berries, Innocent*	1 Bottle/250ml	112.0	0.0	45	0.6	12.0	0.1	2.1
It's Alive, PJ Smoothies*	1 Bottle/250ml	150.0	1.0	60	0.7	13.6	0.3	0.0
Kiwi, Apples & Limes, Innocent*	1 Bottle/250ml	130.0	0.0	52	0.3	11.7	0.1	1.4

	Measure INFO/WEIGHT	per Measure KCAL	FAT	Nutrition Values per 100g / 100ml KCAL	PROT	CARB	FAT	FIBRE

SMOOTHIE

	Measure INFO/WEIGHT	KCAL	FAT	KCAL	PROT	CARB	FAT	FIBRE
Mango & Passion Fruit, Weight Watchers*	1 Serving/90ml	90.0	0.0	100	0.3	23.9	0.1	0.5
Mango Mania, King Parrot Food Company*	1 Drink/450g	248.0	0.0	55	1.3	12.3	0.1	0.4
Mango, Mini-me, Skinny, Boost*	1 Sm/480ml	178.0	1.0	37	0.5	7.7	0.3	0.4
Mangoes & Passion Fruits, Pure Fruit, Innocent*	1 Bottle/250ml	140.0	0.0	56	0.6	14.7	0.2	2.0
Mangoes, Coconuts & Lemongrass, Innocent*	1 Bottle/250ml	172.0	3.0	69	0.6	12.9	1.4	1.2
Orange & Mango, Fruit, Morrisons*	1 Bottle/250ml	145.0	0.0	58	0.5	14.0	0.0	0.7
Orange, Banana & Pineapple, Innocent*	1 Bottle/250ml	120.0	1.0	48	0.6	10.8	0.4	0.0
Orange, Mandarin & Guava, PJ Smoothies*	1 Bottle/250ml	122.0	0.0	49	0.7	10.9	0.0	1.6
Orange, Mango, Banana & Passion Fruit, Asda*	1 Serving/100ml	55.0	0.0	55	0.8	12.0	0.2	1.1
Orange, Strawberry & Guava, Sainsbury's*	1 Serving/300ml	159.0	1.0	53	0.3	12.0	0.2	0.8
Oranges, Bananas & Pineapples, Innocent*	1 Bottle/250ml	142.0	0.0	57	0.6	14.1	0.1	0.0
Peach, Mild & Fruity, Campina*	1 Bottle/330ml	211.0	0.0	64	2.7	13.1	0.0	0.0
Peaches, Bananas & Passionfruit, PJ Smoothies*	1 Bottle/250g	127.0	0.0	51	0.4	12.1	0.1	0.0
Pineapple, Banana & Pear, Asda*	1 Bottle/250ml	147.0	0.0	59	0.5	13.6	0.1	0.3
Pineapple, Banana & Pear, Princes*	1 Bottle/250ml	152.0	0.0	61	0.5	13.9	0.2	0.5
Pineapple, Mango & Passion Fruit, Extra Special, Asda*	½ Bottle/250ml	100.0	0.0	40	0.5	9.0	0.2	1.3
Pineapple, Mango & Passionfruit, 100% Fruit, Sainsbury's*	1 Bottle/250ml	162.0	0.0	65	0.7	15.2	0.1	1.0
Pineapple, Strawberries & Passion Fruit, PJ Smoothies*	1 Bottle/330ml	152.0	0.0	46	0.6	10.8	0.1	1.3
Pineapples, Bananas & Coconuts, Innocent*	1 Bottle/250ml	182.0	3.0	73	0.7	15.3	1.2	1.0
Pomegranate, Raspberry & Cranberry, PJ Smoothies*	1 Bottle/250ml	132.0	0.0	53	1.1	11.6	0.2	0.0
Pomegranates & Raspberries, Innocent*	1 Bottle/250ml	150.0	0.0	60	0.6	15.4	0.1	2.0
Pomegranates, Blueberries & Acai, Superfoods, Innocent*	1 Serving/367ml	250.0	1.0	68	0.5	17.3	0.3	1.2
Raspberry & Bio Yoghurt, M & S*	1 Bottle/500ml	275.0	1.0	55	2.0	10.8	0.3	0.9
Raspberry & Blueberry, Plus, Tesco*	1 Serving/100ml	59.0	0.0	59	2.6	11.6	0.3	0.5
Raspberry & Boysenberry, Shapers, Boots*	1 Bottle/248ml	109.0	0.0	44	0.7	10.0	0.0	1.6
Raspberry & Cranberry, Smoothie Plus, Tesco*	1 Bottle/250ml	140.0	0.0	56	0.6	13.0	0.2	3.0
Raspberry Ripple, King Parrot Food Company*	1 Pack/300g	171.0	2.0	57	1.2	11.9	0.5	0.9
Raspberry, Banana & Peach, Sainsbury's*	1 Bottle/251ml	138.0	0.0	55	0.8	12.8	0.1	1.5
Raspberry, M & S*	1 Bottle/250ml	137.0	1.0	55	1.7	12.2	0.6	1.9
Strawberries & Bananas, PJ Smoothies*	1 Bottle/250ml	117.0	0.0	47	0.4	11.0	0.1	0.0
Strawberries & Bananas, Pure Fruit, Innocent*	1 Bottle/250ml	142.0	0.0	57	0.5	14.4	0.1	1.3
Strawberries & Raspberries, Squeezie, Innocent*	1 Squeezie/40g	16.0	0.0	39	0.3	8.5	0.2	2.1
Strawberries, Blackberries, Raspberries, Kids, Innocent*	1 Carton/180ml	88.0	0.0	49	0.5	11.2	0.1	1.2
Strawberry & Banana, Don Simon, Don Simon*	1 Carton/250ml	132.0	0.0	53	0.6	12.2	0.0	0.3
Strawberry & Banana, Fruit, Finest, Tesco*	1 Bottle/250ml	135.0	1.0	54	0.3	12.5	0.3	0.5
Strawberry & Banana, Fruit, Serious Food Company*	1 Bottle/250ml	135.0	0.0	54	0.5	12.7	0.0	1.3
Strawberry & Banana, Juice, Calypso*	1 Carton/200ml	100.0	0.0	50	0.0	11.9	0.0	0.0
Strawberry & Banana, Tesco*	1 Bottle/250ml	112.0	0.0	45	0.6	10.1	0.2	0.8
Strawberry & Cherry, Organic, M & S*	1 Bottle/250ml	137.0	1.0	55	0.8	12.3	0.3	0.4
Strawberry & Raspberry, Fruity, Sainsbury's*	1 Glass/200ml	106.0	0.0	53	0.6	11.9	0.0	2.4
Strawberry & Raspberry, Rhapsody, M & S*	1 Glass/200ml	90.0	0.0	45	0.6	9.4	0.1	0.9
Strawberry & Raspberry, Shapers, Boots*	1 Bottle/250ml	122.0	0.0	49	0.3	12.0	0.2	0.6
Strawberry & White Chocolate, M & S*	1 Bottle/250ml	100.0	2.0	40	2.5	5.5	1.0	0.1
Strawberry Dairy, Shapers, Boots*	1 Bottle/250ml	120.0	1.0	48	1.7	9.7	0.3	0.5
Strawberry Fields, King Parrot Food Company*	1 Drink/450g	221.0	1.0	49	1.4	10.4	0.2	0.6
Strawberry with Yoghurt, Finest, Tesco*	1 Serving/100ml	62.0	1.0	62	2.1	10.5	1.2	0.6
Strawberry, Raspberry & Banana, Waitrose*	1 Bottle/250ml	122.0	0.0	49	0.7	10.8	0.1	0.8
Strawberry, Raspberry, Apple & Banana, PJ Smoothies*	1 Bottle/250ml	132.0	1.0	53	0.8	11.9	0.3	0.7
Strawberry, Wild Orchard*	1 Bottle/250ml	120.0	0.0	48	0.6	11.8	0.0	1.4
Summer Fruits, Tesco*	1 Bottle/250ml	140.0	0.0	56	0.2	13.8	0.0	0.5
Tangy Apple & Blackcurrant, Sainsbury's*	1 Bottle/250ml	160.0	0.0	64	0.5	14.6	0.0	1.5
Vanilla & Honey, Sainsbury's*	1 Bottle/250ml	237.0	6.0	95	3.2	14.8	2.4	0.3
Vanilla Bean & Honey, Yoghurt, Serious Food Company*	1 Bottle/250ml	250.0	7.0	100	3.7	15.2	2.8	0.0

S

	Measure INFO/WEIGHT	per Measure KCAL	per Measure FAT	Nutrition Values per 100g / 100ml KCAL	PROT	CARB	FAT	FIBRE
SMOOTHIE								
Vanilla Bean, M & S*	1 Bottle/500ml	450.0	13.0	90	3.3	13.9	2.6	0.0
Yoghurt, Vanilla Bean & Honey, Thickie, Innocent*	1 Bottle/250g	235.0	6.0	94	3.5	14.5	2.6	0.0
Zumo Berry, Zumo*	1 Regular/375ml	157.0	2.0	42	1.4	7.8	0.6	0.0
SNACK MIX								
Bowl, Bombay, Tesco*	¼ Bowl/131g	626.0	35.0	477	19.5	40.0	26.6	3.6
Bowl, Oriental Style, Tesco*	¼ Bowl/80g	298.0	1.0	373	7.2	84.2	0.8	1.0
Roasted, Organic, Clearspring*	1 Bag/60g	271.0	17.0	451	37.5	11.1	28.5	14.4
SNACK POT								
Chicken & Sweetcorn Noodles, Morrisons*	1 Pot/246.5g	249.0	1.0	101	4.1	19.8	0.6	1.6
Potato & Vegetable, Quick Snack, Made Up, Tru Free*	1 Pack/245.8g	236.0	7.0	96	1.0	15.0	3.0	1.0
Potato & Vegetable, Wheat & Gluten Free, Trufree*	1 Pot/244.6g	225.0	9.0	92	1.3	13.8	3.5	1.1
Rice & Lentil, Quick Snack, Made Up, Tru Free*	1 Pack/270g	291.0	5.0	108	3.0	20.4	1.8	0.6
SNACK-A-JACKS								
Apple Danish, Jumbo, Quaker Oats*	1 Cake/10g	39.0	0.0	390	5.0	87.0	2.5	1.0
Barbecue, Jumbo, Quaker Oats*	1 Cake/10g	38.0	0.0	380	8.0	83.0	2.0	1.7
Barbecue, Snack, Quaker Oats*	1 Bag/30g	123.0	2.0	410	7.5	81.0	6.0	1.0
Barbeque, Snack-A-Jacks, Quaker Oats*	1 Pack /26g	106.0	2.0	408	7.3	81.1	6.1	0.9
Caramel, Jumbo, Snack-A-Jacks, Quaker Oats*	1 Cake/13g	51.0	0.0	390	5.5	87.0	2.1	1.4
Caramel, Snack, Snack-A-Jacks, Quaker Oats*	1 Bag/30g	121.0	1.0	405	6.0	88.0	3.0	0.8
Cheese & Onion, Snack, Quaker Oats*	1 Bag/30g	120.0	2.0	400	6.7	77.0	7.5	1.5
Cheese, Jumbo, Quaker Oats*	1 Cake/10g	38.0	0.0	380	8.5	81.0	2.5	1.7
Cheese, Snack, Quaker Oats*	1 Bag/26g	108.0	2.0	415	8.5	77.0	8.0	0.9
Chocolate & Caramel, Delights, Quaker Oats*	1 Cake/15g	62.0	1.0	415	6.0	83.0	6.0	1.6
Chocolate & Orange, Delights, Quaker Oats*	1 Cake/15g	59.0	1.0	394	5.5	83.0	4.5	1.0
Chocolate Chip, Jumbo, Snack-A-Jacks, Quaker Oats*	1 Cake/15g	61.0	1.0	410	6.0	81.0	7.0	1.7
Hot Tomato Flavour, Snack-A-Jacks, Quaker Oats*	1 Bag/26g	105.0	2.0	405	7.3	77.1	7.5	1.2
Mini Bites, Mature Cheese & Red Onion, Quaker Oats*	1 Bag/28g	116.0	3.0	415	7.5	76.0	9.0	2.0
Mini Bites, Smoked Ham, Quaker Oats*	1 Bag/28g	114.0	2.0	408	6.5	78.3	7.5	2.0
Mini Bites, Sour Cream & Sweet Chilli, Quaker Oats*	1 Bag/28g	115.0	2.0	410	6.5	78.0	8.0	2.0
Mini Breadsticks, Cheese & Onion, Quaker Oats*	1 Bag/35g	145.0	3.0	414	12.9	71.1	8.9	3.7
Prawn Cocktail, Snack, Quaker Oats*	1 Bag/30g	123.0	2.0	410	7.0	78.0	7.5	0.8
Prawn Cocktail, Snack-A-Jacks, Quaker Oats*	1 Bag/26g	106.0	2.0	408	6.9	78.3	7.5	0.9
Roast Chicken, Snack, Quaker Oats*	1 Bag/30g	124.0	2.0	415	7.0	77.5	8.0	1.0
Salt & Vinegar Flavour, Snack-A-Jacks, Quaker Oats*	1 Bag/30g	123.0	2.0	410	7.0	79.0	7.5	0.9
Salt & Vinegar, Jumbo, Snack-A-Jacks, Quaker Oats*	1 Cake/11g	43.0	1.0	388	7.4	75.4	5.7	1.6
Salt & Vinegar, Snack-A-Jacks, Quaker Oats*	1 Pack/26g	105.0	2.0	404	7.0	77.4	7.4	0.8
Sweet Chilli Flavour, Snack-A-Jacks, Quaker Oats*	1 Packet/26g	107.0	2.0	412	7.3	78.9	7.5	1.1
SNAILS								
in Garlic Butter, Average	6 Snails/50g	219.0	21.0	438	9.7	8.0	41.5	1.0
Raw, Average	1 Snail/5g	4.0	0.0	90	16.1	2.0	1.4	0.0
SNAPPER								
Red, Fried in Blended Oil	*1oz/28g*	*35.0*	*1.0*	*126*	*24.5*	*0.0*	*3.1*	*0.0*
Red, Weighed with Bone, Raw	*1oz/28g*	*25.0*	*0.0*	*90*	*19.6*	*0.0*	*1.3*	*0.0*
SNICKERS								
Cruncher, Mars*	1 Bar/40g	209.0	12.0	523	9.0	57.0	30.0	2.3
Mars*	1 Bar/44g	225.0	13.0	511	9.4	54.5	28.4	1.2
SORBET								
Blackcurrant, Del Monte*	1oz/28g	30.0	0.0	106	0.4	27.1	0.1	0.0
Blackcurrant, Iceland*	¼ Pot/100g	100.0	0.0	100	0.0	25.0	0.0	0.0
Elderflower, Bottle Green*	1 Serving/100g	104.0	0.0	104	0.1	25.6	0.0	0.0
Exotic Fruit, Sainsbury's*	1 Serving/75g	90.0	1.0	120	1.2	24.1	2.0	0.0
Jamaican Me Crazy, Ben & Jerry's*	1 Serving/100g	130.0	0.0	130	0.2	32.0	0.0	0.4
Kiwi & Papaya, World Fruit, Del Monte*	1 Lolly/90ml	61.0	0.0	68	0.2	16.2	0.3	0.0

S

	Measure INFO/WEIGHT	per Measure KCAL	FAT	Nutrition Values per 100g / 100ml KCAL	PROT	CARB	FAT	FIBRE
SORBET								
Lemon	1 Scoop/60g	79.0	0.0	131	0.9	34.2	0.0	0.0
Lemon Harmony, Haagen-Dazs*	1 Serving/90ml	214.0	10.0	238	1.5	32.5	11.3	0.0
Lemon, Asda*	1 Serving/100g	120.0	0.0	120	0.0	30.0	0.0	0.0
Lemon, Del Monte*	1 Sorbet/500g	570.0	0.0	114	0.1	29.2	0.1	0.0
Lemon, Organic, Evernat*	1oz/28g	27.0	0.0	96	0.1	22.8	0.5	0.0
Lemon, Sainsbury's*	¼ Pot/89g	100.0	0.0	112	0.0	28.1	0.0	0.1
Lemon, Sticks, Haagen-Dazs*	1oz/28g	67.0	3.0	238	1.5	32.5	11.3	0.0
Lemon, Tesco*	1 Serving/75g	79.0	0.0	106	0.0	26.2	0.0	0.4
Lemon, The Real Ice Company*	1 Serving/100g	117.0	0.0	117	0.1	29.1	0.1	0.4
Lemon, Zesty, Haagen-Dazs*	1 Serving/125ml	120.0	0.0	96	0.0	24.8	0.0	1.0
Mango Berry Swirl, Ben & Jerry's*	1 Serving/100g	100.0	0.0	100	0.2	25.0	0.0	1.5
Mango Lemon, Fruit Ice, BGTY, Sainsbury's*	1 Lolly/72g	84.0	0.0	116	0.3	28.1	0.3	0.5
Mango, Del Monte*	1 Sorbet/500g	575.0	0.0	115	0.2	29.6	0.1	0.0
Mango, Organic, M & S*	1 Serving/100g	99.0	0.0	99	0.3	24.1	0.1	0.9
Mango, Tesco*	1 Serving/100g	107.0	0.0	107	0.1	26.5	0.0	0.3
Mango, Waitrose*	1 Pot/100g	90.0	0.0	90	0.1	22.1	0.0	0.6
Orange, Del Monte*	1 Sorbet/500g	625.0	0.0	125	0.2	32.1	0.1	0.0
Passion Fruit, Fat Free, M & S*	1 Sorbet/125g	129.0	0.0	103	0.4	25.0	0.0	0.4
Peach & Strawberry, Haagen-Dazs*	1oz/28g	30.0	0.0	108	0.0	27.0	0.0	0.0
Peach & Vanilla Fruit Swirl, HL, Tesco*	1 Pot/73g	93.0	1.0	127	1.1	28.9	0.8	0.5
Pear, Organic, Evernat*	1oz/28g	33.0	0.0	119	0.0	28.3	0.6	0.0
Pineapple, Del Monte*	1 Sorbet/500g	600.0	0.0	120	0.3	30.6	0.1	0.0
Raspberry & Blackberry, Fat Free, M & S*	1 Sorbet/125g	140.0	0.0	112	0.4	27.5	0.0	0.6
Raspberry, Haagen-Dazs*	½ Cup/105g	120.0	0.0	114	0.0	28.6	0.0	1.9
Raspberry, Sticks, Haagen-Dazs*	1oz/28g	28.0	0.0	99	0.2	24.2	0.1	0.0
Raspberry, Tesco*	1 Serving/70ml	97.0	0.0	138	0.5	34.0	0.0	0.0
Raspberry, Waitrose*	1 Pot/750ml	690.0	1.0	92	0.5	22.2	0.1	1.1
Strawberry & Champagne, Sainsbury's*	¼ Pot/89g	95.0	0.0	107	0.2	25.5	0.0	0.6
Strawberry, Fruit Ice, Starburst, Mars*	1 Stick/93ml	99.0	0.0	106	0.1	26.7	0.1	0.0
Strawberry, M & S*	1oz/28g	27.0	0.0	95	0.3	23.4	0.1	0.5
Summer Berry, Swirl, Asda*	¼ Pack/89g	97.0	0.0	109	3.0	26.0	0.4	0.0
Swirl, Raspberry & Blackcurrant, Safeway*	1 Serving/50g	57.0	0.0	115	0.6	27.0	0.0	1.6
SOUFFLE								
Cheese	1oz/28g	71.0	5.0	253	11.4	9.3	19.2	0.3
Cheese, Mini, Waitrose*	1 Souffle/14g	32.0	2.0	232	16.0	2.9	17.4	2.4
Chocolate & Toffee, Gu*	1 Pot/95g	353.0	16.0	372	4.6	46.4	16.6	2.5
Chocolate, Gu*	1 Pot/70g	307.0	25.0	439	6.3	24.4	35.6	2.9
Lemon, Finest, Tesco*	1 Pot/80g	270.0	20.0	338	2.9	24.1	25.6	0.2
Plain	1oz/28g	56.0	4.0	201	7.6	10.4	14.7	0.3
Raspberry & Amaretto, M & S*	1oz/28g	83.0	5.0	298	2.8	33.1	16.7	0.1
Ricotta & Spinach, M & S*	1 Serving/120g	186.0	13.0	155	8.0	6.2	11.1	2.1
Strawberry, M & S*	1 Serving/95g	171.0	10.0	180	1.6	19.5	10.6	0.9
SOUP								
3 Bean & Chorizo, Low Fat, Solo Slim, Rosemary Conley*	1/100g	54.0	1.0	54	4.0	7.6	0.8	5.8
Apple, Carrot, Strawberry, Vie, Knorr*	1 Drink/100g	65.0	1.0	65	0.8	13.0	0.6	1.5
Asparagus & Chicken, Waitrose*	1 Can/415g	166.0	5.0	40	2.1	5.3	1.1	0.7
Asparagus & Creme Fraiche, Morrisons*	½ Pot/300g	186.0	12.0	62	1.3	5.4	3.9	0.5
Asparagus, Fresh, M & S*	1 Serving/300g	135.0	11.0	45	1.1	2.5	3.6	0.9
Asparagus, in a Cup, BGTY, Sainsbury's*	1 Sachet/18g	72.0	1.0	400	1.7	77.8	8.3	2.8
Asparagus, M & S*	1 Serving/300g	180.0	13.0	60	1.1	3.3	4.5	0.7
Asparagus, New Covent Garden Food Co*	½ Carton/300g	132.0	7.0	44	1.5	4.1	2.4	0.9
Asparagus, Slimline, Cup, Waitrose*	1 Sachet/204ml	51.0	1.0	25	0.4	4.3	0.7	0.7
Autumn Vegetable & Lentil, Heinz*	1 Can/400g	184.0	1.0	46	2.3	8.6	0.3	1.0

S

SOUP

INFO/WEIGHT	Measure KCAL	FAT	KCAL	PROT	CARB	FAT	FIBRE
Bean, Italian Style, Tesco*	1 Can/300g	153.0	4.0	51	2.8	7.3	1.2	1.1
Beef & Mushroom, Big Soup, Heinz*	1 Can/515g	216.0	3.0	42	2.3	7.0	0.5	0.7
Beef & Tomato, Cup a Soup, Batchelors*	1 Serving/252g	83.0	2.0	33	0.6	6.3	0.6	0.4
Beef & Vegetable Broth, Chunky, Canned, M & S*	1 Can/415g	166.0	3.0	40	1.9	6.4	0.8	0.6
Beef & Vegetable, Big Soup, Heinz*	1 Can/400g	212.0	4.0	53	3.5	7.5	1.0	0.9
Beef & Vegetable, Chunky, Canned, Sainsbury's*	1 Can/400g	188.0	3.0	47	3.2	6.7	0.8	1.3
Beef & Vegetable, for One, Fresh, Tesco*	1 Pot/300g	102.0	3.0	34	2.9	3.3	1.0	1.1
Beef & Winter Vegetable, Favourites, Baxters*	1 Can/415g	195.0	5.0	47	2.3	6.9	1.1	0.4
Beef Broth, Classic, Heinz*	1 Can/400g	180.0	3.0	45	2.2	7.2	0.7	0.8
Beef Stew & Dumplings, Taste of Home, Heinz*	1 Pot/430g	378.0	14.0	88	3.7	11.1	3.2	0.8
Beef, Mushroom & Red Wine, Farmers Market, Heinz*	1 Can/515g	263.0	9.0	51	2.4	6.4	1.8	0.7
Beef, Spicy, & Tomato, Diet Chef Ltd*	1 Pack/300g	165.0	6.0	55	2.3	7.3	1.9	1.9
Beef, Tripe, In Broth, Flaki, Asda*	1 Jar/520ml	192.0	6.0	37	5.9	1.3	1.2	0.0
Blended Autumn Vegetable, Heinz*	½ Can/200g	114.0	6.0	57	1.2	6.4	3.0	0.7
Blended Leek & Bacon, Heinz*	½ Can/200g	108.0	6.0	54	1.9	5.0	2.9	0.5
Blended Sweetcorn & Yellow Pepper, Heinz*	½ Can/200g	98.0	4.0	49	0.9	6.6	2.1	0.6
Boston Bean & Ham, New Covent Garden Food Co*	½ Carton/300g	171.0	1.0	57	2.4	7.8	0.2	1.6
Broccoli & Cauliflower, Cup-A-Soup, Made Up, Batchelors*	1 Serving/255g	107.0	5.0	42	0.6	5.3	2.0	1.1
Broccoli & Cheddar, Heinz*	1 Can/430g	340.0	24.0	79	2.6	4.4	5.6	0.6
Broccoli & Potato, Organic, Baxters*	1 Can/425g	161.0	3.0	38	1.5	6.2	0.8	0.7
Broccoli & Stilton, Canned, Sainsbury's*	½ Can/200g	108.0	7.0	54	2.0	3.7	3.5	0.6
Broccoli & Stilton, Classics, Fresh, Tesco*	½ Pot/300g	180.0	8.0	60	2.9	5.8	2.8	1.1
Broccoli & Stilton, Fresh, Sainsbury's*	½ Pot/300ml	141.0	10.0	47	2.7	1.8	3.3	1.5
Broccoli & Stilton, New Covent Garden Food Co*	1 Carton/600ml	336.0	26.0	56	2.3	1.8	4.4	0.7
Broccoli with Mustard, New Covent Garden Food Co*	1 Carton/568g	204.0	11.0	36	1.3	3.3	1.9	1.2
Broccoli, Baxters*	1 Can/425g	191.0	8.0	45	1.3	5.9	1.8	0.4
Broth, Ten Vegetable, Morrisons*	1 Pot/600g	240.0	8.0	40	1.7	5.8	1.3	1.1
Butternut Squash & Red Pepper, Baxters*	1 Can/415g	158.0	4.0	38	0.7	6.5	1.0	0.6
Butternut Squash, Creamy, New Covent Garden Food Co*	½ Carton/300g	153.0	7.0	51	0.8	6.4	2.5	0.9
Butternut Squash, Diet Chef Ltd*	1 Pack/300g	135.0	5.0	45	0.8	6.5	1.8	1.6
Butternut Squash, Fresh, Waitrose*	½ Pot/300g	153.0	9.0	51	0.5	5.8	2.9	0.8
Cantonese Hot & Sour Noodle, Baxters*	1 Serving/215g	133.0	3.0	62	1.4	11.1	1.3	0.5
Carrot & Butter Bean, Baxters*	½ Can/207.4g	112.0	4.0	54	1.6	7.7	1.9	1.7
Carrot & Butterbean, Diet Chef Ltd*	1 Pack/300g	174.0	2.0	58	2.7	10.3	0.7	2.8
Carrot & Coriander Soup, Low Fat, Fresh, Sainsbury's*	1 Tub/600g	114.0	4.0	19	0.2	3.2	0.6	1.9
Carrot & Coriander, Baxters*	1 Can/415g	170.0	6.0	41	0.8	6.0	1.5	0.8
Carrot & Coriander, Blended, Heinz*	½ Can/200g	104.0	5.0	52	0.7	6.2	2.7	0.6
Carrot & Coriander, Canned, Tesco*	1 Can/400g	220.0	12.0	55	0.7	5.7	2.9	0.8
Carrot & Coriander, Carton, Campbell's*	1 Serving/250ml	110.0	5.0	44	0.7	5.4	2.2	0.0
Carrot & Coriander, Classic Homestyle, M & S*	1 Can/425g	170.0	8.0	40	0.6	5.6	2.0	0.7
Carrot & Coriander, Fresh, New Covent Garden Food Co*	½ Carton/300g	129.0	7.0	43	0.6	5.2	2.2	1.2
Carrot & Coriander, Fresh, Organic, Simply Organic*	1 Pot/600g	276.0	18.0	46	0.5	4.5	3.0	1.3
Carrot & Coriander, Fresh, Waitrose*	½ Pot/300g	150.0	10.0	50	0.5	4.4	3.4	0.9
Carrot & Coriander, Heinz*	1 Can/400g	196.0	11.0	49	0.5	5.6	2.7	1.0
Carrot & Coriander, Waistline, Crosse & Blackwell*	1 Sachet/300g	111.0	2.0	37	0.7	6.8	0.8	1.0
Carrot & Coriander, with Creme Fraiche, Heinz*	1 Can/515g	232.0	9.0	45	0.7	6.6	1.8	0.9
Carrot & Ginger, Fresh, Sainsbury's*	1 Pot/600g	150.0	5.0	25	0.4	3.9	0.9	1.0
Carrot & Ginger, Perfectly Balanced, Waitrose*	½ Pot/300g	66.0	3.0	22	0.4	3.1	0.9	1.0
Carrot & Lentil, Microwave, Heinz*	1 Can/303g	94.0	0.0	31	1.5	6.1	0.1	0.8
Carrot & Lentil, Weight Watchers*	1 Can/295g	86.0	0.0	29	1.3	5.7	0.1	0.7
Carrot & Orange, Baxters*	1 Can/415g	174.0	2.0	42	1.0	8.3	0.5	0.4
Carrot & Orange, Pouch, Heinz*	½ Pack/300g	165.0	7.0	55	0.6	8.3	2.2	1.0
Carrot with Creme Fraiche, Baxters*	1 Can/415g	170.0	7.0	41	0.5	5.9	1.7	0.7

S

SOUP

Measure INFO/WEIGHT	per Measure KCAL	FAT	Nutrition Values per 100g / 100ml KCAL	PROT	CARB	FAT	FIBRE
Carrot, Onion & Chick Pea, Healthy Choice, Baxters*	1 Can/415ml	170.0	1.0	41	1.9	8.0	0.2	1.2
Carrot, Orange & Coriander, COU, M & S*	1 Pack/415g	145.0	2.0	35	0.6	6.9	0.6	1.2
Carrot, Orange & Ginger, Go Organic*	1 Jar/495g	119.0	4.0	24	0.5	3.6	0.8	1.4
Carrot, Parsnip & Nutmeg, Organic, Baxters*	1 Can/425g	144.0	2.0	34	0.7	6.6	0.5	1.1
Carrot, Parsnip & Sweet Potato, Classic, Baxters*	1 Carton/600g	348.0	17.0	58	0.9	7.2	2.8	1.3
Carrot, Potato & Coriander, Weight Watchers*	1 Can/295g	74.0	0.0	25	0.5	5.5	0.1	0.6
Cauliflower Cheese, Somerfield*	1 Pack/500g	345.0	25.0	69	3.0	3.0	5.0	0.0
Chicken & Bacon, with Pasta, Meal in a Mug, Tesco*	1 Sachet/37g	142.0	3.0	384	9.2	69.5	7.6	2.7
Chicken & Broccoli, Soup a Cups, GFY, Asda*	1 Cup/226ml	52.0	1.0	23	0.5	4.0	0.6	0.4
Chicken & Country Vegetable, Farmers Market, Heinz*	1 Can/342g	229.0	11.0	67	3.2	6.0	3.3	0.5
Chicken & Country Vegetable, Soupfulls, Batchelors*	1 Serving/400g	164.0	4.0	41	5.1	3.0	0.9	1.3
Chicken & Ham, Big, Heinz*	½ Can/200g	92.0	2.0	46	2.3	6.9	1.0	0.7
Chicken & Ham, Chunky, Canned, Sainsbury's*	½ Can/200g	80.0	1.0	40	2.7	6.0	0.6	0.9
Chicken & Herb, Farmers Market, Heinz*	½ Carton/300g	183.0	7.0	61	2.2	7.8	2.3	0.5
Chicken & King Prawn, Noodle, Fresh, Tesco*	1 Pot/400g	180.0	2.0	45	4.7	5.5	0.4	0.4
Chicken & Leek, Big Soup, Heinz*	½ Can/257.5g	162.0	5.0	63	3.0	8.2	2.0	0.6
Chicken & Leek, Cup a Soup, Made Up, Batchelors*	1 Serving/259g	96.0	5.0	37	0.5	4.7	1.8	0.7
Chicken & Mushroom in a Cup, Sainsbury's*	1 Sachet/223ml	107.0	4.0	48	0.7	7.1	1.9	0.1
Chicken & Mushroom, Canned, Tesco*	½ Can/200g	130.0	8.0	65	1.4	5.6	3.8	0.1
Chicken & Mushroom, Extra, Slim a Soup, Batchelors*	1 Serving/257g	90.0	2.0	35	1.4	5.9	0.6	0.3
Chicken & Mushroom, Soup-A-Slim, Asda*	1 Sachet/14g	51.0	1.0	362	10.0	58.0	10.0	4.2
Chicken & Pasta Big, Heinz*	½ Can/200g	68.0	1.0	34	1.8	5.9	0.4	0.8
Chicken & Sweetcorn, Baxters*	1 Can/425g	166.0	4.0	39	1.6	6.2	0.9	0.6
Chicken & Sweetcorn, Canned, BGTY, Sainsbury's*	½ Can/200g	56.0	1.0	28	1.5	4.5	0.4	0.2
Chicken & Sweetcorn, Canned, Tesco*	1 Can/400ml	240.0	6.0	60	1.6	8.2	1.5	0.7
Chicken & Sweetcorn, Cantonese, Fresh, Sainsbury's*	½ Pot/300ml	135.0	1.0	45	2.1	7.9	0.5	0.5
Chicken & Sweetcorn, Cup Soup, Asda*	1 Sachet/200ml	109.0	4.0	54	0.7	8.5	1.9	0.3
Chicken & Sweetcorn, GFY, Asda*	1 Can/400g	108.0	2.0	27	1.5	4.2	0.5	0.2
Chicken & Sweetcorn, Light Choice, Tesco*	½ Can 200g	84.0	1.0	42	1.7	7.9	0.4	0.2
Chicken & Tarragon, Thick & Creamy, Batchelors*	1 Sachet/281g	118.0	6.0	42	0.8	5.7	2.3	0.3
Chicken & Thyme, Diet Chef Ltd*	1 Pack/300g	147.0	9.0	49	2.2	3.4	3.0	0.7
Chicken & Vegetable Broth, Canned, BFY, Morrisons*	½ Can/205g	50.0	0.0	24	1.2	4.5	0.2	0.5
Chicken & Vegetable Casserole, Taste of Home, Heinz*	1 Pot/430g	331.0	17.0	77	3.9	6.7	3.9	0.8
Chicken & Vegetable with Pasta, Select, Campbell's*	1 Can/480ml	220.0	1.0	46	2.9	7.9	0.2	0.8
Chicken & Vegetable, Big Soup, Heinz*	½ Can/200g	104.0	3.0	52	3.3	6.7	1.4	0.8
Chicken & Vegetable, Chunky, Canned, Eat Well, M & S*	½ Can/213g	138.0	4.0	65	4.6	6.9	1.9	1.0
Chicken & Vegetable, Classic, Heinz*	1 Can/400g	132.0	2.0	33	1.1	6.2	0.4	0.6
Chicken & Vegetable, Healthy Choice, Canned, Baxters*	1 Can/415g	162.0	2.0	39	1.9	6.8	0.5	1.7
Chicken & Vegetable, Soup to Go, Asda*	1 Pot/330g	145.0	5.0	44	2.4	5.1	1.5	0.7
Chicken & White Wine, Campbell's*	1 Serving/295g	145.0	10.0	49	1.0	4.0	3.3	0.0
Chicken Broth, Baxters*	1 Can/415g	129.0	2.0	31	1.5	5.4	0.4	0.6
Chicken Curry, Mild, Indian, Soups of the World, Heinz*	1 Can/515g	381.0	21.0	74	3.6	5.9	4.1	0.3
Chicken Leek & Potato Soup, Weight Watchers*	1 Tin/295g	80.0	1.0	27	0.9	5.0	0.4	0.3
Chicken Mulligatawny, Chunky, Meal, Weight Watchers*	1 Pack/340g	163.0	4.0	48	2.2	6.8	1.3	1.5
Chicken Mulligatawny, Perfectly Balanced, Waitrose*	1 Serving/300g	138.0	6.0	46	1.7	5.3	2.0	0.4
Chicken Noodle & Vegetable, Slim a Soup, Batchelors*	1 Serving/203g	55.0	1.0	27	0.8	4.8	0.5	0.6
Chicken Noodle, Batchelors*	1 Pack/284g	71.0	1.0	25	1.6	4.2	0.2	0.3
Chicken Noodle, Canned, Sainsbury's*	½ Can/217g	78.0	1.0	36	1.7	7.4	0.3	0.7
Chicken Noodle, Chunky, Campbell's*	½ Can/200g	86.0	1.0	43	2.8	6.5	0.6	0.0
Chicken Noodle, Classic, Heinz*	1 Can/400g	124.0	1.0	31	1.2	6.0	0.3	0.2
Chicken Noodle, Clear, Weight Watchers*	1 Can/295g	50.0	0.0	17	0.7	3.1	0.1	0.2
Chicken Noodle, Simmer & Serve, Dried, Sainsbury's*	1 Pack/600ml	102.0	1.0	17	0.8	2.9	0.2	0.0
Chicken Noodle, Soup in a Cup, Made Up, Sainsbury's*	1 Serving/200ml	44.0	0.0	22	0.7	4.7	0.1	0.2

S

SOUP

INFO/WEIGHT	Measure KCAL	FAT	Nutrition Values per 100g / 100ml KCAL	PROT	CARB	FAT	FIBRE
Chicken Noodle, with Sweetcorn, Baxters*	1 Can/415g	141.0	2.0	34	1.4	5.8	0.6	0.2
Chicken, Coconut & Lemon Grass, Fresh, Waitrose*	½ Pot/300g	303.0	25.0	101	2.6	4.1	8.3	0.8
Chicken, Condensed, 99% Fat Free, Campbell's*	1 Can/295g	77.0	2.0	26	1.0	3.8	0.7	0.1
Chicken, Cream Of, Canned	1oz/28g	16.0	1.0	58	1.7	4.5	3.8	0.0
Chicken, Cup, Calorie Counter, Dry, Co-Op*	1 Sachet/13g	40.0	1.0	320	6.0	49.0	11.0	7.0
Chicken, Fresh, Sainsbury's*	½ Carton/300g	126.0	6.0	42	2.2	4.0	1.9	0.3
Chicken, Green Thai, Sainsbury's*	1 Pot/600g	366.0	20.0	61	1.9	5.8	3.3	0.3
Chicken, Green Thai, Spiced, M & S*	½ Pot/300g	195.0	11.0	65	2.0	6.3	3.8	0.6
Chicken, in a Cup, Sainsbury's*	1 Serving/221ml	86.0	4.0	39	0.7	5.3	1.7	0.1
Chicken, Leek & Potato, Weight Watchers*	1 Can/400g	108.0	2.0	27	0.9	5.0	0.4	0.3
Chicken, Leek & White Wine, Fresh, Finest, Tesco*	1 Pack/300g	216.0	13.0	72	2.8	5.7	4.2	0.3
Chicken, M & S*	1 Pack/213g	196.0	15.0	92	1.6	5.5	7.2	0.2
Chicken, Moroccan Inspired, Sainsbury's*	1 Bowl/342g	202.0	3.0	59	2.6	10.2	0.9	7.5
Chicken, Mulligatawny, Finest, Tesco*	½ Pot/300g	240.0	12.0	80	4.0	7.0	4.0	0.8
Chicken, Mushroom & Rice, Chilled, M & S*	½ Pot/300g	225.0	10.0	75	3.2	7.3	3.4	1.8
Chicken, Mushroom, & Potato, Big Soup, Heinz*	½ Can/200g	132.0	5.0	66	3.4	8.1	2.3	0.4
Chicken, New Covent Garden Food Co*	1 Carton/600g	510.0	32.0	85	3.8	5.4	5.4	0.6
Chicken, Potato & Bacon, Big Soup, Heinz*	1 Can/515g	278.0	10.0	54	3.1	6.2	1.9	0.5
Chicken, Potato, & Lentil, Weight Watchers*	1 Can/400g	136.0	4.0	34	1.2	5.3	0.9	0.3
Chicken, Red Thai, Chunky, Fresh, Sainsbury's*	½ Pot/300g	165.0	10.0	55	0.9	5.4	3.3	0.9
Chicken, Red Thai, Waitrose*	1 Pot/600g	348.0	19.0	58	3.5	4.1	3.1	1.1
Chicken, Roasted, Canned, Tesco*	1 Can/400g	220.0	11.0	55	1.0	6.6	2.7	0.3
Chicken, Sweetcorn & Potato, Heinz*	1 Can/400g	204.0	11.0	51	1.2	5.4	2.8	0.3
Chicken, Thai Blend, Baxters*	½ Pot/300g	282.0	22.0	94	1.7	5.3	7.3	0.4
Chicken, Thai, Fresh, Finest, Tesco*	½ Tub/300g	255.0	16.0	85	4.1	4.2	5.4	1.1
Chicken, Thai, GFY, Asda*	1 Serving/200g	85.0	3.0	42	1.7	5.5	1.5	0.5
Chicken, Thai, Noodle, Baxters*	1 Serving/430g	400.0	32.0	93	1.6	4.8	7.5	0.3
Chicken, Thai, Spicy, Baxters*	1 Can/415g	278.0	15.0	67	1.8	7.1	3.5	0.3
Chicken, Tomato & Red Pepper, Italian, Big Soup, Heinz*	½ Can/200g	78.0	2.0	39	1.6	6.2	0.9	0.7
Chicken, Weight Watchers*	1 Can/300g	97.0	3.0	32	1.6	4.1	1.0	0.0
Chicken,Noodle, Canned, Asda*	1 Can/400g	148.0	4.0	37	1.7	5.1	1.1	0.7
Chilli Bean, M & S*	½ Carton/300g	150.0	7.0	50	2.5	4.7	2.5	2.7
Chilli Bean, Mexican, Tesco*	1 Carton/600g	270.0	7.0	45	2.2	6.4	1.1	1.9
Chilli Beef, Mighty, Asda*	1 Can/400g	236.0	6.0	59	4.9	6.8	1.4	1.2
Chilli Con Carne, Chunky, Sainsbury's*	½ Can/200g	110.0	2.0	55	3.6	8.0	0.9	1.5
Chilli, Meal, Chunky, Canned, Tesco*	½ Can/200g	120.0	2.0	60	5.0	6.3	1.2	1.6
Chorizo & Bean, TTD, Sainsbury's*	1 Pack/298g	161.0	2.0	54	4.0	7.6	0.8	5.8
Chorizo & Tomato with Vegetables, Canned, Sainsbury's*	½ Can/200g	114.0	6.0	57	2.6	4.9	3.0	0.3
Chowder, Bacon & Corn, M & S*	½ Pot/300g	195.0	11.0	65	2.5	6.0	3.6	1.8
Chowder, Clam, New England, Select, Campbell's*	1 Cup/240ml	221.0	14.0	92	2.5	6.0	6.0	0.8
Chowder, Prawn, Manhattan, Fresh, Sainsbury's*	1 Serving/300g	177.0	7.0	59	1.6	7.9	2.3	0.1
Chowder, Seafood, Baxters*	½ Can/213.3g	160.0	10.0	75	3.3	5.4	4.5	0.4
Chowder, Smoked Haddock, Canned, Sainsbury's*	½ Can/200g	128.0	8.0	64	1.6	5.3	4.0	0.3
Chowder, Sweetcorn & Chicken, Heinz*	1 Serving/200g	148.0	6.0	74	3.3	9.1	2.8	0.6
Chunky Chicken Hotpot, Big Soup, Heinz*	½ Can/258g	126.0	3.0	49	2.3	7.4	1.2	0.8
Cock-A-Leekie, Traditional, Baxters*	1 Can/425g	98.0	2.0	23	1.0	3.7	0.5	0.3
Country Garden, Vegetarian, Canned, Baxters*	1 Can/415g	137.0	2.0	33	1.0	6.0	0.5	0.8
Country Mushroom, Baxters*	1 Pot/600g	378.0	25.0	63	0.9	5.5	4.1	0.1
Country Mushroom, Selection, Campbell's*	1 Serving/250ml	80.0	4.0	32	0.6	3.4	1.8	0.5
Country Vegetable & Herb, Farmers Market, Heinz*	½ Carton/300g	114.0	4.0	38	1.2	5.7	1.2	0.9
Country Vegetable Casserole, Taste of Home, Heinz*	1 Pot/430g	206.0	6.0	48	1.3	7.6	1.4	1.3
Country Vegetable, Asda*	1 Serving/125g	59.0	4.0	47	0.6	4.5	2.9	0.8
Country Vegetable, Chunky, Asda*	½ Pot/300g	138.0	2.0	46	2.0	8.2	0.6	0.5

S

SOUP

INFO/WEIGHT	Measure KCAL	per Measure FAT	KCAL	PROT	CARB	FAT	FIBRE
Country Vegetable, Chunky, Healthy Choice, Baxters*	1 Pot/273.9g	126.0	1.0	46	2.0	8.8	0.3	1.7
Country Vegetable, Fresh, Chilled, Eat Well, M & S*	½ Pot/300g	135.0	6.0	45	1.0	5.2	2.0	1.4
Country Vegetable, Knorr*	1 Pack/500ml	160.0	3.0	32	0.9	5.5	0.7	1.2
Country Vegetable, Weight Watchers*	1 Can/297g	92.0	1.0	31	1.1	6.1	0.2	1.0
Courgette & Parmesan, Fresh, Sainsbury's*	1 Pack/300ml	198.0	17.0	66	1.5	2.5	5.6	0.4
Cream of Asparagus, Baxters*	1 Can/415g	278.0	18.0	67	1.1	6.0	4.3	0.2
Cream of Asparagus, Cup a Soup, Batchelors*	1 Sachet/223g	143.0	6.0	64	0.5	9.2	2.8	0.4
Cream of Asparagus, in a Cup, Sainsbury's*	1 Serving/230ml	129.0	5.0	56	0.7	8.2	2.3	0.1
Cream of Celery, Campbell's*	1 Serving/150g	70.0	5.0	47	0.6	3.2	3.4	0.0
Cream of Chicken & Mushroom, Campbell's*	1 Can/250g	140.0	11.0	56	0.9	3.5	4.4	0.0
Cream of Chicken & Mushroom, Canned, Sainsbury's*	1 Can/400g	248.0	17.0	62	1.8	4.0	4.3	0.4
Cream of Chicken & Mushroom, Heinz*	½ Can/200g	98.0	6.0	49	1.3	4.6	2.9	0.1
Cream of Chicken, Batchelors*	1 Pack/289g	165.0	10.0	57	1.1	5.6	3.3	0.3
Cream of Chicken, Baxters*	½ Can/206.7g	122.0	6.0	59	2.4	5.6	3.0	0.1
Cream of Chicken, Campbell's*	1 Can/590g	283.0	21.0	48	1.1	3.5	3.6	0.0
Cream of Chicken, Classic, Heinz*	1 Can/400g	208.0	12.0	52	1.7	4.7	3.0	0.1
Cream of Chicken, Fresh, Waitrose*	1 Serving/300g	180.0	12.0	60	2.6	3.7	3.9	0.2
Cream of Leek, Baxters*	1 Can/415g	237.0	17.0	57	1.1	3.8	4.2	0.1
Cream of Mushroom, Classics, Heinz*	1 Can/400g	208.0	11.0	52	1.5	5.2	2.8	0.1
Cream of Mushroom, Dry, Knorr*	1 Serving/25g	125.0	8.0	500	5.2	47.8	31.8	1.0
Cream of Mushroom, GFY, Asda*	1 Serving/250g	92.0	1.0	37	2.1	6.0	0.5	0.3
Cream of Mushroom, Soupreme*	1 Serving/200g	100.0	6.0	50	1.4	4.5	2.9	0.3
Cream of Potato & Leek, Canned, Sainsbury's*	½ Can/200g	80.0	3.0	40	0.6	6.1	1.5	0.0
Cream of Sweetcorn, Campbell's*	1 Serving/80g	41.0	2.0	51	0.6	6.2	2.7	0.5
Cream of Vegetable, Velouté De Légumes, Liebig*	1 Portion/200ml	84.0	4.0	42	0.7	5.3	2.0	1.0
Cumberland Sausage & Vegetable, Big Soup, Heinz*	1 Can/515g	211.0	4.0	41	2.1	6.7	0.7	0.8
Egg, Drop, Average	1 Container/500g	470.0	30.0	94	6.0	4.0	6.0	0.0
Farmhouse Vegetable, Canned, BGTY, Sainsbury's*	½ Can/200ml	52.0	2.0	26	0.5	4.4	0.8	0.9
Farmhouse Vegetable, Soup-A-Cup, GFY, Asda*	1 Sachet/219ml	59.0	1.0	27	0.6	4.9	0.5	0.4
Farmhouse Vegetable, Thick, Co-Op*	1 Can/400g	140.0	2.0	35	1.0	7.0	0.4	0.3
Fire Roasted Tomato & Red Pepper, Asda*	½ Tub/265g	114.0	7.0	43	0.7	4.1	2.6	1.0
Flame Roasted Red Pepper & Tomato, Baxters*	½ Can/207g	116.0	6.0	56	0.9	6.8	2.8	0.6
French Onion	1oz/28g	11.0	1.0	40	0.2	5.7	2.1	1.0
French Onion & Cider, Waitrose*	1 Can/425g	93.0	0.0	22	0.5	4.8	0.1	0.4
French Onion & Gruyere Cheese, Fresh, Finest, Tesco*	½ Pot/300g	210.0	15.0	70	1.4	4.7	5.1	0.5
Garden Pea & Wiltshire Cured Ham, Finest, Tesco*	½ Pot/300g	195.0	8.0	65	3.4	5.9	2.7	1.6
Garden Vegetable, Baxters*	1 Serving/200g	70.0	1.0	35	0.9	6.6	0.6	0.8
Garden Vegetable, Heinz*	1 Can/400g	160.0	3.0	40	0.9	7.2	0.8	0.9
Gazpacho, Canned, Average	1 Can/400g	76.0	0.0	19	2.9	1.8	0.1	0.2
Golden Vegetable, Asda*	1 Pack/300g	150.0	6.0	50	1.9	6.0	2.0	0.0
Golden Vegetable, Slim a Soup, Batchelors*	1 Sachet/207g	58.0	2.0	28	0.5	4.7	0.8	0.7
Green Vegetables & Lentil, Lima*	1 Serving/300g	96.0	4.0	32	1.6	3.7	1.2	0.5
Gumbo, Spicy, Fresh, Sainsbury's*	½ Pot/300g	120.0	5.0	40	1.5	4.5	1.8	0.9
Haddock, Smoked, Fresh, Finest, Tesco*	1 Pot/550g	302.0	14.0	55	2.7	5.1	2.5	0.8
Haggis Broth, Baxters*	1 Can/415g	187.0	6.0	45	1.8	6.1	1.5	0.6
Harvest Carrot & Lima Bean, Heinz*	1oz/28g	11.0	0.0	40	0.8	6.9	1.0	1.3
Harvest Vegetable, Soupfull, Batchelors*	1 Can/400g	160.0	0.0	40	1.4	8.4	0.1	1.6
Harvest Vegetable, with Croutons, in a Cup, Sainsbury's*	1 Sachet/226ml	86.0	3.0	38	1.0	5.9	1.2	0.9
Heart Warming, New Covent Garden Food Co*	½ Carton/300g	102.0	3.0	34	1.2	4.7	1.1	1.1
Highlander's Broth, Baxters*	½ Can/206.4g	97.0	3.0	47	1.8	6.5	1.5	0.6
Hot Sweet Piquante Pepper & Carrot, Choices, Baxters*	1 Pouch/300g	135.0	3.0	45	0.8	8.2	1.0	0.6
Italian Bean & Pasta, Healthy Choice, Baxters*	1 Can/415g	170.0	1.0	41	1.7	8.2	0.2	1.3
Italian Chicken Broth, Healthy Choice, Baxters*	½ Can/210g	84.0	2.0	40	1.5	6.6	0.8	0.8

SOUP

INFO/WEIGHT	Measure	per Measure KCAL	per Measure FAT	KCAL	PROT	CARB	FAT	FIBRE
Italian Meatball & Tomato, Soups of the World, Heinz*	1 Can/515g	319.0	15.0	62	2.5	6.4	2.9	1.8
Italian Minestrone, M & S*	1 Can/425g	191.0	2.0	45	2.2	9.0	0.5	0.8
Italian Style Tomato & Basil, Co-Op*	1 Pack/500g	200.0	10.0	40	1.0	4.0	2.0	0.6
Lamb & Cous Cous, M & S*	½ Can/208g	100.0	4.0	48	2.1	6.2	1.8	0.9
Lamb & Vegetable, Big Soup, Heinz*	½ Can/200g	120.0	3.0	60	3.0	9.1	1.3	1.3
Lancashire Lamb Hotpot, Taste of Home, Heinz*	1 Pot/430g	299.0	11.0	70	2.6	8.9	2.6	1.1
Laska, Chicken & Noodle, Simply Fuller Longer, M & S*	1 Pack/385g	289.0	8.0	75	7.0	7.1	2.0	0.9
Leek & Chicken, Knorr*	1 Serving/300ml	82.0	5.0	27	0.6	2.4	1.7	0.1
Leek & Potato, Chunky, Meal, Canned, Tesco*	½ Can/200g	60.0	3.0	30	1.0	3.5	1.3	1.0
Leek & Potato, Creamy, Fresh, Asda*	1 Serving/300g	156.0	10.0	52	2.1	3.7	3.2	0.9
Leek & Potato, Fresh, Tesco*	½ Tub/300g	171.0	10.0	57	1.0	5.3	3.5	0.7
Leek & Potato, in a Cup, BGTY, Sainsbury's*	1 Serving/218ml	59.0	2.0	27	0.3	4.9	0.7	0.2
Leek & Potato, Slim a Soup, Batchelors*	1 Serving/204g	57.0	1.0	28	0.4	5.0	0.7	0.2
Leek & Potato, Smooth, Vie, Knorr*	1 Pack/500ml	155.0	4.0	31	0.9	4.8	0.9	1.0
Leek & Potato, Soup in a Cup, Made Up, Waitrose*	1 Sachet/204ml	47.0	1.0	23	0.3	4.3	0.5	0.5
Leek & Potato, Weight Watchers*	1 Sachet/215ml	58.0	1.0	27	0.5	5.1	0.5	0.1
Lentil & Bacon, Baxters*	1 Can/425g	221.0	4.0	52	3.2	7.7	0.9	0.7
Lentil & Bacon, Canned, Tesco*	1 Serving/200g	96.0	1.0	48	3.2	7.2	0.7	0.5
Lentil & Bean, Spicy, Canned, Organic, Asda*	1 Can/400g	212.0	3.0	53	2.8	8.6	0.8	3.0
Lentil & Chick Pea, Fresh, Organic, Tesco*	1 Serving/300ml	117.0	2.0	39	1.9	6.1	0.8	0.5
Lentil & Pancetta, Tesco*	½ Can/192g	115.0	2.0	60	3.1	8.0	1.3	1.6
Lentil & Parsley, Simply Organic*	1 Pot/600g	390.0	2.0	65	4.4	11.8	0.3	1.4
Lentil & Potato, Spiced, Heinz*	1 Can/295g	118.0	1.0	40	2.0	7.7	0.2	0.7
Lentil & Red Pepper, Sainsbury's*	½ Pot/300g	162.0	4.0	54	3.5	7.4	1.2	1.6
Lentil & Smoked Bacon, Fresh, Tesco*	1 Pack/600g	420.0	11.0	70	3.9	8.5	1.9	1.6
Lentil & Tomato, New Covent Garden Food Co*	½ Pack/284g	162.0	3.0	57	3.6	8.1	1.1	0.7
Lentil & Tomato, Spicy, Chunky, Fresh, Tesco*	½ Pot/300g	195.0	5.0	65	2.6	9.7	1.8	1.3
Lentil & Vegetable Soup, Healthy Choice, Baxters*	1 Can/415g	174.0	1.0	42	2.3	7.8	0.2	1.1
Lentil & Vegetable with Bacon, Organic, Baxters*	½ Can/211g	93.0	1.0	44	1.9	7.6	0.7	1.0
Lentil & Vegetable, Diet Chef Ltd*	1 Pack/300g	156.0	1.0	52	2.6	9.6	0.3	2.1
Lentil & Vegetable, Light Choices, Tesco*	1 Can/400g	188.0	1.0	47	2.5	8.8	0.2	1.1
Lentil, Average	1 Serving/220g	218.0	8.0	99	4.4	12.7	3.8	1.1
Lentil, Bacon & Mixed Bean, Low Fat, Aldi*	1 Serving/400g	260.0	4.0	65	4.7	9.5	0.9	1.6
Lentil, Carrot & Cumin, Canned, BGTY, Sainsbury's*	1 Can/400g	204.0	4.0	51	2.3	8.4	0.9	0.1
Lentil, Low Fat, Amy's Kitchen*	1 Can/411g	242.0	7.0	59	3.1	7.7	1.7	3.6
Lentil, Spicy, Organic, Suma*	1 Can/400g	232.0	5.0	58	2.7	9.0	1.2	1.6
Lentil, Tomato & Vegetable, M & S*	1 Can/415g	170.0	3.0	41	2.0	6.3	0.8	1.4
Lentil, with Red Lentils, Carrots, Potato & Onion, Asda*	1 Can/400g	192.0	1.0	48	1.4	10.2	0.2	1.2
Lincolnshire Sausage Hotpot, Taste of Home, Heinz*	1 Pot/430g	301.0	13.0	70	2.4	7.9	3.1	1.0
Lobster Bisque, Baxters*	1 Can/415g	187.0	9.0	45	3.0	3.6	2.1	0.2
Lobster Bisque, New Covent Garden Food Co*	½ Carton/300g	108.0	2.0	36	3.2	4.4	0.6	0.4
Lobster Bisque, Waitrose*	½ Carton/300g	201.0	14.0	67	0.9	5.5	4.6	0.6
Londoner's Pea Souper, New Covent Garden Food Co*	½ Carton/300g	153.0	6.0	51	4.3	4.1	2.0	1.1
Mediterranean Minestrone, Campbell's*	½ Carton/250ml	95.0	3.0	38	0.9	6.1	1.1	0.6
Mediterranean Tomato & Vegetable, Fresh, Tesco*	½ Pot/300g	105.0	2.0	35	1.0	6.2	0.7	0.7
Mediterranean Tomato, Baxters*	1 Can/415g	129.0	1.0	31	0.9	6.3	0.2	0.7
Mediterranean Tomato, Campbell's*	1 Can/295g	83.0	0.0	28	0.6	6.4	0.0	0.0
Mediterranean Tomato, Instant, Weight Watchers*	1 Serving/200ml	50.0	0.0	25	0.7	5.2	0.1	0.1
Mediterranean Tomato, Slim a Soup, Cup, Batchelors*	1 Serving/208g	56.0	1.0	27	0.5	4.8	0.6	0.4
Mediterranean Vegetable, GFY, Asda*	½ Pot/250g	80.0	4.0	32	0.5	3.6	1.7	1.6
Mediterranean Vegetable, Homepride*	1 Serving/250ml	82.0	3.0	33	0.9	4.3	1.3	0.0
Melon & Carrot, New Covent Garden Food Co*	1 Serving/300g	60.0	1.0	20	0.6	3.6	0.4	0.6
Mexican Bean, Safe To Eat*	1 Pouch/400g	140.0	1.0	35	2.4	4.7	0.3	1.8

SOUP

	Measure INFO/WEIGHT	per Measure KCAL	FAT	Nutrition Values per 100g / 100ml KCAL	PROT	CARB	FAT	FIBRE
Mexican Beef Chilli, Mighty, Asda*	1 Can/400g	192.0	3.0	48	3.3	7.0	0.7	0.9
Mexican Black Bean, Extra Special, Asda*	½ Pot/263g	194.0	11.0	74	2.3	7.0	4.1	1.7
Mexican Chilli Beef & Bean, Soups of the World, Heinz*	1 Can/515g	360.0	9.0	70	4.5	9.0	1.8	1.6
Mexican Spicy Bean, Weight Watchers*	1 Can/400g	160.0	2.0	40	1.4	7.4	0.5	1.0
Minestrone with Wholemeal Pasta, Baxters*	1 Can/400g	136.0	1.0	34	0.9	7.0	0.2	1.0
Minestrone, Average	1 Serving/220g	139.0	7.0	63	1.8	7.6	3.0	0.9
Minestrone, Chunky, Big Soup, Heinz*	½ Can/200g	74.0	2.0	37	1.3	6.2	0.8	1.1
Minestrone, Chunky, Canned, Sainsbury's*	½ Can/200g	80.0	1.0	40	1.5	7.2	0.6	1.2
Minestrone, Chunky, Fresh, Baxters*	1 Serving/250g	95.0	2.0	38	1.5	6.5	0.7	1.1
Minestrone, Chunky, Waitrose*	1 Can/415g	195.0	3.0	47	1.6	8.3	0.8	1.1
Minestrone, Diet Chef Ltd*	1 Pack/300g	123.0	3.0	41	1.4	6.9	0.9	1.2
Minestrone, for One, Heinz*	1 Can/300g	96.0	2.0	32	1.4	5.2	0.7	0.7
Minestrone, Healthy Choice, Baxters*	½ Can/208g	71.0	0.0	34	0.9	7.0	0.2	1.0
Minestrone, Hearty, 99% Fat Free, Campbell's*	1 Can/295g	77.0	0.0	26	0.7	5.6	0.1	0.0
Minestrone, Hearty, Chilled, Farmers Market, Heinz*	½ Carton/300g	123.0	3.0	41	1.4	6.9	0.9	0.5
Minestrone, in a Cup, BGTY, Sainsbury's*	1 Serving/200ml	54.0	0.0	27	0.8	6.0	0.1	0.6
Minestrone, In A Mug, Made Up, Morrisons*	1 Sachet/269g	132.0	2.0	49	1.4	10.4	0.6	0.6
Minestrone, Italian, Canned, Sainsbury's*	1 Can/415g	212.0	7.0	51	2.0	6.6	1.8	1.1
Minestrone, Low Fat, Solo Slim, Rosemary Conley*	1 Serving/100g	41.0	1.0	41	1.4	6.9	0.9	1.2
Minestrone, Organic, M & S*	1 Pack/208g	83.0	1.0	40	1.4	8.9	0.5	1.1
Minestrone, Tuscan, Weight Watchers*	½ Can/200g	86.0	2.0	43	1.1	7.0	1.1	0.9
Minestrone, with Borlotti Beans, Tuscan Style, Heinz*	½ Can/200g	90.0	1.0	45	1.4	8.0	0.7	1.1
Minestrone, with Croutons, Cup a Soup, Batchelors*	1 Serving	93.0	1.0	37	0.7	7.3	0.5	0.3
Minestrone, with Croutons, Slim a Soup, Batchelors*	1 Serving/203g	55.0	1.0	27	0.6	4.8	0.6	0.6
Minted Lamb Hot Pot, Big Soup, Heinz*	1 Can/400g	220.0	5.0	55	2.6	8.5	1.2	1.0
Miso, Instant, Blue Dragon*	1 Sachet/18g	25.0	1.0	139	10.0	14.4	3.9	0.0
Miso, Japanese, Made Up, Yutaka*	1 Serving/250ml	24.0	1.0	10	0.6	1.1	0.3	0.0
Mix, Carrot & Coriander, Fresh Tastes, Asda*	¼ Pack/200g	30.0	0.0	15	0.4	3.1	0.1	1.1
Mixed Bean & Pepper, Organic, M & S*	1 Pack/208g	94.0	1.0	45	2.3	7.7	0.3	1.8
Moroccan Chick Pea, M & S*	1oz/28g	20.0	1.0	70	3.6	8.8	2.1	2.0
Moroccan Chicken, Waitrose*	½ Pot/300g	147.0	4.0	49	3.8	5.4	1.4	4.5
Moroccan Lentil, Waitrose*	½ Pot/300g	153.0	1.0	51	3.5	8.2	0.5	3.4
Mulligatawny	1 Serving/220g	213.0	15.0	97	1.4	8.2	6.8	0.9
Mulligatawny, Classic, Heinz*	1 Can/400g	208.0	7.0	52	2.0	7.1	1.8	0.6
Mulligatawny, in a Cup, Symingtons*	1 Serving/232ml	95.0	1.0	41	0.7	8.3	0.6	0.5
Mushroom & Crouton, Cup Soup, Made Up, Heinz*	1 Cup/200ml	80.0	4.0	40	0.7	4.5	2.1	0.0
Mushroom Potage, Baxters*	1 Can/415g	320.0	22.0	77	1.5	6.1	5.2	0.3
Mushroom, 98% Fat Free, Baxters*	1 Can/425g	170.0	7.0	40	0.9	5.6	1.6	0.3
Mushroom, Canned, HL, Tesco*	1 Can/400g	132.0	6.0	33	0.5	4.4	1.4	0.2
Mushroom, Diet Chef Ltd*	1 Pack/300g	105.0	5.0	35	1.9	3.2	1.7	0.9
Mushroom, Farm Harvest, Green Giant*	1 Pouch/330g	122.0	6.0	37	0.6	5.2	1.8	1.3
Mushroom, Field, Morrisons*	1 Pack/600g	192.0	10.0	32	0.8	3.3	1.7	0.0
Mushroom, for One, Heinz*	1 Can/290g	148.0	8.0	51	1.4	5.1	2.7	0.1
Mushroom, Fresh, M & S*	½ Pack/300g	165.0	12.0	55	1.8	3.5	3.9	0.9
Mushroom, in a Cup, Sainsbury's*	1 Serving/200ml	96.0	4.0	48	0.5	7.0	1.9	0.2
Mushroom, Low Fat, Fresh, Sainsbury's*	½ Pot/300g	132.0	9.0	44	0.7	3.7	2.9	0.6
Mushroom, Simmer & Serve, Dried, Sainsbury's*	½ Pack/600ml	234.0	10.0	39	0.6	5.5	1.6	0.3
Mushroom, Weight Watchers*	1 Can/295g	83.0	2.0	28	1.1	4.5	0.7	0.1
Onion, Ten Calorie, Gourmet Cuisine*	1 Serving/200g	10.0	0.0	5	0.3	0.8	0.1	0.1
Oxtail, Baxters*	1 Can/415g	187.0	5.0	45	1.9	6.4	1.3	0.5
Oxtail, Classic, Heinz*	1 Can/400g	156.0	2.0	39	1.9	6.7	0.5	0.3
Oxtail, Condensed, Classics, Diluted, Campbell's*	1 Can/590g	236.0	9.0	40	1.4	5.3	1.5	0.0
Oxtail, For One, Heinz*	1 Can/300g	117.0	2.0	39	1.7	6.6	0.6	0.3

SOUP

INFO/WEIGHT	Measure	per Measure KCAL	FAT	Nutrition Values per 100g / 100ml KCAL	PROT	CARB	FAT	FIBRE
Oxtail, Simmer & Serve, Dried, Sainsbury's*	1 Pack/600ml	180.0	5.0	30	0.6	4.9	0.9	0.2
Paddestoelen, Cup a Soup, Made Up, Batchelors*	1 Serving/100ml	5.0	0.0	5	0.4	0.6	0.1	0.2
Parsnip & Apple, COU, M & S*	1 Can/415g	187.0	10.0	45	0.7	5.4	2.5	1.2
Parsnip & Chilli, Diet Chef Ltd*	1 Serving /300g	102.0	4.0	34	0.8	4.6	1.4	1.3
Parsnip & Honey, Diet Chef Ltd*	1 Pack/300g	153.0	7.0	51	0.9	6.3	2.5	1.8
Parsnip & Honey, Fresh, Sainsbury's*	½ Carton/300g	192.0	13.0	64	1.1	5.4	4.2	1.5
Parsnip, Fresh, Morrisons*	½ Pot/250g	100.0	4.0	40	0.9	5.8	1.5	1.4
Parsnip, Fresh, VLH Kitchens	1 Serving/400g	180.0	6.0	45	0.9	5.8	1.6	1.4
Parsnip, Honey & Ginger, COU, M & S*	1 Can/415g	124.0	2.0	30	0.7	5.3	0.6	0.7
Parsnip, Leek & Ginger, New Covent Garden Food Co*	1 Carton/600g	162.0	2.0	27	1.2	4.9	0.3	1.3
Parsnip, Mr Bean's*	1 Tin/400g	208.0	8.0	52	1.9	6.7	1.9	0.0
Parsnip, Spicy, Fresh, Tesco*	1 Serving/300g	123.0	6.0	41	0.8	4.6	2.1	1.9
Pasta, Tomato & Basil, Bertolli*	1 Serving/100g	47.0	1.0	47	1.5	7.9	1.1	1.6
Pea & Ham	1 Serving/220g	154.0	5.0	70	4.0	9.2	2.1	1.4
Pea & Ham, Creamy, Chunky, Meal, Weight Watchers*	1 Pack/340g	156.0	4.0	46	2.3	6.8	1.1	2.0
Pea & Ham, Diet Chef Ltd*	1 Portion/300g	138.0	3.0	46	3.2	5.8	1.1	2.6
Pea & Ham, Eat Well, M & S*	½ Can/207g	93.0	2.0	45	3.7	5.1	1.0	2.2
Pea & Ham, Extra Thick, In A Cup, Sainsbury's*	1 Sachet/224ml	85.0	2.0	38	1.1	6.7	0.8	0.4
Pea & Ham, Fresh, Sainsbury's*	½ Pack/300ml	120.0	1.0	40	1.9	7.0	0.5	0.3
Pea & Ham, Low Fat, Solo Slim, Rosemary Conley*	1 Serving/100g	46.0	1.0	46	3.2	5.8	1.1	2.6
Pea & Mint, Baxters*	1 Serving/300g	186.0	10.0	62	2.3	6.1	3.2	1.5
Pea & Mint, Fresh, M & S*	1 Serving/164g	49.0	0.0	30	1.8	6.3	0.1	1.5
Pea & Mint, Fresh, Sainsbury's*	½ Pot/300g	141.0	7.0	47	1.8	4.8	2.3	2.3
Pea & Mint, Fresh, Waitrose*	1 Serving/300g	126.0	4.0	42	2.8	4.7	1.3	2.9
Pea & Mint, New Covent Garden Food Co*	½ Pack/300g	168.0	6.0	56	2.5	7.1	1.9	1.7
Pea & Mint, Tinned, Tesco*	1 Can/400g	180.0	3.0	45	2.0	7.8	0.7	1.3
Pea, Artichoke & Parmesan, The Best, Morrisons*	½ Pot/300g	171.0	8.0	57	2.8	5.6	2.6	1.0
Pea, Organic, Suma*	1 Can /400g	272.0	9.0	68	2.7	9.4	2.2	0.7
Peking Shiitake Mushroom Noodle, Baxters*	1 Serving/215g	90.0	2.0	42	1.3	7.5	0.8	0.2
Pepper & Chorizo, Canned, Sainsbury's*	1 Can/400ml	172.0	4.0	43	7.0	2.0	1.0	0.0
Peppered Steak Casserole, Taste of Home, Heinz*	1 Pot/430g	216.0	4.0	50	2.8	7.7	0.9	0.7
Potato & Leek	1oz/28g	15.0	1.0	52	1.5	6.2	2.6	0.8
Potato & Leek with Peppers & Chicken, Stockmeyer*	½ Can/200g	118.0	5.0	59	2.6	6.7	2.4	0.8
Potato & Leek, Thick and Tasty, Cup Soup, Morrisons*	1 Sachet/226ml	97.0	2.0	43	0.4	8.4	0.9	0.5
Potato & Leek, To Go, Asda*	1 Pot/330g	178.0	9.0	54	1.0	6.5	2.7	0.4
Potato, Leek & Bacon, Fresh, Baxters*	½ Pot/300g	249.0	17.0	83	2.0	6.1	5.6	0.7
Potato, Leek & Chicken, Canned, BGTY, Sainsbury's*	½ Can/200g	62.0	1.0	31	1.6	5.3	0.4	0.4
Potato, Leek & Thyme, Farmers Market, Heinz*	1 Can/515g	294.0	15.0	57	0.9	6.7	3.0	0.6
Pumpkin & Bramley Apple, New Covent Garden Food Co*	½ Carton/300g	99.0	2.0	33	1.1	5.9	0.6	0.8
Pumpkin & Ginger, in a Cup, Symingtons*	1 Serving/200ml	66.0	3.0	33	0.4	4.7	1.4	0.4
Pumpkin, Creamy, Very Special, Heinz*	1 Sm Can/290g	188.0	6.0	65	1.3	9.9	1.9	1.1
Pumpkin, New Covent Garden Food Co*	½ Pint/284ml	97.0	3.0	34	0.4	5.5	1.1	0.6
Pumpkin, Spicy, Fresh, Sainsbury's*	½ Pot/300g	87.0	3.0	29	0.9	4.2	1.0	1.3
Pumpkin, Sweet Potato & Red Pepper, SO, Sainsbury's*	½ Pot/300g	111.0	4.0	37	0.8	5.6	1.3	0.8
Puy Lentil & Tomato, Healthy Choice, Baxters*	½ Can/207g	118.0	1.0	57	3.1	10.5	0.3	2.7
Puy Lentil & Vine Ripened Tomato, Finest, Tesco*	1 Pot/600g	360.0	8.0	60	2.8	9.2	1.3	1.5
Red Lentil & Ham, Waitrose*	½ Pot/300g	147.0	3.0	49	3.9	5.8	1.1	2.0
Red Lentil & Tomato, Canned, Tesco*	½ Can/300g	189.0	4.0	63	4.0	8.9	1.3	1.1
Red Lentil & Vegetable, Favourties, Canned, Baxters*	1 Can/415g	166.0	1.0	40	2.2	7.4	0.2	1.0
Red Pepper & Goats Cheese, Diet Chef Ltd*	1 Pack/300g	138.0	7.0	46	2.2	4.4	2.2	0.9
Red Pepper & Tomato, Canned, Sainsbury's*	1 Can/400g	120.0	4.0	30	0.9	4.1	1.1	1.6
Red Pepper & Tomato, Canned, Weight Watchers*	1 Can /295g	35.0	0.0	12	0.4	2.4	0.1	0.4
Red Pepper, Tomato & Basil, M & S*	1 Can/415g	83.0	1.0	20	1.3	2.7	0.3	0.8

S

SOUP

	INFO/WEIGHT	KCAL	FAT	KCAL	PROT	CARB	FAT	FIBRE
Roasted Red Pepper & Tomato, M & S*	1 Serving/150g	105.0	7.0	70	1.4	5.0	4.9	0.6
Roasted Red Pepper & Tomato, Weight Watchers*	1 Can/400g	136.0	0.0	34	0.7	7.7	0.1	0.6
Roasted Red Pepper, Fresh, Waitrose*	1 Pack/600g	172.0	9.0	29	0.8	3.0	1.5	1.0
Roasted Vegetable, Chunky, M & S*	1 Can/400g	140.0	2.0	35	1.3	5.8	0.6	1.1
Root Vegetable & Barley, Broth, Special, Heinz*	1 Can/400g	188.0	6.0	47	0.9	7.4	1.5	1.1
Sausage & Bean, Spicy, Meal, Canned, Tesco*	1 Can/500g	265.0	7.0	53	2.8	6.4	1.4	1.2
Scotch Broth, Baxters*	1 Can/415g	166.0	4.0	40	1.6	6.4	0.9	0.7
Scotch Broth, British, Sainsbury's*	1 Can/415g	149.0	3.0	36	1.9	5.4	0.7	0.9
Scotch Broth, Classic, Heinz*	1 Can/400g	168.0	5.0	42	1.5	6.0	1.3	0.8
Scotch Broth, Fresh, Baxters*	1 Serving/300g	108.0	2.0	36	1.6	5.9	0.7	0.6
Scotch Broth, Fresh, Tesco*	½ Pack/300g	129.0	5.0	43	1.7	5.0	1.8	1.4
Scotch Broth, M & S*	1 Serving/300g	150.0	7.0	50	2.1	5.1	2.4	1.1
Scottish Vegetable with Lentils & Beef, Heinz*	1 Can/404g	210.0	3.0	52	3.4	8.2	0.7	1.2
Seafood Chowder, Waitrose*	1 Can/415g	224.0	11.0	54	2.1	5.3	2.7	0.8
Smoked Salmon & Dill, Fresh, Finest, Tesco*	½ Carton/300g	240.0	16.0	80	2.2	5.3	5.5	0.6
Spiced Chickpea & Fresh Red Pepper, M & S*	1 Serving/300g	165.0	7.0	55	2.2	5.8	2.3	2.5
Spiced Spinach & Green Lentil, Asda*	½ Pot/250g	122.0	5.0	49	2.7	5.0	2.0	0.0
Spicy Lentil & Vegetable, Chilled, M & S*	½ Serving/600g	300.0	5.0	50	2.7	8.0	0.8	1.1
Spicy Lentil, Chilled, Morrisons*	1 Serving/300ml	271.0	9.0	90	3.9	12.3	2.9	4.0
Spicy Lentil, COU, M & S*	1 Pack/415g	187.0	4.0	45	2.6	6.7	0.9	1.2
Spicy Lentil, In A Mug, Light Choices, Tesco*	1 Sachet/221ml	62.0	0.0	28	1.1	5.9	0.0	0.0
Spicy Lentil, Seeds of Change*	1 Pack/422.2g	190.0	1.0	45	2.5	8.2	0.2	1.9
Spicy Mixed Bean & Vegetable, Eat Smart, Safeway*	1 Can/415g	183.0	2.0	44	2.3	7.5	0.5	3.1
Spicy Mixed Bean, Big Soup, Heinz*	1 Serving/200g	78.0	1.0	39	2.3	6.7	0.3	2.0
Spicy Parsnip, New Covent Garden Food Co*	½ Box/297g	116.0	4.0	39	0.9	5.8	1.3	1.8
Spicy Parsnip, Vegetarian, Baxters*	1 Can/425g	217.0	11.0	51	1.1	6.1	2.5	1.5
Spicy Red Curry, Blue Dragon*	1 Serving/205g	97.0	5.0	47	0.4	5.8	2.5	0.3
Spicy Tomato & Vegetable, Healthy Living, Co-Op*	1 Can/400g	180.0	3.0	45	2.0	8.0	0.8	2.0
Spicy, Three Bean, Tesco*	½ Carton/300g	165.0	4.0	55	2.8	7.3	1.5	2.1
Spinach & Nutmeg, New Covent Garden Food Co*	½ Carton/300g	147.0	7.0	49	1.9	5.3	2.2	1.0
Spinach & Watercress, New Covent Garden Food Co*	½ Carton/298g	60.0	1.0	20	1.3	2.8	0.4	0.8
Spinach, Creme Fraiche, & Nutmeg, Organic, Waitrose*	½ Pot/300g	243.0	23.0	81	0.9	2.3	7.6	1.1
Split Pea & Ham, Asda*	1 Serving/300g	129.0	1.0	43	3.5	6.9	0.2	0.7
Split Peas, Yellow, Simply Organic*	1 Pot/600g	354.0	3.0	59	4.3	10.4	0.5	2.6
Spring Vegetable, Classic, Heinz*	1 Can/400g	136.0	2.0	34	0.8	6.8	0.4	0.7
Squash, Butternut, & Ginger, Waitrose*	½ Pot/300g	210.0	17.0	70	0.9	3.5	5.8	1.0
Squash, Butternut, Curried, & Lentil, Seeds of Change*	1 Pack/400g	164.0	1.0	41	2.3	7.2	0.3	1.9
Steak & Potato, Big Soup, Heinz*	½ Can/258g	129.0	2.0	50	3.0	7.7	0.8	0.8
Steak, Potato & Ale, Chunky, Sainsbury's*	1 Can/400g	152.0	2.0	38	2.2	5.9	0.6	0.8
Stilton & White Port, Baxters*	1oz/28g	25.0	2.0	88	2.5	5.4	6.3	0.3
Stilton, Celery & Watercress, Morrisons*	1 Serving/250g	272.0	23.0	109	3.9	3.1	9.2	0.3
Sun Dried Tomato & Basil, Heinz*	1 Serving/275ml	124.0	5.0	45	0.6	6.5	1.9	0.1
Sun Dried Tomato & Basil, Microwaveable Cup, Heinz*	1 Cup/275ml	118.0	5.0	43	0.6	6.2	1.8	0.1
Sunshine Yellow Tomato, New Covent Garden Food Co*	1 Portion/300g	99.0	2.0	33	0.9	4.9	0.8	1.2
Super Chicken Noodle, Dry, Knorr*	1 Pack/56g	182.0	3.0	325	14.3	56.0	4.9	1.8
Sweet Potato & Coconut, COU, M & S*	1 Can/415g	166.0	5.0	40	0.7	6.7	1.3	0.8
Sweet Potato & Coconut, Diet Chef Ltd*	1 Pack/300g	147.0	9.0	49	0.8	4.9	2.9	0.9
Sweet Potato, Chickpea & Coriander, BGTY, Sainsbury's*	1 Can/400g	188.0	2.0	47	1.4	9.3	0.5	1.3
Sweetcorn & Chilli Chowder, Simply Organic*	½ Pot/300g	126.0	3.0	42	2.2	6.1	0.9	3.8
Sweetcorn & Chilli, COU, M & S*	½ Can/275g	137.0	7.0	50	0.9	6.1	2.4	0.4
Thai Chicken, Diet Chef Ltd*	1 Pack/300g	114.0	4.0	38	1.0	5.1	1.5	1.0
Thai Chicken, New Covent Garden Food Co*	½ Carton/300g	174.0	10.0	58	2.6	4.1	3.5	0.8
Thai Pumpkin Coconut, New Covent Garden Food Co*	1 Carton/568ml	182.0	7.0	32	1.3	3.5	1.3	1.1

SOUP

	Measure INFO/WEIGHT	per Measure KCAL	FAT	Nutrition Values per 100g / 100ml KCAL	PROT	CARB	FAT	FIBRE
Three Bean & Chorizo, Diet Chef Ltd*	1 Pack/300g	162.0	2.0	54	4.0	7.6	0.8	5.8
Three Bean & Smoked Bacon, Farmers Market, Heinz*	1 Can/515g	309.0	10.0	60	2.7	8.1	1.9	1.9
Three Bean & Tomato, Autumn, Farmers Market, Heinz*	½ Carton/300g	132.0	1.0	44	2.3	7.5	0.5	0.9
Three Bean, Chunky, M & S*	1 Can/415g	207.0	5.0	50	2.3	7.5	1.2	1.8
Tomato & Basil with Onion, Waistline, Crosse & Blackwell*	1 Serving/300g	87.0	2.0	29	0.9	5.1	0.6	0.3
Tomato & Basil, Campbell's*	1 Pack/500ml	205.0	6.0	41	0.7	6.7	1.3	1.1
Tomato & Basil, Cup a Soup, Made Up, GFY, Asda*	1 Serving/250ml	50.0	0.0	20	0.4	4.4	0.1	0.2
Tomato & Basil, Diet Chef Ltd*	1 Pack/300g	159.0	5.0	53	1.3	7.7	1.8	1.2
Tomato & Basil, Fresh, Low Fat, Sainsbury's*	½ Carton/300ml	75.0	2.0	25	1.1	4.1	0.6	0.7
Tomato & Basil, Fresh, M & S*	½ Pot/300g	105.0	4.0	35	0.8	5.2	1.2	1.5
Tomato & Basil, GFY, Asda*	1 Serving/250ml	100.0	3.0	40	0.9	6.0	1.4	1.6
Tomato & Basil, Italian, 99% Fat Free, Baxters*	½ Can/208g	119.0	2.0	57	2.6	9.3	1.0	1.1
Tomato & Basil, Loyd Grossman*	½ Pack/210g	97.0	4.0	46	0.8	6.4	1.9	0.2
Tomato & Brown Lentil, Healthy Choice, Heinz*	½ Can/207.5g	112.0	1.0	54	3.1	9.6	0.3	1.5
Tomato & Butterbean, Baxters*	1 Can/415g	166.0	5.0	40	1.2	6.1	1.2	1.0
Tomato & Chorizo, Mediterranean, Tesco*	1 Serving/200g	130.0	7.0	65	2.0	6.1	3.4	0.3
Tomato & Herb, Campbell's*	1 Carton/500ml	180.0	6.0	36	1.0	5.0	1.3	0.0
Tomato & Lentil, M & S*	½ Can/211g	95.0	0.0	45	2.3	8.4	0.2	1.5
Tomato & Lentil, Mediterranean, Weight Watchers*	1 Can/400g	184.0	2.0	46	2.3	7.8	0.6	1.0
Tomato & Lentil, Spicy, Canned, Tesco*	1 Can/400g	180.0	1.0	45	2.1	8.7	0.2	0.8
Tomato & Orange, Baxters*	1 Can/425g	178.0	2.0	42	1.0	8.3	0.5	0.4
Tomato & Pesto, Diet Chef Ltd*	1 Pack/300g	171.0	7.0	57	1.3	7.9	2.2	1.1
Tomato & Puy Lentil, Canned, Tesco*	½ Can/200g	64.0	1.0	32	0.7	6.5	0.3	0.6
Tomato & Red Pepper with Basil, Farmers Market, Heinz*	½ Carton/300g	117.0	4.0	39	1.3	5.2	1.4	0.9
Tomato & Red Pepper, Campbell's*	1 Can/590g	366.0	19.0	62	0.5	7.7	3.3	0.0
Tomato & Red Pepper, to Go, Asda*	1 Pot/330g	102.0	4.0	31	0.6	4.3	1.3	0.6
Tomato & Roasted Red Pepper, COU, M & S*	1 Serving/415g	145.0	0.0	35	1.0	7.6	0.1	0.9
Tomato & Spinach, Organic, Waitrose*	1 Serving/300g	126.0	6.0	42	1.4	4.9	1.9	0.7
Tomato & Three Bean, Canned, BGTY, Sainsbury's*	½ Can/200g	118.0	2.0	59	3.7	9.1	0.9	1.7
Tomato & Vegetable, Cup a Soup, Batchelors*	1 Serving/218g	107.0	3.0	49	1.1	8.5	1.2	0.6
Tomato & Vegetable, Organic, Baxters*	1 Can/400g	200.0	3.0	50	1.6	9.2	0.8	0.8
Tomato Rice, Campbell's*	1oz/28g	13.0	0.0	46	0.9	8.3	1.0	0.0
Tomato, & Lentil, Mediterranean, Weight Watchers*	1 Can/400g	184.0	2.0	46	2.3	7.8	0.6	1.0
Tomato, Basil & Chilli, Microwave, Sainsbury's*	1 Pot/345g	100.0	2.0	29	1.0	5.0	0.6	1.2
Tomato, Canned, HL, Tesco*	½ Can/200g	110.0	4.0	55	0.7	7.4	2.0	0.5
Tomato, Cannellini & Borlotti Bean, M & S*	½ Pot/300g	195.0	10.0	65	2.1	6.7	3.3	2.5
Tomato, Cream Of, Canned	1oz/28g	15.0	1.0	52	0.8	5.9	3.0	0.7
Tomato, Cream Of, Condensed, Batchelors*	1 Can/295g	454.0	19.0	154	1.7	21.9	6.6	0.6
Tomato, Cream Of, Condensed, Prepared, Batchelors*	½ Can/295g	227.0	10.0	77	0.9	11.0	3.3	0.3
Tomato, Cream Of, Microwaveable Cup, Heinz*	1 Cup/275ml	169.0	9.0	61	0.8	6.9	3.4	0.4
Tomato, Cream Of, Organic, Heinz*	1 Can/400g	220.0	10.0	55	1.0	7.0	2.6	0.4
Tomato, Cream Of, Prepared, Campbell's*	½ Can/295g	195.0	9.0	66	0.8	8.5	3.2	0.0
Tomato, Cream Of, with a Hint of Basil, Heinz*	½ Can/200g	114.0	6.0	57	0.9	6.6	3.0	0.4
Tomato, Cream Of, With Red Pepper, Classic, Heinz*	1 Can/400g	232.0	12.0	58	0.9	7.0	2.9	0.6
Tomato, Creme Fraiche & Basil, The Best, Safeway*	1/3 Pot/200g	130.0	8.0	65	1.0	5.0	4.2	1.0
Tomato, Cup a Soup, Made Up, Batchelors*	1 Sachet/256g	92.0	2.0	36	0.3	6.7	0.9	0.3
Tomato, Fire Flamed & Red Onion, Fresh, Sainsbury's*	½ Carton/300ml	129.0	7.0	43	0.8	5.0	2.2	1.0
Tomato, Fresh, Tesco*	1 Serving/100g	44.0	2.0	44	0.7	5.2	2.3	0.4
Tomato, Low Fat, Solo Slim, Rosemary Conley*	1 Serving/100g	56.0	2.0	56	1.3	7.6	2.3	1.2
Tomato, Mediterranean, In A Mug, Light Choices, Tesco*	1 Sachet/220ml	62.0	0.0	28	0.6	6.0	0.2	0.6
Tomato, Mediterranean, Rich, Fresh, Baxters*	1 Carton/600g	318.0	10.0	53	1.8	7.7	1.7	1.1
Tomato, Onion & Basil, GFY, Asda*	1 Can/400g	96.0	3.0	24	1.0	3.4	0.7	1.7
Tomato, Pepper & Basil, Safeway*	1 Can/415g	162.0	7.0	39	0.9	4.8	1.7	1.8

S

	Measure INFO/WEIGHT	per Measure KCAL	FAT	Nutrition Values per 100g / 100ml KCAL	PROT	CARB	FAT	FIBRE
SOUP								
Tomato, Rice & Sweetcorn, Baxters*	1 Serving/400ml	256.0	7.0	64	2.0	9.9	1.8	1.1
Tomato, Simmer & Serve, Dried, Sainsbury's*	1 Serving/200ml	70.0	2.0	35	0.3	6.0	1.1	0.4
Tomato, Sweet Chilli, & Pasta, Classic, Heinz*	½ Can/200g	74.0	0.0	37	0.8	8.0	0.1	0.3
Tomato, Ten Calorie, Gourmet Cuisine*	1 Sachet/200g	10.0	0.0	5	0.3	1.0	0.0	0.1
Tomato, Three Bean & Bacon, Sainsbury's*	½ Can/200g	86.0	2.0	43	3.1	5.4	1.0	3.0
Tomato, Vegetable Garden, Campbell's*	1 Can/310g	240.0	3.0	77	1.6	16.1	0.9	0.0
Tomato, Vine Ripend, Green Giant*	1 Pouch/330g	129.0	3.0	39	0.6	7.7	0.9	1.6
Tomato, Weight Watchers*	1 Can/295g	74.0	1.0	25	0.7	4.5	0.5	0.3
Tuscan Bean, Canned, HL, Tesco*	½ Can/200ml	130.0	4.0	65	3.5	10.3	1.8	1.3
Tuscan Bean, GFY, Asda*	1 Carton/400ml	224.0	4.0	56	2.9	9.0	0.9	0.8
Tuscan Bean, New Covent Garden Food Co*	½ Carton/300g	84.0	2.0	28	1.6	3.7	0.8	1.0
Tuscan Bean, Organic, Fresh, Sainsbury's*	1 Pack/400g	171.0	3.0	43	2.6	6.3	0.8	2.0
Tuscan Bean, Perfectly Balanced, Waitrose*	½ Pot/300g	147.0	5.0	49	2.0	6.1	1.8	1.8
Tuscan Style Bean & Sausage, Chunky, M & S*	1 Can/415g	249.0	9.0	60	2.4	7.7	2.2	1.0
Vegetable & Barley Broth, Canned, Organic, Sainsbury's*	½ Can/200g	48.0	1.0	24	1.4	3.7	0.4	0.9
Vegetable & Chilli, Chunky, Fresh, Sainsbury's*	½ Pot/300g	117.0	2.0	39	1.6	6.9	0.6	2.6
Vegetable & Lentil, Somerfield*	1 Serving/300g	135.0	3.0	45	2.6	6.4	0.9	3.6
Vegetable & Rosemary, Fresh, Sainsbury's*	½ Pack/300g	96.0	3.0	32	0.9	4.9	1.0	1.3
Vegetable Broth, Canned, HL, Tesco*	½ Can/200g	74.0	0.0	37	1.2	7.4	0.2	1.0
Vegetable Broth, M & S*	1 Pack/213g	85.0	3.0	40	1.0	6.3	1.4	0.8
Vegetable Chowder, New Covent Garden Food Co*	½ Carton/300g	159.0	5.0	53	2.9	6.6	1.7	1.1
Vegetable Mulligatawny, Tesco*	½ Pack/300g	210.0	7.0	70	1.9	9.0	2.5	1.1
Vegetable, & Rosemary, Chunky, Tesco*	½ Pot/250g	112.0	5.0	45	1.0	5.8	2.0	1.4
Vegetable, 99% Fat Free, Wattie's*	1 Serving/105g	30.0	0.0	28	0.8	5.9	0.1	0.8
Vegetable, Average	1 Serving/220g	114.0	9.0	52	0.9	3.2	4.0	0.9
Vegetable, Bean & Pasta, Organic, Baxters*	1 Can/415g	212.0	3.0	51	2.2	8.7	0.8	1.4
Vegetable, Canned	1oz/28g	13.0	0.0	48	1.4	9.9	0.6	1.5
Vegetable, Chunky, Canned, Sainsbury's*	1 Can/400g	184.0	3.0	46	1.5	8.3	0.7	1.2
Vegetable, Chunky, Diet Chef Ltd*	1 Pack/300g	105.0	2.0	35	1.9	5.5	0.6	3.0
Vegetable, Chunky, Fresh, Organic, Simply Organic*	½ Tub/300g	153.0	4.0	51	1.9	9.0	1.5	1.4
Vegetable, Chunky, Fresh, Waitrose*	½ Pot/300g	117.0	5.0	39	1.3	4.5	1.8	2.1
Vegetable, Chunky, Organic, Tesco*	½ Pot/300g	150.0	4.0	50	1.7	8.0	1.2	2.1
Vegetable, Chunky, Tesco*	1 Pot/600g	288.0	17.0	48	0.8	5.0	2.9	1.3
Vegetable, Condensed, Campbell's*	1 Can/295g	103.0	2.0	35	0.8	6.2	0.8	0.0
Vegetable, Condensed, Classic, Campbell's*	1 Can/295g	221.0	5.0	75	1.7	13.2	1.7	1.7
Vegetable, Country Garden, Green Giant*	1 Pack/330g	129.0	2.0	39	1.0	7.2	0.6	2.0
Vegetable, Cup Soup, Made Up, Heinz*	1 Cup/200g	50.0	1.0	25	0.4	4.7	0.5	0.2
Vegetable, Extra Thick, Canned, Sainsbury's*	1 Can/400g	184.0	2.0	46	1.5	8.6	0.6	1.4
Vegetable, From Heinz, Canned, Weight Watchers*	1 Can/295g	86.0	1.0	29	0.9	5.6	0.3	0.8
Vegetable, in a Cup, BGTY, Sainsbury's*	1 Sachet/200g	52.0	2.0	26	0.5	4.4	0.8	0.9
Vegetable, in a Cup, Weight Watchers*	1 Serving/100g	57.0	1.0	57	1.2	10.4	1.2	0.5
Watercress & Cream, Soup Chef*	1 Jar/780g	413.0	23.0	53	0.8	5.9	2.9	0.3
Watercress, M & S*	½ Pot/300g	75.0	5.0	25	1.3	1.5	1.7	0.6
SOUP MIX								
Leek & Potato, Made Up, Sainsbury's*	½ Pack/204g	39.0	0.0	19	0.6	3.6	0.2	0.5
Minestrone, Made Up, Sainsbury's*	1 Serving/200ml	44.0	0.0	22	0.3	6.0	0.0	0.3
Pea & Ham, Traditional, King	1 Serving/200ml	66.0	0.0	33	2.2	5.9	0.2	0.0
Scotch Broth, Made Up, Sainsbury's*	1 Serving/175g	31.0	0.0	18	0.2	3.8	0.2	0.6
Scotch Broth, Made Up, Somerfield*	½ Pack/175g	159.0	1.0	91	2.1	19.3	0.6	1.7
Soup & Broth Mix, Wholefoods, Tesco*	¼ Pack/125g	456.0	2.0	365	14.7	71.4	1.9	7.3
SOUTHERN COMFORT								
37.5% Volume	**1 Shot/35ml**	**72.0**	**0.0**	**207**	**0.0**	**0.0**	**0.0**	**0.0**

	Measure INFO/WEIGHT	per Measure KCAL	FAT	Nutrition Values per 100g / 100ml KCAL	PROT	CARB	FAT	FIBRE
SOYA								
Bolognese Style, Sainsbury's*	½ Pack/168g	113.0	1.0	67	3.1	13.9	0.7	2.7
Chunks, Dried, Cooked, Sainsbury's*	1oz/28g	27.0	0.0	98	14.0	9.8	0.3	1.1
Chunks, Protein, Natural, Nature's Harvest*	1 Serving/50g	172.0	0.0	345	50.0	38.0	1.0	4.0
Mince, Dry Weight, Sainsbury's*	1 Serving/50g	164.0	0.0	328	47.2	33.2	0.8	3.6
Mince, Granules	*1oz/28g*	*74.0*	*2.0*	*263*	*43.2*	*11.0*	*5.4*	*0.0*
Mince, Prepared, Sainsbury's*	1 Serving/200g	164.0	0.0	82	11.8	8.3	0.2	0.9
Mince, with Onion, Cooked, Sainsbury's*	½ Pack/180g	122.0	3.0	68	5.4	8.0	1.6	1.8
SOYA MILK								
Banana Flavour, Provamel*	1 Serving/250ml	195.0	5.0	78	3.8	10.4	2.2	0.6
Choco Flavour, Provamel*	1 Serving/250ml	207.0	6.0	83	3.8	11.1	2.4	1.1
Chocolate, So Good Beverages*	1 Serving/250ml	160.0	2.0	64	3.6	10.8	1.0	0.0
Fat Free, Original, So Good Beverages*	1 Serving/250ml	100.0	0.0	40	3.6	6.4	0.1	0.0
Flavoured, Average	1floz/30mls	12.0	1.0	40	2.8	3.6	1.7	0.0
No Added Sugar, Unsweetened, Average	*1 Serving/250ml*	*85.0*	*5.0*	*34*	*3.3*	*0.9*	*1.9*	*0.4*
Omega Original, So Good Beverages*	1 Serving/250ml	130.0	3.0	52	3.6	6.8	1.2	0.0
Omega Vanilla, So Good Beverages*	1 Serving/250ml	130.0	3.0	52	3.6	7.6	1.2	0.0
Original, No Added Sugar, So Good Beverages*	1 Serving/250ml	80.0	2.0	32	3.6	2.0	1.0	0.8
Strawberry Flavour, Provamel*	1 Serving/250ml	160.0	5.0	64	3.6	7.7	2.1	1.2
Strawberry, So Good Beverages*	1 Serving/250ml	160.0	2.0	64	3.6	10.4	1.0	0.0
Sweetened, Average	*1 Glass/200ml*	*93.0*	*4.0*	*47*	*3.4*	*3.7*	*2.1*	*0.4*
Sweetened, Calcium Enriched, Average	1 Glass/200ml	91.0	4.0	46	3.4	3.7	2.0	0.3
Uht, Non Dairy, Alternative to Milk, Waitrose*	1 Serving/250ml	102.0	5.0	41	3.3	2.7	1.9	0.2
Unsweetened, Organic, Waitrose*	1 Serving/60ml	19.0	1.0	31	3.3	0.2	1.9	0.0
Vanilla Flavour, Organic, Provamel*	1 Serving/250ml	150.0	5.0	60	3.8	6.2	2.2	0.6
Vanilla, Fat Free, So Good Beverages*	1 Serving/250ml	140.0	0.0	56	3.6	10.4	0.1	0.0
Vanilla, Organic, Heinz*	1 Serving/200ml	106.0	3.0	53	2.6	6.9	1.6	0.2
Vanilla, So Good Beverages*	1 Serving/250ml	180.0	5.0	72	3.6	10.4	2.0	0.0
SPAGHETTI								
Chicken, BGTY, Sainsbury's*	1 Serving/300g	281.0	3.0	94	9.8	11.6	0.9	2.3
Cooked, Average	*1oz/28g*	*33.0*	*0.0*	*119*	*4.1*	*24.8*	*0.6*	*1.1*
Dried, Waitrose*	1 Serving/75g	256.0	1.0	341	11.5	70.7	1.3	3.7
Dry, Average	*1oz/28g*	*98.0*	*0.0*	*350*	*12.1*	*72.1*	*1.5*	*2.4*
Dry, Carb Check, Heinz*	1 Serving/75g	219.0	2.0	292	52.7	15.2	2.3	20.8
Durum Wheat, Dry, Average	*1oz/28g*	*97.0*	*0.0*	*347*	*12.3*	*71.7*	*0.3*	*1.4*
Fresh, Cooked, Average	*1 Serving/125g*	*182.0*	*2.0*	*146*	*6.1*	*26.9*	*1.7*	*1.8*
Fresh, Dry, Average	*1 Serving/100g*	*278.0*	*3.0*	*278*	*10.8*	*53.0*	*3.0*	*2.2*
in Tomato & Cheese, Sainsbury's*	1 Serving/300g	345.0	10.0	115	4.4	16.8	3.4	1.4
in Tomato Sauce, Canned	1oz/28g	18.0	0.0	64	1.9	14.1	0.4	0.7
in Tomato Sauce, Heinz*	½ Can/200g	120.0	1.0	60	1.7	12.7	0.3	2.4
in Tomato Sauce, HP*	1 Can/410g	247.0	1.0	60	1.5	13.1	0.2	0.4
In Tomato Sauce, Multigrain, Heinz*	½ Can/200g	120.0	1.0	60	1.7	12.7	0.3	2.4
in Tomato Sauce, Organic, Sainsbury's*	½ Can/205g	133.0	0.0	65	1.8	13.9	0.2	1.0
in Tomato Sauce, Whole Wheat, Sainsbury's*	1 Serving/205g	125.0	1.0	61	2.0	11.9	0.6	1.1
TTD, Sainsbury's*	1 Serving/90g	321.0	2.0	357	12.3	73.1	1.7	2.5
Wheat Free, Tesco*	1 Serving/100g	340.0	2.0	340	8.0	72.5	2.0	2.5
Whole Wheat, Cooked, Average	*1oz/28g*	*32.0*	*0.0*	*113*	*4.7*	*23.2*	*0.9*	*3.5*
Whole Wheat, Dry, Average	*1 Serving/100g*	*324.0*	*3.0*	*324*	*13.5*	*62.2*	*2.6*	*8.0*
with Parsley, in Tomato Sauce, Weight Watchers*	1 Sm Can/200g	98.0	0.0	49	1.8	10.0	0.2	0.6
with Sausages, in Tomato Sauce, Heinz*	1 Can/400g	352.0	14.0	88	3.4	10.8	3.5	0.5
with Tomato & Cheese, Tesco*	½ Pack/250g	280.0	6.0	112	4.0	18.1	2.6	1.1
SPAGHETTI & MEATBALLS								
American, Superbowl, Asda*	1 Pack/453g	594.0	18.0	131	11.0	13.0	3.9	1.1
BGTY, Sainsbury's*	1 Pack/300g	249.0	3.0	83	5.9	12.7	0.9	3.1

	Measure INFO/WEIGHT	per Measure KCAL	FAT	Nutrition Values per 100g / 100ml KCAL	PROT	CARB	FAT	FIBRE
SPAGHETTI & MEATBALLS								
Chicken, in Tomato Sauce, Heinz*	1 Can/400g	332.0	9.0	83	4.2	11.3	2.3	0.5
COU, M & S*	1 Pack/400g	360.0	8.0	90	6.0	12.3	2.0	2.6
GFY, Asda*	1 Pack/400g	344.0	6.0	86	7.0	11.0	1.5	1.5
HL, Tesco*	1 Pack/370g	407.0	14.0	110	4.7	13.8	3.9	1.6
Italian Cuisine, Tesco*	1 Pack/400g	500.0	18.0	125	5.9	14.6	4.4	1.7
Italian, Sainsbury's*	1 Pack/450g	495.0	21.0	110	5.0	11.9	4.7	2.7
Sainsbury's*	1 Pack/400g	497.0	18.0	124	6.5	14.2	4.6	2.8
Tesco*	1 Serving/475g	641.0	31.0	135	5.1	14.1	6.5	0.9
SPAGHETTI BOLOGNESE								
Al Forno, Sainsbury's*	1 Pack/400g	460.0	20.0	115	7.8	10.0	4.9	1.1
Average	1 Serving/450g	580.0	25.0	129	7.8	12.5	5.6	0.9
BGTY, Sainsbury's*	1 Pack/400g	416.0	9.0	104	6.3	14.4	2.3	1.1
Canned, Asda*	½ Can/205g	174.0	6.0	85	4.2	10.7	2.8	0.6
Cook*	1 Portion/430g	636.0	25.0	148	7.6	16.2	5.8	1.0
Egg Pasta in Rich Beef Sauce, Waitrose*	1 Pack/400g	404.0	10.0	101	7.6	11.7	2.6	1.0
Frozen, Tesco*	1 Pack/450g	472.0	9.0	105	5.8	15.0	2.0	1.8
GFY, Asda*	1 Pack/400g	352.0	6.0	88	4.9	13.4	1.6	2.2
Good Intentions, Somerfield*	1 Serving/400g	380.0	9.0	95	6.2	12.4	2.3	1.4
Healthy Choice, Iceland*	1 Pack/400g	428.0	4.0	107	6.8	17.8	1.0	1.1
Hidden Veg, Heinz*	1 Can/400g	312.0	6.0	78	3.4	12.6	1.6	0.9
HP*	1 Pack/410g	312.0	8.0	76	3.8	11.3	1.9	0.7
in Tomato & Beef Sauce, Canned, Carlini*	1 Can/410g	324.0	11.0	79	3.7	10.2	2.6	1.2
Italian, Chilled, Tesco*	1 Pack/400g	520.0	17.0	130	6.5	15.9	4.3	1.5
Italiano, Pro-Cuisine, Pro Cuisine*	1 Pack/600g	522.0	11.0	87	5.7	11.7	1.9	0.0
Lean Cuisine, Findus*	1 Pack/320g	275.0	7.0	86	4.5	11.5	2.3	1.1
Meat Free, Heinz*	1 Serving/200g	162.0	3.0	81	3.3	13.1	1.7	0.6
Perfectly Balanced, Waitrose*	1 Pack/400g	380.0	7.0	95	6.7	13.4	1.7	1.1
Quick Pasta, Dry, Sainsbury's*	1 Serving/63g	231.0	3.0	367	10.8	71.0	4.4	3.3
Ross*	1 Serving/320g	288.0	4.0	90	4.2	15.7	1.1	0.9
Vegetarian, Tesco*	1 Pack/340g	374.0	13.0	110	5.1	13.7	3.9	1.2
Weight Watchers*	1 Pack/320g	307.0	7.0	96	5.7	13.1	2.2	0.7
SPAGHETTI CARBONARA								
Chicken & Asparagus, Sainsbury's*	1 Pack/450g	657.0	27.0	146	6.6	16.2	6.1	1.1
Chicken, Mushroom & Ham, Asda*	1 Pack/700g	686.0	14.0	98	10.0	10.0	2.0	1.5
COU, M & S*	1 Pack/330g	346.0	7.0	105	5.7	15.5	2.0	1.8
Free Range Egg, with Italian Bacon, City Kitchen, Tesco*	1 Pack/385g	577.0	30.0	150	4.8	15.5	7.7	1.5
Italian Express*	1 Pack/320g	310.0	12.0	97	4.3	11.6	3.7	1.1
Italian, Chilled, Sainsbury's*	1 Pack/400g	492.0	16.0	123	5.5	16.1	3.9	1.4
Italian, Fresh, Chilled, Tesco*	1 Pack/430g	606.0	26.0	141	7.6	13.9	6.1	1.3
Italian, Tesco*	1 Pack/450g	607.0	27.0	135	5.4	14.1	5.9	0.6
M & S*	1 Pack/360g	630.0	34.0	175	7.6	14.3	9.5	0.1
SPAGHETTI HOOPS								
& Sausages, Tesco*	1 Serving/205g	184.0	7.0	90	3.1	11.9	3.3	0.2
Canned, Smart Price, Asda*	½ Can/205g	127.0	1.0	62	1.7	13.0	0.3	0.4
in Tomato Sauce, Heinz*	½ Can/200g	106.0	0.0	53	1.7	11.1	0.2	0.5
in Tomato Sauce, Hidden Veg, Heinz*	1 Can/400g	244.0	2.0	61	1.7	12.4	0.5	1.1
in Tomato Sauce, Multigrain, Snap Pot, Heinz*	1 Pot/190g	112.0	1.0	59	1.6	12.7	0.3	1.5
in Tomato Sauce, Snap Pot, Heinz*	1 Pot/192g	113.0	1.0	59	1.6	12.7	0.3	1.5
Tesco*	½ Can/205g	123.0	0.0	60	1.6	12.9	0.2	0.5
SPAGHETTI MARINARA								
GFY, Asda*	1 Pack/400g	520.0	17.0	130	8.0	15.0	4.2	0.9
SPAGHETTI RINGS								
in Tomato Sauce, Canned, Sainsbury's*	1 Serving/213g	136.0	1.0	64	1.9	13.3	0.4	0.5

S

	Measure INFO/WEIGHT	per Measure KCAL	FAT	Nutrition Values per 100g / 100ml KCAL	PROT	CARB	FAT	FIBRE
SPAGHETTI WITH								
Cheese & Broccoli Sauce, GFY, Asda*	1 Pack/382g	447.0	7.0	117	3.2	22.0	1.8	0.8
King Prawns, GFY, Asda*	1 Pack/400g	365.0	12.0	91	5.0	11.3	2.9	1.5
Tomato & Mozzarella Sauce, GFY, Asda*	1 Pack/120g	446.0	6.0	372	10.8	70.8	5.0	2.6
SPAGHETTINI								
Wholewheat, Great Stuff, Asda*	1 Serving/100g	99.0	1.0	99	3.4	19.7	0.7	2.4
SPAM*								
Pork & Ham, Chopped, Spam*	1 Serving/100g	296.0	24.0	296	14.5	3.2	24.2	0.0
SPICE BLEND								
Balti, Sharwood's*	1oz/28g	34.0	3.0	122	1.8	7.1	9.6	1.2
Thai, Sharwood's*	1 Pack 260g	424.0	31.0	163	1.8	12.0	11.9	1.0
Tikka, Sharwood's*	1 Pack/260g	263.0	14.0	101	2.7	10.2	5.4	1.7
SPICE MIX								
for Burritos, Old El Paso*	½ Packet/22.5g	68.0	1.0	304	13.0	54.0	4.0	0.0
for Fajitas, Old El Paso*	1 Pack/35g	107.0	2.0	306	9.0	54.0	6.0	0.0
for Mexican Fajitas, Discovery*	½ Pack/15g	34.0	1.0	230	8.0	35.0	6.5	17.5
Tex Mex Chili Con Carne, Schwartz*	1 Sachet/100g	278.0	7.0	278	12.9	66.5	6.6	24.5
SPINACH								
Baby, Average	*1 Serving/90g*	*22.0*	*1.0*	*25*	*2.8*	*1.6*	*0.8*	*2.1*
Boiled Or Steamed, Average	*1 Serving/80g*	*17.0*	*1.0*	*21*	*2.6*	*0.9*	*0.8*	*2.1*
Canned, Average	*1 Serving/80g*	*18.0*	*0.0*	*22*	*3.0*	*1.4*	*0.5*	*2.9*
Chopped, Frozen, Fresh, Somerfield*	1 Serving/90g	22.0	1.0	24	2.8	1.5	0.8	2.7
Chopped, Frozen, Waitrose*	1 Serving/80g	20.0	1.0	25	2.8	1.6	0.8	2.7
Leaf, Frozen, Organic, Waitrose*	1 Serving/80g	20.0	1.0	25	2.8	1.6	0.8	2.1
Raw	*1 Bunch/340g*	*75.0*	*1.0*	*22*	*2.9*	*3.5*	*0.3*	*2.7*
Raw, Average	*1 Serving/80g*	*20.0*	*1.0*	*25*	*2.8*	*1.6*	*0.8*	*2.1*
SPIRA								
Cadbury*	2 Twists/40g	210.0	12.0	525	7.8	56.8	29.4	0.0
SPIRALI								
Dry, Average	*1 Serving/50g*	*176.0*	*1.0*	*351*	*12.1*	*72.5*	*1.6*	*2.7*
SPIRITS								
37.5% Volume	*1 Shot/35ml*	*72.0*	*0.0*	*207*	*0.0*	*0.0*	*0.0*	*0.0*
40% Volume	*1 Shot/35ml*	*78.0*	*0.0*	*222*	*0.0*	*0.0*	*0.0*	*0.0*
SPLENDIPS								
Cheesecake, Philadelphia, Kraft*	1 Pack/85g	200.0	7.0	235	6.1	34.0	8.3	2.9
Chives, Philadelphia, Kraft*	1 Pack/85g	159.0	4.0	187	7.5	27.0	5.2	1.7
Nachos, Philadelphia, Kraft*	1 Pack/85g	150.0	6.0	177	6.4	20.0	7.6	1.0
Poppadoms & Mango Chutney, Light, Philadelphia, Kraft*	1 Pack/76g	131.0	4.0	172	5.1	26.5	4.7	1.9
SPLIT PEAS								
Dried, Average	*1oz/28g*	*89.0*	*0.0*	*319*	*22.1*	*57.4*	*1.7*	*3.1*
Green, Dried, Boiled, Average	*1 Tbsp/35g*	*40.0*	*0.0*	*115*	*8.3*	*19.8*	*0.6*	*3.9*
SPONGE FINGERS								
Boudoir, Sainsbury's*	1 Finger/5g	20.0	0.0	396	8.1	82.8	3.6	0.4
Tesco*	1 Finger/5g	19.0	0.0	386	7.6	80.6	3.7	1.0
SPONGE PUDDING								
Average	1 Portion/170g	578.0	28.0	340	5.8	45.3	16.3	1.1
Banoffee, Heinz*	¼ Can/78g	239.0	10.0	307	2.8	46.6	12.2	0.6
Blackcurrant, BGTY, Sainsbury's*	1 Serving/110g	155.0	1.0	141	2.5	30.7	0.9	3.2
Blackcurrant, Low Fat, Iceland*	1 Pudding/90g	159.0	1.0	177	2.2	39.5	1.1	1.6
Canned, Average	1 Serving/75g	214.0	9.0	285	3.1	45.4	11.4	0.8
Cherry & Chocolate, Eat Smart, Safeway*	1 Serving/86g	150.0	2.0	175	2.7	35.6	2.4	0.8
Chocolate & Sauce, Co-Op*	1 Pack/225g	607.0	29.0	270	5.0	34.0	13.0	0.6
Chocolate, BGTY, Sainsbury's*	1 Pudding/105g	137.0	3.0	131	4.4	23.1	2.4	2.7
Chocolate, Cadbury*	1 Pack/370g	1276.0	73.0	345	4.9	36.7	19.8	0.0

S

SPONGE PUDDING

	Measure INFO/WEIGHT	KCAL	FAT	KCAL	PROT	CARB	FAT	FIBRE
Chocolate, Free From, Sainsbury's*	1 Pudding/110g	388.0	10.0	353	5.2	62.0	9.3	0.3
Chocolate, GFY, Asda*	1 Pudding/105g	187.0	4.0	178	3.0	32.0	4.2	2.6
Chocolate, Heinz*	¼ Pudding/77g	229.0	9.0	298	4.6	44.0	11.5	1.2
Chocolate, HL, Tesco*	1 Serving/125g	239.0	5.0	191	4.4	34.7	3.8	0.9
Chocolate, Less Than 3% Fat, BGTY, Sainsbury's*	1 Pudding/105g	180.0	2.0	171	4.5	34.0	1.9	0.9
Chocolate, M & S*	¼ Pudding/131g	524.0	32.0	400	6.1	38.6	24.6	1.8
Chocolate, Sainsbury's*	¼ Pudding/110g	464.0	28.0	422	5.4	42.3	25.7	0.8
Chocolate, Trufree*	1 Serving/115g	374.0	17.0	325	2.5	44.0	15.0	2.0
Chocolate, Waitrose*	1 Pudding/105g	208.0	2.0	198	4.6	40.0	2.2	1.8
Chocolate, with Cadbury's Caramel Sticky Sauce, Heinz*	1 Serving/200g	762.0	34.0	381	3.5	52.3	16.9	0.6
Circus, & Custard, Weight Watchers*	1 Serving/140g	239.0	4.0	171	4.2	32.1	2.9	0.9
Citrus, BGTY, Sainsbury's*	1 Pudding/110g	230.0	4.0	209	3.5	39.7	4.0	0.7
Forest Fruit, Eat Smart, Safeway*	1 Pot/88g	150.0	2.0	170	4.2	33.5	1.8	2.6
Fruit, Co-Op*	1 Can/300g	1110.0	48.0	370	3.0	53.0	16.0	2.0
Fruited with Brandy Sauce, Sainsbury's*	1 Pudding/125g	261.0	8.0	209	3.6	33.6	6.7	0.8
Fruits of the Forest, Asda*	1 Pudding/115g	323.0	4.0	281	2.8	59.0	3.8	1.3
Ginger, with Plum Sauce, Waitrose*	1 Pudding/120g	424.0	18.0	353	3.1	51.7	14.9	0.7
Golden Syrup, Co-Op*	1 Can/300g	945.0	39.0	315	2.0	47.0	13.0	0.6
Jam & Custard, Co-Op*	1 Pack/244g	598.0	22.0	245	3.0	37.0	9.0	0.3
Jam & Custard, Somerfield*	¼ Pudding/62g	143.0	5.0	231	3.0	38.0	8.0	0.2
Jam, Tesco*	1 Pudding/110g	367.0	13.0	334	3.3	53.3	11.9	0.5
Lemon Curd, Heinz*	¼ Can/78g	236.0	9.0	302	2.6	46.7	11.7	0.6
Lemon, COU, M & S*	1 Pudding/100g	157.0	2.0	157	2.0	32.1	2.3	1.9
Lemon, M & S*	1 Pudding/105g	325.0	16.0	310	4.3	39.4	15.2	2.3
Lemon, Waitrose*	1 Serving/105g	212.0	3.0	202	3.4	41.7	2.4	1.4
Lemon, with Lemon Sauce, Eat Smart, Safeway*	1 Pudding/90g	135.0	2.0	150	2.2	29.0	2.6	1.4
Pear & Ginger, COU, M & S*	1 Pudding/100g	175.0	1.0	175	1.9	39.8	0.7	1.1
Raspberry Jam, Asda*	½ Pudding/147g	481.0	16.0	327	3.1	54.0	11.0	4.1
St Clements, GFY, Asda*	1 Pudding/116g	332.0	5.0	286	2.6	60.0	3.9	1.2
Sticky Toffee, COU, M & S*	1 Pack/150g	277.0	3.0	185	2.5	39.3	1.7	1.8
Sticky Toffee, Microwavable, Heinz*	1 Serving/75g	233.0	9.0	311	3.3	47.4	12.0	0.7
Sticky Toffee, Mini, Somerfield*	1 Pudding/110g	384.0	14.0	349	3.0	54.0	13.0	0.0
Sticky Toffee, Smart Price, Asda*	½ Can/150g	451.0	19.0	301	2.0	44.0	13.0	0.0
Strawberry Jam, Heinz*	¼ Can/82g	230.0	6.0	281	2.6	50.4	7.6	0.6
Strawberry, Co-Op*	1 Can/300g	960.0	39.0	320	2.0	48.0	13.0	0.8
Sultana, with Toffee Sauce, HL, Tesco*	1 Serving/80g	280.0	2.0	350	3.2	60.2	2.7	1.0
Summer Fruits, BGTY, Sainsbury's*	1 Serving/110g	243.0	5.0	221	2.7	42.9	4.3	1.0
Syrup & Custard, Morrisons*	1 Serving/125g	290.0	9.0	232	3.4	39.1	6.9	0.8
Syrup, & Custard, Iceland*	1 Pudding/130g	409.0	21.0	315	3.6	38.8	16.2	0.4
Syrup, BGTY, Sainsbury's*	1 Pudding/110g	338.0	5.0	307	2.8	64.6	4.1	0.4
Syrup, Finest, Tesco*	1 Pudding/115g	330.0	9.0	287	3.1	51.2	7.8	0.6
Syrup, GFY, Asda*	1 Sponge/105g	207.0	4.0	197	2.0	38.0	4.1	2.6
Syrup, Individual, Tesco*	1 Pudding/110g	390.0	15.0	355	3.1	55.6	13.2	0.5
Treacle, Heinz*	1 Serving/160g	445.0	13.0	278	2.5	48.9	8.1	0.6
Treacle, Super Sticky, Heinz*	1 Pudding/110g	318.0	12.0	289	1.9	45.3	11.1	1.6
Treacle, Waitrose*	1 Pudding/105g	385.0	14.0	367	2.8	59.5	13.1	0.5
Treacle, with Custard, Farmfoods*	1 Serving/145g	539.0	33.0	372	3.2	38.4	22.8	0.8
Very Fruity Cherry, M & S*	1 Pot/110g	286.0	11.0	260	3.5	38.6	10.3	1.8
with Dried Fruit	1oz/28g	93.0	4.0	331	5.4	48.1	14.3	1.2
with Jam or Treacle	1oz/28g	93.0	4.0	333	5.1	48.7	14.4	1.0
with Lyles Golden Syrup, Heinz*	½ Pudding/95g	368.0	14.0	386	3.1	53.3	15.1	0.5

SPOTTED DICK

	Measure INFO/WEIGHT	KCAL	FAT	KCAL	PROT	CARB	FAT	FIBRE
Average	1oz/28g	92.0	5.0	327	4.2	42.7	16.7	1.0

	Measure	per Measure		Nutrition Values per 100g / 100ml				
	INFO/WEIGHT	KCAL	FAT	KCAL	PROT	CARB	FAT	FIBRE

SPRATS

Fried	*1oz/28g*	*116.0*	*10.0*	*415*	*24.9*	*0.0*	*35.0*	*0.0*
Raw	*1oz/28g*	*48.0*	*3.0*	*172*	*18.3*	*0.0*	*11.0*	*0.0*

SPREAD

	Measure	KCAL	FAT	KCAL	PROT	CARB	FAT	FIBRE
Butter Me Up, Light, Tesco*	1 Thin Spread/7g	24.0	3.0	350	0.3	0.5	38.0	0.0
Butter Me Up, Tesco*	1 Thin Spread/7g	38.0	4.0	540	0.8	1.2	59.0	0.0
Butterlicious, Vegetable, Sainsbury's*	1 Thin Spread/7g	44.0	5.0	628	0.6	1.1	69.0	0.0
Buttersoft, Light, Reduced Fat, Sainsbury's*	1 Thin Spread/7g	38.0	4.0	544	0.4	0.5	60.0	0.0
Buttery Gold, Somerfield*	1 Thin Spread/7g	44.0	5.0	627	0.5	1.0	69.0	0.0
Buttery Taste, Benecol*	1 Thin Spread/7g	40.0	4.0	575	0.0	0.8	63.3	0.0
Clover, Light, Dairy Crest Ltd*	1 Serving/7g	32.0	3.0	455	0.7	2.9	49.0	0.0
Dairy Free, Organic, Pure Spreads*	1 Thin Spread/7g	37.0	4.0	533	0.5	0.0	59.0	0.0
Diet, Delight*	1 Thin Spread/7g	16.0	2.0	228	3.6	1.6	23.0	0.0
Enriched Olive, Tesco*	1 Thin Spread/7g	38.0	4.0	540	0.2	1.2	59.0	0.0
From Soya, Kallo*	1 Thin Spread/7g	27.0	3.0	380	7.0	6.0	37.0	0.0
Gold, Low Fat, Omega 3, St Ivel*	1 Thin Spread/7g	25.0	3.0	360	0.5	3.1	38.0	0.0
Gold, Low Fat, St Ivel*	1 Thin Spread/7g	23.0	2.0	330	0.5	3.1	35.0	0.0
Gold, Lowest Fat, with Omega 3, St Ivel*	1 Thin Spread/7g	13.0	1.0	192	0.8	4.3	19.0	1.3
Heart, Cholesterol Reducing, Dairygold	1 Thin Spread/7g	24.0	3.0	338	0.7	2.8	36.0	0.0
Irish, Dairy, Original, Low Low*	1 Thin Spread/7g	24.0	3.0	346	0.4	0.5	38.0	0.0
Light, Benecol*	1 Thin Spread/7g	23.0	2.0	333	2.5	0.0	35.0	0.0
Lighter Than Light, Flora*	1 Serving/10g	19.0	2.0	188	5.0	1.6	18.0	0.0
Low Fat, Average	1 Thin Spread/7g	27.0	3.0	390	5.8	0.5	40.5	0.0
Low Fat, Better By Far, Morrisons*	1 Thin Spread/7g	44.0	5.0	627	0.5	1.0	69.0	0.0
Morning Gold, Low Fat, Morrisons*	1 Thin Spread/7g	26.0	3.0	372	7.5	0.0	38.0	0.0
Olive Gold, Reduced Fat, Co-Op*	1 Thin Spread/7g	37.0	4.0	535	0.2	1.0	59.0	0.0
Olive Light, GFY, Asda*	1 Thin Spread/7g	24.0	3.0	345	0.8	0.0	38.0	0.0
Olive Light, Low Fat, BGTY, Sainsbury's*	1 Thin Spread/ 7g	19.0	2.0	265	0.1	0.8	29.0	0.0
Olive Light, Sainsbury's*	1 Thin Spread/7g	24.0	3.0	348	1.5	0.0	38.0	0.0
Olive Oil, 55% Reduced Fat, Benecol*	1 Thin Spread/7g	35.0	4.0	498	0.3	0.5	55.0	0.0
Olive Oil, Bertolli*	1 Thin Spread/7g	38.0	4.0	536	0.2	1.0	59.0	0.0
Olive, Gold, Reduced Fat, Sainsbury's*	1 Thin Spread/7g	38.0	4.0	536	0.1	1.2	59.0	0.0
Olive, Light, Low Fat, HL, Tesco*	1 Thin Spread/7g	24.0	3.0	348	1.5	0.0	38.0	0.0
Olive, Low Fat, Morrisons*	1 Thin Spread/7g	24.0	3.0	346	0.9	0.0	38.0	0.0
Olive, Reduced Fat, Asda*	1 Thin Spread/7g	38.0	4.0	536	0.2	1.1	59.0	0.0
Olive, Reduced Fat, So Organic, Sainsbury's*	1 Thin Spread/7g	38.0	4.0	537	0.1	0.4	59.5	0.0
Olive, Reduced Fat, Somerfield*	1 Thin Spread/7g	38.0	4.0	536	0.1	1.1	59.0	0.0
Olive, Waitrose*	1 Thin Spread/7g	37.0	4.0	534	0.2	0.5	59.0	0.0
Olivite, Low Fat, Weight Watchers*	1 Thin Spread/7g	25.0	3.0	351	0.0	0.2	38.9	0.0
Organic, Dairy Free, M & S*	1 Thin Spread/7g	37.0	4.0	531	0.0	0.0	59.0	0.0
Pure Gold, Light, 65% Less Fat, Asda*	1 Thin Spread/7g	17.0	2.0	239	2.5	1.0	25.0	0.0
Sandwich, Heinz*	1 Tbsp/10ml	22.0	1.0	220	1.0	24.0	13.0	1.0
Sandwich, Light, Heinz*	1 Tbsp/10g	16.0	1.0	161	1.1	18.2	9.2	0.9
Soft, Economy, Sainsbury's*	1 Thin Spread/7g	31.0	3.0	450	0.2	0.9	50.0	0.0
Soft, Reduced Fat, Basics, Sainsbury's*	1 Thin Spread/7g	30.0	3.0	425	0.0	0.0	48.1	0.0
Soft, Reduced Fat, Smart Price, Asda*	1 Thin Spread/7g	32.0	3.0	455	0.2	1.0	50.0	0.0
Soft, Sainsbury's*	1 Thin Spread/7g	44.0	5.0	630	0.1	0.1	70.0	0.0
Soft, Value, Tesco*	1 Thin Spread/7g	30.0	3.0	435	0.0	0.0	48.0	0.0
Sunflower, Asda*	1 Thin Spread/7g	44.0	5.0	635	0.2	1.0	70.0	0.0
Sunflower, Enriched, Light, HL, Tesco*	1 Thin Spread/7g	24.0	3.0	350	0.3	1.0	38.0	0.0
Sunflower, Enriched, Tesco*	1 Thin Spread/7g	37.0	4.0	535	0.1	0.2	59.0	0.0
Sunflower, Light, BFY, Morrisons*	1 Thin Spread/7g	24.0	3.0	342	0.0	0.0	38.0	0.0
Sunflower, Light, BGTY, Sainsbury's*	1 Thin Spread/7g	19.0	2.0	265	0.1	0.8	29.0	0.0
Sunflower, Light, Reduced Fat, Asda*	1 Thin Spread/7g	24.0	3.0	347	0.3	1.0	38.0	0.1

S

	Measure INFO/WEIGHT	per Measure KCAL	FAT	Nutrition Values per 100g / 100ml KCAL	PROT	CARB	FAT	FIBRE
SPREAD								
Sunflower, M & S*	1 Thin Spread/7g	44.0	5.0	630	0.0	0.0	70.0	3.0
Sunflower, Morrisons*	1 Thin Spread/7g	44.0	5.0	631	0.0	0.2	70.0	0.0
Sunflower, Reduced Fat, Suma*	1 Thin Spread/7g	38.0	4.0	537	0.0	0.4	59.5	0.0
Sunflower, Sainsbury's*	1 Thin Spread/7g	37.0	4.0	532	0.1	0.2	59.0	0.0
Sunflower, Value, Tesco*	1 Thin Spread/7g	31.0	3.0	439	0.1	0.4	48.6	0.0
Sunflower, Waitrose*	1 Thin Spread/7g	44.0	5.0	631	0.0	0.2	70.0	0.0
Vegetable, Dairy Free, Free From, Sainsbury's*	1 Thin Spread/7g	44.0	5.0	630	0.0	0.0	70.0	3.0
Vegetable, Soft, Tesco*	1 Thin Spread/7g	46.0	5.0	661	0.1	1.0	73.0	0.0
Vitalite, St Ivel*	1 Thin Spread/7g	35.0	4.0	503	0.0	0.0	56.0	0.8
with Soya, Dairy Free, Pure Spreads*	1 Thin Spread/7g	42.0	5.0	603	0.0	0.0	67.0	0.0
with Sunflower, Dairy Free, Organic, Pure Spreads*	1 Thin Spread/7g	42.0	5.0	603	0.0	0.0	67.0	0.0
SPRING ROLLS								
Cantonese Selection, Sainsbury's*	1 Serving/35g	68.0	3.0	193	4.1	26.9	7.7	1.4
Char Sui Pork & Bacon, M & S*	1 Pack/220g	528.0	21.0	240	4.8	33.9	9.4	0.6
Chicken, & Chilli, Cantonese, Sainsbury's*	1 Roll/51g	85.0	3.0	166	9.7	19.4	5.5	0.6
Chicken, & Chilli, Sainsbury's*	1 Roll/50g	92.0	5.0	185	9.6	15.6	9.3	2.8
Chicken, Asda*	1 Roll/58g	115.0	5.0	199	4.6	25.0	9.0	3.4
Chicken, Finest, Tesco*	1 Roll/60g	118.0	5.0	196	10.1	20.1	8.3	1.0
Chicken, Oriental Snack Selection, Sainsbury's*	1 Roll/15g	38.0	1.0	256	11.5	30.3	9.9	1.7
Chicken, Oriental, Asda*	1 Roll/60g	106.0	4.0	178	3.7	25.0	7.0	0.4
Chicken, Tesco*	1 Roll/50g	115.0	6.0	231	8.1	24.5	11.2	1.5
Chinese Takeaway, Tesco*	1 Roll/50g	100.0	4.0	201	4.4	26.4	8.6	1.5
Dim Sum, Sainsbury's*	1 Roll/12g	26.0	1.0	216	4.1	28.2	9.6	2.9
Duck with Sweet Chilli Sauce, Waitrose*	1 Roll/72g	66.0	1.0	92	5.1	14.0	1.9	0.9
Duck, M & S*	1 Roll/30g	75.0	3.0	250	9.8	27.7	11.2	1.5
Duck, Mini, Asda*	1 Roll/18g	47.0	2.0	259	8.7	32.8	10.3	1.9
Duck, Morrisons*	1 Roll/65g	147.0	7.0	226	6.2	27.2	10.3	1.2
Duck, Party Bites, Sainsbury's*	1 Roll/20g	49.0	2.0	245	10.1	31.4	8.8	1.0
M & S*	1 Pack/180g	333.0	15.0	185	3.5	24.2	8.4	2.3
Mini, Asda*	1 Roll/20g	35.0	1.0	175	3.5	33.6	3.0	1.9
Mini, Sainsbury's*	1 Roll/12g	27.0	1.0	221	4.2	28.7	9.9	1.6
Mini, Veg, Chinese Snack Selection, Morrisons*	1 Roll/25.1g	52.0	2.0	207	3.5	28.8	8.7	2.7
Oriental Vegetable, Tesco*	1 Roll/67.5g	152.0	8.0	225	4.0	25.9	11.3	1.6
Prawn, Cantonese, Sainsbury's*	1 Roll/28g	46.0	2.0	162	6.8	20.3	6.0	2.5
Prawn, Crispy, M & S*	1 Roll/34.1g	75.0	3.0	220	10.0	22.2	9.9	1.3
Prawn, Tesco*	1 Roll/33g	70.0	3.0	211	8.7	22.8	9.4	1.4
Roast Duck, M & S*	1 Roll/31g	85.0	5.0	275	7.8	26.2	15.7	1.4
Thai Prawn, Waitrose*	1 Roll/50g	109.0	5.0	219	8.0	25.4	9.5	2.4
Thai, Sainsbury's*	1 Roll/30g	69.0	3.0	229	2.9	28.8	11.3	3.5
Vegetable & Chicken, Tesco*	1 Roll/60g	110.0	5.0	183	6.1	22.2	7.7	2.5
Vegetable, Asda*	1 Roll/62g	126.0	6.0	203	3.5	27.0	9.0	2.7
Vegetable, Cantonese, Large, Sainsbury's*	1 Roll/63.4g	130.0	6.0	205	3.6	25.3	9.9	1.5
Vegetable, Cantonese, Sainsbury's*	1 Roll/36g	84.0	4.0	233	3.6	28.1	11.7	1.4
Vegetable, Chilled, Tesco*	1 Roll/67.5g	149.0	8.0	221	4.0	25.9	11.3	1.6
Vegetable, Chinese Takeaway, Sainsbury's*	1 Roll/59g	100.0	4.0	170	4.0	24.4	6.3	2.8
Vegetable, Chinese, Sainsbury's*	1 Roll/26g	50.0	2.0	193	4.1	26.9	7.7	1.4
Vegetable, Cocktail, Tiger Tiger*	1 Roll/15g	38.0	2.0	254	6.4	26.7	13.4	2.0
Vegetable, Frozen, Tesco*	1 Roll/60g	123.0	6.0	205	3.5	23.0	10.6	1.3
Vegetable, M & S*	1 Roll/37g	80.0	4.0	215	4.3	27.8	9.6	2.0
Vegetable, Mini, Occasions, Sainsbury's*	1 Roll/24g	52.0	2.0	216	4.1	28.2	9.6	2.9
Vegetable, Mini, Oriental Selection, Waitrose*	1 Roll/18g	35.0	1.0	192	4.2	28.6	6.8	1.7
Vegetable, Mini, Party Food, M & S*	1 Roll/17g	35.0	2.0	205	3.5	26.3	9.7	2.0
Vegetable, Mini, Tesco*	1 Roll/18g	36.0	2.0	205	4.4	26.4	8.6	1.5

S

	Measure INFO/WEIGHT	per Measure		Nutrition Values per 100g / 100ml				
		KCAL	FAT	KCAL	PROT	CARB	FAT	FIBRE
SPRING ROLLS								
Vegetable, Oriental Selection, Party, Iceland*	1 Roll/14.9g	36.0	1.0	241	4.3	34.1	9.7	2.1
Vegetable, Party Delights, Farmfoods*	1 Roll/20g	31.0	1.0	156	4.4	24.8	4.4	1.5
Vegetable, Tempura, M & S*	1 Pack/140g	280.0	12.0	200	2.8	27.9	8.6	1.8
Vegetable, Waitrose*	1 Roll/57g	107.0	5.0	187	3.7	22.1	9.3	3.4
Waitrose*	1 Roll/33g	61.0	3.0	184	3.6	23.1	8.6	2.5
SPRITE								
Sprite*	1 Bottle/500ml	215.0	0.0	43	0.0	10.5	0.0	0.0
Zero, Sprite*	1 Can/330ml	3.0	0.0	1	0.0	0.0	0.0	0.0
SPRITZER								
Rose & Grape, Non Alcoholic, Extra Special, Asda*	1 Bottle/750ml	90.0	0.0	12	0.0	3.0	0.0	0.0
SQUARES								
Rice Krispies, Chewy, Marshmallow, Kellogg's*	1 Lge Bar/28g	116.0	3.0	415	3.0	76.0	11.0	0.9
Rice Krispies, Chocolate & Caramel, Kellogg's*	1 Bar/36g	155.0	5.0	430	4.5	71.0	14.0	2.0
Rice Krispies, Crazy Choc, Kellogg's*	1 Bar/28g	118.0	3.0	422	3.0	76.0	12.0	1.5
SQUASH								
Apple & Blackcurrant, Fruit, Robinson's*	100ml	43.0	0.0	43	0.1	9.7	0.0	0.0
Apple & Blackcurrant, No Added Sugar, Tesco*	1 Serving/30mls	4.0	0.0	15	0.2	2.0	0.0	0.0
Apple & Blackcurrant, Special R, Diluted, Robinson's*	1 fl oz/30ml	2.0	0.0	8	0.1	1.1	0.1	0.0
Apple & Blackcurrant, Special R, Robinson's*	1 Serving/30ml	2.0	0.0	8	0.1	1.1	0.0	0.0
Apple & Cranberry, Fruit Spring, Robinson's*	100ml	39.0	0.0	39	0.0	9.3	0.0	0.0
Apple & Strawberry High Juice, Sainsbury's*	1 Serving/250ml	82.0	0.0	33	0.1	8.2	0.1	0.1
Apple, Blackcurrant, Low Sugar, Diluted, Sainsbury's*	1 Glass/250ml	5.0	0.0	2	0.1	0.2	0.1	0.1
Apple, Cherry & Raspberry, High Juice, Robinson's*	1 Serving/25ml	49.0	0.0	196	0.2	47.6	0.1	0.0
Apple, Hi Juice, Tesco*	1 fl oz/30ml	52.0	0.0	173	0.0	42.5	0.0	0.0
Apple, No Added Sugar, Morrisons*	1 Serving/40ml	8.0	0.0	21	0.1	4.1	0.0	0.0
Blackcurrant, High Juice, M & S*	1 Glass/250ml	50.0	0.0	20	0.1	5.2	0.0	0.1
Blackcurrant, High Juice, Tesco*	1 Serving/75ml	215.0	0.0	287	0.3	70.0	0.0	0.0
Blackcurrant, No Added Sugar, Tesco*	1 Serving/25ml	3.0	0.0	14	0.4	1.7	0.0	0.0
Cherries & Berries, Tesco*	1 Serving/25ml	5.0	0.0	21	0.2	3.2	0.0	0.0
Cranberry, Light, Classic, Undiluted, Ocean Spray*	1 Serving/50ml	31.0	0.0	63	0.2	14.1	0.0	0.0
Dandelion & Burdock, Morrisons*	1 Serving/50ml	1.0	0.0	3	0.0	0.0	0.0	0.0
Forest Fruits, Fruit & Barley, Diluted, Morrisons*	1 fl oz/30ml	4.0	0.0	12	0.1	1.7	0.0	0.0
Forest Fruits, High Juice, Undiluted, Robinson's*	1 Serving/25ml	51.0	0.0	206	0.2	50.0	0.1	0.0
Fruit & Barley Orange, Diluted, Robinson's*	1 Serving/50ml	6.0	0.0	12	0.2	1.7	0.0	0.1
Fruit & Barley, No Added Sugar, Robinson's*	1 fl oz/30ml	4.0	0.0	14	0.3	2.0	0.0	0.0
Fruit & Barley, Tropical, No Added Sugar, Robinson's*	1 fl oz/30ml	4.0	0.0	14	0.3	2.0	0.0	0.0
Grape & Passion Fruit, High Juice, Diluted, Sainsbury's*	1 Serving/250ml	100.0	0.0	40	0.1	9.8	0.1	0.1
Grapefruit, High Juice, No Added Sugar, Sainsbury's*	1 Serving/250ml	1.0	0.0	6	0.1	1.1	0.0	0.0
Lemon, Double Concentrate, Value, Tesco*	1 Serving/25mls	3.0	0.0	11	0.2	0.3	0.0	0.0
Lemon, High Juice, Diluted, Sainsbury's*	1 Glass /250ml	97.0	0.0	39	0.1	9.1	0.1	0.1
Lemon, No Added Sugar, Double Concentrate, Tesco*	1 Serving/25ml	4.0	0.0	16	0.3	0.7	0.0	0.0
Lemon, No Sugar, Asda*	1 Serving/200ml	5.0	0.0	2	0.1	0.3	0.1	0.1
Mixed Fruit, Low Sugar, Sainsbury's*	1 Glass/250ml	5.0	0.0	2	0.1	0.2	0.1	0.1
Mixed Fruit, Tesco*	1 Serving/75ml	13.0	0.0	17	0.0	3.5	0.0	0.0
Orange & Mandarin, Fruit Spring, Robinson's*	1 Serving/440ml	26.0	0.0	6	0.1	0.8	0.0	0.0
Orange & Mango, Low Sugar, Sainsbury's*	1 Serving/250ml	5.0	0.0	2	0.1	0.2	0.1	0.1
Orange & Mango, No Added Sugar, Robinson's*	1 Serving/25ml	2.0	0.0	8	0.2	0.9	0.0	0.0
Orange & Mango, Special R, Diluted, Robinson's*	1 Serving/250ml	20.0	0.0	8	0.2	0.9	0.0	0.0
Orange & Pineapple, Original, Undiluted, Robinson's*	1 Serving/250ml	137.0	0.0	55	1.0	13.0	0.0	0.0
Orange, High Juice, Undiluted, Robinson's*	1 Serving/200ml	364.0	0.0	182	0.3	44.0	0.1	0.0
Orange, No Added Sugar, High Juice, Sainsbury's*	1 Serving/100ml	6.0	0.0	6	0.1	1.1	0.1	0.1
Orange, No Added Sugar, Undiluted, Pennywise, Crystal*	1 Serving/40ml	3.0	0.0	8	0.1	1.2	0.0	0.0
Orange, Sainsbury's*	1 Glass/250ml	7.0	0.0	3	0.1	0.5	0.1	0.1

S

	Measure INFO/WEIGHT	per Measure KCAL	FAT	Nutrition Values per 100g / 100ml KCAL	PROT	CARB	FAT	FIBRE
SQUASH								
Orange, Special R, Diluted, Robinson's*	1 fl oz/30ml	2.0	0.0	8	0.2	0.7	0.1	0.0
Peach, High Juice, Undiluted, Robinson's*	1 fl oz/30ml	54.0	0.0	181	0.5	43.0	0.1	0.0
Pink Grapefruit, High Juice, Diluted, Sainsbury's*	1 Serving/250ml	85.0	0.0	34	0.0	8.1	0.0	0.0
Pink Grapefruit, High Juice, Low Sugar, Tesco*	1 Serving/75ml	12.0	0.0	16	0.2	3.7	0.1	0.0
Pink Grapefruit, High Juice, Tesco*	1 Serving/75ml	135.0	0.0	180	0.2	44.6	0.1	0.0
Pink Grapefruit, High Juice, Undiluted, Robinson's*	1 Glass/250ml	455.0	0.0	182	0.2	43.3	0.1	0.0
Summer Fruit, No Added Sugar, Sainsbury's*	1 Serving/250ml	5.0	0.0	2	0.1	0.2	0.1	0.1
Summer Fruits & Barley, no Added Sugar, Tesco*	1 Serving/50ml	5.0	0.0	11	0.2	1.7	0.0	0.0
Summer Fruits, High Juice, Undiluted, Robinson's*	1 fl oz/30ml	61.0	0.0	203	0.1	49.0	0.1	0.0
Summer Fruits, High Juice, Waitrose*	1 Serving/250ml	102.0	0.0	41	0.0	10.0	0.0	0.0
Summer Fruits, No Added Sugar, Double Strength, Asda*	1 Serving/50ml	1.0	0.0	2	0.0	0.2	0.0	0.0
Summer Fruits, No Added Sugar, Made Up, Morrisons*	1 Glass/200ml	3.0	0.0	1	0.0	0.2	0.0	0.0
Summerfruits. High Juice, Tesco*	1 Serving/50ml	11.0	0.0	23	0.2	4.5	0.0	0.0
Tropical Fruits, Sainsbury's*	1 Serving/250ml	95.0	0.0	38	0.1	9.3	0.1	0.1
Tropical, High Juice, Tesco*	1 Glass/75ml	141.0	0.0	188	0.2	46.6	0.1	0.1
Tropical, No Added Sugar, Diluted, Tesco*	1 Glass/200ml	18.0	0.0	9	0.2	0.9	0.0	0.0
Whole Orange, Spar*	1 Serving/250ml	10.0	0.0	4	0.0	0.8	0.0	0.0
Whole Orange, Tesco*	1 Serving/100ml	45.0	1.0	45	0.2	10.1	1.0	1.0
Winter, Acorn, Baked, Average	*1oz/28g*	*16.0*	*0.0*	*56*	*1.1*	*12.6*	*0.1*	*3.2*
Winter, Acorn, Raw, Average	*1oz/28g*	*11.0*	*0.0*	*40*	*0.8*	*9.0*	*0.1*	*2.3*
Winter, All Varieties, Flesh Only, Raw, Average	*1oz/28g*	*10.0*	*0.0*	*34*	*0.9*	*8.6*	*0.1*	*1.5*
Winter, Butternut, Baked, Average	*1oz/28g*	*9.0*	*0.0*	*32*	*0.9*	*7.4*	*0.1*	*1.4*
Winter, Butternut, Organic, Tesco*	1 Serving/100g	39.0	0.0	39	1.1	8.3	0.1	1.6
Winter, Butternut, Raw, Unprepared, Average	*1 Serving/80g*	*29.0*	*0.0*	*36*	*1.1*	*8.3*	*0.1*	*1.6*
Winter, Butternut, Wedges, Tesco*	1 Pack/300g	108.0	0.0	36	1.1	7.7	0.1	1.6
Winter, Spaghetti, Baked	*1oz/28g*	*6.0*	*0.0*	*23*	*0.7*	*4.3*	*0.3*	*2.1*
Winter, Spaghetti, Including Pips & Rind, Raw	*1oz/28g*	*7.0*	*0.0*	*26*	*0.6*	*4.6*	*0.6*	*2.3*
SQUID								
Calamari, Battered, with Tartar Sauce Dip, Tesco*	1 Pack/210g	573.0	41.0	273	8.9	15.4	19.5	0.6
Dried, Average	*1oz/28g*	*88.0*	*1.0*	*313*	*63.3*	*4.8*	*4.6*	*0.0*
in Batter, Fried in Blended Oil, Average	1oz/28g	55.0	3.0	195	11.5	15.7	10.0	0.5
Pieces in Squid Ink, Palacio De Oriente*	1 Can/120g	274.0	22.0	228	13.0	3.6	18.0	0.0
Raw, Average	*1oz/28g*	*23.0*	*0.0*	*81*	*15.4*	*1.2*	*1.7*	*0.0*
STAR FRUIT								
Average, Tesco	*1oz/28g*	*9.0*	*0.0*	*32*	*0.5*	*7.3*	*0.3*	*1.3*
STARBAR								
Cadbury*	1 Bar/53g	260.0	15.0	491	10.7	49.0	27.9	0.0
STARBURST								
Fruit Chews, Tropical, Mars*	1 Tube/45g	168.0	3.0	373	0.0	76.9	7.3	0.0
Joosters, Mars*	1 Pack/45g	160.0	0.0	356	0.0	88.8	0.1	0.0
Juicy Gums, Mars*	1 Pack/45g	139.0	2.0	309	5.9	71.0	4.1	0.0
Mars*	1 Pack/45g	185.0	3.0	411	0.3	85.3	7.6	0.0
STEAK & KIDNEY PUDDING								
Fray Bentos*	1 Tin/213g	477.0	27.0	224	7.8	19.8	12.6	0.0
M & S*	1 Pudding/121g	260.0	13.0	215	9.2	19.4	11.1	3.2
Somerfield*	1 Pudding/190g	488.0	26.0	257	10.2	23.6	13.5	1.0
Tesco*	1 Serving/190g	437.0	23.0	230	10.0	20.7	11.9	1.2
Waitrose*	1 Pudding/223g	497.0	26.0	223	8.9	20.4	11.7	1.2
STEAMED PUDDING								
Apple & Sultana, BGTY, Sainsbury's*	1 Pudding/110g	294.0	3.0	267	2.9	57.4	2.9	0.8
Apple with Wild Berry Sauce, BGTY, Sainsbury's*	1 Pudding/110g	308.0	4.0	280	2.6	59.7	3.4	1.4
Chocolate Fudge, Less Than 5% Fat, Aunty's*	1 Pudding/110g	329.0	5.0	299	3.0	58.2	4.8	1.6
Golden Syrup, Aunty's*	1 Pudding/110g	324.0	5.0	295	2.9	58.6	4.1	0.7

	Measure INFO/WEIGHT	per Measure KCAL	per Measure FAT	Nutrition Values per 100g / 100ml KCAL	PROT	CARB	FAT	FIBRE
STEAMED PUDDING								
Lemon, BGTY, Sainsbury's*	1 Pudding/110g	307.0	3.0	279	3.0	60.2	2.9	0.7
Sticky Toffee, Aunty's*	1 Pudding/110g	331.0	5.0	301	2.6	58.4	4.8	1.2
Toffee & Date, Aunty's*	1 Pudding/110g	320.0	5.0	291	2.6	59.1	4.6	1.1
STEW								
Beef & Dumplings, Birds Eye*	1 Pack/400g	308.0	8.0	77	4.4	10.0	2.1	0.9
Beef & Dumplings, British Classics, Tesco*	1 Pack/450g	563.0	30.0	125	7.9	8.6	6.6	0.5
Beef & Dumplings, Countryside*	1 Pack/300g	246.0	7.0	82	8.1	7.3	2.3	0.5
Beef & Dumplings, Frozen, Asda*	1 Pack/400g	392.0	13.0	98	6.0	11.0	3.3	0.8
Beef & Dumplings, Frozen, Tesco*	1 Serving/400g	380.0	13.0	95	5.7	10.5	3.2	1.5
Beef & Dumplings, Plumrose*	½ Can/196g	143.0	4.0	73	6.1	9.0	2.0	0.0
Beef & Dumplings, Weight Watchers*	1 Pack/327g	262.0	7.0	80	5.2	10.0	2.1	0.8
Beef with Dumplings, Classic British, Sainsbury's*	1 Pack/450g	531.0	23.0	118	7.7	10.2	5.2	0.5
Beef with Dumplings, COU, M & S*	1 Pack/454g	431.0	12.0	95	8.9	9.1	2.6	0.8
Beef with Dumplings, Sainsbury's*	1 Pack/450g	603.0	27.0	134	9.3	10.5	6.1	0.7
Beef, Asda*	½ Can/196g	178.0	5.0	91	10.0	7.0	2.5	1.5
Beef, Meal for One, M & S*	1 Pack/440g	350.0	8.0	80	7.0	8.7	1.9	2.0
Beef, Value, Tesco*	1 Serving/200g	170.0	10.0	85	4.0	6.2	4.9	1.0
Chicken & Dumplings, Birds Eye*	1 Pack/320g	282.0	9.0	88	7.0	8.9	2.7	0.5
Chicken & Dumplings, Tesco*	1 Serving/450g	567.0	30.0	126	7.6	9.1	6.6	0.7
Chicken, Morrisons*	1 Pack/400g	492.0	8.0	123	17.6	8.9	1.9	0.5
Chickpea, Roast Sweet Potato, & Feta, Stewed!*	½ Pot/250g	187.0	7.0	75	3.3	8.8	2.9	2.7
Irish, Asda*	¼ Can/196g	172.0	8.0	88	6.0	7.0	4.0	1.0
Irish, Diet Chef Ltd*	1 Pack/300g	252.0	8.0	84	8.7	6.3	2.7	1.7
Irish, Morrisons*	1 Can/392g	243.0	5.0	62	3.8	8.9	1.2	0.0
Irish, Plumrose*	1 Can/392g	318.0	10.0	81	7.5	7.2	2.5	0.0
Irish, Sainsbury's*	1 Pack/450g	274.0	9.0	61	5.7	4.8	2.1	0.5
Irish, Tesco*	1 Can/400g	308.0	11.0	77	7.0	5.9	2.8	0.8
Lentil & Vegetable, Organic, Simply Organic*	1 Pack/400g	284.0	6.0	71	3.5	11.0	1.5	1.3
Lentil & Winter Vegetable, Organic, Pure & Pronto*	1 Pack/400g	364.0	10.0	91	3.6	14.0	2.4	4.0
Mixed Vegetable Topped with Herb Dumplings, Tesco*	1 Pack/420g	508.0	26.0	121	1.9	14.5	6.2	1.3
Tuscan Bean, Tasty Veg Pot, Innocent*	1 Pot/400g	320.0	8.0	80	3.1	12.5	1.9	3.6
STIR FRY								
Baby Leaf, Ready Prepared, M & S*	1 Serving/125g	25.0	0.0	20	1.7	4.9	0.1	2.5
Baby Leaf, Waitrose*	1 Pack/265g	50.0	0.0	19	1.7	2.9	0.1	2.0
Baby Vegetable & Pak Choi, Two Step, Tesco*	½ Pack/95g	29.0	1.0	31	2.1	4.0	0.8	2.3
Bean Sprout & Vegetable, with Red Peppers, Asda*	1 Pack/350g	126.0	4.0	36	1.8	4.7	1.1	2.3
Bean Sprout, Chinese, Sainsbury's*	1 Pack/300g	144.0	8.0	48	1.9	5.1	2.8	1.5
Bean Sprout, Ready to Eat, Washed, Sainsbury's*	1 Serving/150g	82.0	6.0	55	1.5	3.3	3.9	1.8
Bean Sprouts & Vegetables, Asda*	½ Pack/173g	107.0	7.0	62	2.0	4.5	4.0	1.8
Bean Sprouts, Asda*	½ Pack/175g	56.0	1.0	32	2.9	4.0	0.5	1.5
Beef, BGTY, Sainsbury's*	½ Pack/125g	156.0	5.0	125	22.0	0.1	4.1	0.0
Beef, Less Than 10% Fat, Asda*	1 Pack/227g	275.0	6.0	121	24.0	0.0	2.8	0.8
Beef, Less Than 3% Fat, BGTY, Sainsbury's*	½ Pack/125g	134.0	3.0	107	22.1	0.0	2.1	0.0
Cabbage, Carrot, Broccoli & Onion, Vegetable, Tesco*	1 Serving/100g	31.0	0.0	31	1.9	4.9	0.4	2.6
Cherry Tomato & Noodle, Waitrose*	1 Pack/400g	304.0	15.0	76	2.1	8.5	3.8	1.5
Chicken Chow Mein, Fresh, HL, Tesco*	1 Pack/400g	312.0	5.0	78	5.7	11.4	1.2	1.3
Chicken Noodle, GFY, Asda*	1 Pack/330g	403.0	11.0	122	7.0	16.0	3.3	2.4
Chicken, Safeway*	1 Serving/200g	204.0	3.0	102	22.0	0.0	1.6	0.0
Chinese Bean Sprout, Sainsbury's*	½ Pack/313g	150.0	9.0	48	1.9	5.1	2.8	1.5
Chinese Chicken, Iceland*	1 Pack/298g	262.0	4.0	88	6.2	12.7	1.4	2.9
Chinese Chicken, Sizzling, Oriental Express*	1 Pack/400g	400.0	8.0	100	6.6	13.8	2.0	1.7
Chinese Exotic Vegetable, Sainsbury's*	1 Pack/350g	133.0	8.0	38	1.7	2.8	2.2	1.8
Chinese Leaf & Mixed Peppers, Cook Asian, M & S*	1 Pack/260g	65.0	1.0	25	1.4	3.4	0.5	1.8

STIR FRY

INFO/WEIGHT	Measure	per Measure KCAL	FAT	Nutrition Values per 100g / 100ml KCAL	PROT	CARB	FAT	FIBRE
Chinese Mushroom, Sainsbury's*	1 Serving/175g	66.0	4.0	38	1.7	2.4	2.4	1.7
Chinese Noodles, Oriental Express*	1oz/28g	20.0	0.0	70	2.7	14.7	0.5	1.4
Chinese Prawn, Asda*	1 Serving/375g	345.0	2.0	92	3.6	18.0	0.6	1.8
Chinese Style Chicken, GFY, Asda*	1 Pack/338g	362.0	6.0	107	6.0	17.0	1.7	1.5
Chinese Style Prawn, GFY, Asda*	1 Pack/400g	324.0	6.0	81	3.6	13.0	1.6	1.6
Chinese Style Rice with Vegetables, Tesco*	1 Serving/550g	495.0	14.0	90	2.2	14.8	2.5	0.3
Chinese Style Turkey, Asda*	½ Pack/210g	321.0	6.0	153	23.8	8.1	2.9	0.8
Chinese Vegetable & Oyster Sauce, Asda*	1 Serving/150g	93.0	4.0	62	1.9	8.0	2.5	0.0
Chinese Vegetables, Oriental Express*	½ Pack/200g	44.0	0.0	22	1.4	3.7	0.2	2.2
Chinese Vegetables, with Chinese Style Sauce, Tesco*	1 Serving/350g	133.0	3.0	38	1.4	5.6	1.0	1.2
Chinese Vegetables, with Oyster Sauce, Tesco*	1 Pack/350g	98.0	1.0	28	2.0	4.6	0.2	1.1
Chinese, Eastern Inspirations*	½ Pack/170g	49.0	1.0	29	2.7	3.5	0.5	1.8
Chinese, Family, Sainsbury's*	1 Serving/150g	60.0	3.0	40	2.3	3.3	2.0	3.6
Chinese, with Oriental Sauce, Tesco*	1 Pack/530g	180.0	2.0	34	2.3	5.4	0.4	1.5
Chinese, With Soy, Garlic & Ginger, Tesco*	1 Pack/150g	90.0	0.0	60	1.5	12.6	0.1	0.5
Classic Medley, Veg Cuisine*	½ Pack/150g	45.0	1.0	30	2.5	4.1	0.4	2.1
Creamy Coconut & Lime, The Best, Safeway*	½ Pack/165g	231.0	12.0	140	3.4	14.4	7.2	2.1
Edamame Bean & Ginger, Tesco*	1 Pack/290g	145.0	5.0	50	4.1	4.9	1.6	2.5
Exotic, Asda*	1 Serving/250g	102.0	4.0	41	2.3	4.2	1.7	2.7
Exotic, Tesco*	1 Pack/191g	42.0	0.0	22	1.3	3.8	0.2	1.5
Family Pack, Vegetables & Beansprouts, Fresh, Tesco*	1 Pack/600g	108.0	1.0	18	2.0	2.2	0.1	2.1
Family, Tesco*	1 Pack/600g	210.0	3.0	35	2.3	5.2	0.5	2.1
Green Vegetable, M & S*	1 Pack/220g	165.0	13.0	75	3.1	2.5	5.9	2.2
Mediterranean Style, Eastern Inspirations*	½ Pack/153g	41.0	1.0	27	1.6	4.0	0.4	2.2
Mediterranean Style, Waitrose*	1 Pack/305g	82.0	1.0	27	1.6	4.6	0.4	2.2
Mixed Pepper, Fresh Tastes, Asda*	½ Pack/160g	75.0	4.0	47	1.4	4.6	2.6	2.0
Mixed Pepper, HL, Tesco*	1 Pack/325g	62.0	0.0	19	1.9	2.6	0.1	1.5
Mixed Pepper, Just Stir Fry, Sainsbury's*	½ Pack/150g	117.0	8.0	67	1.5	4.6	4.8	1.2
Mixed Pepper, Sainsbury's*	1 Pack/300g	201.0	14.0	67	1.5	4.6	4.8	1.2
Mixed Pepper, Tesco*	1/3 Pack/100g	23.0	0.0	23	1.9	3.7	0.1	1.9
Mixed Vegetable, Asda*	1 Serving/200g	96.0	5.0	48	1.7	4.7	2.5	3.0
Mixed Vegetables, Sainsbury's*	½ Pack/140g	70.0	4.0	50	1.7	4.7	2.7	3.0
Mushroom, Just Stir Fry, Sainsbury's*	1 Pack/350g	171.0	9.0	49	2.8	3.3	2.7	2.8
Mushroom, Tesco*	½ Pack/180g	61.0	1.0	34	2.6	3.9	0.5	2.0
Mushroom, Waitrose*	½ Pack/165g	43.0	1.0	26	2.3	3.3	0.4	1.6
Noodles & Bean Sprouts, Tesco*	½ Pack/125g	131.0	3.0	105	4.2	16.1	2.1	0.7
Orient Inspired, M & S*	1 Serving/250g	50.0	1.0	20	1.6	3.4	0.3	1.6
Oriental Chinese, Waitrose*	1 Serving/150g	40.0	1.0	27	2.2	3.9	0.4	1.4
Oriental Leaf, M & S*	½ Pack/125g	25.0	1.0	20	1.9	2.5	0.5	2.2
Oriental Style Pak Choi, M & S*	1 Pack/220g	165.0	13.0	75	2.2	3.5	5.7	2.4
Oriental, Ready Prepared, M & S*	½ Pack/260g	65.0	2.0	25	2.3	2.1	0.6	1.9
Pineapple, Safeway*	1 Pack/300g	237.0	15.0	79	3.6	4.7	5.1	0.9
Singaporean Noodle, Sainsbury's*	½ Pack/160g	202.0	12.0	126	3.2	11.9	7.3	2.4
Smart Price, Asda*	1 Pack/350g	126.0	4.0	36	1.8	4.7	1.1	2.3
Spicy Thai Style Noodle, Tesco*	1 Pack/500g	335.0	13.0	67	2.6	8.4	2.6	1.3
Sweet & Sour Vegetable, Somerfield*	1 Pack/350g	248.0	3.0	71	2.0	14.0	1.0	0.0
Sweet & Sour, Co-Op*	½ Pack/187g	103.0	2.0	55	2.0	10.0	0.9	3.0
Sweet & Sour, Tesco*	1 Pack/350g	161.0	1.0	46	1.8	9.1	0.3	1.3
Sweet Pepper, M & S*	1 Pack/400g	160.0	7.0	40	2.3	3.5	1.8	0.6
Tatsoi & Sugar Snap Pea, M & S*	½ Pack/125g	25.0	0.0	20	2.0	3.0	0.3	1.9
Tender Shoot, Sainsbury's*	½ Pack/126g	113.0	8.0	90	4.4	2.8	6.6	0.8
Thai Style, Eastern Inspirations*	1 Pack/330g	92.0	2.0	28	2.9	3.2	0.5	1.3
Thai Style, M & S*	1 Serving/150g	75.0	4.0	50	2.3	3.0	3.0	1.2

	Measure INFO/WEIGHT	per Measure KCAL	per Measure FAT	Nutrition Values per 100g / 100ml KCAL	PROT	CARB	FAT	FIBRE
STIR FRY								
Thai Style, Tesco*	1 Pack/350g	301.0	18.0	86	3.9	6.2	5.1	1.9
Tomato & Basil, Sundried, Tesco*	1 Pack/325g	205.0	12.0	63	1.6	6.2	3.6	2.2
Turkey, Fresh, Good Intentions, Somerfield*	½ Pack/150g	246.0	7.0	164	31.0	0.0	4.5	0.0
Vegetable & Beansprout, Tesco*	1 Pack/380g	129.0	2.0	34	2.0	5.4	0.5	2.2
Vegetable & Beansprout, Waitrose*	1 Pack/300g	78.0	1.0	26	1.4	4.5	0.3	2.1
Vegetable & Beansprout, with Peanut Sauce, Tesco*	1 Serving/475g	408.0	24.0	86	3.9	6.2	5.0	1.9
Vegetable & Mushroom, Asda*	½ Pack/160g	59.0	2.0	37	2.4	3.4	1.5	3.4
Vegetable & Noodle, Asda*	1 Pack/330g	465.0	15.0	141	4.0	21.0	4.5	3.0
Vegetable Noodles, BGTY, Sainsbury's*	1 Pack/455g	391.0	9.0	86	3.2	14.0	2.0	1.4
Vegetable, Asda*	1 Pack/300g	132.0	7.0	44	1.6	4.2	2.3	3.1
Vegetable, Cantonese, Sainsbury's*	1 Serving/150g	90.0	5.0	60	2.8	4.2	3.5	2.7
Vegetable, Chinese Style, Asda*	1 Pack/300g	81.0	2.0	27	1.6	3.6	0.7	2.8
Vegetable, Chinese Style, Tesco*	1 Pack/360g	79.0	1.0	22	1.9	3.2	0.2	1.4
Vegetable, Crunchy, Sainsbury's*	½ Pack/150g	85.0	6.0	57	1.4	4.1	3.9	2.1
Vegetable, Oriental, Frozen, Freshly, Asda*	1 Serving/100g	25.0	0.0	25	2.2	3.4	0.3	2.0
Vegetable, Oriental, Just Stir Fry, Sainsbury's*	½ Pack/135g	94.0	7.0	70	2.2	3.4	5.3	1.3
Vegetable, Premium, Sainsbury's*	½ Pack/150g	90.0	5.0	60	2.8	4.2	3.5	2.7
Vegetable, Ready Prepared, M & S*	½ Pack/150g	37.0	0.0	25	2.2	3.5	0.3	2.2
Vegetable, Sweet & Crunchy, Waitrose*	1 Pack/300g	69.0	0.0	23	1.8	3.6	0.1	1.4
Vegetable, Thai Style, Tesco*	½ Pack/135g	42.0	1.0	31	2.3	4.2	0.5	2.1
Vegetables, Family Pack, Co-Op*	½ Pack/300g	90.0	1.0	30	2.0	5.0	0.4	2.0
Vegetables, Family, Sainsbury's*	1 Serving/300g	123.0	7.0	41	1.6	3.8	2.2	2.1
Vegetables, Fresh, Asda*	½ Pack/150g	106.0	7.0	71	1.7	4.9	5.0	1.7
Vegetables, Mixed, with Slices of Pepper, Tesco*	1 Pack/300g	57.0	0.0	19	1.9	2.6	0.1	1.5
Vegetables, Sunshine, Tesco*	½ Pack/150g	42.0	0.0	28	1.8	4.6	0.3	2.1
Water Chestnut & Bamboo Shoot, Asda*	½ Pack/175g	61.0	2.0	35	1.4	4.3	1.4	1.7
STOCK								
Beef, As Sold, Stock Pot, Knorr*	1 Serving/5g	5.0	0.0	89	3.0	3.5	7.0	0.7
Beef, Fresh, Tesco*	1 Serving/300ml	54.0	1.0	18	2.1	1.6	0.3	0.5
Beef, Made Up, Stock Pot, Knorr*	1 Serving/100ml	5.0	0.0	5	0.1	0.2	0.4	0.0
Beef, Simply Stock, Knorr*	1 Serving/100ml	6.0	0.0	6	1.4	0.1	0.0	0.0
Beef, Slowly Prepared, Sainsbury's*	1 Serving/100g	7.0	0.0	7	0.7	0.3	0.3	0.5
Chicken, As Sold, Stock Pot, Knorr*	1 Serving/100ml	5.0	0.0	95	2.4	4.9	7.3	0.8
Chicken, Asda*	½ Pot/150g	25.0	1.0	17	1.8	0.7	0.9	0.2
Chicken, Concentrated, M & S*	1 Tsp/5g	16.0	1.0	315	25.6	12.2	18.1	0.8
Chicken, Fresh, Sainsbury's*	½ Pot/142ml	23.0	0.0	16	3.7	0.1	0.1	0.3
Chicken, Fresh, Tesco*	1 Serving/300ml	27.0	0.0	9	1.6	0.5	0.1	0.5
Chicken, Granules, Knorr*	1 Tsp/4.5g	10.0	0.0	232	13.1	36.5	3.7	0.4
Chicken, Made Up, Stock Pot, Knorr*	1 fl oz/30ml	1.0	0.0	5	0.1	0.3	0.4	0.0
Chicken, Prepared, Tesco*	1 Serving/300ml	54.0	0.0	18	2.4	1.8	0.1	0.5
Chicken, Simply Stock, Knorr*	1 Pack/450ml	27.0	0.0	6	1.5	0.1	0.0	0.1
Chicken, Slowly Prepared, Sainsbury's*	1 Pot/300g	27.0	0.0	9	0.6	1.3	0.1	0.5
Fish, Fresh, Finest, Tesco*	1 Serving/100g	10.0	0.0	10	0.6	1.8	0.0	0.5
Fish, Home Prepared, Average	**1 Serving/250ml**	**42.0**	**2.0**	**17**	**2.3**	**0.0**	**0.8**	**0.0**
Fresh, Finest, Tesco*	1 Pot/300g	33.0	0.0	11	1.9	0.8	0.0	0.2
Vegetable, As Sold, Stock Pot, Knorr*	1 Serving/100ml	6.0	0.0	117	2.4	5.7	9.4	1.3
Vegetable, Campbell's*	1 Serving/250ml	37.0	2.0	15	0.3	2.0	0.7	0.0
Vegetable, Concentrated, M & S*	1 Tsp/5g	19.0	1.0	380	3.3	43.0	19.0	1.2
Vegetable, Cooks Ingredients, Waitrose*	1 Pouch/500ml	15.0	0.0	3	0.2	0.4	0.1	0.5
Vegetable, Granules, Knorr*	2 Tsp/9g	18.0	0.0	199	8.5	39.9	0.6	0.9
Vegetable, Made Up, Stock Pot, Knorr*	1 Serving/100ml	6.0	0.0	6	0.1	0.3	0.5	0.1
STOCK CUBES								
Basil, Herb Cubes, Knorr*	1 Cube/10g	47.0	3.0	472	6.1	35.9	33.8	0.6

S

	Measure INFO/WEIGHT	per Measure KCAL	FAT	Nutrition Values per 100g / 100ml KCAL	PROT	CARB	FAT	FIBRE
STOCK CUBES								
Beef Flavour, Made Up, Oxo*	1 Cube/189ml	17.0	0.0	9	0.6	1.3	0.2	0.1
Beef, Dry Weight, Bovril*	1 Cube/5.9g	12.0	0.0	197	10.8	29.3	4.1	0.0
Beef, Dry Weight, Oxo*	1 Cube/5.8	15.0	0.0	265	17.3	38.4	4.7	1.5
Beef, Knorr*	1 Cube/10g	31.0	2.0	310	5.0	19.0	23.0	0.0
Beef, Organic, Kallo*	1 Cube/12g	25.0	1.0	208	16.7	16.7	8.3	0.0
Beef, Smart Price, Asda*	1 Cube/11g	31.0	3.0	279	10.0	8.0	23.0	0.0
Beef, Tesco*	1 Cube/7g	17.0	0.0	260	9.7	48.9	2.8	1.3
Beef, Toro*	1 Cube/60g	90.0	2.0	150	27.0	1.0	4.0	0.0
Beef, Value, Tesco*	1 Cube/10g	19.0	1.0	189	11.2	17.0	8.5	0.1
Chicken	1 Cube/6g	14.0	1.0	237	15.4	9.9	15.4	0.0
Chicken, Dry, Oxo*	1 Cube/7g	17.0	0.0	249	10.9	44.0	3.3	0.9
Chicken, Just Bouillon, Kallo*	1 Cube/12g	30.0	1.0	247	11.8	26.1	10.6	1.0
Chicken, Knorr*	1 Cube/10g	31.0	2.0	310	4.0	29.0	20.0	0.0
Chicken, Made Up, Sainsbury's*	1 Cube/200ml	16.0	0.0	8	0.3	1.4	0.1	0.1
Chicken, Prepared, Oxo*	1 Cube/100ml	9.0	0.0	9	0.4	1.5	0.1	0.1
Chinese, Dry Weight, Oxo*	1 Cube/5.8g	16.0	0.0	274	9.5	42.9	7.2	3.6
Fish, Knorr*	1 Cube/10g	32.0	2.0	321	8.0	18.0	24.0	1.0
Fish, Sainsbury's*	1 Cube/11g	31.0	2.0	282	19.1	7.3	20.0	0.9
Garlic, Dry Weight, Oxo*	1 Cube/6g	18.0	0.0	298	13.4	48.5	5.5	3.6
Ham, Knorr*	1 Cube/10g	31.0	2.0	313	11.8	24.4	18.7	0.0
Indian, Dry Weight, Oxo*	1 Cube/6g	17.0	0.0	291	11.5	43.9	7.7	6.7
Italian, Dry Weight, Oxo*	1 Cube/6g	19.0	0.0	309	11.9	48.9	7.3	4.6
Lamb, Made Up, Knorr*	1 Cube/10g	32.0	2.0	320	11.0	14.0	25.0	0.0
Mexican, Dry Weight, Oxo*	1 Cube/6g	15.0	0.0	248	11.8	36.8	6.0	3.7
Parsley & Garlic, Herb Cubes, Knorr*	1 Cube/10g	42.0	3.0	422	8.6	35.2	27.4	1.8
Vegetable Bouillon, Vegetarian, Amoy*	1 Cube/10g	30.0	2.0	300	0.0	20.0	20.0	0.0
Vegetable Bouillon, Yeast Free, Made Up, Marigold*	1 Serving/250ml	19.0	2.0	8	0.0	0.5	0.6	0.0
Vegetable, Average	1 Cube/7g	18.0	1.0	253	13.5	11.6	17.3	0.0
Vegetable, Dry, Oxo*	1 Cube/6g	17.0	0.0	251	10.4	41.4	4.9	1.4
Vegetable, Knorr*	1 Cube/10g	33.0	2.0	330	10.0	25.0	24.0	1.0
Vegetable, Low Salt, Organic, Made Up, Kallo*	1 Serving/500ml	50.0	3.0	10	0.3	0.7	0.7	0.2
Vegetable, Made Up, Organic, Kallo*	2 Cubes/100ml	7.0	0.0	7	0.1	0.5	0.4	0.1
Vegetable, Made up, Oxo*	1 Cube/100ml	9.0	0.0	9	0.4	1.4	0.2	0.1
Vegetable, Premium, Made Up, Kallo*	1 Serving/125ml	7.0	0.0	6	0.4	0.4	0.3	0.1
Vegetable, Yeast Free, Made Up, Kallo*	1 Cube/500ml	35.0	3.0	7	0.3	0.2	0.6	0.1
STRAWBERRIES								
& Creme Fraiche, Shapers, Boots*	1 Pack/100g	77.0	6.0	77	1.4	5.1	5.7	0.8
Dried, Graze*	1 Pack/35g	131.0	0.0	374	1.0	91.0	0.7	0.0
Dried, Urban Fresh Fruit*	1 Pack/35g	111.0	0.0	318	1.6	77.0	0.4	5.9
Fresh, Raw, Average	*1 Berry/12g*	*3.0*	*0.0*	*28*	*0.8*	*6.0*	*0.1*	*0.9*
in Fruit Juice, Canned, Average	*1/3 Can/127g*	*58.0*	*0.0*	*45*	*0.4*	*11.0*	*0.0*	*1.0*
in Light Syrup, Canned, Drained, Tesco*	1 Can/149g	100.0	0.0	67	0.5	16.0	0.1	0.7
in Raspberry Sauce, WT5, Sainsbury's*	1 Serving/170g	110.0	0.0	65	0.7	15.3	0.1	2.3
TTD, Sainsbury's*	1 Serving/100g	27.0	0.0	27	0.8	6.0	0.1	1.1
STROGANOFF								
Beef & Rice, TTD, Sainsbury's*	1 Pack/410g	595.0	21.0	145	9.6	15.2	5.1	1.7
Beef, Asda*	1 Serving/120g	276.0	20.0	230	16.0	3.3	17.0	0.6
Beef, BGTY, Sainsbury's*	1 Pack/400g	416.0	10.0	104	5.6	14.6	2.6	0.6
Beef, Finest, Tesco*	½ Pack/200g	330.0	13.0	165	9.4	16.2	6.7	0.7
Beef, HL, Tesco*	1 Pack/400g	400.0	9.0	100	7.0	13.0	2.2	1.3
Beef, Sainsbury's*	1 Can/200g	232.0	12.0	116	12.5	3.0	6.0	0.2
Beef, Slow Cooked, With Herby Rice, Sainsbury's*	1 Pack/450g	652.0	23.0	145	9.6	15.2	5.1	1.7
Beef, Weight Watchers*	1 Pack/330g	297.0	8.0	90	4.3	13.0	2.3	0.1

S

	Measure INFO/WEIGHT	per Measure KCAL	FAT	Nutrition Values per 100g / 100ml KCAL	PROT	CARB	FAT	FIBRE
STROGANOFF								
Beef, with Long Grain & Wild Rice, Somerfield*	1 Pack/400g	485.0	16.0	121	7.3	13.8	4.1	1.6
Beef, with Rice 'n' Peppers, Tesco*	1 Pack/450g	562.0	20.0	125	7.5	13.1	4.4	0.4
Beef, with Rice, Naturally Good Food, Tesco*	1 Pack/400g	425.0	9.0	106	7.1	13.9	2.3	1.3
Beef, with White & Wild Rice, Classic, Tesco*	1 Pack/500g	770.0	30.0	154	9.5	15.5	5.9	2.3
Chicken & Mushroom, COU, M & S*	1 Serving/400g	400.0	8.0	100	3.2	16.7	2.0	0.1
Chicken, with Rice, BGTY, Sainsbury's*	1 Pack/415g	448.0	5.0	108	7.0	17.1	1.3	1.1
Mushroom, Diet Chef Ltd*	1 Pack/250g	202.0	15.0	81	2.6	4.5	5.9	1.7
Mushroom, with Rice, BGTY, Sainsbury's*	1 Serving/450g	418.0	7.0	93	3.3	16.6	1.5	1.0
Mushroom, with Rice, Vegetarian, HL, Tesco*	1 Pack/450g	526.0	22.0	117	3.2	15.2	4.8	1.2
STRUDEL								
Apple & Mincemeat, Tesco*	1 Serving/100g	322.0	17.0	322	3.3	39.6	16.7	2.0
Apple, Co-Op*	1 Slice/100g	225.0	12.0	225	3.0	28.0	12.0	3.0
Apple, Frozen, Sainsbury's*	1 Serving/100g	283.0	15.0	283	3.2	32.8	15.4	1.9
Apple, Safeway*	¼ Strudel/150g	414.0	22.0	276	3.1	35.7	14.4	2.4
Apple, Sainsbury's*	1/6 Strudel/90g	255.0	14.0	283	3.2	32.8	15.4	1.9
Apple, Tesco*	1 Serving/150g	432.0	22.0	288	3.3	36.4	14.4	2.8
Apple, with Sultanas, Tesco*	1/6 Strudel/100g	245.0	12.0	245	2.9	30.9	12.0	0.7
Tesco*	1 Serving/150g	370.0	19.0	247	2.9	29.8	12.9	4.7
Woodland Fruit, Sainsbury's*	1/6 Strudel/95g	276.0	15.0	290	3.7	34.0	15.5	2.0
Woodland Fruit, Tesco*	1 Serving/100g	257.0	13.0	257	3.2	31.5	13.1	1.8
STUFFING BALLS								
Pork, Sausagemeat, Aunt Bessie's*	1 Ball/25.9g	55.0	2.0	212	7.2	27.3	8.2	3.0
Sage & Onion, Aunt Bessie's*	1 Ball/26g	63.0	2.0	243	6.4	34.4	8.9	3.1
Sage & Onion, Meat-Free, Aunt Bessie's*	1 Ball/28g	54.0	2.0	193	5.4	28.0	6.7	1.7
Sage & Onion, Tesco*	1 Serving/20g	64.0	4.0	322	10.0	21.1	22.0	1.9
Tesco*	1 Ball/20.6g	65.0	4.0	315	9.6	23.5	20.0	1.4
STUFFING MIX								
Apple & Herb, Special Recipe, Sainsbury's*	1 Serving/41g	68.0	1.0	165	3.8	32.4	2.2	2.2
Apple, Mustard & Herb, Paxo*	1 Serving/50g	83.0	1.0	166	4.2	32.8	2.0	4.0
Chestnut & Cranberry, Celebration, Paxo*	1 Serving/25g	35.0	0.0	141	4.0	26.7	2.0	2.4
Chestnut, Morrisons*	1 Serving/20g	33.0	1.0	165	4.6	29.1	3.4	3.7
Date, Walnut & Stilton, Special Recipe, Sainsbury's*	1 Serving/25g	49.0	2.0	196	5.2	25.0	8.4	2.0
Herb & Onion, Gluten Free, Allergycare*	1 Serving/12g	43.0	0.0	360	7.9	76.8	2.4	0.0
Parsley, Thyme & Lemon, Sainsbury's*	1 Pack/170g	240.0	2.0	141	4.2	28.2	1.3	1.3
Sage & Onion, Asda*	1 Serving/27g	29.0	0.0	107	3.4	22.0	0.6	1.3
Sage & Onion, Co-Op*	1 Serving/28g	94.0	1.0	335	10.0	68.0	2.0	6.0
Sage & Onion, Dry Weight, Tesco*	1 Pack/170g	578.0	4.0	340	10.3	69.3	2.4	6.3
Sage & Onion, Made Up, Paxo*	1 Serving/60g	74.0	1.0	123	3.6	23.0	1.8	1.7
Sage & Onion, Prepared, Tesco*	1 Serving/100g	50.0	0.0	50	1.5	10.1	0.4	0.9
Sage & Onion, Smart Price, Asda*	¼ Pack/75g	262.0	3.0	349	11.0	68.0	3.7	4.7
Sausage Meat, Morrisons*	1 Serving/20g	35.0	1.0	174	6.8	30.8	2.6	2.9
SUET								
Beef, Shredded, Original, Atora*	1 Pack/200g	1592.0	163.0	796	1.1	14.6	81.5	0.5
Beef, Tesco*	1 Serving/100g	854.0	92.0	854	0.6	6.2	91.9	0.1
Vegetable, Average	*1oz/28g*	*234.0*	*25.0*	*836*	*1.2*	*10.1*	*87.9*	*0.0*
SUET PUDDING								
Average	*1oz/28g*	*94.0*	*5.0*	*335*	*4.4*	*40.5*	*18.3*	*0.9*
SUGAR								
Brown, Soft, Average	*1 Tsp/4g*	*15.0*	*0.0*	*382*	*0.0*	*96.5*	*0.0*	*0.0*
Caster, Average	*1 Tbsp/12g*	*48.0*	*0.0*	*399*	*0.0*	*99.8*	*0.0*	*0.0*
Dark Brown, Muscovado, Average	*1 Tsp/7g*	*27.0*	*0.0*	*380*	*0.2*	*94.7*	*0.0*	*0.0*
Dark Brown, Soft, Average	*1 Tsp/5g*	*18.0*	*0.0*	*369*	*0.1*	*92.0*	*0.0*	*0.0*
Demerara, Average	*1 Tsp/5g*	*18.0*	*0.0*	*367*	*0.2*	*99.1*	*0.0*	*0.0*

S

	Measure INFO/WEIGHT	per Measure KCAL	per Measure FAT	Nutrition Values per 100g / 100ml KCAL	PROT	CARB	FAT	FIBRE
SUGAR								
for Making Jam, Silver Spoon*	1oz/28g	111.0	0.0	398	0.0	99.5	0.0	0.0
Fructose, Fruit Sugar, Tate & Lyle*	1 Tsp/4g	16.0	0.0	400	0.0	100.0	0.0	0.0
Golden, Unrefined, Average	*1 Tsp/4g*	*16.0*	*0.0*	*399*	*0.0*	*99.8*	*0.0*	*0.0*
Granulated, Organic, Average	*1 Tsp/4g*	*16.0*	*0.0*	*398*	*0.2*	*99.7*	*0.0*	*0.0*
Light Or Diet, Average	*1 Tsp/4g*	*16.0*	*0.0*	*394*	*0.0*	*98.5*	*0.0*	*0.0*
Muscovado, Light, Average	1 Tsp/5g	19.0	0.0	384	0.0	96.0	0.0	0.0
White, Granulated, Average	*1 Tsp/5g*	*20.0*	*0.0*	*397*	*0.0*	*100.7*	*0.0*	*0.0*
SULTANAS								
Average	*1oz/28g*	*82.0*	*0.0*	*292*	*2.5*	*69.7*	*0.4*	*2.0*
SUMMER FRUITS								
Frozen, Asda*	1 Serving/100g	28.0	0.0	28	0.9	6.0	0.0	2.5
Frozen, Sainsbury's*	1 Serving/80g	43.0	0.0	54	0.9	6.9	0.1	2.0
in Syrup, Sainsbury's*	1 Pudding/289g	188.0	0.0	65	0.5	15.6	0.1	1.2
Mix, Sainsbury's*	1 Serving/80g	26.0	0.0	32	0.9	7.4	0.0	2.4
Tesco*	1 Serving/80g	22.0	0.0	27	1.0	5.4	0.2	3.2
SUNDAE								
Banoffee, Perfectly Balanced, Waitrose*	1 Pot/115g	143.0	2.0	124	3.1	23.6	1.9	0.8
Blackcurrant, M & S*	1 Sundae/53g	212.0	10.0	400	3.0	54.2	19.2	1.9
Blackcurrant, Tesco*	1 Cake/48g	183.0	9.0	385	3.4	52.2	18.1	5.1
Butter Toffee, Mini, Eat Smart, Safeway*	1 Pot/63g	100.0	1.0	160	2.9	32.5	1.8	3.7
Chocolate & Cookie, Weight Watchers*	1 Pot/82g	128.0	3.0	156	2.5	30.3	3.4	2.2
Chocolate & Sticky Toffee, Asda*	1 Sundae/215g	755.0	52.0	351	2.8	31.0	24.0	0.5
Chocolate & Vanilla, HL, Tesco*	1 Sundae/120g	193.0	3.0	161	2.8	31.5	2.6	0.6
Chocolate & Vanilla, Tesco*	1 Sundae/70g	140.0	6.0	199	2.8	27.5	8.6	0.5
Chocolate Brownie, Finest, Tesco*	1 Serving/215g	778.0	57.0	362	2.7	28.7	26.3	2.3
Chocolate Mint, COU, M & S*	1 Pot/90g	108.0	2.0	120	5.4	17.8	2.6	0.5
Chocolate Nut	1 Serving/70g	195.0	11.0	278	3.0	34.2	15.3	0.1
Chocolate, Eat Smart, Safeway*	1 Serving/97g	150.0	3.0	155	3.5	29.0	2.7	4.3
Chocolate, Mini, Asda*	1 Pot/86g	199.0	13.0	231	3.1	21.0	15.0	1.7
Chocolate, Sainsbury's*	1 Pot/140g	393.0	30.0	281	2.5	19.3	21.3	0.6
Galaxy Caramel, Eden Vale*	1 Serving/128g	300.0	16.0	234	4.8	26.5	12.4	0.7
Hot Fudge, Two Scoop, Baskin Robbins*	1 Serving/203g	530.0	29.0	261	3.9	30.5	14.3	0.0
Mango & Passionfruit, Tesco*	1 Pot/78g	112.0	1.0	143	1.1	32.7	0.8	0.4
Peach & Apricot, Perfectly Balanced, Waitrose*	1 Pot/175ml	142.0	1.0	81	1.7	17.7	0.4	0.0
Raspberry, Eat Smart, Safeway*	1 Serving/97g	150.0	2.0	155	3.0	30.9	2.1	2.8
Raspberry, Perfectly Balanced, Waitrose*	1 Pot/175ml	150.0	1.0	86	1.7	18.9	0.6	0.0
Strawberry & Vanilla, Tesco*	1 Serving/68g	120.0	4.0	177	2.0	29.5	5.7	0.1
Strawberry & Vanilla, Weight Watchers*	1 Pot/105g	148.0	2.0	141	1.2	29.1	2.1	0.3
Strawberry, M & S*	1 Sundae/45g	173.0	8.0	385	3.4	53.3	17.8	1.0
Strawberry, Tesco*	1 Sundae/48g	194.0	9.0	408	3.3	57.6	18.3	1.3
Toffee & Vanilla, Tesco*	1 Serving/70g	133.0	5.0	189	2.1	30.7	6.4	0.1
Toffee, Asda*	1 Serving/120g	322.0	19.0	268	2.1	29.0	16.0	0.0
SUNNY DELIGHT*								
Apple & Kiwi Kick, Sunny Delight*	1 Glass/200ml	15.0	0.0	7	0.2	1.3	0.2	0.2
Californian Style, No Added Sugar, Sunny Delight*	1 Serving/200ml	20.0	0.0	10	0.1	1.4	0.2	0.1
Florida Style, Sunny Delight*	1 Serving/200ml	70.0	0.0	35	0.4	7.4	0.1	0.2
Original, Sunny Delight*	1 Glass/200ml	88.0	0.0	44	0.1	10.0	0.2	0.0
SUPPLEMENT								
Ball, Premium Protein, Bounce*	1 Ball/49g	209.0	9.0	426	30.6	40.8	18.4	2.0
Benefiber, Novartis*	1 Sachet/3.5g	7.0	0.0	200	0.1	15.0	0.0	85.0
Cellmass, All Flavours, BSN*	1 Scoop/16g	30.0	0.0	187	43.7	0.0	0.0	0.0
Chocolate, Forever Lite, Ultra, Powder, Forever Living*	1 Scoop/25g	90.0	1.0	360	68.0	16.0	4.0	4.0
Energy Drink, Shape Up & Detox, Arkipharma*	1 Serving/16ml	14.0	0.0	87	0.0	17.5	0.0	0.0

S

	Measure INFO/WEIGHT	per Measure KCAL	FAT	Nutrition Values per 100g / 100ml KCAL	PROT	CARB	FAT	FIBRE
SUPPLEMENT								
Fibre Sure, Protcor & Gamble*	1 Serving/100g	270.0	0.0	270	16.0	0.0	0.1	81.0
Malt Extract, Holland & Barrett*	1 Tbsp/24g	72.0	0.0	300	5.3	70.0	0.0	0.0
Meal, Complex, Cinnamon & Oatmeal, Prolab*	1 Serving/51g	190.0	4.0	373	39.2	39.2	7.8	7.8
Pro Peptide, Cnp*	1 Scoop/32.5g	115.0	2.0	354	69.2	9.2	4.6	0.0
Pro Recover, Cnp*	2 Scoops/80g	297.0	1.0	371	29.5	60.6	1.3	0.0
Protein, Hot Chocolate, Easy Body*	1 Serving/20g	74.0	0.0	370	70.7	19.2	1.2	0.0
Protein, Ultra, 80+, Ultimax*	1 Serving/20g	74.0	0.0	372	80.0	12.5	1.0	1.5
Protein, Vanila, Precision, EAS*	1 Scoop/25.5g	91.0	0.0	357	78.4	4.7	2.0	0.0
Psyllium Husk, Average	1 Tsp/5g	16.0	0.0	330	0.0	80.0	0.0	80.0
Recovery, Gainomax*	1 Carton/250ml	250.0	1.0	100	8.0	16.0	0.5	0.0
Shake, Chocolate, Myoplex, EAS*	1 Serving/76g	279.0	2.0	367	55.0	31.0	2.2	1.1
Shake, Chocolate, Ready to Drink, Myoplex, EAS*	1 Shake/330ml	150.0	3.0	45	7.6	1.5	1.1	0.0
Shake, Strawberry, Max Elle True Diet, My Protein*	1 Scoop/28g	106.0	2.0	378	63.6	14.7	7.4	3.3
Tablet, Berocca*	1 Tablet/4.5g	5.0	0.0	109	0.0	5.7	0.1	0.0
Total Nutrition Today, Plain, Natures Sunshine*	1 Scoop/38g	120.0	1.0	316	2.6	79.0	2.0	32.0
Tropical, Recovery, Powder, Made Up, Sport, Lucozade*	2 Scoops/250ml	147.0	0.0	59	4.1	10.2	0.0	0.0
Vextrago, Carbohydrate, Pvl Fit Foods International*	2 Scoops/75g	280.0	1.0	373	0.7	92.0	0.7	0.0
Whey Protein Isolate, Musashi*	2 Scoop/30g	111.0	0.0	371	88.7	1.2	0.5	0.0
Whey Protein, Body Fortress*	1 Scoop/25g	98.0	2.0	392	70.5	7.9	8.9	2.1
Whey Protein, Define*	1 Serving/40g	165.0	4.0	412	71.5	10.3	9.4	0.5
Whey Protein, Super, Precision*	1 Scoop/24g	94.0	2.0	390	71.5	7.3	8.3	0.0
Whey, Instant, Strawberry Flavour, Reflex Nutrition Ltd*	1 Serving/25g	98.0	1.0	394	80.0	6.0	5.5	0.2
SUSHI								
Aya Set, Waitrose*	1 Pack/110g	200.0	4.0	182	5.4	31.7	3.9	1.5
California Roll Box, M & S*	1 Pack/230g	391.0	12.0	170	7.0	22.0	5.2	1.1
California Set, Waitrose*	1 Pack/120g	223.0	9.0	186	3.8	25.2	7.6	1.7
Californian Roll, Nigiri & Maki Selection, M & S*	1 Pack/210g	294.0	4.0	140	4.4	25.9	2.1	2.2
Californian, Yakatori, M & S*	1 Serving/200g	340.0	9.0	170	6.4	25.0	4.7	1.0
Chicken, M & S*	1 Pack/186g	260.0	4.0	140	6.0	24.4	2.2	1.0
Chicken, Tesco*	1 Pack/147g	243.0	4.0	165	5.2	30.0	2.4	1.0
Classic, Finest, Tesco*	1 Pack/232g	330.0	1.0	142	6.6	27.6	0.4	0.6
Deluxe, Shapers, Boots*	1 Serving/235g	355.0	4.0	151	5.3	29.0	1.5	2.7
Fish & Veg Selection, Tesco*	1 Pack/150g	247.0	3.0	165	6.7	29.2	2.3	0.4
Fish Nigiri, Adventurous, Tesco*	1 Pack/200g	270.0	4.0	135	7.1	21.7	2.2	0.5
Fish Selection, M & S*	1 Pack/210g	346.0	7.0	165	7.4	26.3	3.1	1.4
Fish, Large Pack, Tesco*	1 Pack/284g	469.0	11.0	165	5.5	27.0	3.9	1.5
Fish, Snack, Tesco*	1 Pack/104g	159.0	3.0	153	4.5	28.0	2.5	1.5
Large, Boots*	1 Pack/324g	480.0	6.0	148	5.0	28.0	1.8	0.7
Maki Rolls Box, Sainsbury's*	1 Pack/127g	197.0	2.0	155	4.5	30.5	1.7	0.8
Maki Selection, Shapers, Boots*	1 Pack/158g	225.0	2.0	142	3.5	29.0	1.3	1.1
Nigiri Set, Waitrose*	1 Pack/150g	229.0	4.0	153	6.3	26.0	2.6	0.6
Nigiri, M & S*	1 Serving/190g	303.0	6.0	159	7.3	25.3	3.1	0.6
Nigiri, Selection, Tesco*	1 Pack/152g	236.0	2.0	155	4.6	31.2	1.0	0.6
Nigri, Californian Roll, Maki Roll, Sainsbury's*	1 Pack/195g	283.0	3.0	145	5.3	27.4	1.5	1.9
Oriental Fish Box, M & S*	1 Pack/205g	318.0	8.0	155	6.1	23.3	4.1	0.9
Prawn & Salmon Selection, M & S*	1 Serving/175g	255.0	3.0	146	5.5	27.4	1.7	0.6
Prawn Feast, M & S*	1 Pack/219g	350.0	8.0	160	5.7	25.8	3.7	1.1
Roll Selection, Sainsbury's*	1 Pack/217.4g	363.0	8.0	167	5.0	28.4	3.7	0.5
Roll Selection, Tesco*	1 Pack/214g	327.0	5.0	153	5.0	27.6	2.5	1.2
Rolls, Shapers, Boots*	1 Pack/168g	259.0	4.0	154	4.7	28.0	2.4	0.5
Salmon & Roll Set, Sainsbury's*	1 Serving/101g	167.0	3.0	165	4.9	30.4	2.6	0.8
Salmon Feast Box, M & S*	1 Pack/200g	330.0	6.0	165	5.6	27.0	2.9	1.0
Salmon, Nigri Crayfish, Red Pepper, Sainsbury's*	1 Serving/150g	232.0	4.0	155	5.5	26.4	3.0	1.0

S

	Measure INFO/WEIGHT	per Measure KCAL	per Measure FAT	Nutrition Values per 100g / 100ml KCAL	PROT	CARB	FAT	FIBRE
SUSHI								
Selection, Boots*	1 Pack/268g	434.0	10.0	162	5.5	27.0	3.6	1.6
Tokyo Set, M & S*	1 Pack/150g	240.0	5.0	160	7.3	25.3	3.1	0.6
Tuna, to Snack Selection, Food to Go, M & S*	1 Serving/150g	225.0	4.0	150	5.2	26.4	2.6	2.3
Vegetarian, Snack Selection, Tesco*	1 Pack/85g	106.0	3.0	125	3.7	20.1	3.3	0.6
Vegetarian, with Pickled Vegetables, Waitrose*	1 Pack/135g	244.0	5.0	181	5.0	27.8	3.6	1.7
Veggie, Medium Selection, Tesco*	1oz/28g	38.0	0.0	135	2.5	27.4	1.7	5.0
Yo!, Bento Box, Sainsbury's*	1 Pack/208g	530.0	6.0	255	8.4	48.7	3.0	0.9
Yo!, Salmon Lunch Set, Sainsbury's*	1 Pack/150g	241.0	4.0	161	5.9	28.1	2.8	0.8
SWEDE								
Boiled, Average	*1oz/28g*	*3.0*	*0.0*	*11*	*0.3*	*2.3*	*0.1*	*0.7*
Mash, COU, M & S*	1oz/28g	15.0	0.0	55	1.1	9.5	1.2	2.1
Raw, Unprepared, Average	*1oz/28g*	*6.0*	*0.0*	*21*	*0.8*	*4.4*	*0.3*	*1.9*
SWEET & SOUR								
Beef, Feeling Great, Findus*	1 Pack/350g	385.0	7.0	110	4.0	19.0	2.0	1.5
Beef, Feeling Great, New, Findus*	1 Pack/350g	420.0	9.0	120	4.5	20.0	2.5	1.3
Chicken Balls, Chinese Takeaway, Iceland*	1 Pack/255g	311.0	3.0	122	9.9	17.5	1.3	6.0
Chicken, & Noodles, BGTY, Sainsbury's*	1 Pack/400g	356.0	2.0	89	7.5	13.3	0.6	0.7
Chicken, & Noodles, Chinese Takeaway, Tesco*	1 Pack/350g	350.0	1.0	100	5.7	18.8	0.2	0.2
Chicken, & Rice, Chilled, Tesco*	1 Pack/450g	540.0	6.0	120	4.9	21.9	1.3	0.9
Chicken, & Rice, Mega, Value, Tesco*	1 Pack/500g	675.0	9.0	135	4.4	25.0	1.9	1.9
Chicken, & Rice, Morrisons*	1 Pack/400g	452.0	10.0	113	3.6	18.8	2.6	0.8
Chicken, Breasts, Tesco*	1 Serving/185g	172.0	2.0	93	14.6	6.5	1.0	0.1
Chicken, Canned, Tesco*	1 Can/400g	408.0	6.0	102	9.6	12.4	1.6	1.1
Chicken, Chinese Takeaway, Sainsbury's*	1 Pack/264g	515.0	17.0	195	13.1	21.3	6.4	1.0
Chicken, Crispy, Fillets, Tesco*	1 Pack/350g	507.0	20.0	145	7.2	15.3	5.6	0.9
Chicken, Good Choice, Iceland*	1 Pack/400g	488.0	1.0	122	4.5	25.6	0.2	0.5
Chicken, in Batter, Cantonese, Chilled, Sainsbury's*	1 Pack/350g	560.0	21.0	160	8.9	22.4	6.0	0.9
Chicken, in Crispy Batter, Morrisons*	1 Pack/350g	511.0	14.0	146	10.1	17.6	3.9	1.2
Chicken, M & S*	1 Pack/300g	465.0	11.0	155	6.6	24.4	3.6	0.8
Chicken, Oriental, Tesco*	1 Pack/350g	340.0	4.0	97	9.3	12.2	1.1	0.8
Chicken, Take It Away, M & S*	1 Pack/200g	200.0	2.0	100	9.4	13.2	0.8	1.2
Chicken, Tinned, M & S*	1 Serving/481g	553.0	20.0	115	11.4	7.8	4.2	1.9
Chicken, Waitrose*	1 Serving/300g	372.0	3.0	93	9.8	11.7	0.8	1.4
Chicken, Weight Watchers*	1 Pack/330g	310.0	1.0	94	5.0	17.5	0.4	0.3
Chicken, with Egg Rice, Chilled, HL, Tesco*	1 Pack/450g	499.0	3.0	111	6.8	19.2	0.7	0.6
Chicken, with Rice, Big Eat, Heinz*	1 Pot/350g	329.0	7.0	94	4.4	14.9	1.9	0.6
Chicken, with Rice, Chilled, BGTY, Sainsbury's*	1 Pack/400g	344.0	4.0	86	6.0	13.5	0.9	1.0
Chicken, with Rice, Farmfoods*	1 Pack/300g	324.0	3.0	108	5.9	19.2	0.9	0.7
Chicken, with Rice, Good Intentions, Somerfield*	1 Serving/400g	448.0	2.0	112	6.6	20.1	0.6	0.3
Chicken, with Rice, Nisa, Heritage, Nisa Heritage*	1 Pack/600g	606.0	5.0	101	6.0	17.4	0.8	0.4
Chicken, with Rice, Oriental Express*	1 Pack/340g	350.0	2.0	103	4.4	21.3	0.6	0.7
Chicken, with Rice, Value, Tesco*	1 Pack/300g	348.0	1.0	116	5.9	22.3	0.3	0.7
Chicken, with Rice, Weight Watchers*	1 Pack/400g	352.0	2.0	88	5.4	15.5	0.5	1.4
Chicken, with Vegetable Rice, COU, M & S*	1 Pack/400g	400.0	6.0	100	6.9	14.9	1.4	1.1
Chicken, without Batter, Cantonese, Chilled, Sainsbury's*	1 Pack/350g	409.0	5.0	117	8.5	17.6	1.4	1.0
Pork	1oz/28g	48.0	2.0	172	12.7	11.3	8.8	0.6
Pork, Battered, Sainsbury's*	½ Pack/175g	306.0	9.0	175	7.3	25.1	5.0	0.6
Pork, Cantonese, & Egg Fried Rice, Farmfoods*	1 Pack/327g	520.0	19.0	159	4.8	22.0	5.8	0.1
Roasted Vegetables, Cantonese, Sainsbury's*	1 Pack/348g	327.0	4.0	94	1.1	19.6	1.2	0.9
Vegetables, with Rice, Waitrose*	1 Pack/400g	384.0	4.0	96	1.9	19.5	1.1	1.1
SWEET POTATO								
Baked, Average	*1 Med/130g*	*149.0*	*1.0*	*115*	*1.6*	*27.9*	*0.4*	*3.3*
Boiled in Salted Water, Average	*1 Med/130g*	*109.0*	*0.0*	*84*	*1.1*	*20.5*	*0.3*	*2.3*

S

	Measure INFO/WEIGHT	per Measure		Nutrition Values per 100g / 100ml				
		KCAL	FAT	KCAL	PROT	CARB	FAT	FIBRE
SWEET POTATO								
Raw, Unprepared, Average	1 Med/130g	113.0	0.0	87	1.2	21.3	0.3	2.4
Steamed, Average	1 Med/130g	109.0	0.0	84	1.1	20.4	0.3	2.3
SWEETBREAD								
Lamb, Fried	1oz/28g	61.0	3.0	217	28.7	0.0	11.4	0.0
Lamb, Raw	1oz/28g	37.0	2.0	131	15.3	0.0	7.8	0.0
SWEETCORN								
Baby, Canned, Drained, Average	1 Serving/80g	18.0	0.0	23	2.9	2.0	0.4	1.5
Baby, Frozen, Average	1oz/28g	7.0	0.0	24	2.5	2.7	0.4	1.7
Boiled, Average	1oz/28g	31.0	1.0	111	4.2	19.6	2.3	2.2
Canned, in Water, No Sugar & Salt, Average	½ Can/125g	99.0	1.0	79	2.7	14.9	1.1	1.6
Canned, with Sugar & Salt, Average	½ Can/71g	79.0	1.0	111	3.2	21.9	1.2	1.9
Frozen, Average	1 Sachet/115g	121.0	2.0	105	3.8	17.9	2.1	1.8
Supersweet, Field Fresh, Birds Eye*	1 Portion/80g	67.0	1.0	84	2.6	16.9	0.7	2.4
SWEETENER								
Aspartamo, Artificial Sugar, Zen*	1 Tbsp/2g	8.0	0.0	383	1.8	94.0	0.0	0.0
Canderel*	1 Tbsp/2g	8.0	0.0	379	24.7	7.0	0.0	5.3
Canderel, Spoonful, Canderel*	1 Tsp/0.5g	2.0	0.0	384	2.9	93.0	0.0	0.0
Granulated, Asda*	1 Tsp/1g	4.0	0.0	400	0.0	100.0	0.0	0.0
Granulated, Aspartame, Safeway*	1 Tsp/1g	2.0	0.0	392	3.0	95.0	0.0	0.0
Granulated, Low Calorie, Splenda*	1 Tsp/0.5g	2.0	0.0	391	0.0	97.7	0.0	0.0
Granulated, Silver Spoon*	1 Tsp/0.5g	2.0	0.0	387	1.0	96.8	0.0	0.0
Silver Spoon*	1 Tablet/0.05g	0.0	0.0	325	10.0	71.0	0.0	0.0
Simply Sweet*	1 Tbsp/2g	7.0	0.0	375	1.4	92.3	0.0	0.0
Slendasweet, Sainsbury's*	1 Tsp/1g	4.0	0.0	395	1.8	97.0	0.0	0.1
Spoonfull, Low Calorie, SupaSweet*	1 Tsp/1g	4.0	0.0	392	3.0	95.0	0.0	0.0
Sweet' N Low*	1 Sachet/1g	3.0	0.0	368	0.0	92.0	0.0	0.0
Sweetex*	1oz/28g	0.0	0.0	0	0.0	0.0	0.0	0.0
Tablets, Low Calorie, Canderel*	1 Tablet/0.1g	0.0	0.0	342	13.0	72.4	0.0	0.0
Tablets, Splenda*	1 Tablet/0.1g	0.0	0.0	345	10.0	76.2	0.0	1.6
Tablets, Tesco*	1 Tablet/1g	0.0	0.0	20	2.0	2.0	0.5	0.0
Xylosweet, Xylitol*	1 Serving/4g	10.0	0.0	240	0.0	100.0	0.0	0.0
SWEETS								
Alphabet Candies, Asda*	1 Pack/80g	306.0	0.0	382	0.5	95.0	0.0	0.0
Aquadrops, Citrus & Apple, Mars*	1 Serving/2.5g	6.0	0.0	247	0.1	94.5	1.0	0.0
Banana, Baby Foam, M & S*	1/3 Pack/34g	131.0	0.0	385	4.1	92.7	0.0	0.0
Black Jacks & Fruit Salad, Bassett's*	1 Serving/190g	760.0	12.0	400	0.7	84.9	6.2	0.0
Blackcurrant & Liquorice, M & S*	1 Sweet/8g	32.0	0.0	400	0.6	89.0	4.3	0.0
Bursting Bugs, Rowntree's*	1 Pack/175g	583.0	0.0	333	4.8	78.1	0.2	0.0
Butter Candies, Original, Werther's*	1 Sweet/5g	21.0	0.0	424	0.1	85.7	8.9	0.1
Campino, Oranges & Cream, Bendicks*	1oz/28g	116.0	2.0	416	0.1	85.8	8.1	0.0
Candy Cane, Average	1oz/28g	100.0	0.0	357	3.6	85.7	0.0	0.0
Candy Floss, Asda*	1 Tub/75g	292.0	0.0	390	0.0	100.0	0.0	0.0
Candy Foam Shapes, Fun Fruits, Value, Tesco*	1 Serving/25g	96.0	0.0	384	3.6	94.0	0.3	0.1
Chewitts, Blackcurrant	1 Pack/33.1g	125.0	1.0	378	0.3	86.9	2.7	0.0
Chews, Just Fruit, Fruit-tella*	1 Serving/43g	170.0	3.0	400	0.9	79.5	6.5	0.0
Chews, Strawberry Mix, Starburst*	1 Sweet/3.8g	15.0	0.0	401	0.0	83.9	7.3	0.0
Choco Toffee, Sula*	1 Sweet/7.8g	21.0	1.0	267	3.3	31.7	15.8	0.0
Chocolate Caramels, Milk, Tesco*	1 Sweet/3g	15.0	1.0	444	2.7	72.1	16.1	0.1
Chocolate Eclairs, Cadbury*	1 Sweet/8g	36.0	1.0	455	4.5	68.9	17.9	0.0
Chocolate Limes, Pascall*	1 Sweet/8g	27.0	0.0	333	0.3	77.2	2.5	0.0
Cola Bottles, Fizzy, M & S*	1 Pack/200g	650.0	0.0	325	6.4	75.0	0.0	0.0
Cough, Herbs, Swiss, Orginal, Ricola*	1 Packet/37g	148.0	0.0	400	0.0	98.0	0.0	0.0
Cream Caramel, Sula*	1 Sweet/3g	10.0	0.0	297	0.4	86.1	0.0	0.0

S

	Measure INFO/WEIGHT	per Measure KCAL	FAT	Nutrition Values per 100g / 100ml KCAL	PROT	CARB	FAT	FIBRE
SWEETS								
Crunchies, Fruit, Fruit-tella*	1 Box/23g	90.0	1.0	390	0.7	86.0	5.0	0.0
Dolly Mix, Bassett's*	1 Bag/45g	171.0	1.0	380	3.0	85.1	3.1	0.4
Drops, Lemon & Orange, M & S*	1 Pack42g	97.0	0.0	230	0.0	61.0	0.0	0.0
Drumstick, Matlow's*	1 Pack/40g	164.0	2.0	409	0.4	88.3	5.5	0.0
Flumps, Bassett's*	1 Serving/5g	16.0	0.0	325	4.0	77.0	0.0	0.0
Flumps, Fluffy Mallow Twists, Fat Free, Bassett's*	1 Twist/13g	30.0	0.0	230	4.1	77.1	0.0	0.0
Flying Suacers, Asda*	1 Serving/23g	82.0	1.0	355	0.1	83.0	2.5	0.8
Foamy Mushrooms, Chewy, Asda*	1 Sweet/2.6g	9.0	0.0	347	4.2	82.0	0.2	0.0
Fruit Gums & Jellies	1 Tube/33g	107.0	0.0	324	6.5	79.5	0.0	0.0
Fruit Puffs, Allen's*	1 Serving/25g	91.0	0.0	364	2.2	92.4	0.0	0.0
Fruities, Lemon & Lime, Weight Watchers*	1 Sweet/2g	3.0	0.0	134	0.0	54.0	0.0	33.0
Fruity Babies, Bassett's*	1 Sweet/3g	10.0	0.0	310	4.6	72.7	0.2	0.0
Fruity Chews, Starburst*	1 Sweet/8.3g	34.0	1.0	404	0.0	83.4	7.4	0.0
Fruity Frogs, Rowntree's*	1 Serving/40g	128.0	0.0	321	4.7	74.5	0.2	0.0
Fruity Mallows, Fizzy, Asda*	1 Pack/400g	1252.0	0.0	313	4.3	74.0	0.0	0.0
Gummy Mix, Tesco*	1 Pack/100g	327.0	0.0	327	5.9	75.7	0.1	0.0
Gummy Zingy Fruits, Bassett's*	1 Sm Bag/40g	135.0	0.0	337	5.1	79.2	0.0	0.0
Jelly Babies, Morrisons*	1 Serving/227g	781.0	0.0	344	5.3	80.7	0.0	0.0
Jelly Beans, Tesco*	¼ Bag/63g	243.0	0.0	385	0.1	94.5	0.3	0.3
Kisses, Hershey*	1 Sweet/5g	28.0	2.0	561	7.0	59.0	32.0	0.0
Liquorice and Fruit, Fruit-tella*	1 Sweet/4g	16.0	0.0	395	0.9	83.0	6.5	0.0
Maynards Sours, Bassett's*	1 Pack/52g	166.0	0.0	320	3.9	74.9	0.1	0.0
Milk Chocolate Eclairs, Sainsbury's*	1 Sweet/8g	33.0	1.0	442	2.1	75.7	14.5	0.5
Milk Duds, Hershey*	13 Pieces/33g	170.0	6.0	510	3.0	84.0	18.0	0.0
Parma Violets, Swizzlers*	1 Tube/10g	41.0	0.0	406	0.9	99.1	0.0	0.0
Randoms, Rowntree's*	1 Pack/50g	164.0	0.0	328	4.9	75.7	0.3	0.6
Raspberry Vines, Candy Tree*	1 Pack/75g	267.0	0.0	356	2.0	86.6	0.2	0.0
Rhubarb & Custard, Sainsbury's*	1 Sweet/8g	28.0	0.0	351	0.1	87.7	0.0	0.0
Sherbert Cocktails, Sainsbury's*	1 Sweet/9g	36.0	1.0	400	0.0	83.1	7.5	0.0
Sherbert Lemons, Weight Watchers*	1 Box/35g	84.0	0.0	239	0.0	94.7	0.5	0.0
Sherbet Lemons, Bassett's*	1 Sweet/6.7g	25.0	0.0	375	0.0	93.9	0.0	0.0
Shrimps & Bananas, Sainsbury's*	½ Pack/50g	188.0	0.0	376	2.5	91.3	0.1	0.5
Snakes, Bassett's*	1 Sweet/9.4g	30.0	0.0	320	3.5	76.8	0.1	0.0
Sour Squirms, Bassett's*	1 Serving/7g	21.0	0.0	325	3.1	78.1	0.0	0.0
Squidgy Cars, Shannon's*	1 Sweet/8g	27.0	0.0	342	5.3	80.0	0.1	0.0
Strawberry & Cream, Sugar Free, Sula*	1 Serving/10g	27.0	1.0	267	0.2	90.5	5.4	0.0
Sugar Free, Sula*	1 Sweet/3g	7.0	0.0	231	0.0	96.1	0.0	0.0
Sweetshop Favourites, Bassett's*	1 Sweet/5g	17.0	0.0	340	0.0	84.3	0.0	0.0
Toffo*	1 Tube/43g	194.0	9.0	451	2.2	69.8	22.0	0.0
Tooty Frooties, Rowntree's*	1 Bag/28g	111.0	1.0	397	0.1	91.5	3.5	0.0
Wazzly Wobble Drops, Wonka*	1 Bag/42g	186.0	7.0	443	3.0	71.6	16.1	0.2
Wiggly Worms, Sainsbury's*	1 Serving/10g	32.0	0.0	317	5.6	72.7	0.4	0.2
SWORDFISH								
Grilled, Average	*1oz/28g*	*39.0*	*1.0*	*139*	*22.9*	*0.0*	*5.2*	*0.0*
Raw, Average	*1oz/28g*	*42.0*	*2.0*	*149*	*21.1*	*0.0*	*7.2*	*0.0*
SYRUP								
Balsamic, Merchant Gourmet*	1 Tsp/5g	12.0	0.0	232	0.4	60.0	0.1	0.0
Caramel, for Coffee, Lyle's*	2 Tsps/10ml	33.0	0.0	329	0.0	83.0	0.0	0.0
Corn, Dark, Average	*1 Tbsp/20g*	*56.0*	*0.0*	*282*	*0.0*	*76.6*	*0.0*	*0.0*
Golden, Average	*1 Tbsp/20g*	*61.0*	*0.0*	*304*	*0.4*	*78.2*	*0.0*	*0.0*
Maple, Average	*1 Tbsp/20g*	*52.0*	*0.0*	*262*	*0.0*	*67.2*	*0.2*	*0.0*

S

	Measure INFO/WEIGHT	per Measure KCAL	FAT	Nutrition Values per 100g / 100ml KCAL	PROT	CARB	FAT	FIBRE
TABOULEH								
Average	*1oz/28g*	*33.0*	*1.0*	*119*	*2.6*	*17.2*	*4.6*	*0.0*
TACO SHELLS								
Corn, Crunchy, Old El Paso*	1 Taco/10g	51.0	3.0	506	7.0	61.0	26.0	0.0
Old El Paso*	1 Taco/12g	57.0	3.0	478	7.4	60.8	22.8	0.0
Traditional, Discovery*	1 Taco/11g	55.0	3.0	489	5.7	53.4	28.1	6.0
TAGINE								
Chickpea, Diet Chef Ltd*	1 Pack/300g	237.0	2.0	79	2.9	15.1	0.8	2.7
Spicy Chermoula, Tasty Veg Pot, Innocent*	1 Pot/400g	356.0	10.0	89	3.4	13.8	2.4	5.0
Vegetable, Filo Topped, M & S*	1 Serving/282g	310.0	6.0	110	3.3	18.7	2.3	3.9
TAGLIATELLE								
Basil, M & S*	1 Serving/100g	365.0	3.0	365	15.1	69.0	2.8	4.0
Bicolore, Asda*	¼ Pack/125g	202.0	3.0	162	7.0	28.0	2.4	1.4
Carbonara, Frozen, Tesco*	1 Pack/450g	427.0	9.0	95	5.2	14.1	1.9	0.9
Carbonara, Italiano, Tesco*	1 Serving/325g	757.0	37.0	233	8.6	23.8	11.5	1.2
Carbonara, Naturally Less 5% Fat, Asda*	1 Pack/400g	440.0	10.0	110	4.2	18.0	2.4	0.8
Carbonara, Perfectly Balanced, Waitrose*	1 Pack/350g	357.0	13.0	102	5.3	12.1	3.6	0.7
Carbonara, TTD, Sainsbury's*	1 Pack/405g	644.0	26.0	159	7.8	17.6	6.4	1.6
Chargrilled Chicken & Tomato, Asda*	1 Pack/400g	392.0	12.0	98	5.8	11.7	3.1	1.4
Chicken & Mushroom, GFY, Asda*	1 Pack/400g	359.0	7.0	90	7.2	11.2	1.7	0.7
Chicken & Tomato, Italiano, Tesco*	1 Pack/400g	416.0	8.0	104	6.6	14.8	2.1	0.8
Chicken, Italia, M & S*	1 Pack/360g	342.0	6.0	95	8.1	12.1	1.8	1.2
Chicken, Italian, Sainsbury's*	1 Pack/450g	567.0	16.0	126	6.5	17.0	3.5	2.6
Dry, Average	*1 Serving/100g*	*356.0*	*2.0*	*356*	*12.6*	*72.4*	*1.8*	*1.0*
Egg & Spinach, M & S*	1 Serving/100g	365.0	3.0	365	15.5	69.6	2.7	3.0
Egg & Spinach, Safeway*	1 Serving/83g	289.0	2.0	348	13.2	67.3	2.9	2.9
Egg, Dry, Average	*1 Serving/75g*	*271.0*	*2.0*	*362*	*14.2*	*68.8*	*3.3*	*2.3*
Egg, Fresh, Dry, Average	*1 Serving/125g*	*345.0*	*3.0*	*276*	*10.6*	*53.0*	*2.8*	*2.1*
Fresh, Dry, Average	*1 Serving/75g*	*211.0*	*2.0*	*281*	*11.4*	*53.3*	*2.6*	*2.6*
Garlic & Herb, Fresh, Asda*	½ Pack/151g	202.0	6.0	134	3.5	21.0	4.0	2.1
Garlic & Herb, Fresh, Sainsbury's*	1 Serving/125g	184.0	2.0	147	6.5	26.2	1.8	1.9
Garlic & Herb, Fresh, Waitrose*	1 Serving/125g	327.0	3.0	262	11.8	48.1	2.5	2.1
Garlic & Herb, Italiano, Tesco*	1 Serving/85g	236.0	2.0	278	11.4	52.0	2.7	2.4
Garlic & Herbs, Cooked, Pasta Reale*	1 Pack/250g	390.0	3.0	156	6.2	30.4	1.1	1.0
Garlic Mushroom, BGTY, Sainsbury's*	1 Pack/400g	416.0	9.0	104	4.7	16.2	2.3	2.0
Garlic Mushroom, Italiano, Tesco*	1 Pack/450g	738.0	41.0	164	5.2	15.2	9.1	0.6
Ham & Mushroom, Asda*	1 Pack/340g	469.0	13.0	138	6.0	20.0	3.8	0.2
Ham & Mushroom, BGTY, Sainsbury's*	1 Pack/450g	486.0	14.0	108	5.3	14.5	3.2	0.8
Ham & Mushroom, Light Choices, Tesco*	1 Pack/400g	400.0	9.0	100	6.0	13.8	2.2	1.8
Ham & Mushroom, M & S*	1 Pack/400g	400.0	19.0	100	4.0	15.1	4.7	0.7
Ham & Roasted Mushroom, Finest, Tesco*	1 Pack/450g	562.0	24.0	125	7.3	12.0	5.3	2.4
Mediterranean Style Chicken, Eat Smart, Safeway*	1 Pack/400g	320.0	10.0	80	5.6	8.7	2.5	1.4
Multigrain, BGTY, Uncooked, Sainsbury's*	1 Serving/190g	294.0	5.0	155	7.0	26.0	2.5	3.0
Mushroom & Bacon, BGTY, Sainsbury's*	1 Pack/400g	368.0	10.0	92	4.0	13.5	2.4	1.0
Mushroom & Bacon, Sainsbury's*	1 Pack/450g	585.0	23.0	130	7.1	13.8	5.2	0.5
Mushroom & Ham, GFY, Asda*	1 Pack/398.8g	323.0	9.0	81	5.4	9.6	2.3	0.7
Mushroom & Tomato, Asda*	1 Pack/340g	211.0	4.0	62	2.5	10.0	1.3	1.2
Prawn, Eat Smart, Morrisons*	1 Pack/380g	296.0	7.0	78	6.1	9.4	1.8	0.9
Prawn, Primavera, Sainsbury's*	1 Pack/400g	383.0	6.0	100	6.1	15.3	1.6	1.4
Red Pepper, Organic, Sainsbury's*	½ Bag/125g	182.0	2.0	146	5.4	27.8	1.5	1.4
Salmon & King Prawn, HL, Tesco*	1 Pack/400g	480.0	10.0	120	6.5	17.2	2.4	1.7
Salmon & Prawn, Perfectly Balanced, Waitrose*	1 Pack/401g	341.0	13.0	85	6.8	7.1	3.3	1.1
Salmon, Hot Smoked, HL, Tesco*	1 Packet/400g	420.0	12.0	105	6.0	12.8	2.9	1.4
Salmon, Perfectly Balanced, Waitrose*	1 Pack/400g	376.0	11.0	94	5.4	11.7	2.7	0.8

T

	Measure INFO/WEIGHT	per Measure		Nutrition Values per 100g / 100ml				
		KCAL	FAT	KCAL	PROT	CARB	FAT	FIBRE
TAGLIATELLE								
Smoked Salmon, Ready Meals, M & S*	1 Pack/360g	612.0	40.0	170	6.2	10.6	11.2	0.9
Sundried Tomato, Fresh, Morrisons*	1 Pack/250g	747.0	8.0	299	11.1	56.4	3.3	3.5
Sweet Chilli & Prawn, Tesco*	1 Pack/400g	440.0	12.0	110	5.5	14.9	3.1	1.3
Tomato & Basil Chicken, Weight Watchers*	1 Pack/330g	322.0	4.0	98	7.5	14.1	1.2	0.3
Tricolore, Waitrose*	½ Pack/125g	351.0	4.0	281	12.0	51.6	2.9	1.6
Verdi, Dry, Barilla*	1 Serving/150g	555.0	5.0	370	14.0	70.5	3.5	0.0
Verdi, Fresh, Average	*1 Serving/125g*	*171.0*	*2.0*	*137*	*5.5*	*25.5*	*1.5*	*1.8*
with Chicken & Pancetta, Sainsbury's*	½ Pack/351g	453.0	19.0	129	9.5	10.4	5.5	0.7
with Chicken, Garlic & Lemon, BGTY, Sainsbury's*	1 Pack/450g	409.0	1.0	91	7.8	14.2	0.3	1.7
with Ham & Mushroom, New, BGTY, Sainsbury's*	1 Pack/450g	400.0	10.0	89	5.3	11.8	2.3	1.4
with Roasted Vegetables, Good Intentions, Somerfield*	1 Pack/340g	349.0	8.0	103	3.7	16.6	2.4	1.7
TAHINI PASTE								
Average	*1 Tsp/6g*	*36.0*	*4.0*	*607*	*18.5*	*0.9*	*58.9*	*8.0*
TAMARILLOS								
Fresh, Raw, Average	*1oz/28g*	*8.0*	*0.0*	*28*	*2.0*	*4.7*	*0.3*	*0.0*
TAMARIND								
Leaves, Fresh	*1oz/28g*	*32.0*	*1.0*	*115*	*5.8*	*18.2*	*2.1*	*0.0*
Paste, Barts*	1 Tbsp/15g	20.0	0.0	133	0.9	32.1	0.1	0.0
Pulp	*1oz/28g*	*76.0*	*0.0*	*273*	*3.2*	*64.5*	*0.3*	*0.0*
Whole, Raw, Weighed with Pod, Average	*1oz/28g*	*67.0*	*0.0*	*239*	*2.8*	*62.5*	*0.6*	*5.1*
TANGERINES								
Fresh, Raw	*1oz/28g*	*10.0*	*0.0*	*35*	*0.9*	*8.0*	*0.1*	*1.3*
Weighed with Peel & Pips	*1 Med/70g*	*17.0*	*0.0*	*25*	*0.7*	*5.8*	*0.1*	*0.9*
TANGO*								
Cherry, Britvic*	1 Bottle/500ml	55.0	0.0	11	0.0	2.4	0.0	0.0
Orange, Britvic*	1 Can/330ml	63.0	0.0	19	0.1	4.4	0.0	0.0
TAPIOCA								
Creamed, Ambrosia*	½ Can/213g	159.0	3.0	75	2.6	12.6	1.6	0.2
Raw	*1oz/28g*	*101.0*	*0.0*	*359*	*0.4*	*95.0*	*0.1*	*0.4*
TARAMASALATA								
Average	1oz/28g	141.0	15.0	504	3.2	4.1	52.9	0.0
BGTY, Sainsbury's*	1oz/28g	71.0	6.0	253	4.3	13.5	20.2	0.7
Reduced Fat, Tesco*	½ Pot/85g	256.0	23.0	301	3.8	10.5	27.1	1.5
Reduced Fat, Waitrose*	1 Pack/170g	522.0	48.0	307	4.0	8.9	28.4	1.5
Smoked Salmon, Tesco*	1 Serving/95g	474.0	48.0	499	3.0	7.7	50.7	0.3
Supreme, Waitrose*	1 Serving/20g	84.0	8.0	421	7.4	6.3	40.7	2.9
TARRAGON								
Dried, Ground	*1 Tsp/2g*	*5.0*	*0.0*	*295*	*22.8*	*42.8*	*7.2*	*0.0*
Fresh, Average	*1 Tbsp/3.8g*	*2.0*	*0.0*	*49*	*3.4*	*6.3*	*1.1*	*0.0*
TART								
Apple & Custard, Asda*	1 Tart/84g	227.0	11.0	270	3.1	35.0	13.1	0.1
Apple & Fresh Cream, Asda*	½ Tart/50g	133.0	8.0	267	3.4	33.0	16.0	0.8
Apricot Lattice, Sainsbury's*	1 Slice/125g	321.0	14.0	257	3.4	35.3	11.4	2.6
Assorted, Oakdale Bakeries*	1 Serving/27g	104.0	4.0	386	3.1	62.0	14.0	1.7
Aubergine & Feta, Roast Marinated, Sainsbury's*	1 Serving/105g	227.0	15.0	216	4.8	16.6	14.5	1.7
Bakewell, Average	1 Tart/50g	228.0	15.0	456	6.3	43.5	29.7	1.9
Bakewell, Free From, Tesco*	1 Tart/50g	170.0	5.0	340	1.6	63.0	9.2	4.8
Bakewell, Lemon, Holmefield Bakery*	1 Tart/46g	207.0	11.0	449	4.8	52.9	24.6	0.0
Bakewell, Lyons*	1/6 Tart/52g	205.0	9.0	397	3.8	56.7	17.2	0.9
Bannoffi, Finest, Tesco*	1/6 Tart/87g	291.0	17.0	334	3.0	37.2	19.3	0.5
Blackcurrant Sundae, Asda*	1 Tart/55g	227.0	10.0	413	3.5	57.0	19.0	2.3
Cherry Bakewell, Morrisons*	1 Tart/46g	198.0	10.0	430	4.6	54.9	21.4	1.3
Cherry Tomato & Mascarpone, Extra Special, Asda*	1 Tart/153g	290.0	18.0	190	4.6	16.0	12.0	1.1

T

TART

INFO/WEIGHT	Measure per Measure		Nutrition Values per 100g / 100ml				
	KCAL	FAT	KCAL	PROT	CARB	FAT	FIBRE
Chocolate, Co-Op*	1 Tart/22g	102.0	7.0	465	4.0	42.0	31.0	0.7
Coconut & Cherry, Asda*	1 Serving/50g	215.0	10.0	430	4.4	58.0	20.0	4.0
Coconut & Raspberry, Waitrose*	1 Tart/48g	204.0	12.0	426	5.0	45.0	24.0	3.9
Coconut, M & S*	1 Tart/53g	220.0	10.0	415	5.8	57.8	18.1	3.6
Custard, Individual, Average	1 Tart/94g	260.0	14.0	277	6.3	32.4	14.5	1.2
Date Pecan & Almond, Sticky, Sainsbury's*	1/8 Tart/75g	298.0	10.0	397	5.0	63.5	13.7	1.7
Egg Custard, Asda*	1 Tart/80g	215.0	10.0	269	9.0	29.0	13.0	1.2
Egg Custard, Tesco*	1 Tart/82g	214.0	10.0	261	6.2	31.5	12.2	1.1
Feta Cheese & Spinach, Puff Pastry, Tesco*	1 Tart/108g	306.0	19.0	283	7.1	23.5	17.8	0.9
Filo Asparagus Tartlette, M & S*	1 Serving/15g	45.0	3.0	300	4.4	25.2	20.4	2.1
Frangipane, Chocolate & William Pear, Waitrose*	1/6 Pack/80g	219.0	12.0	274	3.5	29.9	15.5	2.5
Frangipane, Lutowska Cherry Amaretto, Sainsbury's*	1 Serving/66g	264.0	13.0	400	6.0	50.0	19.5	1.3
Fruit, Safeway*	1 Tart/180g	425.0	21.0	236	2.7	30.6	11.4	0.0
Gruyere Pancetta & Balsamic Onion, Finest, Tesco*	1/4 Tart/106.3g	320.0	22.0	301	7.7	21.3	20.6	3.3
Italian Lemon & Almond, Sainsbury's*	1 Slice/49g	182.0	12.0	371	7.4	31.9	23.7	4.1
Jam, Assorted, VLH Kitchens	1 Serving/34g	44.0	5.0	130	3.4	56.0	14.4	1.3
Jam, Average	1 Slice/90g	342.0	13.0	380	3.3	62.0	14.9	1.6
Jam, Real Fruit, Mr Kipling*	1 Tart/35g	136.0	5.0	388	3.8	67.9	14.9	1.7
Jam, Real Fruit, Sainsbury's*	1 Tart/37g	142.0	5.0	383	3.4	60.9	14.0	1.4
Leek & Stilton, Morrisons*	1 Serving/125g	392.0	27.0	314	6.9	23.1	21.5	0.3
Lemon & Raspberry, Finest, Tesco*	1 Tart/120g	360.0	17.0	300	5.2	38.4	14.0	2.9
Lemon Bakewell, Easter, Morrisons*	1 Tart/45g	186.0	7.0	413	3.1	64.8	15.7	1.8
Lemon Curd, Asda*	1 Tart/30g	121.0	5.0	402	2.8	64.0	15.0	2.2
Lemon Curd, Lyons*	1 Tart/30g	122.0	5.0	406	3.7	59.3	17.0	0.0
Lemon, M & S*	1/6 Tart/50g	207.0	15.0	415	5.0	32.7	29.3	0.9
Lemon, Sainsbury's*	1/8 Tart/56g	192.0	8.0	341	5.1	46.8	14.9	2.4
Manchester, M & S*	1oz/28g	104.0	7.0	370	4.1	36.0	23.5	1.1
Mixed Fruit, Waitrose*	1 Tart/146g	318.0	16.0	218	2.3	27.3	11.2	1.0
Normandy Apple & Calvados, Finest, Tesco*	1/6 Tart/100g	256.0	8.0	256	3.2	41.4	7.6	1.9
Raspberry & Blueberry, Tesco*	1 Serving/85g	168.0	7.0	198	2.7	27.0	8.8	2.8
Raspberry Flavoured, Value, Tesco*	1 Tart/29.0g	113.0	5.0	389	3.8	56.6	16.4	1.6
Raspberry, Reduced Sugar, Asda*	1 Tart/34g	129.0	3.0	380	4.6	67.5	10.1	1.2
Red Pepper, Serrano Ham & Goats Cheese, Waitrose*	1 Serving/100g	293.0	19.0	293	8.7	21.3	19.2	3.2
Roasted Vegetable, Finest, Tesco*	1/4 Tart/113g	226.0	13.0	200	3.1	20.6	11.7	2.3
Spinach & Ricotta, Individual, TTD, Sainsbury's*	1 Quiche/170g	466.0	34.0	274	7.5	16.5	19.8	1.4
Strawberries & Cream, Finest, Tesco*	1/6 Tart/74g	210.0	13.0	280	3.4	27.2	17.3	1.5
Strawberry & Fresh Cream, Finest, Tesco*	1 Tart/129g	350.0	19.0	271	3.3	31.1	14.8	1.2
Strawberry Custard, Asda*	1 Tart/100g	335.0	15.0	335	3.1	47.0	15.0	0.0
Strawberry Sundae, Asda*	1 Tart/46g	187.0	8.0	407	3.3	58.0	18.0	1.3
Strawberry, Fresh, M & S*	1 Tart/119.6g	305.0	18.0	255	3.1	26.4	15.4	2.4
Strawberry, Reduced Sugar, Asda*	1 Tart/37g	141.0	4.0	380	4.6	67.5	10.1	1.2
Strawberry, Sainsbury's*	1 Serving/206g	521.0	26.0	253	2.6	32.0	12.7	0.7
Strawberry, Waitrose*	1 Serving/101g	241.0	12.0	239	3.8	29.2	11.9	1.2
Summer Fruit Crumble, Morrisons*	1 Tart/128g	379.0	15.0	296	3.6	43.8	11.8	1.3
Toffee Apple, Co-Op*	1 Tart/20g	69.0	3.0	345	3.0	47.0	16.0	0.7
Toffee Bakewell, Morrisons*	1 Tart/47g	212.0	9.0	451	3.4	69.5	18.2	1.4
Toffee Bakewell, Sainsbury's*	1 Tart/45.0g	200.0	9.0	444	3.4	64.2	19.3	1.1
Toffee Pecan, M & S*	1 Tart/91g	414.0	24.0	455	6.0	48.5	26.5	2.0
Toffee Pecan, Waitrose*	1/4 Tart/133g	564.0	19.0	423	4.3	69.3	14.3	1.6
Tomato, Mozzarella & Basil Puff, Sainsbury's*	1/3 Tart/120g	318.0	25.0	265	9.2	10.2	20.8	0.9
Treacle Lattice, Mr Kipling*	1/6 Tart/70g	255.0	8.0	365	4.4	59.8	12.1	1.1
Treacle, & Custard, Apetito*	1 Pack/142g	330.0	10.0	232	2.0	39.2	7.2	0.8
Treacle, Average	1oz/28g	103.0	4.0	368	3.7	60.4	14.1	1.1

T

	Measure INFO/WEIGHT	per Measure KCAL	FAT	Nutrition Values per 100g / 100ml KCAL	PROT	CARB	FAT	FIBRE
TART								
Treacle, Large, Tesco*	1/6 Tart/59g	237.0	6.0	402	3.3	74.1	10.3	1.7
Treacle, Lattice, Lyons*	1/6 Tart/70g	255.0	8.0	364	4.4	59.3	12.0	1.1
TARTAR								
Cream of, Leavening Agent	**1 Tsp/3g**	**8.0**	**0.0**	**258**	**0.0**	**61.5**	**0.0**	**0.0**
TARTE								
Au Citron, Frozen, Tesco*	1/6 Tarte/81g	255.0	12.0	315	5.4	39.4	14.6	0.7
Au Citron, Waitrose*	1 Tarte/100g	325.0	18.0	325	4.9	35.7	18.1	1.0
Aux Cerises, Finest, Tesco*	1 Serving/98g	219.0	7.0	225	4.9	35.4	7.2	0.6
Bacon, Leek & Roquefort, Bistro, Waitrose*	1/4 Tarte/100g	277.0	18.0	277	8.4	19.8	18.2	0.6
Normande, French Style, M & S*	1/6 Tarte/85g	245.0	16.0	290	3.3	26.8	19.0	0.7
Spinach & Goats Cheese, Flamme, TTD, Sainsbury's*	1/3 Quiche/77g	227.0	17.0	296	6.9	18.1	21.8	5.0
Tatin, Sainsbury's*	1 Serving/120g	244.0	8.0	203	2.9	32.8	6.7	1.9
TARTLETS								
Caramelised Onion & Gruyere, Sainsbury's*	1 Tartlet/145g	381.0	28.0	263	5.8	17.3	19.0	1.3
Cheese & Roast Onion, Asda*	1 Tartlet/50g	135.0	7.0	270	6.0	28.0	15.0	1.9
Cherry & Almond, Go Ahead, McVitie's*	1 Tartlette/46g	165.0	5.0	359	4.1	67.5	9.8	0.7
Cherry Tomato & Aubergine, M & S*	1 Tartlet/160g	320.0	20.0	200	3.1	17.8	12.6	1.7
Mandarin, Mini, M & S*	1 Tartlet/29g	80.0	5.0	280	3.4	30.4	16.3	0.6
Mushroom & Watercress, Waitrose*	1 Tartlet/120g	308.0	25.0	257	8.4	19.1	20.5	2.6
Mushroom Medley, BGTY, Sainsbury's*	1 Serving/80g	134.0	8.0	167	4.7	14.5	10.0	3.4
Potato, Bacon & Cheddar, Tartiflettes, Higgidy*	1 Pie/206g	542.0	34.0	263	9.1	18.9	16.7	0.0
Raspberry, Mini, M & S*	1 Tartlet/27g	90.0	5.0	330	4.3	34.4	19.6	0.5
Red Onion & Goats Cheese, Sainsbury's*	1 Tartlet/113g	335.0	22.0	297	7.0	23.7	19.3	1.5
Redcurrant & Blackcurrant, Mini, M & S*	1 Tartlet/29g	85.0	5.0	290	3.9	30.5	16.8	1.1
Roast Pepper & Mascarpone, Sainsbury's*	1 Tartlet/100g	232.0	16.0	232	3.5	17.7	16.4	1.5
Roasted Red Pepper, BGTY, Sainsbury's*	1 Tartlet/80g	143.0	7.0	179	3.1	21.0	9.2	3.4
Salmon & Watercress, Hot Smoked, Waitrose*	1 Serving/130g	315.0	20.0	242	8.1	18.0	15.3	3.0
Sausage & Tomato, Sainsbury's*	1 Tartlet/135g	323.0	21.0	239	4.8	19.5	15.8	1.6
Spinach Ricotta & Sundried Tomato, Filo, Tesco*	1 Tartlet/135g	358.0	23.0	265	5.2	22.4	17.1	1.9
Tomato & Goats Cheese, Waitrose*	1 Tartlet/130g	295.0	19.0	227	6.6	17.4	14.6	2.0
TASTY VEG POT								
Mexican, Sweet Potato & Chilli, Innocent*	1 Pot/390g	351.0	8.0	90	3.0	14.8	2.1	4.5
Thai Coconut Curry, Innocent*	1 Pot/390g	281.0	11.0	72	3.2	8.8	2.7	3.5
Woodland Mushroom Risotto, Innocent*	1 Pot/380g	342.0	8.0	90	3.0	14.8	2.1	4.5
TEA								
Blackcurrant, Fruit Creations, Typhoo*	1 Cup/100ml	5.0	0.0	5	0.2	0.8	0.0	0.2
Decaf, Tetley*	1 Cup/100ml	1.0	0.0	1	0.0	0.3	0.0	0.0
Earl Grey, Infusion with Water, Average	1 Mug/250ml	2.0	0.0	1	0.0	0.2	0.0	0.0
Fruit Or Herbal, Made with Water, Twinings*	1 Mug/200ml	8.0	0.0	4	0.0	1.0	0.0	0.0
Fruit, Twinings*	1 Mug/227ml	4.0	0.0	2	0.0	0.4	0.0	0.0
Green Tea Pure, Twinings*	1 Serving/100ml	1.0	0.0	1	0.0	0.2	0.0	0.0
Green with Mint, Whittards of Chelsea*	1 Cup/100ml	1.0	0.0	1	0.2	0.1	0.0	0.0
Green, with Citrus, Twinings*	1 Serving/200ml	0.0	0.0	0	1.0	0.2	0.0	0.0
Green, with Jasmine, Twinings*	1 Serving/100ml	1.0	0.0	1	0.0	0.2	0.0	0.0
Green, with Jasmine, Wellbeing Selection, Flavia*	1 Cup/200ml	14.0	0.0	7	0.5	1.2	0.1	0.0
Green, with Lemon, Jackson's*	1 Serving/200ml	2.0	0.0	1	0.0	0.2	0.0	0.0
Green, with Mango, Brewed with Water, Twinings*	1 Cup/200ml	2.0	0.0	1	0.0	0.2	0.0	0.0
Herbal, Wellbeing Blends, Infusions, Twinings*	1 Serving/200ml	4.0	0.0	2	0.0	0.3	0.0	0.0
Iced, Green, Orange, Lipton*	1 Bottle/500ml	100.0	0.0	20	0.0	5.0	0.0	0.0
Iced, Lemon, San Benedetto*	1 Bottle/500ml	170.0	0.0	34	0.1	8.3	0.0	0.0
Iced, Mango, Lipton*	1 fl oz/30ml	10.0	0.0	33	0.0	8.1	0.0	0.0
Iced, Peach, Twinings*	1 Serving/200ml	60.0	0.0	30	0.1	7.3	0.1	0.0
Iced, Pickwick*	1 Serving/250ml	32.0	0.0	13	0.0	3.3	0.0	0.0

T

	Measure INFO/WEIGHT	per Measure KCAL	FAT	Nutrition Values per 100g / 100ml KCAL	PROT	CARB	FAT	FIBRE
TEA								
Iced, with Lemon, Lipton*	1 Bottle/325ml	97.0	0.0	30	0.1	7.2	0.1	0.0
Lemon & Limeflower, Infused, M & S*	1 Bottle/330ml	99.0	0.0	30	0.0	7.8	0.0	0.0
Lemon, Instant, Original, Lift*	1 Serving/15g	53.0	0.0	352	0.0	87.0	0.0	0.0
Lemon, Instant, Tesco*	1 Serving/7g	23.0	0.0	326	1.0	80.5	0.0	0.0
Made with Water	1 Mug/227ml	0.0	0.0	0	0.1	0.0	0.0	0.0
Made with Water with Semi-Skimmed Milk, Average	1 Cup/200ml	14.0	0.0	7	0.5	0.7	0.2	0.0
Made with Water with Skimmed Milk, Average	1 Mug/227ml	14.0	0.0	6	0.5	0.7	0.2	0.0
Made with Water with Whole Milk, Average	1 Cup/200ml	16.0	1.0	8	0.4	0.5	0.4	0.0
Nettle & Peppermint, Twinings*	1 Cup/200ml	2.0	0.0	1	0.0	0.1	0.0	0.0
Peach Flavour, Lift*	1 Cup/15g	58.0	0.0	384	0.3	95.6	0.0	0.0
Red Bush, Made with Water, Tetley*	1 Mug/250ml	2.0	0.0	1	0.0	0.1	0.0	0.0
with Lemon, Lipton*	1 Bottle/591ml	150.0	0.0	25	0.0	6.8	0.0	0.0
TEACAKES								
Average	1 Teacake/60g	178.0	4.0	296	8.0	52.5	7.5	0.0
Caramel, Highlights, Mallows, Cadbury*	1 Teacake/15g	61.0	2.0	408	6.2	69.1	12.4	3.6
Coconut Snowballs, Tunnock's*	1 Cake/30g	116.0	7.0	388	3.9	47.0	21.8	0.0
Currant, Sainsbury's*	1 Teacake/72g	204.0	3.0	284	8.2	53.7	4.0	2.5
Fruited, Co-Op*	1 Teacake/62g	160.0	2.0	258	9.7	46.8	3.2	3.2
Fruited, M & S*	1 Teacake/60g	156.0	1.0	260	8.9	53.4	1.0	2.0
Fruity, Warburton's*	1 Teacake/62g	160.0	2.0	256	8.7	48.0	3.5	2.7
G H Sheldon*	1 Teacake/95g	274.0	3.0	288	8.5	57.4	2.7	0.0
Hovis*	1 Teacake/60g	155.0	2.0	258	9.0	49.9	2.5	3.0
Jam, Castello*	1 Teacake/13g	60.0	2.0	470	5.3	70.1	18.4	1.3
Jam, with Biscuit & Mallow, Chocolate Covered, Burton's*	1 Teacake/13g	57.0	2.0	455	3.8	66.9	19.3	1.1
Lees'*	1 Teacake/19g	81.0	3.0	426	4.2	67.7	15.4	0.0
Mallow, Tesco*	1 Teacake/14g	63.0	3.0	450	4.1	65.4	19.1	1.0
Mallow, Value, Tesco*	1 Teacake/14g	63.0	3.0	450	4.1	65.4	19.1	1.0
Marshmallow, Milk Chocolate, Tunnock's*	1 Teacake/24g	106.0	5.0	440	4.9	61.9	19.2	2.4
Richly Fruited, Waitrose*	1 Teacake/72g	205.0	3.0	285	7.8	55.0	3.7	2.2
Toasted, Average	1 Teacake/60g	197.0	5.0	329	8.9	58.3	8.3	0.0
with Fruit, Morning Fresh, Aldi*	1 Teacake/65g	155.0	2.0	239	7.4	44.6	3.4	2.3
with Orange Filling, M & S*	1 Teacake/20g	80.0	3.0	410	4.5	66.6	14.2	0.9
TEMPEH								
Average	*1oz/28g*	*46.0*	*2.0*	*166*	*20.7*	*6.4*	*6.4*	*4.3*
TEQUILA								
Average	*1 Shot/35ml*	*78.0*	*0.0*	*224*	*0.0*	*0.0*	*0.0*	*0.0*
TERRINE								
Lobster & Prawn, Slices, M & S*	1 Serving/55g	107.0	7.0	195	18.2	0.7	13.4	0.7
Salmon & Crayfish, Slice, Finest, Tesco*	1 Serving/110g	148.0	6.0	135	21.9	0.1	5.2	0.1
Salmon & King Prawn, Waitrose*	1 Serving/75g	97.0	4.0	130	19.3	1.3	5.3	0.0
Salmon & Lemon, Luxury, Tesco*	1 Serving/50g	98.0	8.0	196	10.6	3.2	15.7	0.8
Salmon, Poached, Tesco*	1 Pack/113g	349.0	31.0	309	15.5	0.8	27.1	0.0
Salmon, Reduced Fat, Tesco*	1 Serving/56g	100.0	7.0	179	15.5	1.1	12.5	3.5
Salmon, Three, M & S*	1 Serving/80g	168.0	12.0	210	17.6	0.8	15.3	0.9
Salmon, with Prawn & Lobster, M & S*	1 Serving/55g	107.0	7.0	195	18.2	0.7	13.4	0.7
TEX MEX PLATTER								
M & S*	1 Pack/415g	934.0	61.0	225	12.6	10.5	14.6	0.9
THAI BITES								
Lightly Salted, Jacob's*	1 Bag/25g	94.0	1.0	375	6.9	79.7	3.2	0.1
Mild Thai Flavour, Jacob's*	1 Bag/25g	93.0	1.0	373	6.9	79.0	3.3	1.0
Red Curry & Coriander, Fusions, Jacob's*	1 Bag/30g	110.0	2.0	367	6.0	72.3	6.0	1.0
Roasted Chilli Flavour, Fusions, Jacob's*	1 Bag/30g	109.0	2.0	363	5.5	72.3	5.8	1.2
Seaweed Flavour, Jacob's*	1 Bag/25g	94.0	1.0	377	7.1	80.0	3.2	0.5

T

	Measure INFO/WEIGHT	per Measure KCAL	FAT	Nutrition Values per 100g / 100ml KCAL	PROT	CARB	FAT	FIBRE
THAI BITES								
Sesame & Prawn, Fusions, Jacob's*	1 Bag/25g	91.0	1.0	366	6.3	71.2	5.9	1.3
Sweet Herb, Jacob's*	1 Bag/25g	93.0	1.0	372	7.1	78.8	3.2	0.2
THYME								
Dried, Ground, Average	*1 Tsp/1g*	*3.0*	*0.0*	*276*	*9.1*	*45.3*	*7.4*	*0.0*
Fresh, Average	*1 Tsp/1g*	*1.0*	*0.0*	*95*	*3.0*	*15.1*	*2.5*	*0.0*
TIA MARIA								
Original	*1 Shot/35ml*	*105.0*	*0.0*	*300*	*0.0*	*0.0*	*0.0*	*0.0*
TIC TAC								
Extra Strong Mint, Ferrero*	2 Tic tacs/1g	4.0	0.0	381	0.0	95.2	0.0	0.0
Fresh Mint, Ferrero*	2 Tic Tacs/1g	4.0	0.0	390	0.0	97.5	0.0	0.0
Lime & Orange, Ferrero*	2 Tic Tacs/1g	4.0	0.0	386	0.0	95.5	0.0	0.0
Orange, Ferrero*	2 Tic Tacs/1g	4.0	0.0	385	0.0	95.5	0.0	0.0
Spearmint, Ferrero*	1 Box/16g	62.0	0.0	390	0.0	97.5	0.0	0.0
TIDGY PUDS								
Aunt Bessie's*	4 Puds/17g	55.0	3.0	326	9.6	38.4	14.8	2.1
TIDGY TOADS								
Aunt Bessie's*	1 Serving/45g	125.0	6.0	278	14.7	25.3	13.2	1.1
TIKKA MASALA								
Chicken, & Pilau Basmati Rice, Frozen, Patak's*	1 Pack/400g	580.0	20.0	145	9.9	15.1	5.0	0.2
Chicken, & Pilau Rice, Asda*	1 Pack/400g	608.0	20.0	152	7.0	20.0	4.9	1.5
Chicken, & Pilau Rice, BGTY, Sainsbury's*	1 Pack/400g	380.0	5.0	95	8.1	13.0	1.2	1.1
Chicken, & Pilau Rice, GFY, Asda*	1 Pack/450g	495.0	9.0	110	6.0	17.0	2.0	0.8
Chicken, & Pilau Rice, Waitrose*	1 Pack/500g	797.0	34.0	159	8.2	16.1	6.9	0.8
Chicken, & Rice, Light Choices, Tesco*	1 Pack/450g	472.0	7.0	105	7.9	14.6	1.6	1.3
Chicken, & Rice, M & S*	1 Pack/400g	700.0	35.0	175	7.4	17.0	8.8	1.0
Chicken, & Vegetable, HL, Tesco*	1 Pack/450g	360.0	12.0	80	6.8	6.9	2.7	1.8
Chicken, Asda*	1 Pack/340g	388.0	20.0	114	9.0	6.0	6.0	1.5
Chicken, Birds Eye*	1 Serving/400g	420.0	7.0	105	5.6	16.6	1.8	0.3
Chicken, Boiled Rice & Nan, Meal for One, GFY, Asda*	1 Pack/605g	823.0	19.0	136	6.0	21.0	3.1	0.0
Chicken, Breast, GFY, Asda*	1 Pack/380g	486.0	14.0	128	19.0	4.5	3.8	0.2
Chicken, COU, M & S*	1 Pack/400g	400.0	7.0	100	7.6	14.1	1.7	1.3
Chicken, Feeling Great, Findus*	1 Pack/350g	420.0	12.0	120	5.5	17.0	3.5	2.0
Chicken, Good Choice, Iceland*	1 Pack/398g	486.0	6.0	122	6.6	20.4	1.5	0.6
Chicken, Healthy Choice, Iceland*	1 Pack/399g	431.0	4.0	108	6.5	18.0	1.1	0.9
Chicken, Hot, Sainsbury's*	1 Pack/400g	604.0	37.0	151	13.2	3.6	9.3	1.5
Chicken, Hot, Tesco*	1 Pack/400g	588.0	34.0	147	8.7	8.6	8.6	1.0
Chicken, Indian Meal for One, BGTY, Sainsbury's*	1 Serving/241g	200.0	2.0	83	13.9	5.1	0.8	1.0
Chicken, Indian Takeaway, Iceland*	1 Pack/400g	484.0	28.0	121	8.9	6.0	7.1	1.9
Chicken, Indian Takeaway, Tesco*	1 Serving/125g	100.0	3.0	80	8.9	4.9	2.6	2.1
Chicken, Indian, Medium, Sainsbury's*	1 Pack/400g	848.0	61.0	212	13.2	5.3	15.3	0.1
Chicken, Indian, Tesco*	1 Pack/350g	560.0	33.0	160	11.6	7.2	9.3	0.6
Chicken, Large, Sainsbury's*	1 Pack/650g	1105.0	69.0	170	11.7	7.0	10.6	0.3
Chicken, Low Fat, Iceland*	1 Pack/400g	360.0	4.0	90	7.8	12.5	1.0	0.5
Chicken, Medium Spiced, without Rice, Tesco*	½ Pack/175g	231.0	13.0	132	10.2	5.9	7.5	0.9
Chicken, Mild, Diet Chef Ltd*	1 Pack/300g	291.0	7.0	97	10.4	9.0	2.2	0.6
Chicken, Morrisons*	1 Pack/340g	561.0	35.0	165	12.4	5.9	10.2	1.7
Chicken, Sharwood's*	1 Pack/375g	562.0	25.0	150	7.2	15.1	6.7	0.8
Chicken, Smart Price, Asda*	1 Pack/300g	414.0	18.0	138	13.0	8.0	6.0	1.6
Chicken, Tinned, Asda*	½ Can/200g	238.0	14.0	119	8.0	6.0	7.0	0.9
Chicken, Tinned, M & S*	½ Can/213g	309.0	18.0	145	14.5	2.9	8.5	2.2
Chicken, Waitrose*	½ Pack/200g	298.0	19.0	149	12.8	2.6	9.7	1.6
Chicken, with Fruit & Nut Pilau Rice, Sainsbury's*	1 Pack/500g	885.0	45.0	177	7.6	16.1	9.1	2.8
Chicken, with Golden Rice, Iceland*	1 Pack/500g	885.0	41.0	177	6.2	19.4	8.3	1.1

	Measure INFO/WEIGHT	per Measure KCAL	FAT	Nutrition Values per 100g / 100ml KCAL	PROT	CARB	FAT	FIBRE
TIKKA MASALA								
Chicken, with Pilau Rice, Frozen, Waitrose*	1 Pack/400g	676.0	32.0	169	9.3	14.6	8.1	2.1
Chicken, with Pilau Rice, Perfectly Balanced, Waitrose*	1 Pack/400g	476.0	10.0	119	8.2	15.8	2.5	1.8
Chicken, with Rice & Naan Bread, J D Wetherspoon*	1 Serving/708g	1069.0	36.0	151	7.0	19.9	5.1	1.2
Chicken, with Rice, Sainsbury's*	1 Pack/500g	960.0	41.0	192	8.3	21.2	8.2	0.1
Cooking Sauce, Under 3% Fat, BGTY, Sainsbury's*	¼ Jar/125.8g	83.0	2.0	66	0.8	11.7	1.8	0.6
Green, Asda*	1 Jar/340g	401.0	31.0	118	1.2	8.0	9.0	0.4
King Prawn & Rice, Finest, Tesco*	1 Pack/475g	617.0	30.0	130	6.0	16.6	6.4	1.2
Prawn, COU, M & S*	1 Pack/400g	400.0	6.0	100	6.9	14.7	1.6	1.9
Prawn, King, Perfectly Balanced, Waitrose*	1 Pack/400g	372.0	4.0	93	5.2	16.0	0.9	1.7
Vegetable, Asda*	1 Pack/340g	316.0	21.0	93	2.0	7.4	6.1	1.1
Vegetable, Canned, Waitrose*	1 Can/200g	152.0	4.0	76	3.6	10.5	2.2	0.0
Vegetable, Indian, Tesco*	1 Pack/225g	234.0	13.0	104	2.4	10.4	6.0	2.4
Vegetable, Waitrose*	1 Serving/196g	149.0	4.0	76	3.6	10.5	2.2	3.8
Vegetable, with Rice, Patak's*	1 Pack/298g	247.0	7.0	83	2.9	12.3	2.4	1.4
Vegetable, with Rice, Tesco*	1 Pack/450g	499.0	19.0	111	2.6	15.5	4.3	0.9
Vegetarian, with Pilau Rice, Tesco*	1 Serving/440g	519.0	17.0	118	5.0	15.6	3.9	1.5
TILAPIA								
Raw, Average	*1 Serving/100g*	*95.0*	*1.0*	*95*	*20.0*	*0.0*	*1.0*	*0.0*
TIME OUT								
Break Pack, Cadbury*	1 Serving/20g	108.0	6.0	530	6.2	58.3	30.7	0.0
Chocolate Fingers, Cadbury*	2 Fingers/35g	185.0	11.0	530	6.2	58.3	30.7	0.0
Orange, Snack Size, Cadbury*	1 Finger/11g	61.0	4.0	555	5.0	59.4	32.9	0.0
TIRAMISU								
Asda*	1 Pot/100g	252.0	11.0	252	4.3	34.0	11.0	0.5
BGTY, Sainsbury's*	1 Pot/90g	140.0	2.0	156	4.5	28.3	2.7	0.3
Choc & Mascarpone, Tiramigu, Gu*	1 Pud/90g	316.0	23.0	351	3.3	26.1	25.9	1.0
COU, M & S*	1 Tub/95g	138.0	3.0	145	3.7	26.9	2.7	0.6
Family Size, Tesco*	1 Serving/125g	356.0	18.0	285	4.3	34.5	14.5	4.3
Italian, Co-Op*	1 Pack/90g	229.0	9.0	255	5.0	37.0	10.0	0.4
Light Choices, Tesco*	1 Pot/90g	162.0	4.0	180	7.7	27.6	3.9	2.4
Morrisons*	1 Pot/90g	248.0	10.0	276	4.0	38.0	11.0	0.0
Raspberry, M & S*	1 Serving/84g	197.0	12.0	235	3.8	22.9	14.4	0.2
Sainsbury's*	1 Serving/100g	263.0	10.0	263	4.4	40.2	10.0	0.1
Single Size, Tesco*	1 Pot/100g	290.0	13.0	290	3.8	35.1	12.9	4.5
Trifle, Sainsbury's*	1 Serving/100g	243.0	16.0	243	2.3	23.2	15.7	0.6
Waitrose*	1 Pot/90g	221.0	11.0	246	6.4	27.2	12.4	0.0
TOAD IN THE HOLE								
& Potatoes, M & S*	1 Serving/100g	200.0	13.0	200	6.4	14.6	12.9	0.9
Average	1oz/28g	78.0	5.0	277	11.9	19.5	17.4	1.1
Large, Great Value, Asda*	¼ Pack/81g	238.0	14.0	293	10.0	25.0	17.0	2.3
Vegetarian, Aunt Bessie's*	1 Pack/190.2g	502.0	19.0	264	15.6	27.5	10.2	2.7
Vegetarian, Linda McCartney*	1 Pack/190g	359.0	17.0	189	13.6	13.9	8.8	1.1
Vegetarian, Meat Free, Asda*	1 Serving/173g	407.0	19.0	235	9.0	25.0	11.0	3.1
Vegetarian, Tesco*	1 Pack/190g	471.0	19.0	248	13.1	26.5	10.0	2.8
Vegetarian, Tryton Foods*	1oz/28g	73.0	4.0	262	14.8	18.6	14.2	1.6
with Three Sausages, Asda*	1 Pack/150g	435.0	27.0	290	10.0	22.0	18.0	1.0
TOASTIE								
All Day Breakfast, M & S*	1 Serving/174g	375.0	14.0	215	11.2	25.0	7.9	1.7
Cheese & Ham, Tayto*	1 Serving/50g	259.0	15.0	519	6.8	58.0	29.7	0.0
Cheese & Pickle, M & S*	1 Toastie/136g	320.0	9.0	235	10.4	33.5	6.7	2.6
Ham & Cheddar, British, M & S*	1 Pack/128g	269.0	9.0	210	15.5	22.3	6.7	1.3
Ham & Cheese, Tesco*	1 Serving/138g	388.0	18.0	281	11.5	29.1	13.2	1.0

T

	Measure INFO/WEIGHT	per Measure KCAL	per Measure FAT	Nutrition Values per 100g / 100ml KCAL	PROT	CARB	FAT	FIBRE
TOFFEE APPLE								
Average	1 Apple/141g	188.0	3.0	133	1.2	29.2	2.1	2.3
TOFFEE CRISP								
Biscuit, Nestle*	1 Original/44g	228.0	12.0	519	3.7	62.8	27.6	1.4
Nestle*	1 Bar/44g	227.0	12.0	516	3.7	63.1	27.7	0.0
TOFFEES								
Assorted, Bassett's*	1 Toffee/8g	35.0	1.0	434	3.8	73.1	14.0	0.0
Assorted, Sainsbury's*	1 Sweet/8g	37.0	1.0	457	2.2	76.5	15.8	0.2
Brazil Nut, Diabetic, Thorntons*	1 Serving/20g	93.0	7.0	467	3.2	49.0	35.1	0.5
Butter, Smart Price, Asda*	1 Toffee/8g	37.0	1.0	440	1.3	75.0	15.0	0.0
Chewy, Werther's*	1 Toffee/5g	22.0	1.0	436	3.5	71.3	15.2	0.1
Chocolate Coated, Thorntons*	1 Bag/100g	521.0	31.0	521	3.5	57.9	30.7	0.3
Dairy, Smart Price, Asda*	1 Sweet/9g	37.0	1.0	407	1.3	68.4	14.2	0.0
Dairy, Waitrose*	1 Toffee/14g	64.0	2.0	458	2.0	80.2	14.3	0.5
Devon Butter, Thorntons*	1 Sweet/9g	40.0	2.0	444	1.7	72.2	16.7	0.0
English Butter, Co-Op*	1 Toffee/8g	38.0	2.0	470	2.0	71.0	20.0	0.0
Liquorice, Thorntons*	1 Bag/100g	506.0	29.0	506	1.9	58.8	29.4	0.0
Milk Chocolate Smothered, Thorntons*	1 Pack/125g	655.0	38.0	524	4.3	57.5	30.8	1.1
Mixed, Average	1oz/28g	119.0	5.0	426	2.2	66.7	18.6	0.0
No Added Sugar, Boots*	1 Serving/7g	23.0	1.0	324	1.3	52.0	14.0	0.0
Original, Hard Candies (Sugar Free), Werther's*	1 Pack/90g	260.0	8.0	289	0.2	86.8	8.8	0.1
Original, Thorntons*	1 Bag/100g	514.0	30.0	514	1.8	59.3	30.1	0.0
Squares, No Added Sugar, Russell Stover*	1 Piece/15g	57.0	4.0	380	6.0	49.3	26.0	1.3
TOFU								
Average	**1 Pack/250g**	**297.0**	**16.0**	**119**	**13.4**	**1.4**	**6.6**	**0.1**
Beech Smoked, Organic, Cauldron Foods*	½ Pack/110g	124.0	8.0	113	10.9	1.0	7.1	0.5
Firm Silken Style, Blue Dragon*	1 Pack/216g	134.0	6.0	62	6.9	2.4	2.7	0.0
Fresh, Drained, Kong Nam*	1 Tub/575g	397.0	21.0	69	7.7	1.3	3.7	0.5
Fried, Average	**1oz/28g**	**75.0**	**4.0**	**268**	**28.6**	**9.3**	**14.1**	**0.0**
Smoked, Organic, Evernat*	1oz/28g	36.0	2.0	127	16.3	0.8	6.6	0.0
Traditional Luncheon, Bean Supreme*	1 Serving/100g	210.0	13.0	210	23.4	7.8	13.1	0.0
TOMATILLOS								
Raw	**1 Med/34g**	**11.0**	**0.0**	**32**	**1.0**	**5.8**	**1.0**	**1.9**
TOMATO PASTE								
Average	**1 Tbsp/20g**	**19.0**	**0.0**	**96**	**4.9**	**19.2**	**0.2**	**1.5**
TOMATO PUREE								
Average	**1oz/28g**	**21.0**	**0.0**	**76**	**4.5**	**14.1**	**0.2**	**2.3**
Sun Dried, & Olive Oil & Herbs, GIA*	1 Serving/20g	41.0	4.0	204	2.6	0.5	21.6	0.0
with Garlic, Heinz*	1 Serving/10g	6.0	0.0	57	3.6	10.2	0.2	1.2
TOMATOES								
Cherry, Average	**1 Serving/80g**	**15.0**	**0.0**	**19**	**0.9**	**3.3**	**0.3**	**1.0**
Cherry, Canned, TTD, Sainsbury's*	½ Can/204g	47.0	0.0	23	1.4	4.0	0.2	0.9
Cherry, on the Vine, Average	**1 Serving/80g**	**14.0**	**0.0**	**18**	**0.7**	**3.1**	**0.3**	**1.0**
Cherry, Tinned, Napolina*	1 Can/400g	92.0	2.0	23	1.2	3.3	0.6	0.0
Chopped, Canned, Branded Average	**1 Serving/130g**	**27.0**	**0.0**	**21**	**1.1**	**3.8**	**0.1**	**0.8**
Chopped, Italian, Average	**½ Can/200g**	**47.0**	**0.0**	**23**	**1.3**	**4.4**	**0.1**	**0.9**
Chopped, Italian, with Olive Oil & Garlic, Waitrose*	1 Serving/100g	33.0	2.0	33	1.1	3.6	1.6	0.0
Chopped, Italian, with Olives, Waitrose*	1 Can/400g	184.0	7.0	46	1.4	6.0	1.8	0.8
Chopped, Sugocasa, Premium, Sainsbury's*	¼ Jar/173g	59.0	0.0	34	1.6	6.5	0.2	0.9
Chopped, with Chilli & Peppers, Asda*	1 Pack/400g	92.0	1.0	23	1.0	4.0	0.3	0.0
Chopped, with Chilli, Sainsbury's*	½ Can/200g	44.0	1.0	22	1.0	3.5	0.5	0.9
Chopped, with Garlic, Average	**½ Can/200g**	**43.0**	**0.0**	**21**	**1.2**	**3.8**	**0.1**	**0.8**
Chopped, with Herbs, Average	**½ Can/200g**	**42.0**	**0.0**	**21**	**1.1**	**3.8**	**0.1**	**0.8**
Chopped, with Olive Oil & Roasted Garlic, Sainsbury's*	1 Pack/390g	187.0	8.0	48	1.3	5.9	2.1	1.0

T

	Measure INFO/WEIGHT	per Measure KCAL	FAT	Nutrition Values per 100g / 100ml KCAL	PROT	CARB	FAT	FIBRE
TOMATOES								
Chopped, with Onion & Herbs, Napolina*	1 Can/400g	84.0	0.0	21	1.0	4.0	0.1	0.4
Chopped, with Onions, Italian, Tesco*	½ Can/200g	46.0	0.0	23	1.4	4.0	0.2	0.9
Chopped, with Peppers & Onions, Sainsbury's*	½ Can/200g	40.0	0.0	20	1.2	3.5	0.1	0.9
Chopped, with Sliced Green & Black Olives, Sainsbury's*	1 Pack/390g	183.0	8.0	47	1.3	5.6	2.1	0.7
Creamed, Sainsbury's*	1oz/28g	6.0	0.0	22	1.5	5.0	0.1	1.6
Fried in Blended Oil	1 Med/85g	77.0	7.0	91	0.7	5.0	7.7	1.3
Green Tiger, Raw, M & S*	1 Serving/80g	16.0	0.0	20	0.7	3.1	0.3	1.0
Grilled, Average	1oz/28g	14.0	0.0	49	2.0	8.9	0.9	2.9
Plum, Baby, Average	*1 Serving/50g*	*9.0*	*0.0*	*18*	*1.5*	*2.3*	*0.3*	*1.0*
Plum, in Tomato Juice, Average	*1 Can/400g*	*71.0*	*0.0*	*18*	*0.9*	*3.3*	*0.1*	*0.7*
Plum, in Tomato Juice, Premium, Average	*1 Can/400g*	*93.0*	*1.0*	*23*	*1.3*	*3.8*	*0.3*	*0.7*
Plum, Pomodori d'Oro, TTD, Sainsbury's*	½ Can/200g	42.0	0.0	21	1.1	4.1	0.0	0.5
Pomodorino, TTD, Sainsbury's*	1 Tomato/78g	14.0	0.0	18	0.7	3.1	0.3	1.3
Ripened on the Vine, Average	*1 Med/123g*	*22.0*	*0.0*	*18*	*0.7*	*3.0*	*0.3*	*0.7*
San Marzano, TTD, Sainsbury's*	½ Can/200g	34.0	0.0	17	0.9	3.1	0.1	2.9
Santini, M & S*	1 Serving/80g	16.0	0.0	20	0.7	3.1	0.3	1.0
Stuffed with Rice Based Filling, Average	1oz/28g	59.0	4.0	212	2.1	22.2	13.4	1.1
Sun Dried, Average	*3 Pieces/20g*	*43.0*	*3.0*	*213*	*4.7*	*12.9*	*15.9*	*3.3*
Sun Dried, in Oil, GIA*	1 Serving/10g	15.0	1.0	153	1.9	7.5	13.9	0.0
Sun Dried, in Olive Oil, M & S*	1 Jar/280g	644.0	57.0	230	3.9	7.9	20.4	6.7
Sun Dried, in Sunflower Oil, Deli Express, Asda*	1 Serving/50g	76.0	3.0	153	5.8	15.9	6.0	9.0
Sun Dried, Moist, Waitrose*	1 Serving/25g	44.0	0.0	175	11.8	27.4	2.0	7.2
Sun Dried, with Herbs & Extra Virgin Olive Oil, Waitrose*	1 Serving/50g	72.0	5.0	145	3.4	9.1	10.5	7.1
Sunblush, TTD, Sainsbury's*	¼ Pack/30g	42.0	3.0	140	2.4	8.8	10.6	5.8
Sundried, in Vegetable Oil, Aldi*	1 Serving/50g	76.0	3.0	153	5.8	15.9	6.0	9.0
Sundried, Italian, Merchant Gourmet*	1 Serving/50g	55.0	3.0	111	5.7	20.4	0.7	1.3
Sweet, Aromatico, Extra Special, Extra Special, Asda*	1 Serving/100g	21.0	0.0	21	0.7	3.1	0.5	1.3
Vine, Large, TTD, Sainsbury's*	1 Tomato/78g	14.0	0.0	18	0.7	3.1	0.3	1.3
TONGUE								
Lunch, Average	*1oz/28g*	*51.0*	*3.0*	*181*	*20.1*	*1.8*	*10.6*	*0.0*
Slices, Average	*1oz/28g*	*56.0*	*4.0*	*201*	*18.7*	*0.0*	*14.0*	*0.0*
TONIC WATER								
Average	1 Glass/250ml	82.0	0.0	33	0.0	8.8	0.0	0.0
Diet, Asda*	1 Glass/200ml	2.0	0.0	1	0.0	0.0	0.0	0.0
Indian, Diet, Schweppes*	1 Glass/100ml	1.0	0.0	1	0.0	0.0	0.0	0.0
Indian, Schweppes*	1 Serving/500ml	110.0	0.0	22	0.0	5.1	0.0	0.0
Indian, Slimline, Schweppes*	1 Serving/188ml	3.0	0.0	2	0.4	0.0	0.0	0.0
Indian, with a Hint of Lemon, Low Calorie, Asda*	1 Serving/300ml	3.0	0.0	1	0.0	0.0	0.1	0.0
Light, Royal Club*	1 Glass/250ml	2.0	0.0	1	0.0	0.0	0.0	0.0
Low Calorie, Tesco*	1 Serving/200ml	4.0	0.0	2	0.0	0.5	0.0	0.0
Quinine, Schweppes*	1 Glass/125ml	46.0	0.0	37	0.0	9.0	0.0	0.0
Soda Stream*	1 Glass/100ml	15.0	0.0	15	0.0	3.2	0.0	0.0
TOPIC								
Mars*	1 Bar/47g	234.0	12.0	498	6.2	59.6	26.2	1.7
TOPPING								
Bruschetta, Sainsbury's*	1 Sm Can/230g	60.0	2.0	26	1.2	3.6	0.8	1.1
Bruschetta, Tesco*	1 Can/230g	57.0	2.0	25	1.2	3.2	0.8	1.1
Cake Covering, Milk Chocolate Flavoured, Tesco*	1 Pack/300g	1761.0	116.0	587	2.1	57.3	38.8	2.6
Creamy, Tip Top, Nestle*	1 Serving/50g	53.0	3.0	107	3.5	8.6	6.4	0.1
for Cappuccino, Creamy, Flavia*	1 Serving/15g	38.0	1.0	253	14.7	33.3	6.7	0.0
Ice Cream, Monster Crackin, Silver Spoon*	1 Tbsp/15g	92.0	7.0	612	0.0	50.7	45.5	0.0
Pizza, Italian Tomato & Herb, Sainsbury's*	1/5 Jar/50g	19.0	0.0	38	1.6	7.1	0.4	1.1
Pizza, Tomato with Cheese & Onion, Napolina*	1 Jar/250g	195.0	10.0	78	2.9	7.0	4.0	0.8

T

	Measure INFO/WEIGHT	per Measure KCAL	per Measure FAT	Nutrition Values per 100g / 100ml KCAL	PROT	CARB	FAT	FIBRE
TOPPING								
Pizza, Traditional Tomato with Basil, Napolina*	1 Jar/250g	152.0	6.0	61	1.2	7.8	2.6	0.7
Pizza, with Herbs, Napolina*	1 Serving/100g	49.0	2.0	49	0.9	6.3	2.2	0.6
TORTE								
Chocolate Orange & Almond, Gu*	1 Serving/65g	273.0	20.0	420	5.0	28.2	30.5	2.7
Chocolate Truffle, Waitrose*	1 Serving/116g	359.0	20.0	309	4.6	30.1	17.3	1.4
Chocolate, Half Fat, Waitrose*	1/6 Torte/70g	135.0	4.0	193	5.4	29.7	5.8	2.2
Chocolate, Mint, Weight Watchers*	1 Pot/88g	174.0	4.0	198	4.7	34.3	4.7	5.2
Chocolate, Safeway*	1/6 Torte/55g	122.0	6.0	221	4.1	27.6	10.5	1.5
Chocolate, Tesco*	1 Serving/50g	125.0	6.0	251	3.6	32.3	11.9	1.0
Lemon & Mango, Waitrose*	1 Serving/80g	142.0	2.0	177	3.9	33.6	3.0	0.6
Lemon, Somerfield*	1 Serving/45g	71.0	1.0	157	0.8	32.6	2.6	0.8
Lemon, Tesco*	1 Serving/62g	142.0	6.0	230	2.3	32.9	9.9	0.5
Raspberry, BGTY, Sainsbury's*	1 Serving/100g	154.0	4.0	154	2.6	27.0	3.9	1.2
Raspberry, Safeway*	1/6 Torte/54g	93.0	4.0	172	1.2	25.1	7.4	1.5
TORTELLI								
Gorgonzola & Walnut, Specially Selected, Aldi*	1 Pack/200g	536.0	21.0	268	11.4	32.1	10.4	1.3
TORTELLINI								
3 Cheese, Sainsbury's*	1 Serving/50g	195.0	4.0	391	14.4	63.8	8.7	3.0
Aubergine & Pecorino, Sainsbury's*	½ Pack/150g	354.0	6.0	236	8.9	40.3	4.3	3.2
Beef & Red Wine, Italian, Asda*	½ Pack/150g	242.0	4.0	161	9.0	25.0	2.8	0.0
Beef & Red Wine, Italiano, Tesco*	1 Serving/150g	324.0	5.0	216	11.7	35.3	3.2	3.3
Beef Bolognese, Rich, Italian, Giovanni Ranna*	½ Pack/125g	222.0	9.0	178	7.6	20.6	7.2	4.1
Cheese & Ham, Italiano, Tesco*	½ Pack/150g	396.0	12.0	264	12.8	34.8	8.2	3.0
Cheese, Fresh, Sainsbury's*	½ Pack/180g	329.0	9.0	183	7.6	26.8	5.0	1.7
Cheese, Heinz*	1 Can/395g	233.0	7.0	59	2.1	8.6	1.8	0.5
Cheese, HL, Tesco*	1 Serving/400g	368.0	11.0	92	3.2	13.4	2.8	0.6
Cheese, Tomato & Basil, Tesco*	1 Serving/150g	387.0	8.0	258	13.0	39.5	5.4	3.3
Cheese, Weight Watchers*	1 Can/395g	245.0	6.0	62	2.3	9.7	1.6	0.4
Chicken, Spicy, Big Eat, Heinz*	1 Pot/350g	404.0	23.0	115	2.9	11.2	6.6	0.4
Four Cheese & Tomato, Italian, Asda*	1 Serving/150g	249.0	6.0	166	8.0	25.0	3.8	0.0
Four Cheese with Tomato & Basil Sauce, Tesco*	1 Pack/400g	500.0	15.0	125	6.1	16.9	3.7	0.6
Four Cheese, Italian, Asda*	1 Serving/150g	295.0	7.0	197	8.0	30.0	5.0	3.4
Four Cheese, Tesco*	½ Pack/150g	405.0	12.0	270	12.3	37.3	7.9	3.4
Garlic & Herb, Fresh, Sainsbury's*	½ Pack/150g	364.0	12.0	243	11.1	32.2	7.8	1.8
Garlic, Basil & Ricotta, Asda*	½ Pack/175g	318.0	10.0	182	6.0	26.0	6.0	2.6
Ham & Cheese, Fresh, Asda*	½ Pack/150g	255.0	9.0	170	6.0	23.0	6.0	1.7
Ham & Cheese, Tesco*	1 Serving/225g	578.0	13.0	257	13.5	38.1	5.6	1.8
Italian, Diet Chef Ltd*	1 Pack/300g	234.0	1.0	78	2.3	16.0	0.5	0.2
Meat, Italian, Tesco*	1 Serving/125g	332.0	9.0	266	10.6	38.9	7.6	2.3
Mushroom, Asda*	1 Serving/125g	217.0	5.0	174	6.0	28.0	4.2	2.3
Mushroom, BGTY, Sainsbury's*	½ Can/200g	180.0	6.0	90	2.2	13.2	3.1	0.7
Mushroom, Perfectly Balanced, Waitrose*	1 Pack/250g	572.0	9.0	229	9.4	39.8	3.6	2.4
Pepperoni, Italian, Asda*	½ Pack/150g	250.0	6.0	167	6.7	26.0	4.0	0.0
Pesto & Goats Cheese, Fresh, Sainsbury's*	½ Pack/150g	310.0	12.0	207	8.9	24.6	8.1	2.6
Pork & Beef, BGTY, Sainsbury's*	½ Can/200g	148.0	3.0	74	3.7	11.2	1.5	0.6
Ricotta & Spinach, Giovanni Ranna*	½ Pack/125g	340.0	14.0	272	10.1	34.6	10.9	10.0
Sausage & Ham, Italiano, Tesco*	1 Pack/300g	816.0	28.0	272	13.1	34.0	9.3	3.7
Smoked Bacon & Tomato, Asda*	1 Pack/300g	591.0	15.0	197	9.0	29.0	5.0	0.0
Spicy Pepperoni, Asda*	½ Pack/150g	252.0	6.0	168	7.0	26.0	4.0	0.0
Spinach & Ricotta, Italian, Asda*	½ Pack/150g	189.0	4.0	126	5.0	21.0	2.4	0.6
Spinach & Ricotta, Pasta Reale*	½ Pack/125g	319.0	5.0	255	11.2	45.5	4.2	2.6
Spinach & Ricotta, Verdi, Asda*	1 Serving/125g	186.0	6.0	149	6.0	21.0	4.5	2.4
Spinach & Ricotta, Waistline, Crosse & Blackwell*	1 Serving/300g	219.0	7.0	73	2.9	10.1	2.4	1.3

T

	Measure INFO/WEIGHT	per Measure KCAL	FAT	Nutrition Values per 100g / 100ml KCAL	PROT	CARB	FAT	FIBRE
TORTELLINI								
Tomato & Mozzarella, Fresh, Asda*	½ Pack/150g	235.0	4.0	157	8.0	25.0	2.8	0.0
Tomato & Mozzarella, Fresh, Sainsbury's*	½ Pack/150g	291.0	12.0	194	7.5	23.0	8.0	3.4
Trio, Fresh, Tesco*	½ Pack/125g	322.0	9.0	258	12.8	35.8	7.1	2.0
with Tomato, Basil, & Paprika, Easy Cook, Napolina*	1 Pack/120g	481.0	15.0	401	12.4	60.7	12.1	0.0
TORTELLONI								
Arrabbiata, Sainsbury's*	½ Pack/210g	407.0	12.0	194	7.1	28.8	5.6	2.6
Basil, Mozzarella & Tomato, Weight Watchers*	½ Pack/125g	278.0	3.0	222	9.0	40.5	2.7	4.8
Beef & Chianti, TTD, Sainsbury's*	½ Pack/125g	300.0	8.0	240	11.3	34.3	6.4	1.9
Beef & Pancetta, Aberdeen Angus, Grandi, Budgens*	½ Pack/125g	314.0	5.0	251	12.4	40.5	4.3	2.9
Bell Pepper & Sundried Tomato, Morrisons*	½ Pack/150g	375.0	6.0	250	12.1	40.7	4.3	2.9
Cheese & Smoked Ham, Tesco*	½ Pack/150g	315.0	11.0	210	8.9	26.5	7.1	1.7
Cheese & Smoked Ham, Waitrose*	1 Serving/250g	625.0	17.0	250	11.5	35.8	6.8	1.8
Cheese & Sun Dried Tomato, Fresh, Safeway*	½ Pack/199g	364.0	12.0	183	7.7	24.2	6.2	2.7
Cheese, Garlic & Herb, Co-Op*	1 Serving/125g	331.0	7.0	265	10.0	43.0	6.0	0.0
Cheese, Tomato, & Basil, Sainsbury's*	½ Pack/150g	271.0	10.0	181	8.0	22.7	6.5	1.7
Chicken & Bacon, Italiano, Tesco*	1 Pack/300g	660.0	22.0	220	7.8	29.8	7.3	2.1
Chicken & Ham, Morrisons*	1 Serving/150g	366.0	6.0	244	12.3	38.6	3.9	2.4
Chorizo & Tomato, Morrisons*	1 Serving/150g	447.0	13.0	298	12.8	45.1	8.6	2.6
Five Cheese, Sainsbury's*	1 Serving/125g	285.0	12.0	228	10.8	25.2	9.3	2.9
Four Cheese, Asda*	½ Pack/150g	312.0	13.0	208	7.6	24.9	8.7	1.6
Four Cheese, Express, Dolmio*	1 Pack/220g	411.0	17.0	187	7.6	22.1	7.6	0.0
Four Cheese, Tesco*	1 Serving/200g	390.0	13.0	195	8.0	25.5	6.7	1.8
Four Cheese, Waitrose*	½ Pack/125g	297.0	8.0	238	10.3	34.2	6.7	1.6
Fresh, Ham & Cheese, Asda*	½ Pack/150g	315.0	11.0	210	8.8	26.7	7.6	1.4
Fresh, Morrisons*	1 Serving/150g	430.0	15.0	287	11.2	41.0	9.7	2.4
Garlic & Herb, Cooked, Pasta Reale*	1 Pack/300g	546.0	12.0	182	6.7	30.1	3.9	0.9
Goats Cheese & Basil, Somerfield*	1 Serving/250g	650.0	17.0	260	11.1	38.7	6.8	1.8
Goats Cheese & Red Pepper, Morrisons*	1 Pack/150g	450.0	17.0	300	11.5	38.4	11.1	3.8
Italian Style Sausage & Red Wine, Morrisons*	½ Pack/150g	420.0	11.0	280	11.1	45.5	7.2	2.7
Meat & Cheese, Fresh, Sainsbury's*	½ Pack/125g	304.0	10.0	243	13.5	28.3	8.4	2.6
Meat, Italian, Asda*	½ Pack/150g	265.0	7.0	177	7.0	27.0	4.5	2.4
Mediterranean Vegetable, Perfectly Balanced, Waitrose*	½ Pack/125g	286.0	4.0	229	9.1	40.1	3.6	2.5
Mushroom, Basics, Sainsbury's*	¼ Pack/125g	196.0	6.0	157	6.1	21.8	5.0	3.0
Mushroom, Perfectly Balanced, Waitrose*	½ Pack/125g	300.0	4.0	240	10.9	41.8	3.2	2.2
Olive & Ricotta, Sainsbury's*	½ Pack/175g	403.0	18.0	230	8.8	25.1	10.5	2.3
Pasta, Fresh, Cream Cheese, Garlic & Herb, Morrisons*	1 Serving/150g	400.0	9.0	267	10.3	46.1	6.0	3.2
Pesto, Italian, Tesco*	1 Pack/300g	885.0	34.0	295	10.7	36.7	11.3	3.0
Pesto, Light Choices, Tesco*	½ Pack/150g	277.0	9.0	185	6.5	26.5	5.8	2.0
Potato & Rosemary, Fresh, Sainsbury's*	½ Pack/175g	364.0	15.0	208	5.7	26.6	8.8	2.3
Ricotta & Basil, Asda*	½ Pack/150g	322.0	13.0	215	9.2	25.1	8.6	1.6
Ricotta & Tender Spinach, Cooked, Giovanni Ranna*	½ Pack/189.9g	376.0	12.0	198	7.8	27.0	6.5	3.1
Sausage & Ham, Italiano, Tesco*	1 Serving/150g	285.0	10.0	190	8.5	22.5	7.0	1.8
Sausage, Spicy, Italian, Asda*	½ Pack/150g	339.0	12.0	226	7.4	31.6	7.8	1.5
Sicilian Style & Tuna, Morrisons*	½ Pack/150g	397.0	9.0	265	12.1	43.0	5.9	2.3
Smoked Ham, Bacon & Tomato, Tesco*	½ Packet/150g	450.0	18.0	300	12.0	35.7	11.7	2.5
Spicy Red Pepper & Tomato, Pasta Reale*	½ Pack/125g	310.0	5.0	248	10.0	42.0	4.4	3.3
Spinach & Ricotta, Chilled, Italiano, Tesco*	½ Pack/150g	412.0	13.0	275	10.4	38.1	8.5	3.3
Spinach & Ricotta, Fresh, Waitrose*	½ Pack/125g	327.0	9.0	262	11.3	38.4	7.0	2.4
Spinach & Ricotta, Sainsbury's*	½ Pack/150g	325.0	11.0	217	7.8	30.2	7.2	2.4
Taleggio & Leek, Fresh, Sainsbury's*	½ Pack/175g	450.0	12.0	257	9.7	38.8	7.1	2.6
Tomato & Mozzarella, Sainsbury's*	1 Serving/175g	339.0	14.0	194	7.5	23.0	8.0	3.4
Walnut & Gorgonzola, Fresh, Sainsbury's*	½ Pack/210g	414.0	12.0	197	8.4	27.8	5.8	2.4
Wild Mushroom, Italian, Sainsbury's*	½ Pack/150g	309.0	12.0	206	7.7	25.4	8.2	2.3

T

	Measure INFO/WEIGHT	per Measure KCAL	per Measure FAT	Nutrition Values per 100g / 100ml KCAL	PROT	CARB	FAT	FIBRE
TORTELLONI								
Wild Mushroom, Italian, Tesco*	1 Pack/300g	645.0	24.0	215	6.5	28.5	8.0	2.5
TORTELLONO								
Cheese & Smoked Ham, Italiano, Tesco*	1 Pack/300g	630.0	21.0	210	8.9	26.5	7.1	1.7
TORTIGLIONI								
Dry, Average	**1 Serving/75g**	**266.0**	**1.0**	**355**	**12.5**	**72.2**	**1.9**	**2.1**
TORTILLA								
Spanish Style, M & S*	1 Tortilla/190g	370.0	27.0	195	7.5	8.8	14.2	2.1
TORTILLA CHIPS								
Blazing BBQ, Sainsbury's*	1 Serving/50g	237.0	12.0	474	6.8	58.9	23.5	4.6
Blue, Organic, Sainsbury's*	1 Serving/50g	252.0	12.0	504	7.7	65.8	23.4	5.6
Chilli Flavour, Somerfield*	1 Serving/50g	242.0	12.0	484	6.8	60.1	24.1	5.3
Classic Mexican, Phileas Fogg*	1 Serving/35g	162.0	7.0	464	5.9	67.2	19.1	3.8
Cool Flavour, Sainsbury's*	1 Serving/50g	231.0	9.0	463	5.7	68.1	18.7	3.7
Cool, Salted, Sainsbury's*	1 Serving/50g	253.0	14.0	506	6.5	58.6	27.3	4.3
Cool, Tesco*	1 Serving/40g	190.0	10.0	474	6.3	56.7	24.7	7.8
Easy Cheesy!, Sainsbury's*	1 Serving/50g	249.0	13.0	498	7.1	58.7	26.1	4.5
Hot Chilli Flavour, Weight Watchers*	1 Bag/18g	77.0	3.0	430	5.7	66.7	15.6	5.3
Lightly Salted, M & S*	1 Serving/20g	98.0	5.0	490	7.2	61.5	24.1	4.5
Lightly Salted, Smart Price, Asda*	¼ Bag/50g	251.0	13.0	502	7.0	60.0	26.0	5.0
Lightly Salted, Tesco*	1 Serving/50g	247.0	14.0	495	4.8	56.8	27.6	7.5
Lightly Salted, Waitrose*	1 Serving/40g	187.0	9.0	468	7.1	61.2	21.6	6.5
Lighty Salted, Basics, Sainsbury's*	½ Pack/50g	241.0	12.0	483	6.5	60.7	23.8	5.3
Mexicana Cheddar, Kettle Chips*	1 Serving/50g	249.0	13.0	498	7.9	56.7	26.6	5.1
Nacho Cheese Flavour, M & S*	1 Serving/30g	144.0	7.0	480	7.5	62.0	22.4	4.2
Nacho Cheese Flavour, Mexican Style, Co-Op*	1 Serving/50g	247.0	13.0	495	7.0	58.0	27.0	4.0
Nacho Cheese Flavour, Morrisons*	1 Serving/25g	126.0	7.0	504	7.2	59.4	26.4	3.6
Nacho Cheese Flavour, Weight Watchers*	1 Pack/18g	78.0	3.0	435	6.2	66.8	15.9	4.0
Nachos Kit, Asda*	1 Serving/100g	448.0	24.0	448	7.0	51.0	24.0	0.7
Salsa, Asda*	1 Serving/25g	122.0	6.0	488	6.0	62.0	24.0	6.0
Salsa, M & S*	½ Bag/75g	364.0	19.0	485	5.7	59.1	25.1	6.1
Slightly Salted, Organic, Sainsbury's*	1 Serving/50g	226.0	7.0	453	10.0	73.3	13.3	13.3
Taco, Tesco*	1 Serving/50g	247.0	13.0	495	7.4	59.3	25.4	4.4
TORTILLAS								
Corn, Gluten Free, Discovery*	1 Tortilla/22g	53.0	1.0	243	5.4	53.8	2.3	3.8
Corn, Soft, Old El Paso*	1 Tortilla/37.5g	129.0	3.0	343	10.0	60.0	7.0	0.0
Flour, 10 Pack, Asda*	1 Tortilla/30g	94.0	2.0	315	9.0	54.0	7.0	2.5
Flour, American Style, Sainsbury's*	1 Tortilla/35g	108.0	2.0	313	8.6	53.9	7.0	2.5
Flour, Bakery, Asda*	1 Tortilla/43g	129.0	3.0	303	9.1	50.9	7.1	2.6
Flour, From Dinner Kit, Old El Paso*	1 Tortilla/42g	144.0	5.0	344	8.7	51.1	11.7	0.0
Flour, Mexican Style, Morrisons*	1 Tortilla/33g	103.0	2.0	313	8.6	53.9	7.0	2.5
Flour, Salsa, Old El Paso*	1 Tortilla/41g	132.0	4.0	323	9.0	52.0	9.0	0.0
Flour, Soft, Chilli & Jalapeno, Discovery*	1 Tortilla/39.9g	131.0	5.0	328	7.8	44.8	13.1	2.2
Flour, Soft, Discovery*	1 Tortilla/40g	119.0	3.0	298	8.0	49.6	7.1	2.4
Flour, Soft, Garlic & Coriander, Discovery*	1 Tortilla/40g	116.0	2.0	289	8.1	50.6	6.0	1.7
Flour, Tex "N" Mex 12, Sainsbury's*	1 Tortilla/26g	85.0	2.0	326	8.6	53.9	9.6	2.5
Flour, Wheat, Waitrose*	1 Tortilla/62g	203.0	6.0	327	8.5	51.5	9.8	0.0
Made with Wheat Flour	1oz/28g	73.0	0.0	262	7.2	59.7	1.0	2.4
Mexican Cheese, Phileas Fogg*	1 Pack/278g	1404.0	72.0	505	6.5	61.4	26.0	3.0
Plain, Morrisons*	1 Serving/35g	92.0	1.0	263	8.5	51.2	2.7	2.5
Plain, Wheat, Waitrose*	1 Tortilla/43g	134.0	3.0	311	8.1	51.5	8.1	3.0
Plain, Wraps, HL, Tesco*	1 Wrap/67g	188.0	2.0	280	8.5	54.2	2.8	3.3
Plain, Wraps, Tesco*	1 Tortilla/64g	192.0	4.0	300	8.4	52.2	5.9	2.7
White, Wraps, M & S*	1 Tortilla/64.2g	170.0	2.0	265	7.9	49.0	3.8	1.6

	Measure INFO/WEIGHT	per Measure KCAL	FAT	Nutrition Values per 100g / 100ml KCAL	PROT	CARB	FAT	FIBRE

TORTILLAS

	Measure INFO/WEIGHT	KCAL	FAT	KCAL	PROT	CARB	FAT	FIBRE
Wholewheat, Asda*	1 Tortilla/35g	88.0	3.0	252	9.8	35.7	7.8	7.1
Wholewheat, Magnifico*	1 Tortilla/34.1g	86.0	3.0	252	9.8	35.7	7.8	7.1
Wrap, 8 Pack, Asda*	1 Tortilla/50g	143.0	3.0	286	8.0	50.0	6.0	1.9
Wrap, 8 Pack, Light Choices, Tesco*	1 Tortilla/68g	180.0	2.0	265	8.5	50.7	2.8	3.4
Wrap, Bueno*	1 Tortilla/63g	171.0	4.0	272	6.9	48.2	5.7	2.0
Wrap, Garlic & Parsley, Sainsbury's*	1 Tortilla/60g	166.0	4.0	277	7.2	48.0	6.2	1.8
Wrap, Low Carb, Tesco*	1 Tortilla/17g	77.0	2.0	453	39.4	53.5	8.8	23.5
Wrap, Low Fat, M & S*	1 Serving/180g	225.0	4.0	125	6.3	20.6	2.2	1.9
Wrap, Morrisons*	1 Serving/60g	132.0	2.0	220	6.2	42.0	3.5	1.7
Wrap, Organic, Sainsbury's*	1 Tortilla/56g	167.0	4.0	298	8.6	48.7	7.7	2.1
Wrap, Organic, Tesco*	1 Tortilla/56.6g	173.0	4.0	306	8.1	51.0	7.7	2.0
Wrap, Plain, Mini, Morrisons*	1 Tortilla/34g	91.0	1.0	267	8.1	48.9	4.0	2.8
Wrap, Spicy Tomato, Morrisons*	1 Tortilla/55g	158.0	3.0	288	8.6	50.5	5.7	0.7
Wrap, Spicy Tomato, Tesco*	1 Tortilla/63g	175.0	4.0	278	7.8	49.2	5.6	2.4
Wrap, Tomato & Herb, Tesco*	1 Serving/63g	165.0	3.0	262	7.9	45.1	5.5	2.1
Wrap, Tomato & Herbs, Sainsbury's*	1 Tortilla/52g	157.0	3.0	302	7.8	54.1	6.0	2.4
Wrap, Weight Watchers*	1 Tortilla/42g	102.0	1.0	244	8.3	47.8	2.3	6.9
Wrap, Whole & White, Mini, Kids, Sainsbury's*	1 Tortilla/26g	67.0	1.0	258	9.2	42.9	5.5	6.2
Wraps, Deli, Multigrain, Mission*	1 Tortilla/61g	185.0	4.0	302	8.3	52.6	6.5	3.6
Wraps, Healthy 'n' White, Wrap 'n' Roll, Discovery*	1 Tortilla/40g	161.0	4.0	288	8.0	49.7	6.3	2.6
Wraps, Less Than 3% Fat, BGTY, Sainsbury's*	1 Tortilla/51g	127.0	1.0	250	7.8	50.1	2.2	2.9
Wraps, Mexican, Asda*	1 Tortilla/34g	100.0	3.0	295	7.9	47.2	8.3	3.9
Wraps, Multiseed, Discovery*	1 Tortilla/57g	160.0	3.0	280	8.7	50.1	5.0	3.6
Wraps, Plain, Sainsbury's*	1 Tortilla/56g	167.0	4.0	299	8.1	49.2	7.8	3.6

TREACLE

	Measure INFO/WEIGHT	KCAL	FAT	KCAL	PROT	CARB	FAT	FIBRE
Black, Average	*1 Tbsp/20g*	*51.0*	*0.0*	*257*	*1.2*	*67.2*	*0.0*	*0.0*

TRIFLE

	Measure INFO/WEIGHT	KCAL	FAT	KCAL	PROT	CARB	FAT	FIBRE
Average	1oz/28g	45.0	2.0	160	3.6	22.3	6.3	0.5
Banana & Mandarin, Co-Op*	¼ Trifle/125g	237.0	14.0	190	2.0	21.0	11.0	0.1
Black Forest, Asda*	1 Serving/100g	237.0	9.0	237	3.1	36.0	9.0	0.0
Blackforest, BGTY, Sainsbury's*	1 Pot/125g	171.0	6.0	137	2.1	21.9	4.5	1.6
Caramel, Galaxy, Mars*	1 Pot/100g	255.0	13.0	255	4.5	30.0	13.0	1.0
Cherry & Almond, Somerfield*	1 Trifle/125g	230.0	11.0	184	2.0	23.0	9.0	0.0
Cherry, Finest, Tesco*	¼ Trifle/163g	340.0	19.0	209	2.6	22.9	11.9	0.3
Chocolate, Asda*	1 Serving/125g	272.0	16.0	217	4.1	21.0	13.0	0.5
Chocolate, BGTY, Sainsbury's*	1 Pot/100g	137.0	3.0	137	4.8	23.4	2.7	1.6
Chocolate, Cadbury*	1 Pot/100g	282.0	18.0	282	5.2	24.3	18.5	0.0
Chocolate, HL, Tesco*	1 Serving/150g	189.0	4.0	126	4.0	21.4	2.7	4.6
Chocolate, Light, Cadbury*	1 Pot/90g	166.0	7.0	185	5.5	23.4	7.5	0.0
Chocolate, Tesco*	1 Serving/125g	312.0	19.0	250	4.3	24.0	15.2	0.7
Cream Mandarin, GFY, Asda*	1 Serving/113g	151.0	5.0	134	1.6	27.0	4.4	0.2
Fruit Cocktail, COU, M & S*	1 Trifle/140g	175.0	3.0	125	2.8	23.1	2.3	0.5
Fruit Cocktail, Individual, Shape, Danone*	1 Trifle/115g	136.0	3.0	118	3.2	19.6	2.7	1.6
Fruit Cocktail, Individual, Tesco*	1 Pot/113g	175.0	9.0	155	1.7	19.6	7.8	0.6
Fruit Cocktail, Low Fat, Danone*	1 Pot/115g	140.0	2.0	122	2.2	24.0	1.8	0.4
Fruit Cocktail, Luxury Devonshire, St Ivel*	1 Trifle/125g	211.0	10.0	169	1.9	22.6	7.9	0.2
Fruit Cocktail, M & S*	1 Serving/165g	272.0	14.0	165	2.4	19.6	8.3	0.9
Fruit Cocktail, Sainsbury's*	1 Trifle/150g	241.0	9.0	161	1.8	24.8	6.0	0.4
Fruit, Sainsbury's*	1 Serving/125g	232.0	12.0	186	2.3	21.7	10.0	0.3
Peach & Zabaglione, COU, M & S*	1 Glass/130g	149.0	3.0	115	2.8	20.6	2.3	0.8
Raspberry, Sainsbury's*	1 Pot/125g	204.0	10.0	163	1.7	21.5	7.8	0.6
Raspberry, Tesco*	1 Pot/150g	210.0	10.0	140	1.7	18.5	6.5	1.0
Sainsbury's*	1 Serving/133g	215.0	10.0	162	2.4	20.1	7.5	0.3

	Measure INFO/WEIGHT	per Measure KCAL	FAT	Nutrition Values per 100g / 100ml KCAL	PROT	CARB	FAT	FIBRE
TRIFLE								
Strawberry, BGTY, Sainsbury's*	1 Pot/125g	135.0	3.0	108	2.4	19.9	2.1	0.5
Strawberry, Co-Op*	1 Serving/123g	234.0	14.0	190	2.0	21.0	11.0	0.2
Strawberry, COU, M & S*	1 Pot/140g	154.0	3.0	110	2.8	20.6	2.0	1.2
Strawberry, Individual, Shape, Danone*	1 Pot/115g	137.0	3.0	119	3.3	19.8	2.7	1.6
Strawberry, Individual, Somerfield*	1 Trifle/125g	186.0	8.0	149	1.8	20.5	6.6	0.6
Strawberry, Individual, Waitrose*	1 Pot/150g	205.0	9.0	137	1.8	19.7	5.7	1.0
Strawberry, Low Fat Goodies, Danone*	1 Pot/115g	148.0	2.0	129	2.2	26.0	1.8	0.3
Strawberry, Luxury Devonshire, St Ivel*	1 Trifle/125g	207.0	10.0	166	2.0	21.7	7.9	0.2
Strawberry, Sainsbury's*	¼ Tub/150g	261.0	15.0	174	2.2	18.1	10.3	1.0
Strawberry, St Ivel*	1 Trifle/113g	194.0	10.0	172	2.4	21.0	8.7	0.2
Strawberry, Tesco*	1 Trifle/605	998.0	56.0	165	1.5	19.1	9.2	0.8
Summerfruit, BGTY, Sainsbury's*	1 Trifle/125g	151.0	5.0	121	1.2	19.2	4.4	0.5
Triple Chocolate, Farmfoods*	¼ Trifle/86g	223.0	16.0	259	2.1	21.6	18.2	1.2
TRIFLE MIX								
Strawberry Flavour, Bird's*	1oz/28g	119.0	3.0	425	2.7	78.0	10.5	1.2
TRIFLE SPONGES								
Sainsbury's*	1 Sponge/24g	77.0	0.0	323	5.3	71.9	1.6	1.1
Tesco*	1 Sponge/24g	75.0	1.0	311	5.3	66.6	2.6	1.1
TRIPE &								
Onions, Stewed	1oz/28g	26.0	1.0	93	8.3	9.5	2.7	0.7
TROMPRETTI								
Fresh, Waitrose*	1 Serving/125g	339.0	3.0	271	11.7	50.6	2.4	2.0
Tricolour, Fresh, Tesco*	1 Pack/250g	675.0	8.0	270	11.2	48.6	3.4	4.0
TROUT								
Brown, Steamed, Average	*1 Serving/120g*	*162.0*	*5.0*	*135*	*23.5*	*0.0*	*4.5*	*0.0*
Fillets, Scottish, Hot Smoked, TTD, Sainsbury's*	½ Pack/63g	85.0	3.0	136	20.8	1.0	5.4	0.5
Fillets, Skinless, Chunky, TTD, Sainsbury's*	½ Pack/123g	227.0	13.0	185	22.4	0.1	10.6	0.6
Rainbow, Fillets, with Thyme & Lemon Butter, Asda*	1 Serving/147g	210.0	10.0	143	20.0	0.9	7.0	0.5
Rainbow, Grilled, Average	*1 Serving/120g*	*162.0*	*6.0*	*135*	*21.5*	*0.0*	*5.4*	*0.0*
Rainbow, Raw, Average	*1oz/28g*	*36.0*	*1.0*	*127*	*20.5*	*0.0*	*5.1*	*0.0*
Rainbow, Smoked, Average	*1 Pack/135g*	*190.0*	*8.0*	*140*	*21.7*	*0.7*	*5.6*	*0.0*
Raw, Average	*1 Serving/120g*	*159.0*	*6.0*	*132*	*20.6*	*0.0*	*5.4*	*0.0*
Rosemary Crusted, Finest, Tesco*	1 Fillet/150g	352.0	26.0	235	16.1	3.1	17.5	1.0
Smoked, Average	*2 Fillets/135g*	*187.0*	*7.0*	*138*	*22.7*	*0.3*	*5.2*	*0.1*
TUNA								
Albacore, in Olive Oil, TTD, Sainsbury's*	1 Serving/80g	162.0	9.0	203	26.1	0.0	10.9	0.0
Bluefin, Cooked, Dry Heat, Average	*1 Serving/100g*	*184.0*	*6.0*	*184*	*29.9*	*0.0*	*6.3*	*0.0*
Chunks, in Brine, Average, Drained	*1 Can /130g*	*141.0*	*1.0*	*108*	*25.9*	*0.0*	*0.5*	*0.0*
Chunks, in Spring Water, Average, Drained	*1 Can /130g*	*140.0*	*1.0*	*108*	*25.4*	*0.0*	*0.6*	*0.1*
Chunks, in Sunflower Oil, Average, Drained	*1 Can/138g*	*260.0*	*13.0*	*188*	*26.5*	*0.0*	*9.1*	*0.0*
Chunks, Skipjack, in Brine, Average	*1 Can/138g*	*141.0*	*1.0*	*102*	*24.3*	*0.0*	*0.6*	*0.0*
Coronation Style, Canned, Average	1 Can/80g	122.0	8.0	152	10.2	6.5	9.5	0.6
Coronation, BGTY, Sainsbury's*	1 Can/80g	90.0	2.0	112	16.5	5.7	2.6	1.0
Fillets, in Tomato Sauce, Princes*	1 Can/120g	131.0	3.0	109	19.0	2.5	2.5	0.0
Flakes, in Brine, Average	*1oz/28g*	*29.0*	*0.0*	*104*	*24.7*	*0.0*	*0.5*	*0.0*
French Style, Light Lunch, John West*	1 Pack/240g	221.0	6.0	92	7.9	9.4	2.6	0.9
in a Light Mayonnaise, Slimming World, Princes*	1 Can/80g	96.0	3.0	120	17.3	3.6	4.1	0.0
in a Red Chilli & Lime Dressing, Princes*	1 Sachet/85g	102.0	3.0	120	21.5	1.0	3.3	0.0
in a Tikka Dressing, Slimming World, Princes*	1 Can/80g	108.0	5.0	135	16.8	4.0	5.7	0.0
in Chilli Sauce, Safeway*	1 Serving/100g	158.0	8.0	158	16.8	4.8	7.9	0.5
in Sweet & Sour Sauce, Safeway*	1 Can/185g	148.0	3.0	80	10.9	5.6	1.6	1.0
in Thousand Island Dressing, John West*	1 Can/185g	287.0	13.0	155	18.0	5.1	7.0	0.2
In Thousand Island Dressing, Weight Watchers*	1 Can/78.8g	67.0	2.0	85	8.3	7.8	2.2	0.4

T

	Measure INFO/WEIGHT	per Measure KCAL	FAT	Nutrition Values per 100g / 100ml KCAL	PROT	CARB	FAT	FIBRE
TUNA								
in Water, Average	1 Serving/120g	126.0	1.0	105	24.0	0.1	0.8	0.0
Light Lunch, Indian Style, John West*	1 Pack/240g	401.0	23.0	167	7.7	12.3	9.6	0.6
Light Lunch, Mediterranean Style, John West*	1 Pack/240g	218.0	6.0	91	7.9	9.3	2.5	1.7
Light Lunch, Nicoise Style, John West*	1 Pack/250g	245.0	6.0	98	10.3	9.0	2.3	2.7
Light Lunch, Tomato Salsa Style, John West*	1 Pack/250g	180.0	3.0	72	8.0	7.5	1.1	1.1
Lime & Black Pepper, John West*	1 Serving/85g	133.0	8.0	156	15.6	2.8	9.2	0.0
Puertorican Style, Tinned, Natura*	1 Can/185g	157.0	8.0	85	9.0	1.0	4.5	0.0
Steak, No Drain, in a Little Brine, John West*	1 Can/130g	140.0	0.0	108	26.2	0.0	0.3	0.0
Steaks, Chargrilled, Italian, Sainsbury's*	1 Serving/125g	199.0	8.0	159	25.1	0.2	6.4	0.5
Steaks, in Brine, Average	1 Sm Can/99g	106.0	1.0	107	25.6	0.0	0.5	0.0
Steaks, in Cajun Marinade, Sainsbury's*	1 Steak/100g	141.0	2.0	141	29.8	0.0	2.4	0.0
Steaks, in Olive Oil, Average	1 Serving/111g	211.0	11.0	190	25.8	0.0	9.6	0.0
Steaks, in Oriental Sauce, Good Choice, Iceland*	1 Pack/260g	333.0	2.0	128	22.3	8.1	0.7	0.4
Steaks, in Sunflower Oil, Average	1 Can/150g	276.0	13.0	184	26.7	0.0	8.6	0.0
Steaks, in Water, Average	1 Serving/200g	215.0	1.0	107	25.6	0.0	0.4	0.0
Steaks, Lemon & Herb Marinade, Seared, Sainsbury's*	½ Pack/119g	191.0	9.0	161	23.4	0.1	7.4	0.0
Steaks, Marinated, Sainsbury's*	1 Serving/100g	153.0	5.0	153	25.1	1.3	5.3	0.5
Steaks, Raw, Average	1 Serving/140g	185.0	3.0	132	28.5	0.1	2.0	0.2
Steaks, Skipjack, in Brine, Average	½ Can/75g	73.0	0.0	97	23.2	0.0	0.5	0.0
Steaks, Thai Style Butter, Tesco*	1 Serving/110g	191.0	9.0	174	24.7	0.0	8.3	0.0
Steaks, with Lime & Coriander Dressing, Tesco*	1 Serving/150g	156.0	1.0	104	21.6	3.6	0.4	0.6
Steaks, with Sweet Red Pepper Glaze, Sainsbury's*	1 Steak/100g	135.0	0.0	135	28.5	5.0	0.1	0.1
with a Twist, French Dressing, John West*	1 Pack/85g	135.0	8.0	159	15.2	2.8	9.7	0.1
with a Twist, Oven Dried Tomato & Herb, John West*	1 Pack/85g	129.0	7.0	152	16.1	3.9	8.0	0.1
with Basil Butter, Microwave Easy Steam, Sainsbury's*	1 Pack/170g	292.0	14.0	172	23.3	0.5	8.5	0.1
with Ginger & Soy, Heinz*	1 Can/171g	264.0	12.0	154	22.3	0.9	7.0	0.0
with Onion, John West*	1oz/28g	33.0	1.0	118	19.0	6.0	2.0	0.0
with Salsa Verde, Sainsbury's*	1 Serving/125g	310.0	20.0	248	25.5	0.6	16.0	0.0
Yellowfin, Cooked, Dry Heat, Average	1 Serving/100g	139.0	1.0	139	30.0	0.0	1.2	0.0
Yellowfin, Steak, Chargrilled, in Thai Green Curry, Princes*	1 Pack/140g	151.0	2.0	108	20.5	3.9	1.2	0.0
TUNA MAYONNAISE								
& Sweetcorn, Canned, BGTY, Sainsbury's*	1 Can/80g	78.0	2.0	97	15.2	4.0	2.3	0.7
Garlic & Herb, John West*	½ Can/92g	243.0	20.0	264	12.0	4.0	22.2	0.2
Light, Slimming World*	1 Serving/80g	96.0	3.0	120	17.3	3.6	4.1	0.0
with Sweetcorn & Green Peppers, GFY, Asda*	1 Pack/100g	103.0	3.0	103	14.0	5.0	3.0	0.8
with Sweetcorn, From Heinz, Weight Watchers*	1 Can/80g	114.0	6.0	142	11.5	6.2	7.9	0.1
with Sweetcorn, John West*	½ Can/92g	231.0	19.0	251	12.0	4.5	20.6	0.2
TUNA SNACK POT								
Italian, Weight Watchers*	1 Pot/240g	245.0	9.0	102	9.1	8.5	3.6	0.5
Oriental, Weight Watchers*	1 Pot/240g	269.0	7.0	112	9.0	12.6	2.9	0.3
Provencale, Weight Watchers*	1 Pot/240g	266.0	8.0	111	9.8	10.2	3.4	0.5
TURBOT								
Grilled	1oz/28g	34.0	1.0	122	22.7	0.0	3.5	0.0
Raw	1oz/28g	27.0	1.0	95	17.7	0.0	2.7	0.0
TURKEY								
Breast, Butter Basted, Average	1 Serving/75g	110.0	4.0	146	23.7	1.9	4.9	0.4
Breast, Canned, Average	1 Can/200g	194.0	5.0	97	18.3	0.7	2.3	0.0
Breast, Diced, Healthy Range, Average	1oz/28g	30.0	0.0	107	23.8	0.0	1.3	0.0
Breast, Honey Roast, Sliced, Average	1 Serving/50g	57.0	1.0	114	24.0	1.6	1.3	0.2
Breast, Joint, Lemon & Pepper Basted, Tesco*	¼ Pack/132g	238.0	15.0	180	19.7	0.0	11.2	0.0
Breast, Joint, Raw, Average	1 Serving/125g	134.0	3.0	107	21.3	0.7	2.1	0.6
Breast, Joint, with Sage & Onion Stuffing, Waitrose*	1 Serving/325g	377.0	13.0	116	19.2	1.4	4.1	0.1
Breast, Raw, Average	1oz/28g	33.0	1.0	117	24.1	0.5	2.0	0.1

TURKEY

	Measure INFO/WEIGHT	per Measure KCAL	per Measure FAT	Nutrition Values per 100g / 100ml KCAL	PROT	CARB	FAT	FIBRE
Breast, Roasted, Average	*1oz/28g*	*37.0*	*1.0*	*131*	*24.6*	*0.7*	*3.3*	*0.1*
Breast, Roll, Cooked, Average	*1 Slice/10g*	*9.0*	*0.0*	*92*	*17.6*	*3.5*	*0.8*	*0.0*
Breast, Slices, Cooked, Average	*1 Slice/20g*	*23.0*	*0.0*	*114*	*24.0*	*1.2*	*1.4*	*0.3*
Breast, Smoked, Sliced, Average	*1 Slice/20g*	*23.0*	*0.0*	*113*	*23.4*	*0.7*	*1.9*	*0.0*
Breast, Steaks, in Crumbs, Average	1 Steak/76g	217.0	14.0	286	13.7	16.4	18.5	0.2
Breast, Steaks, Raw, Average	*1oz/28g*	*30.0*	*0.0*	*107*	*24.3*	*0.0*	*1.1*	*0.0*
Breast, Steaks, Thai, Bernard Matthews*	1 Serving/175g	280.0	5.0	160	29.4	4.6	2.7	0.0
Breast, Strips, Chinese Style, Sainsbury's*	¼ Pack/163g	318.0	7.0	196	26.4	12.5	4.5	0.5
Breast, Strips, for Stir Fry, Average	*1 Serving/175g*	*205.0*	*3.0*	*117*	*25.6*	*0.1*	*1.6*	*0.0*
Breast, Stuffed, Just Roast, Sainsbury's*	1 Serving/100g	155.0	7.0	155	21.1	2.9	6.6	0.6
Breast, Wafer Thin, Chinese Style, Bernard Matthews*	1 Pack/100g	110.0	1.0	110	18.0	6.1	1.5	0.0
Butter Roast, TTD, Sainsbury's*	1 Slice/28g	36.0	0.0	127	28.1	0.9	1.2	1.0
Dark Meat, Raw, Average	*1oz/28g*	*29.0*	*1.0*	*104*	*20.4*	*0.0*	*2.5*	*0.0*
Dark Meat, Roasted, Average	*1oz/28g*	*50.0*	*2.0*	*177*	*29.4*	*0.0*	*6.6*	*0.0*
Drummers, Golden, Bernard Matthews*	1 Drummer/57g	147.0	10.0	258	13.1	11.0	18.0	1.1
Drummers, Golden, Grilled, Bernard Matthews*	1 Drummer/50g	147.0	11.0	294	15.6	10.0	21.2	1.0
Drumsticks, Tesco*	1 Serving/200g	272.0	13.0	136	19.9	0.0	6.3	0.0
Fillets, Chinese Marinated, Bernard Matthews*	1 Pack/200g	304.0	7.0	152	23.4	7.2	3.3	0.0
Goujons, Cooked, Bernard Matthews*	4 Goujons/128g	355.0	23.0	277	11.8	16.6	18.2	1.1
Leg, Roast, Uncooked, Bernard Matthews*	1 Serving/283g	317.0	15.0	112	15.4	0.5	5.4	0.0
Light Meat, Raw, Average	*1oz/28g*	*29.0*	*0.0*	*105*	*24.4*	*0.0*	*0.8*	*0.0*
Light Meat, Roasted	*1 Cup/140g*	*220.0*	*5.0*	*157*	*29.9*	*0.0*	*3.2*	*0.0*
Medallions, Tomato Salsa, Morrisons*	½ Pack/125.2g	184.0	3.0	147	30.4	0.8	2.5	0.9
Mince, Average	*1oz/28g*	*45.0*	*2.0*	*161*	*23.9*	*0.0*	*7.2*	*0.0*
Mince, Free Range, TTD, Sainsbury's*	1 Serving/131g	184.0	6.0	141	25.4	0.0	4.4	0.0
Mince, Lean, Healthy Range, Average	*1oz/28g*	*33.0*	*1.0*	*118*	*20.3*	*0.0*	*4.1*	*0.0*
Rashers, Average	*1 Rasher/26g*	*26.0*	*0.0*	*101*	*19.1*	*2.3*	*1.6*	*0.0*
Rashers, Smoked, Average	*1 Serving/75g*	*76.0*	*1.0*	*101*	*19.8*	*1.5*	*1.8*	*0.0*
Ready to Roast, with Stuffing & Bacon, M & S*	1/3 Pack/169g	245.0	10.0	145	20.2	2.1	6.2	1.1
Roast, Meat & Skin, Average	*1oz/28g*	*48.0*	*2.0*	*171*	*28.0*	*0.0*	*6.5*	*0.0*
Roast, Meat Only, Average	*1 Serving/100g*	*157.0*	*3.0*	*157*	*29.9*	*0.0*	*3.2*	*0.0*
Roast, Sugar Marinade, Slices, M & S*	½ Pack/120g	156.0	2.0	130	29.0	0.2	1.6	0.5
Roll, Dinosaur, Cooked, Bernard Matthews*	1 Slice/10g	17.0	1.0	170	13.6	6.0	10.2	1.1
Steaks, Breaded, Bernard Matthews*	1 Steak/110g	319.0	20.0	290	11.0	20.5	18.2	1.5
Sticks, Honey Roast, Mini, Tesco*	1 Serving/90g	101.0	2.0	112	20.0	3.6	1.9	0.0
Strips, Stir-Fried, Average	1oz/28g	46.0	1.0	164	31.0	0.0	4.5	0.0
Thigh, Diced, Average	*1oz/28g*	*33.0*	*1.0*	*117*	*19.6*	*0.0*	*4.3*	*0.0*
Wafer Thin, Cooked, Average	1 Slice/10g	12.0	0.0	122	19.0	3.2	3.7	0.0
Wafer Thin, Honey Roast, Average	1 Slice/10g	11.0	0.0	109	19.2	4.2	1.7	0.2
Wafer Thin, Smoked, Average	1 Slice/10g	12.0	0.0	119	18.1	3.6	3.7	0.0
Whole, Raw, Average	*½ Joint/254g*	*389.0*	*17.0*	*153*	*22.5*	*0.8*	*6.6*	*0.0*

TURKEY DINNER

Roast, Asda*	1 Pack/400g	344.0	6.0	86	7.0	11.0	1.6	2.0
Roast, Iceland*	1 Meal/400g	374.0	7.0	93	8.4	10.9	1.8	1.3
Roast, Meal for One, M & S*	1 Pack/370g	462.0	16.0	125	9.1	12.4	4.4	2.7
Roast, Sainsbury's*	1 Pack/450g	354.0	9.0	79	6.8	8.4	2.0	1.9

TURKEY HAM

Average	*1 Serving/75g*	*81.0*	*3.0*	*108*	*15.6*	*2.8*	*3.9*	*0.0*

TURKISH DELIGHT

Assorted Flavours, Julian Graves*	1 Square/30g	110.0	0.0	366	0.5	91.1	0.1	0.0
Dark Chocolate Covered, Thorntons*	1 Chocolate/10g	39.0	1.0	390	2.7	69.0	11.0	2.0
Fry's*	1 Bar/51g	186.0	4.0	365	2.0	73.3	7.2	0.0
Milk Chocolate, M & S*	1 Pack/55g	220.0	5.0	400	1.6	79.0	8.5	0.0

	Measure INFO/WEIGHT	per Measure KCAL	per Measure FAT	Nutrition Values per 100g / 100ml KCAL	PROT	CARB	FAT	FIBRE
TURKISH DELIGHT								
Sultans*	1 Serving/16g	58.0	0.0	360	0.0	90.0	0.0	0.0
with Mixed Nuts, Hazer Baba*	1 Piece/12g	47.0	0.0	389	1.6	88.5	1.7	0.0
with Rose, Hazer Baba*	1 Square/18g	70.0	0.0	389	1.6	88.6	1.7	0.0
TURMERIC								
Powder	*1 Tsp/3g*	*11.0*	*0.0*	*354*	*7.8*	*58.2*	*9.9*	*0.0*
TURNIP								
Boiled, Average	*1oz/28g*	*3.0*	*0.0*	*12*	*0.6*	*2.0*	*0.2*	*1.9*
Mash, Direct Foods*	½ Pack/190g	49.0	3.0	26	0.6	2.0	1.8	1.9
Raw, Unprepared, Average	*1oz/28g*	*6.0*	*0.0*	*23*	*0.9*	*4.7*	*0.3*	*2.4*
TURNOVER								
Apple, Bramley, Tesco*	1 Turnover/88g	304.0	23.0	346	2.7	25.4	25.9	0.9
Apple, Co-Op*	1 Turnover/77g	308.0	21.0	400	4.0	35.0	27.0	1.0
Apple, Dairy Cream, Safeway*	1 Turnover/92g	349.0	24.0	380	3.8	32.9	25.9	0.9
Apple, Dutch, Sainsbury's*	1 Serving/33g	130.0	6.0	393	3.6	56.9	16.8	1.4
Apple, Fresh Cream, Sainsbury's*	1 Turnover/84g	292.0	21.0	347	4.1	26.9	24.8	2.5
Apple, Tesco*	1 Turnover/88g	294.0	20.0	334	3.2	29.8	22.4	0.9
Mincemeat, Fresh Cream, Tesco*	1 Turnover/83g	334.0	22.0	405	3.1	37.5	26.9	1.1
Raspberry, Fresh Cream, Asda*	1 Turnover/100g	411.0	23.0	411	6.0	45.0	23.0	2.1
Raspberry, Tesco*	1 Turnover/84g	290.0	20.0	345	4.0	27.2	24.1	2.1
TWIGLETS								
Curry, Jacob's*	1 Bag/30g	134.0	6.0	448	8.0	55.7	21.5	6.0
Original, Jacob's*	1 Bag/30g	115.0	3.0	383	12.7	57.0	11.6	11.8
Tangy, Jacob's*	1 Bag/30g	136.0	7.0	454	8.1	55.9	22.0	5.4
TWIRL								
Cadbury*	1 Finger/22g	115.0	7.0	525	8.1	55.9	30.1	0.0
TWISTS								
Apple, Sainsbury's*	1 Serving/10g	37.0	0.0	375	1.7	82.7	3.0	0.1
Black Olive & Basil, Finest, Tesco*	¼ Pack/31g	151.0	8.0	483	11.3	53.1	25.1	3.9
Gruyere & Poppy Seed, TTD, Sainsbury's*	1 Serving/8g	41.0	2.0	509	13.7	50.5	28.0	2.6
Parmesan, All Butter, TTD, Sainsbury's*	1 Serving/8g	38.0	2.0	487	13.8	51.0	25.3	2.8
Strawberry, Sainsbury's*	1 Serving/10g	37.0	0.0	375	1.7	82.7	3.0	0.1
Tomato & Herb, Shapers, Boots*	1 Pack/20g	94.0	4.0	468	3.7	66.0	21.0	3.9
TWIX								
Fun Size, Mars*	1 Bar/21g	103.0	5.0	492	4.7	65.5	23.7	1.5
Standard, Mars*	1 Pack/58g	284.0	14.0	490	4.7	65.5	23.7	1.5
Top, Mars*	1 Bar/28g	143.0	8.0	511	5.2	60.2	27.7	0.0
Twixels, Mars*	1 Finger/6g	31.0	2.0	513	5.0	64.0	26.1	0.0
Xtra, Mars*	1 Pack/85g	416.0	20.0	490	4.7	65.5	23.7	1.5
TZATZIKI								
Average	1oz/28g	18.0	1.0	66	3.7	2.0	4.9	0.2
Greek, Authentic, Total, Fage*	1 Serving/50g	49.0	3.0	99	4.9	4.1	7.0	1.0

T

	Measure INFO/WEIGHT	per Measure KCAL	per Measure FAT	Nutrition Values per 100g / 100ml KCAL	PROT	CARB	FAT	FIBRE
VANILLA								
Bean, Average	*1 pod/2g*	*6.0*	*0.0*	*288*	*0.0*	*13.0*	*0.0*	*0.0*
Flavouring, Supercook*	1 Tsp/4g	2.0	0.0	50	6.2	0.0	0.0	0.0
Madagascan, Extra Special, Asda*	1 Pot/150g	232.0	11.0	155	3.5	19.0	7.2	0.0
VANILLA EXTRACT								
Average	*1 Tbsp/13g*	*37.0*	*0.0*	*288*	*0.1*	*12.6*	*0.1*	*0.0*
Pure, Nielsen Massey Vanillas*	1 Tsp/5mls	8.0	0.0	160	0.1	39.5	0.2	0.1
VEAL								
Chop, Loin, Raw, Weighed with Bone, Average	1 Chop/195g	495.0	28.0	254	29.5	0.0	14.3	0.0
Escalope, Fried, Average	1oz/28g	55.0	2.0	196	33.7	0.0	6.8	0.0
Mince, Raw, Average	*1oz/28g*	*40.0*	*2.0*	*144*	*20.3*	*0.0*	*7.0*	*0.0*
Shoulder, Lean & Fat, Roasted, Average	*1oz/28g*	*52.0*	*2.0*	*183*	*25.5*	*0.0*	*8.2*	*0.0*
Shoulder, Lean Only, Roasted, Average	*1oz/28g*	*46.0*	*2.0*	*164*	*26.1*	*0.0*	*5.8*	*0.0*
Sirloin, Lean & Fat, Roasted, Average	*1oz/28g*	*57.0*	*3.0*	*202*	*25.1*	*0.0*	*10.4*	*0.0*
Sirloin, Lean Only, Roasted, Average	*1oz/28g*	*48.0*	*2.0*	*168*	*26.3*	*0.0*	*6.2*	*0.0*
VEGEMITE								
Australian, Kraft*	1 Tsp/5g	9.0	0.0	173	23.5	19.7	0.0	0.0
VEGETABLE CHIPS								
Beetroot, Carrot & Parsnips, Hand Fried, Tyrells*	½ Pack/25g	103.0	7.0	413	3.9	36.0	28.1	11.5
Cassava, Average	1oz/28g	99.0	0.0	353	1.8	91.4	0.4	4.0
Mixed Root, Tyrells*	1oz/28g	133.0	8.0	476	5.7	35.4	29.8	12.8
Parsnip, Golden, Kettle Chips*	½ Pack/50g	257.0	19.0	515	4.6	39.5	37.6	8.4
Sweet Potato, Kettle Chips*	½ Pack/50g	241.0	16.0	483	2.4	44.4	32.8	9.3
VEGETABLE CRISPS								
Pan Fried, Glennans*	1 Bag/20g	98.0	7.0	490	5.0	42.5	33.5	11.0
VEGETABLE FAT								
Pure, Trex*	1 Tbsp/12g	108.0	12.0	900	0.0	0.0	100.0	0.0
VEGETABLE FINGERS								
Crispy Crunchy, Dalepak*	1 Finger/28g	62.0	3.0	223	4.2	26.7	11.0	15.0
Crispy, Birds Eye*	2 Fingers/60g	107.0	5.0	179	3.2	23.5	8.0	2.3
Sweetcorn, Tesco*	1 Finger/28g	66.0	4.0	236	7.7	23.0	12.6	3.0
VEGETABLE MEDLEY								
& New Potato, Asda*	½ Pack/175g	101.0	4.0	58	2.5	7.0	2.2	5.0
Asda*	1 Pack/300g	84.0	1.0	28	2.8	3.9	0.2	2.9
Asparagus Tips, Perfectly Balanced, Waitrose*	1 Serving/225g	121.0	8.0	54	1.3	4.6	3.4	1.4
Basil & Oregano Butter, Waitrose*	1 Serving/113g	59.0	4.0	52	1.7	3.7	3.4	1.9
Buttered, Sainsbury's*	½ Pack/175g	122.0	7.0	70	1.7	7.0	3.9	1.8
Carrot, Courgette, Fine Bean & Baby Corn, Tesco*	1 Serving/100g	36.0	2.0	36	1.1	2.4	2.4	3.0
Crunchy, M & S*	1 Pack/250g	75.0	2.0	30	3.1	2.8	0.8	2.5
Frozen, M & S*	1 Pack/500g	175.0	4.0	35	3.4	3.9	0.8	3.1
Green, HL, Tesco*	1 Serving/125g	59.0	2.0	47	3.7	4.1	1.8	4.1
Green, M & S*	1 Serving/250g	62.0	1.0	25	3.0	1.8	0.5	1.8
Green, Sainsbury's*	1 Pack/220g	178.0	14.0	81	3.0	2.5	6.5	2.9
HL, Tesco*	1 Serving/100g	23.0	1.0	23	0.8	2.3	1.2	1.3
Mediterranean Style, Asda*	1 Pack/410g	225.0	7.0	55	1.7	8.0	1.8	1.3
Roast, Four Seasons*	1 Pack/375g	202.0	12.0	54	2.8	3.5	3.2	2.7
with Herby Butter, M & S*	1 Pack/300g	225.0	15.0	75	1.5	6.2	5.0	2.6
VEGETABLE SELECTION								
Baby, Tesco*	½ Pack/100g	25.0	0.0	25	1.6	3.7	0.4	1.0
Chefs, M & S*	1 Pack/250g	87.0	1.0	35	2.6	4.5	0.5	2.9
Five, Sainsbury's*	½ Pack/125g	42.0	1.0	34	2.6	4.3	0.8	3.1
Fresh, Finest, Tesco*	1 Pack/250g	182.0	14.0	73	1.9	3.2	5.8	2.2
Garden, Tesco*	1 Pack/275g	124.0	9.0	45	1.2	2.7	3.3	1.2
Lightly Buttered & Seasoned, M & S*	1 Pack/300g	195.0	11.0	65	1.6	6.3	3.6	2.8

	Measure INFO/WEIGHT	per Measure KCAL	per Measure FAT	Nutrition Values per 100g / 100ml KCAL	PROT	CARB	FAT	FIBRE
VEGETABLE SELECTION								
Ready to Cook, Morrisons*	1 Serving/150g	51.0	1.0	34	2.4	4.8	0.6	2.3
Roast, COU, M & S*	1 Serving/250g	95.0	2.0	38	1.2	6.1	0.8	0.6
Winter, M & S*	1 Bag/400g	80.0	0.0	20	2.2	3.2	0.0	3.1
with Chilli & Garlic Dressing, Finest, Tesco*	1 Serving/250g	257.0	12.0	103	2.0	12.8	4.9	1.0
with Herb Butter, Waitrose*	1 Pack/300g	270.0	17.0	90	1.9	8.1	5.6	2.1
VEGETABLES								
Baby Mix, Freshly Frozen, Iceland*	1 Serving/100g	26.0	0.0	26	1.8	3.9	0.3	1.9
Baby, Frozen, Asda*	1 Serving/100g	25.0	0.0	25	1.9	3.7	0.3	1.9
Broccoli & Cauliflower, Layered, M & S*	½ Pack/135g	94.0	5.0	70	1.5	7.6	3.4	1.2
Butternut Squash & Sweet Potato, Fresh Tastes, Asda*	½ Pack/225g	128.0	0.0	57	1.0	12.9	0.2	1.8
Carrot, Broccoli & Cauliflower, Organic, Sainsbury's*	1 Serving/250g	62.0	1.0	25	1.9	3.0	0.6	2.2
Chargrilled with Tomato Sauce, GFY, Asda*	1 Serving/260g	164.0	7.0	63	1.4	8.0	2.8	0.0
Chinese Glazed, Tesco*	1 Pack/200g	110.0	4.0	55	1.3	7.7	2.2	1.2
Chinese Inspired, Crisp, M & S*	1 Pack/250g	62.0	1.0	25	1.7	4.6	0.3	1.9
Crisp & Crunchy, Stir Fry, M & S*	½ Pack/115g	29.0	0.0	25	1.9	3.9	0.2	1.7
Crispy, Asda*	1 Serving/50g	17.0	0.0	35	0.1	8.0	0.3	2.2
Crispy, Ready to Cook, Sainsbury's*	1 Serving/100g	24.0	0.0	24	1.8	3.6	0.3	2.2
Crispy, Tesco*	1 Pack/200g	54.0	1.0	27	1.9	3.9	0.4	2.3
Diamond Sliced, Ready to Cook, Waitrose*	½ Pack/125g	31.0	1.0	25	1.6	3.7	0.5	2.1
Farmhouse Mix, Frozen, Asda*	1 Serving/100g	25.0	1.0	25	2.5	2.2	0.8	0.0
Favourite Five Selection, M & S*	½ Pack/125g	25.0	1.0	20	1.8	2.4	0.6	2.9
for Roasting, M & S*	½ Pack/224g	190.0	13.0	85	1.2	7.7	5.6	2.4
Garden, Washed, Tesco*	1 Bag/250g	65.0	2.0	26	3.0	1.9	0.7	2.0
Grilled, Frozen, Sainsbury's*	1 Serving/80g	42.0	3.0	52	1.2	3.8	3.6	1.5
Italiano Marinated, Roasted, Tesco*	½ Tub/100g	121.0	9.0	121	1.7	9.2	8.6	0.8
Julienne, Tesco*	1 Serving/100g	30.0	0.0	30	1.1	5.7	0.3	1.9
Layered, GFY, Asda*	½ Pack/150g	81.0	4.0	54	1.2	6.0	2.8	2.0
Layered, Tesco*	1 Serving/280g	202.0	15.0	72	1.6	4.8	5.2	1.6
Layered, with Butter, Waitrose*	1 Pack/280g	207.0	16.0	74	1.7	3.6	5.8	2.4
Layered, with Seasoned Butter, Asda*	½ Pack/163g	78.0	3.0	48	1.4	5.9	2.1	3.5
Mediterranean Roasted, Sainsbury's*	1 Serving/150g	118.0	5.0	79	2.2	9.5	3.6	3.4
Mediterranean Style, Asda*	½ Pack/205g	113.0	4.0	55	1.7	7.9	1.8	1.3
Mediterranean Style, COOK!, M & S*	½ Pack/200g	60.0	2.0	30	1.2	5.5	0.9	1.0
Mediterranean Style, M & S*	½ Pack/214g	75.0	2.0	35	1.2	5.5	0.9	1.0
Mediterranean Style, Ready to Roast, Sainsbury's*	½ Pack/200g	138.0	4.0	69	2.3	9.9	2.2	2.2
Mediterranean Style, Roasting, Tesco*	1 Serving/200g	72.0	2.0	36	1.1	5.7	1.0	1.3
Mediterranean, in Tomato Sauce, COU, M & S*	1 Pack/300g	105.0	2.0	35	2.5	4.3	0.7	2.2
Mediterranean, Ready to Roast, Waitrose*	1 Serving/200g	128.0	8.0	64	1.3	5.6	4.0	1.6
Mediterranean, Sainsbury's*	1 Pack/400g	180.0	10.0	45	1.2	4.5	2.4	3.1
Mixed, Farmfoods*	1 Serving/120g	62.0	1.0	52	2.7	8.7	0.7	3.3
Mixed, Frozen, Sainsbury's*	1 Serving/100g	50.0	1.0	50	2.9	7.9	0.7	3.5
Moroccan, COU, M & S*	1 Pack/300g	165.0	4.0	55	2.4	8.2	1.5	1.7
Oriental Inspired, M & S*	1 Pack/260g	78.0	1.0	30	1.9	4.6	0.5	2.7
Oriental Stir Fry, Frozen, Sainsbury's*	½ Pack/225g	142.0	9.0	63	1.5	5.4	3.9	1.5
Oriental, Waitrose*	1 Pack/300g	108.0	1.0	36	0.8	7.8	0.2	1.4
Roast, M & S*	1 Pack/420g	273.0	18.0	65	1.4	4.9	4.2	0.4
Roasted Mediterranean, The Best*	1 Serving/125g	100.0	6.0	80	2.3	7.0	4.6	3.6
Roasted Root, Extra Special, Asda*	½ Pack/205g	160.0	3.0	78	1.1	15.0	1.5	6.0
Roasted Winter, HL, Tesco*	½ Pack/200g	160.0	5.0	80	1.9	12.7	2.5	3.6
Roasted, Italian, M & S*	1 Serving/95g	218.0	20.0	230	1.8	7.1	21.0	1.7
Roasted, Mediterranean, Tesco*	½ Pack/172.7g	95.0	3.0	55	1.3	7.6	1.8	2.0
Roasted, Selection, COU, M & S*	1 Pack/250g	87.0	2.0	35	1.2	6.1	0.8	0.6
Roasting, Tesco*	1 Serving/350g	152.0	2.0	43	1.2	8.0	0.5	3.0

	Measure INFO/WEIGHT	per Measure KCAL	per Measure FAT	Nutrition Values per 100g / 100ml KCAL	PROT	CARB	FAT	FIBRE
VEGETABLES								
Root, Honey Roast, BGTY, Sainsbury's*	½ Pack/150g	174.0	2.0	116	2.5	23.1	1.5	5.5
Root, Honey Roast, Sainsbury's*	1 Pack/400g	748.0	35.0	187	0.0	25.8	8.7	5.2
Root, Ready to Roast, Sainsbury's*	½ Pack/200g	188.0	9.0	94	1.3	13.0	4.3	2.2
Seasonal, Pack, Sainsbury's*	1 Serving/261g	60.0	1.0	23	0.7	4.6	0.3	2.0
Special Mix, Sainsbury's*	1 Serving/80g	54.0	1.0	68	3.4	9.7	1.7	3.2
Steam & Serve, Morrisons*	1 Serving/120g	66.0	1.0	55	2.4	8.8	1.1	2.6
Stew Pack, Budgens*	1 Serving/80g	32.0	0.0	40	0.9	8.4	0.3	1.2
Stir Fry, Frozen, Sainsbury's*	1 Serving/80g	19.0	0.0	24	1.3	3.9	0.3	2.0
Stir Fry, Tesco*	1 Serving/150g	37.0	0.0	25	0.9	5.0	0.1	1.4
Summer, Layered With Butter, Asda*	¼ Pack/80g	50.0	2.0	62	2.6	8.2	2.1	0.0
Summer, Roasting, Tesco*	½ Pack/175g	105.0	7.0	60	1.0	5.1	3.8	1.6
Sun Dried Tomato, Selection, Finest, Tesco*	1 Pack/340g	303.0	17.0	89	1.8	8.9	5.1	1.1
Sweet & Crunchy, Tesco*	1 Serving/50g	21.0	0.0	43	2.3	7.0	0.6	2.4
Sweet Summer, Safeway*	1 Serving/115g	60.0	1.0	52	3.7	7.8	0.7	3.5
Szechuan Style, Ready Prepared, Waitrose*	1 Pack/300g	132.0	4.0	44	2.3	5.7	1.3	1.9
Tender, Green, Medley, Sainsbury's*	½ Pack/88g	35.0	1.0	40	3.6	5.1	0.6	3.3
Vietnamese, Wok, Findus*	1 Serving/100g	25.0	0.0	25	1.5	4.5	0.5	0.0
Winter Crunchy, M & S*	½ Pack/125g	31.0	1.0	25	2.0	3.1	0.8	2.7
Winter, Fresh, Asda*	1 Bag/250g	75.0	2.0	30	3.0	2.2	1.0	2.3
Winter, Ready to Roast, Fresh, Sainsbury's*	1 Pack/272g	226.0	8.0	83	1.2	13.2	2.8	0.0
with Sun Dried Tomato, Roasted, Finest, Tesco*	½ Pack/150g	153.0	11.0	102	1.9	7.3	7.2	1.2
Wok, Chinese, Stir Fry, Classic, Findus*	1 Pack/500g	150.0	2.0	30	1.0	5.0	0.5	3.5
Wok, Thai, Findus*	½ Pack/250g	87.0	1.0	35	1.5	7.0	0.3	0.0
VEGETARIAN								
Chicken Style Pieces, Sainsbury's*	1 Pack/375g	754.0	26.0	201	25.5	9.0	7.0	0.6
Fingers, Fish Style, Breaded, The Redwood Co*	1 Finger/36g	94.0	5.0	262	16.5	16.0	14.5	0.0
Pepperoni Style, Cheatin', The Redwood Co*	1 Slice/10g	28.0	2.0	282	25.3	5.2	17.7	0.2
Roast, Chicken Style, Vegeroast, Realeat*	4 Slices/113.5g	211.0	10.0	186	23.0	3.2	9.0	1.5
Roast, Linda McCartney*	¼ Roast/114g	222.0	10.0	196	19.4	9.4	9.0	1.5
Slices, Sage & Onion, Vegi Deli, The Redwood Co*	1 Slice/10g	23.0	1.0	233	21.4	5.0	14.1	0.5
Slices, Vegetable, Tesco*	1 Slice/165g	452.0	31.0	274	5.6	21.4	18.5	3.3
VEGETARIAN MINCE								
Chicken Style Pieces, Realeat*	¼ Pack/87.5g	119.0	1.0	136	29.0	1.5	1.6	4.4
Easy Cook, Linda McCartney*	1oz/28g	35.0	0.0	126	21.4	9.3	0.4	1.7
Frozen, Meatfree, Sainsbury's*	1oz/28g	49.0	2.0	174	20.0	9.5	6.2	6.0
Meat Free, Asda*	1 Serving/200g	294.0	9.0	147	19.0	7.5	4.5	6.0
Meat Free, Tesco*	1 Serving/76g	113.0	4.0	150	19.0	7.0	5.0	6.0
Safeway*	1 Pack/454g	781.0	43.0	172	17.3	4.5	9.5	1.8
Vegemince, Realeat*	1 Serving/125g	217.0	12.0	174	18.0	3.0	10.0	3.0
VENISON								
Grill Steak, Average	*1 Steak/150g*	*178.0*	*4.0*	*119*	*19.0*	*5.0*	*2.5*	*0.9*
Minced, Cooked, Average	*1 Serving/100g*	*187.0*	*8.0*	*187*	*26.4*	*0.0*	*8.2*	*0.0*
Minced, Raw, Average	*1 Serving/100g*	*157.0*	*7.0*	*157*	*21.8*	*0.0*	*7.1*	*0.0*
Raw, Haunch, Meat Only, Average	1 Serving/100g	103.0	2.0	103	22.2	0.0	1.6	0.0
Roasted, Average	*1oz/28g*	*46.0*	*1.0*	*165*	*35.6*	*0.0*	*2.5*	*0.0*
Steak, Raw, Average	*1oz/28g*	*30.0*	*1.0*	*108*	*22.8*	*0.0*	*1.9*	*0.0*
VENISON IN								
Red Wine & Port, Average	1oz/28g	21.0	1.0	76	9.8	3.5	2.6	0.4
VERMICELLI								
Dry	*1oz/28g*	*99.0*	*0.0*	*355*	*8.7*	*78.3*	*0.4*	*0.0*
Egg, Cooked, Average	*1 Serving/185g*	*239.0*	*3.0*	*129*	*5.0*	*24.0*	*1.4*	*1.0*
VERMOUTH								
Dry	*1 Shot/50ml*	*54.0*	*0.0*	*109*	*0.1*	*3.0*	*0.0*	*0.0*

	Measure INFO/WEIGHT	per Measure KCAL	FAT	Nutrition Values per 100g / 100ml KCAL	PROT	CARB	FAT	FIBRE
VERMOUTH								
Sweet	*1 Shot/50ml*	*75.0*	*0.0*	*151*	*0.0*	*15.9*	*0.0*	*0.0*
VICE VERSAS								
Nestle*	1 Bag/46g	221.0	10.0	485	5.0	69.3	20.9	0.0
VIMTO*								
Cordial, No Added Sugar, Diluted, Vimto Soft Drinks*	1 Glass/250ml	6.0	0.0	2	0.1	0.4	0.1	0.0
Cordial, Original, Diluted, Vimto Soft Drinks*	1 Serving/200ml	60.0	0.0	30	0.0	7.4	0.0	0.0
VINAIGRETTE								
Balsamic Vinegar & Pistachio, Finest, Tesco*	1 Tbsp/15ml	55.0	6.0	370	0.2	2.8	39.2	0.0
Balsamic, Hellmann's*	1 Tbsp/15ml	12.0	0.0	82	0.1	15.3	2.7	0.6
Balsamic, Newman's Own*	1 Serving/20g	67.0	7.0	333	0.5	3.9	35.0	0.0
Blush Wine, Briannas*	2 Tbsp/30ml	100.0	6.0	333	0.0	40.0	20.0	0.0
Fat Free, Hellmann's*	1 Serving/15ml	7.0	0.0	49	0.1	10.9	0.0	0.3
Frank Cooper*	1 Pot/28g	46.0	3.0	163	1.0	14.1	11.4	0.3
French Style, Finest, Tesco*	1 Tbsp/15ml	93.0	10.0	620	0.6	6.3	65.3	0.2
French, Real, Briannas*	2 Tbsp/30ml	150.0	17.0	500	0.0	0.0	56.7	0.0
Luxury French, Hellmann's*	1 Tsp/5ml	15.0	1.0	305	0.8	16.0	26.1	0.4
Olive Oil & Lemon, Amoy*	½ Sachet/15ml	37.0	4.0	250	0.3	3.0	24.0	0.0
Perfectly Balanced, Waitrose*	1 Tsp/5ml	4.0	0.0	89	0.4	20.9	0.4	0.5
Portuguese, Nando's*	1 Tbsp/15g	61.0	7.0	409	1.0	2.0	44.0	0.3
Waistline, 99% Fat Free, Crosse & Blackwell*	1 Tbsp/15ml	1.0	0.0	9	1.0	0.7	0.2	0.2
VINE LEAVES								
Preserved in Brine	*1oz/28g*	*4.0*	*0.0*	*15*	*3.6*	*0.2*	*0.0*	*0.0*
Stuffed with Rice	1oz/28g	73.0	5.0	262	2.8	23.8	18.0	0.0
Stuffed with Rice & Mixed Herbs, Sainsbury's*	1 Leaf/37g	44.0	2.0	120	2.6	16.3	4.9	1.2
Stuffed with Rice, Dolmades, M & S*	1 Leaf/38g	40.0	2.0	105	2.6	14.2	4.1	1.2
Stuffed, Sainsbury's*	1 Parcel/37.5g	46.0	2.0	124	2.9	15.3	5.7	3.1
VINEGAR								
Balsamic, Average	*1 Tsp/5ml*	*4.0*	*0.0*	*88*	*0.5*	*17.0*	*0.0*	*0.0*
Cider	*1 Tbsp/15ml*	*2.0*	*0.0*	*14*	*0.0*	*5.9*	*0.0*	*0.0*
Cyder, Aspall*	1 fl oz/30ml	5.0	0.0	18	0.0	0.1	0.0	0.0
Malt, Average	*1 Tbsp/15g*	*1.0*	*0.0*	*4*	*0.4*	*0.6*	*0.0*	*0.0*
Red Wine, Average	1 Tbsp/15ml	3.0	0.0	19	0.0	0.3	0.0	0.0
Rice, Mizkan*	1 Tbsp/15ml	4.0	0.0	26	0.2	2.6	0.0	0.0
Rice, White, Amoy*	1 Tsp/5ml	0.0	0.0	4	0.0	1.0	0.0	0.0
VODKA								
37.5% Volume	*1 Shot/35ml*	*72.0*	*0.0*	*207*	*0.0*	*0.0*	*0.0*	*0.0*
40% Volume	*1 Shot/35ml*	*78.0*	*0.0*	*222*	*0.0*	*0.0*	*0.0*	*0.0*

V

	Measure INFO/WEIGHT	per Measure KCAL	per Measure FAT	Nutrition Values per 100g / 100ml KCAL	PROT	CARB	FAT	FIBRE
WAFERS								
Apricot & Peach, Highlights, Cadbury*	1 Wafer/19g	80.0	3.0	430	5.2	70.6	14.3	1.4
Cafe Curls, Rolled, Askeys*	1 Wafer/5g	21.0	0.0	422	5.8	80.3	8.6	0.0
Caramel Log, Tunnock's*	1 Wafer/32g	152.0	8.0	474	4.2	64.3	24.0	0.0
Caramel, Dark Chocolate, Tunnock's*	1 Wafer/26g	128.0	7.0	492	5.2	60.7	25.4	0.0
Caramel, Milk Chocolate Coated, Value, Tesco*	1 Wafer/23g	110.0	5.0	475	5.6	67.6	20.2	0.6
Caramel, Milk Chocolate, Farmfoods*	1 Wafer/22g	104.0	5.0	475	5.9	61.9	22.8	3.1
Caramel, Tunnock's*	1 Wafer/26g	116.0	5.0	448	3.6	69.2	17.4	2.5
Cream, Tunnock's*	1 Wafer/20g	103.0	6.0	513	6.6	63.2	28.0	0.0
Filled, Average	1oz/28g	150.0	8.0	535	4.7	66.0	29.9	0.0
Florida Orange, Tunnock's*	1 Wafer/20g	104.0	6.0	519	5.1	64.0	29.0	0.0
for Ice Cream, Askeys*	1 Wafer/1.5g	6.0	0.0	388	11.4	79.0	2.9	0.0
Hazelnut, Elledi*	1 Wafer/8g	38.0	2.0	493	6.3	62.4	24.3	0.0
Milk Chocolate, Sainsbury's*	1 Wafer/10g	51.0	3.0	506	6.2	60.5	26.7	1.4
Orange, Highlights, Cadbury*	1 Wafer/19g	80.0	3.0	430	5.2	70.6	14.3	1.4
WAFFLES								
Belgian, TTD, Sainsbury's*	1 Waffle/25g	122.0	7.0	490	6.0	50.6	29.3	1.2
Caramel, Asda*	1 Waffle/8g	37.0	2.0	459	3.3	62.0	22.0	1.1
Milk Chocolate, Tregroes*	1 Waffle/49g	220.0	21.0	450	4.5	57.0	42.0	0.5
Sweet, American Style, Sainsbury's*	1 Waffle/35.0g	160.0	9.0	457	7.2	50.6	25.3	1.1
Toasting, McVitie's*	1 Waffle/24.9g	118.0	6.0	474	6.0	52.6	25.5	0.6
WAGON WHEEL								
Chocolate, Burton's*	1 Biscuit/39g	165.0	6.0	424	5.3	67.4	14.6	1.9
Jammie, Burton's*	1 Biscuit/40g	168.0	6.0	420	5.1	67.7	14.1	1.9
WALNUT WHIP								
Nestle*	1 Whip/35g	173.0	9.0	494	5.3	61.3	25.2	0.7
The, Classics, M & S*	1 Whip/26g	127.0	7.0	490	7.2	54.9	27.4	1.1
Vanilla, Nestle*	1 Whip/34g	165.0	8.0	486	5.7	60.5	24.6	0.0
WALNUTS								
Average	*6 Halves/20g*	*138.0*	*14.0*	*691*	*15.6*	*3.2*	*68.5*	*3.5*
Halves, Average	*1 Serving/25g*	*167.0*	*16.0*	*669*	*17.4*	*6.3*	*65.0*	*4.7*
WASABI								
Paste, Ready Mixed, Japanese, Yutaka*	1 Tsp/5g	14.0	0.0	286	2.7	53.0	7.0	0.0
WATER								
Berry Blast, Revive, Volvic*	1 Bottle/500ml	9.0	0.0	2	0.3	0.4	0.0	0.0
Blackcurrant Flavour, Still, Danone*	1 Serving/120ml	25.0	0.0	21	0.0	5.0	0.0	0.0
Blackcurrants, Juicy, Innocent*	1 Bottle/420ml	155.0	0.0	37	0.1	8.7	0.1	0.0
Cranberries & Raspberries, Juicy, Innocent*	1 Bottle/380ml	118.0	1.0	31	0.1	6.7	0.3	0.0
Cranberries & Raspberries, Spring Water, This Water*	1 Bottle/420ml	122.0	0.0	29	0.1	6.9	0.1	0.0
Cranberry & Blueberry, Lightly Sparkling, Waitrose*	1 Glass/250mls	10.0	0.0	4	0.0	0.7	0.0	0.0
Elderflower & Pear, Detox, V Water*	1 Bottle/500ml	40.0	0.0	8	0.0	1.9	0.0	0.0
Elderflower Presse, Bottle Green*	1 Serving/250ml	87.0	0.0	35	0.0	8.9	0.0	0.0
Ginger & Mango, Kick, V Water*	1 Bottle/500ml	40.0	0.0	8	0.0	1.9	0.0	0.0
Grapefruit Flavoured, Balanced Lifestyle, Aldi*	1 Serving/100ml	2.0	0.0	2	0.1	0.4	0.0	0.1
Grapefruit, Slightly Sparkling, Tesco*	1 Serving/200ml	4.0	0.0	2	0.0	0.2	0.0	0.0
Green Tea, De-Stress, V Water*	1 Bottle/500ml	40.0	0.0	8	0.0	1.9	0.0	0.0
Lemon & Lime, Shield, V Water*	1 Bottle/500ml	35.0	0.0	7	0.0	1.7	0.0	0.0
Lemon & Lime, Sparkling, M & S*	1 Bottle/500ml	15.0	0.0	3	0.0	0.4	0.0	0.0
Lemon & Lime, Still, M & S*	1 Bottle/500ml	5.0	0.0	1	0.0	0.2	0.0	0.0
Lemon, Vittel*	1 Bottle/500ml	5.0	0.0	1	0.0	0.0	0.0	0.0
Mandarin & Cranberry, Still, M & S*	1 Bottle/500ml	100.0	0.0	20	0.0	5.0	0.0	0.0
Mineral Or Tap	*1 Glass/200ml*	*0.0*	*0.0*	*0*	*0.0*	*0.0*	*0.0*	*0.0*
Mineral, Apple & Elderflower, Hedgerow*	1 Serving/250ml	85.0	0.0	34	0.0	8.2	0.0	0.0
Mineral, Energy, Vittel*	1 fl oz/30ml	7.0	0.0	23	0.0	5.5	0.0	0.0

W

	Measure INFO/WEIGHT	per Measure		Nutrition Values per 100g / 100ml				
		KCAL	FAT	KCAL	PROT	CARB	FAT	FIBRE
WATER								
Orange & Passion Fruit, Vital V, V Water*	1 Bottle/500ml	45.0	0.0	9	0.0	2.1	0.0	0.0
Peach & Lemon, Still, M & S*	1 Bottle/500ml	100.0	0.0	20	0.0	5.0	0.0	0.0
Peach & Raspberry, Still, M & S*	1 Bottle/500ml	10.0	0.0	2	0.0	0.0	0.0	0.0
Pomegranate & Blueberry, Glow, V Water*	1 Bottle/500ml	40.0	0.0	8	0.0	2.0	0.0	0.0
Raspberry & Apple, Still, Shapers, Boots*	1 Serving/250ml	10.0	0.0	4	0.0	0.8	0.0	0.0
Skinny, Bo-Synergy*	1 Bottle/500ml	9.0	0.0	2	0.0	0.3	0.0	0.0
Sparkling, Fruit, Aqua Libra*	1 Glass/200ml	54.0	0.0	27	0.0	5.1	0.0	0.0
Spring, Apple & Blackcurrant, Hadrian*	1 Bottle/365ml	3.0	0.0	1	0.1	0.1	0.0	0.0
Spring, Apple & Cherry Flavoured, Sparkling, Sainsbury's*	1 Glass/250ml	5.0	0.0	2	0.1	0.2	0.1	0.1
Spring, Apple & Lemongrass, Food to Go, M & S*	1 Bottle/500ml	4.0	0.0	1	0.0	0.2	0.0	0.0
Spring, Apple & Mango, Sparkling, Asda*	1 Glass/200ml	2.0	0.0	1	0.0	0.2	0.0	0.0
Spring, Apple & Raspberry Flavoured, Sainsbury's*	1 fl oz/30ml	1.0	0.0	2	0.1	0.1	0.1	0.1
Spring, Apple & Raspberry, Shapers, Boots*	1 Bottle/500mls	10.0	0.0	2	0.0	0.2	0.0	0.0
Spring, Apple & Raspberry, Sparkling, Tesco*	1 Glass/330ml	7.0	0.0	2	0.0	0.5	0.0	0.0
Spring, Elderflower & Pear, Sainsbury's*	1 Glass/250g	5.0	0.0	2	0.1	0.2	0.1	0.1
Spring, Lemon & Lime Flavour, Sparkling, Superdrug*	1 Bottle/500ml	8.0	0.0	2	0.1	0.1	0.1	0.1
Spring, Lemon & Lime Flavoured, Sparkling, Sainsbury's*	1 Glass/250ml	4.0	0.0	2	0.1	0.1	0.1	0.1
Spring, Lemon & Lime, Slightly Sparkling, Tesco*	1 Serving/200ml	4.0	0.0	2	0.1	0.2	0.1	0.1
Spring, Peach, Safeway*	1 Bottle/500ml	10.0	0.0	2	0.1	0.2	0.1	0.1
Spring, Raspberry & Cranberry, Shapers, Boots*	1 Bottle/500ml	10.0	0.0	2	0.0	0.5	0.0	0.0
Spring, Strawberry & Aloe Vera, Botanical, M & S*	1 Bottle/500ml	5.0	0.0	1	0.0	0.2	0.0	0.0
Spring, Strawberry & Kiwi, Still, Shapers, Boots*	1 Glass/250ml	2.0	0.0	1	0.0	0.1	0.0	0.9
Spring, Strawberry & Vanilla, Sainsbury's*	1 Glass/250ml	5.0	0.0	2	0.1	0.2	0.1	0.1
Spring, White Grape & Blackberry, Tesco*	1 Glass/200ml	4.0	0.0	2	0.0	0.5	0.0	0.0
Spring, with a Hint of Orange, Slightly Sparkling, Tesco*	1 Serving/250ml	5.0	0.0	2	0.0	0.2	0.0	0.0
Spring, with Cranberry, Tesco*	1 Glass/250ml	2.0	0.0	1	0.0	0.2	0.0	0.0
Spring, with Grapefruit, Tesco*	1 Serving/200ml	4.0	0.0	2	0.0	0.2	0.0	0.0
Strawberry & Guava, Still, M & S*	1 Glass/250ml	5.0	0.0	2	0.0	0.1	0.0	0.0
Strawberry, Sugar Free, Touch Of Fruit, Volvic*	1 Bottle/500ml	7.0	0.0	1	0.0	0.1	0.0	0.0
WATER CHESTNUTS								
Raw, Average	*1oz/28g*	*10.0*	*0.0*	*34*	*1.0*	*7.8*	*0.0*	*0.1*
Whole, in Water, Drained, Sainsbury's*	1 Can/140g	25.0	0.0	18	0.8	3.4	0.1	0.4
with Bamboo Shoots, Sainsbury's*	1 Serving/50g	29.0	0.0	58	2.0	12.0	0.2	1.1
WATER ICE								
Orange, Iceland*	1 Ice/75ml	73.0	0.0	98	0.2	24.4	0.0	0.2
Pineapple, Iceland*	1 Ice/75ml	64.0	0.0	86	0.0	21.5	0.0	0.2
Raspberry, Iceland*	1 Ice/75ml	67.0	0.0	89	0.0	22.2	0.0	0.2
WATERCRESS								
Morrisons*	1 Pack/85g	19.0	1.0	22	3.0	0.4	1.0	1.5
Raw, Trimmed, Average	*1 Sprig/2.5g*	*1.0*	*0.0*	*22*	*3.0*	*0.4*	*1.0*	*1.5*
WATERMELON								
Flesh Only, Average	*1 Serving/250g*	*75.0*	*1.0*	*30*	*0.4*	*7.0*	*0.3*	*0.4*
Raw	*1 Wedge/286g*	*92.0*	*1.0*	*32*	*0.6*	*7.2*	*0.4*	*0.5*
WHEAT								
Whole Grain, Split, Average	*1 Serving/60g*	*205.0*	*1.0*	*342*	*11.3*	*75.9*	*1.7*	*12.2*
WHEAT BRAN								
Average	*1 Tbsp/7g*	*14.0*	*0.0*	*206*	*14.1*	*26.8*	*5.5*	*36.4*
WHEAT GERM								
Average	*1oz/28g*	*100.0*	*3.0*	*357*	*26.7*	*44.7*	*9.2*	*15.6*
WHELKS								
Boiled	*1oz/28g*	*25.0*	*0.0*	*89*	*19.5*	*0.0*	*1.2*	*0.0*
WHISKEY								
37.5% Volume	*1 Shot/35ml*	*72.0*	*0.0*	*207*	*0.0*	*0.0*	*0.0*	*0.0*

	Measure	per Measure		Nutrition Values per 100g / 100ml				
	INFO/WEIGHT	KCAL	FAT	KCAL	PROT	CARB	FAT	FIBRE
WHISKEY								
40% Volume	*1 Shot/35ml*	*78.0*	*0.0*	*222*	*0.0*	*0.0*	*0.0*	*0.0*
86% Proof	*1 Shot/35ml*	*87.0*	*0.0*	*250*	*0.0*	*0.1*	*0.0*	*0.0*
Jack Daniel's*	1 Shot/35ml	78.0	0.0	222	0.0	0.0	0.0	0.0
Teacher's*	1 Shot/35ml	78.0	0.0	222	0.0	0.0	0.0	0.0
WHISKY								
Scotch, 37.5% Volume	*1 Shot/35ml*	*72.0*	*0.0*	*207*	*0.0*	*0.0*	*0.0*	*0.0*
Scotch, 40% Volume	*1 Shot/35ml*	*78.0*	*0.0*	*222*	*0.0*	*0.0*	*0.0*	*0.0*
WHITE PUDDING								
Average	*1oz/28g*	*126.0*	*9.0*	*450*	*7.0*	*36.3*	*31.8*	*0.0*
WHITEBAIT								
in Flour, Fried	*1oz/28g*	*147.0*	*13.0*	*525*	*19.5*	*5.3*	*47.5*	*0.2*
WHITECURRANTS								
Raw, Average	*1oz/28g*	*7.0*	*0.0*	*26*	*1.3*	*5.6*	*0.0*	*3.4*
WHITING								
in Crumbs, Fried in Blended Oil	1 Serving/180g	344.0	19.0	191	18.1	7.0	10.3	0.2
Raw	*1oz/28g*	*23.0*	*0.0*	*81*	*18.7*	*0.0*	*0.7*	*0.0*
Steamed	*1 Serving/85g*	*78.0*	*1.0*	*92*	*20.9*	*0.0*	*0.9*	*0.0*
WIENER SCHNITZEL								
Average	1oz/28g	62.0	3.0	223	20.9	13.1	10.0	0.4
WINE								
Cherry, Lambrini*	1 Glass/125ml	80.0	0.0	64	0.0	0.0	0.0	0.0
Fruit, Average	*1 Glass/125ml*	*115.0*	*0.0*	*92*	*0.0*	*5.5*	*0.0*	*0.0*
Mulled, Homemade, Average	*1 Glass/125ml*	*245.0*	*0.0*	*196*	*0.1*	*25.2*	*0.0*	*0.0*
Original, Lambrini*	1 Glass/125ml	88.0	0.0	70	0.0	0.0	0.0	0.0
Red, Amarone, Average	1 Glass/125ml	120.0	0.0	96	0.1	3.0	0.0	0.0
Red, Average	*1 Glass/125ml*	*85.0*	*0.0*	*68*	*0.1*	*2.5*	*0.0*	*0.0*
Red, Burgundy, 12.9% Abv, Average	1 Glass/125ml	110.0	0.0	88	0.1	3.7	0.0	0.0
Red, Cabernet Sauvignon, 13.1% Abv, Average	1 Glass/125ml	105.0	0.0	84	0.1	2.6	0.0	0.0
Red, Claret, 12.8% Abv, Average	1 Glass/125ml	105.0	0.0	84	0.1	3.0	0.0	0.0
Red, Gamay, 12.3% Abv, Average	1 Glass/125ml	99.0	0.0	79	0.1	2.4	0.0	0.0
Red, Merlot, 13.3% Abv, Average	1 Glass/125ml	105.0	0.0	84	0.1	2.5	0.0	0.0
Red, Petit Sirah, 13.5% Abv, Average	1 Glass/125ml	107.0	0.0	86	0.1	2.7	0.0	0.0
Red, Pinot Noir, 13% Abv, Average	1 Glass/125ml	104.0	0.0	83	0.1	2.3	0.0	0.0
Red, Sangiovese, 13.6% Abv, Average	1 Glass/125ml	109.0	0.0	87	0.1	2.6	0.0	0.0
Red, Syrah, 13.1% Abv, Average	1 Glass/125ml	105.0	0.0	84	0.1	2.6	0.0	0.0
Red, Zinfandel, 13.9% Abv, Average	1 Glass/125ml	111.0	0.0	89	0.1	2.9	0.0	0.0
Rose, Medium, Average	*1 Glass/125ml*	*89.0*	*0.0*	*71*	*0.1*	*2.5*	*0.0*	*0.0*
Sangria, Average	1 Glass/125ml	95.0	0.0	76	0.1	9.9	0.0	0.1
White, Chenin Blanc, 12% Abv, Average	1 Glass/125ml	101.0	0.0	81	0.1	3.3	0.0	0.0
White, Dry, Average	*1 Glass/125ml*	*82.0*	*0.0*	*66*	*0.1*	*0.6*	*0.0*	*0.0*
White, Fume Blanc, 13.1% Abv, Average	1 Glass/125ml	104.0	0.0	83	0.1	2.3	0.0	0.0
White, Gewurztraminer, 12.6% Abv, Average	1 Glass/125ml	102.0	0.0	82	0.1	2.6	0.0	0.0
White, Late Harvest, 10.6% Abv, Average	1 Glass/125ml	141.0	0.0	113	0.1	13.4	0.0	0.0
White, Medium, Average	*1 Glass/125ml*	*92.0*	*0.0*	*74*	*0.1*	*3.0*	*0.0*	*0.0*
White, Muller-Thurgau, 11.3% Abv, Average	1 Glass/125ml	96.0	0.0	77	0.1	3.5	0.0	0.0
White, Muscat, 11% Abv, Average	1 Glass/125ml	104.0	0.0	83	0.1	5.2	0.0	0.0
White, Non Alcoholic, Ame*	1 Glass/125ml	47.0	0.0	38	0.0	9.5	0.0	0.0
White, Pinot Blanc, 13.3% Abv, Average	1 Glass/125ml	102.0	0.0	82	0.1	0.0	0.0	0.0
White, Pinot Grigio, 13.4% Abv, Average	1 Glass/125ml	105.0	0.0	84	0.1	2.1	0.0	0.0
White, Riesling, 11.9% Abv, Average	1 Glass/125ml	101.0	0.0	81	0.1	3.7	0.0	0.0
White, Sauvignon Blanc, 13.1% Abv, Average	1 Glass/125ml	102.0	0.0	82	0.1	2.0	0.0	0.0
White, Semillon, 12.5% Abv, Average	1 Glass/125ml	104.0	0.0	83	0.1	3.1	0.0	0.0
White, Sparkling, Average	*1 Glass/125ml*	*92.0*	*0.0*	*74*	*0.3*	*5.1*	*0.0*	*0.0*

W

	Measure INFO/WEIGHT	per Measure KCAL	FAT	Nutrition Values per 100g / 100ml KCAL	PROT	CARB	FAT	FIBRE
WINE								
White, Sweet, Average	*1 Glass/125ml*	*113.0*	*0.0*	*94*	*0.2*	*5.9*	*0.0*	*0.0*
WINE GUMS								
Average	1 Av Sweet/6g	19.0	0.0	315	5.0	73.4	0.2	0.1
Haribo*	1 Pack/175g	609.0	0.0	348	0.1	86.4	0.2	0.4
Light, Maynards*	1 Pack/42g	90.0	0.0	215	4.6	48.0	0.2	27.9
Mini, Rowntree's*	1 Sm Bag/36g	125.0	0.0	348	6.7	80.5	0.0	0.0
Sour, Bassett's*	¼ Bag/50g	159.0	0.0	319	3.7	78.0	0.0	0.0
WINKLES								
Boiled	*1oz/28g*	*20.0*	*0.0*	*72*	*15.4*	*0.0*	*1.2*	*0.0*
WISPA								
Bite, with Biscuit in Caramel, Cadbury*	1 Bar/47g	240.0	13.0	510	6.4	56.9	28.6	0.0
Cadbury*	1 Bar/40g	210.0	13.0	525	6.7	53.0	32.2	0.7
Gold, Cadbury*	1 Bar/52g	263.0	15.0	505	5.7	57.0	28.0	0.0
Mint, Cadbury*	1 Bar/50g	275.0	17.0	550	7.0	54.7	33.6	0.0
WONTON								
Prawn, Dim Sum Selection, Sainsbury's*	1 Wonton/10g	26.0	1.0	259	11.3	26.8	11.8	1.3
Prawn, Oriental Selection, Waitrose*	1 Wonton/18g	45.0	2.0	252	9.1	29.2	11.0	1.1
Prawn, Oriental Snack Selection, Sainsbury's*	1 Wonton/20g	53.0	3.0	265	10.6	25.6	13.4	2.0
WOTSITS								
BBQ, Walkers*	1 Bag/21g	108.0	6.0	515	4.5	57.0	30.0	1.3
Flamin' Hot, Walkers*	1 Bag/19g	99.0	6.0	520	5.0	57.0	30.0	1.2
Prawn Cocktail, Walkers*	1 Bag/19g	101.0	6.0	530	5.5	57.0	31.0	1.1
Really Cheesy, Big Eat, Walkers*	1 Bag/36g	196.0	12.0	545	5.5	56.0	33.0	1.1
Really Cheesy, Walkers*	1 Bag/19g	104.0	6.0	545	5.5	56.0	33.0	1.1
WRAP								
All Day Breakfast, M & S*	1 Pack/196g	529.0	31.0	270	10.8	21.2	16.0	1.4
American Deli, Shapers, Boots*	1 Pack/172g	249.0	4.0	145	9.5	21.0	2.6	2.0
Aromatic Duck, Safeway*	1 Pack/180g	376.0	17.0	209	9.1	21.3	9.7	1.6
Beef Fajita, Boots*	1 Pack/200g	352.0	8.0	176	9.5	25.5	4.2	3.1
Beef in Black Bean, M & S*	1 Pack/150g	337.0	17.0	225	10.2	20.5	11.4	1.6
Bombay Potato, Whistlestop*	1 Wrap/180g	343.0	15.0	191	4.2	24.7	8.3	0.3
Brie & Cranberry, M & S*	1 Pack/225g	550.0	28.0	245	6.1	27.3	12.4	1.7
Cajun Chicken, Sandwich King*	1 Pack/138g	386.0	20.0	279	12.3	25.0	14.4	0.0
Cajun Chicken, Tesco*	1 Pack/184g	415.0	17.0	225	9.8	25.1	9.0	1.9
Cajun, GFY, Asda*	1 Pack/176g	231.0	2.0	131	9.0	21.0	1.2	0.9
Chargrilled Chicken, Perfectly Balanced, Waitrose*	1 Pack/230g	361.0	7.0	157	10.3	22.7	2.9	2.9
Cheese & Bean, Tesco*	1 Pack/105g	235.0	9.0	224	7.0	28.6	9.0	1.0
Chicken & Bacon Caesar Salad, Asda*	1 Pack/160g	565.0	35.0	353	18.0	20.8	22.0	0.9
Chicken & Bacon Caesar, COU, M & S*	1 Pack/170g	260.0	4.0	153	10.6	22.0	2.5	2.1
Chicken & Cous Cous, BGTY, Sainsbury's*	1 Pack/230g	359.0	9.0	156	8.8	21.5	3.9	0.0
Chicken & Cous Cous, Moroccan Style, GFY, Asda*	1 Pack/164g	307.0	2.0	187	12.0	32.0	1.2	1.8
Chicken Caesar, HL, Tesco*	1 Pack/200g	296.0	4.0	148	10.2	22.3	2.0	2.2
Chicken Caesar, Tesco*	1 Pack /215g	516.0	24.0	240	11.6	23.0	11.3	1.2
Chicken Fajita, Asda*	1 Pack/180g	369.0	17.0	205	9.4	20.6	9.4	0.4
Chicken Fajita, Daily Bread*	1 Pack/191g	392.0	11.0	205	9.4	29.4	5.5	0.0
Chicken Fajita, Finest, Tesco*	1 Pack/213g	422.0	16.0	198	9.0	24.0	7.3	1.9
Chicken Fajita, Perfectly Balanced, Waitrose*	1 Serving/218g	368.0	6.0	169	10.5	26.0	2.6	1.9
Chicken Fajita, Shapers, Boots*	1 Pack/216g	291.0	5.0	135	14.0	15.0	2.4	3.1
Chicken Fajita, Tesco*	1 Pack/220g	407.0	12.0	185	10.6	23.2	5.3	1.8
Chicken Fajita, VLH Kitchens	1 Serving/170g	311.0	9.0	183	10.6	25.0	5.2	0.0
Chicken Jalfrezi, Boots*	1 Pack/215g	456.0	16.0	212	8.6	28.0	7.3	1.7
Chicken Korma, Patak's*	1 Pack/150g	294.0	14.0	196	7.6	20.0	9.5	0.0
Chicken Louisiana, Benedicts*	1 Pack/250g	410.0	5.0	164	13.4	24.2	2.2	0.0

WRAP

Measure INFO/WEIGHT	per Measure KCAL	FAT	Nutrition Values per 100g / 100ml KCAL	PROT	CARB	FAT	FIBRE
Chicken Nacho, HL, Tesco*	1 Pack/223g	390.0	10.0	175	12.3	21.2	4.5	2.6
Chicken Salad, Roast, Sainsbury's*	1 Pack/214g	443.0	20.0	207	10.0	20.9	9.3	2.5
Chicken Sweet & Sour, Ginsters*	1 Pack/150g	378.0	6.0	252	13.4	40.8	3.9	2.4
Chicken Thai Style, Boots*	1 Pack/156g	290.0	10.0	186	11.0	21.0	6.4	2.2
Chicken Tikka Masala, Patak's*	1 Pack/150g	252.0	10.0	168	7.8	19.3	6.6	0.0
Chicken Tikka, Average	1 Av Wrap/183g	277.0	7.0	151	9.7	18.5	4.0	1.1
Chicken, Barbecue, GFY, Asda*	1 Pack/176g	294.0	4.0	167	9.6	26.4	2.5	1.8
Chicken, Barbecue, Shapers, Boots*	1 Pack/181g	283.0	5.0	156	10.0	23.0	2.7	3.3
Chicken, Cheddar & Peppers, Cajun, Sainsbury's*	1 Pack/242g	535.0	27.0	221	10.4	19.8	11.0	2.1
Chicken, Chilli, GFY, Asda*	1 Pack/194g	277.0	4.0	143	9.1	21.6	2.2	2.3
Chicken, Louisiana Style, GFY, Asda*	1 Pack/195g	355.0	3.0	182	11.0	31.0	1.5	2.0
Chicken, M & S*	1 Pack/247g	530.0	25.0	215	8.2	23.4	10.1	1.6
Chicken, Mediterranean Style, Waitrose*	1 Pack/183g	296.0	11.0	162	8.3	18.6	6.0	2.3
Chicken, Mexican Style, Co-Op*	1 Pack/163g	367.0	15.0	225	11.0	26.0	9.0	3.0
Chicken, Moroccan, BGTY, Sainsbury's*	1 Pack/207g	315.0	3.0	152	9.4	25.3	1.5	0.0
Chicken, Moroccan, Shapers, Boots*	1 Serving/154g	251.0	2.0	163	10.0	27.0	1.5	1.9
Chicken, Nacho, No Mayo, Asda*	1 Pack/183g	392.0	14.0	214	12.0	24.3	7.6	3.1
Chicken, Salsa, Light Choices, Tesco*	1 Pack/219g	340.0	6.0	155	9.7	22.6	2.7	1.9
Chicken, Southern Fried, Fresh for You, Tesco*	1 Pack/206g	485.0	24.0	235	8.6	22.7	11.8	2.0
Chicken, Southern Style, Ginsters*	1 Wrap/210g	527.0	28.0	251	7.4	24.8	13.5	2.2
Chicken, Tasties*	1 Pack/149g	324.0	11.0	218	11.7	26.5	7.1	0.0
Chilli Bean & Cheese, Meat Free, Asda*	1 Wrap/151g	263.0	7.0	174	7.9	25.1	4.7	4.9
Chilli Beef, COU, M & S*	1 Pack/179g	268.0	3.0	150	10.1	23.4	1.6	2.6
Chilli Chicken, BGTY, Sainsbury's*	1 Pack/180g	313.0	4.0	174	10.2	28.0	2.4	0.0
Chinese Chicken, Asda*	1 Pack/200g	404.0	12.0	202	9.0	28.0	6.0	0.0
Chinese Chicken, M & S*	1 Pack/155g	239.0	2.0	154	14.0	22.3	1.0	2.0
Coronation Chicken, Waitrose*	1 Pack/164g	283.0	8.0	173	10.1	21.3	5.1	2.2
Cous Cous, Moroccan Style, Tesco*	1 Serving/240g	370.0	6.0	154	5.3	27.2	2.7	1.2
Crayfish & Rocket, HL, Tesco*	1 Pack/164g	270.0	5.0	165	7.5	25.9	3.1	1.9
Crayfish, Lemon Dressing & Rocket, COU, M & S*	1 Pack/183g	274.0	5.0	150	9.5	22.5	2.7	1.2
Dhansak Prawn, M & S*	1 Pack/208g	385.0	15.0	185	7.1	23.3	7.2	2.4
Duck, Food to Go, M & S*	1 Pack/257g	475.0	14.0	185	8.5	25.5	5.4	1.0
Duck, Hoi Sin, Delicious, Boots*	1 Pack/214g	393.0	11.0	184	10.0	25.0	5.1	1.8
Duck, Hoisin, M & S*	1 Pack/225g	405.0	8.0	180	8.4	27.7	3.7	1.5
Duck, Hoisin, No Mayo, Tesco*	1 Pack/184g	396.0	10.0	215	12.6	28.4	5.6	3.4
Egg Mayonnaise, Tomato & Cress, Sainsbury's*	1 Pack/255g	592.0	38.0	232	7.3	17.7	15.0	0.0
Fajita, Steak, Delicatessen, Waitrose*	1 Pack/232g	489.0	21.0	211	10.5	22.7	9.1	2.7
Feta Cheese Flat Bread, COU, M & S*	1 Pack/180g	225.0	4.0	125	6.3	20.6	2.2	1.9
Feta Cheese, GFY, Asda*	1 Pack/165g	256.0	7.0	155	7.0	22.0	4.3	2.1
Fiery Mexican Cheese, Ginsters*	1 Pack/150g	291.0	11.0	194	7.4	25.0	7.3	1.8
Goats Cheese, & Grilled Pepper, Asda*	1 Serving/75g	194.0	11.0	259	5.0	26.0	15.0	2.1
Greek Feta Salad, Shapers, Boots*	1 Pack/158g	241.0	6.0	153	6.4	24.0	3.6	1.2
Greek Feta, Tortilla, Shapers, Boots*	1 Pack/169g	271.0	5.0	160	6.7	27.0	2.7	1.6
Greek Salad, COU, M & S*	1 Pack/180g	288.0	5.0	160	6.0	27.2	2.7	2.3
Greek Salad, M & S*	1 Pack/179g	250.0	4.0	140	8.1	21.5	2.5	1.0
Greek Salad, Sainsbury's*	1 Pack/167g	242.0	6.0	145	6.7	21.2	3.7	1.8
Green Thai Prawn, BGTY, Sainsbury's*	1 Pack/200g	237.0	3.0	118	7.0	19.2	1.5	1.5
Ham, Cheese & Pickle Tortilla, Weight Watchers*	1 Pack/170g	296.0	5.0	174	10.9	26.4	2.8	1.2
Houmous & Chargrilled Vegetables, Shapers, Boots*	1 Pack/186g	301.0	5.0	162	5.8	29.0	2.7	3.2
Houmous, Royal London Hospital*	1 Pack/200g	318.0	13.0	159	6.3	20.0	6.7	0.0
Houmous, Taste!*	1 Pack/170g	291.0	8.0	171	5.4	26.4	4.9	0.0
King Prawn, Shapers, Boots*	1 Pack/154g	227.0	2.0	147	9.2	24.0	1.4	2.1
Mexican Bean & Potato in Spinach Tortilla, Daily Bread*	1 Pack/196g	329.0	11.0	168	4.9	25.0	5.4	0.0

W

WRAP

	Measure INFO/WEIGHT	KCAL	FAT	KCAL	PROT	CARB	FAT	FIBRE
Mexican Bean, BGTY, Sainsbury's*	1 Pack/216g	341.0	5.0	158	9.2	24.9	2.5	1.5
Mexican Bean, GFY, Asda*	1 Pack/173g	303.0	6.0	175	5.0	31.0	3.4	2.3
Mexican Chicken, M & S*	1 Serving/218g	447.0	22.0	205	8.6	19.7	10.3	1.3
Mexican Three Bean, M & S*	1 Pack/235g	435.0	18.0	185	6.1	21.6	7.8	2.8
Mexican Tortilla, Ainsley Harriott*	1 Pack/230g	421.0	17.0	183	7.1	22.4	7.5	0.0
Mild Chicken Curry, Patak's*	1 Pack/150g	238.0	9.0	159	8.1	21.3	6.0	2.8
Minted Lamb, Darwins Deli*	1 Pack/250g	287.0	6.0	115	3.2	19.9	2.5	0.0
Monterey Jack & Ham, Tesco*	1 Pack/200g	522.0	28.0	261	7.9	25.9	14.1	0.2
Nacho Chicken, COU, M & S*	1 Pack/175g	280.0	4.0	160	10.2	24.4	2.4	2.0
Peking Duck, Average	1 Serving/183g	356.0	10.0	194	9.2	26.5	5.7	1.1
Pepperoni, Tesco*	1 Pack/153g	271.0	7.0	177	6.4	26.9	4.9	1.4
Pork Caribbean Spicy, Ginsters*	1 Pack/150g	396.0	14.0	264	11.3	34.1	9.1	2.3
Red Thai Chicken, BGTY, Sainsbury's*	1 Pack/194g	384.0	8.0	198	11.3	29.3	3.9	1.0
Red Thai Chicken, Shapers, Boots*	1 Pack/172g	234.0	4.0	136	9.5	20.0	2.1	2.4
Roasted Vegetable & Feta, BGTY, Sainsbury's*	1 Serving/200g	318.0	8.0	159	5.8	25.0	4.0	0.0
Selection, Chicken, BBQ Steak, Hoisin Duck, M & S*	1 Pack/334g	685.0	24.0	205	10.9	24.3	7.1	1.7
Sicilian Lemon & Roasted Vegetable, COU, M & S*	1 Pack/178g	240.0	4.0	135	4.9	23.8	2.1	1.9
Soft Cheese & Spinach, to Go*	1 Serving/250g	278.0	7.0	111	4.5	17.4	2.7	0.0
Southern Fried Chicken, Tesco*	1 Pack/213g	395.0	15.0	185	9.9	20.8	6.9	2.1
Sushi Salmon & Cucumber, Waitrose*	1 Pack/180g	299.0	6.0	166	6.3	27.2	3.6	1.6
Sweet Chilli Chicken, Shapers, Boots*	1 Pack/195g	302.0	4.0	155	10.0	24.0	1.9	3.0
Sweet Chilli Chicken, Waitrose*	1 Pack/200g	390.0	15.0	195	10.2	22.0	7.3	2.4
Sweet Chilli Noodle, Sainsbury's*	1 Pack/210g	399.0	10.0	190	10.6	26.1	4.8	2.1
Tandoori Chicken, GFY, Asda*	1 Pack/167g	281.0	5.0	168	10.0	26.0	2.7	1.7
Thai Prawn, COU, M & S*	1 Pack/181g	235.0	3.0	130	8.3	20.4	1.6	1.9
Tortilla, BGTY, Sainsbury's*	1 Tortilla/50g	127.0	1.0	254	7.8	50.1	2.2	2.9
Tortilla, Chicken, Asda*	1 Pack/125g	252.0	2.0	202	9.6	36.9	1.8	3.3
Tortilla, Light Choices, Tesco*	1 Tortilla/64g	166.0	1.0	260	7.1	53.2	2.1	3.5
Tortilla, Vegetable, Asda*	1 Pack/125g	245.0	3.0	196	6.8	37.2	2.2	0.8
Tuna Nicoise, BGTY, Sainsbury's*	1 Pack/181g	273.0	7.0	151	11.0	18.0	3.9	0.0
Tuna, Sweetcorn & Red Pepper, BGTY, Sainsbury's*	1 Pack/178g	306.0	8.0	172	11.5	21.2	4.6	2.1
Turkey, Bacon & Cranberry, COU, M & S*	1 Pack/144g	230.0	2.0	160	9.6	27.1	1.5	2.3
Yellow Thai Prawn, COU, M & S*	1 Pack/171g	266.0	5.0	155	7.6	23.4	2.9	1.7

WRAP KIT

	Measure INFO/WEIGHT	KCAL	FAT	KCAL	PROT	CARB	FAT	FIBRE
Moroccan Style, Sainsbury's*	1 Wrap/62g	205.0	9.0	332	8.0	41.1	15.1	3.6

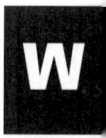

	Measure INFO/WEIGHT	per Measure KCAL	FAT	Nutrition Values per 100g / 100ml KCAL	PROT	CARB	FAT	FIBRE
YAM								
Baked	*1oz/28g*	*43.0*	*0.0*	*153*	*2.1*	*37.5*	*0.4*	*1.7*
Boiled, Average	*1oz/28g*	*37.0*	*0.0*	*133*	*1.7*	*33.0*	*0.3*	*1.4*
Raw	*1oz/28g*	*32.0*	*0.0*	*114*	*1.5*	*28.2*	*0.3*	*1.3*
YEAST								
Active, Dried, Average	1 Tsp/5g	8.0	0.0	169	35.6	3.5	1.5	0.0
Bakers, Compressed	*1oz/28g*	*15.0*	*0.0*	*53*	*11.4*	*1.1*	*0.4*	*0.0*
Dried, Average	*1 Tbsp/6g*	*10.0*	*0.0*	*169*	*35.6*	*3.5*	*1.5*	*0.0*
Extract	*1 Tsp/9g*	*16.0*	*0.0*	*180*	*40.7*	*3.5*	*0.4*	*0.0*
YOGHURT								
Adore Vanilla with Choc Flakes, Ehrmann*	1 Pot/150g	214.0	10.0	143	3.1	17.0	7.0	0.0
Alabama Chocolate Fudge Cake, Crunch Corner, Muller*	1 Pack/150g	249.0	9.0	166	3.3	24.8	5.7	0.2
Apple & Blackberry, Bio, Sainsbury's*	1 Pot/125g	134.0	3.0	107	4.1	16.6	2.7	0.2
Apple & Blackberry, Organic, Yeo Valley*	1 Pot/125g	121.0	4.0	97	4.3	12.5	3.3	0.1
Apple & Cinnamon, COU, M & S*	1 Pot/150g	67.0	0.0	45	4.2	6.1	0.1	0.4
Apple & Cinnamon, Dessert, Low Fat, Sainsbury's*	1 Pot/125g	115.0	2.0	92	4.5	14.7	1.7	0.1
Apple & Custard, Low Fat, Sainsbury's*	1 Pot/125g	116.0	2.0	93	4.3	15.5	1.5	0.2
Apple & Pear, Low Fat, Sainsbury's*	1 Pot/125g	115.0	2.0	92	4.3	15.2	1.5	0.2
Apple & Prune, Fat Free, Yeo Valley*	1 Pot/125g	97.0	0.0	78	5.1	14.1	0.1	0.2
Apple & Spice Bio, Virtually Fat Free, Shape, Danone*	1 Pot/120g	67.0	0.0	56	5.6	7.3	0.1	0.2
Apple Pie, Simply Desserts, Muller*	1 Pot/175g	278.0	8.0	159	4.6	24.7	4.6	0.7
Apple, Light, Muller*	1 Pot/200g	108.0	0.0	54	4.4	9.0	0.1	0.0
Apricot & Mango, Best There Is, Yoplait*	1 Pot/125g	130.0	2.0	104	4.7	17.4	1.6	0.0
Apricot & Mango, Low Fat, Tesco*	1 Pot/125g	126.0	2.0	101	4.9	16.3	1.8	0.0
Apricot & Mango, Thick & Creamy, Sainsbury's*	1 Pot/150g	178.0	5.0	119	4.3	17.3	3.6	0.2
Apricot & Mango, Tropical Fruit, Activ8, Ski, Nestle*	1 Pot/120g	112.0	2.0	93	4.3	15.1	1.7	0.2
Apricot & Nectarine, Sunshine Selection, Sainsbury's*	1 Pot/125g	115.0	2.0	92	4.4	15.3	1.5	0.1
Apricot & Passion Fruit, Fat Free, Yeo Valley*	1 Pot/125g	94.0	0.0	75	5.3	13.2	0.1	0.1
Apricot Tart Style, Sveltesse, Nestle*	1 Pot/125g	97.0	0.0	78	4.8	14.2	0.2	0.1
Apricot, Bio Activia, Danone*	1 Pot/125g	121.0	4.0	97	3.7	13.3	3.2	1.7
Apricot, Bio, Low Fat, Benecol*	1 Pot/125g	98.0	1.0	78	3.9	14.3	0.6	0.0
Apricot, Custard Style, Shapers, Boots*	1 Pot/146g	82.0	1.0	56	3.9	8.3	0.8	0.2
Apricot, Fat Free, Activ8, Ski, Nestle*	1 Pot/120g	88.0	1.0	73	4.5	13.6	0.7	0.2
Apricot, Fat Free, Bio Live, Rachel's Organic*	1 Pot/142g	81.0	0.0	57	3.5	10.5	0.1	0.0
Apricot, French Style Smooth, Tesco*	1 Pot/125g	122.0	4.0	98	3.6	14.1	3.0	0.0
Apricot, Fruity, Mullerlight, Muller*	1 Pot/200g	100.0	0.0	50	4.1	7.5	0.1	0.1
Apricot, HL, Tesco*	1 Pot/125g	67.0	0.0	54	5.1	7.9	0.3	1.1
Apricot, Layered Fruit, Thick & Creamy, Sainsbury's*	1 Pot/125g	141.0	3.0	113	4.1	18.0	2.7	0.2
Apricot, Light, HL, Tesco*	1 Pot/125g	54.0	0.0	43	4.1	6.3	0.2	0.9
Apricot, Low Fat, Organic, Average	1 Serving/100g	84.0	1.0	84	5.8	13.3	1.0	0.6
Apricot, Pro Activ, Flora*	1 Pot/125ml	70.0	1.0	56	4.0	7.9	0.5	1.8
Banana & Custard, Smooth, Mullerlight, Muller*	1 Pot/200g	106.0	0.0	53	4.0	8.4	0.1	0.6
Banana & Orange, Low Fat, 25% Extra Fruit, Asda*	1 Pot/125g	125.0	1.0	100	4.6	18.0	1.1	0.0
Banana Choco Flakes, Crunch Corner, Muller*	1 Pot/150g	214.0	8.0	143	4.1	22.5	5.1	0.3
Banana Smooth, M & S*	1 Pot/150g	165.0	3.0	110	4.8	19.3	1.7	0.2
Banana Toffee, Low Fat, Somerfield*	1 Pot/125g	122.0	1.0	98	4.1	18.0	1.1	0.0
Banana, Custard Style, Asda*	1 Pot/150g	223.0	9.0	149	3.7	20.0	6.0	0.2
Banana, Low Fat, Average	1 Serving/100g	98.0	1.0	98	4.6	16.7	1.4	0.1
Banoffee, Dessert, Low Fat, Sainsbury's*	1 Pot/125g	122.0	2.0	98	4.5	16.1	1.7	0.2
Banoffee, Fat Free, Bio, Eat Smart, Safeway*	1 Pot/125g	69.0	0.0	55	4.7	8.5	0.1	0.0
Banoffee, Low Fat, Asda*	1 Tbsp/125g	126.0	1.0	101	4.6	18.2	1.2	1.0
Bio Fruits with Cherries, 0% Fat, Danone*	1 Pot/125g	65.0	0.0	52	3.6	9.1	0.1	0.0
Black Cherry, Average	1 Serving/100g	96.0	2.0	96	3.4	16.5	2.2	0.1
Black Cherry, Extremely Fruity, Bio, M & S*	1 Pot/150g	165.0	2.0	110	4.9	18.4	1.5	0.2

Y

YOGHURT

	Measure INFO/WEIGHT	per Measure KCAL	per Measure FAT	Nutrition Values per 100g / 100ml KCAL	PROT	CARB	FAT	FIBRE
Black Cherry, Extremely Fruity, M & S*	1 Pot/200g	220.0	3.0	110	4.9	18.4	1.5	0.2
Black Cherry, Greek Style, Corner, Muller*	1 Pot/150g	172.0	4.0	115	5.0	16.2	3.0	0.1
Black Cherry, Live Bio, Perfeclty Balanced, Waitrose*	1 Pot/125g	115.0	0.0	92	4.6	18.3	0.1	0.1
Black Cherry, Low Fat, Average	1 Serving/100g	69.0	1.0	69	3.8	12.2	0.6	0.3
Black Cherry, Swiss, Finest, Tesco*	1 Pot/150g	195.0	9.0	130	3.5	15.7	5.9	0.5
Black Cherry, Thick & Creamy, Waitrose*	1 Pot/125g	139.0	3.0	111	3.7	18.3	2.5	0.4
Black Cherry, Very Cherry, Activ8, Ski, Nestle*	1 Pot/120g	116.0	2.0	97	4.3	16.1	1.7	0.2
Black Cherry, Virtually Fat Free, Shapers, Boots*	1 Pot/125g	71.0	0.0	57	5.3	8.8	0.1	0.1
Black Cherry, VLH Kitchens	1 Serving/150g	188.0	6.0	125	3.7	19.6	3.7	1.0
Blackberry & Apple, BGTY, Sainsbury's*	1 Pot/122g	61.0	0.0	50	4.7	7.2	0.2	0.3
Blackberry & Apple, HL, Tesco*	1 Pot/176g	86.0	0.0	49	2.1	10.0	0.1	1.5
Blackberry & Raspberry, Fruit Corner, Muller*	1 Pot/175g	185.0	7.0	106	3.8	13.1	3.9	1.0
Blackberry, Boysenberry & William Pear, M & S*	1 Pot/150g	187.0	10.0	125	4.0	13.6	6.5	2.4
Blackberry, Farmhouse, BGTY, Sainsbury's*	1 Pot/150g	106.0	1.0	71	3.4	13.5	0.4	1.6
Blackberry, Fat Free, Danone, Shape*	1 Pot/120g	74.0	0.0	62	6.7	8.4	0.2	2.4
Blackberry, Sveltesse, Nestle*	1 Pot/125g	67.0	0.0	54	4.9	8.2	0.1	0.4
Blackberry, Very Berry, Activ8, Ski, Nestle*	1 Pot/120g	114.0	2.0	95	4.4	15.5	1.7	0.7
Blackcurrant with Liquorice, Tesco*	1 Pot/150g	138.0	2.0	92	4.6	15.8	1.1	0.4
Blackcurrant, BGTY, Sainsbury's*	1 Pot/200g	100.0	0.0	50	4.8	7.3	0.2	0.1
Blackcurrant, Bio Live, Rachel's Organic*	1 Serving/225g	166.0	4.0	74	3.6	11.0	1.7	0.0
Blackcurrant, Extra Special, Asda*	1 Pot/100g	163.0	9.0	163	2.6	18.0	9.0	0.0
Blackcurrant, Fat Free, BGTY, Sainsbury's*	1 Pot/125g	64.0	0.0	51	4.6	8.0	0.1	1.6
Blackcurrant, Fruity, Mullerlight, Muller*	1 Pot/200g	102.0	0.0	51	4.1	7.9	0.1	0.8
Blackcurrant, Low Fat, Sainsbury's*	1 Pot/125g	116.0	2.0	93	4.2	15.9	1.4	0.6
Blackcurrant, Munch Bunch, Nestle*	1 Pot/100g	107.0	3.0	107	4.4	15.3	3.1	0.5
Blackcurrant, Probiotic, Organic, Yeo Valley*	1 Pot/150g	151.0	6.0	101	4.1	12.4	3.9	0.2
Blackcurrant, Thick & Creamy, Sainsbury's*	1 Pot/150g	171.0	5.0	114	4.3	15.9	3.6	0.4
Blackcurrant, Virtually Fat Free, Morrisons*	1 Pot/200g	114.0	0.0	57	5.4	8.4	0.2	0.2
Blueberry & Elderberry, with Wholegrains, Bio, Optifit*	1 Pot/250g	150.0	3.0	60	4.9	7.0	1.4	1.6
Blueberry Loganberry, Layered, Bio, Sainsbury's*	1 Pot/125g	134.0	3.0	107	4.0	16.6	2.7	0.2
Blueberry, Extremely Fruity, Low Fat, Probiotic, M & S*	1 Pot/150g	142.0	2.0	95	4.7	14.7	1.4	1.5
Blueberry, Fat Free, Activia, Danone*	1 Pot/125g	64.0	0.0	51	4.7	7.8	0.1	2.4
Blueberry, Fat Free, Probiotic, Organic, Yeo Valley*	1 Serving/100g	73.0	0.0	73	5.1	12.9	0.1	0.4
Blueberry, Fruit Corner, Muller*	1 Pot/175g	184.0	7.0	105	3.8	13.7	3.9	0.4
Blueberry, Low Lactose, Valio*	1 Serving/100g	80.0	2.0	80	3.2	13.0	2.1	0.0
Blueberry, Probiotic, Natural Balance, Asda*	1 Pot/125g	102.0	3.0	82	2.1	13.1	2.3	2.6
Blueberry, Wholemilk, Organic, Sainsbury's*	1 Pot/150g	123.0	5.0	82	3.5	9.2	3.5	0.1
Boysenberry, Low Fat, Yoplait*	1 Pot/100g	49.0	0.0	49	5.3	6.7	0.1	0.0
Caramel & Praline, Indulgent Greek Style, Somerfield*	1 Pot/125g	245.0	10.0	196	4.0	28.0	8.0	0.0
Caramel, Organic, Onken*	1 Serving/50g	55.0	2.0	111	4.6	15.6	3.3	0.0
Caramelised Orange, COU, M & S*	1 Pot/145g	65.0	0.0	45	4.2	6.1	0.1	0.2
Cereals, Fibre, Bio Activia, Danone*	1 Pot/120g	119.0	4.0	99	3.7	13.5	3.4	3.0
Champagne Rhubarb & Vanilla, M & S*	1 Pot/150g	195.0	9.0	130	3.8	15.7	5.8	0.8
Cherry & Vanilla Flavour, Light, Brooklea*	1 Pot/200g	138.0	0.0	69	5.5	11.4	0.1	0.6
Cherry Bakewell Tart Flavour, Muller*	1 Pot/175g	119.0	0.0	68	4.8	11.8	0.2	0.2
Cherry Morello Bio, Tesco*	1 Pot/124g	51.0	0.0	41	4.4	5.4	0.2	0.9
Cherry, 0% Fat, Yoplait*	1 Pot/125g	70.0	0.0	56	3.8	9.8	0.1	0.0
Cherry, 0.1% Fat, Shape, Danone*	1 Pot/120g	56.0	0.0	47	4.6	6.8	0.1	2.1
Cherry, Bio, Low Fat, Benecol*	1 Pot/150g	121.0	1.0	81	3.8	15.2	0.6	0.0
Cherry, Fat Free, Activia, Danone*	1 Pot/125g	71.0	0.0	57	4.7	9.4	0.1	0.9
Cherry, Fruit Corner, Muller*	1 Pot/175g	187.0	7.0	107	3.9	14.0	3.9	0.4
Cherry, Fruit, Biopot, Onken*	1 Serving/100g	110.0	3.0	110	3.9	17.5	2.7	0.3
Cherry, Fruity, Mullerlight, Muller*	1 Pot/200	96.0	0.0	48	4.2	6.9	0.1	0.2

YOGHURT

	Measure INFO/WEIGHT	per Measure KCAL	FAT	Nutrition Values per 100g / 100ml KCAL	PROT	CARB	FAT	FIBRE
Cherry, Greek Style, Shape, Danone*	1 Pot/125g	143.0	3.0	114	6.0	16.4	2.7	0.0
Cherry, Light, Fat Free, Muller*	1 Pot/200g	94.0	0.0	47	4.1	6.7	0.1	0.2
Cherry, Low Fat, Asda*	1 Pot/125g	120.0	1.0	96	4.6	17.0	1.1	0.0
Cherry, Noir De Basle, 0.06% Fat, TTD, Sainsbury's*	1 Pot/150g	195.0	9.0	130	3.7	15.7	5.8	0.3
Chocolate, GFY, Asda*	1 Pot/200g	110.0	1.0	55	4.7	8.0	0.5	0.1
Chocolate, Seriously Smooth, Waitrose*	1 Pot/125g	157.0	3.0	126	6.0	20.1	2.4	0.1
Chocolate, Village Dairy*	1 Pot/125g	181.0	4.0	145	6.3	23.5	3.0	0.0
Chocolate, Vitaline*	1 Pot/125g	102.0	1.0	82	3.5	15.8	0.5	0.0
Citrus Fruit, Tesco*	1 Serving/117g	53.0	0.0	45	4.2	6.5	0.1	0.1
Cranberry, Bio Activia, Danone*	1 Pot/125g	115.0	4.0	92	3.6	12.3	3.2	1.7
Creamy Cranberry & Raspberry, Shapers, Boots*	1 Pot/150g	85.0	2.0	57	4.0	7.0	1.1	1.1
Dessert with Honey, Perfectly Balanced, Waitrose*	1 Pot/125ml	127.0	1.0	102	3.5	19.4	1.2	0.1
Devon Toffee, Low Fat, Sainsbury's*	1 Pot/126g	137.0	2.0	109	4.3	19.6	1.5	0.0
Devonshire Fudge, 0.06% Fat, TTD, Sainsbury's*	1 Pot/150g	219.0	9.0	146	3.5	19.5	6.0	0.0
Exotic Fruits French Set Wholemilk, Asda*	1 Pot/125g	125.0	4.0	100	3.6	14.1	3.2	0.0
Exotic, Alpro*	1 Pot/125g	97.0	2.0	78	3.6	11.1	1.9	0.9
Fig, Bio, Activia, Danone*	1 Pot/125g	121.0	4.0	97	3.7	13.3	3.2	1.6
Forest Fruits, Bio, Activia, Fat Free, Danone*	1 Pot/125g	66.0	0.0	53	4.5	8.5	0.1	1.1
Forest Fruits, Layered Greek Style, Shapers, Boots*	1 Pot/150g	85.0	2.0	57	3.2	7.9	1.4	2.2
Forest Fruits, M & S*	1 Pot/150g	148.0	2.0	99	4.7	16.8	1.6	0.5
French Set, Low Fat, Iceland*	1 Pot/125g	100.0	1.0	80	3.6	13.6	1.2	0.0
French Set, Waitrose*	1 Pot/125g	120.0	4.0	96	3.5	13.4	3.1	0.0
French Style, Whole Milk, Smooth Set, Tesco*	1 Pot/125g	122.0	4.0	98	3.6	14.1	3.0	0.0
Frozen, Cherry Garcia, Low Fat, Ben & Jerry's*	1 Serving/100g	143.0	2.0	143	3.0	26.0	2.4	1.0
Frozen, Choc Fudge Brownie, Low Fat, Ben & Jerry's*	1 Serving/100g	180.0	3.0	180	4.0	34.0	3.0	1.5
Frozen, Strawberry Cheesecake, Low Fat, Ben & Jerry's*	1 Serving/100g	170.0	3.0	170	4.0	31.0	3.0	1.0
Fruit & Nut Layer, Indulgent Greek Style, Somerfield*	1 Pot/125g	214.0	9.0	171	3.0	24.0	7.0	0.0
Fruit Bio, Low Fat, Sainsbury's*	1 Pot/150g	156.0	2.0	104	4.6	18.9	1.1	0.3
Fruit Of The Forest, Zero, Shape, Danone*	1 Pot/120g	73.0	0.0	61	6.0	8.8	0.2	0.9
Fruit Whole Milk	1 Pot/150g	157.0	4.0	105	5.1	15.7	2.8	0.0
Fruit, Low Fat	1 Pot/120g	108.0	1.0	90	4.1	17.9	0.7	0.0
Fruit, Luscious, Low Fat, Bio-Live, Rachel's Organic*	1 Pot/125g	115.0	2.0	92	4.0	15.3	1.6	0.0
Fruits of the Forest, Nestle*	1 Pot/125g	122.0	2.0	98	3.4	16.7	1.6	0.0
Fruity Favourites, Organic, Yeo Valley*	1 Pot/125g	126.0	5.0	101	4.1	12.4	3.9	0.2
Fudge, Devonshire Style, Finest, Tesco*	1 Pot/150g	281.0	14.0	187	3.7	22.4	9.2	0.0
Fudge, Thick & Creamy, Co-Op*	1 Pot/150g	196.0	7.0	131	3.8	17.6	5.0	0.0
Fudge, Thick & Creamy, M & S*	1 Pot/150g	195.0	7.0	130	4.4	17.3	5.0	0.7
Fudge, Thick & Creamy, Waitrose*	1 Pot/150g	196.0	4.0	131	4.4	21.5	3.0	0.0
Garden Fruit, Wholemilk, Bio Live, Rachel's Organic*	1 Pot/125g	109.0	4.0	87	3.5	10.5	3.4	0.0
Get Up & Go, Get Fresh At Home*	1 Pack/100g	113.0	0.0	113	8.0	19.0	0.5	1.9
Goats Whole Milk	*1 Carton/150g*	*94.0*	*6.0*	*63*	*3.5*	*3.9*	*3.8*	*0.0*
Gooseberry, Custard Style, Co-Op*	1 Pot/150g	216.0	8.0	144	3.7	19.3	5.3	0.3
Gooseberry, Custard Style, Shapers, Boots*	1 Pot/151g	106.0	1.0	70	3.9	12.0	0.7	0.2
Gooseberry, Low Fat, Average	1 Serving/100g	90.0	1.0	90	4.5	14.5	1.4	0.2
Greek Style with Honey, Asda*	1 Pot/150g	225.0	13.0	150	4.0	13.9	8.7	0.0
Greek Style with Strawberries, Asda*	1 Pot/125g	159.0	8.0	127	3.2	13.6	6.6	0.2
Greek Style with Strawberry, Morrisons*	1 Pot/125g	162.0	8.0	130	3.3	14.4	6.6	0.0
Greek Style with Toffee & Hazelnuts, Asda*	1 Pot/125g	230.0	11.0	184	3.7	23.1	8.6	0.1
Greek Style with Tropical Fruits, Asda*	1 Pot/125g	164.0	8.0	131	3.3	14.5	6.6	0.3
Greek Style, & Nectarines, Food to Go, M & S*	1 Pack/200g	100.0	4.0	50	2.9	6.3	2.1	1.0
Greek Style, Honey Topped, Tesco*	1 Pot/140g	203.0	12.0	145	3.6	13.4	8.6	0.0
Greek Style, Honey, Selection Pack, Organic, Tesco*	1 Pot/100g	156.0	9.0	156	4.1	15.3	8.7	0.0
Greek Style, Layered, Honey, Shapers, Boots*	1 Pot/150g	136.0	3.0	91	4.2	14.0	2.0	0.0

Y

YOGHURT

Measure INFO/WEIGHT	per Measure KCAL	per Measure FAT	Nutrition Values per 100g / 100ml KCAL	PROT	CARB	FAT	FIBRE
Greek Style, Luxury, Loseley*	1 Pot/175g	226.0	18.0	129	4.8	4.5	10.2	0.0
Greek Style, Natural, Fat Free, Tesco*	½ Pot/100g	55.0	0.0	55	7.5	4.8	0.2	0.4
Greek, 0% Fat, Strained, Authentic, Total, Fage*	¼ Pot/125g	65.0	0.0	52	9.0	4.0	0.0	0.0
Greek, 2% Fat, Strained, Authentic, Total, Fage*	1 Pot/150g	100.0	3.0	67	8.4	3.8	2.0	0.0
Greek, Low Fat, Easiyo*	1 Pot/150g	99.0	2.0	66	5.6	8.4	1.3	0.0
Greek, Strained, Authentic, Original, Total, Fage*	1 Pot/200g	260.0	20.0	130	6.8	3.2	10.0	0.0
Greek, with Honey, Strained, Authentic, Total, Fage*	1 Pot/150g	255.0	12.0	170	5.4	19.0	8.0	0.0
Greek, with Strawberry, 2% Fat, Total, Fage*	1 Pot/150g	139.0	2.0	93	6.7	12.9	1.6	0.0
Guava & Orange, Fat Free, Organic, Yeo Valley*	1 Pot/125g	92.0	0.0	74	5.3	13.0	0.1	0.2
Guava & Passion Fruit, Virtualy Fat Free, Tesco*	1 Pot/125g	56.0	0.0	45	4.2	6.7	0.2	1.2
Hazelnut Crunchy, Jordans*	1 Pot/150g	231.0	6.0	154	5.2	22.2	4.0	1.1
Hazelnut, Low Fat, Average	1 Serving/100g	106.0	2.0	106	4.5	16.9	2.3	0.1
Hazelnut, Sainsbury's*	1 Serving/150g	183.0	3.0	122	5.0	20.3	2.3	0.2
Hazelnut, Yoplait*	1 Pot/125g	166.0	5.0	133	4.6	19.6	4.0	0.0
Hazlenut, Longley Farm*	1 Pot/150g	205.0	8.0	137	5.5	16.0	5.7	0.0
Honey & Ginger, Enhanced, Low Fat, Asda*	1 Pot/150g	150.0	2.0	100	4.6	18.0	1.1	0.0
Honey & Ginger, Tesco*	1 Pot/150g	150.0	2.0	100	4.6	18.0	1.1	0.0
Honey & Ginger, Waitrose*	1 Pot/150g	226.0	11.0	151	3.7	17.0	7.6	0.1
Honey & Muesli, Breakfast Break, Tesco*	1 Pot/170g	207.0	5.0	122	3.9	20.5	2.7	0.6
Honey & Multigrain, Breakfast Selection, Sainsbury's*	1 Pot/125g	126.0	2.0	101	4.4	17.4	1.5	0.2
Honey, Greek Style, Co-Op*	1 Pot/150g	228.0	13.0	152	4.0	13.8	8.5	0.0
Honey, Greek Style, Organic, Sainsbury's*	1 Pot/100g	156.0	9.0	156	4.1	15.3	8.7	0.1
Honey, Low Fat, Asda*	1 Pot/125g	130.0	1.0	104	4.6	19.0	1.1	0.0
Honeyed Apricot, Greek Style, Corner, Muller*	1 Pot/150g	168.0	4.0	112	5.0	15.5	3.0	0.1
Italian Lemon, Amore Luxury, Muller*	1 Pot/150g	219.0	12.0	146	2.8	16.2	7.8	0.1
Jaffa Orange, Morrisons*	1 Pot/150g	133.0	2.0	89	3.6	16.2	1.1	0.0
Kiwi, Activia, Danone*	1 Pot/125g	119.0	4.0	95	3.6	12.7	3.3	0.3
Kiwi, BGTY, Sainsbury's*	1 Pot/125g	61.0	0.0	49	4.6	7.5	0.1	0.2
Kiwi, Cereal, Fibre, Bio Activia, Danone*	1 Pot/120g	124.0	4.0	103	3.8	14.5	3.3	3.0
Lemon & Lime, BGTY, Sainsbury's*	1 Pot/125g	66.0	0.0	53	4.6	8.3	0.1	1.1
Lemon & Lime, Fat Free, Shape, Danone*	1 Pot/120g	61.0	0.0	51	4.5	7.3	0.1	0.1
Lemon Cheesecake, Average	1 Serving/100g	55.0	0.0	55	4.3	8.8	0.2	0.2
Lemon Curd, Indulgent, Dessert, Waitrose*	1 Pot/150g	277.0	14.0	185	4.1	21.5	9.2	0.0
Lemon Lime Mousse, Shapers, Boots*	1 Pot/90g	89.0	4.0	99	4.2	11.0	4.2	0.1
Lemon Meringue, Sveltesse, Nestle*	1 Pot/125g	60.0	0.0	48	4.1	7.7	0.1	0.0
Lemon, COU, M & S*	1 Pot/200g	90.0	0.0	45	4.2	6.6	0.1	0.4
Lemon, Greek Style, GFY, Asda*	1 Pot/150g	124.0	4.0	83	4.1	10.0	2.9	0.1
Lemon, Greek Style, Shape, Danone*	1 Pot/125g	140.0	3.0	112	5.9	15.9	2.7	0.0
Lemon, Low Fat, Average	1 Serving/100g	95.0	1.0	95	4.6	17.3	0.9	0.1
Lemon, Smooth Set French, Low Fat, Sainsbury's*	1 Pot/125g	100.0	1.0	80	3.5	13.6	1.2	0.0
Lemon, Summer, Biopot, Onken*	1 Pot/150g	154.0	4.0	103	3.9	15.9	2.6	0.1
Lemon, Thick & Fruity, Citrus Fruits, Weight Watchers*	1 Pot/120g	49.0	0.0	41	4.0	5.8	0.1	0.1
Light, Fat Free, Apricot, Muller*	1 Pot/200g	98.0	0.0	49	4.1	7.3	0.1	0.1
Loganberry, 0.06% Fat, TTD, Sainsbury's*	1 Pot/150g	186.0	9.0	124	3.7	14.2	5.8	0.8
Loganberry, Low Fat, Sainsbury's*	1 Pot/125g	111.0	2.0	89	4.2	14.5	1.5	0.2
Loganberry, Sainsbury's*	1 Pot/150g	193.0	9.0	129	3.9	14.2	6.2	0.6
Low Calorie	1 Pot/120g	49.0	0.0	41	4.3	6.0	0.2	0.0
Madagascan Vanilla, 0.06% Fat, TTD, Sainsbury's*	1 Pot/150g	210.0	9.0	140	3.7	17.8	6.0	0.0
Madagascan Vanilla, Indulgent, Dessert, Waitrose*	1 Pot/150g	240.0	11.0	160	3.7	19.2	7.6	0.0
Mandarin, Fat Free, Mullerlight, Muller*	1 Pot/190g	103.0	0.0	54	4.2	8.5	0.1	0.0
Mandarin, Low Fat, Asda*	1 Pot/125g	101.0	1.0	81	4.6	13.0	1.2	0.0
Mango & Guava, Sunshine Selection, Sainsbury's*	1 Pot/125g	145.0	2.0	116	5.4	19.3	1.9	0.3
Mango & Passion Fruit, Tropical Fruit, Activ8, Ski, Nestle*	1 Pot/120g	114.0	2.0	95	4.3	15.6	1.7	0.2

YOGHURT

	Measure INFO/WEIGHT	per Measure KCAL	per Measure FAT	Nutrition Values per 100g / 100ml KCAL	PROT	CARB	FAT	FIBRE
Mango & Pineapple, BGTY, Sainsbury's*	1 Pot/124g	63.0	0.0	51	4.6	7.6	0.2	0.2
Mango, Bio Activia, Danone*	1 Pot/125g	121.0	4.0	97	3.7	13.4	3.2	1.6
Mango, Fat Free, Shape Danone*	1 Pot/120g	74.0	0.0	62	6.6	8.6	0.1	2.2
Mango, Light, HL, Tesco*	1 Serving/125g	56.0	0.0	45	4.1	6.6	0.2	0.9
Mango, Light, Muller*	1 Pot/200g	110.0	0.0	55	4.3	9.2	0.1	0.0
Mango, Papaya & Passion Fruit, Summer, Biopot, Onken*	1/5 Pot/100g	101.0	3.0	101	3.9	15.6	2.6	0.2
Mango, Thick & Fruity, Tropical Fruit, Weight Watchers*	1 Pot/120g	49.0	0.0	41	3.9	6.0	0.1	1.1
Mango, Virtually Fat Free, Tesco*	1 Pot/125g	56.0	0.0	45	4.1	6.6	0.2	0.9
Maple & Cinnamon Granola, Low Fat, Natural, Asda*	1 Pot/140g	196.0	5.0	140	6.1	21.5	3.3	0.8
Mixed Seeds, Probiotic, Yoplait*	1 Pot/125g	139.0	6.0	111	4.5	13.2	4.5	3.1
Morello Cherry, Amore Luxury, Muller*	1 Pot/150g	216.0	12.0	144	2.8	16.3	7.8	0.1
Morello Cherry, HL, Tesco*	1 Pot/125g	56.0	0.0	45	4.1	6.6	0.2	0.9
Muesli Nut, Low Fat	1 Pot/120g	134.0	3.0	112	5.0	19.2	2.2	0.0
Natural with Honey, Greek Style, Sainsbury's*	1 Sm Pot/150g	243.0	14.0	162	4.0	15.4	9.4	0.0
Natural, 0.1% Fat, Stirred, Biopot, Onken*	1 Serving/100g	48.0	0.0	48	5.4	6.4	0.1	0.0
Natural, Bio Activia, Individual Pots, Danone*	1 Pot/125g	86.0	4.0	69	4.2	5.5	3.4	0.0
Natural, Bio Life, Easiyo*	1 Pot/150g	95.0	3.0	63	5.0	6.7	1.8	0.0
Natural, Bio Live, Low Fat, Organic, Waitrose*	¼ Pot/125g	81.0	1.0	65	5.8	8.3	1.0	0.0
Natural, Bio Set, Low Fat, Sainsbury's*	1 Pot/150g	78.0	2.0	52	3.9	5.7	1.5	0.0
Natural, Bio, BFY, Morrisons*	1 Serving/100g	65.0	0.0	65	6.5	9.4	0.2	0.0
Natural, Bio, HL, Tesco*	1 Serving/100g	55.0	0.0	55	5.4	7.6	0.1	0.0
Natural, Bio, Light Choices, Tesco*	1 Serving/100g	55.0	0.0	55	5.4	7.6	0.1	0.0
Natural, Bio, Low Fat, Sainsbury's*	1 Serving/100g	48.0	1.0	48	4.0	4.6	1.5	0.0
Natural, Bio, Very Low Fat, Somerfield*	1 Pot/150g	97.0	0.0	65	7.0	9.0	0.0	0.0
Natural, Bio, Virtually Fat Free, HL, Tesco*	1 Serving/100g	47.0	0.0	47	5.5	5.8	0.2	0.1
Natural, Danone*	1 Pot/125g	71.0	4.0	57	3.2	3.8	2.9	0.0
Natural, Fat Free, Rachel's Organic*	1 Pot/500g	180.0	0.0	36	3.9	4.8	0.1	0.0
Natural, Greek Style, Average	1 Serving/100g	138.0	11.0	138	4.7	6.1	10.6	0.0
Natural, Greek Style, Bio Live, Rachel's Organic*	1 Pot/450g	513.0	40.0	114	3.7	4.6	9.0	0.0
Natural, Greek Style, Low Fat, Average	1 Serving/100g	77.0	3.0	77	6.1	7.3	2.7	0.2
Natural, Greek Style, Probiotic, Unsweetened, M & S*	1 Serving/150g	195.0	15.0	130	5.5	4.6	10.1	0.1
Natural, Greek Style, with Cow's Milk, Tesco*	1 Pot/150g	214.0	16.0	143	4.5	6.6	10.9	0.0
Natural, Greek Style, with Honey Sauce, Sainsbury's*	1 Pot/140g	206.0	11.0	147	3.3	15.7	7.9	0.0
Natural, Longley Farm*	1 Pot/150g	118.0	5.0	79	4.8	7.0	3.5	0.0
Natural, Low Fat, Bio, Co-Op*	1 Pot/150g	97.0	1.0	65	6.0	8.0	1.0	0.0
Natural, Low Fat, Bio, Sainsbury's*	1 Pot/125g	85.0	2.0	68	5.6	7.9	1.5	0.0
Natural, Low Fat, Live, Waitrose*	1 Pot/175g	114.0	2.0	65	5.8	8.2	1.0	0.0
Natural, Low Fat, Organic, Average	1 Serving/100g	87.0	1.0	87	5.7	7.7	1.2	0.0
Natural, Low Fat, Stirred, Sainsbury's*	1 Serving/124g	83.0	2.0	67	5.5	7.8	1.5	0.0
Natural, Luxury, Bio Live, Jersey Dairy*	1 Pot/150g	225.0	12.0	150	4.6	8.2	8.0	0.0
Natural, Organic, Evernat*	1 Serving/100g	104.0	4.0	104	3.9	12.9	4.0	0.0
Natural, Organic, Yeo Valley*	1 Pot/150g	120.0	6.0	80	4.7	6.9	3.7	0.0
Natural, Probiotic, Fat Free, Organic, Yeo Valley*	1 Pot/150g	87.0	0.0	58	5.9	8.4	0.1	0.0
Natural, Probiotic, Organic, Yeo Valley*	1 Pot/150g	123.0	6.0	82	4.5	6.6	4.2	0.0
Natural, Set, Asda*	1 Pot/450g	256.0	4.0	57	5.1	6.8	1.0	0.0
Natural, Set, Low Fat, Waitrose*	1 Pot/150g	99.0	2.0	66	5.7	8.1	1.2	0.0
Natural, Very Low Fat, Good Intentions, Somerfield*	1 Serving/125g	66.0	0.0	53	5.4	7.6	0.1	0.0
Natural, Very Low Fat, Longley Farm*	1 Serving/80g	46.0	0.0	57	6.5	7.5	0.1	0.0
Natural, Whole Milk, Set, Biopot, Onken*	1 Pot/150g	108.0	6.0	72	3.9	5.7	3.7	0.0
Natural, Wholemilk, Organic, Sainsbury's*	1 Pot/125g	86.0	5.0	69	3.7	5.0	3.8	0.1
Natural, with Cow's Milk, Greek Style, Sainsbury's*	½ Pot/100g	143.0	11.0	143	4.5	6.6	10.9	0.0
Nectarine & Orange, Best There Is, Yoplait*	1 Pot/122g	131.0	2.0	107	4.7	18.0	1.6	0.0
Nectarine & Orange, Channel Island, M & S*	1 Pot/150g	157.0	5.0	105	4.5	14.7	3.3	0.3

YOGHURT

INFO/WEIGHT	Measure per Measure KCAL	FAT	Nutrition Values per 100g / 100ml KCAL	PROT	CARB	FAT	FIBRE
Nectarine & Orange, Fat Free, Average	1 Serving/100g	46.0	0.0	46	4.4	6.7	0.1	0.0
Nectarine & Orange, M & S*	1 Pot/150g	147.0	2.0	98	4.9	16.0	1.6	0.3
Nectarine & Passion Fruit, BGTY, Sainsbury's*	1 Pot/151g	122.0	1.0	81	3.2	16.3	0.4	0.6
Orange & Lemon, BGTY, Sainsbury's*	1 Pot/125g	62.0	0.0	50	4.7	7.3	0.2	0.2
Orange & Pineapple, Tropical Fruit, Activ8, Ski, Nestle*	1 Pot/120g	112.0	2.0	93	4.4	15.1	1.7	0.2
Orange Blossom Honey, Finest, Tesco*	1 Pot/150g	237.0	11.0	158	3.5	20.1	7.1	0.0
Orange, BGTY, Sainsbury's*	1 Pot/125g	62.0	0.0	50	4.5	7.7	0.1	1.1
Orange, Greek Style, Boots*	1 Pot/140g	207.0	12.0	148	3.7	14.0	8.6	0.2
Orange, Greek Style, Shape, Danone*	1 Pot/125g	140.0	3.0	112	6.0	16.0	2.7	0.1
Orange, Low Fat, Tesco*	1 Pot/125g	114.0	2.0	91	4.3	14.5	1.8	0.0
Orange, Sprinkled with Dark Chocolate, Light, Muller*	1 Pot/165g	84.0	1.0	51	4.0	7.1	0.5	0.1
Passion Fruit with Elderflower Extract, Tesco*	1 Pot/150g	147.0	2.0	98	4.7	17.3	1.1	0.2
Peach & Apricot, 0.1% Fat, Shape, Danone*	1 Pot/120g	55.0	0.0	46	4.6	6.7	0.1	2.1
Peach & Apricot, Fruit Corner, Muller*	1 Pot/175g	191.0	7.0	109	3.9	14.5	3.9	0.3
Peach & Apricot, HL, Tesco*	1 Pot/92g	42.0	0.0	46	4.0	7.4	0.1	1.0
Peach & Apricot, Light, HL, Tesco*	1 Pot/200g	82.0	0.0	41	3.9	6.2	0.1	1.0
Peach & Lemon Balm, Biowild, Onken*	1 Pot/175g	157.0	3.0	90	4.3	14.9	1.5	0.1
Peach & Mango, 0.1% Actimel, Danone*	1 Serving/100g	29.0	0.0	29	2.7	3.6	0.1	0.1
Peach & Mango, Dairy Free, Organic, Yofu, Provamel*	1 Pot/125g	100.0	3.0	80	3.9	10.4	2.2	0.8
Peach & Mango, Thick & Creamy, Waitrose*	1 Pot/125g	136.0	3.0	109	3.7	17.8	2.5	0.3
Peach & Maracuya, Mullerlight, Muller*	1 Pot/200g	102.0	0.0	51	4.5	8.1	0.1	0.0
Peach & Papaya, Fat Free, Yeo Valley*	1 Pot/125g	94.0	0.0	75	5.3	13.1	0.1	0.1
Peach & Papaya, Waitrose*	1 Pot/150g	129.0	0.0	86	4.2	17.1	0.1	0.2
Peach & Passion Fruit, Average	1 Serving/100g	66.0	1.0	66	4.5	10.6	0.7	0.4
Peach & Passion Fruit, Fat Free, Shape, Danone*	1 Pot/120g	74.0	0.0	62	6.6	8.6	0.1	2.3
Peach & Passion Fruit, Fruit Layered, Bio, GFY, Asda*	1 Pot/126g	77.0	1.0	61	4.0	11.0	0.1	0.5
Peach & Passion Fruit, Layers, Mullerlight, Muller*	1 Pot/175g	94.0	0.0	54	3.1	9.7	0.1	0.2
Peach & Passion Fruit, Lite Biopot, Onken*	1/5 Pot/100g	45.0	0.0	45	4.6	6.0	0.2	0.1
Peach & Passionfruit, BGTY, Sainsbury's*	1 Pot/125g	69.0	0.0	55	4.9	8.6	0.1	0.1
Peach & Pear, Seriously Fruity, Low Fat, Waitrose*	1 Pot/125g	110.0	1.0	88	4.5	15.3	1.0	0.3
Peach & Vanilla Flip, Morrisons*	1 Pot/175g	212.0	8.0	121	3.4	16.5	4.6	0.6
Peach & Vanilla, Average, Tesco*	1 Serving/100g	43.0	0.0	43	4.4	6.1	0.1	0.5
Peach & Vanilla, Thick & Creamy, Co-Op*	1 Pot/150g	180.0	7.0	120	3.6	16.0	4.6	0.1
Peach Melba, Low Fat, Average	1 Serving/100g	75.0	1.0	75	2.6	14.5	0.7	0.0
Peach Melba, Value, Tesco*	1 Pot/125g	100.0	1.0	80	2.3	16.0	0.7	0.1
Peach, BGTY, Sainsbury's*	1 Pot/125g	61.0	0.0	49	4.7	7.2	0.2	0.2
Peach, Custard Style, Low Fat, Sainsbury's*	1 Pot/125g	110.0	2.0	88	4.4	14.2	1.5	0.1
Peach, Economy, Sainsbury's*	1 Pot/125g	92.0	0.0	74	2.8	14.7	0.4	0.0
Peach, Fat Free, Activ8, Ski, Nestle*	1 Yogurt/120g	89.0	0.0	74	4.5	13.7	0.1	0.7
Peach, Forbidden Fruits, Rachel's Organic*	1 Pot/125g	156.0	8.0	125	3.4	14.0	6.1	0.0
Peach, Honey & Grain, Eat Smart, Safeway*	1 Serving/200g	120.0	0.0	60	4.7	9.4	0.2	0.3
Peach, Low Fat, Average	1 Serving/100g	86.0	1.0	86	4.5	14.6	1.1	0.1
Peach, Low Fat, Probiotic, Tesco*	1 Pot/125g	106.0	2.0	85	3.9	14.3	1.4	0.3
Peach, Luscious, Low Fat, Rachel's Organic*	1 Pot/125g	112.0	2.0	90	4.0	14.9	1.6	0.2
Peach, Probiotic, Natural Balance, Asda*	1 Pot/125g	107.0	3.0	86	3.1	13.2	2.3	2.5
Peach, Smooth Style, Mullerlight, Muller*	1 Pot/125g	59.0	0.0	47	4.1	6.9	0.1	0.2
Peaches, Farmhouse, BGTY, Sainsbury's*	1 Pot/150g	133.0	1.0	89	3.2	17.8	0.4	0.3
Peach-Nectarine, Bio Activia, Fat Free, Danone*	1 Pot/125g	70.0	0.0	56	4.5	9.3	0.1	1.0
Peanut Toffee, Low Fat, Somerfield*	1 Pot/150g	130.0	1.0	87	4.0	15.0	1.0	0.0
Pear & Butterscotch, Finest, Tesco*	1 Pot/150g	412.0	21.0	275	5.0	32.3	14.0	0.5
Pear & Vanilla, Thick & Creamy, Weight Watchers*	1 Pot/120g	54.0	1.0	45	4.2	5.8	0.5	0.2
Pear, Rosehip & Marigold, Biowild, Onken*	1 Pot/175g	161.0	3.0	92	4.4	15.1	1.5	0.3
Phish Food, Frozen, Lower Fat, Ben & Jerry's*	½ Pot/211g	464.0	11.0	220	4.0	40.0	5.0	1.5

YOGHURT

	Measure INFO/WEIGHT	per Measure KCAL	FAT	Nutrition Values per 100g / 100ml KCAL	PROT	CARB	FAT	FIBRE
Pineapple & Grapefruit, BGTY, Sainsbury's*	1 Pot/125g	67.0	0.0	54	4.4	8.8	0.1	0.1
Pineapple & Passion Fruit, Soya, Light, Alpro*	1 Pot/120g	62.0	1.0	52	2.1	7.3	1.1	0.8
Pineapple & Peach, Fruity, Mullerlight, Muller*	1 Pot/200g	100.0	0.0	50	4.1	7.6	0.1	0.2
Pineapple, Average	1 Serving/100g	73.0	1.0	73	4.4	11.3	1.1	0.5
Pineapple, Bio Activia, Fat Free, Danone*	1 Pot/125g	62.0	0.0	50	4.7	7.5	0.1	1.7
Pineapple, Channel Island, M & S*	1 Pot/150g	165.0	5.0	110	4.3	15.9	3.3	0.3
Pineapple, Extremely Fruity, M & S*	1 Pot/200g	200.0	3.0	100	4.3	17.6	1.4	0.2
Pineapple, Low Fat, Average	1 Serving/100g	89.0	1.0	89	4.6	14.7	1.2	0.0
Pineapple, Thick & Creamy, Waitrose*	1 Pot/125g	136.0	3.0	109	3.6	17.9	2.5	0.2
Pineapple, Virtually Fat Free, Tesco*	1 Pot/125g	55.0	0.0	44	4.1	6.5	0.2	0.9
Pineapple, Vitality, Low Fat, with Omega 3, Muller*	1 Pot/150g	138.0	3.0	92	4.2	13.8	1.9	0.7
Pink Grapefruit, Breakfast Selection, Sainsbury's*	1 Pot/117g	109.0	2.0	93	4.2	15.9	1.4	0.1
Pink Grapefruit, Low Fat, Sainsbury's*	1 Pot/125g	116.0	2.0	93	4.2	15.9	1.4	0.1
Pink Grapefruit, Thick & Fruity, Weight Watchers*	1 Pot/120g	49.0	0.0	41	3.9	6.2	0.1	1.0
Plain, Low Fat, Average	*1 Serving/100g*	*63.0*	*2.0*	*63*	*5.2*	*7.0*	*1.5*	*0.0*
Plain, Whole Milk, Average	*1oz/28g*	*22.0*	*1.0*	*79*	*5.7*	*7.8*	*3.0*	*0.0*
Plum & Hop, Biowild, Onken*	1 Pot/175g	157.0	3.0	90	4.3	14.9	1.5	0.3
Plum, BGTY, Sainsbury's*	1 Pot/125g	69.0	0.0	55	4.8	8.8	0.1	0.1
Plum, Low Fat, Sainsbury's*	1 Pot/125g	117.0	2.0	94	4.5	15.2	1.7	0.1
Plum, Probiotic, Summer Selection, Yeo Valley*	1 Pot/125g	126.0	5.0	101	4.1	12.4	3.9	0.1
Pouring, Strawberry, Activia, Danone*	1 Serving/100g	59.0	2.0	59	3.9	7.3	1.6	0.1
Pouring, Vanilla, Activia, Danone*	1 Serving/100g	62.0	2.0	62	3.9	8.1	1.6	0.0
Probiotic, Low Fat, Organic, Glenisk Organic Dairy Co*	1 Serving/150g	91.0	3.0	61	4.5	6.4	1.9	0.0
Prune, Bio Activia, Danone*	1 Pot/125g	110.0	3.0	88	3.5	12.2	2.8	0.2
Prune, Breakfast Selection, Sainsbury's*	1 Pot/125g	119.0	2.0	95	4.2	16.3	1.4	0.2
Prune, Probiotic, Natural Balance, Asda*	1 Pot/125g	105.0	3.0	84	2.1	13.8	2.3	0.8
Prune, Probiotic, Tesco*	1 Serving/170g	145.0	2.0	85	3.9	14.3	1.4	1.0
Prune, Vitality, Low Fat, with Omega 3, Muller*	1 Pot/150g	144.0	3.0	96	4.7	15.0	1.9	1.1
Rashaka, Plain, Danone*	1 Serving/180ml	88.0	0.0	49	5.5	6.5	0.0	0.0
Raspberry & Blackberry, Rich & Creamy, Spelga*	1 Serving/150g	187.0	7.0	125	3.7	17.2	4.7	0.1
Raspberry & Cranberry, BGTY, Sainsbury's*	1 Pot/125g	65.0	0.0	52	4.4	8.4	0.1	0.5
Raspberry & Cranberry, Fat Free, Mullerlight, Muller*	1 Pot/200g	100.0	0.0	50	4.1	7.6	0.1	0.5
Raspberry & Cranberry, Light, HL, Tesco*	1 Pot/125g	55.0	0.0	44	4.2	6.3	0.2	1.1
Raspberry & Elderberry, Organic, Onken*	1 Serving/50g	53.0	2.0	106	3.8	15.0	3.1	0.0
Raspberry & Orange, Fat Free, Organic, Yeo Valley*	1 Serving/100g	77.0	0.0	77	5.1	13.7	0.1	0.1
Raspberry & Redcurrant, Low Fat, Morrisons*	1 Pot/125g	117.0	2.0	94	4.4	15.4	1.6	0.7
Raspberry & Redcurrant, Low Fat, Sainsbury's*	1 Pot/125g	109.0	2.0	87	4.2	14.5	1.4	0.5
Raspberry Tart, Sveltesse, Nestle*	1 Pot/125g	64.0	0.0	51	4.5	7.1	0.1	0.1
Raspberry, Bio, Activia, Danone*	1 Pot/125g	112.0	3.0	90	3.5	12.8	2.8	2.0
Raspberry, Bio, Activia, Fat Free, Danone*	1 Pot/125g	59.0	0.0	47	4.6	6.9	0.1	2.5
Raspberry, Bio, Low Fat, Benecol*	1 Pot/125g	99.0	1.0	79	3.8	14.5	0.6	0.0
Raspberry, Economy, Sainsbury's*	1 Pot/125g	85.0	1.0	68	3.0	11.9	1.0	0.0
Raspberry, Extremely Fruity, M & S*	1 Pot/200g	190.0	3.0	95	5.0	15.6	1.5	0.5
Raspberry, Fat Free, Average	1 Serving/100g	64.0	0.0	64	4.9	11.0	0.1	1.7
Raspberry, Forbidden Fruit, Rachel's Organic*	1 Pot/125g	155.0	8.0	124	3.4	13.8	6.1	0.1
Raspberry, French Set, Waitrose*	1 Pot/125g	120.0	4.0	96	3.5	13.4	3.1	2.0
Raspberry, Incredibly Fruity, Fat Free, Tesco*	1 Pot/150g	112.0	0.0	75	4.8	13.1	0.1	1.0
Raspberry, Low Fat, Average	1 Serving/100g	83.0	1.0	83	4.1	14.1	1.1	0.8
Raspberry, Organic, Yeo Valley*	1 Pot/150g	151.0	6.0	101	4.2	12.3	3.9	0.4
Raspberry, Probiotic, Live, Yeo Valley*	1 Pot/125g	106.0	1.0	85	5.1	14.0	1.0	0.4
Raspberry, Scottish, The Best, Morrisons*	1 Pot/150g	208.0	10.0	139	3.6	15.6	6.9	1.3
Raspberry, Smooth, Activ8, Ski, Nestle*	1 Pot/120g	113.0	2.0	94	4.6	14.8	1.7	0.7
Raspberry, Smooth, Mullerlight, Muller*	1 Pot/125g	64.0	0.0	51	4.2	7.8	0.1	0.6

Y

YOGHURT

	Measure INFO/WEIGHT	per Measure KCAL	per Measure FAT	Nutrition Values per 100g / 100ml KCAL	PROT	CARB	FAT	FIBRE
Raspberry, Summer, Biopot, Onken*	1/5 Pot/100g	101.0	3.0	101	3.9	15.5	2.6	0.6
Raspberry, Sveltesse, Nestle*	1 Pot/125g	61.0	0.0	49	4.9	7.2	0.1	0.6
Raspberry, Thick & Creamy, Sainsbury's*	1 Pot/150g	178.0	6.0	119	4.4	17.2	3.7	0.2
Raspberry, Thick & Fruity, Probiotic, COU, M & S*	1 Pot/170g	76.0	0.0	45	4.2	6.9	0.1	0.6
Raspberry, Value, Tesco*	1 Serving/125g	100.0	1.0	80	2.3	16.0	0.7	0.1
Raspberry, Vitality, Low Fat, with Omega 3, Muller*	1 Pot/125g	115.0	2.0	92	4.3	13.4	2.0	1.3
Raspberry, Way to Five, Sainsbury's*	1 Pot/151g	104.0	0.0	69	3.3	13.6	0.1	2.1
Raspberry, with Fruit Layer, Bio Activia, Danone*	1 Pot/125g	107.0	3.0	86	3.5	11.6	2.8	2.0
Red Berry, Healthy Balance, Corner, Muller*	1 Pot/150g	178.0	4.0	119	5.0	18.0	2.7	0.5
Red Berry, Vitality, Low Fat, with Omega 3, Muller*	1 Pot/150g	138.0	3.0	92	4.3	13.8	1.9	0.7
Red Cherry, Fat Free, Ski, Nestle*	1 Pot 120g	97.0	0.0	81	4.5	15.6	0.1	0.1
Red Cherry, Fruit Layered, GFY, Asda*	1 Pot/125g	75.0	0.0	60	3.7	11.0	0.1	0.0
Red Cherry, Very Cherry, Activ8, Ski, Nestle*	1 Pot/120	115.0	2.0	96	4.5	15.7	1.7	0.1
Red Fruits, Crumble Style, Sveltesse, Nestle*	1 Pot/125g	100.0	0.0	80	4.9	14.6	0.2	0.4
Rhubarb & Champagne, Truly Irresistible, Co-Op*	1 Pot/150g	195.0	8.0	130	3.5	16.6	5.5	0.2
Rhubarb & Orange, Tesco*	1 Pot/150g	145.0	2.0	97	4.6	17.1	1.1	0.5
Rhubarb & Vanilla, Summer, Biopot, Onken*	1/5 Pot/100g	106.0	3.0	106	3.8	16.9	2.6	0.3
Rhubarb Crumble, Crunch Corner, Muller*	1 Pot/150g	238.0	8.0	159	3.6	23.5	5.6	0.5
Rhubarb, Bio Activia, Danone*	1 Pot/125g	112.0	4.0	90	3.5	11.8	3.2	2.2
Rhubarb, Custard Style, Co-Op*	1 Pot/150g	202.0	8.0	135	3.7	17.2	5.3	0.3
Rhubarb, Extremely Fruity, Low Fat, Probiotic, M & S*	1 Pot/170g	153.0	2.0	90	4.4	15.5	1.0	0.7
Rhubarb, Live Bio, Low Fat, Perfectly Balanced, Waitrose*	1 Pot/150g	114.0	0.0	76	4.2	14.5	0.1	0.4
Rhubarb, Longley Farm*	1 Pot/150g	165.0	6.0	110	4.9	14.3	3.7	0.0
Rhubarb, Low Fat, Average	1 Serving/100g	83.0	1.0	83	4.6	13.3	1.2	0.2
Rhubarb, M & S*	1 Pot/150g	148.0	2.0	99	4.4	17.4	1.4	0.3
Rhubarb, Spiced, Thick & Creamy, COU, M & S*	1 Pot/170g	68.0	0.0	40	4.3	5.8	0.1	0.5
Rich & Creamy, Spelga*	1 Serving/150g	187.0	7.0	125	3.7	17.2	4.7	0.1
Sheep's Milk, Total, Fage*	1 Pot/200g	180.0	12.0	90	4.8	4.3	6.0	0.0
Smooth Vanilla, Eat Smart, Safeway*	1 Pot/125g	69.0	0.0	55	5.0	8.3	0.1	0.0
Soya, Peach, Dairy Free, Organic, Yofu, Provamel*	1 Serving/125g	100.0	3.0	80	3.9	10.3	2.2	0.8
Soya, Plain, Average	*1oz/28g*	*20.0*	*1.0*	*72*	*5.0*	*3.9*	*4.2*	*0.0*
Soya, Red Cherry, Dairy Free, Organic, Yofu, Provamel*	1 Pot/125g	101.0	3.0	81	3.9	10.5	2.2	0.8
Spanish Orange, Amore Luxury, Muller*	1 Pot/150g	226.0	12.0	151	2.9	17.2	7.8	0.1
Spiced Apple, 6% Fat, TTD, Sainsbury's*	1 Pot/15g	16.0	1.0	107	2.7	15.6	3.8	0.5
Spiced Orange, Dessert, Low Fat, Sainsbury's*	1 Pot/125g	121.0	2.0	97	4.5	16.0	1.7	0.1
Sticky Toffee Pudding, Dessert Style, Mullerlight, Muller*	1 Pot/175g	108.0	0.0	62	4.4	9.9	0.2	0.2
Strawberries & Cream, 0.06% Fat, TTD, Sainsbury's*	1 Pot/150g	183.0	8.0	122	3.5	14.7	5.5	0.4
Strawberries & Cream, Finest, Tesco*	1 Pot/150g	205.0	10.0	137	3.4	15.4	6.9	0.5
Strawberry & Cornish Clotted Cream, M & S*	1 Pot/150g	217.0	12.0	145	3.2	15.4	7.7	0.5
Strawberry & French Vanilla, Amore Luxury, Muller*	1 Pot/150g	225.0	12.0	150	2.9	17.0	7.8	0.1
Strawberry & Raspberry, HL, Tesco*	1 Pot/125g	57.0	1.0	46	4.2	7.0	0.1	0.0
Strawberry & Raspberry, Low Fat, Sainsbury's*	1 Pot/125g	109.0	2.0	87	4.2	14.3	1.4	0.2
Strawberry & Raspberry, Probiotic, Organic, Yeo Valley*	1 Pot/125g	125.0	5.0	100	4.2	12.0	3.9	0.1
Strawberry & Rhubarb, Channel Island, M & S*	1 Pot/150g	157.0	4.0	105	3.9	15.4	3.0	0.0
Strawberry & Rhubarb, Low Fat, Sainsbury's*	1 Pot/125g	107.0	2.0	86	4.2	14.1	1.4	0.2
Strawberry & Rhubarb, Onken*	1 Serving/100g	85.0	0.0	85	4.6	16.2	0.1	0.4
Strawberry Crumble, Crunch Corner, Muller*	1 Pot/150g	234.0	8.0	156	3.6	22.9	5.6	0.5
Strawberry Orange Balls. Crunch Corner, Muller*	1 Pot/150g	222.0	8.0	148	4.0	20.8	5.4	0.2
Strawberry Shortcake, Crunch Corner, Muller*	1 Pot/150g	231.0	9.0	154	3.9	21.0	5.7	0.1
Strawberry, & Muesli, Breakfast, Tesco*	1 Pot/170g	192.0	5.0	113	4.1	17.9	2.8	0.5
Strawberry, & Whole Grain, Bio Break, Tesco*	1 Pot/175g	175.0	2.0	100	4.7	17.8	1.1	0.2
Strawberry, Amore for Me, Muller*	1 Pot/150g	216.0	11.0	144	2.6	17.0	7.3	0.2
Strawberry, Bettabuy, Morrisons*	1 Pot/115g	91.0	1.0	79	4.4	12.8	1.3	0.3

YOGHURT

	Measure INFO/WEIGHT	per Measure KCAL	FAT	Nutrition Values per 100g / 100ml KCAL	PROT	CARB	FAT	FIBRE
Strawberry, BGTY, Sainsbury's*	1 Pot/125g	64.0	0.0	51	4.8	7.7	0.1	1.2
Strawberry, Bio Activia, Danone*	1 Pot/125g	117.0	4.0	94	3.5	12.8	3.2	2.0
Strawberry, Bio, Granola, Corner, Muller*	1 Pot/135g	161.0	4.0	119	5.5	17.8	2.6	0.8
Strawberry, Carb Control, Tesco*	1 Pot/125g	61.0	1.0	49	3.7	6.3	1.0	0.2
Strawberry, Cereals, Fibre, Bio Activia, Danone*	1 Pot/120g	113.0	4.0	94	3.7	12.7	3.2	3.0
Strawberry, Custard Style, Shapers, Boots*	1 Pot/150g	117.0	1.0	78	3.9	14.0	0.7	0.5
Strawberry, Eat Smart, Morrisons*	1 Pot/200g	116.0	1.0	58	5.7	8.5	0.3	0.3
Strawberry, Everyday Low Fat, Co-Op*	1 Pot/125g	87.0	1.0	70	3.0	13.0	0.7	0.0
Strawberry, Farmhouse, BGTY, Sainsbury's*	1 Pot/150g	106.0	1.0	71	3.2	13.7	0.4	0.5
Strawberry, Fat Free, Average	1 Serving/100g	66.0	0.0	66	4.9	11.1	0.1	0.6
Strawberry, Fruit Corner, Snack Size, Muller*	1 Pot/95g	108.0	4.0	114	3.9	15.6	4.0	0.4
Strawberry, Fruit 'n' Creamy, Ubley*	1 Pot/151g	167.0	4.0	111	4.3	16.9	2.9	0.3
Strawberry, Fruity, Mullerlight, Muller*	1 Pot/200g	102.0	0.0	51	4.1	7.9	0.1	0.0
Strawberry, Granose*	1 Pot/120g	108.0	2.0	90	4.5	15.5	1.6	0.0
Strawberry, Great Stuff, Asda*	1 Pot/60g	58.0	1.0	97	4.7	14.0	2.5	0.5
Strawberry, Happy Shopper*	1 Pot/150g	130.0	0.0	87	3.0	18.5	0.3	0.0
Strawberry, Healthy Balance, Corner, Muller*	1 Pot/135g	161.0	4.0	119	5.4	17.9	2.6	0.8
Strawberry, Light & Refreshing, Campina*	1 Pot/125g	110.0	1.0	88	2.5	16.9	1.1	0.0
Strawberry, Little Town Dairy*	1 Pot/125g	82.0	2.0	66	2.9	9.9	1.6	0.0
Strawberry, Live, Turners Dairies*	1 Pot/125g	86.0	0.0	69	4.9	11.9	0.3	0.0
Strawberry, Low Fat, Average	1 Serving/100g	81.0	1.0	81	4.5	13.6	1.0	0.2
Strawberry, Luscious, Shapers, Boots*	1 Pot/150g	82.0	2.0	55	4.0	7.3	1.1	0.6
Strawberry, Organic, Yeo Valley*	1 Pot/150g	144.0	5.0	96	4.3	12.4	3.3	0.1
Strawberry, Perfectly Balanced, Waitrose*	1 Pot/150g	136.0	0.0	91	4.6	17.8	0.1	0.1
Strawberry, Petit Filou, Yoplait*	1 Pot/60g	62.0	2.0	104	6.6	12.6	2.9	0.2
Strawberry, Probiotic, Natural Balance, Asda*	1 Pot/125g	109.0	3.0	87	3.1	13.3	2.4	2.4
Strawberry, Probiotic, Organic, Yeo Valley*	1 Pot/125g	125.0	5.0	100	4.4	11.7	4.0	0.1
Strawberry, Redcurrant, Bio Layered, Sainsbury's*	1 Serving/125g	134.0	3.0	107	4.1	16.5	2.7	0.2
Strawberry, Smooth Set French, Low Fat, Sainsbury's*	1 Pot/125g	112.0	4.0	90	3.7	11.8	3.2	0.0
Strawberry, Smooth, Activ8, Ski, Nestle*	1 Pot/120g	113.0	2.0	94	4.6	14.8	1.7	0.7
Strawberry, Soya, Dairy Free, Organic, Yofu, Provamel*	1 Pot/125g	101.0	3.0	81	3.9	10.6	2.2	0.8
Strawberry, Soyage, GranoVita*	1 Pot/145g	112.0	1.0	77	1.8	16.5	0.4	0.0
Strawberry, Thick & Creamy, Co-Op*	1 Pot/150g	181.0	7.0	121	3.6	16.4	4.6	0.1
Strawberry, Thick & Creamy, Waitrose*	1 Pot/125g	135.0	3.0	108	3.7	17.6	2.5	0.4
Strawberry, Thick & Fruity, Fat Free, Weight Watchers*	1 Pot/120g	48.0	0.0	40	4.1	5.7	0.1	0.5
Strawberry, Thick & Fruity, Probiotic, COU, M & S*	1 Pot/170g	76.0	0.0	45	4.1	7.3	0.1	0.4
Strawberry, Very Berry, Activ8, Ski, Nestle*	1 Pot/120g	110.0	2.0	92	4.3	15.0	1.7	0.3
Strawberry, Virtually Fat Free, Average	1 Serving/100g	65.0	0.0	65	4.7	11.3	0.2	0.2
Strawberry, Wholemilk, Organic, Sainsbury's*	1 Pot/150g	123.0	5.0	82	3.5	9.2	3.5	0.1
Strawberry, Yoplait*	1 Pot/125g	61.0	0.0	49	4.2	7.6	0.2	0.9
Summer Fruits, Cool Country*	1 Serving/150g	136.0	2.0	91	3.0	16.3	1.5	0.0
Summer Fruits, Greek Style, Corner, Muller*	1 Pot/165g	181.0	5.0	110	5.0	15.0	3.0	0.5
Summer Fruits, Light, Spelga*	1 Pot/175g	79.0	0.0	45	4.4	7.1	0.2	0.0
Summer Selection, Fat Free, Organic, Yeo Valley*	1 Pot/125g	89.0	0.0	71	5.2	12.3	0.1	0.2
Summer Selection, Thick & Fruity, COU, M & S*	1 Pot/145g	75.0	0.0	52	4.2	7.8	0.1	0.5
Summerfruits Bio, Boots*	1 Pot/150g	139.0	4.0	93	4.1	13.0	2.7	0.4
Summerfruits, Fat Free, Bio Live, Rachel's Organic*	1 Pot/125g	120.0	2.0	96	4.7	15.3	1.8	0.0
Timperley Rhubarb, Seriously Fruity, Waitrose*	1 Pot/150g	127.0	1.0	85	4.6	14.4	1.0	0.0
Timperley Rhubarb, TTD, Sainsbury's*	1 Pot/150g	168.0	7.0	112	3.4	13.6	4.9	0.4
Toffee Apple, COU, M & S*	1 Pot/200g	90.0	0.0	45	4.2	6.3	0.2	0.2
Toffee Flavour, Bio, Virtually Fat Free, Morrisons*	1 Serving/150g	82.0	0.0	55	5.3	8.1	0.2	0.0
Toffee Fudge, Low Fat, Sainsbury's*	1 Pot/125g	146.0	2.0	117	4.3	20.4	2.0	0.0
Toffee Hoops, Crunch Corner, Muller*	1 Pot/150g	232.0	8.0	155	4.0	22.6	5.5	0.2

Y

YOGHURT

	Measure INFO/WEIGHT	per Measure KCAL	FAT	Nutrition Values per 100g / 100ml KCAL	PROT	CARB	FAT	FIBRE
Toffee, Benecol*	1 Pot/125g	124.0	1.0	99	3.8	19.3	0.7	0.0
Toffee, Childrens, Co-Op*	1 Pot/125g	142.0	3.0	114	3.6	18.6	2.8	0.0
Toffee, COU, M & S*	1 Pot/145g	65.0	0.0	45	4.2	7.7	0.2	0.0
Toffee, Economy, Sainsbury's*	1 Pot/126g	91.0	1.0	72	3.0	12.8	1.0	0.0
Toffee, Light, HL, Tesco*	1 Pot/200g	80.0	0.0	40	3.9	5.9	0.1	1.0
Toffee, Live Bio, Perfectly Balanced, Waitrose*	1 Pot/150g	156.0	0.0	104	4.2	21.1	0.3	0.0
Toffee, Low Fat, Co-Op*	1 Pot/150g	124.0	1.0	83	3.8	15.0	0.9	0.2
Toffee, Low Fat, M & S*	1 Pot/150g	180.0	3.0	120	4.9	21.6	1.7	0.0
Toffee, Seriously Smooth, Low Fat, Waitrose*	1 Pot/150g	156.0	3.0	104	4.7	16.5	2.1	0.1
Toffee, Smooth & Creamy, Fat Free, Weight Watchers*	1 Pot/120g	48.0	0.0	40	3.9	5.9	0.1	0.8
Toffee, Smooth, Mullerlight, Fat Free, Muller*	1 Pot/200g	100.0	0.0	50	4.0	7.7	0.1	0.0
Toffee, Virtually Fat Free, Boots*	1 Pot/125g	69.0	0.0	55	5.1	8.3	0.1	0.0
Totally Vanilla, Low Fat, Asda*	1 Pot/150g	133.0	2.0	89	4.7	15.1	1.1	0.0
Treacle Toffee, Dessert, Low Fat, Sainsbury's*	1 Pot/125g	149.0	2.0	119	4.3	21.2	1.9	0.0
Tropical Crunch, Healthy Balance, Fruit Corner, Muller*	1 Pot/150g	169.0	3.0	113	4.7	18.2	2.1	0.5
Tropical Fruit, Bio, Granola, Corner, Muller*	1 Pot/135g	161.0	3.0	119	5.4	18.2	2.4	0.6
Tropical Fruit, Greek Style, Asda*	1 Pot/125g	170.0	9.0	136	3.3	15.0	7.0	0.0
Tropical Fruit, Greek Style, Shapers, Boots*	1 Pot/150g	100.0	2.0	67	3.6	9.8	1.5	0.8
Tropical Fruit, HL, Tesco*	1 Serving/125g	56.0	0.0	45	4.1	6.6	0.2	0.9
Tropical, Luscious, Low Fat, Rachel's Organic*	1 Pot/125g	115.0	2.0	92	4.0	15.3	1.6	0.0
Valencia Orange, Layered, Bio, GFY, Asda*	1 Pot/125g	80.0	0.0	64	3.7	12.0	0.1	0.0
Valencia Orange, Seriously Fruity, Low Fat, Waitrose*	1 Pot/150g	147.0	1.0	98	4.3	18.0	1.0	0.3
Vanilla & Chocolate, Muller*	1 Pot/165g	86.0	1.0	52	4.0	7.2	0.5	0.1
Vanilla & Pineapple, Nestle*	1 Pot/125g	120.0	2.0	96	4.2	16.7	1.5	0.0
Vanilla Choco Balls, Crunch Corner, Muller*	1 Pot/150g	228.0	7.0	152	4.0	22.0	5.0	0.2
Vanilla Flavour, Healthy Living, Light, Tesco*	1 Pot/200g	90.0	0.0	45	4.1	7.0	0.1	0.0
Vanilla Flavour, Organic, Low Fat, Tesco*	1 Pot/125g	114.0	1.0	91	5.3	15.3	1.0	0.0
Vanilla Toffee, Low Fat, Sainsbury's*	1 Pot/125g	145.0	2.0	116	4.3	20.6	1.8	0.0
Vanilla, Average	1 Serving/120g	100.0	5.0	83	4.5	12.4	4.5	0.8
Vanilla, BGTY, Sainsbury's*	1 Pot/200g	98.0	0.0	49	4.5	7.5	0.1	0.0
Vanilla, Bio, BFY, Morrisons*	1 Pot/150g	82.0	0.0	55	5.7	8.4	0.3	0.0
Vanilla, Chocolate, & Black Cherry, Mullerlight, Muller*	1 Pot/165g	97.0	1.0	59	3.1	10.3	0.4	0.3
Vanilla, Creamy, Smarties, Nestle*	1 Pot/120g	200.0	7.0	167	4.1	23.7	6.2	0.0
Vanilla, Fat Free, Onken*	1 Serving/150g	73.0	0.0	49	4.7	7.3	0.1	0.1
Vanilla, Live Bio, Low Fat, Perfectly Balanced, Waitrose*	1 Pot/150g	114.0	0.0	76	4.1	14.7	0.1	0.0
Vanilla, Live, Bio, Bio Green Dairy*	1 Bottle/250ml	262.0	7.0	105	2.5	17.7	2.9	0.0
Vanilla, Low Fat, Bio, Sainsbury's*	1 Pot/150g	147.0	2.0	98	4.8	17.2	1.1	0.0
Vanilla, Low Fat, Probiotic, Organic, M & S*	1 Serving/100g	85.0	2.0	85	6.2	10.9	1.8	0.0
Vanilla, Low Fat, Safeway*	1 Pot/150g	154.0	2.0	103	4.6	18.7	1.1	0.0
Vanilla, Low Fat, Tesco*	1 Pot/125g	125.0	2.0	100	4.9	16.3	1.7	0.0
Vanilla, Organic, Low Fat, Sainsbury's*	1 Pot/125g	114.0	1.0	91	5.3	15.3	1.0	0.0
Vanilla, Organic, Probiotic, Fat Free, Yeo Valley*	1 Pot/500g	400.0	0.0	80	5.4	14.2	0.1	0.0
Vanilla, Smooth & Creamy, Fat Free, Weight Watchers*	1 Pot/120g	50.0	0.0	42	3.9	6.5	0.1	0.1
Vanilla, Smooth, Light, Fat Free, Muller*	1 Pot/200g	100.0	0.0	50	4.3	7.2	0.1	0.0
Vanilla, Soya, Dairy Free, Organic, Yofu, Provamel*	1 Pot/125g	114.0	3.0	91	3.8	13.3	2.2	0.7
Vanilla, Thick & Creamy, Channel Island, M & S*	1 Pot/150g	187.0	7.0	125	4.5	17.5	4.4	1.0
Vanilla, Thick & Creamy, Probiotic, COU, M & S*	1 Pot/170g	76.0	0.0	45	4.5	6.3	0.1	0.5
Vanilla, Virtually Fat Free, Shapers, Boots*	1 Pot/125g	66.0	0.0	53	5.0	7.9	0.1	0.0
Vanilla, Virtually Fat Free, Yeo Valley*	1 Pot/150g	121.0	0.0	81	5.1	15.0	0.1	0.0
Walnut & Greek Honey, Amore Luxury, Muller*	1 Pot/150g	241.0	13.0	161	3.0	17.6	8.7	0.1
White Peach, Seriously Fruity, Waitrose*	1 Pot/150g	151.0	3.0	101	4.8	16.5	1.7	0.2
Wholegrain, Lite, Fig, Date & Grape, Biopot, Onken*	¼ Pot/120g	102.0	0.0	85	4.8	16.0	0.2	1.0
Wholegrain, Lite, Summer Berries, Biopot, Onken*	¼ Pot/120g	100.0	0.0	83	4.6	15.8	0.2	1.4

	Measure INFO/WEIGHT	per Measure KCAL	FAT	Nutrition Values per 100g / 100ml KCAL	PROT	CARB	FAT	FIBRE
YOGHURT								
Wholegrain, Peach, Biopot, Onken*	1 Serving/100g	113.0	3.0	113	4.2	17.9	2.7	0.3
Wholegrain, Strawberry, Biopot, Onken*	1 Serving/100g	109.0	3.0	109	4.2	16.9	2.7	0.3
Wholemilk, Organic, M & S*	1 Pot/454ml	409.0	16.0	90	6.1	7.4	3.6	0.0
Wholemilk, with Maple Syrup, Bio Live, Rachel's Organic*	1 Pot/142g	139.0	5.0	98	3.5	13.0	3.5	0.0
Wicked Wholemilk Vanilla, Bio Live, Rachel's Organic*	1 Pot/125g	125.0	4.0	100	5.2	12.1	3.5	0.0
Wild Blackberry, Seriously Fruity, Waitrose*	1 Pot/125g	120.0	1.0	96	4.4	17.2	1.0	0.4
Wild Blueberry, Finest, Tesco*	1 Pot/150g	211.0	10.0	141	3.4	16.6	6.8	0.5
Wild Blueberry, Light, Fat Free, Muller*	1 Pot/200g	94.0	0.0	47	4.1	6.9	0.1	0.7
Winter Medley, COU, M & S*	1 Pot/150g	67.0	0.0	45	4.2	6.2	0.1	0.1
with Large Fruit Chunks, Bio, Waitrose*	1 Serving/170g	170.0	4.0	100	3.7	15.8	2.4	0.4
Yellow Fruit, Yoplait*	1 Pot/125g	139.0	4.0	111	3.3	18.0	2.9	0.0
Zesty Lemon, Intensley Creamy, Activia, Danone*	1 Pot/120g	119.0	4.0	99	4.8	13.3	3.0	0.1
YOGHURT DRINK								
Actimel, Mixed Fruit, Danone*	1 Bottle/100ml	88.0	1.0	88	2.7	16.0	1.5	0.0
Actimel, Multi Fruit, Danone*	1 Bottle/100g	85.0	1.0	85	2.7	14.4	1.5	0.1
Actimel, Orange, Danone*	1 Bottle/100g	74.0	1.0	74	2.9	11.5	1.5	0.0
Actimel, Original, 0.1% Fat, Danone*	1 Bottle/100g	28.0	0.0	28	2.8	3.3	0.1	1.9
Actimel, Original, Danone*	1 Bottle/100g	80.0	2.0	80	2.8	12.8	1.6	0.0
Actimel, Pineapple, 0.1% Fat, Danone*	1 Bottle/100g	33.0	0.0	33	2.7	5.5	0.0	1.8
Actimel, Strawberry, Danone*	1 Bottle/100g	74.0	1.0	74	2.9	11.5	1.5	0.0
Average	1fl oz/30ml	19.0	0.0	62	3.1	13.1	0.0	0.0
Ayran, Gazi*	1 Can/330ml	34.0	2.0	10	0.5	0.8	0.6	0.0
Banana & Honey, Ski Up & Go, Nestle*	1 Bottle/250g	215.0	2.0	86	0.0	16.0	0.9	0.0
Bioactive, Yagua*	1 Bottle/200ml	84.0	0.0	42	0.4	9.9	0.0	0.0
Blueberry & Blackcurrant, Orchard Maid*	1 Carton/250ml	147.0	0.0	59	1.6	13.6	0.0	0.0
Blueberry, Low Fat, Prebiotic and Probiotic, Muller*	1 Pot/100g	66.0	1.0	66	2.6	10.3	1.4	2.2
Cholesterol Lowering, Asda*	1 Bottle/100g	76.0	1.0	76	2.9	13.0	1.4	1.0
Danacol, Original, Danone*	1 Bottle/100ml	64.0	1.0	64	3.2	10.0	1.0	0.0
Danacol, Strawberry, Danone*	1 Bottle/100g	68.0	1.0	68	3.2	11.2	1.2	0.0
Light, Benecol*	1 Bottle/67.5g	40.0	1.0	60	2.8	7.3	2.1	0.1
Light, Yakult*	1 Bottle/65ml	27.0	0.0	42	1.4	10.2	0.0	1.8
Mixed Berry, Up & Go, Ski, Nestle*	1 Bottle/250g	217.0	2.0	87	3.1	16.0	0.9	0.2
Nectarine, Pfirsich, Light, Bifidus, Emmi*	1 Serving/500ml	245.0	4.0	49	3.0	7.5	0.8	0.0
Omega 3 Plus, Raspberry, Pro Biotic, Flora*	1 Bottle/100g	58.0	2.0	58	2.6	8.5	1.6	0.0
Orange, Banana & Passion Fruit, One a Day, Muller*	1 Bottle/310ml	208.0	0.0	67	2.1	14.1	0.1	0.0
Orchard Maid*	1 Serving/250g	147.0	0.0	59	1.6	13.0	0.0	0.0
Original, Benecol*	1 Serving/70g	62.0	2.0	88	2.6	14.2	2.3	0.0
Peach & Apricot, Benecol*	1 Bottle/67.5g	38.0	1.0	56	2.8	6.2	2.2	0.0
Peach & Mango, Fristi*	1 Carton/330g	191.0	0.0	58	2.6	13.6	0.1	0.0
Pro Activ, Orange, Cholesterol, Flora*	1 Bottle/100g	87.0	3.0	87	2.6	12.5	2.9	0.0
Pro Activ, Original, Blood Pressure, Flora*	1 Bottle/100g	80.0	1.0	80	3.9	12.7	1.5	0.3
Pro Activ, Original, Cholesterol, Flora*	1 Bottle/100g	87.0	3.0	87	2.6	12.5	2.9	0.0
Pro Activ, Strawberry, Blood Pressure, Flora*	1 Bottle/100g	80.0	1.0	80	3.9	12.7	1.5	0.3
Pro Activ, Strawberry, Cholesterol, Flora*	1 Bottle/100g	87.0	3.0	87	2.6	12.5	2.9	0.0
Raspberry & Passion Fruit, Everybody, Yoplait*	1 Bottle/90g	60.0	1.0	67	2.6	12.2	0.9	0.0
Strawberry, Benecol*	1 Bottle/68g	38.0	1.0	56	2.9	6.2	2.2	0.0
Strawberry, Low Fat, Pre & Probiotic, Muller*	1 Pot/100g	67.0	1.0	67	2.5	10.7	1.4	2.4
Strawberry, Yop, Yoplait*	1 Bottle/330g	261.0	4.0	79	2.8	14.0	1.3	0.0
Sveltesse, 0%, Nestle*	1 Pot/125g	61.0	0.0	49	4.8	7.3	0.1	0.1
Yakult*	1 Pot/65ml	51.0	0.0	78	1.4	17.8	0.1	0.0
YORK FRUITS								
Terry's*	1 Sweet/9g	30.0	0.0	328	0.0	81.4	0.0	1.0

Y

	Measure INFO/WEIGHT	per Measure KCAL	FAT	Nutrition Values per 100g / 100ml KCAL	PROT	CARB	FAT	FIBRE
YORKIE								
Honeycomb, Nestle*	1 Bar/65g	331.0	17.0	509	5.7	63.6	25.8	0.0
King Size, Nestle*	1 Bar/83g	445.0	26.0	537	6.1	57.3	31.5	0.0
Original, Nestle*	1 Bar/64.5g	365.0	21.0	537	6.1	57.3	31.5	0.7
Raisin & Biscuit, Nestle*	1 Bar/66.5g	331.0	17.0	497	5.5	59.7	26.2	0.9
YORKSHIRE PUDDING								
3", Baked, Aunt Bessie's*	1 Pudding/36g	91.0	3.0	252	9.0	36.4	7.9	1.7
4 Minute, Aunt Bessie's*	1 Pudding/18g	52.0	2.0	291	10.5	36.6	11.3	2.2
7", Baked, Aunt Bessie's*	1 Pudding/110g	290.0	10.0	264	8.5	37.4	9.0	2.0
Average	1 Pudding/30g	62.0	3.0	208	6.6	24.7	9.9	0.9
Batters, in Foils, Ready to Bake, Frozen, Aunt Bessie's*	1 Pudding/17g	47.0	2.0	276	9.1	32.6	10.8	1.4
Chicken & Vegetable, COU, M & S*	1 Pudding/150g	195.0	3.0	130	12.2	14.3	2.2	1.3
Filled with Beef & Vegetable, Safeway*	1 Pack/300g	396.0	12.0	132	8.6	15.2	4.1	1.3
Filled with Beef, Tesco*	1 Pudding/300g	408.0	16.0	136	6.1	16.2	5.2	1.1
Filled with Chicken, GFY, Asda*	1 Pack/381g	438.0	10.0	115	9.0	14.0	2.6	1.5
Filled with Chicken, Tesco*	1 Pack/300g	366.0	9.0	122	6.5	17.4	2.9	1.3
Filled, with Beef, Morrisons*	1 Serving/350g	514.0	21.0	147	7.4	15.7	6.0	0.5
Filled, with Sausage, Sainsbury's*	1 Pack/300g	576.0	31.0	192	6.9	17.5	10.4	0.9
Frozen, Ovenbaked, Iceland*	1 Pudding/12g	36.0	1.0	290	9.7	45.1	7.9	4.1
Fully Prepared, M & S*	1 Pudding/22g	63.0	3.0	285	9.4	31.6	13.2	1.2
Giant, Aunt Bessie's*	1 Pudding/110g	290.0	10.0	264	8.5	37.4	9.0	2.0
Giant, VLH Kitchens	1 Serving/110g	284.0	11.0	259	8.5	33.6	10.0	2.3
Large, Aunt Bessie's*	1 Pudding/40g	111.0	5.0	277	8.5	35.3	11.4	1.5
Large, Frozen, Co-Op*	1 Pudding/34g	84.0	2.0	250	10.0	36.0	7.0	2.0
Large, The Real Yorkshire Pudding Co*	1 Pudding/34g	103.0	4.0	304	11.5	37.3	12.1	2.5
Made From Batter Mix, Sainsbury's*	1 Pudding/100g	248.0	5.0	248	9.9	40.1	5.3	4.0
Minced Beef Filled, Waitrose*	1 Serving/350g	525.0	25.0	150	7.5	14.1	7.1	1.0
Mini, Co-Op*	1 Serving/16g	50.0	2.0	312	6.2	43.7	12.5	2.5
Mini, Farmfoods*	1 Pudding/3g	8.0	0.0	281	9.6	43.2	7.7	1.9
Premium, Bisto*	1 Pudding/30g	74.0	3.0	248	7.3	30.3	10.9	2.1
Ready Baked, Smart Price, Asda*	1 Pudding/12g	36.0	1.0	297	10.0	44.0	9.0	2.8
Ready to Bake, Aunt Bessie's*	1 Pudding/17g	42.0	1.0	246	8.5	35.1	8.0	1.7
Ready to Bake, Sainsbury's*	1 Pudding/18g	48.0	2.0	263	9.9	35.9	8.9	1.3
Riding Lodge*	1 Pudding/16g	44.0	1.0	276	10.0	41.5	7.8	0.0
Roast Chicken Filled, COU, M & S*	1 Pudding/150g	210.0	4.0	140	12.6	15.7	2.7	0.9
Roberts Bakery*	1 Pudding/18g	48.0	2.0	263	9.9	35.9	8.9	1.3
Safeway*	1 Serving/22g	58.0	2.0	265	8.4	38.9	8.4	2.5
Sage & Onion, Tesco*	1 Pudding/19g	53.0	2.0	280	8.0	35.0	12.0	2.6
Sainsbury's*	1 Pudding/14g	43.0	2.0	309	7.9	37.5	14.1	2.9
Sausage & Onion Gravy Filled, Safeway*	1 Pudding/300g	540.0	28.0	180	6.2	18.0	9.2	1.2
Sausage Filled, Frozen, Tesco*	1 Pack/340g	510.0	20.0	150	6.6	17.8	5.8	1.8
Steak Filled, COU, M & S*	1 Serving/150g	187.0	4.0	125	11.0	14.7	2.5	0.8
The Best, Morrisons*	1 Pudding/22g	60.0	2.0	271	8.3	43.0	8.0	1.6
Traditional Style, Medium, Asda*	1 Pudding/36g	86.0	3.0	241	9.0	31.0	9.0	2.4
Traditional Style, Small, Asda*	1 Pudding/20g	52.0	2.0	262	8.0	35.0	10.0	2.9
Traditional, Giant, Asda*	1 Pudding/110g	310.0	11.0	282	10.0	38.0	10.0	2.3
Unbaked, Iceland*	1 Serving/30.8g	81.0	3.0	263	9.9	35.9	8.9	1.3
Value, Tesco*	1 Pudding/16g	45.0	2.0	282	9.7	34.3	11.8	1.6
YULE LOG								
Chocolate, Sainsbury's*	1/8 Log/49g	186.0	10.0	382	5.1	46.5	19.6	0.7
Christmas Range, Tesco*	1 Serving/30g	131.0	6.0	442	4.9	56.8	21.7	2.8
Mini, M & S*	1 Cake/36g	165.0	8.0	460	5.7	56.9	23.3	1.1

	Measure INFO/WEIGHT	per Measure KCAL	FAT	Nutrition Values per 100g / 100ml KCAL	PROT	CARB	FAT	FIBRE

BAGEL FACTORY

BAGEL

	Measure INFO/WEIGHT	KCAL	FAT	KCAL	PROT	CARB	FAT	FIBRE
Bacon, Bagel Factory*	1 Bagel/100g	613	26.0	613	32.2	62.1	25.9	3.8
Chicken, Tomato & Spinach, Wholemeal, Bagel Factory*	1 Bagel/100g	306	2.0	306	23.0	49.2	1.9	9.1
Salmon & Cream Cheese, Bagel Factory*	1 Serving/300g	515	18.0	172	9.9	19.1	6.1	0.7
with Marmite, Wholemeal, Bagel Factory*	1 Bagel/85g	312	2.0	367	24.4	63.4	1.9	11.6

BURGER KING

5 ALIVE

Berry Blast, Burger King*	1 Serving/250g	62	0.0	25	0.0	6.0	0.0	0.0

APPLE

Fries, Burger King*	1 Serving/60g	28	0.0	47	0.1	12.0	0.1	2.0

BITES

Chicken, Kids, Burger King*	1 Serving/56g	158	7.0	282	16.0	25.0	13.0	2.0

BURGERS

Angus, Burger King*	1 Burger/239g	554	29.0	232	12.0	18.0	12.0	1.0
Angus, Double, Burger King*	1 Burger/323g	795	45.0	246	16.0	14.0	14.0	1.0
Angus, Mini with Cheese, Burger King*	1 Burger/110g	321	15.0	292	15.0	27.0	14.0	1.0
Angus, Mini, Burger King*	1 Burger/97g	272	11.0	280	14.0	31.0	11.0	1.0
Angus, Smoked Bacon & Cheddar, Burger King*	1 Burger/270g	678	38.0	251	14.0	17.0	14.0	1.0
Angus, Smoked Bacon & Cheddar, Double, Burger King*	1 Burger/354g	920	53.0	260	17.0	13.0	15.0	1.0
Bean, Veggie, Kids, Burger King*	1 Burger/116g	278	7.0	240	6.0	42.0	6.0	3.0
Big King, Burger King*	1 Burger/190g	503	27.0	265	15.0	17.0	14.0	1.0
Big King, XL, Burger King*	1 Burger/338g	902	54.0	267	16.0	14.0	16.0	1.0
BK, Veggie Bean Burger, Burger King*	1 Burger/280g	588	20.0	210	6.0	30.0	7.0	3.0
Cheeseburger, Bacon Double, Burger King*	1 Burger/160g	478	26.0	299	19.0	19.0	16.0	1.0
Cheeseburger, Bacon Double, Extra Large, Burger King*	1 Burger/302g	927	54.0	307	21.0	15.0	18.0	1.0
Cheeseburger, Burger King*	1 Burger/123g	320	14.0	260	13.0	25.0	11.0	1.0
Cheeseburger, Double, Burger King*	1 Burger/173g	465	22.0	269	17.0	18.0	13.0	1.0
Cheeseburger, Kids, Burger King*	1 Burger/113g	318	14.0	281	14.0	27.0	12.0	1.0
Chicken Royale, Burger King*	1 Burger/210g	607	31.0	289	11.0	25.0	15.0	1.0
Chicken Royale, Sweet Chilli, Burger King*	1 Burger/210g	542	23.0	258	11.0	28.0	11.0	1.0
Chicken Royale, with Cheese, Burger King*	1 Burger/263g	695	39.0	264	10.6	20.9	14.8	0.4
Chicken, Chargrilled, Mini, Burger King*	1 Burger/109g	214	3.0	196	15.0	28.0	3.0	1.0
Chicken, Piri Piri, Sandwich, Burger King*	1 Sandwich/196g	335	6.0	171	13.0	21.0	3.0	1.0
Hamburger, Burger King*	1 Burger/110g	275	9.0	250	13.0	28.0	8.0	1.0
Hamburger, Kids, Burger King*	1 Serving/100g	272	9.0	272	14.0	31.0	9.0	1.0
Ocean Catch, Burger King*	1 Burger/188g	494	26.0	263	9.0	23.0	14.0	1.0
Whopper, Burger King*	1 Burger/274g	633	36.0	231	11.0	18.0	13.0	1.0
Whopper, Double, Burger King*	1 Burger/355g	877	53.0	247	14.0	14.0	15.0	1.0
Whopper, Double, with Cheese, Burger King*	1 Burger/380g	961	61.0	253	14.0	13.0	16.0	1.0
Whopper, Junior, Burger King*	1 Burger/148g	343	16.0	232	9.0	21.0	11.0	1.0
Whopper, with Cheese, Burger King*	1 Burger/299g	721	42.0	241	11.0	16.0	14.0	1.0
Whopper, with Cheese, Junior, Burger King*	1 Burger/161g	388	19.0	241	10.0	19.0	12.0	1.0

BUTTY

Bacon & Egg, with Heinz Ketchup, Burger King*	1 Butty/140g	362	17.0	259	12.9	25.0	12.1	11.4
Bacon & Egg, with HP Sauce, Burger King*	1 Butty/140g	363	17.0	259	12.9	25.0	12.1	1.4
Bacon, with Heinz Ketchup, Burger King*	1 Butty/77g	221	6.0	287	13.0	41.6	7.8	2.6
Bacon, with HP Sauce, Burger King*	1 Butty/77g	222	6.0	288	13.0	41.6	7.8	2.0
Big Breakfast, with Heinz Ketchup, Burger King*	1 Butty/297g	849	50.0	286	14.0	18.0	17.0	1.0
Big Breakfast, with HP Sauce, Burger King*	1 Butty/297g	852	50.0	287	14.0	18.0	17.0	1.0
Egg & Cheese, with Heinz Ketchup, Burger King*	1 Butty/126g	300	18.0	238	10.3	27.0	14.0	1.6
Egg & Cheese, with HP Sauce, Burger King*	1 Butty/126g	301	13.0	239	10.3	27.0	10.3	1.6
Sausage & Egg, with HP Sauce, Burger King*	1 Butty/182g	454	24.0	249	13.2	19.2	13.2	1.1
Sausage, Cumberland & Egg, with Ketchup, Burger King*	1 Butty/243g	668	39.0	275	11.0	21.0	16.0	1.0

	Measure INFO/WEIGHT	per Measure KCAL	per Measure FAT	Nutrition Values per 100g / 100ml KCAL	PROT	CARB	FAT	FIBRE

BURGER KING

BUTTY
	Measure INFO/WEIGHT	KCAL	FAT	KCAL	PROT	CARB	FAT	FIBRE
Sausage, with Heinz Ketchup, Burger King*	1 Butty/119g	312	13.0	262	13.4	26.9	10.9	1.7
Sausage, with HP Sauce, Burger King*	1 Butty/119g	313	13.0	263	13.4	26.9	10.9	1.7

CHICKEN
Bites, Burger King*	14 Bites/112g	317	15.0	283	16.1	25.0	13.4	0.9

COFFEE
Black, Large, Burger King*	1 Serving/284ml	6	0.0	2	0.0	0.0	0.0	0.0
Black, Regular, Burger King*	1 Reg/200ml	4	0.0	2	0.0	0.0	0.0	0.0
Cappuccino, Large, Burger King*	1 Lge Serving/59g	81	3.0	137	10.0	15.0	5.0	0.0
Cappuccino, Regular, Burger King*	1 Reg Serving/46g	64	2.0	139	9.0	15.0	4.0	0.0
Latte, Large, Burger King*	1 Reg Serving/45g	60	2.0	133	11.0	13.0	4.0	0.0
Latte, Regular, Burger King*	1 Lge Serving/62g	82	3.0	132	10.0	15.0	5.0	0.0

COLA
Coca-Cola, Burger King*	1 Reg/400g	168	0.0	42	0.0	11.0	0.0	0.0
Coca-Cola, Small, Burger King*	1 Sm/300g	126	0.0	42	0.0	11.0	0.0	0.0
Coke, Diet, Burger King*	1 Reg/400g	4	0.0	1	0.0	0.0	0.0	0.0
Coke, Diet, Small, Burger King*	1 Sm/300g	3	0.0	1	0.0	0.0	0.0	0.0

DIP POT
Barbeque Sauce, Heinz, Burger King*	1 Serving/40g	48	0.0	120	0.1	28.0	0.1	0.1
Sweet Chilli, Heinz, Burger King*	1 Pot/40g	96	0.0	240	0.0	60.0	0.0	0.0

DRESSING
French, Burger King*	1 Sachet/40g	7	0.0	17	0.0	2.5	0.0	0.0
Honey & Mustard, Burger King*	1 Sachet/40g	32	1.0	80	2.5	15.0	2.5	0.0

FANTA
Orange, Burger King*	1 Reg/400g	156	0.0	39	0.1	10.0	0.1	0.0
Orange, Small, Burger King*	1 Sm/300g	117	0.0	39	0.1	10.0	0.1	0.0

FRIES
Large, Burger King*	1 Serving/141g	381	18.0	270	3.0	38.0	13.0	4.0
Regular, Burger King*	1 Reg/111g	300	16.0	270	3.0	39.0	14.0	4.0
Small, Burger King*	1 Serving/74g	200	10.0	270	3.0	38.0	14.0	4.0
Super, Burger King*	1 Serving/174g	470	23.0	270	3.0	39.0	13.0	4.0

HASH BROWNS
Large, Burger King*	1 Serving/130g	403	27.0	310	3.0	27.0	21.0	4.0
Regular, Burger King*	1 Serving/102g	316	22.0	310	3.0	27.0	22.0	4.0

KETCHUP
Heinz, Sachet, Burger King*	1 Sachet/10g	10	0.0	100	0.1	20.0	0.1	0.1

MAYONNAISE
Heinz, Sachet, Burger King*	1 Sachet/12g	80	9.0	667	0.0	0.0	75.0	0.0

MILK
Semi Skimmed, Kids, Burger King*	1 Carton/258g	117	4.0	47	3.5	4.6	1.5	0.0

MILK SHAKE
Chocolate, Large, Burger King*	1 Serving/519g	612	10.0	118	3.0	22.0	2.0	0.0
Chocolate, Regular, Burger King*	1 Serving/401g	449	8.0	112	3.0	20.0	2.0	0.1
Chocolate, Small, Burger King*	1 Serving/276g	301	8.0	109	3.0	19.0	3.0	0.1
Strawberry, Large, Burger King*	1 Serving/519g	581	10.0	112	3.0	20.0	2.0	0.0
Strawberry, Regular, Burger King*	1 Serving/401g	433	8.0	108	3.0	19.0	2.0	0.0
Strawberry, Small, Burger King*	1 Serving/276g	293	8.0	106	3.0	18.0	3.0	0.0
Vanilla, Burger King*	1 Serving/124g	124	4.0	100	3.0	16.0	3.0	0.0

ONION RINGS
Large, Burger King*	1 Large/190g	697	36.0	367	6.3	43.2	18.9	4.7
Regular, Burger King*	1 Reg/126g	462	24.0	367	6.3	42.9	19.0	4.8
Super, Burger King*	1 Serving/253g	929	48.0	367	6.3	43.1	19.0	4.7

	Measure INFO/WEIGHT	per Measure KCAL	FAT	Nutrition Values per 100g / 100ml KCAL	PROT	CARB	FAT	FIBRE
BURGER KING								
SALAD								
Chicken, Flame Grilled, Burger King*	1 Salad/240g	127	2.0	53	8.0	3.0	1.0	1.0
Chicken, Flame Grilled, with Dressing, Burger King*	1 Serving/280g	134	3.0	48	7.0	3.0	1.0	1.0
Garden, Burger King*	1 Serving/165g	33	2.0	20	1.0	4.0	1.0	1.0
SPRITE								
Burger King*	1 Reg/400g	148	0.0	37	0.0	9.0	0.0	0.0
TEA								
Regular, White, No Sugar, Burger King*	1 Reg/200ml	22	4.0	11	1.0	1.0	2.0	0.0
CAFFE NERO								
BARS								
Chocolate & Hazelnut, Caffe Nero*	1 Bar/40g	229	15.0	572	8.0	49.5	38.0	1.8
Chocolate, Milk, Caffe Nero*	1 Bar/40g	223	14.0	558	8.0	55.0	34.0	1.0
Fruit & Seed, Caffe Nero*	1 Bar/65g	197	6.0	303	7.5	48.2	8.9	8.7
Granola, Organic, Caffe Nero*	1 Bar/64g	275	13.0	429	6.5	53.7	20.9	4.6
BISCOTTI								
Almond, Organic, Caffe Nero*	1 Pack/52g	202	8.0	388	9.2	53.1	15.3	2.8
BROWNIE								
Chocolate, Belgian, Brownie, Caffe Nero*	1 Brownie/74g	313	15.0	419	4.6	54.6	19.6	2.9
Chocolate, Double, Organic, Gluten Free, Caffe Nero*	1 Brownie/78g	331	16.0	425	4.3	55.4	20.7	2.0
CAKE								
Carrot & Raisin, Slice, Organic, Caffe Nero*	1 Slice/70g	290	18.0	414	4.5	43.4	25.0	3.9
Chocolate Fudge, Caffe Nero*	1 Serving/143g	615	32.0	430	5.3	51.8	22.4	1.3
Lemon Drizzle, Slice, Organic, Caffe Nero*	1 Pack/70g	248	11.0	354	4.2	48.5	15.9	0.8
Passion, Caffe Nero*	1 Slice/125g	518	32.0	414	4.4	42.2	25.3	0.7
CHEESE TWISTS								
Caffe Nero*	1 Serving/76g	316	18.0	416	13.4	36.1	24.2	2.6
CHOCOLATE								
Coin, Caffe Nero*	1 Serving/25g	129	7.0	516	6.3	59.7	27.8	2.1
COFFEE								
Cappuccino, Semi Skimmed Milk, Regular, Caffe Nero*	1 Cup/80g	37	1.0	46	3.5	4.7	1.7	0.0
Cappuccino, Skimmed Milk, Regular, Caffe Nero*	1 Regular/80g	27	0.0	34	3.5	4.8	0.3	0.0
Cappuccino, Soya Milk, Regular, Caffe Nero*	1 Serving/80g	36	2.0	45	3.7	2.5	2.2	0.6
Latte, Caramel, Semi Skimmed Milk, Caffe Nero*	1 Latte/421ml	484	25.0	115	2.3	12.3	6.0	0.0
Latte, Chai, Semi Skimmed Milk, Caffe Nero*	1 Serving/405ml	283	11.0	70	3.8	8.3	2.6	0.0
Latte, Chai, Skimmed Milk, Caffe Nero*	1 Serving/405ml	239	5.0	59	3.8	8.4	1.3	0.0
Latte, Frappe, Semi Skimmed, Caffe Nero*	1 Serving/538ml	302	5.0	56	2.6	9.6	0.9	0.0
Latte, Frappe, Skimmed Milk, Caffe Nero*	1 Serving/533g	277	1.0	52	2.6	10.3	0.2	0.0
Latte, Iced, Caffe Nero*	1 Latte/488g	117	4.0	24	1.8	2.5	0.9	0.0
Latte, Semi Skimmed Milk, Caffe Nero*	1 Regular/150g	69	3.0	46	3.5	4.7	1.7	0.0
Latte, Skimmed Milk, Regular, Caffe Nero*	1 Regular/150g	51	0.0	34	3.5	4.8	0.3	0.0
Latte, Soya Milk, Regular, Caffe Nero*	1 Cup/151g	68	3.0	45	3.7	2.5	2.2	0.6
Mocha, Whipped Cream, SS Milk, Caffe Nero*	1 Cup/180ml	326	19.0	181	4.3	17.2	10.8	0.8
Mocha, White Chocolate, SS Milk, Caffe Nero*	1 Serving/400ml	412	25.0	103	2.4	6.1	6.3	0.0
COFFEE BEANS								
Chocolate Coated, Caffe Nero*	1 Serving/25g	117	7.0	469	8.5	50.0	26.2	11.9
COOKIES								
Chocolate Chip, Organic, Caffe Nero*	1 Cookie/60g	263	12.0	438	4.5	56.6	20.1	1.5
Milk Chocolate Chunk, Caffe Nero*	1 Cookie/71g	338	18.0	470	5.8	55.8	24.9	1.7
Oat & Raisin, Organic, Caffe Nero*	1 Cookie/60g	282	14.0	470	4.4	60.5	23.4	2.6
Triple Chocolate, Caffe Nero*	1 Cookie/72g	333	17.0	463	5.6	55.6	24.3	3.3
CRISPS								
Mature Cheddar & Spring Onion, Caffe Nero*	1 Pack/50g	240	14.0	481	6.1	54.0	28.6	4.4
Sea Salt & Balsamic Vinegar, Caffe Nero*	1 Pack/50g	241	13.0	482	7.0	54.1	26.4	4.0

	Measure INFO/WEIGHT	per Measure KCAL FAT		Nutrition Values per 100g / 100ml				
				KCAL	PROT	CARB	FAT	FIBRE
CAFFE NERO								
CRISPS								
Sea Salt, Caffe Nero*	1 Pack/50g	247	14.0	493	8.0	54.0	27.1	4.5
CROISSANT								
Almond, Caffe Nero*	1 Croissant/90g	379	21.0	422	10.0	41.7	23.9	2.9
Apricot, Caffe Nero*	1 Croissant/104g	286	12.0	273	5.4	37.3	11.3	1.2
Butter, Caffe Nero*	1 Croissant/53g	200	9.0	377	8.9	46.0	17.5	1.9
CUPCAKE								
Chocolate, Caffe Nero*	1 Cupcake/68g	311	19.0	457	3.1	48.7	28.1	0.5
FRUIT SALAD								
Classic, Caffe Nero*	1 Serving/170g	70	0.0	41	0.5	9.8	0.1	1.3
HOT CHOCOLATE								
Milano, Caffe Nero*	1 Cup/240ml	446	24.0	186	3.8	19.4	10.2	2.0
Semi Skimmed Milk, Regular, Caffe Nero*	1 Cup/210ml	280	4.0	133	4.0	25.1	2.0	1.3
Skimmed Milk, No Cream, Regular, Caffe Nero*	1 Cup/210ml	262	2.0	125	4.0	25.5	1.0	1.3
Whipped Cream, Semi Skim Milk, Regular, Caffe Nero*	1 Cup/250ml	432	20.0	173	3.7	21.6	8.2	1.1
JUICE								
Apple & Mango, Caffe Nero*	1 Serving/250ml	125	0.0	50	0.2	12.3	0.0	0.1
Apple, Organic, Caffe Nero*	1 Serving/200ml	94	0.0	47	0.5	11.2	0.0	0.0
Apple, Pressed, 100% Premium Juice, Caffe Nero*	1 Serving/250ml	120	0.0	48	0.1	11.8	0.0	0.0
Orange, 100% Squeezed, Caffe Nero*	1 Bottle/250ml	95	0.0	38	0.5	8.8	0.1	0.0
Orange, Organic, Caffe Nero*	1 Serving/200ml	94	0.0	47	0.5	10.4	0.0	0.0
JUICE DRINK								
Fruit Booster, Mango, Caffe Nero*	1 Drink/644g	219	1.0	34	0.5	8.2	0.1	0.6
Pineapple, Orange & Banana, Fruit Booster, Caffe Nero*	1 Serving/652g	202	1.0	31	0.2	7.9	0.1	0.1
Strawberry & Raspberry, Fruit Booster, Caffe Nero*	1 Drink/638ml	160	1.0	25	0.3	6.4	0.1	0.5
LEMONADE								
Sicilian, Still, Caffe Nero*	1 Serving/250ml	115	0.0	46	0.0	11.2	0.0	0.0
MILKSHAKE								
Banana Frappe, Caffe Nero*	1 Frappe/552ml	447	6.0	81	3.0	14.9	1.1	0.0
Double Chocolate, Semi Skimmed, Frappe, Caffe Nero*	1 Frappe/552ml	469	6.0	85	3.1	16.5	1.0	0.4
Double Chocolate, Skimmed Milk, Frappe, Caffe Nero*	1 Frappe/587g	452	2.0	77	2.8	16.3	0.4	0.4
Mint, Frappe, Caffe Nero*	1 Frappe/553ml	437	6.0	79	3.0	14.6	1.1	0.0
Strawberry, Frappe, Caffe Nero*	1 Frappe/548ml	449	6.0	82	3.0	15.1	1.1	0.0
Vanilla, Frappe, Caffe Nero*	1 Serving/553g	448	6.0	81	3.0	15.1	1.1	0.0
MUFFIN								
Blueberry, Caffe Nero*	1 Muffin/120g	430	23.0	358	4.5	42.7	18.8	1.1
Lemon Poppy Seed, Caffe Nero*	1 Muffin/120g	449	22.0	374	5.7	45.9	18.6	0.9
Raspberry & White Chocolate, Caffe Nero*	1 Muffin/120g	461	24.0	384	5.0	46.0	20.0	0.9
Triple Belgian Chocolate, Caffe Nero*	1 Muffin/120g	488	26.0	407	5.7	46.7	21.9	2.0
PAIN AU CHOCOLAT								
Almond, Caffe Nero*	1 Pain/78g	329	18.0	422	9.8	42.6	23.6	3.6
Caffe Nero*	1 Pain/61g	246	12.0	403	8.9	49.0	19.0	1.9
PAIN AU RAISIN								
Caffe Nero*	1 Pain/95g	325	15.0	342	5.4	45.0	15.6	1.4
PANINI								
All Day Breakfast (New Recipe), Caffe Nero*	1 Serving/224g	432	19.0	193	8.9	19.6	8.7	1.3
Breakfast, Bacon & Tomato Sauce, Caffe Nero*	1 Serving/105g	264	10.0	251	11.1	30.6	9.3	1.4
Breakfast, Gammon Ham & Egg, Caffe Nero*	1 Serving/146g	330	17.0	226	10.8	19.9	11.4	1.2
Chicken Milanese, Caffe Nero*	1 Serving/249g	428	14.0	172	8.5	21.9	5.6	1.2
Chicken, & Creme Fraiche, Spicy, Caffe Nero*	1 Panini/200g	294	7.0	147	9.5	19.4	3.4	1.0
Gammon Ham & Mozzarella, Caffe Nero*	1 Serving/204g	437	18.0	214	12.9	20.9	8.7	1.0
Ham & Egg, Breakfast, Caffe Nero*	1 Panini/141g	362	17.0	257	11.3	26.2	11.9	1.4
Meatball & Mozzarella Napoletana, Caffe Nero*	1 Serving/217.5g	483	22.0	222	10.8	22.2	10.0	1.2

	Measure INFO/WEIGHT	per Measure		Nutrition Values per 100g / 100ml				
		KCAL	FAT	KCAL	PROT	CARB	FAT	FIBRE
CAFFE NERO								
PANINI								
Mozzarella, Red Pepper & Roast Tomato, Caffe Nero*	1 Pack/225g	477	27.0	212	8.1	18.0	11.9	1.5
Mushroom with Gorgonzola Cheese, Caffe Nero*	1 Serving/181g	376	17.0	208	7.0	23.4	9.6	1.5
Napoli Salami & Mozzarella, Caffe Nero*	1 Panini/204g	390	17.0	191	10.5	18.5	8.3	1.0
Pesto Chicken, Caffe Nero*	1 Serving/210g	384	13.0	183	11.8	19.7	6.3	1.1
Roast Beef & Caramelised Onion, Caffe Nero*	1 Serving/189g	365	7.0	193	11.1	29.1	3.5	1.4
Tuna Melt (New Recipe), Caffe Nero*	1 Serving/210g	386	13.0	184	12.7	19.8	6.0	1.0
PENNE								
with Roasted Red Pepper Sauce, Caffe Nero*	1 Serving/341g	317	8.0	93	3.0	14.7	2.4	0.6
PIE								
Mince, Caffe Nero*	1 Pie/100g	386	13.0	386	3.9	62.3	13.5	3.0
PIZZA								
Cheese & Tomato, Caffe Nero*	1 Serving/194g	444	13.0	229	10.4	37.9	6.9	3.3
SALAD								
Chicken, Pasta, with Red Pesto, Caffe Nero*	1 Meal/240g	418	20.0	174	7.0	17.3	8.4	1.8
Tuna, With Herbed Potatoes, Caffe Nero*	1 Pack/247g	254	14.0	103	3.4	9.6	5.8	1.7
SANDWICH								
Bloomer BLT, Caffe Nero*	1 Pack/172g	353	15.0	205	8.1	22.9	9.0	1.8
Bloomer, Cheddar & Pickle, Caffe Nero*	1 Pack/195g	468	23.0	240	11.3	22.4	11.7	2.2
Bloomer, Chicken Salad, Caffe Nero*	1 Pack/185g	401	17.0	217	13.8	20.2	9.0	2.2
Bloomer, Free Range Egg Mayonnaise, Caffe Nero*	1 Serving/165g	342	13.0	207	10.7	23.5	7.8	1.9
Bloomer, Gammon Ham & Cheddar, Caffe Nero*	1 Pack/185g	462	21.0	250	16.6	20.7	11.1	2.0
Bloomer, Tuna Salad, Caffe Nero*	1 Pack/160.5g	297	6.0	185	13.0	24.9	3.7	1.8
SHORTBREAD								
Organic, Caffe Nero*	1 Serving/50g	244	14.0	489	5.4	52.1	28.7	1.5
SLICES								
Caramel, Caffe Nero*	1 Slice/50g	252	15.0	505	4.6	55.5	29.4	2.1
Caramel, Digestive Biscuit, Caffe Nero*	1 Serving/80g	418	24.0	523	4.1	59.2	29.5	1.1
Caramel, Shortcake, Caffe Nero*	1 Slice/98g	514	31.0	524	2.7	49.6	31.1	0.0
Creamed Spinach, Savoury, Pastry, Caffe Nero*	1 Pastry/120g	372	23.0	310	5.7	27.8	19.5	0.0
Ham & Cheese, Savoury, Puff Pastry, Caffe Nero*	1 Pastry/110g	394	25.0	358	11.5	26.9	22.7	0.0
TEA								
Chai Latte, Semi Skimmed Milk, Caffe Nero*	1 Grande/405g	284	11.0	70	3.8	8.3	2.6	0.0
Chai Latte, Skimmed Milk, Caffe Nero*	1 Grande/405g	239	5.0	59	3.8	8.4	1.3	0.0
Chia Latte, Iced, Caffe Nero*	1 Latte/548g	466	11.0	85	3.6	13.7	2.0	0.0
WRAP								
Falafel, Caffe Nero*	1 Pack/157g	424	22.0	270	8.7	29.4	13.9	1.8
YOGHURT								
Blackcurrant, Bio, Caffe Nero*	1 Pot/150g	235	13.0	157	5.3	14.2	8.6	0.2
Blueberry, Brunch Pot, Caffe Nero*	1 Pot/127g	165	6.0	130	1.3	19.8	4.8	1.0
Honey, Bio, Caffe Nero*	1 Serving/149g	231	13.0	155	5.0	14.0	8.7	0.0
Strawberry, Brunch Pot, Caffe Nero*	1 Pot/125g	150	6.0	120	1.3	17.6	4.8	1.1
COSTA								
BISCUITS								
Stem Ginger, Costa*	1 Pack/60g	286	13.0	476	4.8	65.6	21.6	0.0
BROWNIE								
Bites, Costa*	1 Serving/72g	342	22.0	475	5.4	44.3	30.7	0.0
Chocolate, Gluten Free, Costa*	1 Serving/80g	400	25.0	500	7.3	46.2	31.8	0.0
CAKE								
Carrot, Costa*	1 Slice/138g	491	25.0	357	5.1	43.4	18.1	0.0
Chocolate, Costa*	1 Slice/150g	575	24.0	383	4.8	76.7	15.7	0.0
Lemon, Costa*	1 Slice/144g	583	27.0	404	4.3	55.0	18.5	0.0
Victoria Sandwich, Costa*	1 Slice/128g	501	25.0	390	3.2	49.8	19.5	0.0

	Measure INFO/WEIGHT	per Measure KCAL	FAT	Nutrition Values per 100g / 100ml KCAL	PROT	CARB	FAT	FIBRE
COSTA								
COFFEE								
Americano, Massimo, No Added Milk, Costa*	1 Massimo/568ml	11	0.0	2	0.1	0.2	0.0	0.0
Americano, Medio, No Added Milk, Costa*	1 Medio/454ml	8	0.0	2	0.1	0.2	0.0	0.0
Americano, Primo, No Added Milk, Costa*	1 Primo/340ml	5	0.0	1	0.1	0.2	0.0	0.0
Caffe Latte, Full Fat, Massimo, Costa*	1 Massimo/380ml	190	10.0	50	2.6	4.1	2.6	0.0
Caffe Latte, Full Fat, Medio, Costa*	1 Latte/264g	129	7.0	49	2.5	3.8	2.6	0.0
Caffe Latte, Full Fat, Primo, Costa*	1 Cup/190ml	95	5.0	50	1.4	5.0	2.7	0.0
Caffe Latte, Skimmed, Massimo, Costa*	1 Massimo/378ml	102	0.0	27	2.5	4.0	0.1	0.0
Caffe Latte, Skimmed, Medio, Costa*	1 Latte/264ml	71	0.0	27	2.6	3.9	0.1	0.0
Caffe Latte, Soya, Massimo, Costa*	1 Massimo/378ml	185	10.0	49	2.3	4.1	2.6	0.0
Caffe Latte, Soya, Medio, Costa*	1 Medio/261ml	86	4.0	33	2.4	2.4	1.5	0.0
Caffe Latte, Soya, Primo, Costa*	1 Primo/188ml	62	3.0	33	2.5	2.5	1.4	0.0
Cappuccino, Full Fat, Massimo, Costa*	1 Massimo/568g	123	7.0	22	1.1	1.6	1.2	0.0
Cappuccino, Full Fat, Medio, Costa*	1 Medio/454g	102	5.0	22	1.2	2.0	1.0	0.0
Cappuccino, Full Fat, Primo, Costa*	1 Primo/340ml	71	4.0	21	1.1	1.8	1.0	0.0
Cappuccino, Medio, Skimmed Milk, Costa*	1 Medio/454ml	58	0.0	13	1.2	3.5	0.0	0.0
Cappuccino, Skimmed, Massimo, Costa*	1 Mug/280ml	73	1.0	26	2.3	3.5	0.3	0.0
Cappuccino, Skimmed, Medio, Costa*	1 Medio/242g	58	0.0	24	2.2	3.5	0.1	0.0
Cappuccino, Skimmed, Primo, Costa*	1 Primo Cup/183ml	40	0.0	22	1.9	3.1	0.2	0.0
Cappuccino, Soya, Massimo, Costa*	1 Massimo/275g	88	4.0	32	2.3	2.2	1.5	0.0
Cappuccino, Soya, Medio, Costa*	1 Medio/248g	77	3.0	31	2.3	2.6	1.3	0.0
Cappuccino, Soya, Primo, Costa*	1 Primo/181g	47	2.0	26	2.0	1.9	1.1	0.0
Flat White made With Full Fat Milk, Costa*	1 Primo/340ml	191	11.0	56	2.8	3.9	3.3	0.0
Flat White Made with Skimmed Milk, Costa*	1 Cup/340ml	99	1.0	29	3.0	4.1	0.3	0.0
Flat White Made with Soya Milk, Costa*	1 Primo/340ml	122	6.0	36	2.8	2.2	1.6	0.0
Iced, Latte, Full Fat Milk, Medio, Costa*	1 Medio/454ml	114	7.0	25	1.3	1.8	1.4	0.0
Iced, Latte, Full Fat Milk, Primo, Costa*	1 Primo/340ml	79	4.0	23	1.2	1.7	1.3	0.0
Iced, Latte, Skimmed Milk, Medio, Costa*	1 Medio/454ml	62	1.0	14	1.3	1.9	0.1	0.0
Iced, Latte, Skimmed Milk, Primo, Costa*	1 Primo/340ml	43	1.0	13	1.3	1.8	0.1	0.0
Iced, Latte, Soya Milk, Medio, Costa*	1 Medio/454ml	75	3.0	17	1.3	1.1	0.7	0.0
Iced, Latte, Soya Milk, Primo, Costa*	1 Primo/340ml	52	2.0	15	1.2	1.1	0.7	0.0
Latte, Caramel, Full Fat Milk, Massimo, Costa*	1 Massimo/568ml	256	10.0	45	1.7	5.6	1.7	0.0
Latte, Caramel, Full Fat Milk, Medio, Costa*	1 Medio/454ml	181	5.0	40	1.2	4.0	1.2	0.0
Latte, Caramel, Full Fat Milk, Primo, Costa*	1 Primo/340ml	134	5.0	39	0.8	5.6	1.5	0.0
Latte, Caramel, Skimmed Milk, Massimo, Costa*	1 Massimo/568ml	167	0.0	29	1.7	5.5	0.1	0.0
Latte, Caramel, Skimmed Milk, Medio, Costa*	1 Medio/454ml	124	0.0	27	1.5	5.1	0.1	0.0
Latte, Caramel, Skimmed Milk, Primo, Costa*	1 Primo/340ml	91	0.0	27	1.2	5.3	0.1	0.0
Latte, Caramel, Soya Milk, Massimo, Costa*	1 Massimo/568g	251	10.0	44	1.5	5.6	1.7	0.0
Latte, Caramel, Soya Milk, Medio, Costa*	1 Medio/454ml	139	4.0	31	1.4	4.2	0.9	0.0
Latte, Caramel, Soya Milk, Primo, Costa*	1 Primo/340ml	101	3.0	30	1.4	4.3	0.8	0.0
Latte, Cinnamon, Full Fat Milk, Massimo, Costa*	1 Massimo/400ml	255	10.0	64	2.4	7.9	2.4	0.0
Latte, Cinnamon, Full Fat Milk, Medio, Costa*	1 Medio/454ml	181	7.0	40	1.4	5.0	1.5	0.0
Latte, Cinnamon, Skimmed Milk, Massimo, Costa*	1 Massimo/400ml	167	0.0	42	2.4	7.7	0.1	0.0
Latte, Cinnamon, Skimmed Milk, Medio, Costa*	1 Medio/441ml	123	0.0	28	1.6	5.2	0.1	0.0
Latte, Cinnamon, Skimmed Milk, Primo, Costa*	1 Primo/340ml	90	0.0	26	1.2	5.2	0.1	0.0
Latte, Cinnamon, Soya Milk, Massimo, Costa*	1 Massimo/400ml	251	10.0	63	2.2	7.9	2.4	0.0
Latte, Cinnamon, Soya Milk, Medio, Costa*	1 Medio/454ml	139	3.0	31	1.4	4.2	0.6	0.0
Latte, Cinnamon, Soya Milk, Primo, Costa*	1 Primo/340ml	101	3.0	30	1.4	4.2	0.8	0.0
Latte, Gingerbread, Full Fat Milk, Massimo, Costa*	1 Massimo/568ml	258	10.0	45	1.7	5.7	1.7	0.0
Latte, Gingerbread, Full Fat Milk, Medio, Costa*	1 Medio/454ml	183	7.0	40	1.4	5.1	1.5	0.0
Latte, Gingerbread, Full Fat Milk, Primo, Costa*	1 Primo/340ml	136	5.0	40	0.8	5.7	1.5	0.0
Latte, Gingerbread, Skimmed Milk, Massimo, Costa*	1 Massimo/568ml	170	0.0	30	1.7	5.6	0.1	0.0
Latte, Gingerbread, Skimmed Milk, Medio, Costa*	1 Medio/454ml	126	0.0	28	1.5	5.2	0.1	0.0

	Measure INFO/WEIGHT	KCAL	FAT	KCAL	PROT	CARB	FAT	FIBRE
COSTA								
COFFEE								
Latte, Gingerbread, Skimmed Milk, Primo, Costa*	1 Primo/340ml	92	0.0	27	1.2	5.3	0.1	0.0
Latte, Gingerbread, Soya Milk, Massimo, Costa*	1 Massimo/568ml	254	10.0	45	1.5	5.7	1.7	0.0
Latte, Gingerbread, Soya Milk, Medio, Costa*	1 Medio/454ml	141	4.0	31	1.4	4.3	0.9	0.0
Latte, Gingerbread, Soya Milk, Primo, Costa*	1 Primo/340ml	103	3.0	30	1.4	4.3	0.8	0.0
Latte, Iced, Caramel, Full Fat Milk, Medio, Costa*	1 Medio/454ml	167	6.0	37	1.1	5.2	1.3	0.0
Latte, Iced, Caramel, Full Fat Milk, Primo, Costa*	1 Primo/340ml	106	4.0	31	1.1	4.0	1.2	0.0
Latte, Iced, Caramel, Skimmed Milk, Medio, Costa*	1 Medio/454ml	121	1.0	27	1.2	5.2	0.1	0.0
Latte, Iced, Caramel, Skimmed Milk, Primo, Costa*	1 Primo/340ml	73	0.0	21	1.1	4.0	0.1	0.0
Latte, Iced, Caramel, Soya Milk, Medio, Costa*	1 Medio/454ml	132	3.0	29	1.1	4.6	0.6	0.0
Latte, Iced, Caramel, Soya Milk, Primo, Costa*	1 Primo/340ml	81	2.0	24	1.1	3.3	0.6	0.0
Latte, Iced, Hazelnut, Full Fat Milk, Medio, Costa*	1 Medio/454ml	165	6.0	36	1.1	5.1	1.3	0.0
Latte, Iced, Hazelnut, Full Fat Milk, Primo, Costa*	1 Primo/340ml	104	4.0	31	1.1	3.9	1.2	0.0
Latte, Iced, Hazelnut, Skimmed Milk, Medio, Costa*	1 Medio/454ml	118	1.0	26	1.2	5.1	0.1	0.0
Latte, Iced, Hazelnut, Skimmed Milk, Primo, Costa*	1 Primo/340ml	72	0.0	21	1.1	3.9	0.1	0.0
Latte, Iced, Hazelnut, Soya Milk, Medio, Costa*	1 Medio/454ml	130	3.0	29	1.1	4.4	0.6	0.0
Latte, Iced, Hazelnut, Soya Milk, Primo, Costa*	1 Primo/340ml	80	2.0	24	1.1	3.3	0.6	0.0
Latte, Iced, Vanilla, Full Fat Milk, Medio, Costa*	1 Medio/454ml	169	6.0	37	1.1	5.3	1.3	0.0
Latte, Iced, Vanilla, Full Fat Milk, Primo, Costa*	1 Primo/340ml	107	4.0	31	1.1	4.1	1.2	0.0
Latte, Iced, Vanilla, Skimmed Milk, Medio, Costa*	1 Medio/454ml	123	1.0	27	1.2	5.4	0.1	0.0
Latte, Iced, Vanilla, Skimmed Milk, Primo, Costa*	1 Primo/340ml	74	0.0	22	1.1	4.1	0.1	0.0
Latte, Iced, Vanilla, Soya Milk, Medio, Costa*	1 Medio/454ml	134	3.0	30	1.1	4.7	0.6	0.0
Latte, Iced, Vanilla, Soya Milk, Primo, Costa*	1 Primo/340ml	82	2.0	24	1.1	3.5	0.6	0.0
Latte, Roasted Hazelnut, Full Fat Milk, Massimo, Costa*	1 Massimo/568ml	252	10.0	44	1.7	5.5	1.7	0.0
Latte, Roasted Hazelnut, Full Fat Milk, Medio, Costa*	1 Medio/454ml	178	7.0	39	1.4	5.0	1.5	0.0
Latte, Roasted Hazelnut, Full Fat Milk, Primo, Costa*	1 Primo/340ml	132	5.0	39	0.8	5.6	1.5	0.0
Latte, Roasted Hazelnut, Skim Milk, Massimo, Costa*	1 Massimo/568ml	164	0.0	29	1.7	5.4	0.1	0.0
Latte, Roasted Hazelnut, Skimmed Milk, Medio, Costa*	1 Medio/454ml	121	0.0	27	1.5	5.0	0.1	0.0
Latte, Roasted Hazelnut, Skimmed Milk, Primo, Costa*	1 Primo/340ml	89	0.0	26	1.2	5.1	0.1	0.0
Latte, Roasted Hazelnut, Soya Milk, Massimo, Costa*	1 Massimo/568ml	248	10.0	44	1.5	5.5	1.7	0.0
Latte, Roasted Hazelnut, Soya Milk, Medio, Costa*	1 Medio/454ml	136	4.0	30	1.4	4.1	0.9	0.0
Latte, Roasted Hazelnut, Soya Milk, Primo, Costa*	1 Primo/340ml	100	3.0	29	1.4	4.1	0.8	0.0
Latte, Vanilla, Full Fat Milk, Medio, Costa*	1 Medio/454g	183	7.0	40	1.4	5.2	1.5	0.0
Latte, Vanilla, Full Fat Milk, Primo, Costa*	1 Primo/340ml	136	5.0	40	0.8	5.8	1.5	0.0
Latte, Vanilla, Skimmed Milk, Medio, Costa*	1 Medio/454ml	125	0.0	28	1.5	5.2	0.1	0.0
Latte, Vanilla, Skimmed Milk, Primo, Costa*	1 Primo/340ml	92	0.0	27	1.2	5.4	0.1	0.0
Latte, Vanilla, Soya Milk, Massimo, Costa*	1 Massimo/568ml	253	10.0	45	1.5	5.7	1.7	0.0
Latte, Vanilla, Soya Milk, Medio, Costa*	1 Medio/454ml	141	4.0	31	1.4	4.4	0.9	0.0
Latte, Vanilla, Soya Milk, Primo, Costa*	1 Primo/340ml	103	3.0	30	1.4	4.4	0.8	0.0
Mocha Flake, Full Fat, Massimo, Costa*	1 Massimo/332ml	369	24.0	111	2.9	8.7	7.1	0.0
Mocha Flake, Full Fat, Medio, Costa*	1 Medio/288ml	297	19.0	103	2.7	8.1	6.7	0.0
Mocha Flake, Full Fat, Primo, Costa*	1 Primo/234ml	257	17.0	110	2.6	8.1	7.4	0.0
Mocha Flake, Skimmed, Massimo, Costa*	1 Massimo/334ml	338	18.0	101	3.0	10.3	5.3	0.0
Mocha Flake, Skimmed, Medio, Costa*	1 Medio/288ml	262	14.0	91	2.6	9.0	4.9	0.0
Mocha Flake, Skimmed, Primo, Costa*	1 Primo/234ml	227	14.0	97	2.7	8.3	5.9	0.0
Mocha, Full Fat, Massimo, Costa*	1 Massimo/288ml	170	8.0	59	2.6	5.8	2.8	0.0
Mocha, Full Fat, Medio, Costa*	1 Mocha/253ml	153	7.0	60	2.6	6.7	2.6	0.0
Mocha, Full Fat, Primo, Costa*	1 Primo/188ml	113	5.0	60	2.6	6.7	2.5	0.0
Mocha, Skimmed, Massimo, Costa*	1 Massimo/288ml	138	2.0	48	2.8	7.6	0.7	0.0
Mocha, Skimmed, Medio, Costa*	1 Mocha/253ml	119	2.0	47	2.5	7.8	0.6	0.0
Mocha, Skimmed, Primo, Costa*	1 Primo/191ml	84	1.0	44	2.7	7.0	0.6	0.0
Mocha, Soya, Primo, Costa*	1 Primo/340ml	70	2.0	21	1.1	2.5	0.7	0.0
Mocha, Soya, Massimo, Costa*	1 Massimo/568g	200	7.0	35	1.8	4.2	1.2	0.0

	Measure INFO/WEIGHT	per Measure KCAL	FAT	Nutrition Values per 100g / 100ml KCAL	PROT	CARB	FAT	FIBRE
COSTA								
COFFEE								
Mocha, Soya, Medio, Costa*	1 Medio/454ml	173	6.0	38	2.0	4.6	1.3	0.0
COOKIES								
Choc Chunk, Double, Costa*	1 Pack/60g	296	15.0	493	5.2	61.1	25.3	3.7
Fruit & Oat, Costa*	1 Pack/60g	283	13.0	472	5.1	65.2	21.2	2.0
CRISPS								
Sea Salt Flavour, Costa*	1 Pack/50g	251	14.0	503	7.1	55.9	27.9	4.2
CROISSANT								
Almond, Costa*	1 Croissant/88g	336	17.0	382	9.3	43.0	19.2	0.0
Butter, Costa*	1 Croissant/64g	276	17.0	431	8.3	40.6	26.1	0.0
Ham & Cheese, Costa*	1 Serving/100g	337	19.0	337	12.1	28.8	19.3	0.0
Tomato & Emmental, Costa*	1 Serving/98g	342	21.0	349	9.0	30.0	21.4	0.0
CRUMBLE								
Apple, Costa*	1 Slice/100g	469	30.0	469	5.6	46.7	30.1	0.0
CUPCAKES								
Lemon, Costa*	1 Cupcake/97g	435	19.0	448	2.1	64.6	19.9	0.0
Rocky Road, Costa*	1 Cupcake/100g	427	19.0	423	4.6	56.4	18.9	0.0
FLAPJACK								
Fruity, Costa*	1 Serving/85g	353	12.0	415	4.9	67.0	14.2	12.5
Nutty, Costa*	1 Serving/85g	391	20.0	460	7.4	54.8	23.5	5.0
FLATBREAD								
Cajun Chicken, Costa*	1 Pack/168g	310	5.0	184	12.7	26.6	3.0	0.0
Cheddar & Caramelised Onion Chutney, Costa*	1 Pack/118g	340	13.0	288	11.9	34.8	11.3	0.0
Chicken, Green Thai, Costa*	1 Pack/173g	325	6.0	188	12.2	26.6	3.7	0.0
Emmenthal & Mushroom, Costa*	1 Pack/158g	391	16.0	248	13.1	25.9	10.2	0.0
FRESCATO								
Coffee Caramel, Full Fat Milk, Medio, Costa*	1 Medio/454ml	488	8.0	107	1.5	21.5	1.7	0.0
Coffee Caramel, Skimmed Milk, Medio, Costa*	1 Medio/454ml	425	1.0	94	1.6	21.6	0.1	0.0
Coffee Caramel, Skimmed Milk, Primo, Costa*	1 Primo/340ml	289	1.0	85	1.5	19.6	0.1	0.0
Coffee Caramel, Soya Milk, Medio, Costa*	1 Medio/454ml	441	4.0	97	1.5	20.6	0.9	0.0
Coffee Caramel, Soya Milk, Primo, Costa*	1 Primo/340ml	300	3.0	88	1.4	18.6	0.8	0.0
Coffee Mocha, Full Fat Milk, Medio, Costa*	1 Medio/454ml	540	8.0	119	1.6	24.0	1.8	0.0
Coffee Mocha, Full Fat Milk, Primo, Costa*	1 Primo/340ml	380	6.0	112	1.6	22.5	1.7	0.0
Coffee Mocha, Skimmed Milk, Medio, Costa*	1 Medio/454ml	477	1.0	105	1.7	24.1	0.3	0.0
Coffee Mocha, Skimmed Milk, Primo, Costa*	1 Primo/340ml	335	1.0	99	1.6	22.6	0.2	0.0
Coffee Mocha, Soya Milk, Medio, Costa*	1 Medio/454ml	493	4.0	109	1.6	23.1	0.9	0.0
Coffee Mocha, Soya Milk, Primo, Costa*	1 Primo/340ml	346	3.0	102	1.6	21.7	0.9	0.0
Coffee Vanilla, Full Fat Milk, Medio, Costa*	1 Medio/454ml	491	8.0	108	1.5	21.6	1.7	0.0
Coffee Vanilla, Full Fat Milk, Primo, Costa*	1 Primo/340ml	336	6.0	99	1.4	19.6	1.6	0.0
Coffee Vanilla, Skimmed Milk, Medio, Costa*	1 Medio/454ml	427	1.0	94	1.6	21.7	0.1	0.0
Coffee Vanilla, Skimmed Milk, Primo, Costa*	1 Primo/340ml	290	1.0	85	1.5	19.7	0.1	0.0
Coffee Vanilla, Soya Milk, Medio, Costa*	1 Medio/454ml	443	4.0	98	6.7	20.8	0.9	0.0
Coffee Vanilla, Soya Milk, Primo, Costa*	1 Primo/340ml	301	3.0	89	1.4	18.7	0.8	0.0
Coffee, Full fat Milk, Medio (Coffee Only), Costa*	1 Medio/454ml	423	8.0	93	1.5	17.9	1.7	0.0
Coffee, Full Fat Milk, Primo, (Coffee Only), Costa*	1 Primo/340ml	302	6.0	89	1.4	17.1	1.6	0.0
Coffee, Skimmed Milk, Medio (Coffee Only), Costa*	1 Medio/454ml	359	0.0	79	1.6	18.0	0.1	0.0
Coffee, Skimmed Milk, Primo (Coffee Only), Costa*	1 Primo/340ml	256	1.0	75	1.5	17.2	0.1	0.0
Coffee, Soya Milk, Medio (Coffee Only), Costa*	1 Medio/454ml	375	4.0	83	1.5	17.1	0.9	0.0
Coffee, Soya Milk, Primo, (Coffee Only), Costa*	1 Primo/340ml	267	3.0	79	1.4	16.3	0.8	0.0
FRUIT COOLERS								
Mango & Passionfruit, Medio, Costa*	1 Medio/454ml	192	0.0	42	0.1	10.2	0.1	0.0
Mango & Passionfruit, Primo, Costa*	1 Primo/340ml	144	0.0	42	0.1	10.2	0.1	0.0
Red Berry, Medio, Costa*	1 Medio/454ml	282	0.0	62	0.2	14.9	0.1	0.0

	Measure INFO/WEIGHT	per Measure KCAL	per Measure FAT	Nutrition Values per 100g / 100ml KCAL	PROT	CARB	FAT	FIBRE
FRUIT COOLERS								
Red Berry, Primo, Costa*	1 Primo/340ml	211	0.0	62	0.2	14.9	0.1	0.0
Sicilian Lemonade, Medio, Costa*	1 Medio/454ml	264	0.0	59	0.0	14.0	0.0	0.0
Sicilian Lemonade, Primo, Costa*	1 Primo/340ml	197	0.0	58	0.1	14.0	0.1	0.0
GRAPES								
Red, Costa*	1 Serving/91g	58	0.0	64	0.4	15.4	0.1	0.0
HOT CHOCOLATE								
Marshmallows, Whip Cream, Full Fat, Massimo, Costa*	1 Massimo/419ml	423	21.0	101	3.1	11.2	4.9	0.0
Marshmallows, Whip Cream, Full Fat, Medio, Costa*	1 Medio/308ml	321	15.0	104	3.0	11.7	5.0	0.0
Marshmallows, Whip Cream, Full Fat, Primo, Costa*	1 Primo/238ml	285	14.0	120	3.0	13.2	6.1	0.0
Marshmallows, Whip Cream, Skimmed, Massimo, Costa*	1 Serving/418ml	339	11.0	81	3.1	11.2	2.7	0.0
Marshmallows, Whip Cream, Skimmed, Medio, Costa*	1 Medio/309ml	294	11.0	95	3.3	12.4	3.5	0.0
Marshmallows, Whip Cream, Skimmed, Primo, Costa*	1 Primo/238ml	262	11.0	110	3.3	14.0	4.5	0.0
with Frothed Milk, Full Fat, Massimo, Costa*	1 Massimo/376ml	259	11.0	69	3.1	7.6	2.9	0.0
with Frothed Milk, Full Fat, Medio, Costa*	1 Medio/266ml	157	6.0	59	3.0	6.9	2.2	0.0
with Frothed Milk, Full Fat, Primo, Costa*	1 Primo/192ml	121	5.0	63	3.1	6.9	2.5	0.0
with Frothed Milk, Skimmed, Massimo, Costa*	1 Massimo/380ml	175	2.0	46	3.1	7.6	0.4	0.0
with Frothed Milk, Skimmed, Medio, Costa*	1 Medio/265ml	130	1.0	49	3.4	7.7	0.5	0.0
with Frothed Milk, Skimmed, Primo, Costa*	1 Primo/192ml	98	1.0	51	3.4	7.9	0.6	0.0
with Frothed Milk, Soya, Massimo, Costa*	1 Massimo/568ml	298	10.0	52	2.7	6.3	1.7	0.0
with Frothed Milk, Soya, Medio, Costa*	1 Medio/454ml	235	8.0	52	2.7	6.1	1.7	0.0
with Frothed Milk, Soya, Primo, Costa*	1 Primo/340ml	119	4.0	35	1.8	4.2	1.1	0.0
ICE DESSERTS								
Double Choc Flake, Full Fat Milk, Primo, Costa*	1 Primo/340ml	559	25.0	164	1.9	22.9	7.3	0.0
Double Choc Flake, Full Fat Milk, Medio, Costa*	1 Medio/454ml	786	30.0	173	2.1	26.4	6.6	0.0
Double Choc Flake, Skimmed Milk, Medio, Costa*	1 Medio/454ml	722	23.0	159	2.2	26.5	5.0	0.0
Double Choc Flake, Skimmed Milk, Primo, Costa*	1 Primo/340ml	514	20.0	151	2.0	23.0	5.8	0.0
Double Choc Flake, Soya Milk, Medio, Costa*	1 Medio/454ml	738	26.0	163	2.1	25.5	5.7	0.0
Double Choc Flake, Soya Milk, Primo, Costa*	1 Primo/340ml	525	22.0	154	1.9	22.0	6.4	0.0
Simply Vanilla, Full Fat Milk, Medio, Costa*	1 Medio/454ml	421	8.0	93	1.4	17.9	1.7	0.0
Simply Vanilla, Full Fat Milk, Primo, Costa*	1 Primo/340ml	301	6.0	89	1.4	17.1	1.6	0.0
Simply Vanilla, Skimmed Milk, Medio, Costa*	1 Medio/454ml	357	1.0	79	1.5	18.0	0.1	0.0
Simply Vanilla, Skimmed Milk, Primo, Costa*	1 Primo/340ml	255	1.0	75	1.5	17.1	0.1	0.0
Simply Vanilla, Soya Milk, Medio, Costa*	1 Medio/454ml	373	4.0	82	1.4	17.0	0.8	0.0
Simply Vanilla, Soya Milk, Primo, Costa*	1 Primo/340ml	267	3.0	79	1.4	16.2	0.8	0.0
Strawberry Shortcake, Full Fat Milk, Medio, Costa*	1 Medio/454ml	757	26.0	167	1.8	27.1	5.7	0.0
Strawberry Shortcake, Full Fat Milk, Primo, Costa*	1 Primo/340ml	569	24.0	167	1.8	24.3	7.0	0.0
Strawberry Shortcake, Skimmed Milk, Medio, Costa*	1 Medio/454ml	694	19.0	153	1.9	27.2	4.2	0.0
Strawberry Shortcake, Skimmed Milk, Primo, Costa*	1 Primo/340ml	524	19.0	154	1.9	24.4	5.5	0.0
Strawberry Shortcake, Soya Milk, Medio, Costa*	1 Medio/454ml	710	22.0	156	1.8	26.2	4.9	0.0
Strawberry Shortcake, Soya Milk, Primo, Costa*	1 Primo/340ml	535	21.0	157	1.8	23.5	6.2	0.0
MOCHA								
Iced, Full Fat Milk, Medio, Costa*	1 Medio/454ml	209	0.0	46	1.2	7.7	0.0	0.0
Iced, Full Fat Milk, Primo, Costa*	1 Primo/340ml	142	4.0	42	1.1	6.9	1.1	0.0
Iced, Skimmed Milk, Medio, Costa*	1 Medio/454ml	170	1.0	37	1.2	7.7	0.2	0.0
Iced, Skimmed Milk, Primo, Costa*	1 Primo/340ml	115	1.0	34	1.1	7.0	0.2	0.0
Iced, Soya Milk, Medio, Costa*	1 Medio/454ml	180	3.0	40	1.2	7.1	0.7	0.0
Iced, Soya Milk, Primo, Costa*	1 Primo/340ml	122	2.0	36	1.1	6.4	0.6	0.0
MUFFIN								
Banana & Pecan Breakfast Loaf, Costa*	1 Muffin/113g	442	23.0	391	5.1	44.0	20.7	0.0
Blueberry, Costa*	1 Muffin/132g	475	21.0	360	4.0	50.4	15.8	0.0
Chocolate, Mini, Costa*	1 Muffin/19g	73	4.0	383	4.3	44.5	20.5	0.0
Lemon & Orange, Low Fat, Costa*	1 Muffin/135g	319	3.0	236	4.6	49.4	2.3	1.1

COSTA

	Measure INFO/WEIGHT	per Measure KCAL	per Measure FAT	Nutrition Values per 100g / 100ml KCAL	PROT	CARB	FAT	FIBRE
MUFFIN								
Lemon & White Chocolate, Costa*	1 Muffin/129g	472	20.0	366	5.4	52.3	15.8	0.0
Original Breakfast Loaf, Costa*	1 Serving/128g	443	19.0	346	5.0	48.9	14.5	0.0
Raspberry & White Chocolate, Costa*	1 Muffin/135g	511	26.0	376	4.8	46.4	19.1	0.0
Raspberry & White Chocolate, Mini, Costa*	1 Muffin/19g	72	4.0	379	4.1	45.9	19.4	0.0
Triple Chocolate, Costa*	1 Muffin/130g	530	28.0	408	5.3	48.6	21.4	0.0
PAIN AU RAISIN								
Costa*	1 Pastry/119g	356	14.0	299	5.1	43.7	11.5	0.0
PANETTINO								
Chocolate, Costa*	1 Cake/100g	407	20.0	407	8.3	48.4	20.0	0.0
Classic, Costa*	1 Serving/90g	336	14.0	373	7.1	51.5	15.4	0.0
PANINI								
Brie & Tomato Chutney, Costa*	1 Panini/177g	453	16.0	256	9.8	33.3	9.3	2.8
Chicken & Pesto, Costa*	1 Serving/209.5g	419	21.0	200	22.5	57.9	10.2	0.0
Goats Cheese & Pepper, Costa*	1 Serving/197g	424	11.0	215	9.9	30.3	5.6	0.0
Ham & Cheese, Costa*	1 Panini/175g	461	21.0	263	12.5	26.2	12.1	0.0
Mozzarella, Tomato & Basil, Costa*	1 Panini/190g	487	16.0	257	5.3	45.3	8.3	0.0
Ragu Meatball, Costa*	1 Serving/190g	488	16.0	257	5.3	40.3	8.3	0.0
Steak & Cheese, Costa*	1 Serving/228g	492	16.0	216	11.3	25.7	7.2	0.0
Tuna Melt, Costa*	1 Panini/190g	462	14.0	243	14.4	29.5	7.5	0.0
SALAD								
Chargrilled Vegetable & Cous Cous, Costa*	1 Serving/291g	352	8.0	121	3.0	21.5	2.6	0.0
Chicken & Pasta, Costa*	1 Serving/270g	427	11.0	158	8.4	21.9	4.1	0.0
Cous Cous, Moroccan Styles, Costa*	1 Pack/290g	392	7.0	135	3.6	24.6	2.5	2.2
Tuna, Costa*	1 Serving/181.5g	274	4.0	151	10.3	22.6	2.2	0.0
SANDWICH								
Bacon & Tomato Sauce, Tostato, Costa*	1 Tostato/132g	316	7.0	239	8.5	40.2	5.0	0.0
BLT, Costa*	1 Pack/169g	397	16.0	235	11.0	26.8	9.3	0.0
Brie, Apple & Grape, Costa*	1 Serving/225g	535	25.0	238	8.3	28.7	10.9	0.0
Chicken, Coronation, Costa*	1 Pack/258g	600	26.0	232	12.5	23.0	10.1	2.5
Chicken, Roast, Costa*	1 Pack/177g	325	7.0	184	13.0	23.8	4.0	0.0
Club, All Day Breakfast, Costa*	1 Pack/243g	592	21.0	244	11.0	30.6	8.6	0.0
Club, Chicken & Bacon, Costa*	1 Pack/213g	484	13.0	227	13.6	29.3	6.2	0.0
Egg Mayonnaise & Tomato, Free Range, Costa*	1 Pack/174g	389	24.0	223	8.6	18.3	13.8	0.0
Egg, Free Range, Costa*	1 Pack/172g	377	15.0	219	9.7	25.9	8.5	0.0
Houmous, Costa*	1 Pack/165g	263	5.0	160	6.4	25.9	2.8	0.0
Ploughmans, Cheese, Costa*	1 Pack/181g	424	20.0	234	9.3	25.0	10.8	0.0
Prawn, Tiger, with Lime & Chilli Dressing, Costa*	1 Pack/185g	367	19.0	198	8.2	21.2	10.2	0.0
Salmon, & Salad, Poached, Oatmeal, Costa*	1 Pack/151g	224	4.0	148	7.7	22.9	2.8	0.0
Sausage, Chorizo, & Vine Ripened Tomato, Costa*	1 Pack/181g	315	4.0	174	15.5	26.1	2.1	0.0
Tuna, & Salad, Costa*	1 Pack/177g	289	4.0	163	11.9	25.7	2.3	0.0
SCONE								
Fruit, Costa*	1 Serving/110g	370	12.0	336	5.6	55.1	10.7	0.0
SHORTBREAD								
Mini, Bag, Costa*	1 Bag/65g	316	16.0	486	4.1	63.0	24.1	0.0
SHORTCAKE								
Raspberry, Costa*	1 Shortcake/45g	215	11.0	477	2.4	63.5	23.7	0.0
SLICES								
Cheese, Twist, Pastry, Costa*	1 Pastry/103g	346	20.0	336	11.1	29.5	19.8	0.0
Pecan, Pastry, Costa*	1 Pastry/105g	465	30.0	443	5.6	42.1	28.5	3.0
SOUP								
Fish, Bouillabaisse, Costa*	1 Serving/400g	180	6.0	45	5.8	2.2	1.4	0.0

	Measure INFO/WEIGHT	per Measure KCAL	FAT	Nutrition Values per 100g / 100ml KCAL	PROT	CARB	FAT	FIBRE
COSTA								
TEA								
Iced, Lemon, Costa*	1 Bottle/275ml	91	0.0	33	0.0	8.0	0.0	0.0
Iced, Peach, Medio, Costa*	1 Medio/454ml	94	0.0	21	0.0	4.9	0.0	0.0
Iced, Peach, Primo, Costa*	1 Primo/340ml	64	0.0	19	0.0	4.4	0.0	0.0
Iced, Raspberry, Medio, Costa*	1 Medio/454ml	104	0.0	23	0.0	5.5	0.0	0.0
Iced, Raspberry, Primo, Costa*	1 Primo/340ml	70	0.0	21	0.0	5.0	0.0	0.0
TOASTIE								
Bacon, Costa*	1 Toastie/135g	337	9.0	250	12.9	34.4	6.7	5.3
TRAYBAKE								
Chocolate Tiffin Triangle, Costa*	1 Serving/85g	433	26.0	509	4.9	54.6	30.2	0.0
Fruit, Seed, Nut & Honey Bar, Costa*	1 Serving/75g	317	15.0	423	7.5	52.5	20.3	0.0
Raspberry & Almond, Costa*	1 Serving/100g	451	28.0	451	8.5	40.8	28.2	1.0
Shortbread, Caramel, Costa*	1 Serving/77g	426	26.0	553	4.7	55.9	34.4	0.0
WRAP								
Chicken Caesar, Costa*	1 Pack/194g	420	16.0	216	11.8	24.1	8.0	1.4
Spicy Three Bean, Costa*	1 Pack/235g	456	14.0	194	7.1	27.7	6.1	0.0
CRUSSH JUICE BARS								
BREAKFAST CEREAL								
Porridge, Acai & Strawberry, Crussh Juice Bars*	1 Portion/324g	386	9.0	119	2.0	19.7	2.8	3.1
Porridge, Cinnamon, Crussh Juice Bars*	1 Portion/331g	314	7.0	95	3.1	15.7	2.1	1.8
Porridge, Summer, Crussh Juice Bars*	1 Portion/330g	432	14.0	131	4.8	18.8	4.1	1.4
DRESSING								
Crayfish & Yuzu Dressing Salad, Crussh Juice Bars*	1 Portion/150g	36	1.0	24	2.7	2.4	0.4	1.1
Falafel Beet, Crussh Juice Bars*	1 Portion/205g	260	16.0	127	5.5	8.8	7.7	2.2
Greek Dressing (Greek Salad), Crussh Juice Bars*	1 Portion/40g	269	30.0	672	0.1	0.5	74.4	0.2
Green Pesto dressing, Crussh Juice Bars*	1 Portion/16g	115	12.0	716	1.8	5.8	76.2	0.0
Honey Mustard dressing (7-a-day), Crussh Juice Bars*	1 Portion/21g	126	13.0	606	0.4	6.3	64.3	0.0
Summer Crayfish & Yuzu, Crussh Juice Bars*	1 Portion/220g	64	1.0	29	3.8	2.5	0.4	1.3
Sweet Chilli Dressing (Crayfish) Crussh Juice Bars*	1 Portion/40g	102	0.0	255	0.3	61.6	0.3	0.0
Tahini Dressing (Falafel Beet), Crussh Juice Bars*	1 Portion/21g	63	6.0	302	6.4	4.0	28.9	1.5
Yuzu dressing (Crayfish & Yuzu) Crussh Juice Bars*	1 Portion/40g	82	7.0	205	1.4	10.2	17.2	0.3
Zesty dressing (Tuna Nicoise), Crussh Juice Bars*	1 Portion/40g	118	13.0	295	0.4	1.0	32.3	0.0
FRESHLY PRESSED JUICES								
Apple Juice, Crussh Juice Bars*	1 Med Cup/339ml	139	0.0	41	0.1	9.8	0.1	0.0
Carrot Juice, Crussh Juice Bars*	1 Med Cup/340ml	85	0.0	25	0.5	5.4	0.1	0.8
Clean & Lean, Crussh Juice Bars*	1 Med Cup/338ml	159	0.0	47	0.4	11.1	0.1	2.4
Energiser, Crussh Juice Bars*	1 Med Cup/340ml	136	1.0	40	0.5	9.0	0.2	2.9
Green Goddess, Crussh Juice Bars*	1 Med Cup/338ml	132	1.0	39	0.8	8.4	0.3	2.6
Lemon & Ginger Flu Fighter, Crussh Juice Bars*	1 Med Cup/850ml	340	1.0	40	0.3	9.3	0.1	1.0
Love Juice, Crussh Juice Bars*	1 Med Cup/340ml	146	0.0	43	0.6	9.9	0.1	0.5
Orange Juice, Crussh Juice Bars*	1 Med Cup/339ml	112	0.0	33	0.6	7.7	0.0	0.1
Purifier, Crussh Juice Bars*	1 Med Cup/340ml	119	1.0	35	0.6	7.6	0.2	2.8
Spring Zinger , Crussh Juice Bars*	1 Med Cup/341ml	133	0.0	39	0.5	9.0	0.1	1.4
Super Juice, Crussh Juice Bars*	1 Med Cup/338ml	108	1.0	32	0.8	6.5	0.3	2.7
Tropical Crussh, Crussh Juice Bars*	1 Med Cup/340ml	153	1.0	45	0.4	10.5	0.2	2.1
Zinger, Crussh Juice Bars*	1 Med Cup/340ml	119	1.0	35	0.6	7.6	0.2	1.9
HEALTHPOT								
BeetChick & Coriander Healthpot, Crussh Juice Bars*	1 Pot/160g	152	6.0	95	4.6	11.2	3.5	3.1
Butter Bean, Cherry Tom, Parsley , Crussh Juice Bars*	1 Pot/186g	225	13.0	121	3.0	10.1	7.1	1.5
Cactus Guacamole with Veg Sticks, Crussh Juice Bars*	1 Pot/220g	139	11.0	63	1.3	2.7	5.1	2.7
Detox Healthpot, Crussh Juice Bars*	1 Pot/163g	104	5.0	64	3.7	6.0	2.8	1.6
Energy Rice & Cranberry Cashew, Crussh Juice Bars*	1 Pot/165g	246	10.0	149	3.2	20.8	5.8	1.7
Full O' Herbs & Beans Healthpot, Crussh Juice Bars*	1 Pot/120g	197	12.0	164	5.1	12.6	10.4	2.8

CRUSSH JUICE BARS

	Measure INFO/WEIGHT	per Measure KCAL	FAT	Nutrition Values per 100g / 100ml KCAL	PROT	CARB	FAT	FIBRE
HEALTHPOT								
Goats Cheese & Sweet Potato, Crussh Juice Bars*	1 Pot/160g	203	10.0	127	7.1	11.6	6.1	1.9
Great Greens with Avocado, Crussh Juice Bars*	1 Pot/120g	124	8.0	103	5.2	5.4	6.9	2.7
Great Greens, Crussh Juice Bars*	1 Pot/150g	91	4.0	61	6.2	3.4	2.5	4.1
Puy Lentil Healthpot, Crussh Juice Bars*	1 Pot/100g	274	13.0	274	12.5	26.4	13.2	6.8
Spring Tarragon Bean Healthpot, Crussh Juice Bars*	1 Pot/160g	131	6.0	82	3.8	8.2	3.9	2.7
Superfoods, Crussh Juice Bars*	1 Pot/160g	440	24.0	275	10.7	23.9	15.1	4.3
Tuna Lean Bean, Crussh Juice Bars*	1 Pot/160g	214	10.0	134	8.0	11.6	6.1	2.0
Turkish Cous Cous Healthpot, Crussh Juice Bars*	1 Pot/130g	217	8.0	167	5.5	23.0	5.9	1.3
SALAD								
Bang Bang Chicken, Crussh Juice Bars*	1 Portion/273g	202	16.0	74	3.8	4.0	5.7	2.2
Classic Greek Salad, Crussh Juice Bars*	1 Portion/225g	202	17.0	90	3.5	1.8	7.6	1.1
Crayfish & Thai Glass Noodle, Crussh Juice Bars*	1 Portion/240g	132	2.0	55	3.8	8.1	0.8	1.0
Falafel Feta Mezze Salad, Crussh Juice Bars*	1 Portion/200g	190	7.0	95	4.6	11.0	3.6	2.5
Figamajig Stilton Salad Pot, Crussh Juice Bars*	1 Portion/180g	264	13.0	147	6.9	13.9	7.0	3.4
Japanese Detox Noodle Salad, Crussh Juice Bars*	1 Portion/344g	196	7.0	57	4.1	5.8	1.9	7.6
Mix-Me-Up Thai Salad, Crussh Juice Bars*	1 Portion/205g	109	4.0	53	5.2	4.0	1.8	1.7
NY:LON Cobb Salad, Crussh Juice Bars*	1 Portion/215g	230	15.0	107	8.9	1.5	7.2	7.2
O-me-good Salad Pot, Crussh Juice Bars*	1 Portion/255g	446	22.0	175	7.8	16.3	8.7	3.0
Super Greens, Crussh Juice Bars*	1 Portion/230g	78	3.0	34	2.9	2.5	1.3	2.6
Sweet Pepper & Moroccan Chicken, Crussh Juice Bars*	1 Portion/285g	390	21.0	137	6.0	11.9	7.3	0.5
Tuna Nicoise Salad, Crussh Juice Bars*	1 Portion/250g	135	5.0	54	6.7	4.5	2.1	1.2
Wheatfree Roast Vegetable & Pesto, Crussh Juice Bars*	1 Portion/160g	448	10.0	280	9.1	47.6	6.4	3.5
SANDWICH								
5aday Wheat Free, Crussh Juice Bars*	1 Pack/200g	326	15.0	163	4.2	22.2	7.3	1.2
Chicken Avocado & Rocket , Crussh Juice Bars*	1 Pack/190g	367	13.0	193	12.1	20.7	7.0	3.9
Chicken Tarragon & Cucumber, Crussh Juice Bars*	1 Pack/190g	325	10.0	171	10.8	19.7	5.5	3.0
Classic Chicken Club, Crussh Juice Bars*	1 Pack/235g	411	15.0	175	11.8	17.5	6.5	1.3
Egg & Sprout on Genius GF Bread, Crussh Juice Bars*	1 Pack/175g	399	27.0	228	8.6	16.4	15.2	4.6
Egg Mayo & Mustard Cress, Crussh Juice Bars*	1 Pack/318g	369	4.0	116	5.6	20.6	1.3	3.7
Roasted Salmon Dill & Watercress, Crussh Juice Bars*	1 Pack/190g	294	6.0	155	9.5	21.7	3.4	3.3
Smokey Ham Swiss, Crussh Juice Bars*	1 Pack/244g	490	19.0	201	12.1	20.2	7.9	3.0
Tuna Cumber & Mayo, Crussh Juice Bars*	1 Pack/180g	373	17.0	207	11.6	17.3	9.4	2.7
SMOOTHIE								
Bananarama, Crussh Juice Bars*	1 Med Cup/339ml	183	2.0	54	3.7	8.6	0.6	0.4
Blueberry Hill, Crussh Juice Bars*	1 Med Cup/338ml	159	1.0	47	1.8	9.1	0.4	1.6
Crusshberry Blast, Crussh Juice Bars*	1 Med Cup/338ml	159	1.0	47	1.8	9.0	0.4	1.6
Detox Cactus It's Back, Crussh Juice Bars*	1 Med Cup/330ml	221	1.0	67	1.8	14.2	0.2	0.7
Mango Madness, Crussh Juice Bars*	1 Med Cup/340ml	180	1.0	53	1.8	10.6	0.4	0.8
Peach Passion, Crussh Juice Bars*	1 Med Cup/338ml	159	1.0	47	2.0	9.0	0.3	0.6
Pineapple Pleasure, Crussh Juice Bars*	1 Med Cup/338ml	176	1.0	52	1.7	10.5	0.4	0.6
Strawberry Cool, Crussh Juice Bars*	1 Med Cup/339ml	156	1.0	46	1.9	8.9	0.3	0.9
SNACKS & DESSERTS								
Chocolate Cake, Crussh Juice Bars*	1 Portion/115g	469	22.0	408	4.2	54.7	19.4	0.0
Elizabeth Hurley Banana & Choc, Crussh Juice Bars*	1 Portion/26g	99	3.0	381	7.3	60.7	12.6	4.6
Elizabeth Hurley Orange & Choc, Crussh Juice Bars*	1 Portion/26g	98	4.0	376	6.3	58.2	13.7	5.4
Elizabeth Hurley Orange & Cranberry, Crussh Juice Bars*	1 Portion/28g	100	1.0	357	1.3	80.7	3.0	0.8
Elizabeth Hurley Strawberry & Cherry, Crussh Juice Bars*	1 Portion/28g	99	1.0	355	1.3	80.1	2.9	0.6
Natural Wasabi Peas, Crussh Juice Bars*	1 Portion/71g	294	6.0	412	15.7	66.6	8.8	10.8
Orange Crussh Brownie, Crussh Juice Bars*	1 Portion/75g	315	18.0	420	5.4	47.6	23.8	1.3
Organic Choc Chip Hazelnut Cookie, Crussh Juice Bars*	1 Portion/50g	228	13.0	457	5.8	50.3	25.8	2.3
Organic Double Chocolate Cookie, Crussh Juice Bars*	1 Portion/50g	210	9.0	421	5.0	60.8	17.6	2.7
Organic Mince Pie, Crussh Juice Bars*	1 Portion/18g	80	4.0	441	4.5	57.7	21.2	1.9

CRUSSH JUICE BARS

	Measure INFO/WEIGHT	per Measure KCAL	FAT	Nutrition Values per 100g / 100ml KCAL	PROT	CARB	FAT	FIBRE

SNACKS & DESSERTS

	Measure INFO/WEIGHT	KCAL	FAT	KCAL	PROT	CARB	FAT	FIBRE
Organic Oat & Raisin Cookie, Crussh Juice Bars*	1 Portion/50g	203	9.0	406	4.8	55.8	18.2	2.7
Organic Popcorn Honey, Crussh Juice Bars*	1 Portion/30g	135	5.0	449	4.1	75.6	17.3	6.4
Organic Popcorn Sea Salt, Crussh Juice Bars*	1 Portion/30g	118	5.0	394	11.0	64.9	15.8	13.0
Soft Serve Frozen Yoghurt Fat Free, Crussh Juice Bars*	1 Pot/150g	162	0.0	108	33.6	24.0	0.0	0.0

SOUP

	Measure INFO/WEIGHT	KCAL	FAT	KCAL	PROT	CARB	FAT	FIBRE
Beef & Vegetable Pot, Crussh Juice Bars*	1 Med Cup/330g	148	2.0	45	2.9	7.1	0.5	1.2
Beef Bourguignon, Crussh Juice Bars*	1 Med Cup/330g	152	5.0	46	4.1	2.3	1.6	0.6
Beef Chilli, Crussh Juice Bars*	1 Med Cup/329g	240	11.0	73	5.4	5.6	3.2	1.6
Broccoli & Cauliflower Cheese, Crussh Juice Bars*	1 Med Cup/329g	158	8.0	48	2.5	3.9	2.4	0.9
Cajun Black Bean Gumbo, Crussh Juice Bars*	1 Med Cup/329g	125	4.0	38	1.7	4.9	1.3	1.5
Carrot Coriander & Red Pepper, Crussh Juice Bars*	1 Med Cup/330g	175	8.0	53	1.8	6.1	2.5	0.0
Chicken Chilli Stew, Crussh Juice Bars*	1 Med Cup/329g	161	1.0	49	6.1	5.3	0.4	1.5
Chicken, Pumpkin & Jalapeno , Crussh Juice Bars*	1 Med Cup/330g	145	8.0	44	1.8	1.4	2.4	1.0
Chickpea Spinach & Dhal, Crussh Juice Bars*	1 Med Cup/330g	185	6.0	56	3.5	6.6	1.7	1.4
Chorizo Lentil & Bacon, Crussh Juice Bars*	1 Med Cup/330g	231	8.0	70	5.6	6.5	2.4	1.4
Cream of Celeriac, Cheddar, Parsley, Crussh Juice Bars*	1 Med Cup/329g	168	10.0	51	1.5	4.8	3.0	0.8
Egyptian Lentil, Crussh Juice Bars*	1 Med Cup/330g	106	2.0	32	2.3	4.6	0.5	1.2
Fit Meatballs Sicilian Style, Crussh Juice Bars*	1 Med Cup/500g	482	17.0	96	5.3	11.2	3.4	0.9
Ginger Chicken Miso, Crussh Juice Bars*	1 Med Cup/600g	204	7.0	34	2.8	3.3	1.1	0.7
Healthy Italian Vegetable, Crussh Juice Bars*	1 Med Cup/328g	59	1.0	18	1.1	2.4	0.4	1.2
Herb & Chorizo Risotto , Crussh Juice Bars*	1 Med Cup/330g	188	10.0	57	1.8	5.6	3.1	1.0
Hungarian Goulash, Crussh Juice Bars*	1 Med Cup/330g	152	2.0	46	3.8	6.3	0.7	0.9
Indian Chicken Rajah, Crussh Juice Bars*	1 Med Cup/330g	152	2.0	46	2.8	7.7	0.5	1.1
Indian Pea & Cauliflower Dhal, Crussh Juice Bars*	1 Med Cup/330g	211	6.0	64	4.1	8.1	1.8	4.2
Indian Tomato, Crussh Juice Bars*	1 Med Cup/330g	122	7.0	37	1.0	3.4	2.2	0.9
Indonesian Chicken Noodle, Crussh Juice Bars*	1 Med Cup/329g	112	4.0	34	3.7	2.2	1.1	0.3
Italian Minestrone, Crussh Juice Bars*	1 Med Cup/330g	129	1.0	39	2.1	6.8	0.3	2.0
Italian Sun Ripened Tomato & Basil, Crussh Juice Bars*	1 Med Cup/330g	125	6.0	38	0.6	4.6	1.8	1.0
Leek & Potato, Crussh Juice Bars*	1 Med Cup/330g	132	5.0	40	0.9	5.5	1.5	0.7
Lentil & Bacon, Crussh Juice Bars*	1 Med Cup/329g	168	2.0	51	3.1	8.1	0.7	1.3
Lentil & Herbs, Crussh Juice Bars*	1 Med Cup/330g	172	1.0	52	3.8	8.3	0.4	1.7
Louisiana Chicken Gumbo, Crussh Juice Bars*	1 Med Cup/328g	151	8.0	46	3.2	2.9	2.4	1.2
Mediterranean Vegetable, Crussh Juice Bars*	1 Med Cup/331g	116	4.0	35	2.0	4.4	1.1	1.7
Minestrone Alla Ligure, Crussh Juice Bars*	1 Med Cup/330g	56	1.0	17	0.8	3.0	0.2	0.8
Moroccan Lamb Couscous, Crussh Juice Bars*	1 Med Cup/330g	218	7.0	66	3.5	7.8	2.0	1.6
Organic Armenian Dahl, Crussh Juice Bars*	1 Med Cup/330g	262	5.0	79	4.6	11.8	1.5	1.4
Organic Beetroot & Creme Fraiche, Crussh Juice Bars*	1 Med Cup/329g	133	8.0	40	1.1	2.9	2.3	1.9
Organic Carrot & Cardamon, Crussh Juice Bars*	1 Med Cup/331g	116	7.0	35	0.6	3.2	2.2	1.2
Organic Carrot & Coriander, Crussh Juice Bars*	1 Med Cup/331g	88	3.0	27	0.6	4.2	0.8	1.3
Organic Carrot & Creme Fraiche, Crussh Juice Bars*	1 Med Cup/329g	224	13.0	68	1.2	7.3	3.8	1.1
Organic Chickpea, Lentil & Spinach, Crussh Juice Bars*	1 Med Cup/329g	257	10.0	78	4.0	8.9	3.0	1.7
Organic Corn & Sweet Potato, Crussh Juice Bars*	1 Med Cup/330g	360	10.0	109	3.5	17.3	3.1	2.6
Organic Farmhouse Chicken, Crussh Juice Bars*	1 Med Cup/329g	191	9.0	58	3.4	5.2	2.6	3.0
Organic Leek & Potato, Crussh Juice Bars*	1 Med Cup/329g	181	9.0	55	1.2	6.5	2.8	1.0
Organic Mixed Vegetable, Crussh Juice Bars*	1 Med Cup/329g	168	2.0	51	3.5	8.0	0.6	2.0
Organic Moroccan Vegetable, Crussh Juice Bars*	1 Med Cup/331g	86	2.0	26	1.0	4.2	0.7	0.0
Organic Pea, Mint & Lemon , Crussh Juice Bars*	1 Med Cup/330g	123	2.0	37	1.9	4.6	0.6	2.7
Organic Roast Tomato & Thyme, Crussh Juice Bars*	1 Med Cup/330g	99	4.0	30	0.9	4.0	1.1	0.9
Organic Spanish Vegetable, Crussh Juice Bars*	1 Med Cup/330g	132	1.0	40	1.8	5.7	0.2	1.9
Organic Thai Tomato , Crussh Juice Bars*	1 Med Cup/331g	182	11.0	55	1.3	5.7	3.3	1.6
Organic Thai Tomato, Crussh Juice Bars*	1 Med Cup/330g	267	20.0	81	0.9	5.4	6.2	1.6
Organic Tomato & Basil, Crussh Juice Bars*	1 Med Cup/330g	155	10.0	47	0.7	5.2	2.9	0.6

CRUSSH JUICE BARS

SOUP

	Measure INFO/WEIGHT	KCAL	FAT	KCAL	PROT	CARB	FAT	FIBRE
Organic Tomato & Lentil, Crussh Juice Bars*	1 Med Cup/330g	173	3.0	52	2.9	8.3	0.9	11.4
Organic Tuscan Vegetable, Crussh Juice Bars*	1 Med Cup/330g	178	6.0	54	2.8	7.5	1.7	3.1
Organic Wild Mushroom, Crussh Juice Bars*	1 Med Cup/329g	168	10.0	51	1.1	5.3	2.9	0.5
Organic Winter Vegetable, Crussh Juice Bars*	1 Med Cup/330g	122	4.0	37	1.9	5.0	1.1	1.4
Portuguese Caldo Verde, Crussh Juice Bars*	1 Med Cup/329g	102	6.0	31	1.8	2.0	1.7	0.5
Provencale Chicken, Crussh Juice Bars*	1 Med Cup/330g	82	2.0	25	3.2	1.6	0.6	0.6
Red Pepper, Lentil & Tomato , Crussh Juice Bars*	1 Med Cup/329g	135	2.0	41	2.2	6.9	0.5	1.2
Red Thai Chicken & Coconut, Crussh Juice Bars*	1 Med Cup/330g	300	21.0	91	4.0	4.5	6.4	0.5
Smokey Chick Pea & Chorizo, Crussh Juice Bars*	1 Med Cup/330g	165	6.0	50	2.5	5.8	1.9	1.0
Spicy Butternut, Roast Red Pepper, Crussh Juice Bars*	1 Med Cup/330g	155	5.0	47	1.5	6.3	1.6	1.3
Spicy Chicken Tomato & Quinoa, Crussh Juice Bars*	1 Med Cup/330g	181	4.0	55	5.0	6.1	1.1	0.8
Spicy Indonesian Coconut Chicken, Crussh Juice Bars*	1 Med Cup/330g	185	9.0	56	2.2	5.9	2.7	1.1
Spicy Red Lentil & Coriander, Crussh Juice Bars*	1 Med Cup/329g	171	3.0	52	2.7	8.9	0.8	2.8
Spicy Red Lentil & Vegetable, Crussh Juice Bars*	1 Med Cup/330g	214	6.0	65	3.4	8.8	1.8	1.3
Spring Chicken, Crussh Juice Bars*	1 Med Cup/330g	116	3.0	35	3.6	3.0	1.0	0.9
Thai Chicken & Sweet Potato, Crussh Juice Bars*	1 Med Cup/329g	224	7.0	68	4.6	7.6	2.2	2.0
Thai Red Lentil, Crussh Juice Bars*	1 Med Cup/330g	165	10.0	50	1.8	3.8	3.1	0.6
Tomato, Cannellini Bean & Quioa , Crussh Juice Bars*	1 Med Cup/330g	267	9.0	81	3.7	11.1	2.6	3.4
Toulouse Smoked Sausage & Lentil, Crussh Juice Bars*	1 Med Cup/330g	201	12.0	61	2.7	4.7	3.5	1.0
Vegetable Chilli, Crussh Juice Bars*	1 Med Cup/329g	158	5.0	48	2.3	6.3	1.6	2.2
Vegetable Garden, Crussh Juice Bars*	1 Med Cup/330g	188	2.0	57	3.2	10.2	0.5	3.8
Welsh Lamb, Lentil & Vegetable, Crussh Juice Bars*	1 Med Cup/330g	112	5.0	34	3.1	2.1	1.5	0.8

SUPER SMOOTHIES

	Measure INFO/WEIGHT	KCAL	FAT	KCAL	PROT	CARB	FAT	FIBRE
Bliss Blend, Crussh Juice Bars*	1 Med Cup/340ml	163	1.0	48	1.8	9.5	0.3	0.8
Brainstorm, Crussh Juice Bars*	1 Med Cup/339ml	166	1.0	49	1.7	9.8	0.4	1.1
Brazilian, Crussh Juice Bars*	1 Med Cup/339ml	224	2.0	66	1.8	10.1	0.6	0.9
Breakfast Smoothie, Crussh Juice Bars*	1 Med Cup/339ml	346	5.0	102	4.6	17.8	1.4	1.3
Energy Explosion, Crussh Juice Bars*	1 Med Cup/339ml	183	1.0	54	1.7	10.8	0.4	0.9
Fat Burner, Crussh Juice Bars*	1 Med Cup/339ml	156	1.0	46	1.7	9.0	0.4	1.4
Good Morning, Crussh Juice Bars*	1 Med Cup/339ml	166	1.0	49	1.9	9.5	0.2	1.2
Peach Performance, Crussh Juice Bars*	1 Med Cup/346ml	235	5.0	68	12.0	13.8	1.4	0.7
Protein Power, Crussh Juice Bars*	1 Med Cup/346ml	235	4.0	68	9.9	14.0	1.2	0.8
Sporty Spicy, Crussh Juice Bars*	1 Med Cup/329ml	230	1.0	70	1.8	14.8	0.3	0.6
You're CherryFit, Crussh Juice Bars*	1 Med Cup/328ml	243	1.0	74	1.9	11.6	0.2	0.6

SUSHI

	Measure INFO/WEIGHT	KCAL	FAT	KCAL	PROT	CARB	FAT	FIBRE
Avocado Sweet Potato Sushi Wrap, Crussh Juice Bars*	1 Serving/61g	88	1.0	143	2.7	29.0	2.0	1.5
Chicken Salad Sushi Wrap, Crussh Juice Bars*	1 Serving/64g	84	1.0	131	5.7	24.1	1.3	1.2
Salmon Salad Sushi Wrap, Crussh Juice Bars*	1 Serving/71g	96	1.0	135	6.1	24.1	1.5	1.2
Veggie Sushi Salad Box, Crussh Juice Bars*	1 Serving/77g	132	4.0	172	5.8	26.3	5.2	1.6

TOASTIE

	Measure INFO/WEIGHT	KCAL	FAT	KCAL	PROT	CARB	FAT	FIBRE
Cheesy Marmite, Crussh Juice Bars*	1 Toastie/155g	453	17.0	292	18.4	30.6	10.7	0.0
Chilli Cheddar Honey Mustard, Crussh Juice Bars*	1 Toastie/89g	255	11.0	287	14.7	29.6	12.2	0.7
Christmas Turkey, Crussh Juice Bars*	1 Toastie/200g	456	17.0	228	13.3	24.9	8.4	0.2
Jalapeno & Spinach Melt, Crussh Juice Bars*	1 Toastie/150g	403	16.0	269	13.9	29.3	10.7	0.3
Lemon Courgette, Halloumi, Rocket, Crussh Juice Bars*	1 Toastie/105g	226	9.0	215	11.6	23.4	8.3	0.5
Pesto Chicken & Cheddar, Crussh Juice Bars*	1 Toastie/190g	541	27.0	285	17.8	21.7	14.1	0.0
Skinny Ham & Edam, Crussh Juice Bars*	1 Toastie/130g	329	9.0	253	15.4	32.9	6.7	0.0
Tasty Cheddar Cheese, Crussh Juice Bars*	1 Toastie/105g	310	10.0	295	14.5	37.9	9.5	0.0
Tuna Swiss Melt, Crussh Juice Bars*	1 Toastie/170g	379	12.0	223	16.3	24.0	6.8	0.1

WRAP

	Measure INFO/WEIGHT	KCAL	FAT	KCAL	PROT	CARB	FAT	FIBRE
Chipotle Chicken on SunRipe Tom, Crussh Juice Bars*	1 Wrap/300g	588	30.0	196	8.6	17.9	10.1	1.0
Crussh Tricolore & Sun Ripe Tomato, Crussh Juice Bars*	1 Wrap/225g	549	30.0	244	8.1	23.0	13.4	1.0

	Measure INFO/WEIGHT	per Measure KCAL	FAT	Nutrition Values per 100g / 100ml KCAL	PROT	CARB	FAT	FIBRE

CRUSSH JUICE BARS
WRAP

	Measure INFO/WEIGHT	KCAL	FAT	KCAL	PROT	CARB	FAT	FIBRE
Hoummus & Falafel, Crussh Juice Bars*	1 Wrap/178g	318	8.0	179	6.9	27.0	4.7	2.4
Simply Caesar, Crussh Juice Bars*	1 Wrap/190g	538	17.0	283	10.3	40.4	8.8	1.5
Smoked Salmon Royale on Spinach, Crussh Juice Bars*	1 Wrap/220g	453	18.0	206	10.9	21.9	8.3	0.8
Tuna Salad, Crussh Juice Bars*	1 Wrap/210g	365	10.0	174	12.0	20.4	4.9	0.4

CUISINE DE FRANCE
BREAD

Baguette, Demi, Cuisine De France*	1 Serving/140g	360	2.0	257	6.7	56.0	1.4	1.7
Baguette, la Premier, Cuisine De France*	1 Serving/70g	180	1.0	257	7.6	54.3	1.0	1.8
Baguette, Parisien, Cuisine De France*	1 Serving/70g	171	1.0	245	8.5	51.0	0.8	1.9
Baps, Brown, Soft, Cuisine De France*	1 Bap/99g	236	1.0	238	11.5	46.0	0.9	7.3
Ciabattina, Cuisine De France*	1 Roll/120g	299	2.0	249	8.3	50.3	1.6	1.5
French, Cuisine De France*	½ Stick/200g	490	2.0	245	8.5	51.0	0.8	1.9

MUFFIN

Cappuccino, Iced, Luxury, Iced, Cuisine De France*	1 Muffin/105g	457	23.0	435	5.6	54.8	21.5	0.0
Carrot Cake, Cuisine De France*	1 Muffin/105g	373	13.0	355	4.7	56.9	12.0	0.0

DOMINO'S PIZZA
BREAD

Garlic, Pizza, Domino's Pizza*	1 Slice/50.5g	137	5.0	271	16.4	30.3	9.4	2.8

BROWNIES

Chocolate, Squares, Domino's Pizza*	1 Brownie/22g	104	6.0	474	5.9	54.2	25.9	1.8

CHICKEN

Kickers, Domino's Pizza*	7 Kickers/168g	366	15.0	218	18.0	17.0	8.7	0.9
Strippers, Domino's Pizza*	7 Strippers/189g	442	23.0	234	17.0	13.5	12.4	1.1

COLESLAW

Domino's Pizza*	1 Tub/200g	328	30.0	164	1.3	6.6	14.8	1.7

COOKIES

Domino's Pizza*	1 Cookie/40g	175	7.0	438	5.6	66.6	18.0	3.1

DIP

BBQ, Domino's Pizza*	1 Pot/28g	46	0.0	163	0.0	39.5	0.5	0.0
Chocolate Sauce, Domino's Pizza*	1 Pot/28g	88	0.0	313	0.5	76.6	0.4	0.8
Garlic & Herb, Domino's Pizza*	1 Pot/28g	194	21.0	693	1.1	1.9	75.4	0.1
Honey & Mustard, Domino's Pizza*	1 Pot/28g	129	13.0	459	1.8	7.5	46.5	0.2
Mango, Domino's Pizza*	1 Pot/28g	52	0.0	185	0.2	42.5	1.1	0.6
Sweet Chilli, Domino's Pizza*	1 Pot/28g	61	0.0	217	4.0	51.0	0.9	0.6
Toffee, Domino's Pizza*	1 Pot/28g	94	1.0	335	1.5	75.1	3.2	0.1

PIZZA

American Hot, Dominator, Large, Domino's Pizza*	1 Slice/109.5g	306	12.0	279	13.2	31.7	11.0	1.9
American Hot, Regular Crust, Large, Domino's Pizza*	1 Slice/87g	217	8.0	250	13.6	29.0	8.8	2.2
American Hot, Regular Crust, Medium, Domino's Pizza*	1 Slice/79g	194	7.0	245	13.3	28.0	8.9	2.2
American Hot, Regular Crust, Personal, Domino's Pizza*	1 Pizza/244g	644	20.0	264	14.7	32.6	8.3	2.2
American Hot, Regular Crust, Small, Domino's Pizza*	1 Slice/712g	181	7.0	253	14.0	28.5	9.2	2.2
American Hot, Thin Crust, Large, Domino's Pizza*	1 Slice/67g	202	10.0	303	14.7	28.4	14.5	2.2
American Hot, Thin Crust, Medium, Domino's Pizza*	1 Slice/62g	191	9.0	308	15.0	28.4	15.0	2.5
Americano, Large, Domino's Pizza*	1 Slice/114g	334	11.0	293	14.1	37.0	10.0	1.8
Americano, Medium, Domino's Pizza*	1 Slice/103g	346	15.0	336	14.8	36.1	14.7	1.8
Americano, Regular Crust, Large, Domino's Pizza*	1 Slice/91g	268	8.0	295	15.7	37.2	9.3	1.9
Americano, Regular Crust, Medium, Domino's Pizza*	1 Slice/84g	248	8.0	295	15.7	37.2	9.3	1.9
Americano, Regular Crust, Personal, Domino's Pizza*	1 Pizza/257g	738	20.0	287	19.4	35.0	7.7	2.5
Americano, Regular Crust, Small, Domino's Pizza*	1 Slice/76g	224	7.0	295	15.7	37.2	9.3	1.9
Americano, Thin Crust, Large, Domino's Pizza*	1 Slice/71g	257	11.0	362	17.4	39.3	15.0	2.1
Americano, Thin Crust, Medium, Domino's Pizza*	1 Slice/67g	243	10.0	362	17.4	39.3	15.0	2.1
Bacon Dble Cheese, Dominator, Large, Domino's Pizza*	1 Slice/120g	328	13.0	273	14.1	29.3	11.0	1.9

DOMINO'S PIZZA

PIZZA

	Measure INFO/WEIGHT	per Measure KCAL	per Measure FAT	KCAL	PROT	CARB	FAT	FIBRE
Bacon Dble Cheese, Reg Crust, Lge, Domino's Pizza*	1 Slice/97g	240	10.0	247	14.7	24.6	10.0	1.9
Bacon Dble Cheese, Reg Crust, Med, Domino's Pizza*	1 Slice/88g	217	9.0	247	14.7	24.6	10.0	1.9
Bacon Dble Cheese, Regular Crust, Sm, Domino's Pizza*	1 Slice/80g	198	8.0	247	14.7	24.6	10.0	1.9
Bacon Dble Cheese, Thin Crust, Large, Domino's Pizza*	1 Slice/77g	224	12.0	291	16.3	21.8	15.4	2.2
Bacon Dble Cheese, Thin Crust, Med, Domino's Pizza*	1 Slice/71g	215	11.0	303	16.4	24.1	15.6	2.1
Beef & Onion Pie, Dominator, Large, Domino's Pizza*	1 Slice/110g	290	10.0	264	12.5	32.2	9.5	2.1
Beef & Onion Pie, RegCrust, Personal, Domino's Pizza*	1 Pizza/244g	620	19.0	254	14.2	32.3	7.6	2.2
Beef & Onion Pie, Regular Crust, Large, Domino's Pizza*	1 Slice/87g	204	7.0	234	12.7	27.8	8.0	2.2
Beef & Onion Pie, Regular Crust, Med, Domino's Pizza*	1 Slice/79g	185	6.0	234	12.7	27.8	8.0	2.2
Beef & Onion Pie, Regular Crust, Small, Domino's Pizza*	1 Slice/71g	166	6.0	234	12.7	27.8	8.0	2.2
Beef & Onion Pie, Thin Crust, Large, Domino's Pizza*	1 Slice/67g	188	9.0	280	14.0	25.4	13.6	2.6
Beef & Onion Pie, Thin Crust, Medium, Domino's Pizza*	1 Slice/62g	182	9.0	294	14.2	28.1	13.9	2.5
Calypso, Dominator, Large, Domino's Pizza*	1 Slice/106g	279	9.0	263	12.5	33.9	8.7	2.2
Calypso, Double Decadence, Medium, Domino's Pizza*	1 Slice/95g	273	13.0	287	12.1	28.8	13.8	2.4
Calypso, Regular Crust, Large, Domino's Pizza*	1 Slice/80g	185	6.0	231	12.7	29.6	6.9	2.3
Calypso, Regular Crust, Medium, Domino's Pizza*	1 Slice/72g	166	5.0	231	12.7	29.6	6.9	2.3
Calypso, Regular Crust, Personal, Domino's Pizza*	1 Pizza/233g	589	15.0	253	14.2	34.3	6.6	2.2
Calypso, Regular Crust, Small, Domino's Pizza*	1 Slice/65g	150	4.0	231	12.7	29.6	6.9	2.3
Calypso, Thin Crust, Large, Domino's Pizza*	1 Slice/63g	176	8.0	279	14.1	27.8	12.5	2.7
Calypso, Thin Crust, Medium, Domino's Pizza*	1 Slice/59g	132	4.0	223	12.5	28.5	6.6	2.2
Cheese & Tomato, Dominator, Large, Domino's Pizza*	1 Slice/92g	265	9.0	288	13.0	37.6	9.5	2.3
Cheese & Tomato, Reg Crust, Personal, Domino's Pizza*	1 Pizza/201g	559	14.0	278	15.1	38.3	7.2	2.4
Cheese & Tomato, Reg Crust, Small, Domino's Pizza*	1 Slice/56g	148	4.0	264	14.1	34.5	7.8	2.5
Cheese & Tomato, Regular Crust, Lge, Domino's Pizza*	1 Slice/69g	183	5.0	265	14.0	34.7	7.8	2.4
Cheese & Tomato, Regular Crust, Med, Domino's Pizza*	1 Slice/63g	162	5.0	257	13.4	33.6	7.6	2.4
Cheese & Tomato, Thin Crust, Large, Domino's Pizza*	1 Slice/49g	162	7.0	330	15.6	32.9	15.2	3.1
Cheese & Tomato, Thin Crust, Medium, Domino's Pizza*	1 Slice/46g	160	7.0	347	15.7	36.2	15.5	2.9
Chicken Feast, Dble Decadence, Med, Domino's Pizza*	1 Slice/100g	232	7.0	232	14.3	28.9	6.6	2.1
Chicken Feast, Dominator, Large, Domino's Pizza*	1 Slice/112g	289	9.0	258	13.9	32.3	8.2	2.0
Chicken Feast, Reg Crust, Personal, Domino's Pizza*	1 Pizza/248g	613	15.0	247	15.7	32.3	6.1	2.1
Chicken Feast, Regular Crust, Large, Domino's Pizza*	1 Slice/89g	201	6.0	226	14.6	27.8	6.3	2.1
Chicken Feast, Regular Crust, Medium, Domino's Pizza*	1 Slice/81g	183	5.0	226	14.6	27.8	6.3	2.1
Chicken Feast, Regular Crust, Small, Domino's Pizza*	1 Slice/72g	163	5.0	226	14.6	27.8	6.3	2.1
Chicken Feast, Thin Crust, Large, Domino's Pizza*	1 Slice/69g	195	8.0	283	16.5	28.1	11.6	2.4
Chicken Feast, Thin Crust, Medium, Domino's Pizza*	1 Slice/64g	181	7.0	283	16.5	28.1	11.6	2.4
Chicken Tikka, Reg Crust, Personal, Domino's Pizza*	1 Pizza/239g	564	11.0	236	11.7	32.0	4.7	2.4
Chicken Tikka, Regular Crust, Large, Domino's Pizza*	1 Slice/85g	194	6.0	229	13.1	27.8	7.3	2.3
Chicken Tikka, Regular Crust, Medium, Domino's Pizza*	1 Slice/77g	177	6.0	229	13.1	27.8	7.3	2.3
Chicken Tikka, Regular Crust, Small, Domino's Pizza*	1 Slice/69g	158	5.0	229	13.1	27.8	7.3	2.3
Chicken Tikka, Thin Crust, Large, Domino's Pizza*	1 Slice/62g	146	5.0	235	13.6	27.3	7.9	2.4
Chicken Tikka, Thin Crust, Medium, Domino's Pizza*	1 Slice/58g	136	5.0	235	13.6	27.3	7.9	2.4
Deluxe, Double Decadence, Medium, Domino's Pizza*	1 Slice/100g	296	15.0	296	12.5	26.6	15.5	2.3
Deluxe, Regular Crust, Large, Domino's Pizza*	1 Slice/88g	216	8.0	245	13.2	26.9	9.4	2.1
Deluxe, Regular Crust, Medium, Domino's Pizza*	1 Slice/81g	198	8.0	245	13.2	26.9	9.4	2.1
Deluxe, Regular Crust, Personal, Domino's Pizza*	1 Pizza/250g	662	23.0	265	14.4	31.4	9.1	2.1
Deluxe, Regular Crust, Small, Domino's Pizza*	1 Slice/74g	181	7.0	245	13.2	26.9	9.4	2.1
Deluxe, Thin Crust, Large, Domino's Pizza*	1 Slice/68g	199	10.0	292	14.5	24.7	15.1	2.5
Deluxe, Thin Crust, Medium, Domino's Pizza*	1 Slice/64g	196	10.0	307	14.7	27.0	15.5	2.4
Extravaganza, Dble Decadence, Med, Domino's Pizza*	1 Slice/114g	327	18.0	287	13.1	23.7	15.5	2.1
Extravaganza, Dominator, Large, Domino's Pizza*	1 Slice/127g	338	14.0	266	13.3	28.2	11.1	1.9
Extravaganza, Regular Crust, Large, Domino's Pizza*	1 Slice/104g	252	11.0	242	13.7	23.4	10.3	1.9
Extravaganza, Regular Crust, Medium, Domino's Pizza*	1 Slice/95g	230	10.0	242	13.7	23.4	10.3	1.9

	Measure	per Measure		Nutrition Values per 100g / 100ml				
	INFO/WEIGHT	KCAL	FAT	KCAL	PROT	CARB	FAT	FIBRE

DOMINO'S PIZZA

PIZZA

	Measure	per Measure		Nutrition Values per 100g / 100ml				
Extravaganza, Regular Crust, Personal, Domino's Pizza*	1 Pizza/298g	781	31.0	262	15.2	26.7	10.4	1.9
Extravaganza, Regular Crust, Small, Domino's Pizza*	1 Slice/86g	208	9.0	242	13.7	23.4	10.3	1.9
Extravaganza, Thin Crust, Large, Domino's Pizza*	1 Slice/84g	235	13.0	280	15.0	20.7	15.2	2.2
Extravaganza, Thin Crust, Medium, Domino's Pizza*	1 Slice/78g	227	12.0	291	15.1	22.6	15.5	2.1
Farmhouse, Dble Decadence, Medium, Domino's Pizza*	1 Slice/100g	277	13.0	277	12.7	26.5	13.4	2.3
Farmhouse, Dominator, Large, Domino's Pizza*	1 Slice/111g	283	9.0	255	13.0	31.7	8.5	2.0
Farmhouse, Regular Crust, Large, Domino's Pizza*	1 Slice/88g	195	6.0	222	13.4	26.8	6.8	2.1
Farmhouse, Regular Crust, Medium, Domino's Pizza*	1 Slice/81g	180	6.0	222	13.4	26.8	6.8	2.1
Farmhouse, Regular Crust, Personal, Domino's Pizza*	1 Pizza/248g	605	16.0	244	14.8	31.5	6.5	2.1
Farmhouse, Regular Crust, Small, Domino's Pizza*	1 Slice/73g	162	5.0	222	13.4	26.8	6.8	2.1
Farmhouse, Thin Crust, Large, Domino's Pizza*	1 Slice/68g	180	8.0	265	14.8	24.6	11.9	2.5
Farmhouse, Thin Crust, Medium, Domino's Pizza*	1 Slice/63g	175	8.0	277	15.1	26.9	12.2	2.4
Full House, Dble Decadence, Medium, Domino's Pizza*	1 Slice/107g	306	16.0	286	12.4	25.9	14.7	2.2
Full House, Dominator, Large, Domino's Pizza*	1 Slice/119g	312	12.0	262	12.6	31.0	9.7	2.0
Full House, Regular Crust, Large, Domino's Pizza*	1 Slice/96g	231	9.0	241	13.2	27.0	8.9	2.1
Full House, Regular Crust, Medium, Domino's Pizza*	1 Slice/88g	208	8.0	236	13.0	26.0	8.9	2.0
Full House, Regular Crust, Personal, Domino's Pizza*	1 Pizza/280g	666	23.0	238	12.4	28.6	8.3	2.1
Full House, Regular Crust, Small, Domino's Pizza*	1 Slice/80g	190	6.0	238	14.8	27.1	7.8	2.3
Full House, Thin Crust, Large, Domino's Pizza*	1 Slice/76g	210	11.0	276	14.0	23.7	13.9	2.4
Full House, Thin Crust, Medium, Domino's Pizza*	1 Slice/71g	206	10.0	290	14.3	25.9	14.3	2.3
Ham & Pineapple, Dominator, Large, Domino's Pizza*	1 Slice/106g	281	9.0	265	13.2	33.3	8.8	2.0
Ham & Pineapple, Reg Crust, Personal, Domino's Pizza*	1 Pizza/240g	550	13.0	229	12.4	32.3	5.6	2.2
Ham & Pineapple, Regular Crust, Large, Domino's Pizza*	1 Slice/84g	194	6.0	231	13.7	28.5	7.0	2.0
Ham & Pineapple, Regular Crust, Med, Domino's Pizza*	1 Slice/77g	178	5.0	231	13.7	28.5	7.0	2.0
Ham & Pineapple, Regular Crust, Sm, Domino's Pizza*	1 Slice/70g	163	4.0	233	15.7	29.7	5.7	2.3
Ham & Pineapple, Thin Crust, Large, Domino's Pizza*	1 Slice/64g	181	8.0	283	15.4	26.8	12.7	2.5
Ham & Pineapple, Thin Crust, Medium, Domino's Pizza*	1 Slice/60g	175	8.0	292	15.4	29.0	12.7	2.3
Hawaiian, Dominator, Large, Domino's Pizza*	1 Slice/117g	298	10.0	254	13.3	30.4	8.8	1.9
Hawaiian, Double Decadence, Medium, Domino's Pizza*	1 Slice/106g	290	14.0	275	13.0	25.5	13.4	2.1
Hawaiian, Regular Crust, Large, Domino's Pizza*	1 Slice/94g	216	7.0	229	14.1	26.5	7.4	1.9
Hawaiian, Regular Crust, Medium, Domino's Pizza*	1 Slice/86g	192	6.0	223	13.8	25.6	7.3	1.9
Hawaiian, Regular Crust, Personal, Domino's Pizza*	1 Pizza/265g	641	18.0	242	14.9	30.0	6.9	1.9
Hawaiian, Regular Crust, Small, Domino's Pizza*	1 Slice/78.5g	176	5.0	224	15.6	26.7	6.1	2.2
Hawaiian, Thin Crust, Large, Domino's Pizza*	1 Slice/74.5g	195	9.0	262	15.1	23.1	12.1	2.2
Hawaiian, Thin Crust, Medium, Domino's Pizza*	1 Slice/69g	190	9.0	274	15.3	25.3	12.4	2.1
Hawaiian,Regular Crust, Personal, Domino's Pizza*	1 Pizza/265g	588	16.0	222	12.6	29.4	6.0	2.0
Hot & Spicy, Dominator, Large, Domino's Pizza*	1 Slice/107g	284	10.0	264	12.2	33.0	9.2	2.2
Hot & Spicy, Double Decadence, Med, Domino's Pizza*	1 Slice/96g	276	14.0	288	11.8	28.0	14.3	2.4
Hot & Spicy, Regular Crust, Large, Domino's Pizza*	1 Slice/84.5g	201	7.0	238	12.7	29.5	7.7	2.3
Hot & Spicy, Regular Crust, Medium, Domino's Pizza*	1 Slice/76g	178	6.0	232	12.3	28.7	7.6	2.3
Hot & Spicy, Regular Crust, Personal, Domino's Pizza*	1 Pizza/237g	602	17.0	254	13.9	33.3	7.2	2.3
Hot & Spicy, Regular Crust, Small, Domino's Pizza*	1 Slice/69g	163	5.0	237	12.8	29.3	7.7	2.3
Hot & Spicy, Thin Crust, Large, Domino's Pizza*	1 Slice/65g	181	9.0	280	9.3	26.5	13.3	2.7
Hot & Spicy, Thin Crust, Medium, Domino's Pizza*	1 Slice/59.5g	175	8.0	294	13.7	29.2	13.6	2.6
Hot Dog, Dominator, Large, Domino's Pizza*	1 Slice/129g	368	17.0	285	14.0	27.7	13.1	1.9
Hot Dog, Double Decadence, Medium, Domino's Pizza*	1 Slice/117g	358	21.0	306	13.7	23.1	17.6	2.1
Hot Dog, Regular Crust, Large, Domino's Pizza*	1 Slice/106g	323	14.0	305	14.1	31.6	13.5	1.8
Hot Dog, Regular Crust, Medium, Domino's Pizza*	1 Slice/98g	299	13.0	305	14.1	31.6	13.5	1.8
Hot Dog, Regular Crust, Personal, Domino's Pizza*	1 Pizza/284g	784	32.0	276	15.5	27.9	11.3	2.0
Hot Dog, Regular Crust, Small, Domino's Pizza*	1 Slice/90g	274	12.0	305	14.1	31.6	13.5	1.8
Hot Dog, Thin Crust, Large, Domino's Pizza*	1 Slice/86g	265	16.0	308	15.9	20.1	18.1	2.2
Hot Dog, Thin Crust, Medium, Domino's Pizza*	1 Slice/81g	258	15.0	319	16.0	21.8	18.5	2.1

	INFO/WEIGHT	KCAL	FAT	KCAL	PROT	CARB	FAT	FIBRE
DOMINO'S PIZZA								
PIZZA								
House, Dominator, Large, Domino's Pizza*	1 Slice/122g	328	13.0	269	15.0	28.7	10.4	1.9
House, Double Decadence, Medium, Domino's Pizza*	1 Slice/110g	319	16.0	290	14.8	24.1	14.9	2.1
House, Regular Crust, Large, Domino's Pizza*	1 Slice/100g	243	9.0	243	15.8	23.8	9.4	1.9
House, Regular Crust, Medium, Domino's Pizza*	1 Slice/91g	221	9.0	243	15.8	23.8	9.4	1.9
House, Regular Crust, Personal, Domino's Pizza*	1 Pizza/274g	707	24.0	258	16.6	28.4	8.6	1.9
House, Regular Crust, Small, Domino's Pizza*	1 Slice/82g	199	8.0	243	15.8	23.8	9.4	1.9
House, Thin Crust, Large, Domino's Pizza*	1 Slice/80g	227	12.0	284	17.6	21.0	14.4	2.2
House, Thin Crust, Medium, Domino's Pizza*	1 Slice/74g	219	11.0	296	17.8	23.1	14.6	2.1
Jamaican Bombastic, Dominator, Lge, Domino's Pizza*	1 Slice/114g	288	9.0	253	12.5	32.8	7.9	2.2
Jamaican Bombastic, Reg Crust, Lge, Domino's Pizza*	1 Slice/91g	201	6.0	221	12.8	28.7	6.1	2.3
Jamaican Bombastic, Reg Crust, Med, Domino's Pizza*	1 Slice/83g	183	5.0	221	12.8	28.7	6.1	2.3
Jamaican Bombastic, Reg Crust, Small, Domino's Pizza*	1 Slice/75g	166	5.0	221	12.8	28.7	6.1	2.3
Jamaican Bombastic, Thin Crust, Large, Domino's Pizza*	1 Slice/71g	185	8.0	260	14.0	26.7	10.8	2.7
Jamaican Bombastic, Thin Crust, Med, Domino's Pizza*	1 Slice/66g	181	7.0	274	14.2	29.2	11.1	2.6
Meat Lovers, Dble Decadence, Med, Domino's Pizza*	1 Slice/101g	314	16.0	311	14.9	26.3	16.3	2.1
Meat Lovers, Dominator, Large, Domino's Pizza*	1 Slice/111g	320	13.0	288	15.1	31.4	11.3	1.9
Meat Lovers, Regular Crust, Large, Domino's Pizza*	1 Slice/89g	235	9.0	264	16.1	26.5	10.4	1.9
Meat Lovers, Regular Crust, Medium, Domino's Pizza*	1 Slice/81g	214	8.0	264	16.1	26.5	10.4	1.9
Meat Lovers, Regular Crust, Personal, Domino's Pizza*	1 Pizza/244g	683	23.0	280	16.8	31.8	9.4	2.0
Meat Lovers, Regular Crust, Small, Domino's Pizza*	1 Slice/74g	195	8.0	264	16.1	26.5	10.4	1.9
Meat Lovers, Thin Crust, Large, Domino's Pizza*	1 Slice/69g	219	11.0	318	18.3	24.2	16.5	2.3
Meat Lovers, Thin Crust, Medium, Domino's Pizza*	1 Slice/64g	211	11.0	330	18.5	26.5	16.7	2.2
Meat Packer, Dble Decadence, Med, Domino's Pizza*	1 Slice/106g	329	17.0	310	15.5	25.1	16.4	2.0
Meat Packer, Dominator, Large, Domino's Pizza*	1 Slice/116g	334	13.0	288	15.6	30.1	11.6	1.8
Meat Packer, Regular Crust, Large, Domino's Pizza*	1 Slice/94g	249	10.0	265	16.8	25.1	10.9	1.8
Meat Packer, Regular Crust, Medium, Domino's Pizza*	1 Slice/86g	228	9.0	265	16.8	25.1	10.9	1.8
Meat Packer, Regular Crust, Personal, Domino's Pizza*	1 Pizza/264g	739	27.0	280	17.6	29.6	10.1	1.8
Meat Packer, Regular Crust, Small, Domino's Pizza*	1 Slice/79g	209	9.0	265	16.8	25.1	10.9	1.8
Meat Packer, Thin Crust, Large, Domino's Pizza*	1 Slice/74g	234	12.0	316	18.9	22.7	16.6	2.1
Meat Packer, Thin Crust, Medium, Domino's Pizza*	1 Slice/69g	226	12.0	327	19.1	24.7	16.8	2.0
Meatball Mayham, Dominator, Large, Domino's Pizza*	1 Slice/122g	350	13.0	288	11.2	36.1	11.0	1.9
Meatball Mayham, Reg Crust, Medium, Domino's Pizza*	1 Slice/91g	263	10.0	288	12.0	36.0	10.7	2.0
Meatball Mayham, Reg Crust, Personal, Domino's Pizza*	1 Pizza/276g	776	25.0	281	15.9	34.0	9.0	2.5
Meatball Mayham, Regular Crust, Large, Domino's Pizza*	1 Slice/99g	285	11.0	288	12.0	36.0	10.7	2.0
Meatball Mayham, Regular Crust, Small, Domino's Pizza*	1 Slice/84g	241	9.0	288	12.0	36.0	10.7	2.0
Meatball Mayham, Thin Crust, Large, Domino's Pizza*	1 Slice/79g	244	12.0	309	12.0	32.5	14.6	2.0
Meatball Mayham, Thin Crust, Medium, Domino's Pizza*	1 Slice/74g	257	12.0	346	12.7	37.5	16.1	2.2
Meateor, Dominator, Large, Domino's Pizza*	1 Slice/114g	357	14.0	313	13.3	36.6	12.7	1.8
Meateor, Double Decadence, Medium, Domino's Pizza*	1 Slice/103g	368	18.0	356	13.9	35.7	17.5	1.8
Meateor, Regular Crust, Large, Domino's Pizza*	1 Slice/88g	280	11.0	319	14.5	36.7	12.7	1.8
Meateor, Regular Crust, Medium, Domino's Pizza*	1 Slice/81g	258	10.0	319	14.5	36.7	12.7	1.8
Meateor, Regular Crust, Personal, Domino's Pizza*	1 Pizza/266g	825	31.0	310	18.4	32.5	11.8	2.3
Meateor, Regular Crust, Small, Domino's Pizza*	1 Slice/74g	236	9.0	319	14.5	36.7	12.7	1.8
Meateor, Thin Crust, Large, Domino's Pizza*	1 Slice/68g	239	12.0	352	15.3	32.8	17.7	1.7
Meateor, Thin Crust, Medium, Domino's Pizza*	1 Slice/64g	250	12.0	392	16.0	38.6	19.3	2.0
Meatzza Pizza, Dble Decadence, Med, Domino's Pizza*	1 Slice/105g	333	18.0	317	14.6	25.5	17.4	2.1
Meatzza Pizza, Dominator, Large, Domino's Pizza*	1 Slice/115g	338	14.0	294	14.8	30.6	12.5	1.9
Meatzza Pizza, Reg Crust, Personal, Domino's Pizza*	1 Pizza/248g	709	26.0	286	16.4	31.4	10.5	2.0
Meatzza Pizza, Thin Crust, Large, Domino's Pizza*	1 Slice/69g	228	12.0	330	18.5	26.5	16.7	2.2
Mediterranean Spice, Dominator, Large, Domino's Pizza*	1 Slice/129g	306	11.0	237	12.9	27.8	8.3	1.9
Mediterranean Spice, Reg Crust, Large, Domino's Pizza*	1 Slice/106g	218	7.0	206	13.4	22.8	6.8	1.9
Mediterranean Spice, Reg Crust, Med, Domino's Pizza*	1 Slice/97g	200	7.0	206	13.4	22.8	6.8	1.9

DOMINO'S PIZZA

PIZZA	INFO/WEIGHT	KCAL	FAT	KCAL	PROT	CARB	FAT	FIBRE
Mediterranean Spice, Reg Crust, Small, Domino's Pizza*	1 Slice/89g	183	6.0	206	13.4	22.8	6.8	1.9
Mediterranean Spice, Thin Crust, Large, Domino's Pizza*	1 Slice/86g	202	9.0	235	14.3	20.2	10.8	2.1
Mediterranean Spice, Thin Crust, Med, Domino's Pizza*	1 Slice/80g	197	9.0	246	14.7	22.0	11.0	2.0
Mexican Hot, Dble Decadence, Med, Domino's Pizza*	1 Slice/103g	302	16.0	293	12.9	26.2	15.1	2.3
Mexican Hot, Dominator, Large, Domino's Pizza*	1 Slice/114g	308	12.0	270	13.2	31.1	10.2	2.1
Mexican Hot, Regular Crust, Large, Domino's Pizza*	1 Slice/98g	238	9.0	243	13.7	26.4	9.1	2.1
Mexican Hot, Regular Crust, Medium, Domino's Pizza*	1 Slice/90g	219	8.0	243	13.7	26.4	9.1	2.1
Mexican Hot, Regular Crust, Personal, Domino's Pizza*	1 Pizza/252g	655	21.0	260	14.9	31.3	8.3	2.2
Mexican Hot, Regular Crust, Small, Domino's Pizza*	1 Slice/81g	197	7.0	243	13.7	26.4	9.1	2.1
Mexican Hot, Thin Crust, Large, Domino's Pizza*	1 Slice/71g	204	10.0	287	15.1	24.0	14.5	2.5
Mexican Hot, Thin Crust, Medium, Domino's Pizza*	1 Slice/66g	199	10.0	301	15.3	26.4	14.9	2.4
Mighty Meaty, Dble Decadence, Med, Domino's Pizza*	1 Slice/107g	319	17.0	298	13.8	25.1	15.8	2.1
Mighty Meaty, Dominator, Large, Domino's Pizza*	1 Slice/118g	326	13.0	276	14.0	30.0	11.1	1.9
Mighty Meaty, Regular Crust, Large, Domino's Pizza*	1 Slice/95g	243	10.0	256	15.0	26.1	10.2	2.0
Mighty Meaty, Regular Crust, Medium, Domino's Pizza*	1 Slice/87g	218	9.0	251	14.7	25.0	10.3	1.9
Mighty Meaty, Regular Crust, Personal, Domino's Pizza*	1 Pizza/265g	662	24.0	250	13.3	29.1	8.9	2.1
Mighty Meaty, Regular Crust, Small, Domino's Pizza*	1 Slice/80g	202	7.0	253	16.5	26.1	9.1	2.2
Mighty Meaty, Thin Crust, Large, Domino's Pizza*	1 Slice/75g	222	12.0	296	16.2	22.6	15.7	2.3
Mighty Meaty, Thin Crust, Medium, Domino's Pizza*	1 Slice/70g	216	11.0	309	16.5	24.6	16.0	2.1
Mixed Grill, Dominator, Large, Domino's Pizza*	1 Slice/117g	325	14.0	278	13.1	30.0	11.8	1.9
Mixed Grill, Double Decadence, Med, Domino's Pizza*	1 Slice/106g	319	18.0	301	12.8	25.1	16.7	2.2
Mixed Grill, Regular Crust, Large, Domino's Pizza*	1 Slice/94g	240	11.0	255	13.5	25.0	11.2	2.0
Mixed Grill, Regular Crust, Medium, Domino's Pizza*	1 Slice/87g	222	10.0	255	13.5	25.0	11.2	2.0
Mixed Grill, Regular Crust, Personal, Domino's Pizza*	1 Pizza/265g	718	28.0	271	14.8	29.6	10.4	2.0
Mixed Grill, Regular Crust, Small, Domino's Pizza*	1 Slice/79g	201	9.0	255	13.5	25.0	11.2	2.0
Mixed Grill, Thin Crust, Large, Domino's Pizza*	1 Slice/74g	223	12.0	301	14.9	22.5	16.8	2.3
Mixed Grill, Thin Crust, Medium, Domino's Pizza*	1 Slice/70g	220	12.0	314	15.0	24.6	17.3	2.2
New Yorker, Dominator, Large, Domino's Pizza*	1 Slice/110g	307	12.0	279	14.6	31.6	10.5	1.9
New Yorker, Double Decadence, Med, Domino's Pizza*	1 Slice/100g	254	9.0	254	15.1	28.0	9.0	2.0
New Yorker, Regular Crust, Large, Domino's Pizza*	1 Slice/87g	220	8.0	253	15.5	26.7	9.4	2.0
New Yorker, Regular Crust, Medium, Domino's Pizza*	1 Slice/80g	202	8.0	253	15.5	26.7	9.4	2.0
New Yorker, Regular Crust, Personal, Domino's Pizza*	1 Pizza/240g	648	20.0	270	16.3	32.1	8.5	2.0
New Yorker, Regular Crust, Small, Domino's Pizza*	1 Slice/73g	185	7.0	253	15.5	26.7	9.4	2.0
New Yorker, Thin Crust, Large, Domino's Pizza*	1 Slice/67g	212	10.0	317	17.6	26.7	15.5	2.2
New Yorker, Thin Crust, Medium, Domino's Pizza*	1 Slice/63g	200	10.0	317	17.6	26.7	15.5	2.2
Pepperoni Passion, Dominator, Large, Domino's Pizza*	1 Slice/115g	351	15.0	305	16.1	30.4	13.0	1.8
Pepperoni Passion, Reg Crust, Personl, Domino's Pizza*	1 Pizza/272g	830	34.0	305	18.6	28.8	12.5	1.8
Pepperoni Passion, Regular Crust, Lge, Domino's Pizza*	1 Slice/92g	269	11.0	292	17.6	26.5	12.5	1.8
Pepperoni Passion, Regular Crust, Med, Domino's Pizza*	1 Slice/85g	244	11.0	287	17.3	25.4	12.6	1.8
Pepperoni Passion, Regular Crust, Sm, Domino's Pizza*	1 Slice/77g	226	10.0	294	17.9	25.8	12.9	1.9
Pepperoni Passion, Thin Crust, Large, Domino's Pizza*	1 Slice/72g	248	14.0	344	19.6	22.9	18.8	2.1
Pepperoni Passion, Thin Crust, Med, Domino's Pizza*	1 Slice/68g	242	13.0	356	19.8	25.1	19.1	2.0
Piri Piri Pizza, Regular Crust, Large, Domino's Pizza*	1 Slice/60.5g	155	5.0	256	14.7	30.8	8.2	1.9
Piri Piri Pizza, Regular Crust, Medium, Domino's Pizza*	1 Slice/55g	142	5.0	256	14.7	30.8	8.2	1.6
Piri Piri Pizza, Regular Crust, Personal, Domino's Pizza*	1 Pizza/177g	481	16.0	272	17.6	30.0	9.1	1.7
Piri Piri Pizza, Regular Crust, Small, Domino's Pizza*	1 Slice/49g	126	4.0	256	14.7	30.8	8.2	1.6
Piri Piri Pizza, Thin Crust, Large, Domino's Pizza*	1 Slice/41g	126	6.0	310	17.7	26.9	14.7	1.9
Piri Piri Pizza, Thin Crust, Medium, Domino's Pizza*	1 Slice/39g	119	6.0	310	17.7	26.9	14.7	1.9
Premiere, Regular Crust, Large, Domino's Pizza*	1 Slice/83g	213	7.0	257	15.4	30.0	8.3	2.2
Premiere, Regular Crust, Medium, Domino's Pizza*	1 Slice/77g	198	6.0	257	15.4	30.0	8.3	2.2
Premiere, Regular Crust, Small, Domino's Pizza*	1 Slice/69g	177	6.0	257	15.4	30.0	8.3	2.2
Scrummy, Double Decadence, Medium, Domino's Pizza*	1 Slice/119g	369	20.0	310	15.9	23.2	17.1	1.9

DOMINO'S PIZZA

PIZZA

	Measure INFO/WEIGHT	per Measure KCAL	FAT	Nutrition Values per 100g / 100ml KCAL	PROT	CARB	FAT	FIBRE
Scrummy, Regular Crust, Large, Domino's Pizza*	1 Slice/107g	290	13.0	271	17.0	22.8	12.4	1.7
Scrummy, Regular Crust, Medium, Domino's Pizza*	1 Slice/99g	268	12.0	271	17.0	22.8	12.4	1.7
Scrummy, Regular Crust, Personal, Domino's Pizza*	1 Pizza/284g	807	32.0	284	17.7	28.1	11.1	1.8
Scrummy, Regular Crust, Small, Domino's Pizza*	1 Slice/92g	249	11.0	271	17.0	22.8	12.4	1.7
Scrummy, Thin Crust, Large, Domino's Pizza*	1 Slice/87g	283	15.0	325	19.0	22.2	17.8	1.9
Scrummy, Thin Crust, Medium, Domino's Pizza*	1 Slice/82g	266	15.0	324	19.1	21.9	17.8	1.9
Tandoori Hot, Dble Decadence, Med, Domino's Pizza*	1 Slice/101g	275	13.0	273	12.4	26.9	12.9	2.3
Tandoori Hot, Dominator, Large, Domino's Pizza*	1 Slice/112g	280	9.0	250	12.7	31.8	8.0	2.1
Tandoori Hot, Regular Crust, Large, Domino's Pizza*	1 Slice/89g	199	6.0	223	13.4	28.1	6.3	2.2
Tandoori Hot, Regular Crust, Medium, Domino's Pizza*	1 Slice/81g	176	5.0	217	13.0	27.2	6.2	2.2
Tandoori Hot, Regular Crust, Personal, Domino's Pizza*	1 Pizza/248g	541	12.0	218	12.1	31.2	5.0	2.3
Tandoori Hot, Regular Crust, Small, Domino's Pizza*	1 Slice/73g	159	4.0	218	15.0	28.4	4.9	2.4
Tandoori Hot, Thin Crust, Large, Domino's Pizza*	1 Slice/69g	178	8.0	257	14.3	24.9	11.1	2.6
Tandoori Hot, Thin Crust, Medium, Domino's Pizza*	1 Slice/64g	173	7.0	270	14.5	27.4	11.4	2.5
Texas BBQ, Dominator, Large, Domino's Pizza*	1 Slice/110g	312	10.0	284	12.8	37.6	9.2	1.8
Texas BBQ, Double Decadence, Med, Domino's Pizza*	1 Slice/98g	321	14.0	328	13.5	37.0	14.0	1.8
Texas BBQ, Regular Crust, Large, Domino's Pizza*	1 Slice/87g	245	7.0	282	14.1	38.4	8.0	1.9
Texas BBQ, Regular Crust, Medium, Domino's Pizza*	1 Slice/79g	223	6.0	282	14.1	38.4	8.0	1.9
Texas BBQ, Regular Crust, Personal, Domino's Pizza*	1 Pizza/244g	671	16.0	275	18.4	35.6	6.6	2.5
Texas BBQ, Regular Crust, Small, Domino's Pizza*	1 Slice/71g	200	6.0	282	14.1	38.4	8.0	1.9
Texas BBQ, Thin Crust, Large, Domino's Pizza*	1 Slice/67g	206	8.0	307	14.8	34.3	12.2	1.8
Texas BBQ, Thin Crust, Medium, Domino's Pizza*	1 Slice/62g	217	9.0	350	15.5	40.9	13.8	2.1
The Sizzler, Dominator, Large, Domino's Pizza*	1 Slice/117.5g	344	13.0	293	13.7	34.1	11.4	2.1
The Sizzler, Double Decadence, Med, Domino's Pizza*	1 Slice/106g	334	17.0	315	13.5	29.3	16.0	2.3
The Sizzler, Medium, Regular Crust, Domino's Pizza*	1 Slice/75g	172	5.0	230	12.9	29.1	6.9	2.3
The Sizzler, Regular Crust, Large, Domino's Pizza*	1 Slice/95g	270	11.0	285	14.7	31.5	11.2	2.2
The Sizzler, Regular Crust, Medium, Domino's Pizza*	1 Slice/87g	247	10.0	285	14.7	31.5	11.2	2.2
The Sizzler, Regular Crust, Personal, Domino's Pizza*	1 Pizza/261g	707	23.0	271	15.6	32.6	8.7	2.4
The Sizzler, Regular Crust, Small, Domino's Pizza*	1 Slice/78g	223	9.0	285	14.7	31.5	11.2	2.2
The Sizzler, Thin Crust, Large, Domino's Pizza*	1 Slice/75g	227	11.0	303	14.7	28.4	14.5	2.2
The Sizzler, Thin Crust, Medium, Domino's Pizza*	1 Slice/70g	242	12.0	347	16.1	32.1	17.1	2.4
Tuna Delight, Dble Decadence, Med, Domino's Pizza*	1 Slice/97g	279	13.0	288	12.4	28.8	13.8	2.4
Tuna Delight, Dominator, Large, Domino's Pizza*	1 Slice/108g	286	9.0	265	12.8	33.8	8.7	2.1
Tuna Delight, Regular Crust, Large, Domino's Pizza*	1 Slice/80g	186	6.0	233	13.1	29.6	6.9	2.2
Tuna Delight, Regular Crust, Medium, Domino's Pizza*	1 Slice/72g	168	5.0	233	13.1	29.6	6.9	2.2
Tuna Delight, Regular Crust, Personal, Domino's Pizza*	1 Pizza/239g	607	16.0	254	14.5	34.1	6.6	2.2
Tuna Delight, Regular Crust, Small, Domino's Pizza*	1 Slice/65g	151	4.0	233	13.1	29.6	6.9	2.2
Tuna Delight, Thin Crust, Large, Domino's Pizza*	1 Slice/65g	183	8.0	281	14.6	27.8	12.4	2.6
Tuna Delight, Thin Crust, Medium, Domino's Pizza*	1 Slice/60g	177	8.0	295	14.7	30.5	12.7	2.6
Veg-A-Roma, Regular Crust, Large, Domino's Pizza*	1 Slice/86g	240	9.0	279	12.3	34.3	10.4	2.4
Veg-A-Roma, Regular Crust, Medium, Domino's Pizza*	1 Slice/78g	218	8.0	279	12.3	34.3	10.4	2.4
Veg-A-Roma, Regular Crust, Personal, Domino's Pizza*	1 Pizza/242g	641	19.0	265	13.7	34.7	8.0	2.5
Veg-A-Roma, Regular Crust, Small, Domino's Pizza*	1 Slice/70g	195	7.0	279	12.3	34.3	10.4	2.4
Veg-A-Roma, Thin Crust, Large, Domino's Pizza*	1 Slice/66g	180	8.0	273	12.5	29.2	11.8	2.8
Veg-A-Roma, Thin Crust, Medium, Domino's Pizza*	1 Slice/61g	167	7.0	273	12.5	29.2	11.8	2.8
Vegetarian Supreme, Dominator, Large, Domino's Pizza*	1 Slice/111g	274	9.0	247	11.2	32.6	8.0	2.2
Vegetarian Supreme, Reg Crust, Lge, Domino's Pizza*	1 Slice/88g	192	6.0	218	11.5	29.1	6.3	2.3
Vegetarian Supreme, Reg Crust, Med, Domino's Pizza*	1 Slice/80g	170	5.0	213	11.0	28.3	6.1	2.3
Vegetarian Supreme, Reg Crust, Sm, Domino's Pizza*	1 Slice/72g	156	4.0	217	11.5	28.9	6.2	2.3
Vegetarian Supreme, Thin Crust, Large, Domino's Pizza*	1 Slice/68g	171	8.0	252	11.8	26.1	11.1	2.7
Vegetarian Supreme, Thin Crust, Med, Domino's Pizza*	1 Slice/63g	168	7.0	266	12.0	28.7	11.5	2.6
Vegi Lite, Dominator, Large, Domino's Pizza*	1 Slice/108g	270	9.0	250	11.4	32.6	8.2	2.2

	Measure INFO/WEIGHT	per Measure KCAL	FAT	Nutrition Values per 100g / 100ml KCAL	PROT	CARB	FAT	FIBRE

DOMINO'S PIZZA

PIZZA

	Measure INFO/WEIGHT	KCAL	FAT	KCAL	PROT	CARB	FAT	FIBRE
Vegi Lite, Double Decadence, Medium, Domino's Pizza*	1 Slice/97g	266	13.0	274	11.0	27.6	13.3	2.4
Vegi Lite, Regular Crust, Large, Domino's Pizza*	1 Slice/85g	183	5.0	215	11.4	28.2	6.3	2.3
Vegi Lite, Regular Crust, Medium, Domino's Pizza*	1 Slice/77g	166	5.0	215	11.4	28.2	6.3	2.3
Vegi Lite, Regular Crust, Personal, Domino's Pizza*	1 Pizza/239g	569	15.0	238	13.0	32.8	6.1	2.3
Vegi Lite, Regular Crust, Small, Domino's Pizza*	1 Slice/69g	148	4.0	215	11.4	28.2	6.3	2.3
Vegi Lite, Thin Crust, Large, Domino's Pizza*	1 Slice/60g	163	7.0	272	12.5	28.6	11.9	2.7
Vegi Lite, Thin Crust, Medium, Domino's Pizza*	1 Slice/65g	166	7.0	256	12.3	25.8	11.5	2.8
Vegi-Delight, Dble Decadence, Med, Domino's Pizza*	1 Slice/103g	288	15.0	280	11.8	26.4	14.1	2.4
Vegi-Delight, Dominator, Large, Domino's Pizza*	1 Slice/115g	297	11.0	258	12.2	31.1	9.4	2.1
Vegi-Delight, Regular Crust, Large, Domino's Pizza*	1 Slice/92g	209	7.0	227	12.3	26.6	7.9	2.2
Vegi-Delight, Regular Crust, Medium, Domino's Pizza*	1 Slice/84g	191	7.0	227	12.3	26.6	7.9	2.2
Vegi-Delight, Regular Crust, Personal, Domino's Pizza*	1 Pizza/258g	640	19.0	248	13.8	31.3	7.5	2.3
Vegi-Delight, Regular Crust, Small, Domino's Pizza*	1 Slice/75g	170	6.0	227	12.3	26.6	7.9	2.2
Vegi-Delight, Thin Crust, Large, Domino's Pizza*	1 Slice/72g	193	9.0	268	13.4	24.1	13.1	2.6
Vegi-Delight, Thin Crust, Medium, Domino's Pizza*	1 Slice/67g	189	9.0	282	13.6	26.6	13.4	2.5
Vegi-Volcano, Dble Decadence, Med, Domino's Pizza*	1 Slice/102g	282	14.0	276	11.7	26.3	13.7	2.3
Vegi-Volcano, Regular Crust, Large, Domino's Pizza*	1 Slice/91g	202	7.0	222	12.2	26.5	7.4	2.2
Vegi-Volcano, Regular Crust, Medium, Domino's Pizza*	1 Slice/83g	184	6.0	222	12.2	26.5	7.4	2.2
Vegi-Volcano, Regular Crust, Personal, Domino's Pizza*	1 Pizza/254g	617	18.0	243	13.7	31.0	7.1	2.2
Vegi-Volcano, Regular Crust, Small, Domino's Pizza*	1 Slice/75g	166	6.0	222	12.2	26.5	7.4	2.2
Vegi-Volcano, Thin Crust, Large, Domino's Pizza*	1 Slice/72g	189	9.0	262	13.3	23.9	12.5	2.6
Vegi-Volcano, Thin Crust, Medium, Domino's Pizza*	1 Slice/66g	181	8.0	275	13.5	26.5	12.8	2.5

POTATO

Wedges, Domino's Pizza*	1 Serving/190g	298	12.0	157	2.5	21.9	6.5	2.2

POTATO SKINS

Cheese & Bacon, Loaded (3), Domino's Pizza*	1 Skin/56g	99	5.0	176	5.3	19.0	8.8	3.9
Cheese & Onion, Loaded (3), Domino's Pizza*	1 Skin/56g	96	4.0	172	3.8	23.8	6.8	4.1

SAUCE

Hot, Domino's Pizza*	1 Pot/28g	7	0.0	25	0.8	1.8	1.1	1.1

WAFFLES

Domino's Pizza*	1 Serving/104g	491	25.0	472	5.0	58.2	24.4	1.2

EAT

BAGUETTE

Brie, Tomato & Basil, EAT*	1 Baguette/231g	554	24.0	240	9.8	27.0	10.3	1.7
Cheddar, Simple, Kids, EAT*	1 Baguette/95g	311	15.0	327	13.4	32.3	16.0	1.8
Cheddar,& Branston, Farmhouse, Mature, EAT*	1 Baguette/240g	704	34.0	293	10.8	30.7	14.1	1.8
Chicken, Thai, EAT*	1 Baguette/233g	645	30.0	277	13.6	26.6	12.9	1.6
Chorizo & Peppers, EAT*	1 Pack/220g	607	28.0	276	10.8	29.6	12.7	2.0
Goats Cheese, Peppers, & Chilli Jam, Artisan, EAT*	1 Baguette/240g	496	12.0	207	6.5	33.2	5.2	2.3
Ham & Jarlsberg, EAT*	1 Baguette/245g	623	26.0	254	14.9	25.0	10.4	1.5
Ham, Brie & Cranberry, EAT*	1 Baguette/306g	792	41.0	259	10.5	24.0	13.4	1.4
Ham, Simple, Kids, EAT*	1 Baguette/102g	240	7.0	234	12.6	29.9	7.0	1.7
Roast Beef & Rocket, EAT*	1 Baguette/233g	657	30.0	282	14.8	26.5	12.9	1.5
Tuna & Cucumber, EAT*	1 Baguette/260g	637	31.0	245	10.0	24.0	12.1	1.5
Tuna & Cucumber, Kids, EAT*	1 Baguette/130g	318	16.0	245	10.0	24.0	12.1	1.5

BARS

Toffee, EAT*	1 Serving/60g	291	14.0	486	3.7	62.9	24.1	1.4

BREAD

Brown, Chunk, Freshly Baked, EAT*	1 Serving/100g	211	2.0	211	7.4	44.0	1.9	2.7
Cheese Straw, Freshly Baked, EAT*	1 Serving/100g	313	19.0	313	10.6	25.6	19.5	1.7
Rye, Seeded, Wheat Free, EAT*	1 Serving/100g	431	8.0	431	12.5	77.7	7.9	12.4
White, Chunk, Freshly Baked, EAT*	1 Pack/100g	242	4.0	242	7.3	46.4	4.3	1.9

	Measure INFO/WEIGHT	per Measure KCAL	FAT	Nutrition Values per 100g / 100ml KCAL	PROT	CARB	FAT	FIBRE
EAT								
BREAD								
Wholemeal, Chunk, EAT*	1 Serving/67g	138	2.0	206	9.0	37.2	2.4	7.9
BREAKFAST CEREAL								
Muesli, Apple, Almond, & Cinnamon Bircher, EAT*	1 Serving/210g	362	12.0	172	6.1	23.3	5.8	2.3
Muesli, Swiss Bircher, EAT*	1 Serving/205g	246	3.0	120	4.7	21.7	1.5	2.0
Porridge, Plain, EAT*	1 Pack/280g	227	4.0	81	4.5	12.6	1.4	1.0
Porridge, with Apple & Blackberry Compote (12oz), EAT*	1 Pack/331g	291	4.0	88	4.0	15.4	1.2	1.3
Porridge, with Apple & Blackberry Compote, (8oz), EAT*	1 Serving/230g	210	3.0	91	3.7	16.6	1.2	1.5
Porridge, with Banana & Maple Syrup, (12oz Serve), EAT*	1 Serving/324g	295	4.0	91	4.0	15.9	1.2	1.1
Porridge, with Banana, (8oz Serving), EAT*	1 Serving/210g	174	3.0	83	4.0	14.0	1.2	1.2
Porridge, with Banana, EAT*	1 Serving/308g	256	4.0	83	4.2	13.6	1.3	1.1
Porridge, with Maple Syrup (12oz Serving), EAT*	1 Serving/294g	265	4.0	90	4.3	15.2	1.3	0.9
Porridge, with Maple Syrup, (8oz Serving), EAT*	1 Serving/195g	185	3.0	95	4.2	16.5	1.3	0.9
BROWNIE								
Chocolate, EAT*	1 Brownie/50g	341	18.0	682	8.4	80.0	36.4	2.6
CAKE								
Banana & Walnut, EAT*	1 Pack/86g	292	14.0	340	3.8	43.9	16.7	1.7
Carrot, EAT*	1 Slice/90g	329	16.0	365	3.5	46.6	18.1	1.3
Chocolate, EAT*	1 Slice/86g	334	18.0	388	5.4	44.6	20.9	1.5
Lemon, EAT*	1 Slice/84g	326	15.0	388	4.5	51.0	18.3	0.9
White Chocolate, & Raspberry, EAT*	1 Serving/98g	400	20.0	410	4.3	50.4	20.6	1.2
CHEESECAKE								
Lemon, EAT*	1 Serving/115g	454	35.0	395	3.2	26.5	30.3	0.7
COFFEE								
Cappuccino, Skimmed Milk, EAT*	1 Tall/355ml	118	4.0	33	2.4	3.4	1.1	0.0
Cappuccino, Soya Milk, EAT*	1 Tall/355ml	131	5.0	37	3.2	3.5	1.4	0.9
Cappuccino, Whole Milk, EAT*	1 Tall/355ml	168	9.0	47	2.4	3.4	2.6	0.0
Espresso, Macchiato, Skimmed Milk, EAT*	1 Espresso/118ml	8	0.0	7	0.5	0.6	0.3	0.0
Espresso, Macchiato, Soya Milk, EAT*	1 Espresso/118ml	9	0.0	8	0.6	0.7	0.3	0.2
Espresso, Macchiato, Whole Milk, EAT*	1 Espresso/118ml	11	1.0	9	0.5	0.6	0.5	0.0
Latte, Chai, Skimmed Milk, EAT*	1 Tall/355ml	305	1.0	86	3.2	17.7	0.3	0.0
Latte, Chai, Soya Milk, EAT*	1 Tall/355ml	279	5.0	79	2.4	13.9	1.5	0.5
Latte, Chai, Whole Milk, EAT*	1 Tall/355ml	408	13.0	115	3.1	17.5	3.6	0.0
Latte, Chiller, Skimmed Milk, EAT*	1 Tall/355ml	241	3.0	68	3.1	11.9	0.9	0.0
Latte, Chiller, Soya Milk, EAT*	1 Tall/355ml	251	4.0	71	3.7	12.0	1.1	0.7
Latte, Chiller, Whole Milk, EAT*	1 Tall/355ml	412	15.0	116	1.8	17.7	4.2	0.2
Latte, Iced, Skimmed Milk, EAT*	1 Tall/355ml	95	3.0	27	1.9	2.7	0.9	0.0
Latte, Iced, Soya Milk, EAT*	1 Tall/355ml	105	4.0	30	2.5	2.8	1.1	0.7
Latte, Iced, Whole Milk, EAT*	1 Tall/355ml	135	7.0	38	1.9	2.7	2.0	0.0
Latte, Matcha, Skimmed Milk, EAT*	1 Tall/355ml	204	1.0	57	3.0	10.6	0.3	0.3
Latte, Matcha, Soya Milk, EAT*	1 Tall/355ml	201	6.0	57	3.0	7.4	1.6	0.3
Latte, Matcha, Whole Milk, EAT*	1 Tall/355ml	297	12.0	84	3.0	10.4	3.3	0.3
Latte, Skimmed Milk, EAT*	1 Tall/355ml	142	5.0	42	3.0	4.2	1.4	0.0
Latte, Soya Milk, EAT*	1 Tall/355ml	157	6.0	46	4.0	4.3	1.7	1.1
Latte, Whole Milk, EAT*	1 Tall/355ml	202	11.0	59	3.0	4.2	3.2	0.0
Mocha, Chiller, Skimmed Milk, EAT*	1 Tall/355ml	243	3.0	68	2.5	12.6	0.9	0.0
Mocha, Chiller, Soya Milk, EAT*	1 Tall/355ml	253	4.0	71	3.1	12.7	1.1	0.7
Mocha, Chiller, Whole Milk, EAT*	1 Tall/355ml	283	7.0	80	2.5	12.6	2.1	0.0
Mocha, Skimmed Milk, EAT*	1 Tall/355ml	157	5.0	44	3.0	4.8	1.4	0.0
Mocha, Soya Milk, EAT*	1 Tall/355ml	173	6.0	49	4.0	5.0	1.7	1.2
Mocha, Whole Milk, EAT*	1 Tall/355ml	219	11.0	62	3.0	4.8	3.2	0.0
Vanilla Chiller, EAT*	1 Tall /355ml	482	21.0	136	1.8	19.0	5.9	0.1
White, Flat, Skimmed Milk, EAT*	1 Tall/341ml	198	1.0	58	5.8	8.5	0.2	0.0

EAT

	Measure INFO/WEIGHT	per Measure KCAL	FAT	Nutrition Values per 100g / 100ml KCAL	PROT	CARB	FAT	FIBRE
COFFEE								
White, Flat, Soya Milk, EAT*	1 Tall/341ml	205	13.0	60	6.3	0.2	3.7	1.0
White, Flat, Whole Milk, EAT*	1 Tall/341ml	389	20.0	114	5.8	8.2	6.0	0.0
COOKIES								
Chocolate, EAT*	1 Pack/150g	455	23.0	303	3.6	37.9	15.3	0.4
Muesli, EAT*	1 Pack/100g	376	13.0	376	4.5	60.8	12.8	1.8
CROISSANT								
Almond, EAT*	1 Croissant/200g	467	26.0	233	4.8	23.8	13.2	1.5
Chocolate, EAT*	1 Croissant/100g	407	23.0	407	6.7	45.9	23.1	3.0
Plain, EAT*	1 Croissant/100g	274	14.0	274	5.5	32.6	14.2	1.6
CUPCAKES								
Chocolate, EAT*	1 Serving/69g	228	16.0	331	3.7	53.2	23.5	1.3
Strawberry, EAT*	1 Serving/69g	298	16.0	432	3.9	51.9	22.9	1.4
Vanilla, EAT*	1 Pack/69g	257	13.0	373	3.2	59.1	18.5	0.4
DESSERT								
Dark Chocolate, Pot, EAT*	1 Pot/50g	211	17.0	422	2.2	27.0	35.0	2.0
DRIED FRUIT & SEED MIX								
EAT*	1 Pack/50g	224	9.0	448	10.0	61.3	17.8	0.0
FRUIT & NUTS								
Honey & Chilli, EAT*	1 Pack/85g	422	27.0	496	15.9	44.4	31.7	5.6
Honey Toasted, EAT*	1 Pack/50g	226	13.0	453	11.5	44.5	25.5	5.6
FUDGE								
Chocolate, Chunky, EAT*	1 Serving/116g	447	26.0	385	3.3	43.7	22.0	1.5
HOT CHOCOLATE								
Chiller, Whole Milk, EAT*	1 Tall/341ml	562	22.0	165	2.4	24.1	6.6	0.6
Skimmed Milk, EAT*	1 Tall/355ml	171	5.0	48	3.3	5.2	1.5	0.0
Soya Milk, EAT*	1 Tall/355ml	188	7.0	53	4.3	5.4	1.9	1.3
Whole Milk, EAT*	1 Tall/355ml	239	12.0	67	3.3	5.2	3.5	0.0
ICE CREAM								
Belgian Chocolate, Haagen Das, EAT*	1 Serving/100g	227	18.0	227	3.9	23.8	18.4	1.7
Cookies & Cream, Haagen Das, EAT*	1 Serving/100g	225	14.0	225	3.7	20.0	14.4	0.7
Strawberry, Haagen Das, EAT*	1 Serving/100g	221	14.0	221	3.5	20.0	14.1	0.3
Vanilla, Haagen Das, EAT*	1 Serving/100g	225	15.0	225	3.8	18.1	15.2	0.0
JELLY								
Berry & Elderflower, EAT*	1 Pack/135g	105	0.0	78	2.1	16.9	0.0	0.8
JUICE DRINK								
Mango & Lime, Blast, EAT*	1 Tall/355ml	253	0.0	71	0.3	17.7	0.1	0.1
Peach & Mint, Blast, EAT*	1 Tall/355ml	216	0.0	61	0.2	15.1	0.1	0.0
Wild Berry, Blast, EAT*	1 Tall/355ml	330	0.0	93	0.2	23.5	0.1	0.5
MILK								
Skimmed, Steamed, EAT*	1 Tall/355ml	169	6.0	48	3.5	4.9	1.6	0.0
Soya, Steamed, EAT*	1 Tall/355ml	187	7.0	53	4.5	5.0	1.9	1.3
Whole, Steamed, EAT*	1 Tall/355ml	241	13.0	68	3.4	4.9	3.7	0.0
MUFFIN								
Bacon Butty, EAT*	1 Serving/90g	279	11.0	310	15.8	34.5	11.9	2.3
Bacon Butty, Large, EAT*	1 Muffin/190g	577	20.0	304	14.3	37.7	10.3	3.4
Blueberry, Low Fat, EAT*	1 Muffin/100g	280	3.0	280	5.7	58.1	2.7	2.3
Breakfast, Full English, EAT*	1 Pack/293g	714	29.0	244	10.5	26.1	10.0	2.4
Breakfast, Full Scottish (Scotland Only), EAT*	1 Pack/297g	711	28.0	239	10.5	27.3	9.3	2.3
Chocolate, Belgian, EAT*	1 Muffin/100g	511	26.0	511	6.2	60.6	26.4	2.6
Cumberland Sausage, EAT*	1 Muffin/110g	323	15.0	293	10.9	27.3	13.2	2.0
Egg, Mushroom & Cheddar, EAT*	1 Pack/135g	289	11.0	214	8.9	26.8	7.8	2.0
Eggs Benedict, EAT*	1 Muffin/120g	290	12.0	241	10.2	26.5	10.3	1.6

	Measure INFO/WEIGHT	per Measure KCAL	FAT	Nutrition Values per 100g / 100ml KCAL	PROT	CARB	FAT	FIBRE
EAT								
MUFFIN								
Sunshine, EAT*	1 Muffin/100g	498	25.0	498	7.1	58.5	25.2	4.7
NOUGAT								
EAT*	1 Pack/30g	132	3.0	440	3.7	86.3	9.0	0.7
PAIN AU CHOCOLAT								
EAT*	1 Pain/120g	460	19.0	383	6.6	28.6	15.8	2.4
PASTRY								
Cinnamon Whirl, EAT*	1 Serving/100g	406	24.0	406	4.5	38.3	24.0	2.3
Maple Pecan Plait, EAT*	1 Serving/100g	435	27.0	435	5.0	41.3	26.8	3.1
PEAS								
Wasabi, EAT*	1 Pack/92g	136	5.0	148	1.3	22.4	5.9	7.9
PIE								
Banoffee, EAT*	1 Pie/114g	409	26.0	359	3.7	34.4	23.0	1.6
Beef, Chorizo, & Butterbean, EAT*	1 Pie/270g	683	38.0	253	8.5	23.3	14.0	0.0
Cheddar Cheese, Potato & Onion, EAT*	1 Pie/270g	672	35.0	249	6.2	26.9	12.9	0.0
Chicken & Mushroom, EAT*	1 Pie/280g	597	28.0	213	8.4	24.1	10.1	0.0
Chicken, Ham & Leek, EAT*	1 Pie/270g	615	30.0	228	9.3	22.7	11.1	0.0
Steak & Ale, EAT*	1 Pie/270g	613	30.0	227	8.0	27.0	11.0	0.0
Three Bean Chilli, EAT*	1 Pie/270g	618	25.0	229	5.7	30.7	9.3	0.0
SALAD								
Chicken Noodles, Spicy, EAT*	1 Pack/285g	394	10.0	138	9.5	17.3	3.4	0.9
Christmas Lunch, with Dressing, EAT*	1 Serving/332g	645	34.0	194	8.1	17.5	10.1	2.0
Christmas Lunch, Without Dressing, EAT*	1 Serving/307g	549	26.0	179	8.8	16.8	8.5	2.1
Crayfish Noodles, Spicy, EAT*	1 Pack/288g	371	10.0	129	5.9	18.6	3.4	0.7
Ham, & Potato, with Dressing, EAT*	1 Pack/326g	489	37.0	150	6.6	5.0	11.5	0.9
Ham, & Potato, without Dressing, EAT*	1 Box/305g	412	30.0	135	6.9	4.7	9.8	0.9
Mezze, with Dressing, EAT*	1 Serving/347g	486	34.0	140	3.6	9.8	9.7	2.4
Mezze, without Dressing, EAT*	1 Serving/322g	390	26.0	121	3.8	8.5	8.1	2.6
Noodle, Thai, EAT*	1 Pack/198g	533	18.0	269	7.6	42.3	9.2	2.1
Prawn Cocktail, Side, EAT*	1 Pack/192g	325	31.0	169	4.4	1.9	15.9	1.1
Rainbow Sprouted, Side Salad, with Dressing, EAT*	1 Pack/186g	324	15.0	174	7.5	17.9	8.2	2.7
Rainbow Sprouted, Side Salad, without Dressing, EAT*	1 Pack/161g	218	6.0	135	8.6	17.2	3.8	3.1
Superfood, without Dressing, EAT*	1 Pack/300g	396	21.0	132	8.2	9.7	6.9	4.3
Tuna, & Bean, with Dressing, Side, EAT*	1 Pack/209g	276	10.0	132	8.8	12.2	4.7	4.4
Tuna, & Bean, without Dressing, EAT*	1 Serving/184g	207	3.0	112	10.0	13.1	1.5	4.9
SANDWICH								
BLT, EAT*	1 Pack/204g	510	30.0	250	10.4	19.8	14.5	1.8
Bombay Bhaji, EAT*	1 Pack/237g	543	8.0	229	5.2	25.6	3.5	1.0
Chicken, & Bacon, EAT*	1 Pack/244g	547	28.0	224	12.4	17.0	11.5	1.5
Chicken, Avocado, Basil, EAT*	1 Pack/232g	597	37.0	257	11.5	16.7	16.1	2.5
Chicken, Basil Pesto & Pine Nuts, EAT*	1 Pack/228g	577	27.0	253	11.0	25.5	11.7	4.2
Chicken, Lemon & Black Pepper, EAT*	1 Pack/237g	522	19.0	220	12.0	24.7	8.2	3.9
Chicken, Salad, Simple, EAT*	1 Pack/203g	339	9.0	167	12.1	19.2	4.3	1.7
Chicken, Thai Citrus, EAT*	1 Pack/213g	415	14.0	195	12.9	21.5	6.4	1.6
Club, EAT*	1 Pack/285.5g	768	46.0	269	14.2	16.7	16.2	1.3
Coriander & Lemon Houmous, EAT*	1 Pack/244g	487	23.0	199	5.6	26.2	9.6	5.8
Crayfish, Lemon, & Rocket, EAT*	1 Pack/198g	336	13.0	170	7.3	19.9	6.7	1.5
Egg Mayo, & Cress, Free Range, EAT*	1 Pack/182g	409	21.0	224	8.7	21.6	11.4	1.8
Egg Mayo, & Tomato, Free Range, Bloomer, EAT*	1 Pack/260g	627	37.0	241	7.1	20.0	14.4	1.6
Egg Mayo, & Watercress, Free Range, Chunky, EAT*	1 Pack/203g	462	25.0	227	8.8	20.0	12.4	1.7
Falafel, & Houmous, EAT*	1 Sandwich/255g	393	11.0	154	5.9	23.6	4.5	3.4
Ham, & Mustard Salad, EAT*	1 Pack/85g	363	10.0	427	26.8	54.9	11.2	6.1
Ham, Cheddar & Real Ale Pickle, EAT*	1 Pack/273g	554	27.0	203	10.3	18.4	9.8	1.4

EAT

	Measure INFO/WEIGHT	per Measure KCAL	per Measure FAT	Nutrition Values per 100g / 100ml KCAL	PROT	CARB	FAT	FIBRE
SANDWICH								
Ham, Tomato, & Mustard, EAT*	1 Pack/203g	394	17.0	194	9.8	19.3	8.6	1.6
Mature Cheddar, & Bramley Apple, EAT*	1 Pack/238g	618	36.0	260	9.8	20.7	15.3	1.6
Mature Cheddar, & Chilli Jam, EAT*	1 Pack/239g	580	30.0	243	9.7	21.9	12.6	1.5
New York Pastrami, EAT*	1 Pack/224g	358	11.0	160	9.9	18.6	5.1	1.3
Pork, Apple, Sage, & Onion Bloomer, EAT*	1 Pack/245g	520	15.0	212	13.1	25.5	6.1	1.5
Prawn Cocktail, EAT*	1 Pack/198g	432	25.0	218	7.3	19.3	12.4	1.6
Smoked Chicken, Tomato, & Pesto Bloomer, EAT*	1 Pack/263g	507	19.0	193	11.8	19.2	7.3	1.6
Superfood, EAT*	1 Pack/324g	490	28.0	151	7.6	10.9	8.7	3.9
Toastie, Cheese, & Onion, Small, EAT*	1 Pack/155g	530	33.0	342	15.0	23.2	21.3	1.5
Toastie, Chicken, & Basil, Smoked, EAT*	1 Pack/255g	777	43.0	305	13.9	24.1	16.9	1.6
Toastie, Chicken, Mushroom, & Emmental, EAT*	1 Pack/263g	654	29.0	249	12.8	23.8	11.0	1.9
Toastie, Ham & Cheese, Simply, EAT*	1 Pack/250g	760	42.0	304	13.9	24.2	16.8	1.5
Toastie, Steak & Cheese Melt, EAT*	1 Pack/290g	853	48.0	294	13.0	23.7	16.4	1.7
Toastie, Tuna, & Cheddar, Melt, EAT*	1 Pack/250g	782	44.0	313	14.9	23.9	17.5	1.5
Tuna, Ginger & Wasabi, EAT*	1 Pack/224g	516	28.0	230	10.3	19.3	12.5	2.1
Tuna, Mediterranean, EAT*	1 Pack/234g	472	17.0	202	8.7	26.3	7.1	4.7
Tuna, No Mayo, Very Small, The Amazing, EAT*	1 Pack/253g	331	11.0	131	10.2	16.2	4.5	1.7
Turkey, & Cranberry, EAT*	1 Pack/218g	384	9.0	176	9.9	25.1	4.1	1.3
Wensleydale, & Apricot Chutney, EAT*	1 Pack/203g	490	23.0	241	7.4	27.2	11.4	1.9
SLICE								
Coconut, EAT*	1 Pack/150g	688	42.0	459	6.1	45.2	28.1	4.4
SOUP								
Bean, Mexican, Big Serving, EAT*	1 Big/400g	196	7.0	49	2.7	5.6	1.8	1.9
Bean, Mexican, Small Serving, EAT*	1 Small/300g	159	7.0	53	2.9	5.6	2.2	1.9
Bean, Mexican, Very Big Serving, EAT*	1 Very Big/800g	368	12.0	46	2.6	5.5	1.5	1.9
Beef, Chilli & Ginger Pho, EAT*	1 Pot/850g	323	8.0	38	3.1	4.4	0.9	0.4
Cauliflower Cheese, EAT*	1 Small/300g	222	14.0	74	2.6	4.9	4.7	1.1
Chicken & Egg Noodles, Old Fashioned, EAT*	1 Small/300g	93	1.0	31	4.8	2.1	0.4	0.6
Chicken & Garden Vegetable, Broth, EAT*	1 Small/300g	150	2.0	50	6.1	5.0	0.7	1.3
Chicken Laksa, EAT*	1 Small/300g	276	15.0	92	5.8	6.1	5.0	0.8
Chicken Pho, EAT*	1 Pot/860g	327	5.0	38	4.0	4.2	0.6	0.4
Chicken Pot Pie, EAT*	1 Small/300g	282	13.0	94	5.8	7.8	4.4	1.2
Chicken, Creamy, EAT*	1 Small/300g	237	15.0	79	4.1	4.5	5.0	0.8
Chicken, Leek & Bacon Risotto, EAT*	1 Sm/301g	319	18.0	106	5.9	6.9	6.0	0.4
Chilli Con Carne, Texan, Big Serving, EAT*	1 Big/400g	376	18.0	94	6.6	7.5	4.4	2.0
Chilli Con Carne, Texan, Small Serving, EAT*	1 Small/300g	297	15.0	99	6.6	6.9	4.9	2.0
Chilli Con Carne, Texan, Very Big Serving, EAT*	1 Very Big/800g	720	32.0	90	6.5	6.9	4.0	2.0
Chorizo & Chickpea, EAT*	1 Small/300g	282	14.0	94	5.6	7.4	4.6	1.5
Courgette & Coriander, EAT*	1 Lge/454g	164	5.0	36	1.6	4.6	1.1	0.9
Cream of Corn, EAT*	1 Small/300g	288	23.0	96	1.5	5.6	7.6	1.1
Dal, Gujarati, EAT*	1 Small/300g	186	1.0	62	4.3	9.7	0.5	1.0
Dal, Red, Gujarati, with Raita, Big Serving, EAT*	1 Big/400g	144	5.0	36	2.0	4.4	1.2	0.7
French Onion, EAT*	1 Small/300g	174	7.0	58	1.9	7.2	2.2	0.6
Garden Vegetable, EAT*	1 Small/300ml	153	9.0	51	0.8	5.4	2.9	1.2
Gazpacho, EAT*	1 Sm/350ml	78	2.0	22	0.6	3.6	0.6	0.9
Goan Potato, EAT*	1 Big Soup/401g	293	16.0	73	1.7	7.6	4.1	1.7
Goulash, Hungarian, EAT*	1 Small/300g	213	6.0	71	7.2	6.0	1.9	1.0
Ham, Pea, & Mint, EAT*	1 Small/300g	180	0.0	60	4.6	6.7	0.1	1.2
Hoisin Duck, Gyoza Dumpling, Pot, EAT*	1 Pot/875g	420	6.0	48	2.1	8.3	0.7	0.6
Leek, Potato & Chive, EAT*	1 Small/300g	159	9.0	53	1.2	5.7	2.9	1.0
Mexican Chicken Tortilla, EAT*	1 Small/300g	165	6.0	55	4.2	4.7	1.9	1.2
Mexican Chicken Tortilla, without Garnish, EAT*	1 Small/300g	123	2.0	41	4.2	3.6	0.8	1.0

	Measure INFO/WEIGHT	per Measure KCAL	FAT	per 100g KCAL	PROT	CARB	FAT	FIBRE
EAT								
SOUP								
Minestrone, with Pesto, Chunky, EAT*	1 Small/300g	159	8.0	53	1.9	4.6	2.8	1.5
Mushroom, Wild, Forest, EAT*	1 Small/300g	144	9.0	48	2.0	3.6	2.9	0.9
Parsnip, & Apple, EAT*	1 Small/300g	162	3.0	54	1.2	8.7	0.9	3.0
Parsnip, Spiced, EAT*	1 Small/300g	141	8.0	47	1.0	5.2	2.6	1.9
Prawn, Tom Yum, EAT*	1 Pot/835g	292	8.0	35	1.8	4.8	0.9	0.6
Pumpkin, Roast, EAT*	1 Small/300g	156	9.0	52	0.8	5.8	2.9	1.1
Red Pepper, Roasted, & Tomato, EAT*	1 Small/300g	75	2.0	25	0.9	4.1	0.6	1.0
Smokey Bacon & Lentil, EAT*	1 Small/300g	111	3.0	37	2.6	4.3	1.1	0.6
Steak, & Ale Pot Pie, EAT*	1 Small /300g	300	9.0	100	8.4	9.0	3.1	1.2
Thai Butternut Squash, EAT*	1 Small/300g	144	7.0	48	0.8	6.2	2.2	1.6
Tomato, Slow Roasted, EAT*	1 Small/300g	243	18.0	81	1.4	5.2	6.1	1.4
Tomato, Spicy, & Basil, EAT*	1 Small/300g	63	1.0	21	0.9	3.8	0.3	1.0
Vegetarian Gyoza Dumpling, EAT*	1 Large Pot/865g	441	10.0	51	2.2	7.9	1.2	0.7
SUSHI								
Fish, EAT*	1 Pack/222	349	3.0	157	4.8	32.0	1.5	1.6
Vegetarian, EAT*	1 Pack/165g	252	2.0	153	2.5	33.4	1.4	1.6
TOASTIE								
Ham, Cheese & Mustard, EAT*	1 Pack/250g	593	28.0	237	12.5	21.9	11.1	1.9
WRAP								
Falafel, Moroccan, EAT*	1 Pack/204g	367	12.0	180	5.3	26.6	5.9	2.7
Mexican Chicken, EAT*	1 Pack/224g	410	15.0	183	10.7	20.9	6.5	1.4
Peking Duck, EAT*	1 Pack/208g	426	17.0	205	10.6	22.3	8.1	1.9
YOGHURT								
& Granola, EAT*	1 Serving/210g	348	12.0	166	6.4	22.0	5.9	2.3
Banana, Honey & Grapenut, EAT*	1 Pot/249g	378	6.0	152	4.7	28.1	2.4	1.0
with Apple & Blackberry (Small), EAT*	1 Small Pot/135g	139	4.0	103	4.4	15.1	2.9	1.0
with Apple & Blackberry Compote, EAT*	1 Pack/210g	366	11.0	174	5.2	27.4	5.0	3.1
with Blueberry & Pomegranate Compote, EAT*	1 Pot/135g	150	4.0	111	4.5	17.0	2.9	0.9
with Muesli & Mixed Berries, EAT*	1 Pack/210g	290	6.0	138	4.7	24.1	2.7	2.1
GREGGS								
BAGUETTE								
Cheese & Ham, Greggs*	1 Serving/224g	580	20.0	259	13.8	31.5	8.7	0.0
Chicken Club, Greggs*	1 Serving/273g	680	27.0	249	10.8	29.1	9.9	0.0
Chicken Pesto, Greggs*	1 Serving/226g	530	12.0	235	11.1	35.0	5.3	0.0
Chicken Tikka, Greggs*	1 Serving/250g	440	6.0	176	9.4	29.8	2.4	0.0
Egg Mayonnaise & Tomato, Greggs*	1 Serving/237g	530	16.0	224	8.4	30.4	7.0	0.0
Tuna Crunch, Greggs*	1 Serving/240g	560	18.0	233	10.6	30.4	7.5	0.0
BAKE								
Chicken, Greggs*	1 Serving/138g	440	28.0	319	8.3	26.1	20.3	0.0
Steak, Greggs*	1 Serving/139g	420	25.0	302	9.3	26.3	17.6	0.0
BLOOMER								
Chicken Mango, on Brown, Greggs*	1 Serving/255g	560	13.0	220	13.1	29.8	5.3	0.0
Chicken Mango, on White, Greggs*	1 Serving/255g	540	16.0	212	12.0	26.9	6.1	0.0
Chicken, Bacon & Sweetcorn on Brown, Greggs*	1 Serving/268g	670	27.0	250	11.4	28.5	10.1	0.0
Chicken, Bacon & Sweetcorn on White, Greggs*	1 Serving/268g	600	21.0	224	12.7	25.2	7.8	0.0
Egg & Bacon on Brown, Greggs*	1 Serving/248g	640	25.0	258	12.1	29.6	9.9	0.0
Ham, Cheese & Pickle on Brown, Greggs*	1 Serving/266g	620	19.0	233	12.2	29.5	7.3	0.0
Ham, Cheese & Pickle on White, Greggs*	1 Serving/266g	590	20.0	222	13.3	25.2	7.5	0.0
Tuna Crunch, on Brown, Greggs*	1 Serving/255g	520	15.0	204	10.8	27.6	5.7	0.0
Tuna Crunch, on White, Greggs*	1 Serving/255g	490	12.0	192	11.2	25.5	4.9	0.0
COFFEE								
Black, Regular, Greggs*	1 Serving/455g	23	1.0	5	0.1	0.6	0.1	0.0

GREGGS

	Measure INFO/WEIGHT	per Measure KCAL	FAT	Nutrition Values per 100g / 100ml KCAL	PROT	CARB	FAT	FIBRE
COFFEE								
Black, Small, Greggs*	1 Serving/340g	17	0.0	5	0.0	0.9	0.1	0.0
Cappuccino, No Chocolate Topping, Small, Greggs*	1 Serving/340g	140	5.0	41	2.6	4.1	1.4	0.0
Latte, Regular, Greggs*	1 Serving/455g	190	7.0	42	2.7	4.4	1.5	0.0
Latte, Small, Greggs*	1 Serving/340g	140	5.0	41	2.8	4.0	1.5	0.0
Regular Cappuccino No Chocolate Topping, Greggs*	1 Serving/455g	190	7.0	42	2.6	4.2	1.5	0.0
White, Regular, Greggs*	1 Serving/455g	91	4.0	20	0.2	3.3	0.8	0.0
White, Small, Greggs*	1 Serving/340g	68	2.0	20	0.6	3.2	0.7	0.0
COLA								
Coca Cola, Diet, Greggs*	1 Serving/500ml	3	0.0	1	0.0	0.0	0.0	0.0
Coca Cola, Greggs*	1 Serving/500ml	210	0.0	42	0.0	10.6	0.0	0.0
DR PEPPER								
Greggs*	1 Serving/500ml	210	0.0	42	0.0	2.1	0.0	0.0
DRINKING CHOCOLATE								
Regular, Greggs*	1 Serving/455g	250	7.0	55	0.9	9.4	1.6	0.0
Small, Greggs*	1 Serving/340g	140	4.0	41	0.6	7.1	1.2	0.0
FANTA								
Orange, Greggs*	1 Serving/500ml	150	0.0	30	0.0	7.1	0.0	0.0
IRON BRU								
Diet, Greggs*	1 Serving/330ml	2	0.0	1	0.0	0.0	0.0	0.0
Greggs*	1 Serving/500ml	215	0.0	43	0.0	10.5	0.0	0.0
JUICE								
Apple, Fairtrade, Greggs*	1 Serving/500ml	220	0.0	44	0.0	11.0	0.0	0.0
Orange, Fairtrade, Greggs*	1 Serving/500ml	220	0.0	44	0.1	10.2	0.0	0.0
JUICE DRINK								
Caprisun, Greggs*	1 Serving/330ml	143	0.0	43	0.0	10.5	0.0	0.0
Citrus Punch, Oasis, Greggs*	1 Serving/500ml	90	0.0	18	0.0	4.1	0.0	0.0
Ribena, Greggs*	1 Serving/500ml	215	0.0	43	0.0	10.5	0.0	0.0
Summer Fruits, Oasis, Greggs*	1 Serving/500ml	90	0.0	18	0.0	4.2	0.0	0.0
LUCOZADE								
Orange, Energy, Greggs*	1 Serving/500ml	350	0.0	70	0.0	17.2	0.0	0.0
Sport, Greggs*	1 Serving/500ml	140	0.0	28	0.0	6.4	0.0	0.0
MELT								
Sausage, Bean & Cheese, Greggs*	1 Serving/140g	460	28.0	329	7.5	28.6	20.0	0.0
PASTY								
Cheese & Onion, Greggs*	1 Serving/125g	380	23.0	304	6.8	28.0	18.4	0.0
Cornish, Greggs*	1 Serving/175g	460	26.0	263	6.6	24.9	15.1	0.0
PIZZA								
Cheese & Tomato, Greggs*	1 Serving/111g	330	13.0	297	10.8	37.8	11.7	0.0
ROLL								
Oval Bites, Chargrill Chicken, Greggs*	1 Serving/207g	430	16.0	208	11.8	22.2	8.0	0.0
Oval Bites, Cheese Ploughmans, Greggs*	1 Serving/202g	450	20.0	223	8.9	24.5	10.1	0.0
Oval Bites, Ham Salad, Greggs*	1 Serving/173g	310	9.0	179	9.0	22.8	5.5	0.0
Oval Bites, Mexican Chicken, Greggs*	1 Serving/175g	390	15.0	223	13.1	23.7	8.6	0.0
SANDWICH								
BLT, Greggs*	1 Serving/201g	520	22.0	259	10.9	28.4	11.2	0.0
Cheese & Tomato, Greggs*	1 Serving/173g	450	16.0	260	12.4	31.5	9.2	0.0
Cheese Savoury, Greggs*	1 Serving/174g	470	17.0	270	11.5	33.0	9.8	0.0
Chicken & Stuffing, Greggs*	1 Serving/191g	500	17.0	262	12.3	32.2	9.2	0.0
Chicken Salad, Greggs*	1 Serving/218g	480	18.0	220	11.0	25.9	8.3	0.0
Egg Mayonnaise, Greggs*	1 Serving/174g	430	16.0	247	10.9	30.2	8.9	0.0
Prawn Mayonnaise, Greggs*	1 Serving/166g	430	16.0	259	10.8	32.8	9.3	0.0
Tuna Mayonnaise, Greggs*	1 Serving/201g	440	14.0	219	11.7	28.1	6.7	0.0

	Measure INFO/WEIGHT	per Measure KCAL	FAT	Nutrition Values per 100g / 100ml KCAL	PROT	CARB	FAT	FIBRE
GREGGS								
SAUSAGE ROLL								
Greggs*	1 Serving/92g	320	22.0	348	8.1	27.2	23.4	0.0
SMOOTHIE								
Mango & Orange, Greggs*	1 Serving/250ml	145	0.0	58	0.6	13.2	0.0	0.0
Raspberry & Banana, Greggs*	1 Serving/250ml	135	0.0	54	0.6	12.2	0.0	0.0
SPRITE								
Greggs*	1 Serving/500ml	220	0.0	44	0.0	10.6	0.0	0.0
TEA								
White, Regular, Greggs*	1 Serving/455g	23	1.0	5	0.0	0.9	0.2	0.0
White, Small, Greggs*	1 Serving/340g	17	0.0	5	0.0	0.8	0.0	0.0
WATER								
Cranberry & Raspberry, Greggs*	1 Serving/500ml	5	0.0	1	0.0	0.0	0.0	0.0
Greggs*	1 Serving/500ml	0	0.0	0	0.0	0.0	0.0	0.0
ITSU								
BEANS								
Edamame, Raw, Cold, Itsu*	1 Pack/80g	100	3.0	125	10.7	12.0	4.0	5.3
DESSERT								
If Bounty Went to Heaven, Itsu*	1 Pot/80g	347	23.0	434	5.9	24.2	28.2	3.7
Valrhona Chocolate Shot, Itsu*	1 Serving/44g	134	2.0	305	7.7	21.1	3.9	0.0
FROZEN YOGHURT								
Skinny, Original, Itsu*	1 Pot/166g	180	0.0	108	3.6	24.1	0.0	0.0
Yo Cream, Itsu*	1 Pot/166g	166	0.0	100	3.0	20.0	0.0	0.0
NUTS								
Squirrel's Dream, Itsu*	1 Pack/70g	210	24.0	300	9.1	40.3	34.0	0.0
PEAS								
Wasabi, Itsu*	1 Pack/70g	301	21.0	430	13.9	15.4	30.7	0.0
RICE CRACKERS								
Peanut, Itsu*	1 Pack/70g	232	10.0	331	12.6	39.6	13.7	0.0
SALAD								
Chicken, Chilli, with Greens, Itsu*	1 Pack/210g	270	8.0	129	10.2	13.0	3.9	2.6
Chicken, Sesame, Itsu*	1 Box/297g	482	25.0	162	9.7	12.1	8.3	2.5
Graze & Dazzle, Itsu*	1 Pack/125g	264	11.0	211	5.9	26.6	8.8	2.2
Gulfstream, Itsu*	1 Pack/356g	402	6.0	113	14.8	9.5	1.8	1.1
Hip, Humble & Healthy, Itsu*	1 Box/314g	336	16.0	107	4.3	11.2	5.2	5.6
Salmon, Skinny, Itsu*	1 Salad/182g	272	13.0	149	11.4	9.7	7.2	1.5
Salmon, Special, Itsu*	1 Box/473g	514	17.0	109	5.7	13.4	3.5	1.5
Sirloin Steak & Noodles, Itsu*	1 Box/397g	367	15.0	92	7.4	8.8	3.7	1.6
Superfood, Itsu*	1 Box/314g	336	16.0	107	4.2	11.1	5.2	5.6
Tuna, Asian Seared, Itsu*	1 Box/100g	212	0.0	212	34.0	18.0	0.5	1.0
Tuna, Yellow Fin, Line Caught, Itsu*	1 Box/328g	401	16.0	122	9.0	10.6	4.8	1.9
SOUP								
Chicken Teriyaki Noodles, Itsu*	1 Serving/805g	453	3.0	56	3.8	9.2	0.4	1.2
Dynamite, Detox, Itsu*	1 Pot/425g	153	1.0	36	0.6	8.1	0.1	0.6
Dynamite, Duck, Itsu*	1 Pot/474g	263	4.0	55	2.1	7.7	0.8	0.6
Dynamite, Itsu*	1 Serving/425g	133	0.0	31	0.3	7.4	0.1	0.4
Dynamite, Salmon, Sense, Itsu*	1 Pot/482g	179	6.0	37	2.6	3.8	1.3	0.7
Miso, Forever Young, Itsu*	1 Serving/395g	86	3.0	22	2.5	1.1	0.8	1.5
Miso, Skinny, Itsu*	1 Serving/500ml	19	0.0	4	0.0	0.0	0.1	0.0
Spicy Dumpling Noodles, Itsu*	1 Serving/782g	589	18.0	75	2.8	10.7	2.3	1.4
SUSHI								
Caviar, Sashimi & Salmon, Itsu*	1 Pack/362g	398	18.0	110	15.1	0.8	5.0	7.5
Health & Happiness, Itsu*	1 Pack/384g	453	21.0	118	8.1	8.9	5.5	3.7
Maki Roll, Chicken, Free Range, Itsu*	1 Pack/221g	241	10.0	109	6.0	11.2	4.6	1.2

	Measure INFO/WEIGHT	per Measure KCAL	FAT	Nutrition Values per 100g / 100ml KCAL	PROT	CARB	FAT	FIBRE
ITSU								
SUSHI								
Maki Roll, Duck Hoi Sin, Itsu*	1 Box/162g	171	4.0	106	5.4	14.4	2.5	0.8
Maki Roll, Salmon & Avocado, Itsu*	1 Box/211g	239	13.0	113	4.6	9.3	6.3	1.5
Maki Roll, Spicy Crab, Itsu*	1 Box/202g	238	13.0	118	4.3	9.8	6.7	0.8
Maki Roll, Tuna, Itsu*	1 Serving/98g	152	3.0	155	5.1	24.0	3.6	0.0
Maki Roll, Vegetarian Sunrise, Itsu*	1 Box/222g	213	11.0	96	1.8	10.9	4.9	1.9
Prawn, Itsu*	1 Portion/98g	151	2.0	154	6.0	28.5	1.8	0.0
Salmon Rushdie, Itsu*	1 Box/400g	488	16.0	122	5.2	16.5	3.9	0.0
Salmon Sashimi, Itsu*	1 Portion/48g	53	2.0	110	15.5	0.8	5.0	0.0
Salmon Supreme, Omega 3, Itsu*	1 Pack/340g	509	25.0	150	7.4	13.6	7.2	1.1
Salmon, Itsu*	1 Portion/64g	129	4.0	202	8.3	26.4	6.9	0.0
Salmon, Super, 3 Ways, Itsu*	1 Pack/391g	451	21.0	115	7.9	8.7	5.4	4.4
Tuna & Salmon, Itsu*	1 Pack/282g	315	7.0	112	7.5	14.2	2.6	0.3
Tuna & Salmon, Junior, Itsu*	1 Pack/175g	181	6.0	103	9.5	9.0	3.2	8.1
Tuna, Avocado & Chives, Itsu*	1 Pack/210g	234	10.0	111	6.4	11.5	4.8	1.5
TEA								
Green, Beautiful Detox, Itsu*	1 Bottle/500ml	58	0.0	12	0.0	2.7	0.0	0.0
YOGHURT								
Fruit & Goji Berries, Itsu*	1 Pack/70g	320	11.0	457	44.0	0.0	16.0	0.0
IXXY'S								
BAGEL								
Chicken & Bacon, Ixxy's*	1 Serving/215g	589	27.0	274	12.8	29.3	12.5	0.0
Chicken, Caesar, Ixxy's*	1 Pack/200g	530	25.0	265	12.9	24.7	12.7	1.7
Cranberry & Honey, Multigrain, Mini, Ixxy's*	1 Bagel/34g	95	1.0	278	9.2	49.7	3.8	5.3
Ham & Rosemary Ricotta Cheese, Ixxy's*	1 Pack/215g	372	7.0	173	11.1	25.0	3.2	0.3
Plain, Mini, Ixxy's*	1 Bagel/45g	120	1.0	266	9.6	53.6	1.5	3.0
Salt Beef & Dill Pickle, Ixxy's*	1 Bagel/213g	403	10.0	189	11.1	25.5	4.7	1.8
Sesame, Mini, Ixxy's*	1 Bagel/49g	133	2.0	271	9.6	51.0	3.2	3.6
Smoked Salmon & Soft Cheese, Ixxy's*	1 Pack/192g	474	18.0	247	11.3	28.8	9.6	1.6
Soft Cheese & Tomato, Low Fat, Ixxy's*	1 Serving/191g	332	3.0	174	7.2	33.1	1.4	0.0
Tuna & Cucumber, Ixxy's*	1 Bagel/260g	390	4.0	150	11.3	23.1	1.4	0.0
Tuna Mayonnaise, Ixxy's*	1 Serving/220g	462	15.0	210	11.1	26.1	6.8	1.4
J D WETHERSPOON								
BAGUETTE								
BLT, Malted Grain, J D Wetherspoon*	1 Baguette/399g	823	46.0	206	8.3	17.8	11.4	1.3
Chicken, South'n Fried, Creole Mayo, J D Wetherspoon*	1 Meal/250g	817	36.0	327	12.6	37.7	14.3	2.0
Club, Malted Grain, J D Wetherspoon*	1 Baguette/388g	768	37.0	198	9.8	18.5	9.5	1.4
Crayfish, Malted Grain, J D Wetherspoon*	1 Baguette/314g	594	25.0	189	6.1	23.2	8.1	1.7
Hot Sausage & Tomato Chutney, J D Wetherspoon*	1 Meal/250g	839	33.0	336	14.1	40.7	13.4	3.8
Mature Cheddar, Pickle, Malt Grain, J D Wetherspoon*	1 Baguette/361g	696	30.0	193	7.9	21.9	8.3	1.6
Ploughmans, Lloyds, J D Wetherspoon*	1 Baguette/346g	778	34.0	225	8.6	25.5	9.9	2.2
Tuna Mayonnaise, Malted Grain, J D Wetherspoon*	1 Baguette/401g	710	31.0	177	8.9	18.1	7.8	1.3
Wiltshire Ham, J D Wetherspoon*	1 Baguette/346g	536	13.0	155	9.9	20.4	3.8	1.5
BEEF DINNER								
Roast Potatoes, Yorkshire Pud & Veg, J D Wetherspoon*	1 Portion/836.5g	1305	63.0	156	6.1	17.7	7.5	2.3
BHAJI								
Onion, J D Wetherspoon*	1 Bhaji/30g	43	2.0	143	5.3	18.7	7.3	5.7
BIRYANI								
Chicken, Naan, Curry Club Dinner, J D Wetherspoon*	1 Meal/706g	897	27.0	127	5.1	18.1	3.8	1.3
Chicken, without Naan, J D Wetherspoon*	1 Meal/614g	700	25.0	114	4.7	14.8	4.0	1.3
BREAD								
Garlic, Ciabatta, J D Wetherspoon*	1 Serving/142g	406	18.0	286	8.0	1.0	12.6	1.5
Naan, J D Wetherspoon*	1 Naan/90g	197	3.0	219	7.6	41.0	2.8	1.4

	Measure INFO/WEIGHT	per Measure KCAL	FAT	Nutrition Values per 100g / 100ml KCAL	PROT	CARB	FAT	FIBRE

J D WETHERSPOON

BREAKFAST

	Measure INFO/WEIGHT	KCAL	FAT	KCAL	PROT	CARB	FAT	FIBRE
Baguette, Quorn Sausage, J D Wetherspoon*	1 Baguette/285g	622	18.0	218	10.5	29.4	6.4	3.4
Blueberry Muffin, J D Wetherspoon*	1 Muffin/124g	467	26.0	374	4.7	43.2	20.7	0.4
Bran, Fruit & Nut Muffin, J D Wetherspoon*	1 Serving/145g	571	32.0	394	7.2	43.0	21.9	1.1
Children's, J D Wetherspoon*	1 Serving/341g	613	37.0	180	10.4	10.8	10.9	2.3
Chocolate Muffin, J D Wetherspoon*	1 Muffin/125g	490	28.0	392	5.0	43.6	22.7	4.8
Farmhouse, with Toast, J D Wetherspoon*	1 Serving/796g	1647	102.0	207	9.4	14.0	12.8	1.9
Morning Roll, with Bacon, J D Wetherspoon*	1 Roll/183g	546	35.0	298	11.1	21.7	18.9	1.1
Morning Roll, with Fried Egg, J D Wetherspoon*	1 Roll/143g	400	21.0	280	9.7	27.8	14.9	1.4
Morning Roll, with Quorn Sausage, J D Wetherspoon*	1 Roll/143g	367	16.0	257	10.1	29.5	11.3	2.6
Morning Roll, with Sausage, J D Wetherspoon*	1 Roll/158g	517	28.0	327	13.8	30.1	17.7	2.3
Sandwich,Sausage, Bacon & Egg, J D Wetherspoon*	1 Sandwich/357g	840	56.0	235	12.6	11.3	15.6	1.5
Scrambled Egg, on Toast, J D Wetherspoon*	1 Serving/265g	503	25.0	190	8.4	17.4	9.4	1.1
Toast & Preserves, J D Wetherspoon*	1 Serving/148g	420	15.0	284	5.7	41.8	10.3	3.2
Traditional, J D Wetherspoon*	1 Breakfast/523g	904	60.0	173	8.4	9.4	11.5	1.8
Vegetarian, J D Wetherspoon*	1 Breakfast/562g	804	47.0	143	6.7	10.2	8.4	2.1

BROWNIES

Chocolate, Fudge, Vanilla Ice Cream, J D Wetherspoon*	1 Portion/108g	334	18.0	309	4.5	35.6	16.2	1.5

BURGERS

Beef, Dble, Bacon, Cheese, & Chips, J D Wetherspoon*	1 Serving/729g	1891	119.0	259	18.1	9.4	16.4	0.4
Beef, Double, & Chips, J D Wetherspoon*	1 Serving/598g	1382	82.0	231	16.8	11.4	13.6	0.5
Beef, Double, Cheese, & Chips, J D Wetherspoon*	1 Serving/654g	1565	91.0	239	17.2	10.7	14.0	0.5
Beef, with Bacon, Cheese & Chips, J D Wetherspoon*	1 Serving/531g	1295	79.0	244	15.2	12.6	14.8	0.5
Beef, with Cheese, & Chips, J D Wetherspoon*	1 Serving/456g	966	54.0	212	13.7	13.8	11.8	0.5
Beef, with Chips, J D Wetherspoon*	1 Serving/428g	881	46.0	206	12.8	15.7	10.8	0.6
Chicken, Fillet, with Chips, J D Wetherspoon*	1 Serving/465g	727	17.0	156	10.9	16.7	3.7	0.8
Lamb, Double, Minted, with Chips, J D Wetherspoon*	1 Serving/598g	1077	47.0	180	14.6	14.1	7.9	0.9
Lamb, Minted, with Chips, J D Wetherspoon*	1 Serving/428g	712	28.0	166	11.3	17.2	6.5	0.9
Vegetable, with Chips, J D Wetherspoon*	1 Meal/488g	839	26.0	172	4.7	27.2	5.3	2.0

BUTTY

Bacon & Egg, Brown Bloomer, J D Wetherspoon*	1 Serving/269g	702	31.0	261	18.2	21.0	11.6	1.4
Bacon & Egg, White Bloomer, J D Wetherspoon*	1 Serving/269g	689	33.0	256	16.7	20.9	12.2	1.2
Bacon, Brown Bloomer, J D Wetherspoon*	1 Serving/309g	869	40.0	281	23.3	18.3	12.8	1.2
Chip & Cheese, Brown Bloomer, J D Wetherspoon*	1 Serving/232g	593	24.0	256	9.7	31.4	10.5	1.6
Chip & Cheese, White Bloomer, J D Wetherspoon*	1 Serving/232g	580	26.0	250	7.9	31.3	11.2	1.4
Chip, Brown Bloomer, J D Wetherspoon*	1 Serving/204g	478	15.0	234	7.6	35.7	7.2	1.9
Chip, White Bloomer, J D Wetherspoon*	1 Serving/204g	465	16.0	228	5.6	35.6	8.0	1.6
Sausage & Egg, Brown Bloomer, J D Wetherspoon*	1 Serving/331g	885	49.0	267	16.8	20.8	14.8	1.3
Sausage & Egg, White Bloomer, J D Wetherspoon*	1 Serving/331g	872	51.0	263	11.4	20.7	15.3	1.1

CAKE

Chocolate Fudge, & Ice Cream, J D Wetherspoon*	1 Serving/239g	822	47.0	344	4.0	37.6	19.8	0.4

CAULIFLOWER CHEESE

J D Wetherspoon*	1 Portion/220g	275	15.0	125	4.1	3.6	6.9	0.8

CHEESECAKE

Chocolate Chip, J D Wetherspoon*	1 Serving/100g	270	11.0	270	4.9	36.8	11.5	0.5
White Chocolate & Raspberry, J D Wetherspoon*	1 Serving/175g	656	37.0	375	5.6	40.8	21.1	0.9

CHICKEN

Wings, Buffalo, J D Wetherspoon*	1 Portion/328g	636	43.0	194	15.2	4.0	13.1	0.5

CHICKEN ALFREDO

Pasta, with Dressed Side Salad, J D Wetherspoon*	1 Meal/576g	950	52.0	165	8.7	12.0	9.1	0.3
Pasta, with Garlic Bread, J D Wetherspoon*	1 Meal/501g	1007	48.0	201	10.8	13.0	9.5	0.3
Pasta, without Garlic Bread, J D Wetherspoon*	1 Meal/430g	804	39.0	187	11.3	15.0	9.0	0.1

J D WETHERSPOON

	Measure INFO/WEIGHT	per Measure KCAL	FAT	Nutrition Values per 100g / 100ml KCAL	PROT	CARB	FAT	FIBRE
CHICKEN DINNER								
Roast Potatoes, Yorkshire Pud & Veg, J D Wetherspoon*	1 Meal/993g	1529	64.0	154	10.8	14.6	6.4	2.1
CHICKEN FORESTIERRE								
J D Wetherspoon*	1 Serving/684g	626	26.0	91	7.7	8.7	3.8	1.0
CHICKEN PHAAL								
Meal, J D Wetherspoon*	1 Serving/720g	1234	46.0	171	7.5	21.0	6.4	1.6
CHICKEN ROAST								
& Chips, Peas, Toms, Mushrooms, J D Wetherspoon*	1 Meal/742g	904	39.0	122	13.0	5.6	5.2	1.2
Dressed Side Salad & BBQ Sauce, J D Wetherspoon*	1 Meal/666g	913	46.0	137	12.2	6.0	6.9	0.9
with BBQ Sauce, J D Wetherspoon*	1 Meal/742g	948	37.0	128	11.3	9.2	5.0	0.6
with Chips & BBQ Sauce, J D Wetherspoon*	1 Meal/768g	1183	53.0	154	11.5	12.2	6.9	0.9
with Chips & Salad, J D Wetherspoon*	1 Meal/695g	983	52.0	141	13.1	5.9	7.5	0.6
with Jacket Potato, Salad, & Salsa, J D Wetherspoon*	1 Meal/785g	1193	57.0	152	12.2	10.2	7.3	1.3
with Piri Piri Sauce, J D Wetherspoon*	1 Serving/994g	994	47.0	100	8.4	5.8	4.7	0.8
CHICKEN VINDALOO								
J D Wetherspoon*	1 Meal/500g	704	19.0	141	6.4	21.0	3.8	1.3
CHILLI								
Con Carne, Rice, & Tortilla Chips, J D Wetherspoon*	1 Serving/585g	744	20.0	127	6.5	17.8	3.4	1.6
Five Bean, Rice & Tortilla Chips, J D Wetherspoon*	1 Portion/390g	511	9.0	131	3.6	24.0	2.3	1.7
CHIPS								
Bowl, J D Wetherspoon*	1 Serving/300g	750	30.0	250	3.5	36.5	10.1	2.9
with Cheese, J D Wetherspoon*	1 Serving/501g	1002	52.0	200	5.2	21.9	10.3	1.8
with Roast Gravy, J D Wetherspoon*	1 Serving/400g	392	12.0	98	2.5	17.6	3.1	0.0
CHUTNEY								
Mango, J D Wetherspoon*	1 Serving/25g	47	0.0	188	0.4	44.8	0.8	0.4
CIABATTA								
BBQ Chicken & Bacon Melt, J D Wetherspoon*	1 Ciabatta/333g	716	34.0	215	11.3	20.4	10.1	1.8
BLT, J D Wetherspoon*	1 Ciabatta/390g	789	47.0	202	8.2	15.4	12.1	1.5
Club, J D Wetherspoon*	1 Ciabatta/378g	734	39.0	194	9.7	16.1	10.2	1.6
Crayfish, J D Wetherspoon*	1 Ciabatta/305g	561	27.0	184	5.8	20.3	9.0	1.9
Mature Cheddar Cheese & Pickle, J D Wetherspoon*	1 Ciabatta/350g	662	32.0	189	7.8	19.4	9.0	1.7
Tuna Mayonnaise, J D Wetherspoon*	1 Ciabatta/391g	676	33.0	173	8.8	15.8	8.4	1.5
Wiltshire Ham, J D Wetherspoon*	1 Ciabatta/335g	503	15.0	150	9.8	17.7	4.4	1.7
CRUMBLE								
Apple, Pear, & Raspberry, Custard, J D Wetherspoon*	1 Serving/372g	648	24.0	174	2.5	26.3	6.4	0.0
Apple, Pear, & Raspberry, Ice Cream, J D Wetherspoon*	1 Serving/300g	579	24.0	193	2.6	27.0	8.1	2.1
CURRY								
Beef, Malaysian, Rendang, no Naan, J D Wetherspoon*	1 Meal/615g	947	38.0	154	6.7	17.0	6.2	1.0
Beef, Malaysian, Rendang, with Naan, J D Wetherspoon*	1 Meal/706g	1144	41.0	162	6.8	20.1	5.8	1.1
Goan, Vegetable, without Naan, J D Wetherspoon*	1 Meal/748g	1017	42.0	136	3.1	18.3	5.6	1.3
Kashmiri, Lamb, with Naan, J D Wetherspoon*	1 Meal/704g	1021	33.0	145	7.2	19.5	4.7	1.2
Kashmiri, Lamb, without Naan, J D Wetherspoon*	1 Meal/615g	824	31.0	134	7.1	16.3	5.0	1.1
Kerala, Fish, with Naan, J D Wetherspoon*	1 Meal/706g	1066	36.0	151	7.0	20.0	5.1	1.0
Kerala, Fish, without Naan, J D Wetherspoon*	1 Meal/616g	869	33.0	141	6.9	16.9	5.4	0.9
Mushroom Dopiaza, no Naan Bread, J D Wetherspoon*	1 Meal/617g	580	14.0	94	2.6	16.7	2.3	1.4
Mushroom Dopiaza, with Naan Bread, J D Wetherspoon*	1 Serving/719g	899	24.0	125	3.5	21.5	3.4	1.5
Royal Thali, with Naan, J D Wetherspoon*	1 Meal/948g	1336	48.0	141	7.1	16.8	5.1	1.3
Thai, Green Chicken, without Naan, J D Wetherspoon*	1 Meal/617g	1037	47.0	168	7.5	17.6	7.6	0.5
Vegetable, Goan, with Naan Bread, J D Wetherspoon*	1 Meal/707g	1032	37.0	146	3.6	21.2	5.2	1.3
Vegetarian, Thali, with Naan, J D Wetherspoon*	1 Meal/950g	1320	43.0	139	5.3	20.3	4.5	2.4
DHANSAK								
Lamb, Meal, J D Wetherspoon*	1 Serving/720g	983	26.0	137	7.2	19.6	3.6	0.8

J D WETHERSPOON

	Measure INFO/WEIGHT	per Measure KCAL	FAT	Nutrition Values per 100g / 100ml KCAL	PROT	CARB	FAT	FIBRE
FISH & CHIPS								
Haddock, J D Wetherspoon*	1 Meal/496g	806	41.0	162	7.2	14.4	8.2	2.4
Plaice, Breaded, & Peas, J D Wetherspoon*	1 Serving/460g	550	16.0	120	6.8	15.0	3.4	1.7
Traditional, J D Wetherspoon*	1 Serving/495g	804	41.0	162	7.2	14.4	8.2	2.4
FISH CAKES								
Salmon & Lime, with Tartare Sauce, J D Wetherspoon*	1 Serving/355g	569	31.0	160	5.8	14.5	8.8	1.0
GAMMON								
Egg, Chips & Side Salad, J D Wetherspoon*	1 Meal/593g	801	42.0	135	10.2	9.0	7.0	0.3
Egg, Jacket & Dressed Side Salad, J D Wetherspoon*	1 Meal/707g	1040	45.0	147	10.1	13.1	6.4	1.3
Egg, Jacket, Peas, Tom & Mushroom, J D Wetherspoon*	1 Meal/660g	963	39.0	146	10.8	13.5	5.9	1.3
Eggs, Chips & Pineapple, J D Wetherspoon*	1 Meal/609g	1036	52.0	170	13.4	10.2	8.5	0.8
Pineapple, Chips & Dressed Salad, J D Wetherspoon*	1 Meal/654g	830	42.0	127	9.3	9.3	6.4	0.3
Pineapple, Jacket & Dressed Salad, J D Wetherspoon*	1 Meal/697g	767	36.0	110	8.8	8.3	5.1	0.4
GAMMON &								
Chips, Peas, Tomato, & Egg, J D Wetherspoon*	1 Meal/564g	844	41.0	150	15.0	6.7	7.3	1.3
Chips, Peas, Tomato, & Pineapple, J D Wetherspoon*	1 Meal/575g	799	36.0	139	13.6	7.8	6.3	1.4
HAGGIS								
with Neeps & Tatties, J D Wetherspoon*	1 Meal/682g	982	53.0	144	4.6	15.0	7.7	1.9
HAM								
& Eggs, J D Wetherspoon*	1 Serving/396g	253	13.0	64	4.9	3.5	3.2	0.0
ICE CREAM								
Bombe, Mint Chocolate, J D Wetherspoon*	1 Portion/135g	300	13.0	222	2.6	30.6	9.9	0.8
Chocolate, Bomb, J D Wetherspoon*	1 Portion/100g	259	13.0	259	5.9	34.3	13.4	5.4
Neopolitan, Movenpick, J D Wetherspoon*	1 Bowl/100g	181	10.0	181	3.0	20.0	9.6	0.0
JALFREZI								
Chicken, Meal, with Naan Bread, J D Wetherspoon*	1 Meal/705g	916	20.0	130	6.8	19.9	2.8	1.3
Chicken, without Naan Bread, J D Wetherspoon*	1 Meal/614.5g	719	17.0	117	6.7	16.9	2.8	1.3
KORMA								
Chicken, Meal, without Naan, J D Wetherspoon*	1 Meal/617g	944	38.0	153	6.4	17.0	6.2	0.8
Chicken, with Naan, J D Wetherspoon*	1 Meal/704g	1141	41.0	162	6.6	20.1	5.8	0.9
LAMB								
Braised, with Mash & Vegetables, J D Wetherspoon*	1 Meal/844g	1114	67.0	132	8.9	6.8	7.9	1.0
LASAGNE								
Al Forno with Dressed Side Salad, J D Wetherspoon*	1 Meal/658g	823	41.0	125	5.5	11.4	6.2	0.8
MASALA								
Chicken, Hot, with Naan, J D Wetherspoon*	1 Meal/707g	1033	31.0	146	6.9	20.1	4.4	1.2
Chicken, Hot, without Naan, J D Wetherspoon*	1 Meal/614g	835	28.0	136	6.8	17.1	4.6	1.1
Prawn, Sri Lankan, with Naan, J D Wetherspoon*	1 Meal/708g	1027	36.0	145	5.7	19.7	5.1	0.8
Prawn, Sri Lankan, without Naan, J D Wetherspoon*	1 Meal/617g	827	33.0	134	5.4	16.6	5.4	1.0
Vegetable, Tandoori, Meal, J D Wetherspoon*	1 Serving/720g	1020	36.0	142	3.4	20.7	5.0	2.3
MEATBALLS								
with Linguine Pasta, J D Wetherspoon*	1 Serving/512g	614	24.0	120	6.3	13.1	4.7	1.9
MELT								
BBQ Chicken, & Chips, & Salad, J D Wetherspoon*	1 Serving/643g	849	42.0	132	10.4	8.2	6.6	0.4
MIXED GRILL								
with Chips, & Dressed Side Salad, J D Wetherspoon*	1 Serving/784g	1324	87.0	169	12.0	5.6	11.1	0.3
MOUSSAKA								
Vegetarian, J D Wetherspoon*	1 Serving/555g	582	39.0	105	2.7	7.6	7.0	2.7
NACHOS								
J D Wetherspoon*	1 Serving/366g	1139	67.0	311	7.0	29.2	18.4	3.2
with Chilli Con Carne, J D Wetherspoon*	1 Meal/570g	1505	89.0	264	8.6	22.2	15.6	1.8
with Fajita Chicken, J D Wetherspoon*	1 Serving/486g	1225	70.0	252	5.7	24.7	14.5	2.9
with Five Bean Chilli, J D Wetherspoon*	1 Serving/571g	1399	81.0	245	7.3	21.8	14.2	2.7

	Measure INFO/WEIGHT	per Measure KCAL	FAT	Nutrition Values per 100g / 100ml KCAL	PROT	CARB	FAT	FIBRE
J D WETHERSPOON								
PANINI								
BBQ Chicken & Bacon, Melt, J D Wetherspoon*	1 Panini/337g	650	28.0	193	9.9	19.9	8.2	1.7
Cheese & Tuna, J D Wetherspoon*	1 Panini/221g	551	22.0	249	15.5	24.9	10.1	0.7
Cheese, Tomato, & Bacon, J D Wetherspoon*	1 Panini/261g	630	29.0	241	14.3	21.6	11.1	0.8
Club, J D Wetherspoon*	1 Panini/378g	734	39.0	194	9.7	16.1	10.2	1.6
Fajita Chicken, J D Wetherspoon*	1 Panini/235g	359	6.0	153	4.4	28.8	2.6	1.7
Mature, Cheddar Cheese & Tomato, J D Wetherspoon*	1 Panini/330g	750	27.0	227	10.4	18.0	8.2	1.7
Pepperoni & Mozzarella, J D Wetherspoon*	1 Panini/205g	617	33.0	301	11.6	27.5	16.3	1.0
Tomato, Mozzarella & Green Pesto, J D Wetherspoon*	1 Panini/245g	502	23.0	205	7.3	23.0	9.3	1.4
Wiltshire Ham & Cheddar, J D Wetherspoon*	1 Panini/354g	868	50.0	245	12.7	16.7	14.1	1.5
PASTA								
5 Cheese & Bacon, & Dressed Salad, J D Wetherspoon*	1 Meal/544g	506	29.0	93	2.3	9.1	5.3	1.3
5 Cheese & Bacon, & Garlic Ciabatta, J D Wetherspoon*	1 Meal/469g	563	23.0	120	3.6	9.7	5.0	1.5
Veg, Chargrilled & Sundried Tomato, J D Wetherspoon*	1 Meal/500g	600	2.0	120	3.6	15.2	0.5	0.7
PASTA BAKE								
Mediterranean, J D Wetherspoon*	1 Serving/450g	577	22.0	128	4.3	16.4	4.9	0.9
PEAS								
& Ham, White Poppy Seed Bloomer, J D Wetherspoon*	1 Portion/456g	474	18.0	104	4.4	12.5	3.9	2.0
PIE								
Aberdeen Angus, Chips, & Veg J D Wetherspoon*	1 Serving/780g	1356	87.0	174	5.5	15.7	11.1	0.9
Beef & Abbot Ale, Chips, Veg & Gravy, J D Wetherspoon*	1 Meal/850g	1258	68.0	148	4.0	14.9	8.0	1.0
Cottage, with Chips & Peas, J D Wetherspoon*	1 Meal/682g	846	33.0	124	3.7	15.6	4.9	1.9
Fish, Carrot & Broccoli, in Herb Butter, J D Wetherspoon*	1 Serving/550g	612	38.0	111	4.6	9.7	6.9	2.4
Scotch, J D Wetherspoon*	1 Serving/145g	302	15.0	208	13.1	7.8	10.6	0.9
Scotch, with Chips & Beans, J D Wetherspoon*	1 Serving/435g	603	22.0	139	6.8	14.9	5.1	1.5
PLATTER								
Italian Style, J D Wetherspoon*	1 Platter/1020g	1985	75.0	195	10.4	22.9	7.4	0.6
Mexican, Chilli, Sour Cream, J D Wetherspoon*	1 Platter/1062g	2560	141.0	241	7.5	22.6	13.3	2.8
Mexican, with Five Bean Chilli, J D Wetherspoon*	1 Platter/1002g	2358	123.0	235	6.2	25.6	12.3	3.6
Western, J D Wetherspoon*	1 Platter/1454g	2973	169.0	204	16.9	9.1	11.6	0.4
POPPADOMS								
& Dips, J D Wetherspoon*	1 Serving/134g	425	11.0	317	4.6	28.4	8.1	2.5
J D Wetherspoon*	1 Poppadom/12g	35	0.0	281	6.7	45.0	1.9	10.0
PORK DINNER								
Roast Potatoes, Yorkshire Pud & Veg, J D Wetherspoon*	1 Meal/1022g	1543	63.0	151	10.4	14.6	6.2	2.1
POTATO BOMBAY								
J D Wetherspoon*	1 Serving/300g	285	15.0	95	1.8	10.8	4.9	2.5
POTATO SKINS								
Cheese & Bacon, Loaded, J D Wetherspoon*	1 Serving/439g	949	58.0	216	8.9	15.2	13.3	1.5
Cheese & Red Onion, Loaded, J D Wetherspoon*	1 Serving/414g	835	51.0	202	6.0	16.5	12.4	1.6
Chilli Con Carne, Loaded, J D Wetherspoon*	1 Serving/503g	735	36.0	146	5.0	15.7	7.1	1.9
POTATO WEDGES								
Spicy, J D Wetherspoon*	1 Serving/270g	434	16.0	161	2.2	27.7	5.8	1.8
Spicy, with Sour Cream, J D Wetherspoon*	1 Serving/330g	558	27.0	169	2.3	23.4	8.3	1.5
POTATOES								
Baked, Jacket, Coleslaw, J D Wetherspoon*	1 Meal/596g	918	49.0	154	2.3	17.1	8.2	1.8
Jacket, Baked Beans, & Salad, J D Wetherspoon*	1 Meal/575g	725	25.0	126	3.3	19.6	4.3	2.4
Jacket, Chilli, Sour Cream & Salad, J D Wetherspoon*	1 Meal/615g	775	30.0	126	4.4	17.0	4.9	1.9
Jacket, Crayfish, Marie Rose Dressing, J D Wetherspoon*	1 Meal/524g	796	41.0	152	3.5	18.2	7.8	1.7
Jacket, Mature, Cheddar Cheese, J D Wetherspoon*	1 Meal/496g	858	45.0	173	5.6	18.7	9.0	1.8
Jacket, with 5 Bean Chilli, & Salad, J D Wetherspoon*	1 Meal/597g	705	26.0	118	3.0	17.9	4.3	2.4
Jacket, with Tuna Mayo, & Salad, J D Wetherspoon*	1 Meal/645g	845	40.0	131	5.4	14.6	6.1	1.3
Mashed, Creamy, J D Wetherspoon*	1 Portion/279g	349	21.0	125	1.5	15.0	7.6	1.1

J D WETHERSPOON

Measure INFO/WEIGHT	per Measure KCAL	FAT	Nutrition Values per 100g / 100ml KCAL	PROT	CARB	FAT	FIBRE

POTATOES

	Measure INFO/WEIGHT	KCAL	FAT	KCAL	PROT	CARB	FAT	FIBRE
Roast, J D Wetherspoon*	1 Portion/200g	290	9.0	145	2.5	23.0	4.7	2.3
RIBS								
Double, J D Wetherspoon*	1 Serving/350g	767	41.0	219	16.7	11.9	11.7	0.4
Double, with Chips, J D Wetherspoon*	1 Serving/500g	949	46.0	190	12.5	14.9	9.3	0.3
Double, with Jacket Potato, J D Wetherspoon*	1 Serving/590g	1159	51.0	196	11.4	19.2	8.6	1.3
RICE								
Basmati, Yellow, J D Wetherspoon*	1 Portion/200g	286	1.0	143	3.4	31.1	0.6	0.2
J D Wetherspoon*	1 Serving/200g	274	0.0	137	2.9	30.9	0.2	0.2
ROGAN JOSH								
Lamb, Meal, without Naan, J D Wetherspoon*	1 Meal/617g	820	28.0	133	7.1	17.0	4.5	1.0
Lamb, with Naan, J D Wetherspoon*	1 Meal/706g	1017	30.0	144	7.2	20.1	4.3	1.1
SALAD								
Caesar, Chicken, J D Wetherspoon*	1 Meal/230g	507	36.0	220	14.3	5.1	15.8	0.8
Caesar, J D Wetherspoon*	1 Meal/211g	448	38.0	212	6.8	5.8	18.0	1.1
Chicken & Bacon, Warm, J D Wetherspoon*	1 Meal/426g	600	41.0	141	9.8	3.8	9.7	0.6
Chicken, BBQ, Croutons & Dressing, J D Wetherspoon*	1 Portion/350g	315	8.0	90	9.4	7.5	2.4	0.8
Crayfish, J D Wetherspoon*	1 Meal/317g	247	18.0	78	4.4	2.7	5.7	0.6
Side, No Dressing, J D Wetherspoon*	1 Salad/195g	125	4.0	64	2.0	8.9	2.3	1.1
Side, with Dressing & Croutons, J D Wetherspoon*	1 Portion/140g	221	18.0	158	2.1	8.6	13.1	1.1
Side, with Dressing & No Croutons, J D Wetherspoon*	1 Portion/129g	145	14.0	112	1.0	3.2	10.8	0.9
Side, with Dressing, J D Wetherspoon*	1 Salad/215g	263	20.0	122	2.2	8.1	9.1	1.0
Side, without Croutons, J D Wetherspoon*	1 Portion/111g	157	11.0	141	9.8	3.8	9.7	0.6
Thai Noodle, J D Wetherspoon*	1 Portion/394g	433	21.0	110	2.7	12.7	5.4	1.4
Thai Noodle, with Chicken, J D Wetherspoon*	1 Meal/554g	637	28.0	115	9.2	9.6	5.0	1.4
Tiger Prawn, Dressing, & Chilli Jam, J D Wetherspoon*	1 Portion/340g	500	33.0	147	4.7	10.1	9.7	0.9
Tuna, with Eggs, Olives, & Croutons, J D Wetherspoon*	1 Portion/395g	679	52.0	172	10.3	3.2	13.1	0.7
SALMON & SALAD								
Watercress, Creme Fraiche, Chips, J D Wetherspoon*	1 Meal/585g	912	56.0	156	6.7	10.7	9.6	1.1
Watercress, Creme Fraiche, Jacket, J D Wetherspoon*	1 Meal/655g	995	51.0	152	6.8	14.5	7.8	1.4
SAMOSAS								
Lamb, J D Wetherspoon*	1 Samosa/90g	160	4.0	178	7.9	29.9	4.2	3.9
Vegetable, J D Wetherspoon*	1 Samosa/50g	92	3.0	184	5.4	28.4	6.2	2.2
SANDWICH								
Beef, Hot, Brown Bloomer, J D Wetherspoon*	1 Sandwich/299g	618	27.0	207	11.4	19.9	9.1	1.3
Beef, Hot, White Poppy Seed Bloomer, J D Wetherspoon*	1 Sandwich/299g	605	29.0	202	10.0	19.8	9.6	1.1
BLT, Brown Bloomer, J D Wetherspoon*	1 Sandwich/404g	885	40.0	219	18.0	14.6	9.8	1.2
BLT, White Bloomer, J D Wetherspoon*	1 Sandwich/404g	872	33.0	216	17.0	14.6	8.1	1.0
Cheddar, & Pickle, Brown Bloomer, J D Wetherspoon*	1 Sandwich/260g	665	32.0	256	11.0	25.4	12.3	1.9
Cheddar, & Pickle, White Bloomer, J D Wetherspoon*	1 Sandwich/260g	638	33.0	245	9.2	0.0	12.6	1.5
Chicken, Cheese, Bacon, Mayo, White, J D Wetherspoon*	1 Sandwich/312g	710	40.0	228	13.5	18.8	12.7	1.2
Chicken, Half Fat Mayo, Brown, Hot, J D Wetherspoon*	1 Sandwich/289g	628	28.0	217	11.8	20.7	9.8	1.7
Chicken, Half Fat Mayo, White, Hot, J D Wetherspoon*	1 Sandwich/289g	615	30.0	213	11.3	20.6	10.3	1.5
Egg Mayonnaise, Brown Bloomer, J D Wetherspoon*	1 Sandwich/295g	704	40.0	239	10.1	19.7	13.4	1.3
Egg Mayonnaise, White Bloomer, J D Wetherspoon*	1 Sandwich/295g	692	41.0	235	8.7	19.6	13.9	1.1
Ham, & Tomato, Brown Bloomer, J D Wetherspoon*	1 Sandwich/239g	514	17.0	215	11.4	24.4	7.2	1.8
Ham, & Tomato, White Bloomer, J D Wetherspoon*	1 Sandwich/239g	501	19.0	210	9.7	24.4	7.8	1.5
Prawn Mayonnaise, Brown Bloomer, J D Wetherspoon*	1 Sandwich/244g	579	27.0	237	11.0	23.8	10.9	1.6
Prawn Mayonnaise, White Bloomer, J D Wetherspoon*	1 Sandwich/244g	567	28.0	232	9.3	23.7	11.6	1.4
Salmon, Lemon Mayo, Brown Bloomer, J D Wetherspoon*	1 Sandwich/229g	637	34.0	278	11.4	25.4	14.7	1.7
Salmon, Lemon Mayo, White Bloomer, J D Wetherspoon*	1 Sandwich/229g	625	35.0	273	9.6	25.2	15.4	1.4
Tuna Mayo, Half Fat Mayo, White, J D Wetherspoon*	1 Sandwich/389g	828	47.0	213	11.2	15.6	12.1	1.0

J D WETHERSPOON

	Measure INFO/WEIGHT	per Measure KCAL	per Measure FAT	Nutrition Values per 100g / 100ml KCAL	PROT	CARB	FAT	FIBRE
SAUSAGE & MASH								
with Red Wine Gravy, J D Wetherspoon*	1 Portion/677g	887	51.0	131	6.0	10.2	7.5	1.8
SAUSAGES WITH								
Bacon & Egg, J D Wetherspoon*	1 Serving/582g	1040	58.0	179	11.7	11.3	9.9	1.0
Chips & Beans, J D Wetherspoon*	1 Meal/554g	897	43.0	162	7.3	16.4	7.7	2.3
SCAMPI								
Breaded, Chips, Peas, Tartare Sauce, J D Wetherspoon*	1 Serving/561g	987	44.0	176	5.2	19.9	7.8	2.3
SORBET								
Mango & Passionfruit, J D Wetherspoon*	1 Serving/135g	115	0.0	85	0.2	20.0	0.1	0.2
SOUP								
Leek & Potato, & Malt Grain Baguette, J D Wetherspoon*	1 Bowl/490g	490	9.0	100	3.2	17.9	1.8	1.7
Leek & Potato, no Bread & Butter, J D Wetherspoon*	1 Bowl/420	105	1.0	25	0.9	5.1	0.2	1.0
Mushroom, no Bread, J D Wetherspoon*	1 Serving/305g	252	16.0	83	2.8	5.5	5.4	0.4
Mushroom, with Brown Bloomer, J D Wetherspoon*	1 Serving/429g	561	24.0	131	3.4	16.0	5.5	1.2
Mushroom, with White Bloomer, J D Wetherspoon*	1 Serving/429g	549	25.0	128	3.4	15.9	5.9	1.1
Tomato & Basil, Organic, J D Wetherspoon*	1 Serving/491g	584	23.0	119	2.9	15.8	4.7	1.2
Tomato & Basil, Organic, no Bread, J D Wetherspoon*	1 Bowl/350g	199	15.0	57	0.7	3.0	4.3	0.6
Tomato, no Bread, J D Wetherspoon*	1 Serving/305g	198	14.0	65	0.9	3.9	4.6	0.6
Tomato, with Brown Bloomer, J D Wetherspoon*	1 Serving/429g	576	26.0	134	3.7	15.7	6.0	1.3
Tomato, with White Bloomer, J D Wetherspoon*	1 Serving/429g	563	27.0	131	2.8	15.6	6.4	1.2
SPONGE PUDDING								
Treacle, with Hot Custard, J D Wetherspoon*	1 Serving/515g	1267	71.0	246	2.3	41.8	13.8	0.2
SQUASH								
Butternut, Roast Dinner, J D Wetherspoon*	1 Meal/847g	1211	56.0	143	4.9	17.5	6.6	2.9
STEAK								
Ribeye, Chips & Side Salad, J D Wetherspoon*	1 Meal/562g	1006	72.0	179	8.0	8.9	12.8	0.3
Ribeye, Chips, Peas, Tom, Mushroom, J D Wetherspoon*	1 Portion/531g	945	64.0	178	9.3	9.3	12.0	0.3
Ribeye, Jacket & Dressed Side Salad, J D Wetherspoon*	1 Meal/620g	850	43.0	137	8.2	10.1	7.0	1.1
Ribeye, Jacket, Peas, Tom & Mushrm, J D Wetherspoon*	1 Meal/674g	1253	154.0	186	7.8	11.5	22.8	1.9
Ribeye, Prawns, Chips, & Salad, J D Wetherspoon*	1 Meal/714g	1093	56.0	153	11.0	7.7	7.9	0.3
Ribeye, Prawns, Jacket & Side Salad, J D Wetherspoon*	1 Meal/727g	1178	57.0	162	10.8	7.7	7.9	0.3
Rump, Chips & Dressed Salad, J D Wetherspoon*	1 Meal/787g	1283	72.0	163	14.3	6.3	9.1	0.2
Rump, Chips, Peas, Tom & Mushroom, J D Wetherspoon*	1 Meal/759g	1268	71.0	167	14.9	6.5	9.3	0.2
Rump, Jacket & Dressed Side Salad, J D Wetherspoon*	1 Meal/867g	1466	71.0	169	13.6	10.7	8.2	1.0
Rump, Jacket, Peas, Tom & Mushroom, J D Wetherspoon*	1 Meal/839g	1451	70.0	173	14.1	11.0	8.3	1.1
T-Bone, Jacket & Dressed Salad, J D Wetherspoon*	1 Meal/756g	1496	97.0	198	9.1	12.3	12.8	1.2
T-Bone, Jacket, Peas, Tom & Mushroom, J D Wetherspoon*	1 Meal/722g	1481	95.0	205	9.5	12.7	13.2	1.2
T-Bone, Chips, & Dressed Salad, J D Wetherspoon*	1 Meal/673g	1313	98.0	195	9.4	7.4	14.5	0.2
STEW								
Irish, J D Wetherspoon*	1 Serving/600g	516	23.0	86	7.3	5.6	3.9	0.9
STUFFING BALLS								
Sage & Onion, J D Wetherspoon*	1 Portion/70g	137	1.0	196	6.6	32.3	1.6	3.6
TART								
Apple, with Ice Cream, J D Wetherspoon*	1 Serving/235g	464	20.0	197	1.6	29.8	8.5	0.4
TIKKA								
Mixed Grill, Starter, J D Wetherspoon*	1 Portion/374g	460	24.0	123	13.4	3.2	6.4	0.9
TIKKA MASALA								
Chicken, with Rice & No Naan Bread, J D Wetherspoon*	1 Meal/614g	872	33.0	142	6.9	16.9	5.4	1.2
WAFFLES								
Belgian, Ice Cream & Maple Syrup, J D Wetherspoon*	1 Serving/395g	934	34.0	236	13.8	28.4	8.5	0.8
WRAP								
Caesar Wetherwrap & Potato Wedges, J D Wetherspoon*	1 Serving/289g	687	40.0	238	5.0	25.2	13.9	1.6
Caesar Wetherwrap, J D Wetherspoon*	1 Wrap/159g	478	33.0	301	7.0	23.1	20.5	1.5

J D WETHERSPOON
WRAP

Caesar Wetherwrap, Tortillas & Salsa, J D Wetherspoon*	1 Serving/244g	624	39.0	256	5.7	23.4	15.9	1.6
Chicken & Cheese, J D Wetherspoon*	1 Wrap/271g	553	26.0	204	10.7	19.6	9.7	1.4
Chicken, Cheese, & Potato Wedges, J D Wetherspoon*	1 Serving/401g	762	34.0	190	8.0	22.2	8.5	1.5
Chicken, Cheese, Tortilla Chips, Salsa, J D Wetherspoon*	1 Serving/356g	699	32.0	196	8.8	20.6	9.1	1.5
Chicken, Guacamole, Potato Wedges, J D Wetherspoon*	1 Serving/318g	537	18.0	169	7.2	23.7	5.8	2.0
Chicken, Guacamole, Tortillas, Salsa, J D Wetherspoon*	1 Serving/273g	474	17.0	174	8.2	21.9	6.2	2.0
Chicken, Southern Fried, Creole Mayo, J D Wetherspoon*	1 Wrap/320g	553	30.0	173	7.1	16.3	9.4	1.4
Chicken, with Chicken Breast, J D Wetherspoon*	1 Wrap/292g	450	22.0	154	9.4	14.5	7.4	1.5
Chicken, with Potato Wedges, J D Wetherspoon*	1 Serving/373g	647	24.0	173	6.7	23.9	6.5	1.7
Chicken, with Tortilla Chips & Salsa, J D Wetherspoon*	1 Serving/328g	584	23.0	178	7.5	22.3	7.0	1.6
Club Wetherwrap, Tortilla Chips, Salsa, J D Wetherspoon*	1 Serving/336g	759	42.0	226	12.2	17.1	12.5	1.1
Club Wetherwrap, with Potato Wedges, J D Wetherspoon*	1 Serving/381g	822	43.0	216	10.9	19.2	11.3	1.2
Club, J D Wetherspoon*	1 Wrap/286g	711	40.0	249	12.1	19.2	14.1	1.0
Fajita Chicken, J D Wetherspoon*	1 Wrap/228g	345	14.0	151	3.8	21.2	6.2	1.9
Fajita Chicken, Tortilla Chips, Salsa, J D Wetherspoon*	1 Serving/313g	491	20.0	157	3.5	21.9	6.5	1.9
Fajita Chicken, with Potato Wedges, J D Wetherspoon*	1 Serving/358g	554	22.0	155	3.2	23.5	6.1	1.9
Poached Salmon & Prawn Salad, J D Wetherspoon*	1 Wrap/355g	512	34.0	144	9.8	4.5	9.6	0.5
Poached Salmon, Tortilla Chips, Salsa, J D Wetherspoon*	1 Serving/203g	573	33.0	282	9.9	25.8	16.2	1.6
Poached Salmon, with Potato Wedges, J D Wetherspoon*	1 Serving/298g	656	34.0	220	7.1	24.2	11.5	1.5

YORKSHIRE PUDDING

J D Wetherspoon*	2 Puddings/56g	132	5.0	236	8.2	32.9	8.2	1.1

KFC
BEANS

BBQ, Regular, KFC*	1 Serving/130g	200	1.0	154	6.1	30.0	1.1	6.9

BURGERS

Fillet Tower Burger, KFC*	1 Burger/163g	617	21.0	378	24.3	41.4	12.9	0.0
Fillet, KFC*	1 Burger/245g	479	20.0	196	11.1	19.5	8.1	0.0
Fillet, Mini, KFC*	1 Burger/114g	275	11.0	241	14.8	23.9	9.8	0.0
Mini Fillet, Kids, KFC*	1 Burger/114g	253	6.0	222	15.8	27.0	5.6	0.0
Tower, KFC*	1 Burger/210g	628	21.0	299	15.9	30.0	9.9	0.0
Tower, Zinger, KFC*	1 Burger/264g	655	33.0	248	11.2	24.3	12.4	0.0
Zinger, Fillet, KFC*	1 Serving/185g	445	20.0	241	13.9	22.4	10.6	1.4
Zinger, KFC*	1 Burger/219g	481	21.0	220	12.2	22.0	9.5	0.0

CHEESECAKE

Boysenberry, Chateau, KFC*	1 Serving/85g	196	9.0	230	4.0	30.0	11.0	0.0
Cookies & Cream, KFC*	1 Serving/80g	261	17.0	326	4.3	29.1	21.4	0.0

CHICKEN

Breast, Original Recipe, KFC*	1 Breast/137g	285	13.0	207	24.9	5.6	9.7	0.0
Drumsticks, Original Recipe, KFC*	1 Drumstick/95g	161	9.0	170	11.9	9.1	10.0	0.0
Fillet, Mini, Not In a Bun, KFC*	1 Fillet/50g	116	4.0	232	26.6	14.0	8.0	0.0
Popcorn, Kids, KFC*	1 Portion/66g	144	8.0	219	14.1	13.2	12.7	0.0
Popcorn, Large, KFC*	1 Serving/188.5g	494	30.0	262	17.5	13.5	15.8	0.0
Popcorn, Regular, KFC*	1 Serving/122g	307	19.0	251	16.8	12.9	15.2	0.0
Ribs, Original Recipe, KFC*	1 Rib/126g	238	13.0	188	19.8	4.1	10.6	0.0
Strips, Crispy, KFC*	1 Strip/46g	112	5.0	243	15.4	20.4	11.7	0.0
Thighs, Original Recipe, KFC*	1 Thigh/134g	218	14.0	162	12.6	4.4	10.6	0.0
Wings, Hot, KFC*	1 Wing/58g	102	7.0	175	9.4	7.5	12.1	0.0
Wings, Original Recipe, KFC*	1 Wing/48g	126	4.0	262	25.0	8.3	8.0	0.0

COLESLAW

Large, KFC*	1 Serving/200g	268	22.0	134	0.8	9.5	11.2	0.0
Regular, KFC*	1 Serving/100g	134	11.0	134	0.8	9.5	11.2	0.0

	Measure INFO/WEIGHT	per Measure KCAL	FAT	Nutrition Values per 100g / 100ml KCAL	PROT	CARB	FAT	FIBRE
KFC								
CORN								
Cobs, Cobette, KFC*	1 Serving/70g	141	8.0	201	4.3	20.1	12.1	0.0
DRESSING								
Caesar, KFC*	1 Sachet/35g	103	11.0	295	19.2	2.7	31.1	0.0
French, KFC*	1 Sachet/45g	30	1.0	66	0.2	2.9	2.9	0.0
Vinaigrette, Low Fat, KFC*	1 Sachet/35g	21	1.0	59	0.5	8.9	2.2	0.0
Yoghurt, Coriander & Chilli, KFC*	1 Sachet/45g	166	16.0	369	2.2	9.3	36.0	0.0
FRIES								
Large, KFC*	1 Serving/162g	375	19.0	231	3.1	32.4	11.9	0.0
Regular, KFC*	1 Serving/111g	257	13.0	232	3.1	32.4	11.9	0.0
GRAVY								
Large, KFC*	1 Serving/204g	144	8.0	71	2.3	7.3	3.9	0.0
Regular, KFC*	1 Serving/102g	72	4.0	71	2.3	7.3	3.9	0.0
ICE CREAM								
Avalanche, KFC*	1 Pot/28g	114	5.0	407	10.4	51.4	18.2	0.0
Soft, KFC*	1 Serving/110g	171	7.0	155	3.7	20.6	6.4	0.0
PIE								
Apple Slice, Colonel's Pies, KFC*	1 Slice/113g	310	14.0	274	1.7	38.9	12.3	0.0
Strawberry Creme, Slice, KFC*	1 Slice/78g	279	15.0	358	5.4	41.0	19.2	2.5
SALAD								
Chicken, Original Recipe, No Dressing, KFC*	1 Salad/292g	270	10.0	92	9.0	7.0	3.3	0.0
Chicken, Zinger, No Dressing, KFC*	1 Salad/285g	307	15.0	108	7.8	8.0	5.2	0.0
Potato, KFC*	1 Portion/160g	229	14.0	143	2.5	14.3	8.7	1.8
WRAP								
Twister, Salsa, Toasted, KFC*	1 Wrap/222g	516	25.0	232	8.7	24.6	11.2	0.0
Twister, Toasted, KFC*	1 Wrap/217g	509	25.0	235	8.9	24.6	11.5	0.0
Wrapstar, KFC*	1 Wrapstar/239g	642	37.0	269	11.4	25.9	15.3	0.0
KRISPY KREME								
DOUGHNUT								
Chocolate, Glazed, Krispy Kreme*	1 Doughnut/80g	309	14.0	387	4.0	55.0	17.0	3.0
Vanilla, Krispy Kreme*	1 Doughnut/80g	315	14.0	391	4.0	57.0	17.0	2.0
DOUGHNUTS								
Blueberry, Powdered, Filled, Krispy Kreme*	1 Doughnut/86g	307	17.0	357	7.0	36.0	20.0	5.0
Chocolate Iced, Creme Filled, Krispy Kreme*	1 Doughnut/87g	339	17.0	390	6.0	47.0	20.0	4.0
Chocolate Iced, Custard Filled, Krispy Kreme*	1 Doughnut/87g	307	15.0	353	6.0	43.0	17.0	2.0
Chocolate Iced, Glazed, Krispy Kreme*	1 Doughnut/66g	270	13.0	410	5.0	51.0	20.0	3.0
Chocolate Iced, with Creme Filling, Krispy Kreme*	1 Doughnut/87g	350	21.0	402	3.0	42.0	24.0	1.0
Chocolate Iced, with Sprinkles, Krispy Kreme*	1 Doughnut/71g	293	13.0	413	5.0	56.0	19.0	3.0
Cinnamon Apple, Filled, Krispy Kreme*	1 Doughnut/81g	269	15.0	332	7.0	37.0	18.0	5.0
Cruller, Glazed, Krispy Kreme*	1 Doughnut/54g	254	16.0	471	4.0	49.0	29.0	4.0
Glazed, with a Creme Filling, Krispy Kreme*	1 Doughnut/86g	309	15.0	359	5.0	44.0	18.0	4.0
Lemon Filled, Glazed, Krispy Kreme*	1 Doughnut/66g	218	11.0	331	5.0	41.0	16.0	4.0
Maple Iced, Krispy Kreme*	1 Doughnut/66g	279	15.0	422	5.0	49.0	23.0	3.0
Original, Glazed, Krispy Kreme*	1 Doughnut/52g	217	13.0	417	6.0	43.0	25.0	4.0
Raspberry, Glazed, Krispy Kreme*	1 Doughnut/86g	307	14.0	357	6.0	47.0	16.0	4.0
Sour Cream, Krispy Kreme*	1 Doughnut/80g	340	18.0	425	4.0	53.0	23.0	1.0
Strawberry Filled, Powdered, Krispy Kreme*	1 Doughnut/74g	248	13.0	335	7.0	36.0	18.0	5.0
LEON RESTAURANTS								
DINNER								
Brown Rice, Leon Restaurants*	1 Serving/165g	312	8.0	189	4.3	32.4	4.7	0.0
Malay Red Curry, Leon Restaurants*	1 Portion/245g	256	11.0	104	4.6	11.5	4.6	0.0
Pork Jambalaya, Leon Restaurants*	1 Portion/245g	165	7.0	67	1.2	6.7	2.9	0.0
Slaw, Leon Restaurants*	1 Serving/115g	179	15.0	156	3.4	6.4	13.0	0.0

	Measure INFO/WEIGHT	per Measure KCAL	FAT	Nutrition Values per 100g / 100ml KCAL	PROT	CARB	FAT	FIBRE
LEON RESTAURANTS								
JUICE								
Blackcurrant, Leon Restaurants*	1 Portion/300g	120	0.0	40	0.1	9.8	0.0	0.0
LUNCH								
Red Bean & Squash Chilli, Leon Restaurants*	1 Serving/225g	153	10.0	68	0.6	3.5	4.4	0.0
Superfood Salads, Grilled Chicken, Leon Restaurants*	1 Serving/400g	619	34.0	155	13.5	6.2	8.6	0.0
LUNCH, HOT DISHES								
Chilli Chicken, Leon Restaurants*	1 Serving/494g	815	42.0	165	8.1	13.8	8.6	0.0
LUNCH, SPECIALS								
Chilli Con Carne, Leon Restaurants*	1 Serving/499g	732	34.0	147	5.6	15.8	6.7	0.0
SMOOTHIE								
Strawberry Power Shake, Leon Restaurants*	1 Serving/300g	348	14.0	116	4.1	14.1	4.8	0.0
WRAP								
Chicken & Chorizo, Leon Restaurants*	1 Serving/286g	420	17.0	147	13.4	17.5	6.0	0.0
Slow Cooked Shredded Pork, Leon Restaurants*	1 Wrap/280g	449	12.0	160	10.0	20.7	4.3	0.0
WRAPS								
Grilled Chicken, Leon Restaurants*	1 Wrap/280g	429	11.0	153	12.9	17.5	4.0	0.0
Sweet Potato Falafel, Leon Restaurants*	1 Wrap/281g	441	10.0	157	4.9	28.0	3.6	0.0
MCDONALD'S								
BAGEL								
Plain, Toasted, McDonald's*	1 Bagel/85g	210	1.0	248	9.0	50.0	1.0	3.0
Toasted, with Strawberry Jam, McDonald's*	1 Bagel/105g	260	1.0	248	8.0	52.0	1.0	3.0
with Bacon, Egg & Cheese, McDonald's*	1 Bagel/173g	455	22.0	263	13.0	26.0	13.0	2.0
with Butter & Jam, McDonald's*	1 Bagel/122g	399	10.0	326	5.9	58.8	8.3	2.2
with Flora & Jam, McDonald's*	1 Bagel/120g	369	7.0	305	6.0	59.4	5.7	2.2
with Philadelphia, McDonald's*	1 Bagel/125g	317	6.0	254	7.7	47.5	4.7	2.1
with Sausage & Egg, McDonald's*	1 Bagel/207g	551	27.0	266	13.3	23.3	12.8	1.6
with Sausage, Egg & Cheese, McDonald's*	1 Bagel/203g	540	28.0	266	14.0	22.0	14.0	2.0
BREAKFAST								
Big Breakfast Bun, McDonald's*	1 Bun/242g	571	32.0	236	13.0	15.1	13.3	0.9
Big Breakfast, McDonald's*	1 Breakfast/264g	595	37.0	225	11.0	15.0	14.0	1.0
BREAKFAST CEREAL								
Porridge, Oatso Simple, & Jam, McDonald's*	1 Serving/232g	246	5.0	106	4.0	17.0	2.3	0.9
Porridge, Oatso Simple, & Sugar, McDonald's*	1 Serving/215g	205	5.0	95	4.3	13.7	2.5	0.9
Porridge, Oatso Simple, Plain, McDonald's*	1 Serving/212g	195	4.0	92	5.0	13.0	2.0	1.0
BROWNIE								
Belgian Bliss, McDonald's*	1 Serving/85g	390	22.0	459	6.0	51.0	26.0	2.0
BURGERS								
Big Mac, McDonald's*	1 Burger/214g	491	26.0	229	13.0	19.0	12.0	2.0
Big Mac, No Sauce, No Cheese, McDonald's*	1 Sandwich/181g	400	16.0	221	12.1	23.8	8.8	1.1
Big Tasty, McDonald's*	1 Burger/346g	835	52.0	241	13.0	14.0	15.0	1.0
Big Tasty, with Bacon, McDonald's*	1 Burger/359g	890	57.0	248	14.0	14.0	16.0	1.0
Bigger Big Mac, McDonald's*	1 Burger/324.5g	714	34.0	220	12.9	18.5	10.5	1.6
Cheeseburger, Bacon, McDonald's*	1 Burger/127g	336	15.0	264	16.0	24.0	12.0	2.0
Cheeseburger, Double, McDonald's*	1 Burger/169g	440	24.0	260	17.0	19.0	14.0	1.0
Cheeseburger, McDonald's*	1 Burger/119g	300	12.0	253	14.3	26.2	10.1	2.5
Chicken Legend, with Bacon, Cool Mayo, McDonald's*	1 Burger/227g	590	23.0	260	15.0	27.0	10.0	2.0
Filet-O-Fish, McDonald's*	1 Burger/150g	350	18.0	232	10.0	24.0	12.0	1.0
Filet-O-Fish, No Tartar Sauce, McDonald's*	1 Burger/124g	290	9.0	234	12.1	30.6	7.3	0.8
Hamburger, McDonald's*	1 Burger/104g	250	8.0	240	13.0	29.0	8.0	2.0
Mayo Chicken, McDonald's*	1 Burger/122g	310	13.0	254	10.0	30.0	11.0	2.0
McChicken Sandwich, McDonald's*	1 Sandwich/171g	385	17.0	224	9.0	26.0	10.0	2.0
Quarter Pounder, Bacon with Cheese, McDonald's*	1 Burger/230g	592	33.0	259	16.5	15.4	14.5	1.3
Quarter Pounder, Deluxe, McDonald's*	1 Burger/253g	521	27.0	206	11.4	16.1	10.6	1.7

MCDONALD'S

	Measure INFO/WEIGHT	per Measure KCAL	per Measure FAT	Nutrition Values per 100g / 100ml KCAL	PROT	CARB	FAT	FIBRE
BURGERS								
Quarter Pounder, Double, with Cheese, McDonald's*	1 Burger/275g	710	40.0	259	19.5	12.2	14.7	1.1
Quarter Pounder, McDonald's*	1 Burger/178g	424	19.0	238	14.5	20.9	10.7	2.1
Quarter Pounder, with Cheese, McDonald's*	1 Burger/194g	490	25.0	252	16.0	19.0	13.0	2.0
The M with Bacon, McDonald's*	1 Serving/249g	620	32.0	249	17.0	18.0	13.0	1.0
The M, McDonald's*	1 Serving/240g	580	29.0	242	16.0	18.0	12.0	1.0
BURGERS VEGETARIAN								
Vegetable, Deluxe, McDonald's*	1 Burger/181g	411	16.0	227	6.0	30.0	9.0	6.0
BUTTER								
Country Life, McDonald's*	1 Pack/11g	85	9.0	752	0.0	0.0	80.0	0.0
CADBURY BYTE								
McMini, McDonald's*	1 Byte/14g	67	3.0	478	6.5	64.7	20.7	1.7
CAKE								
Birthday, McDonald's*	1 Portion/158g	640	23.0	405	2.7	65.4	14.3	1.0
CARROTS								
Sticks, McDonald's*	1 Bag/80g	30	0.0	38	0.0	8.0	0.0	2.0
CHEESE								
Soft, Philadelphia, Light, McDonald's*	1 Serving/35g	55	4.0	157	9.0	3.0	11.0	0.0
CHICKEN								
McNuggets, 4 Pieces, McDonald's*	4 Pieces/70g	170	9.0	243	13.0	19.0	13.0	1.0
McNuggets, 6 Pieces, McDonald's*	6 Pieces/105g	250	14.0	238	13.0	19.0	13.0	1.0
McNuggets, 9 Pieces, McDonald's*	9 Pieces/157g	375	20.0	239	13.0	19.0	13.0	1.0
Selects, 3 Pieces, McDonald's*	3 Pieces/130g	365	20.0	280	16.0	20.0	15.0	1.0
Selects, 5 Pieces, McDonald's*	5 Pieces/219g	612	33.0	280	16.0	20.0	15.0	1.0
COFFEE								
Black, Large, McDonald's*	1 Serving/428ml	0	0.0	0	0.0	0.0	0.0	0.0
Cappuccino, Large, McDonald's*	1 Serving/307ml	120	3.0	39	3.0	4.0	1.0	0.0
Cappuccino, Regular, McDonald's*	1 Serving/231ml	90	2.0	39	3.0	4.0	1.0	0.0
Latte, Large, McDonald's*	1 Serving/451ml	185	5.0	41	3.0	4.0	1.0	0.0
Latte, Regular, McDonald's*	1 Serving/337ml	135	3.0	40	3.0	4.0	1.0	0.0
White, Large, McDonald's*	1 Serving/428ml	30	0.0	7	0.0	1.0	0.0	0.0
White, Regular, McDonald's*	1 Serving/313ml	25	0.0	8	1.0	1.0	0.0	0.0
COLA								
Coca-Cola, Diet, McDonald's*	1 Med/405ml	4	0.0	1	0.0	0.0	0.0	0.0
Coca-Cola, McDonald's*	1 Med/405ml	170	0.0	42	0.0	10.0	0.0	0.0
Coke, Zero, McDonald's*	1 Small/200ml	2	0.0	1	0.0	0.0	0.0	0.0
CREAMER								
Uht, McDonald's*	1 Cup/14ml	17	1.0	123	4.2	4.2	10.0	0.0
CROUTONS								
McDonald's*	1 Sachet/14g	60	2.0	426	11.8	63.4	14.0	2.7
DIP								
BBQ, McDonald's*	1 Pot/50g	83	0.0	166	0.0	37.0	0.0	0.0
Caramelised Onion, McDonald's*	1 Dip/31g	45	2.0	144	3.0	19.0	6.0	3.0
Sour Cream & Chive, McDonald's*	1 Pot/50g	150	16.0	300	2.0	2.0	32.0	4.0
Sweet Chilli, McDonald's*	1 Pot/31g	80	1.0	256	0.0	58.0	3.0	0.0
DOUGHNUTS								
Chocolate Donut, McDonald's*	1 Donut/79g	345	16.0	437	5.7	43.8	20.5	1.0
Chocolate Donut, McMini, McDonald's*	1 Donut/17g	64	3.0	375	6.8	46.9	17.8	1.6
Cinnamon Donut, McDonald's*	1 Donut/72g	302	18.0	419	5.1	43.1	25.1	3.8
Sugared Donut, McDonald's*	1 Donut/49g	205	15.0	418	6.0	35.0	30.0	4.0
DRESSING								
Balsamic, Low Fat, McDonald's*	1 Sachet/33g	20	1.0	60	0.0	9.0	3.0	0.0
Caesar, Low Fat, McDonald's*	1 Sachet/80g	55	2.0	68	2.0	10.0	2.0	0.0

MCDONALD'S

	Measure INFO/WEIGHT	per Measure KCAL	FAT	Nutrition Values per 100g / 100ml KCAL	PROT	CARB	FAT	FIBRE
DRESSING								
French, Low Fat, McDonald's*	1 Serving/22g	13	1.0	58	0.5	7.1	2.6	1.0
FANTA								
Orange, McDonald's*	1 Super/750ml	315	0.0	42	0.0	10.0	0.0	0.0
FISH FINGERS								
McDonald's*	3 Fingers/84g	195	9.0	232	15.0	19.0	11.0	1.0
FRIES								
French, Large, McDonald's*	1 Serving/160g	460	22.0	288	3.0	38.0	14.0	4.0
French, Medium, McDonald's*	1 Serving/114g	330	16.0	289	3.0	37.0	14.0	4.0
French, Small, McDonald's*	1 Serving/80g	230	11.0	288	2.0	38.0	14.0	4.0
FRUIT								
Bag, McDonald's*	1 Pack/80g	40	1.0	50	0.0	12.0	1.0	2.0
FRUIT SHOOT								
Robinsons, McDonald's*	1 Bottle/200ml	10	0.0	5	0.0	1.0	0.0	0.0
HASH BROWNS								
McDonald's*	1 Hash Brown/54g	130	7.0	241	2.0	26.0	13.0	2.0
HOT CHOCOLATE								
McDonald's*	1 Serving/330ml	164	4.0	50	0.7	8.8	1.1	0.0
HOT DOG								
& Ketchup, McDonald's*	1 Serving/116g	296	15.0	255	9.6	25.8	12.6	1.3
ICE CREAM								
Smartie, McDonald's*	1 Pot/120g	260	10.0	216	3.4	33.3	7.9	1.0
ICE CREAM CONE								
McDonald's*	1 Cone/90g	141	5.0	156	4.5	24.4	5.0	0.0
with Flake, McDonald's*	1 Cone/107g	204	8.0	191	4.8	27.0	7.2	0.0
JAM								
Strawberry, McDonald's*	1 Pack/20g	50	0.0	250	0.0	60.0	0.0	0.0
JUICE								
Tropicana, McDonald's*	1 Bottle/250ml	107	0.0	43	1.0	9.0	0.0	0.4
KETCHUP								
Tomato, McDonald's*	1 Portion/23g	25	0.0	109	0.0	26.0	0.0	0.0
LEMONADE								
Sprite, Z, McDonald's*	1 Lge/500ml	5	0.0	1	0.0	0.0	0.0	0.0
MARGARINE								
Flora, Original, McDonald's*	1 Portion/10g	55	6.0	550	0.0	0.0	60.0	0.0
MCFLURRY								
After Eight, McDonald's*	1 McFlurry/204g	381	11.0	187	2.8	31.4	5.4	0.5
Cadbury, Shortcake, Limited Edition, McDonald's*	1 McFlurry/205g	385	14.0	187	3.0	28.0	7.0	1.0
Chocolate, Cornetto, McDonald's*	1 Serving/207g	400	17.0	193	3.0	29.0	8.0	1.0
Creme Egg, Cadbury's, McDonald's*	1 McFlurry/203g	381	13.0	188	2.9	29.8	6.3	0.5
Crunchie, McDonald's*	1 McFlurry/185g	330	11.0	178	3.0	28.0	6.0	1.0
Dairy Milk, McDonald's*	1 McFlurry/184g	340	13.0	184	3.0	28.0	7.0	1.0
Dairy Milk, with Caramel, McDonald's*	1 McFlurry/206g	385	13.0	187	2.9	29.1	6.3	0.0
Jammie Dodger, McDonald's*	1 McFlurry/128g	256	8.0	200	3.9	33.6	6.4	0.3
Rolo, McDonald's*	1 McFlurry/205g	390	13.0	190	4.0	29.2	6.5	0.1
Strawberry, Cornetto, McDonald's*	1 McFlurry/207g	375	12.0	181	3.0	29.0	6.0	0.0
Toffee Swirl, Oreo Cookie, McDonald's*	1 McFlurry/206ml	400	12.0	194	3.0	31.0	6.0	1.0
Yorkie, McDonald's*	1 McFlurry/204g	379	15.0	186	3.4	27.0	7.3	0.8
MCMUFFIN								
Bacon & Egg, Double, McDonald's*	1 McMuffin/161g	395	21.0	244	15.0	16.0	13.0	1.0
Bacon & Egg, McDonald's*	1 McMuffin/143g	340	17.0	237	14.0	18.0	12.0	1.0
Sausage & Egg, Double, McDonald's*	1 McMuffin/222g	560	36.0	252	16.0	12.0	16.0	1.0
Sausage & Egg, McDonald's*	1 McMuffin/174g	420	24.0	242	14.0	16.0	14.0	1.0

MCDONALD'S

	Measure INFO/WEIGHT	per Measure KCAL	FAT	Nutrition Values per 100g / 100ml KCAL	PROT	CARB	FAT	FIBRE
MCMUFFIN								
Scrambled Egg, McDonald's*	1 McMuffin/147g	294	14.0	200	10.9	17.5	9.6	1.3
MELT								
Toasted Ham & Cheese, McDonald's*	1 Serving/100g	239	8.0	239	11.2	30.6	8.0	1.8
MILK								
Fresh, Portion, McDonald's*	1 Portion/14ml	10	0.0	69	0.0	7.0	0.0	0.0
Organic, McDonald's*	1 Bottle/250ml	117	5.0	47	4.0	5.0	2.0	0.0
MILKSHAKE								
Banana, Large, McDonald's*	1 Serving/432ml	545	13.0	126	3.0	21.0	3.0	0.0
Banana, Medium, McDonald's*	1 Serving/338ml	425	10.0	126	3.0	21.0	3.0	0.0
Banana, Small, McDonald's*	1 Serving/178ml	226	5.0	127	3.0	21.0	3.0	0.0
Cadbury Dairy Milk, Caramel Flavour, Small, McDonald's*	1 Serving/177ml	220	5.0	124	3.0	20.0	3.0	1.0
Cadburys Dairy Milk, Caramel, Large, McDonald's*	1 Serving/417ml	505	17.0	121	3.0	19.0	4.0	1.0
Cadburys Dairy Milk, Caramel, Medium, McDonald's*	1 Serving/394ml	480	16.0	122	3.0	19.0	4.0	1.0
Chocolate, Large, McDonald's*	1 Serving/431ml	530	13.0	123	3.0	20.0	3.0	0.0
Chocolate, Small, McDonald's*	1 Serving/177ml	225	5.0	127	3.0	21.0	3.0	0.0
Strawberry, Large, McDonald's*	1 Serving/432ml	540	13.0	125	3.0	21.0	3.0	0.0
Strawberry, Medium, McDonald's*	1 Serving/336ml	420	10.0	125	3.0	21.0	3.0	0.0
Strawberry, Small, McDonald's*	1 Serving/177ml	220	5.0	124	3.0	21.0	3.0	0.0
Vanilla, Large, McDonald's*	1 Serving/431ml	535	13.0	124	3.0	21.0	3.0	0.0
MOZZARELLA								
Dippers, McDonald's*	3 Dippers/85g	265	14.0	312	13.0	27.0	16.0	1.0
MUFFIN								
Blueberry, Low Fat, McDonald's*	1 Muffin/126g	300	4.0	238	5.0	50.0	3.0	2.0
Double Chocolate, McDonald's*	1 Muffin/123g	515	28.0	419	6.0	46.0	23.0	2.0
ONION RINGS								
McDonald's*	1 Serving/99g	245	12.0	247	4.0	31.0	12.0	3.0
PANCAKE								
& Sausage, with Syrup, McDonald's*	1 Portion/223g	615	20.0	275	8.0	42.0	9.0	2.0
& Syrup, McDonald's*	1 Pack/175g	515	14.0	294	4.0	52.0	8.0	2.0
PIE								
Apple, McDonald's*	1 Pie/80g	231	13.0	289	2.0	35.0	16.0	0.0
POTATO WEDGES								
McDonald's*	1 Portion/177g	349	18.0	197	3.3	23.3	10.0	2.8
QUORN*								
Burger, Premiere, McDonald's*	1 Burger/210g	311	6.0	148	9.1	24.2	2.9	2.7
ROLL								
Bacon, McBacon, McDonald's*	1 Roll/122g	349	14.0	286	13.5	30.5	11.5	1.7
Bacon, with Brown Sauce, McDonald's*	1 Roll/126g	350	9.0	278	15.0	37.0	7.0	2.0
Bacon, with Tomato Ketchup, McDonald's*	1 Roll/126g	345	9.0	273	15.0	36.0	7.0	2.0
SALAD								
Chicken, No Bacon, Grilled, McDonald's*	1 Salad/255g	115	3.0	45	7.0	2.0	1.0	1.0
Chicken, with Bacon, Grilled, McDonald's*	1 Salad/266g	164	5.0	62	9.0	2.0	2.0	1.0
Crispy Chicken, No Bacon, McDonald's*	1 Salad/281g	270	11.0	96	8.0	6.0	4.0	1.0
Crispy Chicken, with Bacon, McDonald's*	1 Serving/292g	326	15.0	111	10.0	7.0	5.0	1.0
Garden, Side, No Dressing, McDonald's*	1 Salad/91g	10	0.0	11	1.0	2.0	0.0	1.0
Garden, Side, with Balsamic Dressing, McDonald's*	1 Salad/128g	91	4.0	71	1.0	11.0	3.0	1.0
SANDWICH								
Deli, Chicken & Bacon, McDonald's*	1 Sandwich/192g	405	13.0	211	10.0	27.0	7.0	2.0
Deli, Chicken, Salad, McDonald's*	1 Sandwich/216g	350	9.0	162	7.0	24.0	4.0	2.0
Deli, Chicken, Sweet Chilli, McDonald's*	1 Sandwich/250g	570	22.0	228	12.0	28.0	9.0	2.0
Deli, Spicy Veggie, McDonald's*	1 Sandwich/216g	555	22.0	257	6.0	36.0	10.0	4.0

	Measure INFO/WEIGHT	per Measure KCAL	FAT	Nutrition Values per 100g / 100ml KCAL	PROT	CARB	FAT	FIBRE
MCDONALD'S								
SAUCE								
Barbeque, McDonald's*	1 Portion/50g	85	1.0	170	0.0	38.0	2.0	0.0
Curry, Sweet, McDonald's*	1 Portion/29g	50	1.0	171	0.0	38.0	3.0	3.0
Mustard, Mild, McDonald's*	1 Portion/30g	64	4.0	212	1.0	24.8	12.1	0.0
Sweet & Sour, McDonald's*	1 Portion/29g	50	0.0	172	0.0	38.0	0.0	0.0
SUNDAE								
Hot Caramel, McDonald's*	1 Sundae/189g	357	8.0	189	3.8	33.9	4.4	0.0
Hot Fudge, McDonald's*	1 Sundae/187g	352	11.0	188	4.5	30.0	5.7	0.0
No Topping, McDonald's*	1 Sundae/149g	219	8.0	147	4.2	21.6	5.1	0.0
Strawberry, McDonald's*	1 Sundae/214g	360	9.0	168	2.0	33.0	4.0	0.0
Toffee, McDonald's*	1 Sundae/182g	350	9.0	192	3.0	34.0	5.0	1.0
SYRUP								
Pancake, McDonald's*	1 Pot/55g	190	0.0	345	0.0	84.0	0.0	0.0
TEA								
with Milk, McDonald's*	1 Serving/333ml	10	3.0	3	0.0	1.0	1.0	0.0
WRAP								
Chicken Fajita, McDonald's*	1 Wrap/259g	647	31.0	250	8.9	26.7	12.0	1.2
Chicken, Cajun, McDonald's*	1 Wrap/222g	585	33.0	263	9.0	22.0	15.0	2.0
Chicken, Grilled, Salad, McDonald's*	1 Wrap/221g	335	11.0	152	7.2	19.9	5.0	1.8
Chicken, Snack, McDonald's*	1 Wrap/112g	266	11.0	237	10.0	29.0	10.0	2.0
Garlic & Herb, Snack, McDonald's*	1 Serving/121g	335	18.0	276	12.0	25.0	15.0	2.0
Oriental, Snack, McDonald's*	1 Wrap/127g	265	10.0	209	10.0	25.0	8.0	2.0
PIZZA HUT								
BACON BITS								
Pizza Hut*	1 Serving/12g	60	4.0	496	8.3	48.7	29.8	0.0
BEETROOT								
Pizza Hut*	1 Portion/25g	14	0.0	55	0.9	12.0	0.1	0.0
BISCUIT								
Cafe Curls, Dessert, Pizza Hut*	1 Biscuit/9g	38	1.0	422	5.8	80.3	8.6	0.0
BREAD								
Ciabatta, Garlic, Pizza Hut*	2 Pieces/253g	820	32.0	324	9.1	43.4	12.7	0.0
Garlic, Dipsters, Pizza Hut*	1 Piece/90g	308	14.0	342	6.8	43.1	15.8	0.0
Garlic, Pizza Hut*	1 Slice/30g	95	5.0	318	6.8	38.1	15.4	0.0
Garlic, with Cheese, Pizza Hut*	4 Pieces/187g	569	34.0	304	16.0	19.1	18.2	0.0
BREADSTICKS								
Garlic, Pizza Hut*	1 Stick/50g	173	7.0	347	9.8	46.9	13.4	1.0
BRUSCHETTA								
Light Lunch, Pizza Hut*	3 Pieces/211g	369	16.0	175	4.1	22.4	7.6	0.0
CAKE								
Chocolate Fudge, Dessert, Pizza Hut*	1 Piece/178g	684	32.0	384	4.2	51.4	17.9	0.0
CARBONARA								
Ham, Buffet, Pizza Hut*	1 Portion/200g	180	5.0	90	3.4	14.4	2.3	0.0
CHEESE								
4 & Vegetable, Buffet, Pizza Hut*	1 Portion/200g	210	9.0	105	4.0	12.6	4.3	0.0
Hard, Grated, Pizza Hut*	1 Serving/30g	121	9.0	404	33.0	0.1	30.0	0.0
CHEESECAKE								
Chocolate, Pizza Hut*	1 Serving/63g	228	11.0	360	5.6	44.9	17.5	0.0
Clotted Cream, Pizza Hut*	1 Serving/63.5g	205	10.0	323	4.6	39.3	16.4	0.0
Lemon & Ginger, Pizza Hut*	1 Serving/63.5g	205	10.0	323	4.2	42.4	15.2	0.0
New York Style, Baked, Pizza Hut*	1 Slice/113g	442	16.0	391	6.6	62.3	14.3	0.0
Vanilla, Madagascan, Dessert, Pizza Hut*	1 Serving/133g	397	18.0	298	4.8	39.2	13.6	0.0
CHICKEN								
Cheesy Jalapeno Poppers, Pizza Hut*	6 Pieces/150g	408	20.0	272	5.2	32.8	13.3	0.0

PIZZA HUT

	Measure INFO/WEIGHT	per Measure KCAL	per Measure FAT	Nutrition Values per 100g / 100ml KCAL	PROT	CARB	FAT	FIBRE
CHICKEN								
Dippin, Pizza Hut*	1 Serving/155g	332	14.0	214	15.7	17.1	9.3	0.0
Goujons, Pizza Hut*	5 Pieces/169g	311	14.0	184	17.0	11.0	8.0	1.5
Strips, Breaded, Pizza Hut*	5 Pieces/200g	368	16.0	184	17.0	11.0	8.0	0.0
Strips, Hot n Kicking, Pizza Hut*	7 Pieces/140g	276	13.0	197	17.0	12.0	9.0	0.0
Wings, BBQ, (Delivery Only), Pizza Hut*	6 Pieces/184g	412	25.0	224	21.0	4.5	13.5	0.0
Wings, BBQ, Pizza Hut*	6 Pieces/184g	427	16.0	232	31.5	6.9	8.6	0.0
Wings, BBQ, Saucy, Pizza Hut*	6 Wings/159g	355	22.0	223	21.4	3.6	13.7	0.0
Wings, Buffalo, Saucy, Pizza Hut*	6 Wings/181g	380	22.0	209	21.0	3.7	12.2	0.0
Wings, Spicy, Crunch, (Delivery Only), Pizza Hut*	1 Portion/218g	510	31.0	234	17.0	10.0	14.0	0.0
Wings, with Sour Cream & Chive Dip, Pizza Hut*	1 Pack/178g	680	56.0	382	22.8	1.9	31.5	1.3
CHICKEN STRIPS								
Breaded, with Wedges, 3, Kids, Pizza Hut*	1 Serving/265g	451	14.0	170	8.1	22.2	5.4	0.0
Breaded, with Wedges, 2, Kids, Pizza Hut*	1 Serving/231g	386	12.0	167	6.7	23.9	5.0	0.0
Breaded, Wrap Factory, 2, Kids, Pizza Hut*	1 Serving/247g	434	12.0	176	8.3	24.8	4.9	0.0
Breaded, Wrap Factory, 3, Kids, Pizza Hut*	1 Serving/325g	617	18.0	190	9.2	25.9	5.5	0.0
COLESLAW								
Pizza Hut*	1 Pot/38g	54	5.0	143	0.9	7.1	12.3	0.0
Pot, Pizza Hut*	1 Serving/200g	268	22.0	134	0.8	7.4	11.2	0.0
CREAM								
Pizza Hut*	1 Serving/45.5g	153	16.0	336	2.1	3.2	35.0	0.0
Single, Dessert, Pizza Hut*	1 Serving/40g	75	7.0	188	2.6	3.9	18.0	0.0
UHT, Dessert, Pizza Hut*	1 Serving/12.5g	46	4.0	367	2.3	3.4	28.4	0.0
UHT, Portion, Pizza Hut*	1 Portion/12g	23	2.0	188	2.7	3.9	18.0	0.0
CROUTONS								
Pizza Flavoured, Pizza Hut*	1 Serving/12g	23	3.0	196	10.1	55.2	26.1	0.0
Salad, Large, Pizza Hut*	1 Portion/20g	94	4.0	470	11.0	59.1	21.1	0.0
DESSERT								
Cherries in Sauce, Pizza Hut*	1 Serving/20g	28	0.0	142	0.5	34.9	0.1	0.0
Chocolate Obsession, Pizza Hut*	1 Serving/100g	157	7.0	157	2.0	22.1	6.8	0.0
Cookie Dough, Pizza Hut*	1 Serving/145g	650	30.0	448	5.9	59.4	20.7	0.0
Toffee Apple Meltdown, Pizza Hut*	1 Serving/120g	325	11.0	271	3.3	43.7	9.2	0.0
Vanilla Ice Cream Pots, Pizza Hut*	1 Serving/55g	110	6.0	200	2.8	19.9	11.6	0.0
DIP								
BBQ Sauce, Pizza Hut*	1 Serving/28g	34	0.0	123	1.3	29.3	0.1	0.0
BBQ Tabasco, Pizza Hut*	1 Serving/25g	36	0.0	142	1.2	33.6	0.2	0.0
BBQ, Tabasco, (Delivery Only), Pizza Hut*	1 Serving/25g	35	0.0	142	1.2	33.6	0.2	0.0
Garlic & Herb, Pizza Hut*	1 Serving/28g	93	9.0	331	1.4	7.6	32.6	0.0
Sour Cream & Chive, Pizza Hut*	1 Serving/28g	82	1.0	294	0.9	4.1	4.0	0.0
Sweet Chilli Sauce, Pizza Hut*	1 Serving/28g	48	0.0	172	0.3	32.9	0.8	0.0
Tomato Ketchup, Pizza Hut*	1 Serving/28g	39	0.0	141	1.4	34.1	0.1	0.0
DRESSING								
1000 Island, Pizza Hut*	1 Serving/38g	107	10.0	280	0.7	11.5	25.5	0.0
Blue Cheese, Pizza Hut*	1 Serving/35g	91	8.0	258	1.7	11.5	22.7	0.0
Caesar, Pizza Hut*	1 Serving/40g	27	1.0	68	1.5	8.9	2.8	0.0
Ranch, Pizza Hut*	1 Serving/32g	163	18.0	510	1.2	1.5	56.4	0.0
Vinaigrette, Low Fat, Pizza Hut*	1 Serving/30ml	23	0.0	77	0.3	17.2	0.5	0.0
FRIES								
Seasoned, Savoury, (Express Only), Pizza Hut*	1 Portion/145g	247	11.0	171	2.3	23.0	7.7	0.0
FRUIT								
Frozen, Dessert, Pizza Hut*	1 Serving/20g	7	0.0	34	1.0	12.1	0.3	0.0
FUDGE BROWNIE								
Pizza Hut*	1 Serving/105g	418	16.0	398	4.3	60.1	15.6	0.0

PIZZA HUT

	Measure INFO/WEIGHT	per Measure KCAL	per Measure FAT	Nutrition Values per 100g / 100ml KCAL	PROT	CARB	FAT	FIBRE
ICE CREAM								
Coco Mango, Pizza Hut*	1 Serving/100g	88	2.0	88	0.6	17.3	1.8	0.0
Cookie Craving, Pizza Hut*	1 Serving/100g	149	7.0	149	1.6	20.1	6.9	0.0
Dairy, Dessert, Pizza Hut*	1 Portion/142g	272	13.0	192	4.6	23.3	8.9	0.2
Mix, Pizza Hut*	1 Serving/100g	147	6.0	147	4.0	18.8	6.2	0.0
Traditional, Dessert, Pizza Hut*	1 Serving/130g	251	14.0	193	2.6	22.4	10.4	0.0
Traditional, Kids, Pizza Hut*	1 Serving/89g	171	9.0	193	2.6	22.4	10.4	0.0
Traditional, Pizza Hut*	1 Serving/132g	254	14.0	193	2.6	22.4	10.4	0.0
Vanilla, Pots, Ice Cream Factory, (Delivered), Pizza Hut*	1 Portion/55g	110	6.0	200	2.8	19.9	11.6	0.0
KETCHUP								
Heinz, Pizza Hut*	1 Serving/12g	14	0.0	119	0.5	28.4	0.1	0.0
Tomato, Sachet, Heinz, (express Only), Pizza Hut*	1 Sachet/12g	14	0.0	119	0.0	28.4	0.1	0.0
MACARONI CHEESE								
Pizza Hut*	1 Serving/41g	57	2.0	140	4.9	16.6	6.0	
MARSHMALLOWS								
Mini, Ice Cream Factory, Pizza Hut*	1 Serving/30g	96	0.0	320	5.4	74.3	0.0	0.0
MAYONNAISE								
Heinz, Pizza Hut*	1 Serving/12g	88	10.0	731	1.3	1.8	81.2	0.0
MEATBALLS								
in Pomodoro Sauce, Light Lunch, Pizza Hut*	1 Portion/253g	342	18.0	135	6.6	11.0	7.2	0.0
MILK								
Half Fat, Portions, Millac Maid, Pizza Hut*	1 Portion/14g	6	0.0	45	6.0	5.1	1.6	0.0
MILKSHAKE								
Strawberry Cheesecake, Pizza Hut*	1 Serving/236g	371	14.0	157	3.4	22.3	5.9	0.0
The Chocoholic, Pizza Hut*	1 Serving/248g	442	20.0	178	3.6	22.8	8.2	0.0
Toffee Banoffee Shake, Pizza Hut*	1 Serving/404g	763	23.0	189	2.4	32.3	5.6	0.0
MUFFIN								
Cheesecake, Sicilian Lemon, Pizza Hut*	1 Portion/130g	508	24.0	391	5.1	50.9	18.6	0.0
Double Choc Chip, Pizza Hut*	1 Muffin/108g	442	23.0	409	6.4	48.7	21.0	0.0
Fruity, Pizza Hut*	1 Serving/115g	366	14.0	318	4.1	48.4	11.9	0.0
Mixed Berry, Pizza Hut*	1 Muffin/108g	402	23.0	372	4.4	41.6	20.9	0.0
Triple Choc Chip, Pizza Hut*	1 Serving/130g	497	22.0	382	5.0	52.5	16.9	0.0
Triple Choc, Pizza Hut*	1 Portion/130g	497	29.0	382	5.0	52.5	22.0	0.0
MUSHROOMS								
Breaded, Pizza Hut*	6 Mushrooms/180g	410	14.0	228	4.5	26.1	8.0	0.0
Garlic, Crispy Coated, Pizza Hut*	1 Portion/135g	240	10.0	178	4.1	23.4	7.5	0.0
Garlic, Pizza Hut*	1 Serving/230g	570	43.0	248	7.9	6.9	18.9	0.0
Garlic, with BBQ Dip, Pizza Hut*	1 Portion/112g	263	11.0	234	6.2	30.5	10.0	3.4
Garlic, with Sour Cream & Chive Dip, Pizza Hut*	1 Portion/112g	426	35.0	380	6.4	20.0	30.8	3.4
NACHOS								
Chilli, Pizza Hut*	1 Serving/190g	550	33.0	289	8.8	27.2	17.4	0.0
Pizza Hut*	1 Serving/222g	669	40.0	301	7.7	30.2	18.1	0.0
OLIVES								
Mixed, Pizza Hut*	1 Serving/70g	140	9.0	200	1.5	19.6	12.8	0.0
ONION								
Chilli, Rings, (Delivery Only), Pizza Hut*	1 Ring/12.5g	26	1.0	212	3.2	28.2	9.6	0.0
ONION RINGS								
Chilli, Pizza Hut*	8 Rings/100g	212	10.0	212	3.2	28.2	9.6	0.0
ONIONS								
White, Pizza Hut*	1 Serving/24g	10	0.0	42	1.0	10.0	0.0	0.0
PANCAKE								
Fruity, Kids, Pizza Hut*	1 Serving/155.5g	227	3.0	146	1.9	30.6	2.1	0.0

	INFO/WEIGHT	KCAL	FAT	KCAL	PROT	CARB	FAT	FIBRE
PIZZA HUT								
PASTA								
3 Cheese & Vegetable, Pizza Hut*	1 Serving/300g	315	13.0	105	4.0	12.6	4.3	0.0
4 Cheese, Sharing, Pizza Hut*	1 Serving/1200g	1860	102.0	155	6.1	13.5	8.5	0.0
Alfredo, Chicken, Sharing, (Delivery Only), Pizza Hut*	1 Pack/1200g	1680	41.0	140	8.1	19.1	3.4	0.0
Alfredo, Light Lunch, Pizza Hut*	1 Portion/226g	294	5.0	130	4.1	23.3	2.2	0.0
Alfredo, Pizza Hut*	1 Serving/400g	520	9.0	130	4.1	23.3	2.2	0.0
Arrabiata, Light Lunch, Pizza Hut*	1 Portion/226g	221	7.0	98	2.9	15.0	2.9	0.0
Arrabiata, Pizza Hut*	1 Serving/450g	441	13.0	98	2.9	15.0	2.9	0.0
Bolognese, Sharing, Pizza Hut*	1 Serving/1200g	1500	65.0	125	7.2	11.9	5.4	0.0
Cannelloni, Spinach & Ricotta, Pizza Hut*	1 Serving/404g	565	27.0	140	6.2	13.1	6.8	0.0
Ham & Mushroom, Pizza Hut*	1 Serving/450g	473	10.0	105	4.2	17.0	2.3	0.0
Lasagne, Traditional, Pizza Hut*	1 Serving/461g	589	27.0	128	5.9	13.0	5.8	0.0
Macaroni Cheese, Kids, Pizza Hut*	1 Serving/251g	333	16.0	133	4.0	14.8	6.5	0.0
Mezzaluna, Tomato & Mozzarella, Pizza Hut*	1 Serving/350.5g	340	10.0	97	3.1	14.7	2.9	0.0
Spaghetti Bolognese, Kids, New, Pizza Hut*	1 Serving/234g	211	4.0	90	7.6	14.6	1.5	0.0
Spaghetti Bolognese, Pizza Hut*	1 Portion/475g	745	31.0	157	6.2	17.8	6.6	0.0
Tagliatelle, Alla Carbonara, Pizza Hut*	1 Serving/400g	548	32.0	137	5.6	10.4	8.1	0.0
Tagliatelle, Meatball, Italian Recipe, Pizza Hut*	1 Portion/240g	324	11.0	135	6.9	16.6	4.4	0.0
Tomato & Pepperoni, Pizza Hut*	1 Serving/300g	312	8.0	104	3.6	16.3	2.7	0.0
PASTA BAKE								
Salmon, Pizza Hut*	1 Portion/400g	692	43.0	173	7.9	11.3	10.7	0.0
PASTA SALAD								
Sweetcorn & Pepper, Pizza Hut*	1 Serving/47g	75	3.0	159	4.6	23.1	5.3	0.0
Tomato & Basil, Pizza Hut*	1 Serving/50g	50	1.0	100	3.7	17.8	1.5	0.0
PENNE								
Mediterranean Vegetable, Pizza Hut*	1 Portion/448g	592	20.0	132	3.7	18.3	4.4	0.0
PEPPERS								
Red & Green Wedges, Pizza Hut*	1 Serving/40g	6	0.0	15	0.8	2.6	0.3	0.0
PIE								
Banoffee, Dessert, Pizza Hut*	1 Serving/125g	428	25.0	340	2.5	37.3	20.1	0.0
Banoffee, Pizza Hut*	1 Serving/100g	350	21.0	350	4.2	34.9	21.5	0.0
PIZZA								
BBQ Deluxe, Cheesy Bites, Pizza Hut*	1 Slice/143g	358	12.0	251	11.7	34.4	8.1	0.0
BBQ Deluxe, Italian, Individual, Pizza Hut*	1 Serving/78g	185	6.0	238	10.9	34.3	7.9	0.0
BBQ Deluxe, Italian, Large, Pizza Hut*	1 Slice/95g	239	8.0	252	14.3	29.7	8.4	0.0
BBQ Deluxe, Italian, Medium, Pizza Hut*	1 Slice/105g	253	8.0	241	12.0	31.1	7.6	0.0
BBQ Deluxe, Pan, Individual, Pizza Hut*	1 Serving/79g	200	8.0	253	12.7	28.0	10.0	0.0
BBQ Deluxe, Pan, Large, Pizza Hut*	1 Serving/122g	306	12.0	251	11.8	28.6	9.9	0.0
BBQ Deluxe, Pan, Medium, Pizza Hut*	1 Serving/107g	276	11.0	257	11.7	28.8	10.5	0.0
BBQ Deluxe, Stuffed Crust, Pizza Hut*	1 Slice/155g	337	10.0	217	11.6	31.9	6.7	0.0
Cajun Chicken, Hot One, Italian, Medium, Pizza Hut*	1 Slice/100g	250	9.0	250	12.5	29.1	9.3	0.0
Cajun Chicken, Hot One, Pan, Large, Pizza Hut*	1 Slice/125g	321	15.0	257	12.9	24.7	11.8	0.0
Cajun Chicken, Hot One, Pan, Medium, Pizza Hut*	1 Slice/105g	273	12.0	259	12.7	25.6	11.7	0.0
Cajun Chicken, Hot One, Stuffed Crust, Pizza Hut*	1 Slice/135g	331	11.0	245	13.3	30.0	8.0	0.0
Cheese Feast, Italian, Medium, Pizza Hut*	1 Slice/96g	260	11.0	272	12.3	29.1	11.8	0.0
Cheese Feast, Stuffed Crust, Pizza Hut*	1 Slice/132g	361	14.0	273	14.3	30.5	10.4	0.0
Chicken Feast, Pan, Medium, Pizza Hut*	1 Slice/109g	283	12.0	259	15.5	24.6	11.0	0.0
Chicken Feast, Stuffed Crust, Pizza Hut*	1 Slice/133g	337	13.0	254	14.8	27.3	9.5	0.0
Chicken Supreme, Cheesy Bites, Delivery, Pizza Hut*	1 Serving/113g	247	8.0	218	11.8	29.5	6.8	0.0
Chicken Supreme, Cheesy Bites, Pizza Hut*	1 Slice/148g	322	10.0	218	11.8	29.5	6.8	0.0
Chicken Supreme, Italian, Individual, Pizza Hut*	1 Serving/74g	169	4.0	229	10.7	35.4	5.9	0.0
Chicken Supreme, Italian, Large, Delivery, Pizza Hut*	1 Serving/74g	158	5.0	213	11.1	30.7	6.6	0.0
Chicken Supreme, Italian, Large, Pizza Hut*	1 Slice/111g	217	6.0	196	9.8	29.3	5.8	0.0

PIZZA HUT

PIZZA

	Measure INFO/WEIGHT	per Measure KCAL	FAT	Nutrition Values per 100g / 100ml KCAL	PROT	CARB	FAT	FIBRE
Chicken Supreme, Italian, Medium, Delivery, Pizza Hut*	1 Serving/65.5g	133	4.0	203	10.9	28.3	6.5	0.0
Chicken Supreme, Italian, Medium, Pizza Hut*	1 Slice/102g	220	6.0	215	10.3	31.9	6.2	0.0
Chicken Supreme, Pan, Individual, Pizza Hut*	1 Serving/80.5g	186	8.0	231	11.6	26.9	9.9	0.0
Chicken Supreme, Pan, Large Pizza Hut*	1 Serving/124g	271	12.0	219	10.9	26.1	9.4	0.0
Chicken Supreme, Pan, Large, Delivery, Pizza Hut*	1 Serving/99g	216	9.0	219	10.9	26.1	9.4	0.0
Chicken Supreme, Pan, Medium, Delivery, Pizza Hut*	1 Serving/86g	189	7.0	219	11.2	26.6	8.6	0.0
Chicken Supreme, Pan, Medium, Pizza Hut*	1 Serving/115g	251	10.0	219	11.2	26.6	8.6	0.0
Chicken Supreme, Stuffed Crust, Delivery, Pizza Hut*	1 Serving/122g	293	9.0	240	11.6	34.8	7.2	0.0
Chicken Supreme, Stuffed Crust, Pizza Hut*	1 Slice/153g	367	11.0	240	11.6	34.8	7.2	0.0
Chicken, Hi Light, Medium, Pizza Hut*	1 Slice/83g	189	6.0	230	13.2	29.2	6.7	0.0
Country Feast, Italian, Medium, Pizza Hut*	1 Slice/109g	252	10.0	232	9.7	28.6	8.8	0.0
Country Feast, Pan, Medium, Pizza Hut*	1 Slice/115g	279	12.0	243	11.4	25.8	10.5	0.0
Country Feast, Stuffed Crust, Pizza Hut*	1 Slice/144g	326	11.0	227	11.5	28.4	7.5	0.0
Express, Chicken Supreme, Pizza Hut*	1 Serving/65g	143	6.0	221	10.1	28.1	9.0	0.0
Express, Hawaiian, Pizza Hut*	1 Serving/60g	147	6.0	245	10.5	29.9	10.6	0.0
Express, Supreme, Pizza Hut*	1 Serving/68g	165	8.0	242	10.7	27.8	11.2	0.0
Farmhouse, Cheesy Bites, Delivery, Pizza Hut*	1 Serving/106g	266	10.0	250	13.2	30.7	9.5	0.0
Farmhouse, Cheesy Bites, Pizza Hut*	1 Slice/133g	332	13.0	250	13.2	30.7	9.5	0.0
Farmhouse, Hi Light, Medium, Pizza Hut*	1 Slice/82g	184	5.0	225	12.1	29.1	6.7	0.0
Farmhouse, Italian, Individual, Pizza Hut*	1 Serving/74g	188	6.0	253	11.8	33.1	8.1	0.0
Farmhouse, Italian, Large, Delivery, Pizza Hut*	1 Serving/62g	141	5.0	225	11.5	32.1	7.7	0.0
Farmhouse, Italian, Large, Pizza Hut*	1 Slice/92g	206	7.0	224	10.2	34.0	7.3	0.0
Farmhouse, Italian, Medium, Delivery, Pizza Hut*	1 Serving/56g	126	4.0	226	10.7	33.0	7.1	0.0
Farmhouse, Italian, Medium, Pizza Hut*	1 Slice/84g	192	5.0	229	10.2	35.7	6.4	0.0
Farmhouse, Pan, Individual, Pizza Hut*	1 Serving/70g	180	7.0	256	11.3	31.6	10.6	0.0
Farmhouse, Pan, Large, Delivery, Pizza Hut*	1 Serving/85g	206	9.0	242	11.4	29.7	10.4	0.0
Farmhouse, Pan, Large, Pizza Hut*	1 Serving/106g	257	11.0	242	11.4	29.7	10.4	0.0
Farmhouse, Pan, Medium, Delivery, Pizza Hut*	1 Serving/75g	182	8.0	242	11.3	28.6	10.4	0.0
Farmhouse, Pan, Medium, Pizza Hut*	1 Serving/100g	242	10.0	242	11.3	28.6	10.4	0.0
Farmhouse, Stuffed Crust, Delivery, Pizza Hut*	1 Serving/106g	235	8.0	222	11.8	30.0	7.6	0.0
Farmhouse, Stuffed Crust, Pizza Hut*	1 Slice/132g	387	10.0	293	11.8	30.0	7.6	0.0
Happy Hour, Chicken & Mushroom, Pizza Hut*	1 Serving/80g	165	5.0	207	9.6	27.6	6.8	0.0
Happy Hour, Ham & Sweetcorn, Pizza Hut*	1 Serving/86g	174	6.0	202	9.4	27.0	6.5	0.0
Happy Hour, Margherita, Pizza Hut*	1 Serving/78g	183	7.0	234	10.5	28.6	8.8	0.0
Happy Hour, Pepper & Tomato, Pizza Hut*	1 Serving/86g	163	5.0	189	8.0	26.1	6.3	0.0
Happy Hour, Pepperoni & Onion, Pizza Hut*	1 Serving/80g	179	7.0	224	9.4	28.2	8.6	0.0
Hawaiian, Cheesy Bites, Delivery, Pizza Hut*	1 Serving/109g	253	9.0	232	11.6	31.2	7.8	0.0
Hawaiian, Cheesy Bites, Pizza Hut*	1 Slice/136g	316	11.0	232	11.6	31.2	7.8	0.0
Hawaiian, Italian, Individual, Pizza Hut*	1 Serving/71g	164	4.0	229	9.8	37.9	5.8	0.0
Hawaiian, Italian, Large, Delivery, Pizza Hut*	1 Serving/68g	148	5.0	217	10.6	31.1	7.3	0.0
Hawaiian, Italian, Large, Pizza Hut*	1 Slice/99g	221	7.0	223	10.0	33.2	7.1	0.0
Hawaiian, Italian, Medium, Delivery, Pizza Hut*	1 Serving/60g	131	4.0	219	10.0	33.8	6.5	0.0
Hawaiian, Italian, Medium, Pizza Hut*	1 Slice/92g	201	6.0	219	9.8	33.3	6.1	0.0
Hawaiian, Pan, Individual, Pizza Hut*	1 Serving/73g	175	6.0	240	10.9	32.2	8.9	0.0
Hawaiian, Pan, Large, Delivery, Pizza Hut*	1 Serving/89g	234	10.0	262	10.6	32.6	11.4	0.0
Hawaiian, Pan, Large, Pizza Hut*	1 Serving/112g	293	13.0	262	10.6	32.6	11.4	0.0
Hawaiian, Pan, Medium, Delivery, Pizza Hut*	1 Serving/82g	184	7.0	224	10.1	28.5	8.9	0.0
Hawaiian, Pan, Medium, Pizza Hut*	1 Serving/109g	245	10.0	224	10.1	28.5	8.9	0.0
Hawaiian, Stuffed Crust, Delivery, Pizza Hut*	1 Serving/113g	245	8.0	217	11.0	30.7	7.3	0.0
Hawaiian, Stuffed Crust, Pizza Hut*	1 Slice/141g	306	10.0	217	11.0	30.7	7.3	0.0
Hot 'n' Spicy, Cheesy Bites, Pizza Hut*	1 Slice/127g	331	13.0	261	12.6	33.7	9.9	0.0
Hot 'n' Spicy, Italian, Individual, Pizza Hut*	1 Slice/66g	180	7.0	272	11.0	36.5	10.4	0.0

PIZZA HUT

PIZZA

INFO/WEIGHT	Measure	KCAL	FAT	KCAL	PROT	CARB	FAT	FIBRE
Hot 'n' Spicy, Italian, Large, Pizza Hut*	1 Slice/93g	236	9.0	254	11.2	32.7	10.1	0.0
Hot 'n' Spicy, Italian, Medium, Pizza Hut*	1 Slice/86g	222	8.0	259	11.0	34.5	9.8	0.0
Hot 'n' Spicy, Pan, Individual, Pizza Hut*	1 Slice/71g	183	8.0	259	10.9	30.4	11.2	0.0
Hot 'n' Spicy, Pan, Large, Pizza Hut*	1 Slice/105g	266	11.0	254	12.0	30.2	10.9	0.0
Hot 'n' Spicy, Pan, Medium, Pizza Hut*	1 Slice/93g	237	11.0	254	11.5	29.2	11.4	0.0
Hot 'n' Spicy, Stuffed Crust, Pizza Hut*	1 Slice/139g	329	11.0	236	11.8	33.1	7.9	0.0
Margherita, Cheesy Bites, Delivery, Pizza Hut*	1 Serving/103g	270	10.0	263	12.8	33.1	10.1	0.0
Margherita, Cheesy Bites, Pizza Hut*	1 Serving/128g	337	13.0	263	12.8	33.1	10.1	0.0
Margherita, Fingers, Kids, Pizza Hut*	1 Serving/94.5g	258	12.0	273	11.0	28.4	12.8	0.0
Margherita, Italian, Individual, Pizza Hut*	1 Slice/67g	177	5.0	264	11.9	39.2	8.0	0.0
Margherita, Italian, Large, Delivery, Pizza Hut*	1 Serving/61g	154	6.0	251	12.2	31.8	9.5	0.0
Margherita, Italian, Large, Pizza Hut*	1 Slice/91g	229	9.0	252	10.4	34.2	9.5	0.0
Margherita, Italian, Medium, Delivery, Pizza Hut*	1 Serving/54g	138	5.0	257	10.6	35.6	9.4	0.0
Margherita, Italian, Medium, Pizza Hut*	1 Slice/80g	205	7.0	256	11.0	35.7	8.8	0.0
Margherita, Pan, Individual, Pizza Hut*	1 Serving/70.5g	189	8.0	268	11.6	32.4	11.5	0.0
Margherita, Pan, Large, Delivery, Pizza Hut*	1 Serving/84g	219	10.0	261	11.6	29.8	11.9	0.0
Margherita, Pan, Large, Pizza Hut*	1 Serving/105g	273	12.0	261	11.6	29.8	11.9	0.0
Margherita, Pan, Medium, Delivery, Pizza Hut*	1 Serving/72.5g	192	9.0	265	11.6	30.6	11.8	0.0
Margherita, Pan, Medium, Pizza Hut*	1 Serving/97g	256	11.0	265	11.6	30.6	11.8	0.0
Margherita, Stuffed Crust, Delivery, Pizza Hut*	1 Serving/103g	255	9.0	248	14.0	31.6	8.8	0.0
Margherita, Stuffed Crust, Pizza Hut*	1 Serving/128g	318	11.0	248	14.0	31.6	8.8	0.0
Margherita, Thick, Kids, Pizza Hut*	1 Serving/202g	506	18.0	251	9.0	33.0	8.9	0.0
Meat Feast, Cheesy Bites, Delivery, Pizza Hut*	1 Serving/114g	310	13.0	272	13.9	30.3	11.4	0.0
Meat Feast, Cheesy Bites, Pizza Hut*	1 Slice/142g	387	16.0	272	13.9	30.3	11.4	0.0
Meat Feast, Italian, Individual, Pizza Hut*	1 Serving/81.5g	220	9.0	270	13.9	32.3	10.8	0.0
Meat Feast, Italian, Large, Delivery, Pizza Hut*	1 Serving/74.5g	187	8.0	251	12.5	29.6	10.7	0.0
Meat Feast, Italian, Large, Pizza Hut*	1 Slice/111g	279	13.0	251	12.9	27.3	11.4	0.0
Meat Feast, Italian, Medium, Delivery, Pizza Hut*	1 Serving/66g	169	7.0	257	12.0	29.8	11.2	0.0
Meat Feast, Italian, Medium, Pizza Hut*	1 Slice/100g	257	11.0	258	13.0	30.0	11.0	0.0
Meat Feast, Pan, Individual, Pizza Hut*	1 Serving/84g	220	10.0	262	13.3	27.6	11.8	0.0
Meat Feast, Pan, Large, Delivery, Pizza Hut*	1 Serving/100g	275	13.0	277	12.6	29.1	13.2	0.0
Meat Feast, Pan, Large, Pizza Hut*	1 Serving/124g	344	16.0	277	12.6	29.1	13.2	0.0
Meat Feast, Pan, Medium, Delivery, Pizza Hut*	1 Serving/84g	221	10.0	262	12.2	28.0	12.4	0.0
Meat Feast, Pan, Medium, Pizza Hut*	1 Serving/112g	294	14.0	262	12.2	28.0	12.4	0.0
Meat Feast, Stuffed Crust, Delivery, Pizza Hut*	1 Serving/122g	301	13.0	247	13.5	28.0	10.4	0.0
Meat Feast, Stuffed Crust, Pizza Hut*	1 Slice/152g	376	16.0	247	13.5	28.0	10.4	0.0
Meaty BBQ, Cheesy Bites, Delivery, Pizza Hut*	1 Serving/115g	282	11.0	245	11.3	31.1	9.4	0.0
Meaty BBQ, Italian, Large, Delivery, Pizza Hut*	1 Serving/81g	176	6.0	217	11.1	29.4	7.4	0.0
Meaty BBQ, Italian, Medium, Delivery, Pizza Hut*	1 Serving/70g	154	5.0	220	10.9	30.0	7.2	0.0
Meaty BBQ, Pan, Large, Delivery, Pizza Hut*	1 Serving/111g	313	9.0	282	10.7	26.4	8.3	0.0
Meaty BBQ, Pan, Medium, Delivery, Pizza Hut*	1 Serving/92g	215	9.0	234	11.1	25.9	9.5	0.0
Meaty BBQ, Stuffed Crust, Delivery, Pizza Hut*	1 Serving/122g	259	9.0	213	12.0	28.3	7.4	0.0
Meaty, The Edge, Medium, Pizza Hut*	1 Slice/36g	110	6.0	308	17.0	20.4	16.1	0.0
Mediterranean Meat Deluxe, Cheesy Bites, Pizza Hut*	1 Slice/201g	547	22.0	272	13.5	33.0	10.7	0.0
Mediterranean Meat Deluxe, Italian, Individual, Pizza Hut*	1 Slice/72g	206	9.0	288	12.6	34.7	12.3	0.0
Mediterranean Meat Deluxe, Italian, Large, Pizza Hut*	1 Slice/95g	267	11.0	280	12.4	33.0	12.0	0.0
Mediterranean Meat Deluxe, Italian, Medium, Pizza Hut*	1 Slice/91g	245	9.0	270	12.8	33.5	10.4	0.0
Mediterranean Meat Deluxe, Pan, Individual, Pizza Hut*	1 Slice/75g	212	10.0	284	13.5	29.5	13.9	0.0
Mediterranean Meat Deluxe, Pan, Large, Pizza Hut*	1 Slice/108g	285	13.0	262	11.6	29.2	11.9	0.0
Mediterranean Meat Deluxe, Pan, Medium, Pizza Hut*	1 Slice/98g	245	11.0	249	11.7	28.1	11.4	0.0
Mediterranean Meat Deluxe, Stuffed Crust, Pizza Hut*	1 Slice/143g	382	16.0	268	13.4	31.9	11.1	0.0
Mountain Fantastico, Cheesy Bites, Pizza Hut*	1 Slice/140.5g	340	11.0	242	10.9	33.5	8.0	0.0

	Measure INFO/WEIGHT	per Measure		Nutrition Values per 100g / 100ml				
		KCAL	FAT	KCAL	PROT	CARB	FAT	FIBRE
PIZZA HUT								
PIZZA								
Mountain Fantastico, Italian, Individual, Pizza Hut*	1 Slice/75g	183	6.0	245	9.3	36.4	8.5	0.0
Mountain Fantastico, Italian, Large, Pizza Hut*	1 Slice/94g	222	9.0	235	10.0	32.6	9.0	0.0
Mountain Fantastico, Italian, Medium, Pizza Hut*	1 Slice/102g	247	9.0	242	9.6	33.1	9.1	0.0
Mountain Fantastico, Pan, Individual, Pizza Hut*	1 Slice/74g	181	7.0	244	10.7	31.4	9.9	0.0
Mountain Fantastico, Pan, Large, Pizza Hut*	1 Slice/113g	295	14.0	261	10.6	29.1	12.5	0.0
Mountain Fantastico, Pan, Medium, Pizza Hut*	1 Slice/106g	273	14.0	258	9.6	28.9	12.8	0.0
Mountain Fantastico, Stuffed Crust, Pizza Hut*	1 Slice/151g	327	11.0	217	10.5	30.8	7.5	0.0
Pepperoni Feast, Cheesy Bites, Delivery, Pizza Hut*	1 Serving/108g	306	13.0	284	15.8	29.6	12.4	0.0
Pepperoni Feast, Cheesy Bites, Pizza Hut*	1 Serving/134.5g	382	17.0	284	15.8	29.6	12.4	0.0
Pepperoni Feast, Italian, Individual, Pizza Hut*	1 Serving/73g	205	8.0	282	11.4	36.3	11.6	0.0
Pepperoni Feast, Italian, Large, Delivery, Pizza Hut*	1 Serving/68g	195	10.0	286	12.0	30.8	14.0	0.0
Pepperoni Feast, Italian, Large, Pizza Hut*	1 Slice/103g	286	13.0	278	12.2	30.9	12.9	0.0
Pepperoni Feast, Italian, Medium, Delivery, Pizza Hut*	1 Serving/63g	171	8.0	270	12.4	30.6	11.9	0.0
Pepperoni Feast, Italian, Medium, Pizza Hut*	1 Slice/93g	254	10.0	273	12.3	35.0	10.5	0.0
Pepperoni Feast, Pan, Individual, Pizza Hut*	1 Serving/79g	227	11.0	286	12.3	30.3	13.6	0.0
Pepperoni Feast, Pan, Large, Delivery, Pizza Hut*	1 Serving/92g	278	16.0	302	12.0	26.4	17.6	0.0
Pepperoni Feast, Pan, Large, Pizza Hut*	1 Serving/115g	347	20.0	302	12.0	26.4	17.6	0.0
Pepperoni Feast, Pan, Medium, Delivery, Pizza Hut*	1 Serving/80g	223	12.0	279	12.6	26.2	14.9	0.0
Pepperoni Feast, Pan, Medium, Pizza Hut*	1 Serving/106.5g	297	16.0	279	12.6	26.2	14.9	0.0
Pepperoni Feast, Stuffed Crust, Delivery, Pizza Hut*	1 Serving/115g	300	13.0	261	13.1	30.4	11.3	0.0
Pepperoni Feast, Stuffed Crust, Pizza Hut*	1 Slice/143g	375	16.0	261	13.1	30.4	11.3	0.0
Seafood Fantastico, Italian, Individual, Pizza Hut*	1 Slice/81g	173	5.0	213	15.3	25.1	5.7	0.0
Seafood Fantastico, Italian, Large, Pizza Hut*	1 Slice/106g	228	7.0	215	15.1	24.6	6.2	0.0
Seafood Lovers, Cheesy Bites, Pizza Hut*	1 Serving/128g	328	12.0	257	11.6	33.7	9.1	0.0
Seafood Lovers, Italian, Individual, Pizza Hut*	1 Serving/66g	170	5.0	258	9.8	38.4	8.2	0.0
Seafood Lovers, Italian, Large, Pizza Hut*	1 Slice/90g	215	7.0	239	10.2	35.3	7.6	0.0
Seafood Lovers, Italian, Medium, Pizza Hut*	1 Slice/82g	202	7.0	245	10.1	35.3	8.0	0.0
Seafood Lovers, Pan, Individual, Pizza Hut*	1 Serving/69g	160	6.0	232	10.7	31.3	8.7	0.0
Seafood Lovers, Pan, Large, Pizza Hut*	1 Serving/106g	260	12.0	245	10.4	28.2	11.3	0.0
Seafood Lovers, Pan, Medium, Pizza Hut*	1 Serving/98g	233	10.0	237	9.7	28.3	10.6	0.0
Seafood Lovers, Stuffed Crust, Pizza Hut*	1 Slice/131g	314	11.0	239	12.3	31.8	8.3	0.0
Spicy, Hot One, Pan, Medium, Pizza Hut*	1 Slice/115g	274	13.0	239	11.2	23.1	11.3	0.0
Spicy, Hot One, Stuffed Crust, Pizza Hut*	1 Slice/141g	352	14.0	249	13.0	27.6	9.6	0.0
Stuffed Crust, Cheesy Bites, Delivery, Pizza Hut*	1 Serving/129.5g	312	13.0	241	11.9	29.0	9.8	0.0
Stuffed Crust, Italian, Large, Delivery, Pizza Hut*	1 Serving/85g	198	9.0	234	11.7	26.9	10.2	0.0
Stuffed Crust, Italian, Medium, Delivery, Pizza Hut*	1 Serving/76g	170	8.0	225	11.0	25.3	10.3	0.0
Stuffed Crust, Pan, Large, Delivery, Pizza Hut*	1 Serving/120g	289	15.0	241	10.9	25.0	12.1	0.0
Stuffed Crust, Pan, Medium, Delivery, Pizza Hut*	1 Serving/100g	234	12.0	234	11.6	22.9	12.0	0.0
Super Supreme, Cheesy Bites, Pizza Hut*	1 Serving/162g	393	16.0	242	12.4	26.9	10.0	0.0
Super Supreme, Italian, Individual, Pizza Hut*	1 Serving/97g	260	11.0	267	13.9	27.3	11.3	0.0
Super Supreme, Italian, Large, Pizza Hut*	1 Slice/128g	281	13.0	219	10.6	24.4	10.3	0.0
Super Supreme, Italian, Medium, Pizza Hut*	1 Slice/119g	267	12.0	225	11.1	26.3	9.7	0.0
Super Supreme, Pan, Individual, Pizza Hut*	1 Serving/96g	228	11.0	237	11.9	24.8	11.3	0.0
Super Supreme, Pan, Large, Pizza Hut*	1 Serving/148g	346	18.0	234	11.4	22.5	12.0	0.0
Super Supreme, Pan, Medium, Pizza Hut*	1 Serving/127g	323	18.0	255	11.4	22.8	14.6	0.0
Super Supreme, Stuffed Crust, Pizza Hut*	1 Serving/165g	366	16.0	222	11.9	25.2	10.0	0.0
Supreme, Cheesy Bites, Delivery, Pizza Hut*	1 Serving/118g	296	12.0	251	12.6	29.9	9.8	0.0
Supreme, Cheesy Bites, Pizza Hut*	1 Slice/147g	369	14.0	251	12.6	29.9	9.8	0.0
Supreme, Italian, Individual, Pizza Hut*	1 Serving/81g	204	7.0	251	10.9	33.5	9.2	0.0
Supreme, Italian, Large, Delivery, Pizza Hut*	1 Serving/74g	178	8.0	240	11.4	28.7	10.3	0.0
Supreme, Italian, Large, Pizza Hut*	1 Slice/113g	264	11.0	233	9.7	29.6	9.7	0.0
Supreme, Italian, Medium, Delivery, Pizza Hut*	1 Serving/69g	155	6.0	224	10.0	28.8	9.1	0.0

PIZZA HUT

PIZZA

Supreme, Italian, Medium, Pizza Hut*	1 Slice/110g	286	12.0	261	12.2	28.9	10.7	0.0
Supreme, Pan, Individual, Pizza Hut*	1 Serving/84g	209	10.0	248	11.0	28.0	11.4	0.0
Supreme, Pan, Large, Delivery, Pizza Hut*	1 Serving/106g	242	12.0	228	10.4	24.0	11.6	0.0
Supreme, Pan, Large, Pizza Hut*	1 Serving/132.5g	302	15.0	228	10.4	24.0	11.6	0.0
Supreme, Pan, Medium, Delivery, Pizza Hut*	1 Serving/90g	232	12.0	259	10.5	27.0	13.1	0.0
Supreme, Pan, Medium, Pizza Hut*	1 Serving/120g	310	16.0	259	10.5	27.0	13.1	0.0
Supreme, Stuffed Crust, Delivery, Pizza Hut*	1 Serving/128g	297	11.0	232	11.9	29.7	8.6	0.0
Supreme, Stuffed Crust, Pizza Hut*	1 Slice/160g	371	14.0	232	11.9	29.7	8.6	0.0
The Sizzler, Cajun Chicken, Cheesy Bites, Pizza Hut*	1 Serving/114g	265	9.0	232	11.4	33.1	7.7	0.0
The Sizzler, Cajun Chicken, Italian, Large, Pizza Hut*	1 Serving/83g	177	6.0	213	11.2	28.1	7.4	0.0
The Sizzler, Cajun Chicken, Italian, Medium, Pizza Hut*	1 Serving/67g	147	5.0	220	11.8	30.2	7.2	0.0
The Sizzler, Cajun Chicken, Pan, Large, Pizza Hut*	1 Serving/90g	215	8.0	238	10.8	27.2	8.8	0.0
The Sizzler, Cajun Chicken, Pan, Medium, Pizza Hut*	1 Serving/75g	166	7.0	221	10.3	27.3	9.3	0.0
The Sizzler, Cajun Chicken, Stuffed Crust, Pizza Hut*	1 Serving/114g	270	10.0	236	11.7	31.7	8.6	0.0
The Sizzler, Spicy Beef, Cheesy Bites, Pizza Hut*	1 Serving/112g	266	10.0	238	12.1	30.4	9.2	0.0
The Sizzler, Spicy Beef, Italian, Large, Pizza Hut*	1 Serving/80g	179	6.0	223	9.6	33.1	7.4	0.0
The Sizzler, Spicy Beef, Italian, Medium, Pizza Hut*	1 Serving/68g	163	6.0	240	10.9	31.6	9.0	0.0
The Sizzler, Spicy Beef, Pan, Large, Pizza Hut*	1 Serving/96g	240	11.0	250	10.5	29.1	11.5	0.0
The Sizzler, Spicy Beef, Pan, Medium, Pizza Hut*	1 Serving/76g	173	8.0	228	10.3	32.0	10.1	0.0
The Sizzler, Spicy Beef, Stuffed Crust, Pizza Hut*	1 Serving/117.5g	275	9.0	234	11.1	32.5	8.0	0.0
The Sizzler, Spicy Mushroom, Cheesy Bites, Pizza Hut*	1 Serving/112g	257	9.0	229	10.4	32.0	7.9	0.0
The Sizzler, Spicy Mushroom, Italian, Large, Pizza Hut*	1 Serving/79g	165	6.0	209	9.3	31.2	7.0	0.0
The Sizzler, Spicy Mushroom, Italian, Medium, Pizza Hut*	1 Serving/65.5g	146	5.0	223	10.5	30.1	8.2	0.0
The Sizzler, Spicy Mushroom, Pan, Large, Pizza Hut*	1 Serving/92g	207	9.0	225	9.1	28.9	9.7	0.0
The Sizzler, Spicy Mushroom, Pan, Medium, Pizza Hut*	1 Serving/78g	174	7.0	224	9.3	27.9	9.6	0.0
The Sizzler, Spicy Mushroom, Stuffed Crust, Pizza Hut*	1 Serving/116g	244	8.0	210	9.7	31.7	6.8	0.0
The Works, The Edge, Medium, Pizza Hut*	1 Slice/64g	150	7.0	235	12.7	19.5	10.4	0.0
Tortilla, Thin, Kids, Pizza Hut*	1 Serving/108g	264	14.0	245	9.1	20.9	13.4	0.0
Tuscani Caprina, Pizza Hut*	1 Pizza/474g	990	45.0	209	9.0	20.6	9.6	0.0
Tuscani, Chicken & Mushroom, Pizza Hut*	1 Serving/491g	1032	55.0	210	10.5	16.9	11.2	0.0
Tuscani, Mediterranean Meats, Pizza Hut*	1 Serving/379g	1065	57.0	281	13.6	21.8	15.0	0.0
Tuscani, Rocket & Proscuitto, Pizza Hut*	1 Serving/434g	829	37.0	191	9.2	19.2	8.5	0.0
Tuscani, Verde, Pizza Hut*	1 Serving/460g	878	42.0	191	8.0	18.6	9.2	0.0
Vegetable Supreme, Cheesy Bites, Delivery, Pizza Hut*	1 Serving/116g	250	8.0	215	10.0	30.7	6.9	0.0
Vegetable Supreme, Cheesy Bites, Pizza Hut*	1 Serving/145g	312	10.0	215	10.0	30.7	6.9	0.0
Vegetable Supreme, Italian, Individual, Pizza Hut*	1 Serving/77g	160	5.0	207	8.7	32.4	6.1	0.0
Vegetable Supreme, Italian, Large, Delivery, Pizza Hut*	1 Serving/74g	143	5.0	193	8.4	27.9	6.5	0.0
Vegetable Supreme, Italian, Large, Pizza Hut*	1 Slice/111g	222	6.0	200	7.4	32.5	5.7	0.0
Vegetable Supreme, Italian, Medium, Delivery, Pizza Hut*	1 Serving/66g	129	4.0	196	7.8	30.6	5.9	0.0
Vegetable Supreme, Italian, Medium, Pizza Hut*	1 Slice/99g	196	6.0	198	8.3	30.7	6.1	0.0
Vegetable Supreme, Pan, Individual, Pizza Hut*	1 Serving/84g	180	8.0	214	8.6	27.7	9.0	0.0
Vegetable Supreme, Pan, Large, Delivery, Pizza Hut*	1 Serving/101g	206	9.0	204	8.1	25.7	9.2	0.0
Vegetable Supreme, Pan, Large, Pizza Hut*	1 Serving/126.5g	258	12.0	204	8.1	25.7	9.2	0.0
Vegetable Supreme, Pan, Medium, Delivery, Pizza Hut*	1 Serving/82g	197	8.0	241	9.9	30.0	10.3	0.0
Vegetable Supreme, Pan, Medium, Pizza Hut*	1 Serving/109g	263	11.0	241	9.9	30.0	10.3	0.0
Vegetable Supreme, Stuffed Crust, Delivery, Pizza Hut*	1 Serving/125g	246	9.0	197	9.3	27.8	6.9	0.0
Vegetable Supreme, Stuffed Crust, Pizza Hut*	1 Serving/156g	308	11.0	197	9.3	27.8	6.9	0.0
Vegetarian Hot One, Cheesy Bites, Pizza Hut*	1 Slice/142g	302	10.0	212	9.8	30.3	7.1	0.0
Vegetarian Hot One, Italian, Individual, Pizza Hut*	1 Serving/77g	164	5.0	211	8.1	34.6	5.8	0.0
Vegetarian Hot One, Italian, Large, Pizza Hut*	1 Slice/114g	165	7.0	145	7.5	19.1	5.9	0.0
Vegetarian Hot One, Italian, Medium, Pizza Hut*	1 Slice/98g	188	5.0	192	9.3	29.5	5.5	0.0
Vegetarian Hot One, Pan, Individual, Pizza Hut*	1 Serving/82.5g	174	6.0	211	8.8	29.6	7.3	0.0

PIZZA HUT

	Measure INFO/WEIGHT	per Measure KCAL	FAT	Nutrition Values per 100g / 100ml KCAL	PROT	CARB	FAT	FIBRE
PIZZA								
Vegetarian Hot One, Pan, Large, Pizza Hut*	1 Serving/125.5g	290	12.0	231	9.4	29.7	9.6	0.0
Vegetarian Hot One, Pan, Medium, Pizza Hut*	1 Serving/115g	234	10.0	204	8.4	26.6	8.6	0.0
Vegetarian Hot One, Stuffed Crust, Pizza Hut*	1 Serving/160g	334	11.0	208	10.1	30.2	6.9	0.0
Vegetarian, Hi Light, Medium, Pizza Hut*	1 Slice/77g	170	5.0	221	10.3	30.0	6.6	0.0
Veggie, The Edge, Medium, Pizza Hut*	1 Slice/60g	136	5.0	227	11.2	22.2	9.0	0.0
POTATO SKINS								
Jacket, Loaded, with Cheese, Pizza Hut*	1 Portion/267g	571	34.0	214	13.6	11.2	12.8	0.0
Jacket, Pizza Hut*	1 Portion/ 223.5g	571	37.0	255	3.4	23.0	16.6	2.1
Jacket, with Sour Cream & Chive Dip, Pizza Hut*	1 Portion/224g	311	24.0	139	1.4	9.3	10.8	0.8
POTATO WEDGES								
Pizza Hut*	1 Serving/260g	380	16.0	146	2.5	20.3	6.1	0.0
POTATOES								
Savoury Seasoned Fries, Pizza Hut*	1 Serving/144g	238	12.0	165	2.4	20.8	8.0	0.0
PROFITEROLES								
Dessert, Pizza Hut*	1 Serving/100g	381	31.0	381	4.6	20.1	31.3	0.0
PUDDING								
Sticky Toffee, Pizza Hut*	1 Serving/105g	400	18.0	380	5.5	50.6	17.3	0.0
RAISINS								
Chocolate, Ice Cream Factory, Pizza Hut*	1 Serving/30g	121	4.0	405	5.4	63.3	14.2	0.0
SALAD								
4 Leaf Mix, Pizza Hut*	1 Serving/100g	14	0.0	14	0.8	1.7	0.5	0.0
Caesar, Chicken, Light Lunch, Small, Pizza Hut*	1 Portion/172g	263	13.0	153	14.1	7.4	7.4	0.0
Caesar, Classic, Light Lunch, Small, Pizza Hut*	1 Portion/97g	183	12.0	189	7.2	13.0	11.9	0.0
Caesar, Classic, Pizza Hut*	1 Portion/194g	367	23.0	189	7.2	13.0	11.9	0.0
Caesar, Pizza Hut*	1 Salad/195g	344	20.0	177	6.0	14.8	10.4	0.0
Caesar, Prawn, Light Lunch, Small, Pizza Hut*	1 Portion/172g	229	12.0	133	9.6	7.6	7.0	0.0
Chicken & Bacon, Pizza Hut*	1 Serving/323g	514	32.0	159	10.3	6.9	9.9	0.0
Chicken Caesar, Pizza Hut*	1 Serving/174g	296	15.0	170	11.5	11.7	8.5	0.0
Chicken Caesar, with Bacon, Pizza Hut*	1 Serving/374.5g	588	30.0	157	14.4	6.8	7.9	0.0
Dressed, Pasta, Tomato, Med, Pizza Hut*	1 Serving/100g	112	1.0	112	3.5	21.2	1.5	0.0
Dressed, Tabbouleh, Pizza Hut*	1 Serving/100g	189	8.0	189	4.2	24.9	8.1	0.0
Fresh, Apple & Grape, Mix, Pizza Hut*	1 Portion/80g	39	1.0	49	0.4	12.0	1.0	0.0
Fresh, Carrot, Grated, Pizza Hut*	1 Serving/17g	5	0.0	30	0.7	6.0	0.5	0.0
Fresh, Cucumber, Slices, Pizza Hut*	1 Serving/80g	8	0.0	10	0.7	1.5	0.1	0.0
Fresh, Onion, Red, Slices, Pizza Hut*	1 Portion/80g	29	0.0	36	1.2	7.9	0.2	0.0
Fresh, Seasonal, Pizza Hut*	1 Serving/80g	12	0.0	15	0.7	1.8	0.6	0.0
Fresh, Tomatoes, Cherry, Pizza Hut*	1 Serving/80g	15	0.0	19	0.8	3.0	0.4	0.0
Goats Cheese, Pizza Hut*	1 Serving/341g	525	40.0	154	7.5	4.4	11.8	0.0
Leaf Mix, Pizza Hut*	1 Serving/41g	7	0.0	17	2.9	6.3	1.1	0.0
Mozzarella & Tomato, Pizza Hut*	1 Serving/188g	387	31.0	206	12.3	2.4	16.3	0.0
Olive & Feta, Pizza Hut*	1 Portion/406g	345	26.0	85	3.8	3.6	6.4	0.0
Potato, Whole, Pizza Hut*	1 Serving/100g	154	10.0	154	1.6	13.5	10.1	0.0
Prawn, Caesar, Pizza Hut*	1 Portion/345g	459	24.0	133	9.6	7.6	7.0	0.0
Tuna, Pizza Hut*	1 Portion/461g	378	9.0	82	10.4	5.9	1.9	2.0
Warm Chicken, Pizza Hut*	1 Salad/342g	403	17.0	118	11.0	6.8	5.1	0.0
SALAD BAR								
Adults Pasta, Pizza Hut*	1 Serving/100g	250	11.0	250	5.7	16.8	10.9	0.0
Apple & Grape Mix, Fresh, Pizza Hut*	1 Serving/80g	39	0.0	49	0.4	12.0	0.1	0.0
Baby Potatoes, Pizza Hut*	1 Serving/80g	63	1.0	79	1.2	14.6	1.8	0.0
Beetroot & Carrot, with Balsamic Vinaigrette, Pizza Hut*	1 Serving/80g	24	0.0	30	1.1	5.7	0.3	0.0
Carrot Batons, Fresh, Pizza Hut*	1 Serving/80g	28	0.0	35	0.6	7.9	0.3	0.0
Coleslaw, Pizza Hut*	1 Serving/80g	149	15.0	186	1.1	4.5	18.2	0.0

	Measure INFO/WEIGHT	per Measure KCAL	FAT	Nutrition Values per 100g / 100ml KCAL	PROT	CARB	FAT	FIBRE
PIZZA HUT								
SALAD BAR								
Cos Lettuce, Fresh, Pizza Hut*	1 Serving/80g	10	0.0	13	0.7	1.9	0.3	0.0
Cous Cous, Pizza Hut*	1 Serving/100g	219	9.0	219	5.0	30.0	9.0	0.0
Gemelli Pasta, Pizza Hut*	1 Serving/100g	155	4.0	155	4.3	26.0	4.4	0.0
Kids Pasta, Pizza Hut*	1 Serving/100g	180	9.0	180	6.9	16.5	9.4	0.0
Melon Pieces, Fresh, Pizza Hut*	1 Serving/80g	27	0.0	34	0.8	8.2	0.0	0.0
Potato Salad, Pizza Hut*	1 Serving/80g	123	10.0	154	1.7	10.0	11.9	0.0
Sweetcorn, Fresh, Pizza Hut*	1 Serving/80g	63	1.0	79	1.8	16.8	0.8	0.0
Tomato Pasta, Pizza Hut*	1 Serving/80g	149	7.0	186	3.7	21.8	9.3	0.0
Tomato Slices, Fresh, Pizza Hut*	1 Serving/80g	14	0.0	17	0.7	3.1	0.3	0.0
SAUCE								
Caramel, Ice Cream Factory, Pizza Hut*	1 Serving/25g	77	1.0	307	0.7	67.2	3.9	0.0
Chocolate, Ice Cream Factory, Pizza Hut*	1 Serving/25g	74	1.0	298	2.0	66.8	2.5	0.0
Lemon, Ice Cream Factory, Pizza Hut*	1 Serving/25g	70	0.0	280	0.1	69.0	0.0	0.0
Strawberry, Ice Cream Factory, Pizza Hut*	1 Serving/25g	70	0.0	280	0.0	69.5	0.0	0.0
SMOOTHIE								
BananaBerry Split, Pizza Hut*	1 Serving/171g	258	0.0	151	1.5	33.6	0.2	0.0
Truly Tropical, Pizza Hut*	1 Serving/239g	234	0.0	98	0.6	24.0	0.1	0.0
Very Berry, Pizza Hut*	1 Serving/220g	189	0.0	86	0.6	20.4	0.1	0.0
SUNDAE								
Double Chocolate, Pizza Hut*	1 Sundae/145g	307	16.0	212	3.1	27.0	11.2	0.0
TIRAMISU								
Delivery, Pizza Hut*	1 Serving/75g	223	10.0	297	3.9	39.5	13.7	0.0
Pizza Hut*	1 Serving/83.5g	248	11.0	297	3.9	39.5	13.7	0.0
TOFFEE APPLE								
Meltdown, Ice Cream Factory, (Delivery Only), Pizza Hut*	1 Portion/300g	813	28.0	271	3.3	43.7	9.2	0.0
TOMATO								
Spicy & Red Pepper, Buffet, Pizza Hut*	1 Portion/200g	170	2.0	85	3.1	16.7	0.9	0.0
TOPPINGS								
Caramel Sauce, Pizza Hut*	1 Serving/100g	307	4.0	307	0.7	67.2	3.9	0.0
Chocolate Raisins, Pizza Hut*	1 Serving/100g	405	14.0	405	5.4	63.3	14.2	0.0
Chocolate Sauce, Pizza Hut*	1 Serving/100g	298	2.0	298	2.0	66.8	2.5	0.0
Coated Chocolate Beans, Pizza Hut*	1 Serving/100g	475	18.0	475	5.5	72.2	18.1	0.0
Frozen Fruits, Pizza Hut*	1 Serving/21g	7	0.0	34	1.0	12.1	0.3	0.0
Lemon Sauce, Pizza Hut*	1 Serving/100g	280	0.0	280	0.1	69.0	0.0	0.0
Mini Marshmallows, Pizza Hut*	1 Serving/100g	320	0.0	320	5.4	74.3	0.0	0.0
Strawberry Sauce, Pizza Hut*	1 Serving/100g	280	0.0	280	0.0	69.5	0.0	0.0
UHT Cream, Pizza Hut*	1 Serving/12.5g	46	4.0	367	2.3	3.4	28.4	0.0
TORTIZZA								
Margherita, Pizza Hut*	1 Serving/209g	573	28.0	274	13.7	25.1	13.2	0.0
TUSCANI PLATTER								
Pizza Hut*	1 Serving/461.5g	1223	90.0	265	8.8	13.2	19.4	0.0
PRET A MANGER								
BAGUETTE								
Brie, Tomato, & Whole Leaf Basil, Pret a Manger*	1 Serving/232g	432	18.0	186	7.7	21.1	7.9	1.6
Cheddar & Pickle, Posh, Artisan, Pret a Manger*	1 Slim Pret/148g	390	20.0	264	10.1	25.7	13.2	1.8
Chicken, Sweet Chilli , Pret a Manger*	1 Baguette/210g	390	11.0	186	10.2	23.8	5.4	1.5
Egg Mayo, & Bacon, Breakfast, Pret a Manger*	1 Baguette/138g	333	15.0	242	12.2	24.5	10.6	0.3
Egg Mayo, Roasted Tomato, Breakfast, Pret a Manger*	1 Baguette/147g	327	16.0	222	8.2	22.4	11.2	1.2
Italian Tricolore, Pret a Manger*	1 Baguette/227g	514	26.0	226	8.2	22.2	11.6	2.1
Prosciutto, Artisan, Italian, Pret a Manger*	1 Baguette/288g	636	29.0	221	9.3	23.5	9.9	2.0
Retro Prawn, on Artisan, Pret a Manger*	1 Baguette/249g	492	13.0	198	10.5	27.5	5.1	2.0
Smoked Salmon & Egg Breakfast, Pret a Manger*	1 Baguette/153g	349	16.0	229	10.9	23.0	10.4	2.2

	Measure INFO/WEIGHT	per Measure KCAL	FAT	Nutrition Values per 100g / 100ml KCAL	PROT	CARB	FAT	FIBRE
PRET A MANGER								
BAGUETTE								
Soup Bread, Artisan , Pret a Manger*	1 Roll/80g	175	1.0	219	7.2	45.6	0.7	2.0
Tuna, Pole & Line Caught, Pret a Manger*	1 Baguette/232g	477	23.0	206	9.0	20.4	9.8	1.2
Wiltshire Cured Ham, & Greve, Pret a Manger*	1 Baguette/225g	540	25.0	240	14.0	21.3	11.0	1.5
BARS								
Chocolate, Brownie, Pret a Manger*	1 Serving/65g	289	17.0	445	4.6	47.7	26.2	1.4
Chocolate, Pret a Manger*	1 Serving/105g	555	39.0	529	5.0	44.3	36.8	2.6
Love, Pret a Manger*	1 Serving/72g	324	18.0	450	6.0	49.2	25.4	3.5
Pret, Pret a Manger*	1 Serving/65g	265	16.0	408	6.8	41.4	24.0	6.2
BEANS								
Edamame Bowl, Pret a Manger*	1 Serving/125g	94	4.0	75	6.3	4.9	3.4	0.0
BREAKFAST CEREAL								
Granola, Hot & Cold, Pret a Manger*	1 Serving/226g	579	20.0	256	6.4	38.4	8.8	3.5
Muesli, Bircher, Pret a Manger*	1 Serving/206g	304	10.0	148	6.3	20.2	4.7	1.4
Porridge, Pret a Manger*	1 Serving/300g	242	8.0	81	3.0	9.6	2.8	1.7
Porridge, with Compote, Pret a Manger*	1 Serving/324g	267	8.0	82	2.8	10.8	2.6	1.7
Porridge, with Honey, Pret a Manger*	1 Serving/321g	307	8.0	96	2.8	14.0	2.6	1.6
CAKE								
Apple, Slice, Pret a Manger*	1 Slice/100g	303	15.0	303	3.8	38.8	14.7	1.9
Banana, Slice, Pret a Manger*	1 Slice/103g	345	18.0	335	4.6	39.0	17.8	1.9
Carrot, Indulgent, Pret a Manger*	1 Slice/90g	310	17.0	344	4.3	38.6	19.3	2.8
Carrot, Slice, Pret a Manger*	1 Slice/112g	402	22.0	359	4.0	41.0	19.9	2.3
Chocolate, Slice, Pret a Manger*	1 Slice/88g	354	21.0	402	5.3	41.7	23.7	1.4
Lemon, Slice, Pret a Manger*	1 Slice/100g	330	15.0	330	4.2	44.0	15.1	0.9
CHEESECAKE								
Lemon Pot, Pret a Manger*	1 Serving/120g	390	26.0	325	2.7	29.3	21.6	1.4
COFFEE								
Cappuccino, Pret a Manger*	1 Serving/340ml	106	6.0	31	1.7	2.2	1.7	0.0
Latte, Pret a Manger*	1 Serving/340ml	194	11.0	57	3.1	3.9	3.3	0.0
Mocha, Pret a Manger*	1 Serving/340ml	243	11.0	71	2.8	7.6	3.4	0.0
COOKIES								
Chocolate, Chunk, Pret a Manger*	1 Cookie/90g	319	12.0	354	4.8	52.6	13.6	3.7
Harvest, Pret a Manger*	1 Cookie/90g	344	13.0	382	7.4	49.4	14.6	5.6
CRISPS								
Croxton Manor, & Red Onion, Pret a Manger*	1 Pack/40g	181	10.0	452	6.5	50.5	24.7	7.0
Maldon Sea Salt, Pret a Manger*	1 Pack/40g	184	10.0	460	5.5	51.2	26.0	7.5
Parsnip, Beetroot, & Carrot, Pret a Manger*	1 Pack/25g	120	9.0	480	4.4	38.4	34.4	15.2
Sea Salt, & Organic Cider Vinegar, Pret a Manger*	1 Pack/40g	178	10.0	445	5.2	52.0	24.2	7.0
Spicy Piri Chilli, Pret a Manger*	1 Pack/40g	190	10.0	475	5.2	56.7	25.2	5.2
Sweet Potato, & Chipotle Chilli, Pret a Manger*	1 Pack/25g	123	8.0	492	5.2	44.8	32.8	9.6
CROISSANT								
Almond, Pret a Manger*	1 Croissant/100g	365	21.0	365	8.8	34.9	21.1	1.1
Chocolate, Pret a Manger*	1 Croissant/95g	406	24.0	427	7.9	45.2	25.6	3.6
Egg, & Bacon, Pret a Manger*	1 Croissant/167g	483	20.0	289	11.3	20.6	12.0	1.8
French Butter, Pret a Manger*	1 Croissant/80g	304	16.0	380	8.5	41.7	19.9	2.6
Ham, Bacon, & Cheese, Pret a Manger*	1 Croissant/110g	352	23.0	320	13.2	20.6	20.5	1.5
Mozzarella, & Tomato, Pret a Manger*	1 Croissant/110g	373	25.0	339	13.4	20.2	22.4	1.3
Pain au Raisin, Pret a Manger*	1 Croissant/110g	311	14.0	283	5.1	37.5	12.3	1.6
DRIED FRUIT								
Mango, Pret a Manger*	1 Serving/60g	200	0.0	333	1.5	84.5	0.3	3.7
FRUIT								
Mango, & Lime, Pret a Manger*	1 Pack/135g	70	0.0	52	0.7	12.0	0.2	2.3
Pot, Kids, Pret a Manger*	1 Pack/140g	43	0.0	31	0.5	7.4	0.1	1.0

	INFO/WEIGHT	KCAL	FAT	KCAL	PROT	CARB	FAT	FIBRE
PRET A MANGER								
FRUIT								
Salad, Pret a Manger*	1 Pack/250g	98	0.0	39	0.6	8.8	0.2	1.1
Superfruit Bowl, Pret a Manger*	1 Pack/155g	71	0.0	46	0.8	11.0	0.1	2.0
Tropical Sticks, Pret a Manger*	1 Pack/200g	78	0.0	39	0.6	8.9	0.2	1.4
Very Berry, Breakfast Bowl, Pret a Manger*	1 Pack/219g	368	15.0	168	5.2	20.3	6.9	1.4
Very Berry, Pret Pot, Pret a Manger*	1 Pack/148g	147	5.0	99	6.0	11.6	3.2	0.2
GINGER BEER								
Pure Pret, Pret a Manger*	1 Serving/330ml	152	0.0	46	0.0	11.4	0.0	0.0
GINGERBREAD								
Man, Godfrey, Pret a Manger*	1 Serving/54g	198	8.0	367	4.8	55.7	13.9	1.9
HOT CHOCOLATE								
Hot Chocolate, Pret a Manger*	1 Serving/340ml	309	12.0	91	3.0	11.6	3.6	0.0
JELLY								
Mango, & Pomegranate, Pret a Manger*	1 Serving/135g	112	0.0	83	0.4	20.0	0.0	0.7
JUICE								
Apple, Pret a Manger*	1 Serving/250ml	120	0.0	48	0.1	11.8	0.1	0.0
Carrot, Pret a Manger*	1 Serving/250ml	60	0.0	24	0.5	5.7	0.1	0.0
Orange, Large, Pret a Manger*	1 Serving/520ml	229	0.0	44	0.6	11.0	0.0	0.1
Orange, Pret a Manger*	1 Serving/260ml	114	0.0	44	0.6	11.0	0.0	0.1
JUICE DRINK								
Apple, Pure Pret, Pret a Manger*	1 Serving/330ml	159	0.0	48	0.0	11.6	0.0	0.0
Grape, & Elderflower, Pure Pret, Pret a Manger*	1 Serving/330ml	146	0.0	44	0.0	10.6	0.0	0.0
Orange, Pure Pret, Pret a Manger*	1 Serving/330ml	200	0.0	61	0.1	3.1	0.0	0.0
Yoga Bunny, Pure Pret, Pret a Manger*	1 Serving/330ml	132	0.0	40	0.0	9.7	0.0	0.0
MOUSSE								
Chocolate, Pret a Manger*	1 Serving/100g	506	39.0	506	3.7	23.3	39.0	1.7
MUFFIN								
Double Berry, Pret a Manger*	1 Muffin/140g	521	32.0	372	7.4	35.2	22.6	3.2
High Fibre, Pret a Manger*	1 Muffin/130g	455	23.0	350	7.2	36.0	18.0	7.4
POPCORN								
Chocolate Crackle, Topcorn, Pret a Manger*	1 Serving/55g	220	8.0	400	5.1	59.6	15.3	7.1
Double Cheddar, & Onion, Pret a Manger*	1 Serving/25g	123	6.0	492	8.0	55.6	26.0	9.6
Rock Salt, Topcorn, Pret a Manger*	1 Serving/23g	115	6.0	500	8.3	53.5	26.5	10.4
Sweet & Salt, Topcorn, Pret a Manger*	1 Serving/25g	123	6.0	492	5.6	60.0	24.8	8.8
PRETZELS								
Plain, Sesame, or Poppy, Pret a Manger*	1 Serving/120g	371	8.0	309	10.9	51.6	6.5	2.5
SALAD								
Chef's Italian Chicken, Pret a Manger*	1 Pack/311g	322	23.0	104	6.8	2.7	7.3	1.9
Crayfish, & Avocado, No Bread, Pret a Manger*	1 Pack/206g	182	15.0	88	4.7	1.5	7.3	2.2
Humous, Super, Pret a Manger*	1 Pack/354g	332	19.0	94	4.1	7.1	5.4	1.6
Pesto Pasta, Pret a Manger*	1 Pack/259g	337	15.0	130	5.1	12.4	5.8	2.6
Tuna, Simple, Pret a Manger*	1 Pack/245g	120	3.0	49	7.4	1.7	1.4	0.8
SANDWICH								
Beech Smoked BLT, Pret a Manger*	1 Pack/248g	496	29.0	200	8.5	15.4	11.6	1.6
Cheese & Butter, Kids, Pret a Manger*	1 Pack/132g	418	22.0	317	14.4	27.8	16.6	2.1
Chicken, Avocado, Pret a Manger*	1 Pack/244g	444	23.0	182	8.7	15.8	9.4	2.9
Chicken, Ham, & Swiss, Club, Pret a Manger*	1 Pack/318g	498	21.0	157	11.6	12.9	6.5	1.3
Crayfish, & Rocket, Pret a Manger*	1 Slim Pret/97g	185	9.0	192	8.4	19.6	8.9	1.7
Egg Mayo, Free Range , Pret a Manger*	1 Pack/185g	426	23.0	231	9.1	19.9	12.7	1.6
Egg Salad, Cracking , Pret a Manger*	1 Pack/262g	439	24.0	168	6.6	15.1	9.0	1.5
Egg, Bloomin Marvellous, Bloomer, Pret a Manger*	1 Pack/227g	467	23.0	206	7.4	22.2	10.0	2.5
Emmental Salad, Pret a Manger*	1 Pack/239g	494	28.0	207	8.3	16.9	11.8	1.8
Famous All Day Breakfast, Pret a Manger*	1 Pack/329g	652	38.0	198	9.9	14.1	11.4	1.4

	Measure INFO/WEIGHT	per Measure		Nutrition Values per 100g / 100ml				
		KCAL	FAT	KCAL	PROT	CARB	FAT	FIBRE

PRET A MANGER

SANDWICH

	Measure INFO/WEIGHT	KCAL	FAT	KCAL	PROT	CARB	FAT	FIBRE
Ham & Butter, Kids, Pret a Manger*	1 Pack/127g	289	8.0	228	13.4	28.9	6.5	2.2
Ham, & Eggs, Classic, Bloomer , Pret a Manger*	1 Pack/225g	550	25.0	244	14.1	21.3	11.3	2.0
King Prawn, & Avocado, Pret a Manger*	1 Pack/240g	458	24.0	191	8.7	16.7	10.1	2.8
Mature Cheddar, & Pickle, Pret a Manger*	1 Pack/292g	588	34.0	201	8.8	15.6	11.6	1.5
Mozzarella, Pesto, Bloomer, Pret a Manger*	1 Pack/270g	564	28.0	209	8.7	18.8	10.4	2.0
Salmon, Scottish, Smoked , Pret a Manger*	1 Pack/158g	348	11.0	220	16.5	21.8	7.3	1.7
Simply Ham & Mustard, Pret a Manger*	1 Pack/180g	417	18.0	232	14.9	15.2	9.9	1.6
Sweet Potato Falafel, Pret a Manger*	1 Pack/214g	451	19.0	211	5.5	26.7	9.0	1.9
The New Yorker, Bloomer, Pret a Manger*	1 Pack/223g	513	22.0	230	11.9	25.2	9.9	2.5
Tuna Mayo, Kids, Pret a Manger*	1 Pack/150g	372	17.0	248	10.9	24.9	11.5	1.9
Tuna, & Rocket, Pole & Line, Bloomer, Pret a Manger*	1 Baguette/232g	484	23.0	209	9.1	20.7	9.9	1.2
Tuna, & Rocket, Pole & Line, Bloomer, Pret a Manger*	1 Pack/237g	523	26.0	221	10.4	20.6	11.1	2.1

SHORTBREAD

	Measure INFO/WEIGHT	KCAL	FAT	KCAL	PROT	CARB	FAT	FIBRE
Millionaire's, Pret a Manger*	1 Pack/70g	330	20.0	471	2.3	51.0	28.9	1.0

SMOOTHIE

	Measure INFO/WEIGHT	KCAL	FAT	KCAL	PROT	CARB	FAT	FIBRE
Mango, Pret a Manger*	1 Serving/250ml	143	0.0	57	0.6	13.7	0.2	1.2
Strawberry, Pret a Manger*	1 Serving/250ml	128	1.0	51	0.9	11.2	0.3	0.0
Vitamin Volcano, Pret a Manger*	1 Serving/250ml	135	1.0	54	4.6	12.4	0.3	2.3

SOUP

	Measure INFO/WEIGHT	KCAL	FAT	KCAL	PROT	CARB	FAT	FIBRE
Carrot, & Coriander, Pret a Manger*	1 Serving/370g	219	10.0	59	2.5	5.8	2.7	0.7
Celeriac Mash, Pret a Manger*	1 Serving/370g	148	10.0	40	0.9	2.4	2.7	1.0
Chicken, & Mushroom, Pret a Manger*	1 Serving/370g	229	12.0	62	3.6	4.4	3.3	0.7
Chicken, Malaysian, Pret a Manger*	1 Serving/370g	243	12.0	66	2.5	7.3	3.3	0.9
Chicken, Moroccan , Pret a Manger*	1 Serving/370g	205	8.0	55	3.8	5.6	2.2	1.7
Chilli Beef, & Rice, Pret a Manger*	1 Serving/370g	270	9.0	73	5.4	7.3	2.5	2.8
Italian Meatball, Pret a Manger*	1 Serving/370g	361	16.0	98	2.4	5.8	4.2	1.0
Leek, & Potato, Pret a Manger*	1 Serving/370g	204	11.0	55	1.3	5.7	3.0	1.0
Lentil, & Bacon, Pret a Manger*	1 Serving/370g	272	12.0	74	5.9	6.3	3.1	1.2
Mushroom Risotto, Pret a Manger*	1 Serving/347g	202	9.0	58	1.5	7.0	2.7	1.2
Sag-Aloo, Pret a Manger*	1 Serving/375g	248	12.0	66	1.6	8.0	3.1	0.2
Tomato, Pret Classic, Pret a Manger*	1 Serving/370g	225	14.0	61	1.5	4.6	3.8	1.2

SUSHI

	Measure INFO/WEIGHT	KCAL	FAT	KCAL	PROT	CARB	FAT	FIBRE
Deluxe, Pret a Manger*	1 Serving/250g	380	7.0	152	5.5	25.2	2.7	4.0
Maki, & Nigiri, Pret a Manger*	1 Serving/200g	314	8.0	157	5.4	23.4	4.2	1.0
Vegetable, Pret a Manger*	1 Serving/193g	277	5.0	144	3.4	25.9	2.8	5.6

TART

	Measure INFO/WEIGHT	KCAL	FAT	KCAL	PROT	CARB	FAT	FIBRE
Bakewell, Pret, Pret a Manger*	1 Serving/68g	315	18.0	463	7.2	50.0	26.0	2.2

TOASTIE

	Measure INFO/WEIGHT	KCAL	FAT	KCAL	PROT	CARB	FAT	FIBRE
Cheese, & Onion, Pret a Manger*	1 Serving/190g	580	30.0	305	17.1	25.3	15.7	2.4
Ham, Cheese, & Mustard, Pret a Manger*	1 Serving/242g	696	38.0	288	18.1	20.0	15.5	1.9
Mozzarella, & Pesto, Pret a Manger*	1 Serving/233g	496	23.0	213	9.7	21.2	9.9	2.2
New York Deli, Pret a Manger*	1 Serving/233g	575	28.0	247	14.6	22.0	11.9	2.4
Tuna Melt, Pret a Manger*	1 Serving/218g	550	25.0	252	16.2	22.0	11.5	2.4

WRAP

	Measure INFO/WEIGHT	KCAL	FAT	KCAL	PROT	CARB	FAT	FIBRE
Avocado, & Herb Salad, Pret a Manger*	1 Wrap/252g	461	30.0	183	4.8	14.1	12.0	2.7
Hoisin Duck, Pret a Manger*	1 Wrap/211g	433	20.0	205	9.5	20.7	9.5	1.4
Humous Salad, Chunky, Pret a Manger*	1 Wrap/208g	345	18.0	166	5.1	16.2	8.8	1.3
Italian Pizza Hot, Pret a Manger*	1 Serving/203g	381	16.0	188	9.1	20.4	7.7	2.0
Swedish Meatball Ragu Hot, Pret a Manger*	1 Serving/219g	566	26.0	259	13.3	24.9	11.9	2.2

YOGHURT

	Measure INFO/WEIGHT	KCAL	FAT	KCAL	PROT	CARB	FAT	FIBRE
Bunny Breakfast Bowl, Pret a Manger*	1 Serving/233g	198	5.0	85	5.2	10.9	2.1	1.0
Honey, & Granola, Pret Pot, Pret a Manger*	1 Pot/133g	263	8.0	198	7.3	28.8	5.9	1.3

	Measure INFO/WEIGHT	per Measure KCAL	FAT	Nutrition Values per 100g / 100ml KCAL	PROT	CARB	FAT	FIBRE
PRET A MANGER								
YOGHURT								
Nuts, Pret a Manger*	1 Serving/75g	430	33.0	573	6.9	29.7	44.3	6.9
YOGHURT DRINK								
Vanilla Bean, & Honey, Pret a Manger*	1 Serving/250ml	233	5.0	93	4.0	14.5	2.1	0.0
STARBUCKS								
BAGEL								
Cheese, & Jalapeno, Starbucks*	1 Bagel/115g	292	4.0	254	10.8	45.8	3.1	1.5
Cheesy, Starbucks*	1 Bagel/90g	253	7.0	281	11.9	41.7	7.3	2.2
Cinnamon & Raisin, Starbucks*	1 Bagel/83g	190	1.0	229	44.8	9.4	1.4	1.3
Fruity, Starbucks*	1 Bagel/90g	338	16.0	376	9.7	44.5	17.9	3.4
BARS								
Almond, Cranberry & Yoghurt, Starbucks*	1 Bar/50g	220	13.0	440	6.6	46.0	25.5	10.2
Chocolate, Milk, Starbucks*	1 Bar/45g	252	17.0	559	8.4	48.8	36.7	0.0
Granola, Starbucks*	1 Bar/80g	348	20.0	435	7.3	46.4	24.6	4.4
Mango, Pistachio & Cashew, Fruit & Nut, Starbucks*	1 Bar/50g	200	11.0	401	7.7	45.0	21.1	16.9
Rocky Road, Starbucks*	1 Bar/65g	366	27.0	563	4.2	46.6	41.1	2.2
BISCOTTI								
Almond, Starbucks*	1 Biscuit/27g	120	5.0	446	10.4	61.6	17.6	11.4
BISCUITS								
Ginger Snaps, Organic, Starbucks*	3 Biscuits/60g	267	9.0	445	4.8	71.9	15.4	1.5
Golden Crunch, Starbucks*	1 Biscuit/30g	144	7.0	481	5.1	65.4	22.1	2.0
BREAD								
Fruit, Luxury, Starbucks*	1 Serving/145g	486	12.0	335	7.0	58.0	8.3	2.3
BREAKFAST CEREAL								
Porridge, Dried Fruit, Made with Full Fat Milk, Starbucks*	1 Serving/244g	344	10.0	141	4.3	23.1	3.9	1.6
Porridge, Dried Fruit, Made with Skim Milk, Starbucks*	1 Serving/243g	292	3.0	120	4.4	23.3	1.4	1.6
Porridge, Dried Fruit, Made with Soy Milk, Starbucks*	1 Serving/244g	307	6.0	126	4.3	21.6	2.6	2.0
Porridge, Dried Fruit, with Semi Skim Milk, Starbucks*	1 Serving/244g	320	6.0	131	4.4	23.3	2.5	1.6
CAKE								
Banana & Date, Skinny, Starbucks*	1 Slice/120g	300	3.0	250	3.9	52.1	2.9	2.5
Banana Date & Raisin, Wholemeal, Low Fat, Starbucks*	1 Slice/70g	169	2.0	242	5.0	49.1	2.9	3.4
Butterfly, Starbucks*	1 Slice/80g	361	18.0	451	3.4	58.2	22.7	0.5
Carrot & Valencia Orange, Low Fat, Starbucks*	1 Slice/80g	200	2.0	250	3.3	53.0	3.0	3.0
Carrot Loaf, Starbucks*	1 Slice/100g	352	20.0	352	4.7	38.4	19.9	2.3
Carrot, Skinny, Starbucks*	1 Slice/75g	192	2.0	256	4.0	54.1	3.3	2.1
Chocolate Decadence, Starbucks*	1 Slice/170g	717	41.0	422	4.4	46.9	24.1	1.4
Chocolate Orange, Starbucks*	1 Slice/70g	276	15.0	395	5.7	45.4	21.2	1.9
Chocolate, Fairtrade, Starbucks*	1 Serving/70g	330	20.0	471	10.9	40.7	28.3	4.6
Coconut & Raspberry, Starbucks*	1 Cake/62g	267	15.0	430	4.0	49.9	23.6	1.6
Fruit, Starbucks*	1 Slice/80g	236	7.0	295	3.6	50.1	8.7	2.8
Ginger, Square, Starbucks*	1 Square/45g	202	13.0	450	3.8	45.0	28.2	0.9
Iced Fancies, Starbucks*	1 Cake/81g	307	11.0	379	2.3	63.7	13.0	0.6
Marshmallow, Chocolate, Twizzle, Starbucks*	1 Cake/35g	143	3.0	410	4.2	78.6	8.3	2.2
Marshmallow, with Coloured Strands, Twizzle, Starbucks*	1 Cake/35g	136	2.0	390	2.5	85.0	4.4	0.5
Orange, Summer Valencia, no Wheat & Dairy, Starbucks*	1 Slice/70g	190	10.0	271	7.6	28.9	14.0	2.9
Orange, Wheat & Gluten Free, Starbucks*	1 Serving/55g	138	7.0	251	7.4	25.8	13.2	3.3
Passion, Starbucks*	1 Slice/145g	528	32.0	364	4.3	37.2	22.0	1.8
Victoria Sponge, Classic, Starbucks*	1 Slice/127g	490	25.0	385	3.2	48.4	19.7	0.8
Victoria Sponge, Mini, Starbucks*	1 Cake/65g	243	12.0	375	3.7	47.5	18.8	0.9
Yoghurt & Berry Loaf, Low Fat, Starbucks*	1 Slice/94g	254	5.0	270	5.3	50.8	5.1	1.7
CHEESECAKE								
Blueberry Swirl, Starbucks*	1 Slice/155g	463	30.0	299	5.6	24.1	19.7	0.9
Chocolate, Starbucks*	1 Serving/185g	723	50.0	391	6.9	30.5	26.8	0.8

STARBUCKS

COFFEE

	Measure INFO/WEIGHT	per Measure KCAL	FAT	Nutrition Values per 100g / 100ml KCAL	PROT	CARB	FAT	FIBRE
Brewed, Grande, Starbucks*	1 Cup/473ml	5	0.0	1	0.1	0.0	0.0	0.0
Brewed, Short, Starbucks*	1 Cup/236ml	3	0.0	1	0.1	0.0	0.1	0.0
Brewed, Tall, Starbucks*	1 Cup/254ml	4	0.0	2	0.2	0.0	0.0	0.0
Brewed, Venti, Starbucks*	1 Cup/591ml	6	0.0	1	0.1	0.0	0.0	0.0
Caffe Americano, Grande, Starbucks*	1 Cup/473ml	17	0.0	4	0.2	0.6	0.0	0.0
Caffe Americano, Short, Starbucks*	1 Cup/236ml	6	0.0	3	0.2	0.4	0.0	0.0
Caffe Americano, Tall, Starbucks*	1 Cup/335ml	11	0.0	3	0.1	0.3	0.0	0.0
Caffe Americano, Venti, Starbucks*	1 Cup/591ml	23	0.0	4	0.2	0.7	0.0	0.0
Caffe Latte, Grande, Semi Skimmed Milk, Starbucks*	1 Cup/473ml	188	7.0	40	2.6	4.0	1.5	0.0
Caffe Latte, Grande, Skimmed Milk, Starbucks*	1 Cup/473ml	131	0.0	28	2.7	4.0	0.1	0.0
Caffe Latte, Grande, Soy, Starbucks*	1 Cup/473ml	148	5.0	31	2.2	2.7	1.1	0.3
Caffe Latte, Grande, Whole Milk, Starbucks*	1 Cup/473ml	223	11.0	47	2.6	3.8	2.4	0.0
Caffe Latte, Short, Semi Skimmed Milk, Starbucks*	1 Cup/236ml	95	3.0	40	2.7	3.8	1.5	0.0
Caffe Latte, Short, Skimmed Milk, Starbucks*	1 Cup/236ml	67	0.0	28	2.7	4.2	0.0	0.0
Caffe Latte, Short, Soy, Starbucks*	1 Cup/236ml	75	3.0	32	2.2	3.0	1.1	0.3
Caffe Latte, Short, Whole Milk, Starbucks*	1 Cup/236ml	113	6.0	48	2.6	3.8	2.5	0.0
Caffe Latte, Tall, Semi Skimmed Milk, Starbucks*	1 Cup/335ml	148	6.0	44	2.9	4.2	1.7	0.0
Caffe Latte, Tall, Skimmed Milk, Starbucks*	1 Cup/335ml	102	0.0	30	3.0	4.5	0.1	0.0
Caffe Latte, Tall, Soy, Starbucks*	1 Cup/335ml	116	4.0	35	2.4	3.0	1.3	0.3
Caffe Latte, Tall, Whole Milk, Starbucks*	1 Cup/335ml	176	9.0	53	2.8	4.2	2.7	0.0
Caffe Latte, Venti, Semi Skimmed Milk, Starbucks*	1 Cup/591ml	242	9.0	41	2.7	4.1	1.5	0.0
Caffe Latte, Venti, Skimmed Milk, Starbucks*	1 Cup/591ml	210	0.0	36	2.8	4.2	0.1	0.0
Caffe Latte, Venti, Soy, Starbucks*	1 Cup/591ml	190	7.0	32	2.3	2.7	1.2	0.3
Caffe Latte, Venti, Whole Milk, Starbucks*	1 Cup/591ml	289	15.0	49	2.6	3.9	2.5	0.0
Caffe Misto, Cafe Au Lait, Grande, Skim Milk, Starbucks*	1 Cup/473ml	73	0.0	15	1.5	2.1	0.0	0.0
Caffe Misto, Cafe Au Lait, Grande, Soy, Starbucks*	1 Cup/473ml	82	3.0	17	1.2	1.3	0.7	0.2
Caffe Misto, Cafe Au Lait, Grande, SS Milk, Starbucks*	1 Cup/473ml	106	4.0	22	1.5	2.1	0.9	0.0
Caffe Misto, Cafe Au Lait, Grande, Wh. Milk, Starbucks*	1 Cup/473ml	126	7.0	27	1.5	1.9	1.4	0.0
Caffe Misto, Cafe Au Lait, Short, SkimMilk, Starbucks*	1 Cup/236ml	37	0.0	16	1.6	2.1	0.0	0.0
Caffe Misto, Cafe Au Lait, Short, Soy, Starbucks*	1 Cup/236ml	42	2.0	18	1.3	1.3	0.7	0.2
Caffe Misto, Cafe Au Lait, Short, SS Milk, Starbucks*	1 Cup/236ml	54	2.0	23	1.5	2.1	0.9	0.0
Caffe Misto, Cafe Au Lait, Short, Whole Milk, Starbucks*	1 Cup/236ml	65	3.0	28	1.5	2.1	1.5	0.0
Caffe Misto, Cafe Au Lait, Tall, Skimmed Milk, Starbucks*	1 Cup/335ml	56	0.0	17	1.7	2.4	0.1	0.0
Caffe Misto, Cafe Au Lait, Tall, Soy, Starbucks*	1 Cup/335ml	63	2.0	19	1.3	1.5	0.7	0.2
Caffe Misto, Cafe Au Lait, Tall, SS Milk, Starbucks*	1 Cup/335ml	81	3.0	24	1.6	2.1	1.0	0.0
Caffe Misto, Cafe Au Lait, Tall, Whole Milk, Starbucks*	1 Cup/335ml	97	5.0	29	1.6	2.1	1.5	0.0
Caffe Misto, Cafe Au Lait, Venti, Skim Milk, Starbucks*	1 Cup/591ml	92	0.0	16	1.6	2.2	0.0	0.0
Caffe Misto, Cafe Au Lait, Venti, Soy, Starbucks*	1 Cup/591ml	104	4.0	18	1.3	1.3	0.7	0.2
Caffe Misto, Cafe Au Lait, Venti, SS Milk, Starbucks*	1 Cup/591ml	134	5.0	23	1.5	2.0	0.9	0.0
Caffe Misto, Cafe Au Lait, Venti, Whole Milk, Starbucks*	1 Cup/591ml	160	9.0	27	1.5	2.0	1.5	0.0
Caffe Misto, Skimmed Milk, Starbucks*	1 Tall/354ml	64	0.0	18	1.8	2.5	0.0	0.0
Caffe Misto, Whole Milk, Starbucks*	1 Grande/442ml	134	7.0	30	1.6	2.3	1.6	0.0
Caffe Mocha, Skimmed Milk, Starbucks*	1 Tall/354ml	175	1.0	49	0.3	9.3	0.4	0.4
Caffe Mocha, Skimmed Milk, with Whip, Starbucks*	1 Grande/473ml	324	12.0	68	3.0	9.3	2.4	0.4
Caffe Mocha, Whole Milk, Starbucks*	1 Tall/354ml	233	9.0	66	2.8	8.8	2.6	0.4
Caffe Mocha, Whole Milk, with Whip, Starbucks*	1 Tall/354ml	313	17.0	88	2.8	9.0	4.9	0.4
Caffe Mocha, with Whip, Grande, Skim Milk, Starbucks*	1 Cup/473ml	288	10.0	61	2.8	9.3	2.0	0.4
Caffe Mocha, with Whip, Grande, Soy, Starbucks*	1 Cup/473ml	302	14.0	64	2.4	8.0	2.9	0.6
Caffe Mocha, with Whip, Grande, SS Milk, Starbucks*	1 Cup/473ml	335	15.0	71	2.8	9.1	3.2	0.4
Caffe Mocha, with Whip, Grande, Whole Milk, Starbucks*	1 Cup/473ml	364	19.0	77	2.7	8.9	3.9	0.4
Caffe Mocha, with Whip, Short, Skimmed Milk, Starbucks*	1 Cup/236ml	160	6.0	68	2.9	9.3	2.7	0.4
Caffe Mocha, with Whip, Short, Soy, Starbucks*	1 Cup/236ml	167	8.0	71	2.5	8.5	3.6	0.6

	Measure INFO/WEIGHT	per Measure KCAL	per Measure FAT	Nutrition Values per 100g / 100ml KCAL	PROT	CARB	FAT	FIBRE

STARBUCKS
COFFEE

	Measure INFO/WEIGHT	KCAL	FAT	KCAL	PROT	CARB	FAT	FIBRE
Caffe Mocha, with Whip, Short, SS Milk, Starbucks*	1 Cup/236ml	184	9.0	78	2.8	9.3	3.9	0.4
Caffe Mocha, with Whip, Short, Whole Milk, Starbucks*	1 Cup/236ml	198	11.0	84	2.8	9.3	4.7	0.4
Caffe Mocha, with Whip, Tall, Semi Skimmed, Starbucks*	1 Cup/254ml	266	12.0	105	4.1	13.0	4.9	0.5
Caffe Mocha, with Whip, Tall, Skimmed Milk, Starbucks*	1 Cup/335ml	228	8.0	68	3.2	10.1	2.4	0.4
Caffe Mocha, with Whip, Tall, Soy, Starbucks*	1 Cup/254ml	239	11.0	94	3.6	11.4	4.5	0.9
Caffe Mocha, with Whip, Tall, Whole Milk, Starbucks*	1 Cup/335ml	290	16.0	87	3.0	9.8	4.6	0.4
Caffe Mocha, with Whip, Venti, Skimmed Milk, Starbucks*	1 Cup/591ml	347	10.0	59	2.9	9.3	1.7	0.4
Caffe Mocha, with Whip, Venti, Soy, Starbucks*	1 Cup/591ml	366	16.0	62	2.5	8.1	2.7	0.6
Caffe Mocha, with Whip, Venti, SS Milk, Starbucks*	1 Cup/591ml	409	17.0	69	2.9	9.1	3.0	0.4
Caffe Mocha, with Whip, Venti, Whole Milk, Starbucks*	1 Cup/591ml	448	23.0	76	2.8	9.0	3.8	0.4
Cappuccino, Grande, Semi Skimmed Milk, Starbucks*	1 Cup/473ml	115	4.0	24	1.6	2.5	0.9	0.0
Cappuccino, Grande, Soy, Starbucks*	1 Cup/473ml	92	3.0	19	1.3	1.7	0.7	0.2
Cappuccino, Grande, Whole Milk, Starbucks*	1 Cup/473ml	136	7.0	29	1.6	2.3	1.4	0.0
Cappuccino, Short, Semi Skimmed Milk, Starbucks*	1 Cup/236ml	78	3.0	33	2.2	3.4	1.2	0.0
Cappuccino, Short, Skimmed Milk, Starbucks*	1 Cup/236ml	55	0.0	23	2.2	3.4	0.0	0.0
Cappuccino, Short, Soy, Starbucks*	1 Cup/236ml	62	2.0	26	1.8	2.5	0.9	0.2
Cappuccino, Short, Whole Milk, Starbucks*	1 Cup/236ml	92	5.0	39	2.1	3.4	2.0	0.0
Cappuccino, Tall, Semi Skimmed Milk, Starbucks*	1 Cup/335ml	91	3.0	27	1.8	2.7	1.0	0.0
Cappuccino, Tall, Skimmed Milk, Starbucks*	1 Cup/335ml	64	0.0	19	1.8	2.7	0.0	0.0
Cappuccino, Tall, Soy, Starbucks*	1 Cup/335ml	72	3.0	21	1.5	1.8	0.8	0.2
Cappuccino, Tall, Whole Milk, Starbucks*	1 Cup/335ml	108	6.0	32	1.8	2.7	1.7	0.0
Cappuccino, Venti, Semi Skimmed Milk, Starbucks*	1 Cup/591ml	155	6.0	26	1.7	2.5	1.0	0.0
Cappuccino, Venti, Skimmed Milk, Starbucks*	1 Cup/591ml	109	0.0	18	1.8	2.7	0.0	0.0
Cappuccino, Venti, Soy, Starbucks*	1 Cup/591ml	123	4.0	21	1.5	1.9	0.7	0.2
Cappuccino, Venti, Whole Milk, Starbucks*	1 Cup/591ml	184	9.0	31	1.7	2.5	1.6	0.0
Caramel Macchiato, Grande, Skimmed Milk, Starbucks*	1 Cup/473ml	193	1.0	41	2.3	7.4	0.2	0.0
Caramel Macchiato, Grande, Soy, Starbucks*	1 Cup/473ml	207	5.0	44	1.9	6.1	1.1	0.2
Caramel Macchiato, Grande, SS Milk, Starbucks*	1 Cup/473ml	240	7.0	51	2.2	7.2	1.4	0.0
Caramel Macchiato, Grande, Whole Milk, Starbucks*	1 Cup/473ml	269	11.0	57	2.2	7.2	2.2	0.0
Caramel Macchiato, Short, Semi Skim Milk, Starbucks*	1 Cup/236ml	122	4.0	52	2.3	6.8	1.6	0.0
Caramel Macchiato, Short, Skimmed Milk, Starbucks*	1 Cup/236ml	97	1.0	41	2.4	7.2	0.4	0.0
Caramel Macchiato, Short, Soy, Starbucks*	1 Cup/236ml	104	3.0	44	1.9	5.9	1.3	0.2
Caramel Macchiato, Short, Whole Milk, Starbucks*	1 Cup/236ml	137	6.0	58	2.2	6.8	2.4	0.0
Caramel Macchiato, Skimmed Milk, Starbucks*	1 Tall/354ml	173	1.0	49	3.1	8.5	0.2	0.0
Caramel Macchiato, Tall, Semi Skimmed Milk, Starbucks*	1 Cup/335ml	178	5.0	53	2.4	7.5	1.6	0.0
Caramel Macchiato, Tall, Skimmed Milk, Starbucks*	1 Cup/335ml	142	1.0	42	2.4	7.5	0.3	0.0
Caramel Macchiato, Tall, Soy, Starbucks*	1 Cup/335ml	153	4.0	46	2.0	6.3	1.2	0.3
Caramel Macchiato, Tall, Whole Milk, Starbucks*	1 Cup/335ml	201	8.0	60	2.3	7.2	2.4	0.0
Caramel Macchiato, Venti, Semi Skim Milk, Starbucks*	1 Cup/591ml	299	8.0	51	2.2	7.3	1.4	0.0
Caramel Macchiato, Venti, Skimmed Milk, Starbucks*	1 Cup/591ml	239	1.0	40	2.3	7.4	0.2	0.0
Caramel Macchiato, Venti, Soy, Starbucks*	1 Cup/591ml	256	7.0	43	1.9	6.3	1.1	0.2
Caramel Macchiato, Venti, Whole Milk, Starbucks*	1 Cup/591ml	337	13.0	57	2.2	7.1	2.2	0.0
Caramel Macchiato, Whole Milk, Starbucks*	1 Tall/354ml	244	10.0	69	2.8	7.9	2.9	0.0
Espresso Con Panna, Doppio, Starbucks*	1 Cup/60ml	36	3.0	60	1.5	5.0	4.2	0.0
Espresso Con Panna, Solo, Starbucks*	1 Cup/30ml	31	2.0	103	1.7	6.7	8.3	0.0
Espresso Macchiato, Doppio, Skimmed Milk, Starbucks*	1 Cup/60ml	13	0.0	22	1.7	3.3	0.0	0.0
Espresso Macchiato, Doppio, Soy, Starbucks*	1 Cup/60ml	13	0.0	22	1.5	3.3	0.2	0.0
Espresso Macchiato, Doppio, SS Milk, Starbucks*	1 Cup/60ml	14	0.0	23	1.5	3.3	0.2	0.0
Espresso Macchiato, Doppio, Whole Milk, Starbucks*	1 Cup/60ml	15	0.0	25	1.5	3.3	0.3	0.0
Espresso Macchiato, Solo, Semi Skim Milk, Starbucks*	1 Cup/30ml	8	0.0	27	1.7	3.3	0.3	0.0
Espresso Macchiato, Solo, Skimmed Milk, Starbucks*	1 Cup/30ml	7	0.0	23	1.7	3.3	0.0	0.0
Espresso Macchiato, Solo, Soy, Starbucks*	1 Cup/30ml	7	0.0	23	1.7	3.3	0.3	0.0

STARBUCKS

	Measure INFO/WEIGHT	per Measure KCAL	FAT	Nutrition Values per 100g / 100ml KCAL	PROT	CARB	FAT	FIBRE

COFFEE

	Measure INFO/WEIGHT	KCAL	FAT	KCAL	PROT	CARB	FAT	FIBRE
Espresso Macchiato, Solo, Whole Milk, Starbucks*	1 Cup/30ml	8	0.0	27	1.7	3.3	0.7	0.0
Espresso, Doppio, Starbucks*	1 Doppio/60ml	11	0.0	18	1.2	3.3	0.0	0.0
Espresso, Solo, Starbucks*	1 Solo/30ml	6	0.0	20	1.3	3.3	0.0	0.0
Hazelnut Mocha, with Whip, Grande, Soy, Starbucks*	1 Cup/473ml	369	13.0	78	2.3	12.0	2.8	0.6
Hazelnut Mocha, with Whip, Grande, SS Milk, Starbucks*	1 Cup/473ml	399	15.0	84	2.6	12.9	3.1	0.4
Hazelnut Mocha, with Whip, Grande, Wh. Milk, Starbucks*	1 Cup/473ml	425	18.0	90	2.6	12.7	3.8	0.4
Hazelnut Mocha, with Whip, Short, Skim Milk, Starbucks*	1 Cup/236ml	197	6.0	83	2.8	13.6	2.6	0.4
Hazelnut Mocha, with Whip, Short, Soy, Starbucks*	1 Cup/236ml	201	8.0	85	2.3	12.3	3.5	0.6
Hazelnut Mocha, with Whip, Short, SS Milk, Starbucks*	1 Cup/236ml	216	9.0	92	2.7	13.1	3.8	0.4
Hazelnut Mocha, with Whip, Short, Wh. Milk, Starbucks*	1 Cup/236ml	229	11.0	97	2.6	13.1	4.5	0.4
Hazelnut Mocha, with Whip, Tall, Skim Milk, Starbucks*	1 Cup/335ml	277	8.0	83	3.0	13.7	2.4	0.4
Hazelnut Mocha, with Whip, Tall, Soy, Starbucks*	1 Cup/335ml	288	11.0	86	2.6	12.5	3.3	0.7
Hazelnut Mocha, with Whip, Tall, SS Milk, Starbucks*	1 Cup/335ml	312	12.0	93	2.9	13.7	3.6	0.4
Hazelnut Mocha, with Whip, Tall, Whole Milk, Starbucks*	1 Cup/335ml	334	15.0	100	2.9	13.4	4.4	0.4
Hazelnut Mocha, with Whip, Venti, Skim Milk, Starbucks*	1 Cup/591ml	430	10.0	73	2.7	13.0	1.7	0.4
Hazelnut Mocha, with Whip, Venti, Soy, Starbucks*	1 Cup/591ml	448	15.0	76	2.4	11.8	2.6	0.6
Hazelnut Mocha, with Whip, Venti, SS Milk, Starbucks*	1 Cup/591ml	487	17.0	82	2.7	12.9	2.8	0.4
Hazelnut Mocha, with Whip, Venti, Wh. Milk, Starbucks*	1 Cup/591ml	523	21.0	88	2.6	12.7	3.6	0.4
Iced, Caffe Americano, Tall, Starbucks*	1 Cup/335ml	11	0.0	3	0.2	0.6	0.0	0.0
Iced, Caffe Latte, Grande, Semi Skim Milk, Starbucks*	1 Cup/473ml	126	4.0	27	1.8	2.7	0.9	0.0
Iced, Caffe Latte, Grande, Skimmed Milk, Starbucks*	1 Cup/473ml	90	0.0	19	1.8	2.7	0.0	0.0
Iced, Caffe Latte, Grande, Soy, Starbucks*	1 Cup/473ml	104	4.0	22	1.5	1.9	0.8	0.2
Iced, Caffe Latte, Grande, Whole Milk, Starbucks*	1 Cup/473ml	149	8.0	31	1.7	2.5	1.6	0.0
Iced, Caffe Latte, Tall, Semi Skimmed Milk, Starbucks*	1 Cup/335ml	97	4.0	29	1.9	3.0	1.1	0.0
Iced, Caffe Latte, Tall, Skimmed Milk, Starbucks*	1 Cup/335ml	68	0.0	20	1.9	3.0	0.1	0.0
Iced, Caffe Latte, Tall, Soy, Starbucks*	1 Cup/335ml	80	3.0	24	1.7	2.1	0.9	0.2
Iced, Caffe Latte, Tall, Whole Milk, Starbucks*	1 Cup/335ml	115	6.0	34	1.8	2.7	1.8	0.0
Iced, Caffe Latte, Venti, Semi Skimmed Milk, Starbucks*	1 Cup/591ml	142	5.0	24	1.6	2.4	0.9	0.0
Iced, Caffe Latte, Venti, Skimmed Milk, Starbucks*	1 Cup/591ml	100	0.0	17	1.6	2.5	0.0	0.0
Iced, Caffe Latte, Venti, Soy, Starbucks*	1 Cup/591ml	118	4.0	20	1.4	1.9	0.7	0.2
Iced, Caffe Latte, Venti, Whole Milk, Starbucks*	1 Cup/591ml	168	9.0	28	1.5	2.4	1.4	0.0
Iced, Caffe Mocha, with Whip, Grande, Soy, Starbucks*	1 Cup/473ml	300	16.0	63	1.8	7.6	3.4	0.5
Iced, Caffe Mocha, with Whip, Grande, SS Milk, Starbucks*	1 Cup/473ml	316	17.0	67	2.0	8.0	3.5	0.4
Iced, Caffe Mocha, with Whip, Tall, Soy, Starbucks*	1 Cup/335ml	221	12.0	66	2.0	8.1	3.5	0.6
Iced, Caffe Mocha, with Whip, Tall, SS Milk, Starbucks*	1 Cup/335ml	234	12.0	70	2.1	8.7	3.7	0.4
Iced, Caffe Mocha, with Whip, Tall, Whole Milk, Starbucks*	1 Cup/335ml	248	14.0	74	2.1	8.4	4.2	0.4
Iced, Caffe Mocha, with Whip, Venti, Skim Milk, Starbucks*	1 Cup/591ml	310	13.0	52	1.8	7.8	2.2	0.4
Iced, Caffe Mocha, with Whip, Venti, Soy, Starbucks*	1 Cup/591ml	322	16.0	54	1.6	7.1	2.7	0.5
Iced, Caffe Mocha, with Whip, Venti, SS Milk, Starbucks*	1 Cup/591ml	340	17.0	58	1.8	7.6	2.8	0.4
Iced, Caffe Mocha, with Whip, Venti, Wh. Milk, Starbucks*	1 Cup/591ml	358	19.0	61	1.7	7.6	3.2	0.4
Iced, Caramel Macchiato, Grande, Skim Milk, Starbucks*	1 Cup/473ml	188	1.0	40	2.1	7.2	0.3	0.0
Iced, Caramel Macchiato, Grande, Soy, Starbucks*	1 Cup/473ml	206	5.0	44	1.8	6.3	1.1	0.2
Iced, Caramel Macchiato, Grande, SS Milk, Starbucks*	1 Cup/473ml	231	6.0	49	2.0	7.0	1.3	0.0
Iced, Caramel Macchiato, Grande, Whole Milk, Starbucks*	1 Cup/473ml	257	10.0	54	2.0	7.0	2.1	0.0
Iced, Caramel Macchiato, Tall, Skimmed Milk, Starbucks*	1 Cup/335ml	139	1.0	41	2.1	7.5	0.4	0.0
Iced, Caramel Macchiato, Tall, Soy, Starbucks*	1 Cup/335ml	152	4.0	45	1.8	6.6	1.2	0.2
Iced, Caramel Macchiato, Tall, SS Milk, Starbucks*	1 Cup/335ml	171	5.0	51	2.1	7.2	1.5	0.0
Iced, Caramel Macchiato, Tall, Whole Milk, Starbucks*	1 Cup/335ml	191	8.0	57	2.0	7.2	2.2	0.0
Iced, Caramel Macchiato, Venti, Skim Milk, Starbucks*	1 Cup/591ml	215	1.0	36	1.8	6.8	0.2	0.0
Iced, Caramel Macchiato, Venti, Soy, Starbucks*	1 Cup/591ml	234	6.0	40	1.6	5.9	1.0	0.2
Iced, Caramel Macchiato, Venti, SS Milk, Starbucks*	1 Cup/591ml	262	7.0	44	1.8	6.6	1.1	0.0
Iced, Caramel Macchiato, Venti, Whole Milk, Starbucks*	1 Cup/591ml	291	11.0	49	1.7	6.6	1.8	0.0

	Measure	per Measure		Nutrition Values per 100g / 100ml				
	INFO/WEIGHT	KCAL	FAT	KCAL	PROT	CARB	FAT	FIBRE

STARBUCKS

COFFEE

	Measure INFO/WEIGHT	KCAL	FAT	KCAL	PROT	CARB	FAT	FIBRE
Iced, Grande, Starbucks*	1 Cup/473ml	4	0.0	1	0.1	0.0	0.0	0.0
Iced, Hazelnut Mocha, with Whip, Grande, Soy, Starbucks*	1 Cup/473ml	437	19.0	92	2.2	11.8	4.1	0.1
Iced, Hazelnut Mocha, with Whip, Tall, Sk Milk, Starbucks*	1 Cup/335ml	316	12.0	94	2.6	13.1	3.7	0.0
Iced, Hazelnut Mocha, with Whip, Tall, Soy, Starbucks*	1 Cup/335ml	325	14.0	97	2.4	12.5	4.3	0.1
Iced, Hazelnut Mocha, with Whip, Tall, SS Milk, Starbucks*	1 Cup/335ml	337	15.0	101	2.5	12.8	4.4	0.0
Iced, Hazelnut Mocha, with Whip, Venti, Soy, Starbucks*	1 Cup/591ml	578	22.0	98	2.4	13.7	3.8	0.1
Iced, Latte, Vanilla, Grande, Skimmed Milk, Starbucks*	1 Cup/473ml	155	0.0	33	1.6	6.5	0.0	0.0
Iced, Latte, Vanilla, Grande, Soy, Starbucks*	1 Cup/473ml	168	3.0	36	1.3	5.7	0.7	0.2
Iced, Latte, Vanilla, Grande, SS Milk, Starbucks*	1 Cup/473ml	187	4.0	40	1.5	6.3	0.8	0.0
Iced, Latte, Vanilla, Grande, Whole Milk, Starbucks*	1 Cup/473ml	207	6.0	44	1.5	6.3	1.4	0.0
Iced, Latte, Vanilla, Tall, Semi Skimmed Milk, Starbucks*	1 Cup/335ml	142	3.0	42	1.7	6.9	0.9	0.0
Iced, Latte, Vanilla, Tall, Skimmed Milk, Starbucks*	1 Cup/335ml	121	0.0	36	1.8	7.2	0.0	0.0
Iced, Latte, Vanilla, Tall, Soy, Starbucks*	1 Cup/335ml	128	3.0	38	1.5	6.0	0.7	0.2
Iced, Latte, Vanilla, Tall, Whole Milk, Starbucks*	1 Cup/335ml	158	5.0	47	1.6	6.6	1.5	0.0
Iced, Latte, Vanilla, Venti, Semi Skimmed Milk, Starbucks*	1 Cup/591ml	218	4.0	37	1.4	6.1	0.7	0.0
Iced, Latte, Vanilla, Venti, Skimmed Milk, Starbucks*	1 Cup/591ml	182	0.0	31	1.4	6.3	0.0	0.0
Iced, Latte, Vanilla, Venti, Soy, Starbucks*	1 Cup/591ml	197	3.0	33	1.2	5.6	0.6	0.1
Iced, Latte, Vanilla, Venti, Whole Milk, Starbucks*	1 Cup/591ml	240	7.0	41	1.3	6.1	1.2	0.0
Iced, Tall, Starbucks*	1 Cup/335ml	3	0.0	1	0.1	0.0	0.0	0.0
Mocha, Peppermint, Skimmed, Grande, Starbucks*	1 Cup/473ml	304	2.0	64	2.9	13.3	0.5	0.4
Mocha, Peppermint, Skimmed, Tall, Starbucks*	1 Cup/354ml	237	1.0	67	3.1	13.6	0.4	0.4
Mocha, Peppermint, Skimmed, Venti, Starbucks*	1 Cup/591ml	385	3.0	65	3.0	13.4	0.5	0.4
Mocha, Peppermint, Skimmed, Whip, Grande, Starbucks*	1 Cup/473ml	405	21.0	86	2.9	13.7	4.4	0.4
Mocha, Peppermint, Skimmed, Whip, Tall, Starbucks*	1 Cup/354ml	317	9.0	90	3.1	13.8	2.7	0.4
Mocha, Peppermint, Skimmed, Whip, Venti, Starbucks*	1 Cup/591ml	486	12.0	82	3.0	13.7	2.1	0.4
Mocha, Peppermint, Whole, Grande, Starbucks*	1 Cup/473ml	372	11.0	79	2.7	12.9	2.4	0.4
Mocha, Peppermint, Whole, Tall, Starbucks*	1 Cup/354ml	293	9.0	83	2.8	13.3	2.5	0.4
Mocha, Peppermint, Whole, Venti, Starbucks*	1 Cup/591ml	475	15.0	80	2.8	12.9	2.6	0.4
Mocha, Peppermint, Whole, Whip, Grande, Starbucks*	1 Cup/473ml	473	21.0	100	2.7	13.3	4.4	0.4
Mocha, Peppermint, Whole, Whip, Tall, Starbucks*	1 Cup/354ml	373	17.0	105	2.8	13.6	4.8	0.4
Mocha, Peppermint, Whole, Whip, Venti, Starbucks*	1 Cup/591ml	576	25.0	97	2.8	13.2	4.2	0.4
Vanilla Latte, Grande, Semi Skimmed Milk, Starbucks*	1 Cup/473ml	251	6.0	53	2.4	7.6	1.3	0.0
Vanilla Latte, Grande, Skimmed Milk, Starbucks*	1 Cup/473ml	199	0.0	42	2.5	7.8	0.1	0.0
Vanilla Latte, Grande, Soy, Starbucks*	1 Cup/473ml	214	5.0	45	2.0	6.5	1.0	0.2
Vanilla Latte, Grande, Whole Milk, Starbucks*	1 Cup/473ml	284	11.0	60	2.4	7.6	2.2	0.0
Vanilla Latte, Short, Semi Skimmed Milk, Starbucks*	1 Cup/236ml	127	3.0	54	2.5	7.6	1.4	0.0
Vanilla Latte, Short, Skimmed Milk, Starbucks*	1 Cup/236ml	101	0.0	43	2.5	8.0	0.0	0.0
Vanilla Latte, Short, Soy, Starbucks*	1 Cup/236ml	108	3.0	46	2.1	6.8	1.1	0.2
Vanilla Latte, Short, Whole Milk, Starbucks*	1 Cup/236ml	144	5.0	61	2.4	7.6	2.3	0.0
Vanilla Latte, Tall, Semi Skimmed Milk, Starbucks*	1 Cup/335ml	195	5.0	58	2.7	8.1	1.5	0.0
Vanilla Latte, Tall, Skimmed Milk, Starbucks*	1 Cup/335ml	152	0.0	45	2.8	8.4	0.1	0.0
Vanilla Latte, Tall, Soy, Starbucks*	1 Cup/335ml	165	4.0	49	2.3	6.9	1.2	0.3
Vanilla Latte, Tall, Whole Milk, Starbucks*	1 Cup/335ml	221	9.0	66	2.7	8.1	2.6	0.0
Vanilla Latte, Venti, Semi Skimmed Milk, Starbucks*	1 Cup/591ml	321	9.0	54	2.5	7.8	1.4	0.0
Vanilla Latte, Venti, Skimmed Milk, Starbucks*	1 Cup/591ml	252	0.0	43	2.6	7.9	0.1	0.0
Vanilla Latte, Venti, Soy, Starbucks*	1 Cup/591ml	272	7.0	46	2.1	6.6	1.1	0.3
Vanilla Latte, Venti, Whole Milk, Starbucks*	1 Cup/591ml	364	14.0	62	2.5	7.6	2.4	0.0
Vanilla, with Whip, Grande, Starbucks*	1 Cup/473ml	364	14.0	77	1.2	11.4	3.0	0.0
Vanilla, with Whip, Tall, Starbucks*	1 Cup/335ml	284	10.0	85	1.3	13.1	3.1	0.0
Vanilla, with Whip, Venti, Starbucks*	1 Cup/591ml	412	14.0	70	1.1	11.2	2.3	0.0
White Mocha, with Whip, Grande, Skim Milk, Starbucks*	1 Cup/473ml	425	13.0	90	3.2	13.5	2.7	0.0
White Mocha, with Whip, Grande, Soy, Starbucks*	1 Cup/473ml	439	17.0	93	2.8	12.3	3.6	0.2

STARBUCKS

COFFEE

	Measure INFO/WEIGHT	KCAL	FAT	KCAL	PROT	CARB	FAT	FIBRE
White Mocha, with Whip, Grande, SS Milk, Starbucks*	1 Cup/473ml	471	18.0	100	3.1	13.3	3.9	0.0
White Mocha, with Whip, Grande, Whole Milk, Starbucks*	1 Cup/473ml	500	22.0	106	3.1	13.1	4.7	0.0
White Mocha, with Whip, Short, Skimmed Milk, Starbucks*	1 Cup/236ml	229	8.0	97	3.3	13.6	3.4	0.0
White Mocha, with Whip, Short, Soy, Starbucks*	1 Cup/236ml	236	10.0	100	2.9	12.7	4.3	0.2
White Mocha, with Whip, Short, SS Milk, Starbucks*	1 Cup/236ml	252	11.0	107	3.2	13.6	4.6	0.0
White Mocha, with Whip, Short, Whole Milk, Starbucks*	1 Cup/236ml	267	13.0	113	3.2	13.6	5.4	0.0
White Mocha, with Whip, Tall, Skimmed Milk, Starbucks*	1 Cup/335ml	331	10.0	99	3.5	14.3	3.1	0.0
White Mocha, with Whip, Tall, Soy, Starbucks*	1 Cup/335ml	342	14.0	102	3.1	13.1	4.1	0.3
White Mocha, with Whip, Tall, SS Milk, Starbucks*	1 Cup/335ml	369	15.0	110	3.5	14.3	4.5	0.0
White Mocha, with Whip, Tall, Whole Milk, Starbucks*	1 Cup/335ml	392	18.0	117	3.4	14.0	5.4	0.0
White Mocha, with Whip, Venti, Skimmed Milk, Starbucks*	1 Cup/591ml	518	14.0	88	3.3	13.5	2.4	0.0
White Mocha, with Whip, Venti, Soy, Starbucks*	1 Cup/591ml	537	20.0	91	2.9	12.3	3.4	0.2
White Mocha, with Whip, Venti, SS Milk, Starbucks*	1 Cup/591ml	581	22.0	98	3.2	13.4	3.7	0.0
White Mocha, with Whip, Venti, Whole Milk, Starbucks*	1 Cup/591ml	619	27.0	105	3.2	13.2	4.5	0.0

COOKIES

Chocolate, Chunk, Starbucks*	1 Cookie/90g	396	12.0	440	6.8	69.7	13.3	0.3

CORNFLAKE

Chocolate, Belgian, Square, Starbucks*	1 Slice/62g	285	13.0	460	4.0	63.7	20.5	2.5

CREPE

Ham, Mushroom & Tomato, Starbucks*	1 Pack/153g	148	5.0	97	4.3	14.0	3.1	1.0

CRISPS

Strong Cheese & Onion, Starbucks*	1 Bag/50g	227	11.0	455	7.1	56.2	22.6	4.0

CROISSANT

Almond, Starbucks*	1 Croissant/92g	389	20.0	423	7.0	48.2	21.9	2.2
Butter, Starbucks*	1 Croissant/70g	279	17.0	398	6.9	39.5	23.6	1.4
Cheese, & Ham, Starbucks*	1 Pack/114g	359	21.0	315	13.2	24.9	18.1	0.8

CUPCAKES

Banana & Chocolate Chip, Starbucks*	1 Cupcake/80g	342	15.0	428	4.7	57.8	18.6	0.5
Lemon, Sicilian, Starbucks*	1 Cake/80g	350	18.0	437	3.3	55.3	22.5	0.5
Strawberry, Starbucks*	1 Cupcake/83g	385	21.0	464	4.1	55.9	25.1	0.6

DOUGHNUT

Chocolate & Custard, Mini, Starbucks*	1 Doughnut/25g	77	3.0	307	5.8	39.8	13.8	1.6
Jam, Mini, Starbucks*	1 Doughnut/24g	77	3.0	323	6.2	49.6	11.1	1.4

DRIED FRUIT

Starbucks*	1 Serving/30g	88	0.0	294	2.2	75.3	0.4	1.4

FLAPJACK

Banana & Caramel, Starbucks*	1 Serving/70g	301	15.0	430	3.3	54.4	22.0	2.5

FRAPPUCCINO

Caramel Cream, Grande, Starbucks*	1 Grande/473ml	339	5.0	72	2.8	12.7	1.1	0.0
Caramel Cream, Tall, Starbucks*	1 Tall/354ml	261	4.0	74	2.8	13.0	1.1	0.0
Caramel Cream, Venti, Starbucks*	1 Venti/591ml	409	6.0	69	2.6	12.3	1.0	0.0
Caramel Cream, with Whip, Grande, Starbucks*	1 Grande/473ml	431	14.0	91	2.6	13.5	3.0	0.0
Caramel Cream, with Whip, Tall, Starbucks*	1 Tall/254ml	329	10.0	130	3.6	19.7	4.1	0.0
Caramel Cream, with Whip, Venti, Starbucks*	1 Venti/591ml	489	14.0	83	2.4	13.0	2.3	0.0
Caramel, Grande, Starbucks*	1 Grande/473ml	294	4.0	62	0.0	12.5	0.8	0.0
Caramel, Light, Grande, Starbucks*	1 Grande/473ml	158	2.0	33	1.3	6.3	0.3	0.5
Caramel, Light, Tall, Starbucks*	1 Cup/335ml	129	1.0	39	1.4	7.5	0.4	0.6
Caramel, Light, Venti, Starbucks*	1 Cup/591ml	192	2.0	32	1.2	6.4	0.3	0.5
Caramel, Tall, Starbucks*	1 Tall/354ml	228	3.0	64	0.0	12.7	0.9	0.0
Caramel, Venti, Starbucks*	1 Venti/591ml	370	5.0	63	0.0	12.7	0.8	0.0
Caramel, with Whip, Grande, Starbucks*	1 Cup/473ml	382	15.0	81	1.2	12.0	3.1	0.0
Caramel, with Whip, Tall, Starbucks*	1 Cup/335ml	302	11.0	90	1.3	13.7	3.3	0.0

STARBUCKS

FRAPPUCCINO

INFO/WEIGHT	KCAL	FAT	KCAL	PROT	CARB	FAT	FIBRE
Caramel, with Whip, Venti, Starbucks*	1 Cup/591ml	431	14.0	73	1.1	11.7	2.4	0.0
Chocolate, Grande, Starbucks*	1 Cup/473ml	338	6.0	71	3.0	12.7	1.2	0.0
Chocolate, Tall, Starbucks*	1 Cup/354ml	260	4.0	73	3.0	13.0	1.3	0.0
Chocolate, Venti, Starbucks*	1 Cup/591ml	413	7.0	70	2.8	12.7	1.2	0.0
Chocolate, with Whip, Grande, Starbucks*	1 Cup/473ml	469	18.0	99	3.0	13.1	3.8	0.1
Chocolate, with Whip, Tall, Starbucks*	1 Cup/354ml	354	13.0	100	3.0	13.6	3.7	0.2
Chocolate, with Whip, Venti, Starbucks*	1 Cup/591ml	544	19.0	92	2.8	13.0	3.3	0.2
Coffee, Grande, Starbucks*	1 Cup/473ml	239	3.0	51	1.1	10.1	0.7	0.0
Coffee, Light, Grande, Starbucks*	1 Cup/473ml	128	1.0	27	1.3	5.3	0.2	0.5
Coffee, Light, Tall, Starbucks*	1 Cup/335ml	91	1.0	27	1.3	5.4	0.2	0.5
Coffee, Light, Venti, Starbucks*	1 Cup/591ml	151	1.0	26	1.2	4.9	0.2	0.5
Coffee, Tall, Starbucks*	1 Cup/254ml	184	2.0	72	1.5	14.6	0.9	0.0
Coffee, Venti, Starbucks*	1 Cup/591ml	278	4.0	47	1.0	9.5	0.6	0.0
Cream, Caramel, with Whip, Tall, Starbucks*	1 Cup/335ml	329	10.0	98	2.7	14.9	3.1	0.0
Cream, Chocolate Chip, with Whip, Grande, Starbucks*	1 Cup/473ml	498	18.0	105	2.8	15.6	3.8	0.3
Cream, Chocolate Chip, with Whip, Tall, Starbucks*	1 Cup/335ml	368	13.0	110	3.0	16.7	3.8	0.4
Cream, Chocolate Chip, with Whip, Venti, Starbucks*	1 Cup/591ml	562	19.0	95	2.6	14.9	3.2	0.4
Cream, Chocolate, with Whip, Grande, Starbucks*	1 Cup/473ml	425	14.0	90	2.7	13.5	3.0	0.1
Cream, Chocolate, with Whip, Tall, Starbucks*	1 Cup/335ml	322	10.0	96	2.9	14.6	3.1	0.2
Cream, Chocolate, with Whip, Venti, Starbucks*	1 Cup/591ml	480	14.0	81	2.5	13.0	2.4	0.2
Cream, Vanilla, with Whip, Tall, Starbucks*	1 Cup/335ml	310	10.0	93	2.7	14.0	2.9	0.0
Cream, Vanilla, with Whip, Venti, Starbucks*	1 Cup/591ml	470	13.0	80	2.3	12.7	2.2	0.0
Espresso, Grande, Starbucks*	1 Cup/473ml	209	3.0	44	1.0	8.9	0.6	0.0
Espresso, Tall, Starbucks*	1 Cup/335ml	146	2.0	44	1.0	8.7	0.6	0.0
Espresso, Venti, Starbucks*	1 Cup/591ml	243	3.0	41	0.9	8.1	0.5	0.0
Java Chip, with Whip, Grande, Starbucks*	1 Cup/473ml	456	19.0	96	1.5	14.6	3.9	0.3
Java Chip, with Whip, Tall, Starbucks*	1 Cup/335ml	345	14.0	103	1.7	16.1	4.1	0.4
Java Chip, with Whip, Venti, Starbucks*	1 Cup/591ml	520	20.0	88	1.4	14.0	3.3	0.4
Mango Passion, Grande, Starbucks*	1 Cup/473ml	191	0.0	40	0.2	9.7	0.1	0.3
Mango Passion, Tall, Starbucks*	1 Cup/335ml	157	0.0	47	0.2	11.3	0.1	0.3
Mango Passion, Venti, Starbucks*	1 Cup/591ml	228	0.0	39	0.1	9.3	0.0	0.2
Mocha, Light, Grande, Starbucks*	1 Cup/473ml	144	1.0	30	1.3	6.1	0.3	0.6
Mocha, Light, Tall, Starbucks*	1 Cup/335ml	113	1.0	34	1.5	6.9	0.3	0.7
Mocha, Light, Venti, Starbucks*	1 Cup/591ml	184	2.0	31	1.3	6.3	0.3	0.6
Mocha, White Chocolate, with Whip, Grande, Starbucks*	1 Cup/473ml	408	16.0	86	1.4	12.9	3.3	0.0
Mocha, White Chocolate, with Whip, Venti, Starbucks*	1 Cup/591ml	481	16.0	81	1.4	13.0	2.7	0.0
Mocha, with Whip, Grande, Starbucks*	1 Cup/473ml	378	15.0	80	1.3	12.0	3.1	0.1
Mocha, with Whip, Tall, Starbucks*	1 Cup/335ml	283	11.0	84	1.4	12.8	3.2	0.1
Mocha, with Whip, Venti, Starbucks*	1 Cup/591ml	428	15.0	72	1.3	11.7	2.5	0.1
Raspberry Tea, Grande, Starbucks*	1 Cup/473ml	200	0.0	42	0.1	11.0	0.0	0.2
Raspberry Tea, Tall, Starbucks*	1 Cup/354ml	144	0.0	41	0.1	10.4	0.0	0.2
Raspberry Tea, Venti, Starbucks*	1 Cup/591ml	261	0.0	44	0.1	11.3	0.0	0.2
Raspberry, Black Currant, Zen Tea, Grande, Starbucks*	1 Cup/473ml	192	0.0	41	0.1	9.9	0.0	0.1
Raspberry, Black Currant, Zen Tea, Tall, Starbucks*	1 Cup/335ml	158	0.0	47	0.1	11.6	0.0	0.2
Raspberry, Black Currant, Zen Tea, Venti, Starbucks*	1 Cup/591ml	229	0.0	39	0.1	9.5	0.0	0.1
Strawberries & Cream, Grande, Starbucks*	1 Cup/473ml	424	5.0	90	2.9	17.3	1.1	0.0
Strawberries & Cream, Tall, Starbucks*	1 Cup/354ml	299	4.0	84	2.7	16.4	1.0	0.0
Strawberries & Cream, Venti, Starbucks*	1 Cup/591ml	543	7.0	92	3.0	17.6	1.1	0.0
Strawberries & Cream, with Whip, Grande, Starbucks*	1 Cup/473ml	494	13.0	104	2.5	17.5	2.8	0.1
Strawberries & Cream, with Whip, Tall, Starbucks*	1 Cup/254ml	374	10.0	147	3.5	24.8	3.8	0.1
Strawberries & Cream, with Whip, Venti, Starbucks*	1 Cup/591ml	548	13.0	93	2.2	16.2	2.2	0.1
Tazo Chai, Grande, Starbucks*	1 Cup/473ml	405	5.0	86	2.9	16.5	1.1	0.0

STARBUCKS
FRAPPUCCINO

	Measure INFO/WEIGHT	per Measure KCAL	FAT	KCAL	PROT	CARB	FAT	FIBRE
Tazo Chai, Tall, Starbucks*	1 Cup/354ml	294	4.0	83	2.9	15.8	1.1	0.0
Tazo Chai, Venti, Starbucks*	1 Cup/591ml	487	6.0	82	2.7	16.1	1.0	0.0
Tazo Chai, with Whip, Grande, Starbucks*	1 Cup/473ml	536	17.0	113	2.9	16.9	3.7	0.0
Tazo Chai, with Whip, Tall, Starbucks*	1 Cup/354ml	388	12.0	110	2.9	16.4	3.5	0.0
Tazo Chai, with Whip, Venti, Starbucks*	1 Cup/591ml	618	18.0	105	2.7	16.4	3.1	0.0
Tropical Citrus Tea, Grande, Starbucks*	1 Cup/473ml	178	0.0	38	0.3	9.3	0.1	0.3
Tropical Citrus Tea, Tall, Starbucks*	1 Cup/354ml	128	0.0	36	0.3	9.0	0.1	0.3
Tropical Citrus Tea, Venti, Starbucks*	1 Cup/591ml	232	0.0	39	0.3	9.8	0.1	0.3
Vanilla, with Whip, Grande, Starbucks*	1 Cup/473ml	364	14.0	77	1.2	11.4	3.0	0.0
Vanilla, with Whip, Tall, Starbucks*	1 Cup/254ml	284	10.0	112	1.7	17.3	4.1	0.9
Vanilla, with Whip, Venti, Starbucks*	1 Cup/591ml	412	14.0	70	1.1	11.2	2.3	0.0
White Chocolate Mocha, with Whip, Tall, Starbucks*	1 Cup/335ml	319	12.0	95	1.5	14.6	3.5	0.0

FRUIT SALAD

	Measure INFO/WEIGHT	per Measure KCAL	FAT	KCAL	PROT	CARB	FAT	FIBRE
Starbucks*	1 Salad/170g	66	0.0	39	0.6	9.5	0.2	1.2

HOT CHOCOLATE

	Measure INFO/WEIGHT	per Measure KCAL	FAT	KCAL	PROT	CARB	FAT	FIBRE
Signature, with Whip, Grande, Skimmed Milk, Starbucks*	1 Cup/473ml	505	27.0	107	3.3	12.5	5.7	1.4
Signature, with Whip, Grande, Soy, Starbucks*	1 Cup/473ml	515	30.0	109	3.0	11.8	6.3	1.6
Signature, with Whip, Grande, SS Milk, Starbucks*	1 Cup/473ml	537	31.0	114	3.2	12.5	6.5	6.5
Signature, with Whip, Grande, Whole Milk, Starbucks*	1 Cup/473ml	556	33.0	118	3.2	12.5	7.1	1.4
Signature, with Whip, Short, Skimmed Milk, Starbucks*	1 Cup/236ml	267	15.0	113	3.3	12.7	6.4	1.4
Signature, with Whip, Short, Soy, Starbucks*	1 Cup/236ml	272	16.0	115	3.0	11.9	6.9	1.6
Signature, with Whip, Short, SS Milk, Starbucks*	1 Cup/236ml	283	17.0	120	3.3	12.7	7.2	1.4
Signature, with Whip, Short, Whole Milk, Starbucks*	1 Cup/236ml	293	18.0	124	3.2	12.7	7.7	1.4
Signature, with Whip, Tall, Semi Skimmed Milk, Starbucks*	1 Cup/335ml	418	24.0	125	3.5	13.4	7.2	1.5
Signature, with Whip, Tall, Skimmed Milk, Starbucks*	1 Cup/335ml	393	21.0	117	3.5	13.7	6.4	1.5
Signature, with Whip, Tall, Soy, Starbucks*	1 Cup/335ml	401	23.0	120	3.2	12.8	7.0	1.7
Signature, with Whip, Tall, Whole Milk, Starbucks*	1 Cup/335ml	433	26.0	129	3.5	13.4	7.8	1.5
Signature, with Whip, Venti, Skimmed Milk, Starbucks*	1 Cup/591ml	624	32.0	106	3.3	12.7	5.5	1.4
Signature, with Whip, Venti, Soy, Starbucks*	1 Cup/591ml	637	36.0	108	3.0	12.0	6.1	1.6
Signature, with Whip, Venti, SS Milk, Starbucks*	1 Cup/591ml	665	37.0	113	3.3	12.7	6.3	1.4
Signature, with Whip, Venti, Whole Milk, Starbucks*	1 Cup/591ml	690	40.0	117	3.2	12.5	6.8	1.4
Skimmed Milk, Grande, Starbucks*	1 Cup/473ml	261	2.0	55	3.3	10.6	0.5	0.4
Skimmed Milk, Tall, Starbucks*	1 Cup/354ml	209	1.0	59	3.5	11.3	0.4	0.4
Skimmed Milk, Venti, Starbucks*	1 Cup/591ml	340	3.0	58	3.3	11.2	0.5	0.4
White, Skimmed Milk, Grande, Starbucks*	1 Cup/442ml	361	17.0	82	3.8	13.9	3.8	0.0
White, Skimmed Milk, Tall, Starbucks*	1 Cup/354ml	301	4.0	85	4.1	14.4	1.1	0.0
White, Skimmed Milk, Venti, Starbucks*	1 Cup/591ml	493	7.0	83	4.0	14.2	1.2	0.0
White, Skimmed Milk, with Whip, Grande, Starbucks*	1 Cup/443ml	456	14.0	103	3.8	14.4	3.2	0.0
White, Skimmed Milk, with Whip, Tall, Starbucks*	1 Cup/354ml	381	12.0	108	4.1	14.7	3.4	0.0
White, Skimmed Milk, with Whip, Venti, Starbucks*	1 Cup/553ml	556	15.0	101	4.0	14.5	2.8	0.0
White, Whole Milk, Grande, Starbucks*	1 Cup/443ml	449	17.0	101	3.5	13.3	3.8	0.0
White, Whole Milk, Tall, Starbucks*	1 Cup/354ml	377	14.0	106	3.8	13.8	4.0	0.0
White, Whole Milk, Venti, Starbucks*	1 Cup/591ml	618	24.0	105	3.7	13.5	4.1	0.0
White, Whole Milk, with Whip, Grande, Starbucks*	1 Cup/443ml	543	25.0	123	3.5	13.7	5.7	0.0
White, Whole Milk, with Whip, Tall, Starbucks*	1 Cup/354ml	457	22.0	129	3.8	14.1	6.3	0.0
White, Whole Milk, with Whip, Venti, Starbucks*	1 Cup/553ml	673	31.0	122	3.7	13.9	5.6	0.0
Whole Milk, Grande, Starbucks*	1 Cup/473ml	347	14.0	73	3.0	9.9	3.0	0.4
Whole Milk, Tall, Starbucks*	1 Cup/354ml	277	11.0	78	3.1	10.7	3.0	0.4
Whole Milk, Venti, Starbucks*	1 Cup/591ml	448	18.0	76	3.0	10.7	3.0	0.4
Whole Milk, with Whip, Grande, Starbucks*	1 Cup/443ml	420	22.0	95	3.0	10.4	5.0	0.4
Whole Milk, with Whip, Tall, Starbucks*	1 Cup/354ml	357	19.0	101	3.1	11.0	5.3	0.4
Whole Milk, with Whip, Venti, Starbucks*	1 Cup/553ml	514	25.0	93	3.0	11.0	4.6	0.4

	Measure INFO/WEIGHT	per Measure KCAL	per Measure FAT	Nutrition Values per 100g / 100ml KCAL	PROT	CARB	FAT	FIBRE
STARBUCKS								
HOUMOUS								
with Tomato, Vegetables, Red Pepper, Starbucks*	1 Pack/218g	405	14.0	186	5.4	26.2	6.6	2.0
with Vegetable Sticks, Starbucks*	1 Pot/150g	96	4.0	64	2.9	7.3	2.6	4.5
JUICE								
Orange, Starbucks*	1 Bottle/250ml	112	0.0	45	0.8	11.4	0.1	0.3
MILK								
Steamed, Semi Skimmed, Grande, Starbucks*	1 Cup/473ml	203	8.0	43	2.8	4.0	1.7	0.0
Steamed, Semi Skimmed, Short, Starbucks*	1 Cup/236ml	103	4.0	44	2.9	4.2	1.7	0.0
Steamed, Semi Skimmed, Tall, Starbucks*	1 Cup/254ml	168	7.0	66	4.4	6.4	2.6	0.0
Steamed, Semi Skimmed, Venti, Starbucks*	1 Cup/591ml	258	10.0	44	2.9	4.1	1.7	0.0
Steamed, Skimmed, Grande, Starbucks*	1 Cup/473ml	257	1.0	54	5.4	7.9	0.1	0.0
Steamed, Skimmed, Short, Starbucks*	1 Cup/236ml	70	0.0	30	2.9	10.0	0.2	0.0
Steamed, Skimmed, Tall, Starbucks*	1 Cup/254ml	114	0.0	45	4.4	6.4	0.1	0.0
Steamed, Skimmed, Venti, Starbucks*	1 Cup/591ml	175	0.0	30	2.9	4.4	0.1	0.0
Steamed, Soy, Grande, Starbucks*	1 Cup/473ml	157	6.0	33	2.3	2.7	1.3	0.3
Steamed, Soy, Short, Starbucks*	1 Cup/236ml	80	3.0	34	2.4	2.5	1.3	0.0
Steamed, Soy, Tall, Starbucks*	1 Cup/254ml	120	5.0	47	3.3	3.9	1.8	0.5
Steamed, Soy, Venti, Starbucks*	1 Cup/591ml	199	8.0	34	2.4	2.7	1.3	0.3
Steamed, Whole, Grande, Starbucks*	1 Cup/473ml	244	25.0	52	5.2	7.1	5.2	0.0
Steamed, Whole, Short, Starbucks*	1 Cup/236ml	123	7.0	52	2.8	3.8	2.8	0.0
Steamed, Whole, Tall, Starbucks*	1 Cup/254ml	187	10.0	74	3.9	5.5	4.0	0.0
Steamed, Whole, Venti, Starbucks*	1 Cup/591ml	309	17.0	52	2.8	3.9	2.8	0.0
MUFFIN								
Banana & Walnut, Starbucks*	1 Muffin/125g	469	25.0	375	5.7	42.9	20.1	4.2
Blueberry, Starbucks*	1 Muffin/125g	561	23.0	449	5.8	46.5	18.4	1.1
Chocolate, with Belgian Choc Sauce Centre, Starbucks*	1 Muffin/135g	551	29.0	408	6.2	49.5	21.3	2.5
Raspberry, with White Chocolate Icing, Starbucks*	1 Muffin/121g	397	18.0	328	4.9	43.2	15.1	1.1
Skinny Blueberry, Starbucks*	1 Muffin/130g	323	6.0	249	4.3	51.7	4.3	1.6
Skinny Peach & Raspberry, Starbucks*	1 Muffin/140g	321	5.0	229	4.4	49.0	3.3	1.6
Skinny Sunrise, Starbucks*	1 Muffin/131g	255	4.0	194	4.6	36.7	3.0	1.3
Skinny, Ginger Iced, Starbucks*	1 Muffin/140g	405	5.0	289	3.9	62.3	3.4	0.9
Skinny, Lemon, Poppy Seed, Starbucks*	1 Muffin/140g	393	6.0	281	4.3	56.2	4.3	4.2
Sunrise, Starbucks*	1 Muffin/150g	592	35.0	395	5.5	40.8	23.1	1.9
PAIN AU CHOCOLAT								
Starbucks*	1 Pastry/70g	296	17.0	423	6.7	43.8	24.4	2.8
PAIN AU RAISIN								
Starbucks*	1 Pastry/120g	445	22.0	371	5.3	45.6	18.5	1.8
PANINI								
Beef Pastrami & Roast Chicken, Starbucks*	1 Panini/220g	443	13.0	201	12.3	25.1	5.7	1.4
Cheese & Marmite, Breakfast, Starbucks*	1 Serving/115g	298	10.0	259	14.5	30.3	8.8	1.7
Chicken & Green Pesto, Starbucks*	1 Panini/203g	351	9.0	173	12.3	21.2	4.4	1.2
Chicken, Mediterranean, with Green Pesto, Starbucks*	1 Panini/224g	387	9.0	173	11.4	22.6	4.1	1.3
Croque Monsieur, Starbucks*	1 Panini/190g	441	17.0	232	12.4	25.3	9.0	1.2
Egg Mayo, Breakfast, Starbucks*	1 Panini/146g	327	12.0	224	12.3	25.4	8.1	1.7
Egg, Bacon & Mushroom , Breakfast, Starbucks*	1 Pack/153g	269	9.0	176	10.4	20.3	5.9	0.3
Falafel, Starbucks*	1 Pack/213g	384	7.0	180	6.8	30.9	3.3	2.7
Grilled Chicken Salsa, Lightly Spiced, Starbucks*	1 Panini/238g	385	8.0	162	7.9	25.0	3.4	2.0
Grilled Chicken Salsa, with Creme Fraiche, Starbucks*	1 Panini/180g	385	8.0	214	10.4	32.9	4.5	0.0
Ham, Cheese & Roasted Vegetable, Starbucks*	1 Panini/217g	388	8.0	179	11.0	25.4	3.7	1.4
Mozzarella & Slow Roast Tomato, Starbucks*	1 Panini/180g	461	21.0	256	11.1	27.1	11.5	2.1
Pesto Chicken, with Sunblush Tomato, Starbucks*	1 Panini/208g	399	10.0	192	13.1	24.1	4.8	3.0
Roasted Vegetable & Taw Valley Cheddar, Starbucks*	1 Panini/225g	485	20.0	215	9.2	25.1	8.8	1.7
Roasted Vegetables & Cheese, Starbucks*	1 Panini/215g	542	32.0	252	8.7	20.6	15.1	0.0

STARBUCKS

	Measure INFO/WEIGHT	per Measure KCAL	FAT	Nutrition Values per 100g / 100ml KCAL	PROT	CARB	FAT	FIBRE
PANINI								
Sausage, Egg & Baked Bean, Starbucks*	1 Panini/100g	395	10.0	395	16.9	59.8	9.8	1.5
Steak & Cheese, Starbucks*	1 Panini/219g	451	15.0	206	12.3	24.2	6.7	1.3
Tuna Melt, Starbucks*	1 Panini/197g	486	21.0	247	13.5	24.1	10.8	1.6
SALAD								
Chicken Caesar, Starbucks*	1 Pack/233g	403	18.0	173	8.7	18.0	7.9	1.2
Chicken, Roasted, Starbucks*	1 Pack/157g	165	10.0	105	7.1	5.1	6.5	1.2
Minted Pea & Potato Salad, Starbucks*	1 Packet/290g	276	13.0	95	5.4	8.5	4.4	2.2
Mozzarella & Cherry Tomato, Starbucks*	1 Pack/172g	322	29.0	187	5.5	2.9	17.0	17.0
Pasta, Chicken & Red Pesto, Starbucks*	1 Pack/300g	390	13.0	130	7.1	15.3	4.4	1.2
Salmon & Dill, Starbucks*	1 Pack/260g	614	35.0	236	7.8	21.0	13.4	1.0
Salmon Nicoise, Starbucks*	1 Pack/260g	291	18.0	112	6.9	7.2	7.0	1.0
Tuna & Bean Salad, Starbucks*	1 Pack/326g	254	4.0	78	7.1	9.9	1.1	2.5
Tuna Nicoise, Starbucks*	1 Pack/184g	175	10.0	95	7.8	4.6	5.3	1.2
SANDWICH								
Atlantic Prawn, Starbucks*	1 Pack/185g	348	12.0	188	10.1	22.0	6.7	2.7
BLT, Starbucks*	1 Pack/181g	483	27.0	267	9.6	22.9	15.2	1.9
Cheddar Cheese & Pickle, Starbucks*	1 Pack/190g	504	30.0	265	10.2	20.5	15.7	1.6
Cheddar, & Italian Style Roasted Vegetables, Starbucks*	1 Pack/223g	553	31.0	248	5.3	25.8	13.7	0.0
Cheese, & Tomato, & Apple Chutney, Half Fat, Starbucks*	1 Pack/200g	318	8.0	159	8.8	21.3	4.2	0.0
Chicken, & Bacon, Club, Starbucks*	1 Pack/252g	590	39.0	234	11.5	12.8	15.3	0.0
Chicken, Club, Starbucks*	1 Pack/206g	422	19.0	205	12.6	17.8	9.4	1.7
Chicken, in Lemon Pepper Dressing, Starbucks*	1 Pack/198g	307	7.0	155	11.8	19.4	3.5	1.6
Chicken, Lightly Spiced, Starbucks*	1 Pack/200g	286	5.0	143	11.2	18.2	2.4	0.0
Chicken, Roasted, with Tomato & Herb Mayo, Starbucks*	1 Pack/201g	323	7.0	161	11.5	20.6	3.6	1.8
Egg Mayonnaise, & Cress, Starbucks*	1 Pack/200g	410	20.0	205	10.5	17.4	10.2	1.9
Egg Mayonnaise, on Gluten Free Bread, Starbucks*	1 Pack/227g	340	12.0	150	6.2	20.3	5.1	2.9
Falafel & Houmous, in Flatbread, Starbucks*	1 Pack/250g	467	9.0	187	7.0	34.8	3.8	3.6
Ham, & Tomato, Smoked, Starbucks*	1 Pack/206g	297	8.0	144	5.2	22.0	3.9	0.0
Ham, Yorkshire, Starbucks*	1 Pack/208g	374	11.0	180	10.0	23.0	5.3	2.3
Houmous, with Crunchy Vegetables, Starbucks*	1 Pack/219g	359	10.0	164	4.7	26.4	4.4	2.9
Prawn, Mayo, Starbucks*	1 Sandwich/183g	386	20.0	211	9.8	18.3	11.0	1.6
Salmon, Oak Smoked & Soft Cheese, Starbucks*	1 Pack/221g	523	24.0	236	9.6	12.6	10.9	1.9
Soft Cheese, & Tomato, Extra Light, Starbucks*	1 Pack/186g	283	5.0	152	8.0	24.0	2.7	3.1
Tuna, Mayonnaise, Starbucks*	1 Pack/184g	333	11.0	181	9.4	22.8	5.8	1.8
Turkey, & Salad, Smoked, Starbucks*	1 Pack/198g	303	5.0	153	10.8	22.3	2.4	1.5
Turkey, Pork & Herb, Starbucks*	1 Pack/198g	465	21.0	235	11.7	22.6	10.8	2.1
SCONE								
Berry, Starbucks*	1 Scone/90g	301	15.0	335	5.6	40.3	16.3	2.1
Blueberry, Starbucks*	1 Scone/128g	460	18.0	359	3.9	53.1	14.1	2.3
Extremely Fruity, Starbucks*	1 Scone/100g	325	8.0	325	5.7	57.1	8.5	2.3
Raisin, Jumbo, Starbucks*	1 Scone/150g	564	22.0	376	5.9	54.9	14.8	2.1
SHORTBREAD								
Chocolate Caramel, Starbucks*	1 Bar/62g	319	18.0	515	3.7	59.0	29.3	0.8
Chocolate, Chunk, Fairtrade, Starbucks*	1 Serving/90g	484	28.0	538	5.7	57.9	31.5	1.4
SLICES								
Apricot, Pastry, Starbucks*	1 Pastry/115g	279	15.0	243	4.7	26.1	13.3	1.1
Belgian Chocolate & Orange, Swirl, Pastry, Starbucks*	1 Pastry/140g	525	18.0	375	7.5	57.4	13.2	2.6
Cheese, Savoury, Pastry, Starbucks*	1 Pastry/120g	497	31.0	414	11.8	32.2	26.2	1.2
Cinnamon Swirl, Pastry, Starbucks*	1 Pastry/140g	434	8.0	309	7.0	57.9	5.5	2.8
SYRUP								
Bar Mocha, 1 Pump, Starbucks*	1 Pump/17g	26	1.0	153	3.5	35.3	3.5	5.9
Flavoured, 1 Pump, Starbucks*	1 Pump/10g	20	0.0	200	0.0	50.0	0.0	0.0

STARBUCKS

INFO/WEIGHT	Measure	per Measure KCAL	per Measure FAT	Nutrition Values per 100g / 100ml KCAL	PROT	CARB	FAT	FIBRE
TEA								
Brewed, Grande, Starbucks*	1 Cup/473ml	0	0.0	0	0.0	0.0	0.0	0.0
Chai, Latte, Tazo, Grande, Skim Milk, Starbucks*	1 Cup/473ml	204	0.0	43	1.6	9.3	0.0	0.0
Chai, Latte, Tazo, Grande, Soy, Starbucks*	1 Cup/473ml	213	3.0	45	1.3	8.7	0.7	0.2
Chai, Latte, Tazo, Grande, SS Milk, Starbucks*	1 Cup/473ml	236	4.0	50	1.6	9.3	0.8	0.0
Chai, Latte, Tazo, Grande, Whole Milk, Starbucks*	1 Cup/473ml	255	6.0	54	1.5	9.1	1.4	0.0
Chai, Latte, Tazo, Short, Skim Milk, Starbucks*	1 Cup/236ml	103	0.0	44	1.6	9.3	0.0	0.0
Chai, Latte, Tazo, Short, Soy, Starbucks*	1 Cup/236ml	108	2.0	46	1.4	8.5	0.7	0.2
Chai, Latte, Tazo, Short, SS Milk, Starbucks*	1 Cup/236ml	119	2.0	50	1.6	9.3	0.8	0.0
Chai, Latte, Tazo, Short, Whole Milk, Starbucks*	1 Cup/236ml	129	3.0	55	1.6	9.3	1.4	0.0
Chai, Latte, Tazo, Tall, Skimmed Milk, Starbucks*	1 Cup/335ml	154	0.0	46	1.7	9.8	0.1	0.0
Chai, Latte, Tazo, Tall, Soy, Starbucks*	1 Cup/335ml	162	2.0	48	1.4	9.2	0.7	0.2
Chai, Latte, Tazo, Tall, SS Milk, Starbucks*	1 Cup/335ml	179	3.0	53	1.7	9.8	0.9	0.0
Chai, Latte, Tazo, Tall, Whole Milk, Starbucks*	1 Cup/335ml	194	5.0	58	1.6	9.8	1.5	0.0
Chai, Latte, Tazo, Venti, Skim Milk, Starbucks*	1 Cup/591ml	256	0.0	43	1.6	9.5	0.0	0.0
Chai, Latte, Tazo, Venti, Soy, Starbucks*	1 Cup/591ml	268	4.0	45	1.3	8.6	0.7	0.2
Chai, Latte, Tazo, Venti, SS Milk, Starbucks*	1 Cup/591ml	297	5.0	50	1.6	9.3	0.8	0.0
Chai, Latte, Tazo, Venti, Whole Milk, Starbucks*	1 Cup/591ml	322	8.0	54	1.5	9.3	1.4	0.0
Iced, Chai, Latte, Tazo, Grande, Skim Milk, Starbucks*	1 Cup/473ml	205	0.0	43	1.6	9.3	0.0	0.0
Iced, Chai, Latte, Tazo, Grande, Soy, Starbucks*	1 Cup/473ml	219	3.0	46	1.4	8.7	0.7	0.2
Iced, Chai, Latte, Tazo, Grande, SS Milk, Starbucks*	1 Cup/473ml	238	4.0	50	1.6	9.3	0.9	0.0
Iced, Chai, Latte, Tazo, Grande, Whole Milk, Starbucks*	1 Cup/473ml	259	7.0	55	1.5	9.3	1.5	0.0
Iced, Chai, Latte, Tazo, Tall, Semi Skimmed, Starbucks*	1 Cup/335ml	176	3.0	53	1.6	9.8	0.9	0.0
Iced, Chai, Latte, Tazo, Tall, Skimmed Milk, Starbucks*	1 Cup/335ml	152	0.0	45	1.6	9.8	0.1	0.0
Iced, Chai, Latte, Tazo, Tall, Whole Milk, Starbucks*	1 Cup/335ml	191	5.0	57	1.6	9.5	1.5	0.0
Iced, Chai, Latte, Tazo, Venti, Skimmed Milk, Starbucks*	1 Cup/591ml	242	0.0	41	1.4	9.0	0.0	0.0
Iced, Chai, Latte, Tazo, Venti, Soy, Starbucks*	1 Cup/591ml	256	3.0	43	1.2	8.5	0.6	0.2
Iced, Chai, Latte, Tazo, Venti, SS Milk, Starbucks*	1 Cup/591ml	277	4.0	47	1.3	9.0	0.7	0.0
Iced, Chai, Latte, Tazo, Venti, Whole Milk, Starbucks*	1 Cup/591ml	299	7.0	51	1.3	9.0	1.2	0.0
TOASTIE								
Ham & Cheese, Mini, Starbucks*	1 Pack/126g	328	11.0	260	13.3	31.7	8.8	1.8
TOPPING								
Caramel, Starbucks*	1 Serving/4g	15	1.0	375	0.0	50.0	15.0	0.0
Chocolate, Starbucks*	1 Serving/4g	6	0.0	150	2.5	25.0	2.5	2.5
Whipped Cream, Cold, Grande Beverage, Starbucks*	1 Serving/35g	114	11.0	326	1.7	8.6	32.0	0.0
Whipped Cream, Cold, Tall Beverage, Starbucks*	1 Serving/25g	81	8.0	324	1.6	8.0	32.0	0.0
Whipped Cream, Cold, Venti Beverage, Starbucks*	1 Serving/32g	104	10.0	325	1.9	9.4	31.9	0.0
Whipped Cream, Hot, Grande/venti, Starbucks*	1 Serving/22g	72	7.0	327	1.8	9.1	31.8	0.0
Whipped Cream, Hot, Short Beverage, Starbucks*	1 Serving/16g	52	5.0	325	1.9	6.2	31.9	0.0
Whipped Cream, Hot, Tall Beverage, Starbucks*	1 Serving/19g	62	6.0	326	1.6	10.5	32.1	0.0
TZATZIKI								
with Vegetable Sticks, Starbucks*	1 Tub /140g	73	4.0	52	2.0	4.8	2.8	1.7
WAFFLES								
Caramel, Starbucks*	1 Waffle/30g	140	6.0	467	4.3	66.7	20.3	1.3
WRAP								
Chicken with Salad, Starbucks*	1 Wrap/223g	362	10.0	162	10.1	21.9	4.3	2.1
Chicken, Breast, in Honey Mustard, Starbucks*	1 Pack/200g	332	8.0	166	7.3	25.8	3.9	1.4
Chicken, Chargrilled, Tomato & Pepper Salsa, Starbucks*	1 Pack/187g	320	8.0	171	10.4	22.5	4.4	1.6
Chicken, Roasted, Starbucks*	1 Pack/197g	374	13.0	190	11.6	21.2	6.6	2.2
Emmental Cheese, & Roasted Aubergines, Starbucks*	1 Pack/225g	517	26.0	230	8.9	22.3	11.4	0.0
Greek Salad, Starbucks*	1 Pack/181.5g	265	7.0	146	6.1	21.5	4.0	2.0
Houmous & Roasted Vegetable, Starbucks*	½ Pack/102g	205	7.0	200	6.2	29.2	6.7	3.5
Houmous & Falafel, Starbucks*	1 Wrap/213g	383	9.0	180	6.4	30.0	4.0	2.8

	Measure INFO/WEIGHT	per Measure		Nutrition Values per 100g / 100ml				
		KCAL	FAT	KCAL	PROT	CARB	FAT	FIBRE
STARBUCKS								
WRAP								
Prawn Caesar, Starbucks*	1 Pack/173g	464	27.0	268	11.4	20.2	15.7	1.1
Roasted Chicken Salad, with Mange Tout, Starbucks*	1 Pack/184g	294	4.0	160	12.2	23.5	2.0	1.7
YOGHURT								
Blueberry with Mixed Seeds, Organic, Starbucks*	1 Pot/180g	194	6.0	108	3.6	15.1	3.6	0.6
Blueberry, Starbucks*	1 Pot/130g	116	0.0	89	4.4	17.8	0.0	0.0
Greek, with Crunchy Granola & Honey, Starbucks*	1 Pot/150g	267	15.0	178	1.7	20.5	10.0	1.1
Strawberry with Mixed Seeds, Organic, Starbucks*	1 Pot/180g	178	6.0	99	3.6	12.6	3.6	1.1
Strawberry, Starbucks*	1 Pot/180g	176	6.0	98	3.6	12.4	3.6	1.7
SUBWAY								
BACON								
Strips, Subway*	2 Strips/9g	40	3.0	444	33.3	0.0	32.2	0.0
BREAD								
Roll, Hearty Italian, 6", Subway*	1 Roll/79g	191	2.0	242	10.1	45.6	2.0	2.2
Roll, Honey Oat, 6", Subway*	1 Roll/91g	228	2.0	251	9.9	44.0	2.6	3.0
Roll, Italian Herbs & Cheese, 6", Subway*	1 Roll/86g	223	5.0	259	11.6	40.7	5.2	2.2
Roll, Wheat, 6", Subway*	1 Roll/80g	187	2.0	234	10.0	42.5	2.0	2.7
Roll, White, Italian, 6", Subway*	1 Roll/75g	180	1.0	240	9.3	45.3	1.9	1.6
CHEESE								
American, Subway*	1 Serving/11g	40	4.0	364	18.2	0.0	32.7	0.0
Monterey Cheddar, Subway*	1 Serving/14g	55	4.0	393	25.0	2.1	31.4	0.0
COLA								
Coke, Subway*	1 Serving/455ml	191	0.0	42	0.0	10.6	0.0	0.0
Diet Coke, Subway*	1 Serving/455ml	2	0.0	0	0.0	0.0	0.0	0.0
COOKIES								
Chocolate Chip, Subway*	1 Cookie/45g	218	10.0	484	4.4	64.4	22.9	2.4
Chocolate Chunk, Subway*	1 Cookie/45g	224	12.0	498	4.4	62.2	26.0	2.0
Double Choc Chip, Subway*	1 Cookie/45g	221	12.0	491	4.4	60.0	26.0	2.7
Oatmeal Raisin, Subway*	1 Cookie/45g	190	9.0	422	4.4	55.6	19.6	4.2
Rainbow, Subway*	1 Cookie/45g	215	10.0	478	4.4	62.2	23.1	2.0
Sugar, Subway*	1 Cookie/45g	231	12.0	513	4.4	64.4	26.2	1.3
White Chip Mac Nut, Subway*	1 Cookie/45g	222	12.0	493	4.4	60.0	26.0	1.6
CRISPS								
Melted Cheese Nachos, Subway*	1 Serving/126g	411	24.0	326	8.7	28.6	19.3	2.0
DOUGHNUTS								
Chocolate, Subway*	1 Doughnut/55g	243	16.0	442	7.3	38.2	28.2	2.2
Sugared, Subway*	1 Doughnut/49g	207	12.0	422	6.1	42.9	23.7	1.0
FANTA								
Orange, Subway*	1 Serving/455ml	136	0.0	30	0.0	7.1	0.0	0.0
MEATBALLS								
Bowl, Subway*	1 Serving/206g	315	20.0	153	9.4	8.9	9.6	1.4
MUFFIN								
Blueberry, Subway*	1 Muffin/111g	352	21.0	317	4.5	36.0	18.6	2.7
Chocolate Chunk, Subway*	1 Muffin/111g	394	23.0	355	5.4	39.6	20.6	2.6
Double Chocolate Chunk, Subway*	1 Muffin/111g	389	22.0	350	5.4	40.5	19.8	2.8
SALAD								
Garden, Side, Subway*	1 Serving/135g	21	0.0	16	1.0	1.9	0.1	1.3
SANDWICH								
Beef, Kids Pack, Subway*	1 Sub/156g	182	2.0	117	9.6	16.0	1.3	1.4
Ham, Kids Pack, Subway*	1 Sub/147g	164	2.0	112	7.5	17.0	1.4	1.5
Sub, Bacon Egg, & Cheese, Wheat Bread, 6", Subway*	1 Sub/135g	331	13.0	245	12.6	25.9	10.0	1.7
Sub, Bacon, Wheat Bread, Breakfast, 6", Subway*	1 Sub/98g	268	7.0	273	15.3	34.7	7.7	2.2
Sub, Beef, Wheat Bread, 6", Subway*	1 Sub/221g	271	3.0	123	10.0	16.7	1.4	1.4

SUBWAY

	Measure INFO/WEIGHT	per Measure KCAL	FAT	Nutrition Values per 100g / 100ml KCAL	PROT	CARB	FAT	FIBRE
SANDWICH								
Sub, Chicken Breast, Wheat Bread, 6", Subway*	1 Sub/235g	297	4.0	126	11.5	16.2	1.7	1.4
Sub, Chicken Tikka, Wheat Bread, 6", Subway*	1 Sub/247g	360	11.0	146	11.3	15.4	4.3	1.2
Sub, Chicken, Bacon Ranch, & Cheese, 6", Subway*	1 Sub/294g	491	20.0	167	12.6	13.3	6.8	1.1
Sub, Ham, Wheat Bread, 6", Subway*	1 Sub/221g	258	4.0	117	8.6	17.2	1.7	1.4
Sub, Italian BMT, & Cheese, Wheat Bread, 6", Subway*	1 Sub/239g	425	20.0	178	10.0	11.7	8.5	1.3
Sub, Meatball & Cheese, Wheat Bread, 6", Subway*	1 Sub/319g	506	21.0	159	8.5	17.2	6.5	1.9
Sub, Mega, Wheat Bread, Breakfast, 6", Subway*	1 Sub/211g	507	25.0	240	13.3	20.4	11.7	1.5
Sub, Onion Chicken Teriyaki, Wheat Bread, 6", Subway*	1 Sub/278g	352	4.0	127	9.7	18.0	1.5	1.3
Sub, Sausage, Egg, & Cheese, Wheat Bread, 6", Subway*	1 Sub/202g	467	22.0	231	12.4	21.3	10.7	1.6
Sub, Sausage, Wheat Bread, Breakfast, 6", Subway*	1 Sub/156g	364	13.0	233	12.8	26.9	8.1	1.9
Sub, Spicy Italian, & Cheese, Wheat Bread, 6", Subway*	1 Sub/235g	501	29.0	213	10.2	15.7	12.3	1.4
Sub, Steak & Cheese, Wheat Bread, 6", Subway*	1 Sub/247g	332	9.0	134	10.1	15.8	3.6	1.5
Sub, Subway Club, Wheat Bread, 6", Subway*	1 Sub/254g	298	4.0	117	11.0	15.0	1.6	1.3
Sub, Subway Melt, & Cheese, Wheat Bread, 6", Subway*	1 Sub/251g	346	10.0	138	10.8	11.2	4.1	1.3
Sub, Tuna, & Cheese, Wheat Bread, 6", Subway*	1 Sub/247g	398	18.0	161	8.5	15.8	7.2	1.3
Sub, Turkey Breast & Ham, Wheat Bread, 6", Subway*	1 Sub/230g	266	4.0	116	9.1	16.1	1.6	1.4
Sub, Turkey Breast, Wheat Bread, 6", Subway*	1 Sub/221g	256	3.0	116	9.0	16.7	1.4	1.4
Sub, Veggie Delite, Wheat Bread, 6", Subway*	1 Sub/164g	202	2.0	123	5.5	22.0	1.1	2.0
Sub, Veggie Patty, & Cheese, Wheat Bread, 6", Subway*	1 Sub/261g	409	12.0	157	8.8	17.6	4.8	1.2
Tuna with Cheese, Kids Pack, Subway*	1 Sub/165g	254	11.0	154	7.9	15.8	6.7	1.3
Turkey Breast, Kids Pack, Subway*	1 Sub/156g	172	2.0	110	8.3	16.0	1.3	1.4
SAUCE								
BBQ, Subway*	1 Serving/21g	40	0.0	190	1.0	45.7	0.5	0.5
Chipotle Southwest Sauce, Subway*	1 Serving/21g	88	9.0	419	0.0	9.5	42.9	1.0
Honey Mustard Sauce, Subway*	1 Serving/21g	32	0.0	152	0.0	33.3	1.0	0.5
Light Mayonnaise, Subway*	1 Serving/15g	56	6.0	373	0.0	6.7	40.0	0.0
Ranch Dressing, Subway*	1 Serving/21g	44	4.0	210	0.0	4.8	21.4	0.0
Sweet Onion Sauce, Subway*	1 Serving/21g	38	0.0	181	0.0	42.9	1.0	0.5
SOUP								
Beef Goulash, Subway*	1 Serving/250g	199	12.0	80	3.3	6.0	4.7	0.9
Carrot & Coriander, Subway*	1 Serving/250g	81	2.0	32	0.9	5.6	0.7	1.1
Country Chicken & Vegetable, Subway*	1 Serving/250g	168	11.0	67	2.7	4.2	4.4	0.2
Cream of Chicken, Subway*	1 Serving/250g	160	11.0	64	2.7	3.1	4.5	0.0
Cream of Mushroom, Subway*	1 Serving/250g	150	11.0	60	1.0	4.4	4.3	0.3
Highland Vegetable, Subway*	1 Serving/250g	73	0.0	29	1.5	5.5	0.1	0.9
Leek & Potato, Subway*	1 Serving/250g	124	3.0	50	1.7	8.0	1.2	1.1
Lentil & Bacon, Subway*	1 Serving/250g	182	5.0	73	4.4	9.3	2.0	1.1
Minestrone, Subway*	1 Serving/250g	81	3.0	32	0.7	4.4	1.3	0.7
Red Pepper & Tomato, Subway*	1 Serving/250g	96	3.0	38	1.4	5.0	1.4	0.9
Thai Style Vegetable, Subway*	1 Serving/250g	87	1.0	35	1.1	6.7	0.4	0.8
Tomato, Subway*	1 Serving/250g	103	4.0	41	0.8	6.1	1.5	0.3
Wild Mushroom, Subway*	1 Serving/250g	101	5.0	40	1.0	4.1	2.2	0.3
SPRITE								
Subway*	1 Serving/455ml	200	0.0	44	0.0	10.6	0.0	0.0
TOASTIE								
Cheese, Subway*	1 Serving/66g	200	10.0	303	16.2	26.5	14.4	0.9
Pepperoni, Pizza, Subway*	1 Serving/95g	241	13.0	254	12.3	21.7	13.4	0.9
WRAP								
Beef, Subway*	1 Wrap/356g	121	3.0	34	4.5	1.7	0.7	1.1
Chicken Breast, Subway*	1 Wrap/371g	146	3.0	39	5.7	1.9	0.9	1.1
Ham, Subway*	1 Wrap/356g	108	3.0	30	3.7	2.0	0.8	1.1
Subway Club, Subway*	1 Wrap/390g	147	3.0	38	5.6	1.8	0.9	1.0

	Measure INFO/WEIGHT	per Measure KCAL	per Measure FAT	Nutrition Values per 100g / 100ml KCAL	PROT	CARB	FAT	FIBRE
SUBWAY								
WRAP								
Sweet Onion Teriyaki, Subway*	1 Wrap/413g	201	4.0	49	5.1	4.8	0.9	1.1
Turkey Breast & Ham, Subway*	1 Wrap/366g	115	3.0	31	4.1	1.9	0.8	1.1
Turkey Breast, Subway*	1 Wrap/356g	105	3.0	29	3.9	1.7	0.7	1.1
Veggie Delite, Subway*	1 Wrap/300g	52	1.0	17	1.0	2.0	0.3	1.3
Wrap, Subway*	1 Wrap/101g	328	7.0	325	7.8	59.4	6.5	2.0
THE REAL GREEK FOOD COMPANY LTD								
COLD MEZE								
Crudites, The Real Greek Food Co. Ltd*	1 Serving/231g	37	0.0	16	0.6	3.1	0.2	1.6
Dolmades, The Real Greek Food Co. Ltd*	1 Serving/131g	254	16.0	194	2.9	18.8	12.0	0.8
Flatbread, Greek, The Real Greek Food Co. Ltd*	1 Serving/200g	615	16.0	307	6.6	52.6	7.8	7.4
Gigandes Plaki, The Real Greek Food Co. Ltd*	1 Serving/210g	183	12.0	87	2.3	7.4	5.6	2.5
Htipiti, The Real Greek Food Co. Ltd*	1 Serving/140g	305	25.0	218	8.0	7.8	17.7	3.5
Hummus, The Real Greek Food Co. Ltd*	1 Serving/140g	298	19.0	213	7.6	15.6	13.6	5.2
Koliosalata, The Real Greek Food Co. Ltd*	1 Serving/140g	506	48.0	361	12.1	1.6	34.1	0.3
Melitzanasalata, The Real Greek Food Co. Ltd*	1 Serving/140g	236	22.0	168	1.2	7.1	15.5	3.2
Revithia, The Real Greek Food Co. Ltd*	1 Serving/160g	286	20.0	179	4.8	11.9	12.6	4.0
Salad, Melon, Mint, Feta, The Real Greek Food Co. Ltd*	1 Serving/192g	102	8.0	53	1.9	2.6	4.0	0.2
Salad, Tabouleh, The Real Greek Food Co. Ltd*	1 Serving/165g	117	8.0	71	1.3	6.3	5.0	1.9
Taramasalata, The Real Greek Food Co. Ltd*	1 Serving/140g	913	99.0	652	2.5	2.1	70.7	0.0
Tzatziki, The Real Greek Food Co. Ltd*	1 Serving/141g	163	14.0	116	3.5	3.1	10.0	0.4
DIPS								
Aioli, Parsley, The Real Greek Food Co. Ltd*	1 Serving/34g	176	19.0	504	2.3	2.3	53.8	0.6
HOT MEZE								
Asparagus, Grilled, The Real Greek Food Co. Ltd*	1 Serving/110g	140	10.0	127	3.3	9.3	8.9	2.3
Bifteki with Yoghurt, The Real Greek Food Co. Ltd*	1 Serving/250g	252	60.0	101	21.6	3.7	24.2	0.0
Chicken, Skewer, The Real Greek Food Co. Ltd*	1 Serving/144g	177	8.0	123	3.1	1.3	5.3	0.7
Cod, Salt, The Real Greek Food Co. Ltd*	1 Serving/152g	346	1.0	227	21.1	34.2	1.0	0.6
Lamb, Cutlets, The Real Greek Food Co. Ltd*	1 Serving/260g	881	79.0	339	16.3	0.0	30.4	0.0
Lamb, Kefte, The Real Greek Food Co. Ltd*	1 Serving/216g	344	25.0	159	12.0	2.2	11.5	0.3
Lamb, Skewer, The Real Greek Food Co. Ltd*	1 Serving/166g	255	19.0	154	11.8	1.1	11.3	0.6
Octopus, Grilled, The Real Greek Food Co. Ltd*	1 Serving/128g	447	25.0	349	39.3	3.2	19.8	0.3
Pork, Skewer, The Real Greek Food Co. Ltd*	1 Serving/165g	281	22.0	170	11.8	1.1	13.1	0.6
Sardines, Grilled, The Real Greek Food Co. Ltd*	1 Serving/360g	619	33.0	172	22.2	0.3	9.1	0.1
Squid, Kalamari, Grilled, The Real Greek Food Co. Ltd*	1 Serving/140g	286	135.0	203	12.4	1.6	96.1	0.2
Tiropitakia, The Real Greek Food Co. Ltd*	1 Serving/120g	416	21.0	344	10.0	37.3	17.5	1.3
NIBBLES								
Bread, Olive & Dukkah, The Real Greek Food Co. Ltd*	1 Serving/129g	538	32.0	417	6.4	41.3	25.1	6.3
Olive, The Real Greek Food Co. Ltd*	1 Serving/110g	317	33.0	288	1.7	2.4	30.2	4.3
TOBY CARVERY								
BEEF								
Tewkesbury, Toby Carvery*	1 Serving/100g	176	6.0	176	31.4	0.1	5.6	0.0
DRESSING								
Sauce, Mint, Toby Carvery*	1 Serving/100g	67	0.0	67	1.1	15.6	0.1	0.0
Sauce, Parsley, Toby Carvery*	1 Serving/100g	42	1.0	42	1.6	5.9	1.3	0.0
GRAVY								
Beef, Toby Carvery*	1 Serving/100g	22	0.0	22	0.6	4.5	0.2	0.0
Caramelised Onion, Toby Carvery*	1 Serving/100g	80	1.0	80	1.7	16.4	0.8	0.0
Poultry, Toby Carvery*	1 Serving/100g	29	0.0	29	1.1	6.1	0.1	0.0
Vegetarian, Toby Carvery*	1 100g/100g	18	0.0	18	1.2	3.2	0.1	0.0
PORK								
Horseshoe of, Toby Carvery*	1 Serving/100g	203	8.0	203	31.7	0.1	8.4	0.0

	Measure INFO/WEIGHT	per Measure KCAL	FAT	Nutrition Values per 100g / 100ml KCAL	PROT	CARB	FAT	FIBRE
TOBY CARVERY								
POTATOES								
Mashed, Toby Carvery*	1 Serving/100g	70	2.0	70	1.3	10.8	2.4	0.0
New, Toby Carvery*	1 Spoonful/100g	73	0.0	73	1.8	15.4	0.5	0.0
Roasted, Toby Carvery*	1 Serving/80g	137	4.0	171	2.7	28.9	4.6	0.0
TURKEY								
with Orange Glaze, Toby Carvery*	1 Serving/100g	145	2.0	145	32.0	0.1	1.8	0.0
VEGETABLES								
Broccoli, Toby Carvery*	1 Spoon/100g	60	2.0	60	2.7	7.6	2.1	0.0
Cabbage, Toby Carvery*	1 Serving/80g	34	1.0	43	1.7	6.0	1.4	0.0
Carrots, Toby Carvery*	1 Serving/100g	46	1.0	46	1.1	3.0	1.1	0.0
Leeks, Toby Carvery*	1 Serving/100g	32	0.0	32	0.8	7.1	0.1	0.0
YORKSHIRE PUDDING								
New Muffin Style, Toby Carvery*	1 Serving/100g	330	12.0	330	15.3	41.0	11.7	0.0
WIMPY								
BREAKFAST								
Bacon & Egg Breakfast Roll, Wimpy*	1 Roll/194g	368	12.0	190	13.4	18.3	6.2	0.0
Bacon Breakfast Roll, Wimpy*	1 Roll/144g	278	5.0	193	13.3	24.7	3.5	0.0
Banger Breakfast, Wimpy*	1 Serving/212g	391	26.0	184	12.9	4.2	12.4	0.0
Sausage & Egg Breakfast Roll, Wimpy*	1 Roll/211g	527	28.0	250	11.8	20.3	13.5	0.0
Sausage Breakfast Roll, Wimpy*	1 Roll/161g	437	22.0	271	11.3	26.6	13.4	0.0
The Country Breakfast, Wimpy*	1 Serving/261g	325	17.0	125	8.6	7.7	6.5	0.0
The Great Wimpy Breakfast, Wimpy*	1 Serving/439g	779	41.0	177	9.7	13.6	9.4	0.0
Wimpy Breakfast, Wimpy*	1 Serving/297g	437	25.0	147	10.7	6.7	8.4	0.0
Wimpy Club, Wimpy*	1 Serving/310g	639	26.0	206	13.5	19.4	8.5	0.0
Wimpy Hashbrown Breakfast, Wimpy*	1 Serving/424g	542	41.0	128	4.1	9.0	9.7	0.0
BURGERS								
BBQ Burger, Wimpy*	1 Burger/236g	646	30.0	274	14.2	26.1	12.8	0.0
Bender in a Bun with Cheese, Wimpy*	1 Burger/170g	423	23.0	249	9.9	22.0	13.7	0.0
Chicken & Bacon Melt, Wimpy*	1 Burger/172g	443	20.0	258	12.6	25.4	11.7	0.0
Chicken Fillet, Wimpy*	1 Burger/327g	380	17.0	116	6.7	11.1	5.1	0.0
Chicken in a Bun, Wimpy*	1 Burger/154g	408	21.0	265	10.0	26.9	13.5	0.0
Classic Bacon Cheeseburger, Wimpy*	1 Burger/192g	405	19.0	211	13.6	16.8	9.9	0.0
Classic Kingsize, Wimpy*	1 Burger/227g	551	31.0	243	16.2	14.2	13.7	0.0
Classic with Cheese, Wimpy*	1 Burger/171g	378	18.0	221	12.8	18.8	10.8	0.0
Classic, Wimpy*	1 Burger/159g	337	15.0	212	12.4	19.9	9.5	0.0
Halfpounder with Bacon & Cheese, Wimpy*	1 Burger/276g	859	46.0	311	21.4	18.9	16.8	0.0
Mega Burger, Wimpy*	1 Burger/206g	594	36.0	288	15.3	18.0	17.5	0.0
Quarterpounder with Bacon & Cheese, Wimpy*	1 Burger/191g	596	27.0	312	19.2	27.3	14.1	0.0
Quarterpounder with Cheese, Wimpy*	1 Burger/213g	578	35.0	271	15.1	17.2	16.2	0.0
Quarterpounder, Wimpy*	1 Burger/200g	538	31.0	269	15.0	18.0	15.6	0.0
CHICKEN								
Chicken Chunks with Chips, Wimpy*	1 Serving/333g	779	47.0	234	8.3	19.0	14.1	0.0
DESSERT								
Brown Derby with Dairy Ice Cream, Wimpy*	1 Serving/125g	399	21.0	319	5.4	36.9	16.6	0.0
Cheese Cake, Wimpy*	1 Serving/144g	412	18.0	286	4.5	38.5	12.7	0.0
Chocolate Fudge Cake, Wimpy*	1 Serving/100g	371	12.0	371	4.7	60.2	12.4	0.0
Chocolate Waffle with Dairy Ice Cream, Wimpy*	1 Serving/178g	691	37.0	388	5.1	45.3	20.8	0.0
Chocolate Waffle with Squirty Cream, Wimpy*	1 Serving/158g	667	37.0	422	5.1	47.7	23.4	0.0
Dairy Ice Cream with Chocolate Sauce, Wimpy*	1 Serving/88g	200	8.0	227	3.4	32.5	9.2	0.0
Dairy Ice Cream with Strawberry Sauce, Wimpy*	1 Serving/88g	199	8.0	226	3.0	34.3	9.0	0.0
Deep Filled Apple Tart, Wimpy*	1 Serving/164g	339	10.0	207	1.7	36.2	6.2	0.0
Half Chocolate Waffle with Dairy Ice Cream, Wimpy*	1 Serving/116g	395	19.0	341	4.0	44.7	16.2	0.0
Mini Knickerbocker Glory with Dairy Ice Cream, Wimpy*	1 Serving/194g	190	8.0	98	1.6	13.2	4.4	0.0

	Measure INFO/WEIGHT	per Measure KCAL	FAT	Nutrition Values per 100g / 100ml KCAL	PROT	CARB	FAT	FIBRE
DESSERT								
Spotted Dick Pudding, Wimpy*	1 Serving/130g	400	17.0	308	4.1	44.2	12.7	0.0
Treacle Sponge Pudding, Wimpy*	1 Serving/130g	504	21.0	388	3.9	56.1	16.4	0.0
EXTRAS								
Chips Large Portion, Wimpy*	1 Portion/143g	333	17.0	233	3.0	30.4	12.0	0.0
Chips Standard Portion, Wimpy*	1 Portion/114g	267	14.0	234	3.0	30.5	12.0	0.0
Heinz Baked Beans, Wimpy*	1 Portion/110g	83	0.0	75	4.7	13.6	0.2	0.0
Mushrooms, Wimpy*	1 Portion/114g	179	18.0	157	2.4	0.3	16.2	0.0
Onion Rings Large (12), Wimpy*	1 Portion/180g	401	23.0	223	3.2	23.6	12.9	0.0
Onion Rings Standard (6), Wimpy*	1 Portion/90g	201	12.0	223	3.2	23.6	12.9	0.0
Peas, Wimpy*	1 Portion/50g	35	0.0	70	6.0	9.8	1.0	0.0
Side Salad, Wimpy*	1 Portion/145g	44	0.0	30	1.4	6.1	0.2	0.0
FISH								
Haddock, Peas & Chips, Wimpy*	1 Serving/314g	676	38.0	215	6.6	21.3	12.1	0.0
Scampi & Chips, Wimpy*	1 Serving/250g	589	32.0	236	6.5	25.1	12.9	0.0
GRILL								
Classic Bacon Grill, Wimpy*	1 Serving/321g	722	45.0	225	11.5	14.0	14.1	0.0
Classic Grill, Wimpy*	1 Serving/314g	755	51.0	240	11.1	14.1	16.2	0.0
Gourmet Chicken Platter, Wimpy*	1 Serving/412g	607	31.0	147	10.9	9.4	7.5	0.0
Sausage, Egg & Chips, Wimpy*	1 Serving/244g	597	39.0	245	9.0	17.4	15.9	0.0
Steak Platter, Wimpy*	1 Serving/424g	719	38.0	170	9.9	12.9	9.0	0.0
The International Grill, Wimpy*	1 Serving/400g	895	59.0	224	12.8	11.2	14.7	0.0
Wimpy All-Day Breakfast, Wimpy*	1 Serving/410g	731	40.0	178	8.3	14.5	9.7	0.0
ICE CREAMS								
Banana Longboat with Soft Ice Cream, Wimpy*	1 Serving/209g	260	6.0	124	2.3	23.9	2.9	0.0
Brown Derby with Dairy Ice Cream, Wimpy*	1 Serving/125g	397	20.0	318	5.6	38.9	15.8	0.0
Choc Nut Sundae, Wimpy*	1 Serving/83g	196	6.0	236	4.6	38.4	7.5	0.0
Fruit & Nut Sundae, Wimpy*	1 Serving/83g	138	6.0	166	4.2	23.3	7.0	0.0
Ice Cream Portion, Soft with Chocolate Sauce, Wimpy*	1 Serving/71g	137	3.0	193	2.8	36.1	4.5	0.0
Ice Cream Portion, Soft with Strawberry Sauce, Wimpy*	1 Serving/71g	137	3.0	193	2.4	38.3	4.2	0.0
Knickerbockerglory with Soft Ice Cream, Wimpy*	1 Serving/138g	196	6.0	142	2.7	24.7	4.3	0.0
Triple Strawberry Sundae with Soft Ice Cream, Wimpy*	1 Serving/170g	123	3.0	72	1.4	13.1	1.9	0.0
KIDS								
Cheese Toastie with Chips, Wimpy*	1 Serving/235g	541	18.0	230	7.0	35.3	7.7	0.0
Cheese Toastie with Salad, Wimpy*	1 Serving/250g	367	9.0	147	5.9	24.2	3.5	0.0
Cheeseburger Meal with Chips, Wimpy*	1 Serving/196g	498	23.0	254	9.6	28.3	11.9	0.0
Cheeseburger Meal with Salad, Wimpy*	1 Serving/211g	323	14.0	153	8.2	15.7	6.6	0.0
Chicken Chunks Meal with Chips, Wimpy*	1 Serving/172g	440	17.0	256	8.4	9.2	9.8	0.0
Chicken Chunks Meal with Salad , Wimpy*	1 Serving/187g	265	14.0	142	6.8	10.0	7.6	0.0
Fish Bites Meal with Chips , Wimpy*	1 Serving/160g	380	21.0	237	6.7	24.7	13.1	0.0
Fish Bites Meal with Salad , Wimpy*	1 Serving/175g	205	12.0	117	5.2	9.8	6.6	0.0
Hamburger Meal with Chips, Wimpy*	1 Serving/184g	457	20.0	248	9.0	29.9	10.9	0.0
Hamburger Meal with Salad, Wimpy*	1 Serving/199g	283	11.0	142	7.5	16.4	5.4	0.0
Sausage Meal with Chips, Wimpy*	1 Serving/160g	428	28.0	267	8.9	19.9	17.3	0.0
Sausage Meal with Salad , Wimpy*	1 Serving/175g	253	18.0	145	7.1	5.5	10.5	0.0
Wimpy Hot Dog with Chips, Wimpy*	1 Serving/226g	599	31.0	265	8.2	28.3	13.5	0.0
Wimpy Hot Dog with Salad, Wimpy*	1 Serving/241g	425	21.0	176	7.0	17.3	8.8	0.0
MUFFIN								
Giant Blueberry, Wimpy*	1 Muffin/108g	470	26.0	435	5.9	48.9	23.7	0.0
Giant Choc Chunk, Wimpy*	1 Muffin/108g	473	27.0	438	5.5	49.7	24.6	0.0
PANINI								
Cheese & Tomato , Wimpy*	1 Panini/225g	548	21.0	244	11.3	29.0	9.2	0.0
Ham & Cheese, Wimpy*	1 Panini/235g	596	22.0	254	14.6	27.5	9.4	0.0

	Measure INFO/WEIGHT	per Measure KCAL	FAT	Nutrition Values per 100g / 100ml KCAL	PROT	CARB	FAT	FIBRE
WIMPY								
PANINI								
Ham, Tomato & Cheese, Wimpy*	1 Panini/275g	602	22.0	219	12.6	23.9	8.1	0.0
Steak, Cheese & Onion , Wimpy*	1 Panini/285g	589	29.0	207	14.7	23.1	10.1	0.0
POTATO JACKET								
with Baked Beans, Wimpy*	1 Serving/452g	547	8.0	121	3.8	23.8	1.7	0.0
with Beans & Cheese, Wimpy*	1 Serving/577g	1067	52.0	185	8.5	18.7	8.9	0.0
with Butter, Wimpy*	1 Serving/327g	453	8.0	139	3.5	27.7	2.3	0.0
with Coleslaw, Wimpy*	1 Serving/452g	776	41.0	172	2.9	21.2	9.0	0.0
with Grated Cheese, Wimpy*	1 Serving/452g	973	51.0	215	9.5	20.1	11.3	0.0
with Tuna Mayo, Wimpy*	1 Serving/452g	776	36.0	172	5.9	20.6	7.9	0.0
RIBS								
Pork Rib, Wimpy*	1 Rib/189g	463	22.0	245	13.0	21.6	11.9	0.0
ROLL								
Bacon in a Bun, Wimpy*	1 Roll/105g	212	3.0	202	12.5	29.0	3.3	0.0
Wimpy Club, Wimpy*	1 Roll/310g	639	26.0	206	13.5	19.4	8.5	0.0
SALAD								
Fish, Wimpy*	1 Serving/356g	389	21.0	109	4.6	9.9	6.0	0.0
Gourmet Chicken, Wimpy*	1 Serving/383g	254	4.0	66	11.1	2.7	1.1	0.0
Hot & Spicy Chicken, Wimpy*	1 Serving/315g	285	15.0	90	5.6	6.3	4.8	0.0
Scampi, Wimpy*	1 Serving/356g	376	19.0	106	4.2	10.7	5.4	0.0
Spicy Beanburger, Wimpy*	1 Serving/334g	406	23.0	122	1.5	13.6	6.9	0.0
Steak, Wimpy*	1 Serving/350g	329	17.0	94	10.1	2.7	4.8	0.0
TEACAKE								
with Butter, Wimpy*	1 Teacake/62g	237	9.0	382	8.1	56.3	14.5	0.0
TOAST								
with Jam, Wimpy*	1 Serving/89g	276	8.0	310	7.3	52.6	9.3	0.0
VEGETARIAN								
Lemon Pepper Quorn, Wimpy*	1 Serving/239g	586	27.0	245	8.0	29.2	11.1	0.0
Spicy Beanburger, Wimpy*	1 Serving/233g	593	29.0	255	5.4	30.8	12.5	0.0

Useful Resources

Beating Bowel Cancer
Beating Bowel Cancer is a leading UK charity for bowel cancer patients, working to raise awareness of symptoms, promote early diagnosis and encourage open access to treatment choice for those affected by bowel cancer.
Tel: 08450 719301   Email: nurse@beatingbowelcancer.org
Website: http://www.beatingbowelcancer.org

Cancer Research
Cancer Research UK is the leading UK charity dedicated to research, education and fundraising for all forms of cancer.
Tel: 0207 242 0200 Email: via their website
Website: www.cancerresearchuk.org

Diabetes Advice
Diabetes UK is the leading charity working for people with diabetes. Their mission is to improve the lives of people with diabetes and to work towards a future without diabetes
Tel : 0845 120 2960 Email: info@diabetes.org.uk
Website: www.diabetes.org.uk

Dietary Advice
The British Dietetic Association has helpful food fact leaflets and information on how to contact a registered dietitian.
Tel: 0121 200 8080 Email: webmaster@bda.uk.com
Website: www.bda.uk.com

Exercise Equipment for Home
Diet and Fitness Resources has a range of equipment for exercise at home, from pedometers to treadmills and fitballs to weights. As well as diet tools such as food diaries, a weight loss kit and diet plates.
Tel: 01733 345592   Email: helpteam@dietandfitnessresources.co.uk
Website: www.dietandfitnessresources.co.uk

Healthy Eating
The British Nutrition Foundation has lots of in depth scientifically based nutritional information, knowledge and advice on healthy eating for all ages.
Tel: 0207 404 6504 Email: postbox@nutrition.org.uk
Website: www.nutrition.org.uk

Healthy Heart

The British Heart Foundation provides advice and information for all on all heart aspects from being healthy, to living with heart conditions, research and fundraising.

Tel: 0207 554 000   Email: via their website
Website: www.bhf.org.uk

Safety and Standards

The Food Standards Agency is an independent watchdog, set up to protect the public's health and consumer interests in relation to food.

Tel: 0207 276 8829 Email: helpline@foodstandards.gsi.gov.uk
Website: www.food.gov.uk

Weight Loss

Weight Loss Resources is home to the UK's largest calorie and nutrition database along with diaries, tools and expert advice for weight loss and health.

Tel: 01733 345592 Email: helpteam@weightlossresources.co.uk
Website: www.weightlossresources.co.uk

Feedback

If you have any comments or suggestions about The Calorie, Carb & Fat Bible, or would like further information on Weight Loss Resources, please call, email, or write to us:

Tel: 01733 345592
Email: helpteam@weightlossresources.co.uk
Address: Pat Wilson,
            Weight Loss Resources Ltd,
            29 Metro Centre,
            Woodston,
            Peterborough,
            PE2 7UH.

Reviews for The Calorie Carb & Fat Bible

'What a brilliant book. I know I'll be sinking my teeth into it.'
GMTV Nutritionist Amanda Ursell, BSc RD

'To help you make low-cal choices everyday, invest in a copy.'
ZEST magazine

'There is no doubt that the food listings are extremely helpful
for anyone wishing to control their calorie intake in order to lose
pounds or maintain a healthy weight.'
Women's Fitness magazine

'Useful if you don't want to exclude any overall food groups.'
Easy Living magazine

'Quite simply an astonishing achievement by the authors.'
Evening Post, Nottingham

'The book gives you all the basic information so you can work out
your daily calorie needs.'
Woman magazine

'This is a welcome resource in view of the 'national epidemic of obesity.'

Bryony Philip, Bowel Cancer UK

'The authors seem to understand the problems of slimming.'

Dr John Campion

'Jam-packed with info on dieting, and full to bursting point with the calorie, carbohydrate and fat values of thousands of different foods, it's the perfect weight loss tool.'

Evening Express, Aberdeen

'Excellent resource tool - used by myself in my role as a Practice Nurse.'

Pam Boal, Sunderland

'I recently bought your book called the Calorie, Carb & Fat Bible and would love to tell you what a brilliant book it is. I have recently started a weight management programme and I honestly don't know where I'd be without your book. It has helped me a lot and given me some really good advice.'

Rachel Mitchell

About Weight Loss Resources

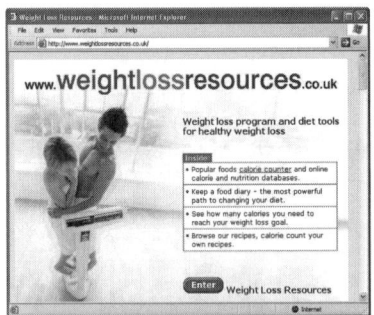

"What this does is put you in control with no guilt, no awful groups and no negativity! Fill in your food diary, get support on the boards and watch it fall off!"

LINDAB, Weight Loss Resources Member

How Does It Work?

Weight Loss Resources is home to the UK's biggest online calorie and nutrition database. You simply tap in your height, weight, age and basic activity level - set a weight loss goal, and the programme does all the necessary calculations.

What Does It Do?

The site enables you to keep a food diary which keeps running totals of calories, fat, fibre, carbs, proteins and portions of fruit and veg. You can also keep an exercise diary which adds the calories you use during exercise. At the end of a week, you update your weight and get reports and graphs on your progress.

How Will It Help?

You'll learn a great deal about how your eating and drinking habits affect your weight and how healthy they are. Using the diaries and other tools you'll be able to make changes that suit your tastes and your lifestyle. The result is weight loss totally tailored to your needs and preferences. A method you can stick with that will help you learn how to eat well for life!

Try It Free!

Go to **www.weightlossresources.co.uk** and take a completely free, no obligation, 24 hour trial. If you like what you see you can sign up for membership from £7.95 per month.